Complexities in Colorectal Surgery

Scott R. Steele • Justin A. Maykel
Bradley J. Champagne • Guy R. Orangio
Editors

Complexities in Colorectal Surgery

Decision-Making and Management

Springer

Editors
Scott R. Steele, MD
Division of Colon and Rectal Surgery
Department of Surgery
Madigan Army Medical Center
Fort Lewis, WA
USA

Justin A. Maykel, MD
Division of Colorectal Surgery
Department of Surgery
UMass Memorial Medical Center
University of Massachusetts Medical School
Worcester, MA
USA

Bradley J. Champagne, MD
Division of Colon and Rectal Surgery
Department of Surgery
Case Western Reserve University
School of Medicine
University Hospitals
Cleveland, OH
USA

Guy R. Orangio, MD
Division of Colon and Rectal Surgery
Department of Surgery
Louisiana State University Health Science Center
LSU School of Medicine
New Orleans, LA
USA

Videos to this book can be accessed at http://www.springerimages.com/videos/978-1-4614-9021-0

Corrected at 2nd printing 2014

ISBN 978-1-4614-9021-0 ISBN 978-1-4614-9022-7 (eBook)
DOI 10.1007/978-1-4614-9022-7
Springer New York Heidelberg Dordrecht London

Library of Congress Control Number: 2014930571

Printed on acid-free paper

Springer is part of Springer Science+Business Media (www.springer.com)

Foreword

Fifty years ago, with the publication of *Surgery of the Anus, Rectum and Colon*, John Goligher set the modern standard for textbooks of colorectal surgery. Several outstanding textbooks in the Goligher mold have followed, and a few of these have become classics in their own right. So it is fair to ask: why one more?

The answer becomes evident with the present work. *Complexities in Colorectal Surgery: Decision-Making and Management* in many ways starts where standard texts begin to leave off: with an up-to-date view of some of the most vexing problems in intestinal surgery. A quick review of the chapters provides the general idea. It's not "Diverticular Disease" but "Diverticulitis: Beyond the Basics;" not "Rectal Cancer" but "Recurrent Rectal Cancer;" not "The Ileal Pouch" but "Ileal Pouch Complications." Difficult problems such as the failed anastomosis, pelvic bleeding, and chronic pain are addressed head on. There is a strong focus on technical advances, such as TEMS and TAMIS for the local treatment of rectal cancer and robotics, SILS and CLER approaches to abdominal surgery. Finally, there is material to address the difficult personal and social aspects of surgery that traditionally receive little or no discussion in textbooks: facing our failures, balancing clinical and research practice, medicolegal and ethical dilemmas, economic considerations, and knowing when to say "when."

The editors are to be commended for assembling a truly outstanding roster of authors, each a recognized authority at the cutting edge of his or her field. As for the editorial team itself, Scott Steele, Justin Maykel, Brad Champagne, and Guy Orangio are exceptional surgeons and surgical educators, representative of the new generation of innovative colorectal surgical leaders who stand ready to challenge conventional wisdom and push our field boldly into the future. With this book, they take a giant step in that direction.

Minneapolis, MN, USA — Robert D. Madoff, MD

Preface

There is a simplicity that exists on the far side of complexity....

–P. Buchanan

Merriam-Webster's Dictionary defines complex as "a whole made up of complicated or interrelated parts." For surgeons, this could not be more accurate, as there remains a seemingly never-ending assortment of *complex* patient disease processes and complications that permeate colorectal surgery and precisely illustrate this definition. Even when the technical challenges of surgery are managed successfully, the preoperative evaluation and decision-making can be demanding, and postoperative functional changes may impact short- and long-term quality of life. Furthermore, the economic implications of care for the patient, family, and the healthcare system must be considered.

Despite extensive training and a wealth of clinical experience, surgeons are often consumed with an internal struggle over how to provide the best patient-centered care and formulate optimal approaches for complex clinical scenarios. Beyond the simple application of knowledge lie deeper questions about the ideal "next step" in patient management, especially for those who have experienced postoperative complications. Unfortunately, in many situations algorithms of care do not exist or are not founded in reliable evidence-based recommendations. Rather, we rely on experience and pragmatic advice from experts who have spent a career discerning their "best" approach. Hence, our goal with *Complexities* is to provide a unique, practical guide that covers the strategic evaluation, specific approaches, and detailed management techniques utilized by expert colorectal surgeons caring for patients with complex problems.

With *Complexities* we sought to understand the intricate thought process behind each author's proposed approach and treatment strategy. When possible, this involved incorporating evidence-based recommendations. Our experts also lend their personal insight into situations where data is sparse, yet their individual but extensive experience becomes the cornerstone of making sound decisions and optimizing patient outcomes. What is the optimal algorithm for patients with fecal incontinence with or without a sphincter injury? How do we manage and time surgery for the patient with metastatic cancer? When do we operate on smoldering diverticulitis? What is the best option for a failing J-pouch or low rectal anastomosis? Surgery is an art rooted in scientific principles. This book attempts to bridge that gap.

Not every surgeon can independently accrue the years and volume of experience that result from a specialty practice at a high-volume referral center. Therefore, by covering all aspects from the assessment of risk to the medical and surgical treatment for abdominal, pelvic, and anorectal disease, the authors focus on the details that make these situations challenging. Additionally, beyond the clinical aspects of colorectal surgery, we have highlighted aspects that pertain to the true essence of being a surgeon, from the importance of the first encounter to the medical-legal, ethical, and economic challenges surgeons face. In these situations, there is little evidence but abundant practical advice to guide us. Furthermore, while disease and complications of treatment inflict a tremendous physical and emotional burden on patients, we examine something rarely discussed among providers—the psychological and emotional impact complications have on surgeons, and how they may impact subsequent care. Finally, we confront one of the most difficult personal decisions surgeons will face—knowing when to say "when"—and dealing with our transition out of clinical medicine.

Since inception, it has been our privilege and pleasure to work with this tremendous gathering of authors, as their unique contributions have come together to make this textbook a reality. We would like to personally thank each one of them for their invaluable insights. It is our wish that Complexities serves as a resource for this and future generations of surgeons who find themselves faced with complex clinical and professional challenges.

Internet Access to Video Clip

The owner of this text will be able to access these video clips through Springer with the following Internet link: http://www.springerimages.com/videos/978-1-4614-9021-0.

Olympia, WA, USA Scott R. Steele, MD
Worcester, MA, USA Justin A. Maykel, MD
Cleveland, OH, USA Bradley J. Champagne, MD
New Orleans, LA, USA Guy R. Orangio, MD

Acknowledgments

Scott Steele, MD
We would first like to thank our outstanding Developmental Editor, Elektra McDermott, for her extraordinary efforts in overseeing this edition and ensuring its timely completion and thoroughness. I personally would like to thank my fellow editors for their tremendous vision and hard work throughout this entire process, as well as all of my mentors in colorectal surgery for guiding me and giving me such incredible opportunities. Finally, and most importantly, thank you to my family for supporting and encouraging me throughout this endeavor.

Justin Maykel, MD
I would like to thank all of the teachers at Tufts Medical School who introduced me to the field of surgery, the attendings at Beth Israel Deaconess Medical Center who shared their skills and passion for surgery, and my mentors at the University of Minnesota who helped shape my independence as a surgeon. Finally, thank you to my family for supporting me through this entire process.

Bradley Champagne, MD
I would like to thank my mentors at Albany Medical Center and Georgia Colorectal Surgical Associates for their incredible teaching and patience during my training. I would also like to thank my wife, Christina, for providing balance in my life and for her exceptional support in all of my endeavors.

Guy Orangio, MD
I want to express my gratitude and appreciation to Drs. Victor Fazio, Ian Lavery, and David Jagelman. I had the privilege and honor to be trained by probably the greatest master colon and rectal surgeons in the world. Thank you for setting a standard as a surgeon, physician, and professional that I strive toward every day. To all of the fellows that I had the privilege of training at Georgia Colon and Rectal Surgical Associates, you have given me more than I could have ever given to you. Thank you all.

Contents

Contributors

Herand Abcarian, MD, FACS Division of Colon and Rectal Surgery, Department of Surgery, University of Illinois at Chicago, John Stroger Hospital of Cook County, Chicago, IL, USA

Kenneth S. Azarow, MD Division of Pediatric Surgery, Department of Surgery, Oregon Health Science University, Portland, OR, USA

Oregon Health Science University, Doernbecher Children's Hospital, Portland, OR, USA

H. Randolph Bailey, MD, FACS Division of Colon and Rectal Surgery, The University of Texas Health Science Center, Methodist Hospital, Houston, TX, USA

Amir L. Bastawrous, MD, MBA, FACS, FASCRS Department of Colorectal Surgery, Swedish Colon and Rectal Clinic, Swedish Hospital Medical Center, Madison, Seattle, WA, USA

Nancy N. Baxter, MD, PhD, FRCSC, FACS Division of General Surgery, University of Toronto, St Michael's Hospital, Toronto, ON, Canada

David E. Beck, MD, FACS, FASCRS Department of Colon and Rectal Surgery, Ochsner Clinic Foundation, New Orleans, LA, USA

Willem A. Bemelman, MD, PhD Department of Surgery, Academic Medical Center, University of Amsterdam, Amsterdam, WZ, The Netherlands

Anton Bilchik, MD, PhD, FACS Department of Surgery, John Wayne Cancer Institute, Santa Monica, CA, USA

Richard P. Billingham, M.D., FACS, FASCRS Department of Colorectal Surgery, Swedish Colon and Rectal Clinic, Swedish Hospital Medical Center, Madison, Seattle, WA, USA

Joshua I. S. Bleier, MD, FACS, FASCRS Division of Colon and Rectal Surgery, Department of Surgery, Pennsylvania Hospital/Hospital of the University of Pennsylvania, University of Pennsylvania, Philadelphia, PA, USA

Marja M. Boermeester, MD, PhD Department of Surgery, Academic Medical Center, University of Amsterdam, Amsterdam, AZ, The Netherlands

Liliana Bordeianou, MD, MPH Department of Surgery, Massachusetts General Hospital and Harvard Medical School, Boston, MA, USA

Robin P. Boushey, BSc, MD, PhD, CIP, FRCSC Department of Surgery, The Ottawa Hospital, Ottawa, ON, Canada

Carlos V.R. Brown, MD, FACS Department of Surgery, University of Texas Southwestern – Austin, Austin, TX, USA

Björn L.D.M. Brücher, MD, PhD, FRCS (Engl), FACS
Department of Surgery, Bon Secours Cancer Institute, Richmond, VA, USA

INCORE = International Consortium of Research of the Theodor-Billroth-Academy®, Richmond, VA, USA

W. Donald Buie, MD, MSC, FRCSC, FACS Department of Surgery, University of Calgary, Foothills Medical Centre, Calgary, AB, Canada

Peter Cataldo, MD Department of Surgery, Fletcher Allen Health Center, University of Vermont, Burlington, VT, USA

Bradley J. Champagne, MD Division of Colon and Rectal Surgery, Department of Surgery, Case Western Reserve University School of Medicine, University Hospitals, Cleveland, OH, USA

Robert A. Cusick, MD Department of Pediatric Surgery, Children's Hospital and Medical Center, Omaha and University of Nebraska Medical Center, Omaha, NE, USA

Bradley Davis, MD Division of Colon and Rectal Surgery, Department of Surgery, University of Cincinnati, Cincinnati, OH, USA

Conor P. Delaney, MD, MCh, PhD, FRCSI, FACS, FASCRS Division of Colorectal Surgery, Department of Surgery, University Hospitals Case Medical Center, Case Western Reserve University, Cleveland, OH, USA

Jonathan E. Efron, MD Ravitch Division, Department of Surgery, Johns Hopkins University, Baltimore, MD, USA

Victor W. Fazio, AO, MB, MS, FRACS, FACS, FRCS (Ed Hon), MD (Pol Hon), FRCSI (Hon) Division of Colorectal Surgery, Department of Surgery, Cleveland Clinic Lerner College of Medicine of Case Western University, Cleveland Clinic Foundation, Cleveland, OH, USA

James W. Fleshman, MD Department of Surgery, Baylor University Medical Center, Dallas, TX, USA

Todd D. Francone, MD, MPH Division of Surgery, Department of Colon and Rectal Surgery, Lahey Clinic, Burlington, MA, USA

Robert D. Fry, MD, FACS, FASCRS Division of Colon and Rectal Surgery, Department of Surgery, Pennsylvania Hospital, University of Pennsylvania, Philadelphia, PA, USA

Stanley Goldberg, MD Division of Colorectal Surgery, Department of Surgery, University of Minnesota, Minneapolis, MN, USA

Angelita Habr-Gama, MD Department of Colorectal Surgery, Angelita and Joaquim Gama Institute, Sao Paulo, Brazil

Department of Gastroenterology, University of São Paulo School of Medicine, Sao Paulo, Brazil

Dana M. Hayden, MD, MPH Department of General Surgery, Loyola University Medical Center, Maywood, IL, USA

Stefan. D. Holubar, MD, MS, FACS Section of Colon and Rectal Surgery, Dartmouth-Hitchcock Medical Center, Geisel School of Medicine at Dartmouth, The Dartmouth Institute for Health Policy Research, Lebanon, NH, USA

Tracy L. Hull, MD Department of Colon and Rectal Surgery, Digestive Disease Institute, The Cleveland Clinic Foundation, Cleveland, OH, USA

Leif Hultén, MD, PhD, FACS, ACGBI (Hon), ISUCRS (Hon), SICCR (Hon) The Colorectal Unit, Department of Surgery, Sahigrenska University Hospital SU/O, Goteborg, Sweden

Jennifer Lynn Irani, MD Department of Surgery, Harvard Medical School, Brigham and Women's Hospital, Boston, MA, USA

Terah C. Isaacson, MD Department of Colon and Rectal Surgery, Methodist Houston, Houston, TX, USA

Avital Itzhak, MD, FACS Department of Surgery, Bon Secours Cancer Institute, Richmond, VA, USA

Uniformed Services University of the Health Sciences, Bethesda, MD, USA

Eric K. Johnson, MD, FACS, FASCRS Department of Surgery, Madigan Healthcare System, Uniformed Services University of the Health Sciences, Tacoma, WA, USA

Deborah S. Keller, MD Division of Colorectal Surgery, Department of Surgery, University Hospitals, Case Medical Center, Cleveland, OH, USA

Jason D. Keune, MD, MBA Department of Surgery, Washington University School of Medicine, Barnes-Jewish Hospital, St. Louis, MO, USA

Ravi Pokala Kiran, MBBS, MS (Gen Surgery), FRCS (Eng), FRCS (Glas), FACS, MSc (EBM) Division of Colorectal Surgery, Department of Surgery, New York-Presbyterian/Columbia University Medical Center, New York, NY, USA

Ira J. Kodner, MD, FACS Department of Surgery, Washington University School of Medicine, Barnes-Jewish Hospital, St. Louis, MO, USA

Anjali S. Kumar, MD, MPH, FACS Section of Colon and Rectal Surgery, Medstar Washington Hospital Center, Georgetown University, Washington, DC, USA

Sang W. Lee, MD, FACS, FASCRS Division of Colon and Rectal Surgery, Department of Surgery, Weill Cornell Medical College, New York, NY, USA

Ann C. Lowry, MD Division of Colorectal Surgery, Department of Surgery, University of Minnesota, Minneapolis, MN, USA

Anthony R. MacLean, MD, FRCSC, FACS Department of Surgery, University of Calgary, Foothills Medical Centre, Calgary, AB, Canada

Helen MacRae, MD, FRCSC, FACS, FASCRS Department of Surgery, Mount Sinai Hospital and University of Toronto, Toronto, ON, Canada

Lillias Holmes Maguire, MD Division of Gastrointestinal Surgery, Massachusetts General Hospital, Boston, MA, USA

John H. Marks, MD, FACS, FASCRS Division of Colorectal Surgery, Department of Surgery, Main Line Health Systems, Lankenau Medical Center, Wynnewood, PA, USA

Division of Colorectal Surgery, Lankenau Medical Center, Wynnewood, PA, USA

Matthew J. Martin, MD, FACS Department of Surgery, Legacy Emanuel Medical Center, Portland, OR, USA

Department of Surgery, Madigan Army Medical Center, Tacoma, WA, USA

Justin A. Maykel, MD Division of Colorectal Surgery, Department of Surgery, UMass Memorial Medical Center, University of Massachusetts Medical School, Worcester, MA, USA

Amit Merchea, MD Division of Colon and Rectal Surgery, Department of Surgery, College of Medicine, Mayo Clinic, Jacksonville, FL, USA

Steven Mills, MD Department of Surgery, University of California, Irvine, Orange, CA, USA

Matthew G. Mutch, MD Department of Surgery, Section of Colon and Rectal Surgery, Washington University School of Medicine, St. Louis, MO, USA

Helge E. Myrvold, MD, PhD, SEC (Hon) Department of Cancer Research and Molecular Medicine, Norwegian University of Science and Technology, Trondheim, Norway

Aviram Nissan, MD, FACS Department of Surgery, Hadassah-Hebrew University, Jerusalem, Israel

United States Military Cancer Institute, Bethesda, MD, USA

Guy R. Orangio, MD Division of Colon and Rectal Surgery, Department of Surgery, Louisiana State University Health Science Center, LSU School of Medicine, New Orleans, LA, USA

Rodrigo O. Perez, MD, PhD Division of Colorectal Surgery, Department of Gastroenterology, University of São Paulo School of Medicine, São Paulo, Brazil

Angelita and Joaquim Gama Institute, São Paulo, Brazil

Janice F. Rafferty, MD Division of Colon and Rectal Surgery, Department of Surgery, University of Cincinnati, Cincinnati, OH, USA

Harry Reynolds, MD, FACS, FASCRS Colon and Rectal Cancer Surgery, Case Western Reserve University, University Hospitals Case Medical Center, Cleveland, OH, USA

David E. Rivadeneira, MD, MBA, FACS, FASCRS Division of Colorectal Surgery, Huntington and Southside Hospitals Northshore/LIJ Health System, Hofstra University School of Medicine, Huntington, NY, USA

Patricia L. Roberts, MD Division of Surgery, Department of Colon and Rectal Surgery, Lahey Clinic, Tufts University School of Medicine, Burlington, MA, USA

Howard M. Ross, MD, FACS, FASCRS Division of Colon and Rectal Surgery, Department of Clinical Surgery, Temple University Health System, Red Bank, NJ, USA

David A. Rothenberger, MD, FACS, FASCRS Department of Surgery, University of Minnesota Medical Center, Fairview, Minneapolis, MN, USA

David J. Schoetz Jr., MD Division of Surgery, Department of Colon and Rectal Surgery, Lahey Clinic, Tufts University School of Medicine, Burlington, MA, USA

Adrian Seah, MD Department of Surgery, Fletcher Allen Health Care, University of Vermont, Burlington, VT, USA

Anthony J. Senagore, MD, MS, MBA Division of Colorectal Surgery, Department of Surgery, Central Michigan College of Medicine, Saginaw, MI, USA

Joongho Shin, MD Department of Surgery, New York-Presbyterian/Weill Cornell Medical Center, New York, NY, USA

Nathan Smallwood, MD Department of Surgery, Baylor University Medical Center, Dallas, TX, USA

Lee E. Smith, MD, FACS, FASCRS Section of Colon and Rectal Surgery, MedStar Washington Hospital Center, Georgetown University, Washington, DC, USA

Michael J. Stamos, MD Department of Surgery, University of California, Irvine, Orange, CA, USA

Benjamin W. Starnes, MD Division of Vascular Surgery, Department of Surgery, University of Washington, Seattle, WA, USA

Scott R. Steele, MD Division of Colon and Rectal Surgery, Department of Surgery, Madigan Army Medical Center, Fort Lewis, WA, USA

Alexander Stojadinovic, MD, FACS Department of Surgery, Bon Secours Cancer Institute, Richmond, VA, USA

Uniformed Services University of the Health Sciences, Bethesda, MD, USA

United States Military Cancer Institute, Bethesda, MD, USA

Tiffany Tanner, MD Department of Surgery, University of Nebraska Medical Center, Omaha, NE, USA

Alan G. Thorson, MD, FACS Division of Colon and Rectal Surgery, Department of Surgery, Creighton University School of Medicine, The University of Nebraska College of Medicine, Omaha, NE, USA

H. David Vargas, MD Department of Colon and Rectal Surgery, Ochsner Clinic Foundation, New Orleans, LA, USA

Martin R. Weiser, MD Department of Surgery, Memorial Sloan-Kettering Cancer Center, New York, NY, USA

Mark Lane Welton, MD, MHCM, FACS, FASCRS Department of Colon and Rectal Surgery, Stanford University School of Medicine, Stanford Hospital and Clinics, Stanford, CA, USA

Steven D. Wexner, MD, PhD (Hon), FACS, FRCS, FRCS(Ed) Department of Colorectal Surgery, Cleveland Clinic Florida, Weston, FL, USA

Alia Whitehead, MD Department of Surgery, Fletcher Allen Health Center, University of Vermont, Burlington, VT, USA

Bruce G. Wolff, MD Division of Colon and Rectal Surgery, Department of Surgery, College of Medicine, Mayo Clinic, Rochester, MN, USA

Ilun Yang, MD, FRCSC Department of Surgery, McMaster University, Hamilton, ON, Canada

Nathan P. Zwintscher, MD Department of Surgery, Madigan Healthcare System, Tacoma, WA, USA

Part I

Preoperative

The First Encounter

1

Lee E. Smith and Anjali S. Kumar

Key Points

- Honesty, humility, and communication are the keys to success in establishing a solid relationship with your patient at the first encounter.
- Advocating for the patient by providing extra support services will endear you to your patients.
- Patients have difficult yet predictable questions. Know the answers beforehand in order to ease the encounter.
- Making yourself available by phone and Internet, and making time for face-to-face meetings, will make you approachable and popular among referring providers.
- Approaching each situation as if you were the patient is always the best practice.
- While it is important to educate and counsel your patients, it is often much more important to be a good listener.

Introduction

Key Concept: Draw upon your own personal experiences and background to form a solid base for your patient interactions. While your goals may vary depending on the stage of your career, each patient interaction is often unique, and approaching things from the patient's perspective is a good rule of thumb.

This chapter may seem unusual for a textbook of surgery. How does one create an atmosphere of trust with patients? As with all human interactions, first impressions are key, and this chapter is a subjective look at the topic from the perspective of two surgeons at opposite ends of their careers. The topic is quite subjective, so we draw heavily from our experiences in order to provide the perspective of both a senior surgeon with 40 years of experience in the field of colon and rectal surgery (*LE Smith*) and that of a junior surgeon just starting her colorectal surgery specialty practice (*AS Kumar*). We preface our individual statements with our respective voices.

(*LE Smith*) In writing this chapter, I reflect on more than 40 years of seeing patients in military, academic, and non-profit private hospitals. The patients in each type of hospital vary to some degree, but certain universal principles exist to help enlist the patient as an ally in solving his or her problem. One principle that has guided me throughout life is worth sharing, because it applies to surgery as it does to life. As a child in grammar school, I was given a cheap 12-in. ruler, which had printed on the side: "Do unto others as you would have them do unto you." Even as a child during the depression and the emotionally charged days of World War II, I recognized the wisdom of this succinct rule and permanently fixed it in my mind. It has served me well in my surgical career.

(*AS Kumar*) In working with Dr. Smith to craft this chapter, I reflect on my first 3 years building a practice and a referral base within our region. I was hired to help Dr. Smith retire, but soon found that his referral network consisted of physicians of his generation who thought an older, more experienced physician would be better suited to care for their patients than someone who was just starting out of fellowship.

L.E. Smith, MD, FACS, FASCRS (✉)
A.S. Kumar, MD, MPH, FACS
Section of Colon and Rectal Surgery,
MedStar Washington Hospital Center,
Georgetown University, 106 Irving St NW St 2100 N,
Washington, DC 20010, USA
e-mail: caroleandlee@rcn.com; askumarmd@gmail.com

S.R. Steele et al. (eds.), *Complexities in Colorectal Surgery*,
DOI 10.1007/978-1-4614-9022-7_1, © Springer Science+Business Media New York 2014

My success, therefore, relied more on my accessibility and visibility for in-hospital consults, my presence on the Internet, and my ability to connect with recent graduates of other referring medical fellowships (such as interventional gastroenterologists and medical oncologists with emphases on gastrointestinal cancers). Once securing an appointment with a new patient, it is essential that I give the best of care, be well liked and well respected by my patients, no matter what the circumstances. I quickly found that patients would refer their friends and families to me if they saw me as a passionate advocate for their health.

Keep in mind that someday roles may reverse, and you could be the patient. In the first encounter and the succeeding ones, imagine yourself on the receiving end of whatever it is that you are dispensing—an unfavorable pathologic result, the terminal sentence of a chronic disease, the news of a permanent, potentially disfiguring procedure that offers the best chance for a cure, or even a lubricated finger.

Prior to the Encounter

Key concept: The patient's first encounter with you and your team sets the stage for their entire work-up, management, and follow-up. Make it as easy as possible (within reason) for your patients and your referring physicians to gain access to you, whether it is through the phone, e-mail, or in person.

The team—every member of it—must be competent and convey this sense to the patient. The selection of your patient-oriented team is, therefore, critical. Regardless of how thoughtful, competent, well-trained, and skilled you are, the patient will ultimately judge you and the hospital by the qualities of your entire team.

The teamwork begins with the first telephone call the patient makes to schedule an appointment. In most practices, the telephone is the main interface with patients and referring physicians; therefore, this initial telephone conversation must be answered promptly with a friendly and helpful attitude. The receptionist must discreetly find the reason for the requested visit and make a decision about urgency. Generally, patients with pain, an abscess, or a presumed cancer need early or urgent appointments. The receptionist must have a medical professional—a nurse or a doctor—whom they can call upon if the course of action is uncertain. More importantly, they should recognize *when* they should "bump up" the request to a more authoritative, more experienced triaging assistant. Sometimes, patients may be reluctant to discuss anorectal problems on the phone. If hesitancy is recognized, it is often wise not to question further, and instead turn the discussion toward sending or bringing records from the referring physician. The patient's needs for the first visit should be explained verbally and repeated back by the patient if there is any question of the ability to understand or hear. If there is time, the confirmation of the appointment and what is required should be sent by mail. The patient needs to know that in order to accomplish as much as possible during the first visit, he or she needs to provide pertinent records, such as color copies of colonoscopy reports, operative reports, digital files of imaging studies, laboratory reports, pathology reports, and sometimes even pathology slides. If a mailing goes out, forms for demographics, insurance, and medical history could be included in order to save time during the registration process. No patient wants to get lost, so providing a map for travel, parking, and public transportation is useful. Figure 1.1 provides an example of what the radiology department at our hospital uses to remind patients of the preparation they need to undertake before coming for their appointment, and where on a map the appointment is. Tangible and clear communications like these convey to the patient the sense of a plan being formed.

Choosing a staff member for telephone scheduling and counseling is no trivial matter. A person who is rude, abrupt, or slow will have an outsized impact on your patient's experience. Consider splitting the task between several people; the receptionist's job is repetitive and tiring, and it is helpful to find ways to relieve stress and burnout. Maintaining a caring and friendly attitude is in everyone's interest. Whatever attitude the patient is greeted with, or whatever frustrations they harbor from the obstacles they had to surmount to get to you, will be present when you begin your evaluation.

Referring doctors handle their patients' referrals in different ways. Some will have the patient call and make an appointment without providing any information. Others will give the patient background records and studies to pass on, and some may even send a cover letter requesting the referral with records and studies included. Sometimes, a referring physician may be the first person to call regarding the patient and his problem. To aid the referring physician, the recording that usually greets him or her must be short and include the option to go quickly to a "live person" who can put him or her in contact with the surgeon. Listening to a long and time-consuming recorded message can lead to a hang-up and the loss of a referral. In recent years, we have maintained a separate telephone line, the "back line", for physicians. It is provided to referring physicians who call frequently. The referring doctors message needs to be conveyed to the surgeon whether he or she is in the office or the operating room. A good experience for referring physicians makes it more likely they will call again. If the surgeon cannot be reached, staff should arrange an appointment for the patient and promise that the surgeon will be alerted so that a return call can be made.

(*AS Kumar*) I am in contact with many of my referring physicians by e-mail. Through my hospital's secure network, they are able to send me the patient's pertinent medical records as PDF attachments, and I am able to ask them the necessary questions to ascertain the urgency of the appointment. Often, especially if I get a sense that the patient will need

PARKING AND DIRECTIONS TO MRI

Washington Hospital Center
110 Irving Street, NW
Suite G-104
Washington, DC 20010
Office: 202-877-5903
Fax: 202-877-5335

PARKING IS FREE FOR OUR MRI PATIENTS
From Michigan or Irving Street turn onto First Street. Follow MRI signs to the patient parking lot #5.

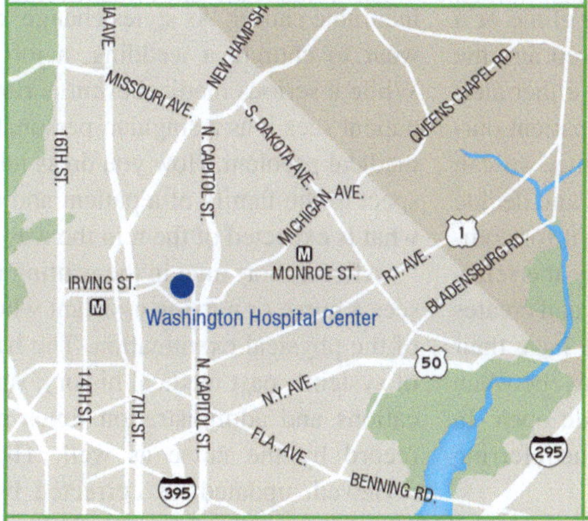

PATIENT PREP INSTRUCTIONS:

- Please arrive 15 minutes prior to appointment
- Bring insurance card, photo ID, doctor's orders and any referral if applicable
- No jewelry, no make-up, no hair pieces, hair pins, wigs, ornaments, etc.
- Breast imaging exams: bring prior mammography film(s)

SMALL BOWEL TEST PREP INSTRUCTIONS:

- If your appointment is in the morning, do not eat breakfast
- If your appointment is in the afternoon, do not eat lunch

Start prep 3 hrs. prior to test:

- Mix 2 teaspoonfuls of Metamucil in 16 oz. of water

Drink as follows:

- First Cup, 3 hours prior to test
- Second Cup, 2 hours prior to test
- Third Cup, 1 hour prior to test
- Fourth Cup will be administered by MRI clinical staff

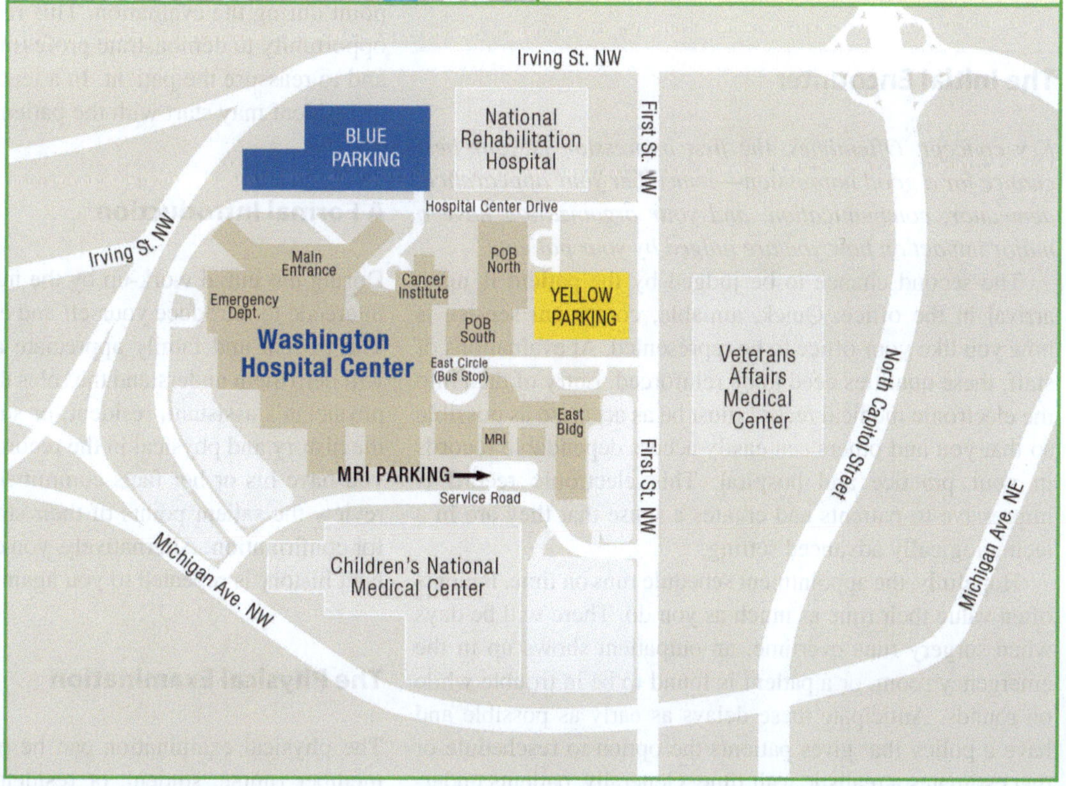

Fig. 1.1 An appointment confirmation notice with a map can be extremely helpful to patients

minor surgery (e.g., a recent finding of anal dysplasia), I appreciate having control over my clinical schedule to get them triaged in time for an open, convenient slot in my operating room schedule. My referring providers appreciate how rapidly I get the issue settled. They enjoy knowing that the loop is closed. Often, the e-mail interaction with the referring physician is simply a quick reply that is forwarded to my front desk staff to schedule the appointment. On occasion, my front desk staff has been willing to e-mail the patient for additional information. Some practices rely almost exclusively on new patient referral requests coming through the Internet and hire staff specifically with this intent.

We look at the appointment schedule to review new patients and their diagnoses. We grew accustomed to doing so in residency when preparing for an upcoming clinic or a case. If we see that a neoplasm or pain is involved and the appointment seems to be too far in the future, we either alert a nurse to get more information or telephone the patient ourselves to hear an abbreviated history. At that time, we can reassert the need to bring the appropriate records and decide if it is best to move the appointment up, or delay it for completion of studies that may have been ordered by the referring physician, or that we think to order. A simple call creates an early bond that reassures the patient that you have their interest at heart and that communication lines between patient, the referring physician, and you are wide open. In addition, word of this call may be transmitted to the referring doctor, who will be appreciative of your efforts.

The Initial Encounter

Key concept: Oftentimes, the first impression is your best chance for a good impression—remember your appearance, demeanor, communication, and your organization have a major impact on how you are judged by your patients.

The second chance to be judged by the patient is upon arrival in the office. Quick, amiable, competent service is how you like your office to be represented. At evaluations of staff, these qualities need to be reinforced. Entry of data into the electronic medical record must be as accurate as possible so that you and others can easily access dependable records in your practice and hospital. This electronic record is impressive to patients and creates a sense that they are in a technologically advanced setting.

Hopefully, the appointment schedule runs on time. Patients often value their time as much as you do. There will be days when surgery runs overtime, an outpatient shows up in the emergency room, or a patient is found to be in trouble while on rounds. Anticipate these delays as early as possible and have a policy that gives patients the option to reschedule or that estimates a realistic wait time. Generally, patients understand unexpected situations and delays in a hospital; they imagine that if it were them that needed urgent attention, they would appreciate the priority. Your desire to excel in the operating room is self-evident to your staff and patients. Apologize to the long-waiting patient when you arrive late, but only the briefest explanation of what detained you is necessary.

How you dress is a sign of respect for your patient. What is in fashion has changed, and there has been a trend toward informality. An exception is the military and uniform of the day. Sometimes, you or the staff wear surgical scrubs in order to save time when rushing to get to the office. This should be a rare occurrence because, with good planning, the office schedule should not be a reason to hurry an operation. We encourage dressing with the respect that is warranted when you tell a patient he has a chronic disease or a late-stage or incurable cancer. As styles change, consider what you would wear to church, a wedding, a job interview, or a funeral. While a serious medical event is run-of-the-mill for you, the patient sees it as a singular, personal, and even life-changing medical problem. How you dress telegraphs respect or disrespect to the family of a patient and also lets your staff know what is expected of them in the way of appearance.

After a short time in the waiting room, the patient usually sees a nurse or nursing assistant who takes vital signs as part of the physical examination. The basic forms for the review of systems, past medical history, surgical history, and medications and administration times may be entered into the record by the nurse as well. These records need to be reviewed, updated, or corrected by the surgeon at a later point during the evaluation. This record handling is another opportunity to demonstrate professionalism and competency and to reassure the patient. In a teaching setting, the student or resident may start with the patient to gather a history.

A Formal Introduction

During the initial work-up by the nurse, student, or resident, intercede to introduce yourself and explain your team's roles. The patient and family appreciate a formal introduction. It will help them understand the roles that the nurse practitioner, physician's assistant, resident, or student plays in filling out the history and physical in the record. To let the patient know you have his or her facts committed to memory, you might review the salient points of their story back to them, asking for confirmation. Alternatively, you can request that the pertinent history is repeated to you again to seal it in your mind.

The Physical Examination

The physical examination can be performed with the team member (nurse, student, or resident) and surgeon together. Usually, this will be the abdominal examination, digital rectal examination, anoscopy, and sigmoidoscopy. To explain why so many people are involved, say "It's good to have multiple sets of eyes on this so we don't miss anything" or "I'm going to need a hand with some of the instruments so I have a few helpers." For male physicians, it is often good practice to have a female member of the team present during the pelvic and anorectal exams of women patients. A team-oriented physical examination also helps to sell your team as a competent unit.

If a sink is in the examination room, wash your hands in front of the patient both before and after the examination. Patients appreciate this after so much publicity regarding the safety promoted by hand washing. Patients do not like to have their bare bottoms exposed, so try to position the table so that the patient's head faces the door. If you traditionally examine the patient in the knee-chest position, consider installing a curtain to be drawn in front of the exam room door.

Patients feel vulnerable not being able to see what you are about to do. Talk the patient through every part of the examination. Predict what the patient may experience and give a warning that a finger is entering the anus or vagina, or estimate and verbalize the size of an instrument relative to your finger. Let them know that an urgency to defecate is normal and not to move if a cramp occurs. We have found that a letter sent to the patient prior to the appointment which explains that a rectal exam is a standard part of a colorectal first encounter, helps establish a sense of preparedness for this intimate and sometimes uncomfortable part of the exam. Also, suggest to patients that they consider clearing their rectal vault of any contents by self-administering an over-the-counter saline enema 2 h prior to the visit. This is something that, when done in the privacy of home, helps the patient mentally prepare for what may ensue during your examination.

If pain is elicited, perform the painful examination only once. If there is no perception of pain, the step may be repeated by the other examiner, with the introduction "you are going to feel another finger now." Depending upon the working diagnosis, pain may be predicted with some manipulations, while some exams should not be painful. In any case, an effort to minimize pain will endear you to your patient. For example, lubricate the finger or instrument liberally and be gentle. If you see an obvious fissure, do not feel obligated to perform a digital rectal examination or anoscopy on the first visit. Sometimes, asking the patient to push out against your finger not only relaxes the muscles but gives the patient an action to focus on so that he or she will not immediately tense up when sensing your hand nearby.

Conveying Pathology Results

When biopsies are taken or a biopsy result is outstanding, have the patient schedule an appointment within the week to come back and learn the result and plan the ensuing steps. If the pathology is favorable, consider telephoning the patient to relay the good news. This demonstrates to the patient that you are thinking of him or her. Do not put off the call. Often, the patient is anxious and waiting by the phone. If a weekend is near, and the result is favorable, telephone them with the happy result, even if it is late on Friday night. Waiting and not knowing a pathology result exacerbates patient anxiety. Hearing from you during the "off-hours" especially impresses a patient. If the pathology is foreboding, wait for the scheduled appointment or move the appointment sooner.

(*AS Kumar*) I employ e-mail to communicate with many patients about their pathology. After taking a biopsy and before leaving the patient's side, I discuss the option of receiving the results by e-mail. In an era of exorbinent outpatient co-pays, I sympathize with the patient's interest in avoiding another face-to-face encounter. If e-mail is an option, we can spend a few extra minutes at the initial encounter itself, talking through the potential next steps based on the outcomes of the pathology report. The e-mail that I ultimately send encloses a digital version of their entire report and includes a summary of my impressions. I ask the patient to reply with a phone number and a good time for me to call to discuss it further. This step empowers the patient, since many like to keep shadow copies of their medical records and also like the opportunity to share the diagnoses with the primary care provider. Sophisticated electronic personal health systems employ a web portal where patients log in to see their personal health record and interact with their physicians. This allows them to access their laboratory and pathology reports and correspond with their physicians via the secure portal (Fig. 1.2) [1]. Nonetheless, I am careful to get the patient's permission before sending an e-mail, since the Internet is not a fully private environment. Many institutions' e-mail servers provide a disclaimer statement (Fig. 1.3) that underscores that your e-mail is a confidential communication to them. I take the extra step of committing e-mails to and from patients in the electronic health record (EHR) under the "letter" or "correspondence" sections. Similar to a "phone note," this step makes your electronic conversation with the patient or providers an integral part of the medical chart.

The Team and Teaching

Key concept: Each member of the team plays a critical role—ensure the patient understands who everyone is and what that role encompasses. Have several different platforms (i.e., *brochures, videos, online links, support groups*) *of educational resources available for your patients.*

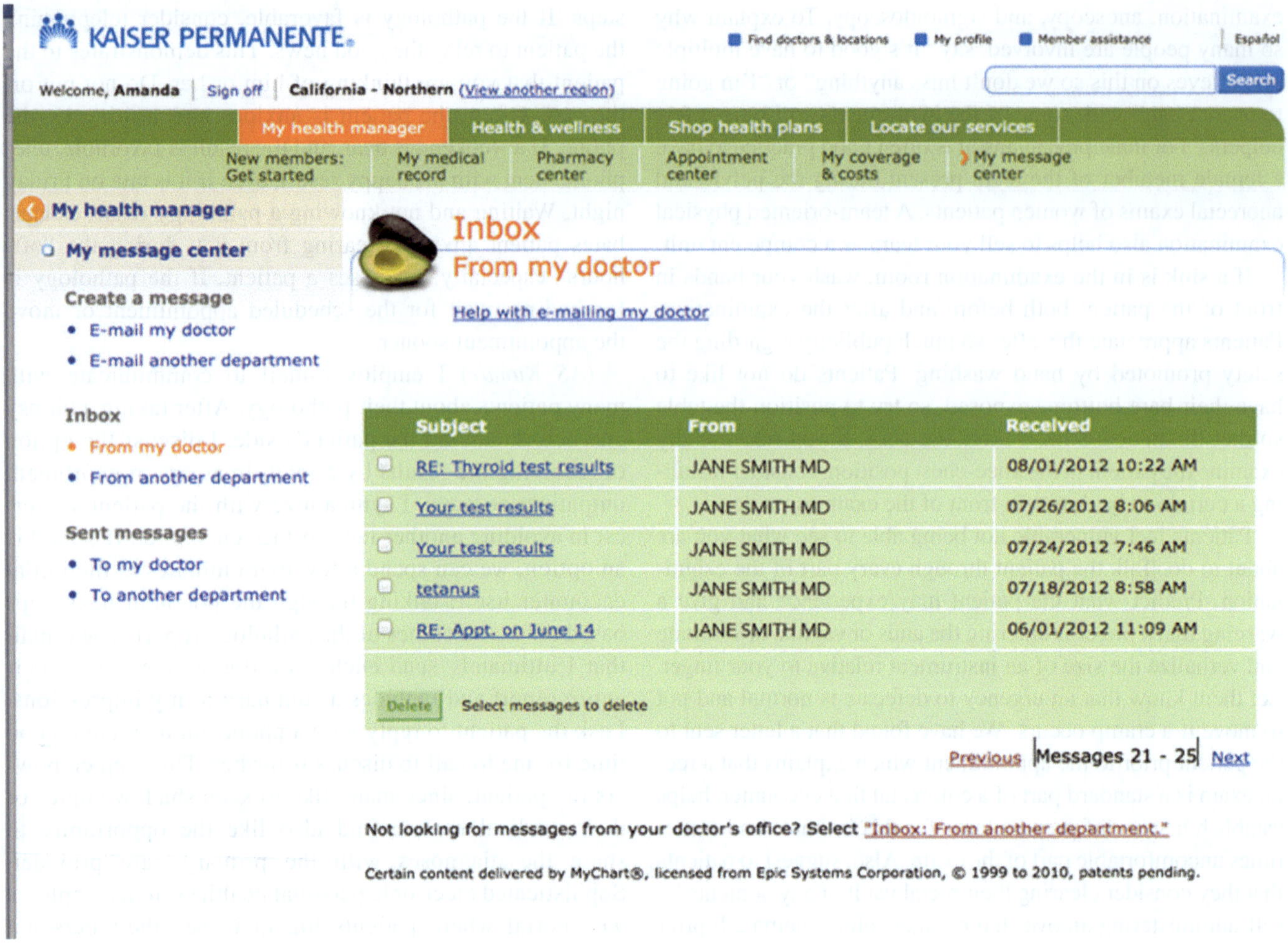

Fig. 1.2 Internet portals can allow patients to access their personal health records (*With permission from Kaiser Permanente* [1])

MedStar Health
CONFIDENTIAL: The information contained in this communication, including its attachments may contain confidential information and is intended only for the individual (s) or entity (ies) to whom it is addressed. The information contained in this communication may also be protected by legal privilege, federal law or other applicable law. If you are not the intended recipient of this communication, you are hereby notified that any distribution, dissemination or duplication of this communication is strictly prohibited. If you have received this communication in error please immediately delete and destroy all copies of this message and please immediately notify us of the error by separate communication. Thank you.

a

Memorial Sloan Kettering
Please note that this e-mail and any files transmitted from Memorial Sloan-Kettering Cancer Center may be privileged, confidential, and protected from disclosure under applicable law. If the reader of this message is not the intended recipient, or an employee or agent responsible for delivering this message to the intended recipient, you are hereby notified that any reading, dissemination, distribution, copying, or other use of this communication or any of its attachments is strictly prohibited. If you have received this communication in error, please notify the sender immediately by replying to this message and deleting this message, any attachments, and all copies and backups from your computer.

b

Chesapeake Potomac Regional Cancer Center
The PHI (Protected Health Information) contained in this FAX/email is HIGHLY CONFIDENTIAL. It is intended for the exclusive use of the addressee. It is to be used only to aid in providing specific healthcare services to this patient. Any other use is a violation of Federal Law (HIPAA) and will be reported as such. If you have received this FAX/email in error please destroy/delete it immediately.

c

Fig. 1.3 Confidentiality statements employed by institutions' Internet transmissions at (**a**) MedStar Health (**b**) Memorial Sloan Kettering and (**c**) Chesapeake Potomac Regional Cancer Center

The Team's Role

At a convenient break during the first outpatient visit, explain that the team consists of a nurse, nurse practitioner, physician's assistant, residents, other surgeons, ostomy nurses, or others who will be working with the patient and emphasize that these same people may be present at the hospital or during follow-up. For example, you may volunteer that they might be speaking to the nurse by telephone to answer questions, to residents or partners for hospital rounds, or to nurse

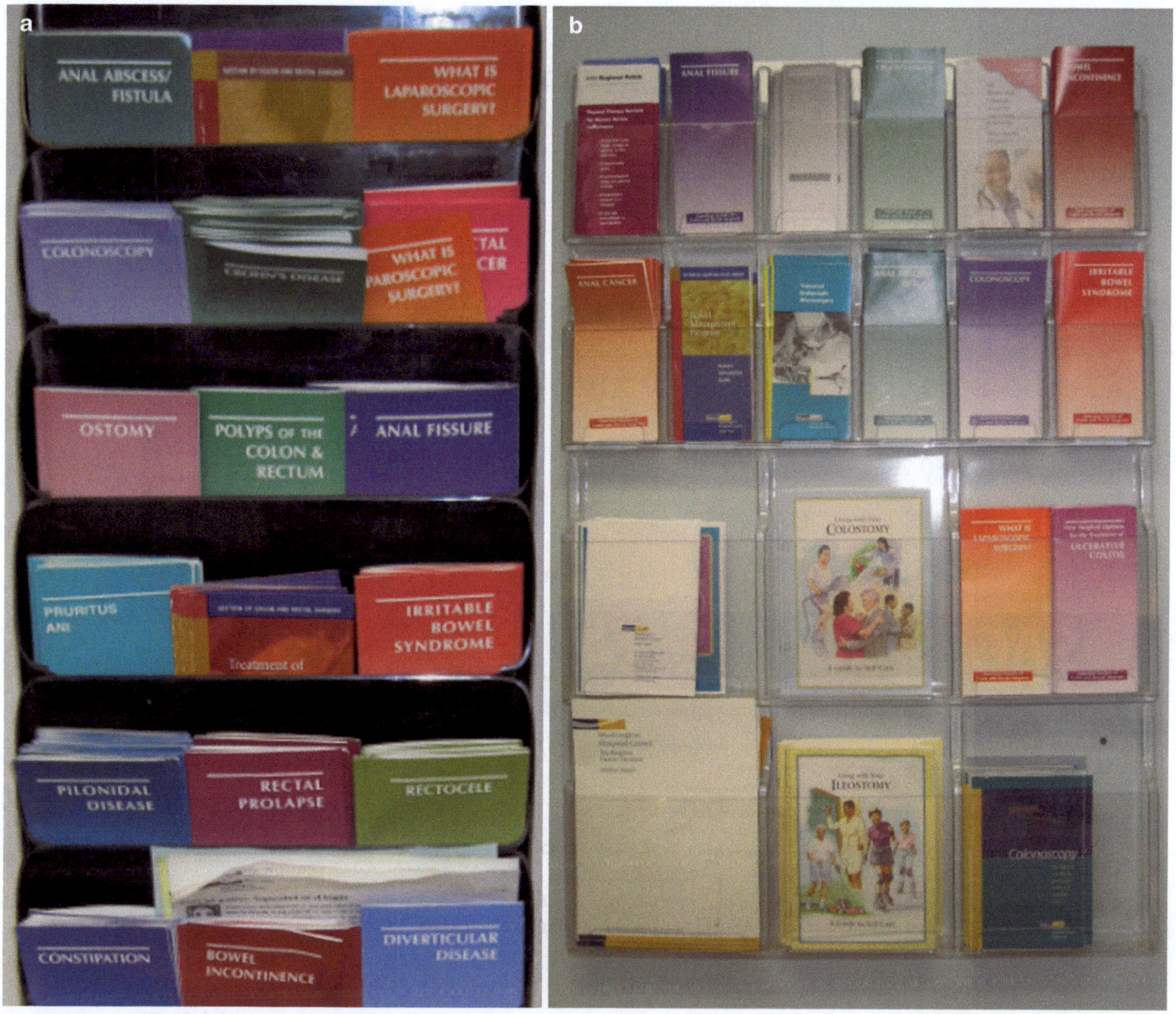

Fig. 1.4 Brochure racks are a simple and affordable solution for patient education. (**a**) An example of what is displayed in a patient exam room; (**b**) in our nurses' room, information about ostomies is also provided

practitioners or physician's assistants during follow-up. This never frees you as the surgeon from your ultimate responsibility—rounds and follow-up are a part of your primary obligation to your patients.

The patient may wonder why there are so many people involved. You can assure them that each team member plays a valuable role, that many minds are dedicated to their problem, and that not a step will be missed. It also serves to keep everyone educated. For a colon and rectal surgery resident or a chief resident, you can add that they are a trained (often board certified) general surgeon or are about to finish a rigorous general surgery-training program. The residents provide an additional observer of progress or problems and a level of continuity if surgery and hospitalization are contemplated.

Educational and Informational Resources for Patients

Repetition is a form of teaching. Direct your patient to the many resources for more information, such as pamphlets or videos. Educational aids are readily available from several sources. The American Society of Colon and Rectal Surgeons (ASCRS) and the Society of American Gastrointestinal and Endoscopic Surgeons (SAGES) have brochures and videos that address the various diseases and surgeries of the colon, rectum, and anus. Such educational references can set up as hyperlinks on your practice's website. Putting up a brochure rack (Fig. 1.4) is a small investment, but videos and customized websites may be costlier. As an alternative, provide the patient with the links to websites you trust. Both ASCRS and

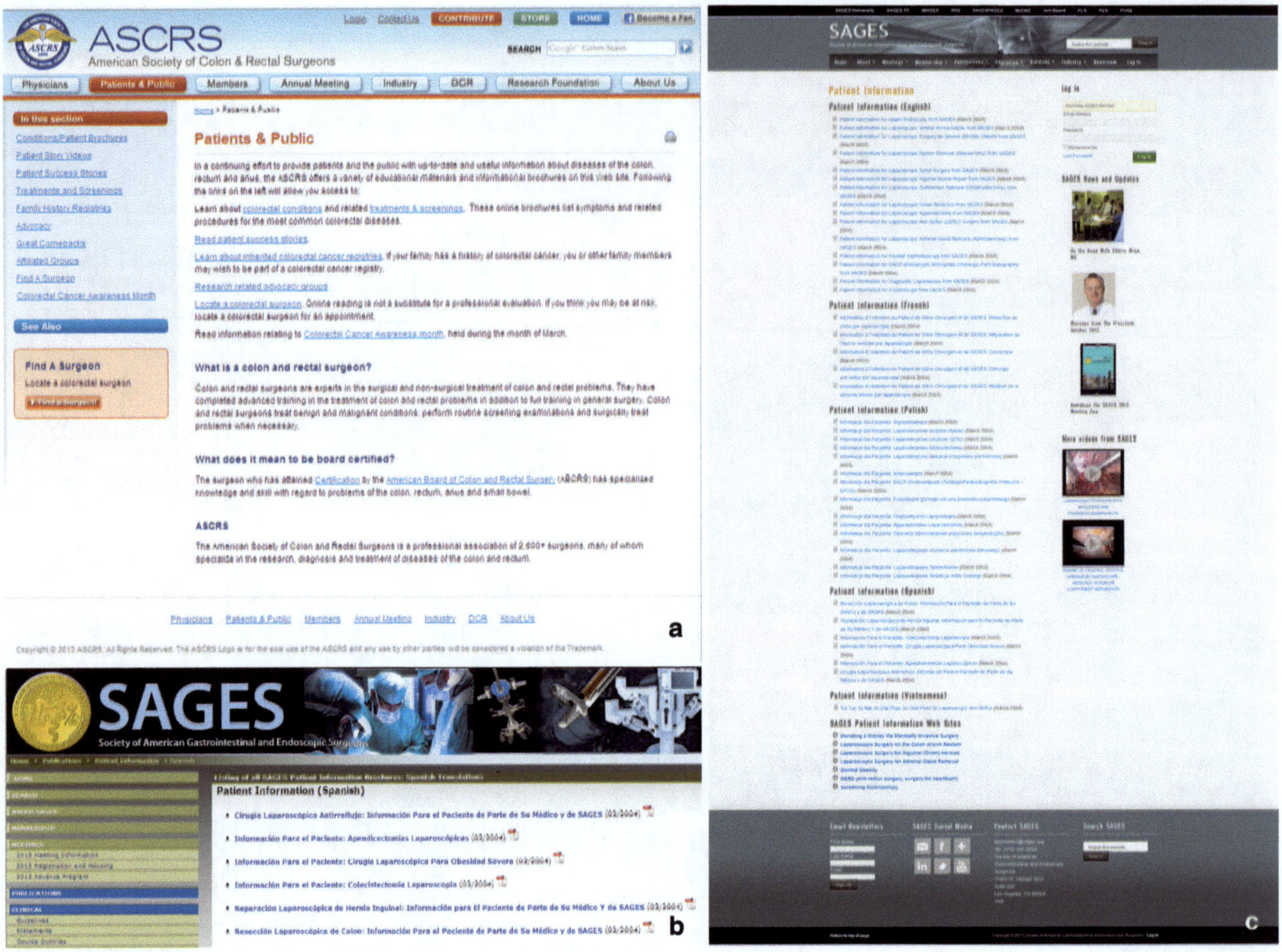

Fig. 1.5 Specialty society websites provide patient information. (**a**) American Society of Colon and Rectal Surgeons (ASCRS) (*With permission* [2]); (**b**) Society of Gastrointestinal and Endoscopic Surgeons (SAGES) (*With permission* [3]); (**c**) SAGES Patient information in multiple languages (*With permission* [3])

SAGES have patient-specific links (Fig. 1.5a–c) [2, 3], which also include written and video testimonies from patients who have had specific colorectal issues [4]. Take a few minutes to browse the web for materials relevant to the patient's situation. An endorsement from you will be more productive than leaving your patient adrift on Internet search engines.

Support Groups and Personal Resources

We sometimes encounter patients who declare, "I will never have an ostomy," and this is always a tricky conversation. What helps is to acknowledge their desires but also ask that he or she investigate and get all the information. As necessary, they can then revisit the issue with you, or if there is a misunderstanding, then schedule a revisit for a repeat discussion. It is an overwhelming decision to choose a permanent ostomy on the first encounter with you, especially if their primary care provider has not previously broached the subject. In cases like these, it is best to introduce the *possibility* of an ostomy, and then give some time for the news to sink in. Then patients can check in with their support systems, as well as others that you may suggest. Many communities have support groups. Our region has several ostomy help groups, which have trained ostomates to share their situations and show that they are able to go about their lives. It is reassuring for a potential ostomy patient to see someone who is a match in disease, gender, and age and who is living well. An educated patient is your ally and will work with you to get the best outcome. Also, linking an ostomy nurse to your practice is a valuable asset in instructing a patient about the practical use of an ostomy. A patient will learn more readily before surgery than after when postoperative pain and anxiety may interfere with concentration.

Counseling and Consent

Key concept: An upfront, open, and honest discussion regarding the risks, benefits, and alternatives to your planned management is the key to successful counseling and managing expectations.

After the history, physical, review of the available studies, and a call to the referring physician (if necessary), a plan is formulated. The patient should not leave the office without this plan firmly in mind. Missing pieces such as additional studies or communication with other doctors must be filled in. Release-of-information forms must be signed, studies ordered and scheduled, and follow-up arranged. Accounting for each step conveys to the patient a sense of efficiency and relief that a plan is in motion. Many term this concept "one-stop shopping". If information is complete enough, the management discussion can start. If the course is surgery, the informed consent requires a discussion of risks, benefits, and alternatives, the procedure(s) recommended, and the possible complications. In communicating potential risks and complications, we counter the inevitable fears by offering that permanent morbidity or mortality is statistically possible, but usually not a great probability. A cancer diagnosis means that therapy needs to begin within a month, i.e., chemotherapy, radiation, or surgery. Document everything you recommend.

Honesty is the key to successful counseling. Your training, postgraduate education, and experience reinforce the standards of care that you live by. If your opinion differs from that of another physician, explain the standard of care for colon and rectal surgery as you honestly know it. Educate the patient and family in clear, simple terms. This brings them to the point where they can understand you and make informed decisions. We do not routinely offer our volumes of similar operations, outcomes, or experiences unless patients ask. Seldom do we know these numbers unless a targeted effort has been made to collect the data. As electronic data collection becomes uniform (such as in the case of the Surgeon Specific Registry [5]), more of your case data, and comparisons to national standards, will be available (Fig. 1.6) [5]. In the days of an implicit trust in the healthcare system and its practitioners, more patients just said, "do what you need to do." In recent years, patients are emboldened to ask more questions. Patient's rights need be honored. An informed patient is an understanding patient. If your recommendations are not within the standard of care, the plan could be deemed research or experimental, and a protocol should be reviewed by the investigational review board (IRB) of your hospital. If it is research, the elements of a research informed consent need to be included as per the IRB.

Counseling is one thing, and critical instructions are another. For example, with a patient who needs a colonoscopy, the surgeon must review possible complications and stress the need for good colon preparation. Critical instructions are needed for other procedures or studies. The colonoscopy scheduler and the person who goes over the preparation of the colon may not emphasize the importance of a perfectly clean colon, so a word from you may be necessary. Explain that a poorly prepared colon hinders your ability to see and may force cancellation of the colonoscopy. Also keep in mind that patients often flout the rules and overestimate their abilities after discharge, assuming that they can take a taxi alone or find their own way home on public transportation. Many institutions require that if sedation is received, an escort is required. Make it clear to the patient that the absence of an escort may result in procedure cancellation, which is especially frustrating to a patient who has completed a bowel preparation. We have found that we cannot always rely on our schedulers to convey this critical piece of information, so we take a few moments to go over it personally.

Difficulties at the First Encounter

Key concept: Recognize potential barriers to your patient's overall care, be prepared for the difficult questions, and, again, rely upon an open and honest discussion in educating and counseling your patients.

Physical, Psychological, or Language Barriers

Some patient difficulties are apparent immediately, such as obesity, difficulty walking, shortness of breath, or pallor, but others do not emerge until the patient starts to talk. Language barriers, limits on mental capacity, anxieties, denial, and inappropriate expectations are among the obstacles you will encounter.

The patient may not be fluent in English, so have an interpreter available. Since Spanish is frequently a first language, a Spanish-speaking employee can provide a valuable bridge while arrangements are made for an interpreter. Often, the patient recognizes the language problem and brings a friend or relative who can interpret. The initial phone call usually alerts your receptionist to the language situation, and arrangements can be made in advance. Similar arrangements need to be made if the patient is a minor, needs a guardian, is mentally compromised, or needs consultation via a power of attorney.

The Internet: A Double-Edged Sword

Patients, friends, and relatives all go online to learn about the disease. At the same time, they may use the Internet to read about you. Being board certified equates with "better" in many patient's minds. Since your education is usually listed, you may need to be ready to discuss where you studied and why or why you have stayed in the area or moved so many times.

(*AS Kumar*) Many surgeons view free online profiles such as healthgrades.com or vitals.com [6, 7] as a nuisance, but in fact, this can be a tremendous marketing advantage if you take some time to feed the sites correct information and a photo [8]. If your practice does not have or cannot afford a web presence, these sites could help promote your practice and yourself. As

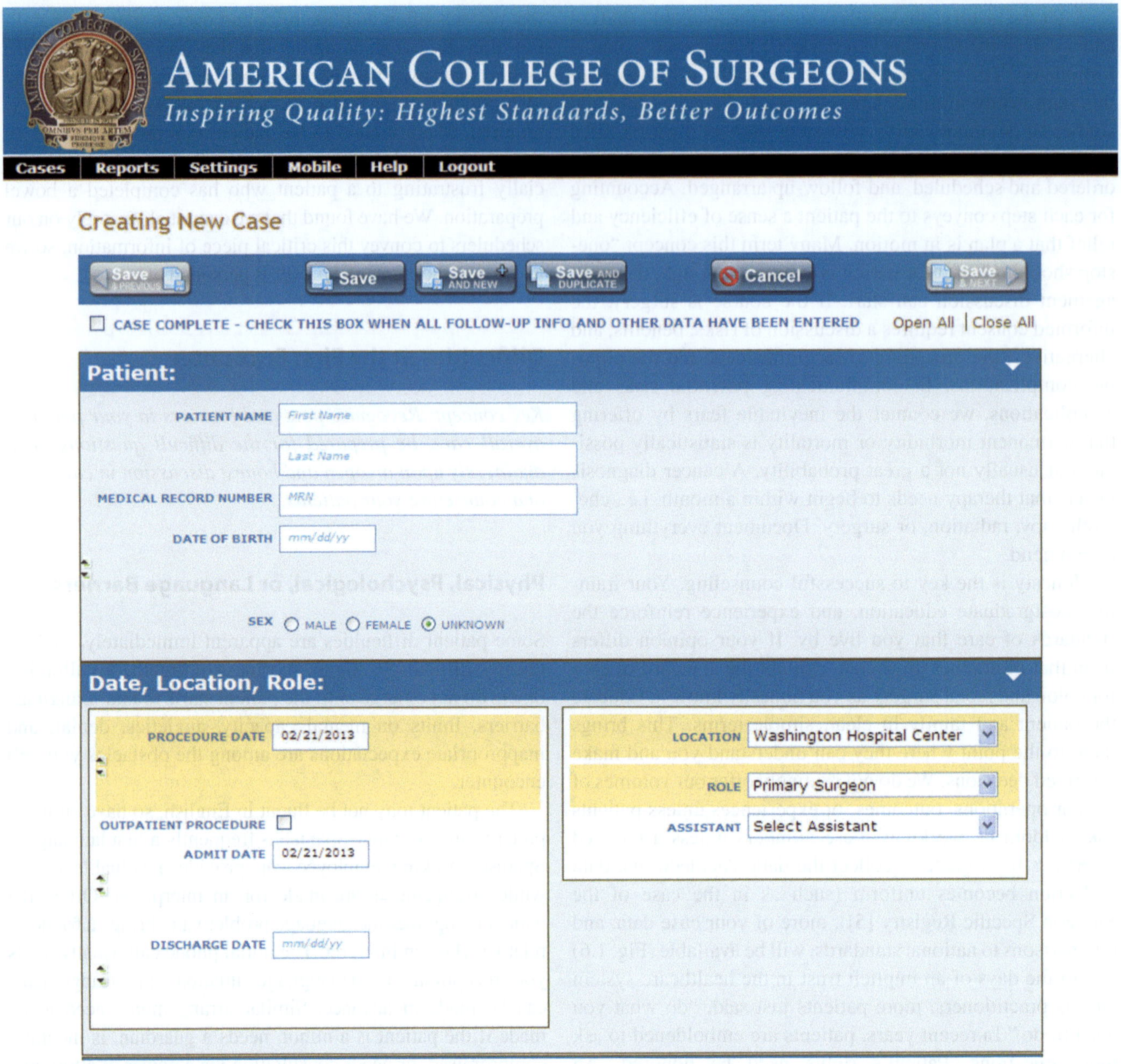

Fig. 1.6 The ACS Case Log Portal allows surgeons to record their cases and track their outcomes compared to national trends (*With permission* [5])

a young surgeon, half of the patients come from my referral network in the region and half is self-referred. It is common for me to ask a new patient, "How did you find me?" and hear that my Internet presence is the answer [9].

However, much of what is available about colon and rectal surgery on the Internet will fall short of your own expertise. Be prepared for the patient who comes armed with a printout of his or her personal research and one that disagrees with your diagnoses or course of actions. The ensuing discussion needs to be honest, thorough enough for a layperson to understand, and consistent with standards of care in colon and rectal surgery. Repeat that you believe your plan is best and that your plan is similar to what would be proposed by other specialists in colon and rectal disease. It is seldom necessary to point out your education and training, but be prepared and rehearse what you might say if such a statement becomes necessary.

Navigating a Litany "To Dos"

In taking on the care of a patient, you become the patient's advocate. Your plan may include phone calls to other doctors, investigations of comorbidities, laboratory studies, imaging studies, physiological testing, endoscopy, or a referral to an ostomy nurse, a medical oncologist, a radiation oncologist, a geneticist, a psychiatrist, an infectious disease specialist, an interventional gastroenterologist, etc. This is a daunting list of "to dos" for a patient who is elderly or has a physical or mental limitation. Therefore, you and your team become the advocate. You, after all, are an expert at navigating the barriers that build up in hospital policies and routines. Cutting through the red tape on the patient's behalf endears the patient to you. The patient should not leave the office until each step in the plan is arranged or the means to accomplish it is clear to the patient and family. If a barrier is encountered by the patient that seems insurmountable, offer that the patient can always call you or your team for help. Such helpfulness adds to the bond between the patient, you, and your team. If your schedule affords it, calling to make some of the patients' appointments while the patient is in your office is especially appreciated. If possible, use a speakerphone; it will allow the patient to learn how smoothly a request is entertained when made by a physician personally or how even a physician must contend with red tape. When a patient witnesses you navigating phone trees and other roadblocks in scheduling, it humanizes you.

Difficult Questions Posed to You

Often, one of the first patient responses is "how soon can we have surgery?" It is especially difficult to win patients over to neoadjuvant chemoradiation and its long time frame. First, the patient wonders how long she or he has had the cancer. The answer is months to years. As surgeons, we know, from our experience of rectal cancer, that a relatively short delay is worthwhile to shrink the tumor, reduce the local recurrence rate, and "sterilize" the lymph nodes. We create realistic expectations by telling our patients that they will be seeing us for the next year. Now the team includes a medical oncologist and radiation oncologist.

"Can't you do it any sooner?" is another awkward question. Some patients will have had an issue for many years, but the moment they see you, they are suddenly inspired to have their elective surgery occur immediately. This puts a surgeon in the challenging position of wanting to please the patient, on the one hand, and on the other hand wanting to optimize the clinical and operative schedule.

(*AS Kumar*) Early in my practice, I was very accommodating with patients, especially because my operating room schedule was still a blank slate. As I have become more clinically busy and more involved academically, I have learned to negotiate patient requests more gingerly, in order to keep my schedule manageable and efficient. The "bad news" that surgery will not be for another month can be blunted if imaging, laboratory tests, or clearance letters are required before the operation. In the case of outpatient anorectal cases on healthy, uncomplicated patients, it is often useful to schedule surgery for them all on one day, even if that given day is only once a month. A patient is generally satisfied with the explanation, "I only do this type of case on a specific day." You can assure him or her that if anything opens up earlier, you will let them know. For patients who are negotiating their work or vacation schedules, I explain that it is easier to offer them a selection of times and then for them to coordinate with the schedulers to get the time or date to their liking. At many institutions, it is easier to cancel or reschedule a case than to book it from scratch. I ask the patients to understand that hospitals usually function at capacity and that many entities stand to lose when cases are unexpectedly cancelled. This instills a respect for the effort it takes for something as serious as surgery to be scheduled. While I had a very high no-show or last-minute cancellation rate in the first year of my practice, it has since greatly reduced, in part due to my modified counseling methods. On the other hand, when I see a patient in the office whose surgery cannot necessarily wait a month (i.e., an anal abscess or a chronic, unresponsive anal fissure), I adjust accordingly while explaining to the patient that surgery is demanded sooner or urgently. A high level of trust is created from an extraordinarily brief encounter.

"Doctor, how many of these procedures have you done?" Again, honesty must prevail. (*LE Smith*) Someone like me, who has been in practice for several years, may be able to say that the answer is many. But if this is the first such procedure I have ever done, I tell them so. For instance, my first sphincterotomy for fissure presented in the first month after my residency. Sphincterotomy made more sense than the fissurectomy that I had been trained to do in residency. Before IRBs were introduced, I was obliged to tell a patient that he would be my first anal manometry patient and that I had created an anal catheter by gluing together several narrow tubes with a balloon at the tip, and from several sources assembled a water infusion pump, pressure recorder, and transducers. Likewise, my first patients with an ileoanal pouch, an end-to-end stapled anastomosis, laser treatment, transanal endoscopic microsurgery, and laparoscopy were informed that they were the first. No one walked away, but I was mentally prepared for the conversation.

(*AS Kumar*) The challenge of a young surgeon is that he or she can seem inexperienced to the patient and family. This puts a burden on the young surgeon to educate and to create bonding and trust. The educational discussion and the likely ensuing questions may take longer for the young surgeon. Emphasize that your recent training exposed you to the most modern practices and techniques. When I am asked how many of "Procedure X" I have done, I understand that the patient is not just seeking reassurance of my competence, but looking to judge my humility and honesty. I recount that I have been in the field for 10 years (include the start of your general surgery training to present date) and in my specialty for 4 years (include the start of your fellowship training to present date). I describe the rigors of the Accreditation Council of Graduate Medical Education (ACGME) specialty training programs and the tough standards of our boards of surgery and medical licensing authorities. I have ready access to my case logs from practice and from fellowship and can immediately provide them with not only my personal numbers if they are still interested but also the number of similar cases that my practice as a whole does per year. I reassure them that I have the advantage of a group practice where I can call on the expertise of my partners if needed. Sometimes, it introduces levity when I mention that youth gives me the advantage of bountiful energy and stamina for longer procedures (i.e., laparoscopic colectomy or transanal endoscopic operations). At this point, I am usually comfortable enough with the patient that I can say in all honesty, "You have every right to seek care from whomever you choose, and if you would like to see one of my partners for a second opinion, I can easily arrange that for you. We often operate together and having two surgeons involved in your case is an option if that makes you more comfortable." Booking a case to be "double-scrubbed" can often be cumbersome on both your and your partner's schedule. But sometimes all that is needed is for your partner to greet the patient with you in the preoperative area and then scrub during the critical portion of the case. It is reassuring both to me and to my patients that I have expert partners just a phone call away. This conversation conveys to the patient that his or her need is my utmost priority and that my ego does not factor into my decision-making.

Preemptive Discussion of Potential Complications

Although the patient seeks reassurance, never promise a cure or a complication-free recovery. You cannot predict which patient will have a recurrence, a leak, a wound infection, pulmonary embolus, or even death.

(*LE Smith*) Even for something as seemingly simple as a hemorrhoidectomy, it is bad practice to tell a patient that the risk of complication, ostomy, or death is nil. I do not mention death as a complication of anorectal disease or anorectal surgeries, but I also never promise that something untoward will not happen. I can remember almost every patient who died during the admission for my surgery. Interestingly, most were young and expected to tolerate surgery well; all this is perhaps the reason I remember them. For example, a 39-year-old woman with ulcerative colitis was to have a proctocolectomy with ileostomy when there was an uncontrollable intraoperative hemorrhage in the pelvis, cardiac arrest on the operating table, closed chest massage with liver laceration, and finally exsanguination and death. Bleeding and death were discussed during consent, but this does not make telling her husband and small children that she died any easier. Yet it would have been worse if nothing had been said about the possibility preoperatively. Another example was a 41-year-old man, who had a pouch procedure without technical problems, but in the early morning of the second postoperative day, he died due to an unexpected myocardial infarction. The consent and documentation included the risk of death and had been discussed with both the patient and his wife, but it is still an incredibly difficult and emotional situation for everyone involved.

The Patient's Family

Key concept: The family plays a crucial role in all aspects of your patient's recovery. Be sure the accompanying person/family member understands the plan just as well or better than your patient.

A family member, or several, may accompany the patient. Often, the patient is insecure being alone or may be elderly and concerned about not understanding what is being explained. The anxious patient is unable to concentrate, and the elderly may have short-term memory failures. This relative or friend is your ally, serving as a liaison if the patient questions details of your counseling later.

The patient usually wants to tell you what has happened. Family members sometimes interrupt to tell the history even when the patient is willing and able to do so. Return the conversation back to the patient and look him or her in the eye when you are talking. This concentration alerts the patient that you recognize their fears and that you will be their advocate through the illness. Thereafter, the family may add information that they think has been omitted. Do not cut the patient or family off before they have completed reporting the history as they want you to hear it. Listen. The most important concept we can pass on to you is to become a good listener.

(*LE Smith*) I believe that the willingness to listen (and good documentation) kept me out of legal action for my entire career.

Occasionally, the family is overbearing, unreasonable, or lacks consensus. This can become a significant and difficult obstacle, and sometimes we have appointed one of the more thoughtful members to serve as spokesperson. Through this, however, the patient still has the deciding vote. If you have been honest and dedicated to providing all the information, the patient will almost always accept your recommendations.

The family often is the most important support for post-hospital care. Asking where the patient might go after leaving the hospital starts the family thinking about a plan.

When the family does not accompany a patient who needs an extensive surgery, or for whom you foresee a complicated recovery, it is imperative to include the family in the preoperative discussion, even if that discussion needs to be scheduled for another time. Occasionally, we will employ speakerphone to include absent family members. The patient sees that you understand the big picture and that you are anticipating their future needs.

Often, as you finish your session with the family, someone asks, "What would you do if this was one of your family members?" This has been an easy question for us and hopefully for you, because the correct answer is, "I would do the same thing if I were the patient, or for you if you were my family member." One young patient of ours with advanced rectal cancer faced the decision to undergo an abdominoperineal resection with permanent end colostomy. In an example like this, spend some time thinking about how you would face such a decision and answer yourself honestly about what you would choose, knowing that pelvic recurrence could cost you your life. It is an intimate and personal decision that only the patient can make. But as a leading authority on this subject, your judgment may carry more weight than the patient's own.

Communicating with Other Physicians

Key concept: Stay in contact with your referring providers about not only patient care but also developments in colorectal surgery (i.e., *new technology*). *Take advantage of the different ways to keep the lines of communication open, especially those face-to-face interactions.*

Sometimes, the patient has seen another surgeon, and you are the second opinion. The opinion may be the same or very similar. At this point, the patient often returns to the original surgeon. We do not make any effort to "steal" the patient; however, the patient may be impressed with you and your team and want to stay. In this case, the patient should personally cancel future appointments with the other surgeon, if scheduled. It is wise to write a letter to the primary care doctor, the gastroenterologist, and the original surgeon including your recommendations. Inform all parties that the patient requested to remain with your practice, and note that this was not by your suggestion. For the other surgeon, however, the loss will be remembered. Keep the lines of communication open by asking the surgeon if he or she wants to see the operative notes, pathology reports, and discharge summaries of the patient's subsequent care. If referrals to oncologists are required, the original surgeon's recommendations could be solicited, especially if the patient wishes his or her care to be in a geographic area that you are not familiar with.

If a difference in opinion exists between you and another surgeon, explain to the patient that this is the standard of care as you know it, point out that you have kept up with your education, and support your opinion with the latest, best knowledge and experience. On the other hand, if the patient or family wants a second opinion after visiting you—or if a visit to another surgeon is already scheduled—do not be offended, but welcome it as a chance to gain the insight of another trained professional.

In either case, regional societies are a venue to interact with your specialty's colleagues. Apart from the weather, the stock market, or the latest in sports, there is no easier topic of conversation than mutual patients. The phenomenon of "doctor shopping" is now frequent, and all doctors are aware of it.

Another set of parties to keep in mind is the referring physician and primary care doctor. Good practice demands that you write a letter after the first encounter regarding your diagnosis and recommendations. This has been aided by electronic medical records, which usually permits a link to send an automated letter to the referring doctors. Consider reinforcing your letter with a telephone call; doing so befriends the referring physician and makes it easier to follow-up in case of an infection, a leak, a change in diagnosis, or, worst of all, death. The referring doctor feels responsible for complications after having recommended you to the patient.

Letters, e-mails, and telephone conversations simply cannot substitute for face-to-face interactions with your referral network. If opportunities do not currently exist in your region for these meetings, seek to start one, such as a monthly dinner for case discussion. Continuing medical education (CME) credit can often be awarded and will be a draw for referring providers. Alternatively, give a luncheon talk at your referring physicians' practice. For young physicians just starting out, this is an excellent way to get to know the region, make contact with the referral base, and educate physicians about your unique areas of interest, technologies, and techniques. An educational talk is an excellent strategy when faced with a particular referral network that has the habit of sending you mismanaged cases. Often word from you is all the push they need to get you in the loop earlier.

Conclusion

As surgeons caring for patients with complex colorectal diseases, we are in the unique position of assisting patients to a diagnosis of a chronic, lifelong illness (such as Crohn's), discussing potentially disfiguring procedures (such as abdominoperineal resections, permanent ostomies, and sacrectomies), and counseling those with unresectable carcinoma of the colon or rectum. These are the worst-case scenarios. We also care for benign, bread-and-butter, anorectal disorders, those with polyps amenable to advanced endoscopic techniques, curable cancers with little to no external incisions, and those with chronic but significant quality of life issues such as constipation or incontinence.

Part of why we choose this specialty is that we are drawn to the vast array of diagnostic and clinical complexities. However, patients and referring providers carry their own quirks and challenges that must also be carefully navigated, often all at the first encounter.

In our practice, we have found it helpful to prepare for the encounter prior to the visit, provide formal introductions of ourselves and our team members when the patient is fully clothed, prepare the patient adequately for the examination (especially if it involves an inspection of their genitalia), and finally allow the patient to dress, use the toilet if necessary, and come to our office or a conference room to discuss the next steps in their care. Including the family in person or by speakerphone during this review is especially useful and forms a bond with the people who will provide the patient their necessary postoperative support. Delineating, in writing, the next steps in their care is essential, as patients are often overwhelmed by all that is attempted to be accomplished in one visit and details are bound to be missed. Advocating for your patient by making the referral appointments you deem necessary will quickly endear your patients to you. Equipping your patients with brochures, diagrams, and Internet resources that you endorse will further help them understand the nature of their disease and the procedure you propose. Finally, having excellent communication with your referral network will keep you in their good graces and elevate you as a respected member of your region's surgical community.

Summary Pearls

- Having a patient-oriented team is critical because the patient's first encounter with you and your team sets the stage for everything that follows. The right receptionist is crucial, as is the right gateway for referring providers.
- Adroit use of e-mail and phone calls make the surgeon efficient and generate patient trust and repeated referrals.
- The clinic atmosphere must be designed for maximum efficiency, not just because it creates the best outcome, but because it also creates an impression of competence. A respectful style of dress matters. So does a proper introduction of the team.
- The physical examination can be a vulnerable time for patients, so explanation of what to expect during each step of the exam is important. The same goes for conveying pathology results, where simple attention to detail makes for a dramatically different patient experience.
- Educate the patient about his or her disease, and the options for treatment, with repetitive and consistent messages. Guide the patient to the right support groups and online resources.
- Honesty is the key to successful counseling. When it comes to critical instructions, make sure that the patient brings the necessary information, so neither the patient's nor the physician's time is wasted.
- Use the Internet as a means to provide confirmatory information to patients, to generate trust and referrals.
- Be the advocate for your patient as he or she navigates the obstacles of healthcare.
- Use understandable language to answer your patient's questions, as it sets the stage for efficient management and patient cooperation.
- Managing a patient's family wisely can turn them into allies.
- Respect is the key when other physicians wind up treating your patients or you end up treating theirs.

Acknowledgment The authors gratefully acknowledge the contributions of Kirthi Kolli, MBBS, who provided invaluable editorial assistance in the completion of this work.

References

1. Kaiser Permanente. Create a message, email my doctor [Internet] editorial policies last updated 27 Sept 2011 [cited 21 Feb 2013]. Available from: https://healthy.kaiserpermanente.org/health/mycare/consumer/my-health-manager/message-center/from-my-doctor.
2. American Society of Colon and Rectal Surgeons. Patients and public [Internet] Copyright © 2013 ASCRS [cited 21 Feb 2013]. Available from: http://www.fascrs.org/patients/.
3. Listing of all SAGES Patient Information Brochures, English, Spanish [Internet] Content on this site is Copyright © 1995–2013 [cited 21 Feb 2013]. Available from: https://www.sages.org/publications/patient_information/ and https://www.sages.org/publications/patient_information/spanish.php.
4. American Society of Colon and Rectal Surgeons. Patients and public [Internet] Copyright © 2013 ASCRS [cited 21 Feb 2013]. Available from: http://www.fascrs.org/patients/patient_stories/.
5. American College of Surgeons, American College of Surgeons Surgeon Specific Registry (Case Log) [Internet] Copyright ©2005–2012 Resilience Software, Inc. [cited 21 Feb 2013]. Available from: https://acspbls.resiliencesoftware.com/.
6. Health Grades. Find doctors [Internet] Copyright 2013 Health Grades, Inc [cited 21 Feb 2013]. Available from: http://www.healthgrades.com/.
7. Vitals, find doctors by name, specialty or condition. [Internet] Copyright © 2006–2013 Vitals.com & MDx Medical, Inc. [cited 21 Feb 2013]. Available from: http://www.vitals.com/.
8. Steven Schwaitzberg. Webpages, Facebook, and social media: marketing your practice in 2012; young surgeons' symposium. In: 2012 annual scienting meeting, San Antonio. The American Society of Colon & Rectal Surgeons. [Course ID: ASCRS1226B].
9. MedStar Washington Hospital Center Colon and Rectal Surgery, Our Team, Dr. Anjali Kumar [Internet] 2009 Nov 1 [cited 21 Feb 2013]. Available from: http://www.whcenter.org/colorectal-kumar.

Perioperative Risk Assessment

2

W. Donald Buie and Anthony R. MacLean

Key Points

- Understand the goals (and limitations) of a perioperative risk assessment and how it is ultimately used clinically.
- Tailor your preoperative laboratory tests to your particular patient, even if it means not checking any labs.
- You (the surgeon) are the one who "clears" your patient for surgery.
- The urgency of the clinical situation will often determine the (in) ability to obtain and extent of a preoperative risk assessment.
- Wound infections are common in colorectal surgery; however, you need to have a system in place to reduce their occurrence, and pathways with several components are the best way to achieve this goal.

Introduction

Key Concept: Colorectal surgery has inherent risks. It is ultimately your responsibility, as the surgeon, to ensure that your patients have been completely and thoroughly evaluated prior to surgery.

While no surgery can be completely risk-free, a thorough preoperative evaluation serves to identify and control perioperative risk as much as possible. Major advances in surgery and anesthesia and improvements in preoperative risk assessment and management have led to a dramatic decrease in perioperative morbidity and mortality. This, in turn, has expanded the eligible patient population for major surgical procedures to include patients who would not have been considered surgical candidates in the past.

Perioperative risk assessment has three fundamental goals: (1) to identify previously undetected comorbid conditions or factors, (2) to evaluate known conditions or factors that may increase the risk of perioperative complications, and (3) to optimize medical conditions preoperatively to reduce perioperative risk. Perioperative risk can be classified into three categories: patient-specific risk, procedure-specific risk, and anesthetic-specific risk. Although these categories exist as distinct concepts, in practical terms, they are not independent and must be considered in concert when patients are being evaluated for surgery.

This chapter will focus on the role of the colorectal surgeon in assessing perioperative risk, obtaining appropriate consultation and synthesizing the information to provide safe surgery for patients.

Risk Stratification

Key Concept: There is no validated perioperative risk assessment tool that combines all three categories of risk. You must integrate several sources to obtain an overall preoperative risk assessment for each individual patient. The ability to formulate a composite risk assessment is an essential component of a good clinical judgment.

Assessing a Procedure-Specific Risk

Key Concept: Several aspects (and potential outcomes) of a colorectal procedure need to be considered to more accurately determine the procedure-specific risk.

The AHA/ACC 2007 perioperative guidelines [1] classify procedure-specific risk into high, intermediate, and low-risk surgery (Fig. 2.1). Based on the Revised Cardiac Risk Index (RCRI), most colorectal procedures fall into the intermediate

W.D. Buie, MD, MSC, FRCSC, FACS (✉)
A.R. MacLean, MD, FRCSC, FACS
Department of Surgery,
University of Calgary, Foothills Medical Centre,
1403-29th Street NW, Calgary, AB T2N-2T9, Canada
e-mail: wdbuie@ucalgary.ca; tony.maclean@albertahealthservices.ca

S.R. Steele et al. (eds.), *Complexities in Colorectal Surgery*,
DOI 10.1007/978-1-4614-9022-7_2, © Springer Science+Business Media New York 2014

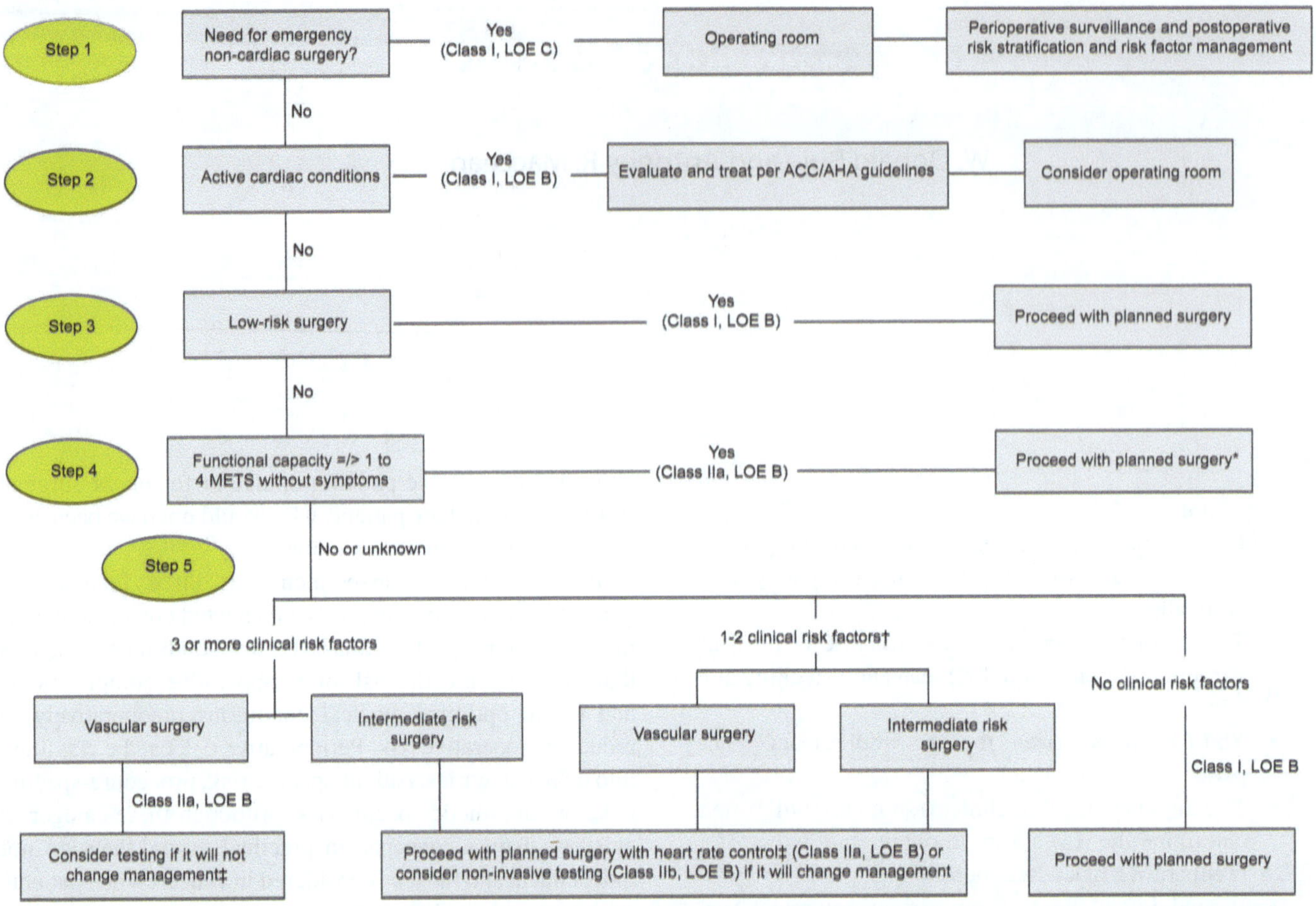

Fig. 2.1 Cardiac evaluation and cardiac care prior to noncardiac surgery. *Noninvasive testing may be considered before surgery in specific patients with risk factors if it will change the management. †Clinical risk factors include ischemic heart disease, compensated or prior heart failure, diabetes mellitus, renal insufficiency, and cerebrovascular disease. ‡Consider perioperative beta-blockade for populations in which this has been shown to reduce cardiac morbidity/mortality. *LOE* level of evidence, *MET* metabolic equivalent (Modified from Fleisher et al. [2])

(i.e., abdominal procedures) and low-risk categories (i.e., ambulatory perianal, endoscopy), with an associated estimated risk of cardiac morbidity of 1–5 and <1 %, respectively. Patients in the low-risk category normally require minimal workup and do not require preoperative cardiac testing [2]. However, an estimation of cardiac risk based solely on this classification system may under- or overestimate risk, as these values are independent of preexisting comorbidities and do not include an estimate of surgical complexity. For example, an elderly otherwise healthy 80-year-old undergoing an extended low anterior resection for rectal cancer may have an estimated risk of 1–5 % of having cardiac event based on the RCRI index. Yet, from your (i.e., the surgeon's) point of view, the risk of anastomotic leak is potentially much greater, and it may result in a significant cardiac morbidity.

Surgical complexity is difficult to quantify. The NICE guidelines for surgical stress has four categories in order to help group procedures by the amount of physiological stress that may result (Table 2.1) [3]. Colonic resection is considered grade 4 (major +) along with total joint replacement, lung operations, neurosurgery, and cardiac surgery. This division is somewhat arbitrary, as even within each category, not all procedures are equal. When evaluating surgical stress, the surgeon must also take into account the effect of body habitus, fluid shifts, the potential for blood loss, and prolonged surgery. Re-operative surgery also adds to complexity, which in turn is affected by the surgeon's level of expertise and experience. When there is more than one procedure available as in rectal prolapse, you may opt for a less invasive approach in a high-risk patient. Although often implied, there is no evidence that a laparoscopic approach presents a lower risk to patients, and stress level alone does not appear to have affected the uptake of laparoscopy in colorectal cancer [4].

What is clear, however, is that any patient who requires emergency surgery is at a higher risk for complications regardless of the presence or absence of any other variables. This is especially true in the elderly population [5]. Unfortunately, in most cases, you will have little opportunity

Table 2.1 National Institute for Health and Care Excellence (NICE) classification of surgical stress

Grade 1	Minor	Excision of lesion of skin; drainage of breast abscess
Grade 2	Intermediate	Primary repair of inguinal hernia; excision of varicose vein(s) of leg; tonsillectomy; adenotonsillectomy; knee arthroscopy
Grade 3	Major	Total abdominal hysterectomy; endoscopic resection of prostate; lumbar discectomy; thyroidectomy
Grade 4	Major+	Total joint replacement; lung operations; colonic resection; radical neck dissection; neurosurgery; cardiac surgery

From: Reynolds et al. [3]

to modify even known risk factors in this setting. It requires tremendous coordination between you and the anesthesiologist in the perioperative setting, along with the critical care team postoperatively, to follow these patients closely, anticipate potential problems based on their risk factors, and hopefully mitigate or manage them early as they arise.

Assessing an Anesthesia-Specific Risk

Key Concept: *Anesthetic risk is a combination of the effects of the anesthetic agents and, in large part, the skill level of the anesthesiologist.*

Modern anesthesia is typically very safe, with an estimated risk of death from anesthesia at 1 per 200,000–300,000 anesthetics [6]. Based on the American Society of Anesthesiologists (ASA) physical status classification system, a normal healthy ASA class 1 patient has a mortality rate of less than 0.03 %. The rate increases to 0.2 % for class 2 patients, 1.2 % for class 3 patients, 8 % for class 4 patients, and 34 % for class 5 patients [7]. Significant perioperative morbidity is also related to ASA status, with a relative risk of 2.2 and 4.4 for ASA classes 3 and 4, respectively [8].

A number of meta-analyses have shown that overall mortality is lower in patients receiving neuraxial anesthesia (epidural or spinal) when compared to general inhalation anesthesia. Much of this difference is due to lower rates of thromboembolic disease, pneumonia, and respiratory depression [9–11]. In general, there is no difference in the rate of cardiac events between general and neuraxial anesthesia, though every effort is made to support the blood pressure during induction of general anesthesia. Patients who are being considered for neuraxial anesthesia for postoperative pain control may also gain additional benefits from the point of view of enhanced recovery, although this has not been consistent in the literature [12].

Several special devices are at the disposal of (and often used by) the anesthesiologist to enhance intraoperative monitoring. These include central venous catheters for volume status, arterial catheter for continuous blood pressure monitoring and frequent blood gas analysis, and pulmonary artery catheterization to monitor cardiac output, pulmonary artery pressure, and pulmonary vascular resistance. Perhaps surprisingly, there is no good evidence that any of these interventions decrease the incidence of perioperative complications. The routine use of pulmonary artery catheters for high-risk patients undergoing noncardiac surgery is not recommended [13, 14]. On the other hand, transesophageal echocardiography is increasingly being used in high-risk patients undergoing high-risk procedures to promote goal-directed therapy [15]. However, the indications for this technology are still evolving and oftentimes anesthesia dependent.

Assessing a Patient-Specific Risk

Key Concept: *Healthy patients can be screened with a simple questionnaire that includes age, exercise tolerance, social habits, medications, and problems with previous anesthetics. In general, selective preoperative testing should be based on a focused history and physical examination.*

The Healthy Patient

The goal in evaluating the healthy patient is to identify previously unrecognized conditions or factors that may increase perioperative risk. When a healthy patient is seen in the office regarding surgery, we have them fill out a short questionnaire regarding their medical history. With respect to perioperative risk, we are specifically interested in a basic screen focused on cardiac and respiratory symptoms to elucidate occult disease. These two systems are responsible for most of the significant postoperative morbidity. In addition, there is level I data for effective preventative strategies geared towards them. As such, we consider 5 factors: *patient age, exercise capacity, social habits (alcohol and smoking), medication use, and problems with previous anesthetics.*

Age

Much of the age-related risk is due to the increasing prevalence of comorbidities that occur with advancing age. In a large study of 1.2 million Medicare patients undergoing elective surgery, the operative mortality for patients ≥80 years was more than twice that of patients 65–69 years of age [16]. In another study of 50,000 elderly patients undergoing elective surgery, operative mortality increased from 1.3 % in patients less than 60 years of age to 11.3 % in patients 80–89 years of age [17]. With respect to pulmonary events, a large systematic review found that age was one of the most important independent predictors for complications, even after adjusting for comorbidities [18]. Despite these negative findings, improvements in anesthetic and surgical care have reduced age-related differences such that some authors state age should not be used as the sole criteria to withhold a surgical procedure [19], while others disagree [20]. Despite the disagreement, it is not uncommon to successfully perform major abdominal procedures in relatively healthy nonagenarians and even have >90-year-old patients recover well from emergency surgery [21, 22].

Exercise Tolerance

Patients with unlimited exercise tolerance are generally at low risk for perioperative cardiopulmonary complications. A general assessment of exercise tolerance has been defined as the ability to walk two blocks on level ground without symptoms or carry two bags of groceries up one flight of stairs without symptoms [23, 24]. When these simple criteria were used prospectively in a study of 600 patients undergoing major surgery, patients with poor exercise capacity suffered twice as many postoperative complications (20 % vs. 10 %) and twice as many cardiovascular complications (10 % vs. 5 %) when compared to patients with good exercise capacity [25]. In a study of 847 patients undergoing elective abdominal surgery, poor exercise capacity was a stronger predictor of mortality than the individual risk factors comprising the Revised Cardiac Risk Index (RCRI) [26]. It is an easy question to ask and get an overall feel for the patient's tolerance.

Social Habits

The association between social habits and increased perioperative risk is well described, and generally bad habits lead to bad outcomes. In a study of US veterans, a validated questionnaire on alcohol use administered within 1 year prior to surgery was able to stratify patients for risk of surgical site infections, overall infections, and cardiopulmonary complications [27]. Another small trial of patients undergoing colorectal surgery reported a beneficial effect of alcohol cessation prior to surgery on postoperative complications. Although the optimal time for cessation of alcohol is unknown, the earlier, the better [28]. You should note, however, that stopping in a time frame where acute withdrawal is likely to occur (i.e., DTs) would not be ideal.

Smoking is strongly associated with postoperative morbidity, especially pulmonary and wound complications, and mortality [29]. Yet, there is something you can do about it, *if* you can get your patient to quit. A recent meta-analysis of 6 randomized trials and 15 observational studies demonstrated a significantly lower overall risk of postoperative complications with cessation of smoking [30]. In contrast to alcohol use, complication rates were inversely proportional to longer smoke-free periods; thus, preoperative counseling and adjunctive measures to stop smoking should be encouraged.

Medications

In addition to a complete list of prescription medications and allergies, a medication screen must include information on both over-the-counter and alternative medications. Aspirin and other nonsteroidal anti-inflammatory medications are commonly used and potentially effect hemostasis. Patients often forget to include them as medications, except if directly asked by name. Some alternative medicines are associated with an increased risk of perioperative complications, but because they are "natural," patients may only provide information on direct questioning. A complete list of these medications is beyond the scope of this review. However, there are several excellent reviews of the common alternative medications and their potential perioperative effects [31].

Anesthetic Issues

Likely, the most important question you can ask in this category relates to their past history with anesthetics. Patients who have had problems with previous surgery or anesthetics should receive a preoperative anesthesia consult. This includes a family history of anesthetic problems, which may mandate additional preoperative investigations or intraoperative precautionary measures. Other anatomical factors that must be considered include the finding of a potentially difficult airway due to limitations on mouth opening, micrognathia, obesity, and limitations of neck extension in patients with cervical arthritis. Furthermore, patients who are undergoing a laparotomy require a thorough preoperative discussion of the options for postoperative pain control.

The initial preoperative screen is supplemented with a thorough physical examination. Based on any positive findings from either the history or physical examination, selective investigations are ordered, and if appropriate, a medical consult is organized.

Preoperative Testing

Key Concept: *Preoperative testing should be selective and based on positive findings from a focused history and physical examination.*

There is ample evidence that nonselective testing of healthy patients rarely results in a positive test that in turn is unlikely to result in a significant adverse event [32–35]. Because of the low incidence of significant abnormalities in healthy patients, the positive predictive value of specific tests is also very low. You should remember that nonselective testing actually increases the rate of false-positive results, which then necessitate further testing, increased expense, inconvenience, and a possible delay of surgery. Furthermore, a normal test does not necessarily reduce the risk of an adverse perioperative event [36].

This is not to say that you should never order tests. Baseline preoperative tests may be indicated when the proposed surgery is expected to significantly alter values

Table 2.2 Revised Cardiac Risk Index (RCRI)

Predictors	Number of predictions	Risk (cardiac death, nonfatal myocardial infarction, and nonfatal cardiac arrest) (%)
History of ischemic heart disease	0	0.4
History of congestive heart failure	1	1.0
History of cerebrovascular disease (stroke or transient ischemic attack)	2	2.4
History of diabetes requiring preoperative insulin use	3	5.4
Chronic kidney disease (creatinine >2 mg/dL)	>3	5.4
Undergoing suprainguinal vascular, intraperitoneal, or intrathoracic surgery		

Modified from Lee et al. [40]

(i.e., large operation in a patient with baseline mild renal insufficiency—see below) or if an asymptomatic patient is in a high-risk group for a specific condition. There should be an expectation of an abnormal result that is relevant for anesthesia or surgical care.

At the present time, we check a baseline hemoglobin in healthy patients who are at risk of significant blood loss such as colonic resection or in patients with a high chance of anemia due to their underlying disease process. We do not routinely check electrolytes, blood glucose, liver function, hemostasis, or urinalysis in healthy patients undergoing either a colonic resection (moderate risk) or outpatient low-risk surgery. We do get a serum Cr in patients over 50 years of age undergoing colonic resection and in all patients suspected of having renal dysfunction (see below). We do not order a routine ECG unless patients are over 60 years of age or have other specific clinical indications such as asthma or smoking. Routine preoperative chest X-rays are not ordered in healthy patients. They may also be part of a workup for malignant disease when a chest CT has not been performed (Table 2.2).

The Comorbid Patient

Key Concept: Patients with newly recognized or known comorbidities require preoperative consultation with system evaluation and the institution of preoperative strategies to minimize risk and maximize safety.

Consultation

The preoperative evaluation of specific comorbidities and anesthetic risks requires consultation. Good communication is paramount. The surgeon should provide all the essential history and physical findings, diagnostic imaging, and laboratory results. The consult should be centered on a very specific question usually regarding specific comorbidities. *Asking for the patient to be cleared for surgery is not sufficient.* In addition, the urgency of the surgery should be indicated; is the condition emergent, urgent, or elective? For complicated or emergent cases, we try to discuss the case directly with the internist prior to the consult. It is sometimes helpful for the internist to understand the surgical options and the potential compromises that may have to be made depending on the degree of patient-specific risk. In high-risk non-emergent situations, the patient may see the internist prior to a final decision regarding surgery, especially when the preoperative assessment is an important part of the decision to operate.

Try to direct the consult to the specialist who is best equipped to provide not only an answer but also specific treatment and postoperative support should a complication arise. If a patient has a single-system disease with a previously established relationship (i.e., cardiology or nephrology only), we use that consultant and reserve the general internist for those with multisystem disease.

In complex cases or patients at very high risk due to extensive comorbidities or high procedural risk, arrangements should be made in advance for ICU support. While open units have been the norm in the past, most hospitals are moving towards closed ICUs. A frank discussion with the patient regarding the potential for ICU admission, ventilator dependency, and the level of acceptable resuscitative measures must occur and must be communicated preoperatively to the ICU team.

Cardiovascular Risk Assessment and Risk Reduction

Key Concept: Cardiovascular risk is best assessed using one of the well-defined cardiac risk indices. High-risk patients with significant cardiovascular disease may require preoperative stabilization with medical therapy, and in some cases, preoperative revascularization to decrease risk.

Cardiovascular risk assessment is based on an evaluation of specific predictive clinical variables, exercise capacity, and surgery-specific risk. The algorithm for cardiovascular risk assessment is reproduced in Fig. 2.1 [1]. Patients at high risk of cardiovascular events who require emergency surgery may not have time to be fully evaluated or medically optimized due to the urgency of their surgical problem. In this situation, clinical conditions should be documented for monitoring with management and stabilization occurring intraoperatively and in the postoperative period.

In the urgent or elective situation, there are several factors that increase the risk of significant postoperative cardiac events such as myocardial infarction (MI), heart failure, and death. These factors include unstable angina, severe angina or recent MI (within 30 days), decompensated heart failure, significant arrhythmias, and severe valvular heart disease. When these factors are present (especially in combination), a very careful preoperative evaluation is required and may justify a delay in, or even preclude proceeding with, surgery. In addition, there are a number of secondary clinical variables that include a history of ischemic heart disease, cerebral vascular disease, compensated heart failure or prior heart failure, diabetes mellitus, and renal insufficiency, which are also predictive for cardiovascular morbidity [37]. While many of them are incorporated into the clinical risk indexes outlined below to give an overall risk score for the patient, they do have independent associations with worse outcomes as well.

An evaluation of patient-specific risk also includes an assessment of exercise tolerance. As noted previously, poor exercise tolerance has been defined as the inability to walk two to four blocks or climb two flights of stairs at a normal pace due to the development of dyspnea, angina, or excessive fatigue. This translates to a metabolic equivalent of ~4 (4 MET), and failure to achieve this is predictive of in-hospital perioperative risk. Additional activities with a similar metabolic equivalent include carrying objects of 15–20 lb and playing golf or doubles tennis.

The overall perioperative cardiovascular risk for each individual patient is determined using one of several cardiac risk indexes. In 1977, Goldman was one of the first to develop a cardiac risk index using nine variables to predict the development of cardiac complications [38]. Since then, several others have come along—some cardiac-specific, and others more general (i.e., ASA Classification [39, 70]; Table 2.3). Earlier, we introduced the Revised Cardiac Risk Index (RCRI) or Lee Index, as it is one of the most widely used due to its simplicity and clinical utility [40] (Table 2.2). It is the primary index applied at our center and is based on the presence or absence of six predictive factors: *high-risk surgery, ischemic heart disease, congestive heart failure, cerebrovascular disease, diabetes mellitus, and renal dysfunction*. Patients receive one point for each risk factor that is present to give a cumulative index score. The rate of development of a major cardiac event—defined as myocardial infarction, pulmonary edema, ventricular fibrillation/cardiac arrest, and complete heart block—is estimated to be 0.4 % (95 % CI 0.1–0.8 %), 1 % (95 % CI 0.5–1.4 %), 2.4 % (95 % CI 1.3–3.5 %), and 5.4 % (95 % CI 2.8–7.9 %) for scores of 0, 1, 2, and ≥3, respectively [41, 42]. Using the AHA algorithm, patients at high risk for cardiac complications (score ≥3) should undergo noninvasive cardiac (stress) testing. If severe myocardial ischemia is identified, coronary revascularization should be considered prior to planned surgery (if possible), in addition to preventative medical strategies outlined below.

Recently, a new predictive risk model for perioperative myocardial infarction/cardiac arrest was constructed from the American College of Surgeons National Surgery Quality Improvement Program (NSQIP) database [43]. This model is based on a very large patient cohort where more recent preventive and interventional cardiac strategies were applied. On multivariate regression analysis, significant predictive variables included type of surgery, dependent functional class, abnormal creatinine, ASA class, and increased age. This model is not as well known; thus, many internists are not comfortable using it. However, when compared directly to the RCRI model, it demonstrated higher predictive accuracy. An online calculator has been created which makes it easy to apply by the surgeon to determine individual risk [44].

Perioperative medical therapy for cardiac risk reduction includes B-blockers, statins, and aspirin. High-risk patients or those who take these medications preoperatively require medical consultation. Based on recent evidence, preoperative B-blocker use has been limited to specific risk groups and must be introduced gradually. Despite good evidence for the beneficial effect of B-blockers and statins [45, 46], the evidence for the perioperative use of aspirin and/or thienopyridine for the reduction of cardiac risk is less clear due to an increased risk of perioperative bleeding. While aspirin alone is safe, the combination of aspirin with thienopyridine is associated with an increased risk of perioperative bleeding and transfusion. To reduce the risk of bleeding, thienopyridine should be discontinued 5–7 days prior to surgery and restarted as soon as the risk of postoperative bleeding has decreased.

Table 2.3 American Society of Anesthesiologists (ASA) classification

ASA1	A normal healthy patient
ASA 2	A patient with mild systemic disease
ASA 3	A patient with severe systemic disease
ASA 4	A patient with severe systemic disease that is a constant threat to life
ASA 5	A moribund patient who is not expected to survive without the operation
ASA 6	A declared brain-dead patient whose organs are being removed for donor purposes

Modified from the American Society of Anesthesiologists (ASA) [70]
There are modifications—the addition of "E" for an emergency and the addition of "P" for pregnancy

High-risk patients with severe cardiac ischemia may be candidates for preoperative coronary revascularization. Patients with left main stem or three-vessel CAD associated with poor left ventricular function have a recognized survival advantage with either coronary artery bypass (CABG) or percutaneous coronary intervention (PCI) including balloon angioplasty and/or stent placement. The benefits and risks of revascularization must be factored into the decision-making process. CABG has a higher procedural risk than PCI. However, PCI with stent placement is associated with an increased risk of perioperative bleeding due to the use of dual antiplatelet agents, which, if stopped prematurely, may result in stent occlusion. Ideally, colorectal surgery should be delayed ~30–45 days after placement of a bare metal stent and 1 year following a drug-eluding stent. This may not be practical in a patient with a near obstructing cancer or in the situation of a narrow therapeutic window following chemoradiation. Patients who require surgery within a month of coronary revascularization should undergo either an angioplasty without stent placement or, in select circumstances, a CABG. The colorectal surgeon must be involved in these complex decisions, especially when determining the urgency of the situation.

Pulmonary Risk Assessment and Risk Reduction

Key Concept: Perioperative pulmonary complications are common and predictable and can be minimized with good perioperative care.

Pulmonary complications are a major source of postoperative morbidity and mortality. In a large systematic review by Smetana, the overall rate of significant postoperative pulmonary complications was 6.8 % [18]. These included atelectasis, pneumonia, bronchitis, respiratory failure (with or without a need for mechanical ventilation), an exacerbation of underlying chronic lung disease, and bronchospasm [18, 47].

Pulmonary risk assessment is based on patient-specific factors and procedure-related factors. Recognized patient-related factors include age >50 years, chronic obstructive lung disease, congestive heart failure, obstructive sleep apnea, poor general health (ASA >2), pulmonary hypertension, low oxygen saturation, and serum albumin <35 g/L [18, 48, 49]. Additional variables that are contributory, but not as well defined, include hypocapnea, abnormal chest X-ray, smoking within the previous 8 weeks, and an active upper respiratory tract infection. From a procedural point of view, patients undergoing emergency surgery or prolonged major abdominal surgery (>3 h) such as a colon resection are considered to be at high risk of postoperative pulmonary complications [50, 51]. If you are prone to using a Pfannenstiel incision for many of your abdominal cases, it is worth noting that lower abdominal incisions are associated with a decreased risk from a pulmonary standpoint. Additionally, a Cochrane analysis of short-term outcomes in laparoscopic vs. open colon surgery demonstrated improved pulmonary function with the laparoscopic approach [52].

A complete history and physical examination is the cornerstone of preoperative evaluation for pulmonary disease. You should look for signs and symptoms of occult respiratory disease, a recent exacerbation of known disease, and symptoms of uncontrolled disease. The American College of Physicians has published guidelines for preoperative evaluation and perioperative management of pulmonary risk [53]. Preoperative use of chest radiography and spirometry may be indicated in patients with chronic obstructive lung disease (COPD) or asthma, but have not been shown to predict the risk of postoperative pulmonary complications. Patients with acute or chronic pulmonary illness should, in general, have surgery postponed until their pulmonary disease is stabilized. What can help to a certain degree are a few straightforward things. First, excellent perioperative pain control is paramount to encourage deep breathing and early mobilization. This may take the form of patient-controlled anesthesia or an epidural and should be discussed with anesthesia preoperatively. Second, we try to get patients mobilizing as soon as possible, often within the first 6–12 h postoperatively. All patients undergoing abdominal procedures are instructed preoperatively in deep breathing exercises and/or incentive spirometry. While these may seem trivial, there is likely no better thing you can get your patient to do other than get out of bed and breathe. In contrast, there is no evidence to support the use of pulmonary artery catheterization or total parenteral nutrition to reduce the risk of pulmonary complications.

Chronic Renal Failure Risk Assessment and Risk Reduction

Key Concept: When dealing with patients with chronic renal failure, you must be careful to avoid exacerbating their renal function with contrast imaging, ill-guided perioperative fluid management, and/or medications. These patients also have higher rates of postoperative morbidity and mortality and should be counseled accordingly.

The rate of chronic renal failure in patients over the age of 60 is approximately 25 % [54]. Chronic renal failure (CRF) includes a broad spectrum of diseases that can range from a decrease in a patient's glomerular filtration rate (GFR) below 60 mL/min to end-stage renal failure with dialysis dependence. Important issues to consider in these patients include avoiding situations that will worsen renal function (particularly in those who are not dialysis dependent), recognizing the potential for additional comorbidities (i.e., ischemic heart disease), and identifying the increased risk of perioperative morbidity and mortality.

Although an unenhanced CT scan provides far less information, we generally try to avoid intravenous contrast, whenever possible, in patients with renal failure who are not dialysis dependent but with underlying borderline renal insufficiency. Options include non-contrast CT scans, MRI, and/or ultrasound. When a contrast-enhanced scan is necessary in a patient with a GFR below 60 mL/min, and especially below 45 mL/min, nephrotoxic medications (including metformin) should be held for 48 h pre- and post-contrast (if at all possible). Intravenous hydration prior to the scan provides additional protection. Of note, *N*-acetylcysteine is now proven to be largely unhelpful and should not be relied upon in isolation to decrease the risk of contrast-induced nephropathy [55]. In patients who are already on dialysis, we generally utilize IV contrast if indicated and arrange for the patient to undergo dialysis post-contrast.

If a bowel preparation is required, it is important to provide clear instructions to these patients to avoid the risk of preoperative dehydration. We typically utilize a split dose polyethylene glycol preparation in these situations and make sure that patients understand the need to consume regular amounts of oral fluids in addition to the prep.

Patients with chronic renal failure often have multiple comorbid illnesses and thus require careful and complete preoperative assessment to optimize their safety. We feel that all of these patients require a preoperative internal medicine consultation. In patients with CRF who do not have known cardiac disease, the clinician should have a high index of suspicion of subclinical ischemic heart disease. We and others have demonstrated a higher risk for perioperative morbidity and mortality [56]. In this cohort, it is worth noting that mortality following elective colorectal surgery is ~5–10 % and can range up to 40 % following emergency colorectal surgery. These risks must be taken into consideration when consenting patients with chronic renal failure for surgery.

Diabetes Mellitus Risk Assessment and Risk Reduction

Key Concept: Diabetic patients have high rates of additional comorbidity and are more likely to be asymptomatic. Therefore, keep a high degree of suspicion. Diabetics also have higher rates of surgical site infection, which can be minimized by good glycemic control.

Diabetic patients also have a spectrum of disease, ranging from mild diet-controlled diabetes to type 1 insulin-dependent diabetes. Greater than 8 % of the US population are now diabetics. Approximately 50 % of diabetics will require surgery at some point in their lifetime, and it's estimated that 20 % of surgical patients have diabetes. A study using the National Inpatient Sample showed that 15 % of patients undergoing screening for colorectal cancer between 1998 and 2005 were diabetic [57].

Patients with long-standing diabetes often have additional comorbidity, which is sometimes occult. Diabetics have higher rates of cardiovascular disease, and more concerning, diabetic patients who have ischemic heart disease are more likely to be asymptomatic than nondiabetics. Thus, you need to have a high degree of suspicion, and a lower threshold, for formal preoperative cardiac evaluation in this cohort. Diabetic patients also have higher rates of nephropathy, so care needs to be exercised when using potentially nephrotoxic medications and contrast agents.

When possible, we have our diabetic patients scheduled as the first case in the morning to minimize the duration of their fast and the disruption to their diabetic routine. Patients on oral hypoglycemic medications can generally hold their medication in the morning of surgery. Insulin-dependent diabetics can generally be advised to take half of their regular morning dose. It is often helpful to have the patient's primary care physician or a consulting general internist make specific recommendation for their diabetic medications perioperatively. Patients with type 1 diabetes are insulin deficient and prone to developing ketosis and acidosis, so they need long-acting insulin regardless of where their glucose readings lie. If they will be unable to eat, they also require glucose in their IV fluids (we typically use D5/0.45NS +20 mEq/L KCl).

Finally, diabetic patients are at higher risk of surgical site infections following colorectal surgery [58]. This is particularly true for patients whose HbA1C levels are greater than 7 %. Both the American Diabetes Association and the Canadian Diabetes Association have clinical practice guidelines that suggest keeping random glucose readings below 180 mg/dL (10 mmol/L). While we do not necessarily change our practice (as we are diligent about wound care in all patients), wound redness in a diabetic is likely a problem and may need to be opened, cultured, and given antibiotics as indicated.

Hepatic Failure Risk Assessment and Risk Reduction

Key Concept: Patients with cirrhosis who require colorectal surgery are at increased risk of perioperative morbidity and mortality. When assessing a patient with known cirrhosis for surgery, it is critical to take into consideration the natural history of the disease state in question, the life expectancy of the patient, and whether the patient is a candidate for liver transplantation. Most importantly, both the surgeon and the patient should have a realistic expectation of the morbidity and mortality risk associated with the surgery.

While the number of patients with cirrhosis who require colorectal surgery is currently low, that number will likely increase significantly in the near future. In addition to the known conditions that lead to cirrhosis, the increasing prevalence of obesity has led to approximately one-third of the US population having nonalcoholic fatty liver disease, of which about 20 % will develop nonalcoholic steatohepatitis (NASH). This in turn will likely lead to many more patients with significant liver disease, as approximately 20–30 % of adults with NASH will develop cirrhosis.

There are two clinical scoring systems that are commonly used to estimate a cirrhotic patient's perioperative mortality risk: the Child-Turcotte-Pugh classification, which was initially used to estimate risk in patients undergoing portosystemic shunt procedures, but more recently has been shown to be valid in other abdominal surgery [59] and the Model for End-Stage Liver Disease or MELD score [60]. The MELD score is complex to calculate without electronic means, but is the result of the following formula: $MELD = 3.78 \times (\text{bilirubin mg/dL}) + 11.2 \times INR + 9.57 \times \text{creatinine mg/dL} + 6.43$. Fortunately, several websites are available where patient values can be inputted and a risk estimate can be immediately provided, including that of the authors of the original paper at the Mayo Clinic [61].

One of the more difficult situations in colorectal surgery is the discovery of a colorectal cancer in a patient waiting for liver transplantation. The presence of a malignancy automatically removes the patient from the transplant list. To be eligible for reinstatement, a 5-year disease-free period is required. This requires a thorough evaluation of the risks, potential morbidity and mortality, as well as the life expectancy of the patient with respect to the tumor and the hepatic failure (both with and without the transplant). A multidisciplinary discussion including the surgeon, the transplant team, and the hepatologist, along with the patient, is required so that proper and realistic decisions can be made on an individual basis.

Surgical Site Infection (SSI) Risk Assessment and Reduction

Key Concept: Surgical site infections are common following colorectal surgery. Steps to minimize the risk, particularly in the high-risk patient, are essential.

Colorectal surgery is associated with a relatively high rate of SSI. A few (of several) factors that have been shown to increase the risk include DM, obesity, open surgery, longer operative time, and emergency surgery [62]. While most of the factors associated with SSI are not modifiable, it is important to recognize the risks and to use the best practice patterns to minimize the likelihood of SSI in these patients.

Important components of SSI prevention include preoperative antibiotics, appropriate skin preparation, maintenance of normothermia, avoiding hyperglycemia, and good postoperative care [63]. Likely one of the easiest, yet often missed, is ensuring the prophylactic antibiotics are administered within 1 h of the skin incision. We typically use cefazolin and metronidazole. In patients with *B*-lactam allergy, gentamicin can be substituted for cefazolin. Patients known to be colonized with MRSA require vancomycin instead of cefazolin. Cefazolin should be re-dosed in cases lasting greater than 3 h or with significant blood loss. Metronidazole is typically re-dosed for cases lasting longer than 8 h.

For skin preparation, avoidance of shaving is important, especially the night prior. If hair removal is required, clippers should be used in the operating room prior to surgery. Although chlorhexidine wash has been recommended, the results of a Cochrane analysis showed that chlorhexidine preparation did not demonstrate a significant reduction in SSIs [64]. There is also conflicting evidence for the use of wound protectors, though data does support its use for decreasing SSI in colorectal surgery [65]. Our standard practice includes the routine use of clippers for hair removal, chlorhexidine-alcohol skin prep, when possible, and selective use of wound protectors.

Maintenance of normothermia is an important component for SSI prevention. Two randomized controlled trials have demonstrated a significantly reduced incidence of SSI in patients who are kept normothermic by active warming methods, and they are generally a component of most pathways aimed at reducing SSIs [66]. We use warmed fluids and forced air warmers to maintain normothermia. In addition, there is an emerging body of literature for colorectal patients that supplemental and high FiO_2 is associated with lower rates of SSI [67]. Finally, as stated above, it is imperative to maintain tight glucose control pre- and perioperatively to help reduce the risk of infection.

Anastomotic Leak: Risk Assessment and Risk Reduction

Key Concept: Diverting stomas decrease both the incidence and the consequences of high-risk anastomoses and should be considered in distal rectal anastomoses.

While there is a detailed review on anastomotic leak by Dr. Fleshman elsewhere in this text, a few brief notes are worth mentioning in the context of risk assessment (and mitigating it). There are many situations where an anastomosis is considered to be at increased risk of leak. Aside from technical issues at the time of surgery, commonly implicated patient factors include prolonged operative time, significant blood loss or need for transfusion, low rectal anastomosis, male sex, steroid use, weight loss, low albumin, obesity,

ASA class >3, smoking, COPD, and emergency surgery [68]. When more than one of these factors is present, the risk of anastomotic leak is increased.

Diverting stomas had previously been felt to decrease the consequences of a leak, but not the incidence. However, a Cochrane review by Montedori and colleagues in 2010 demonstrated that a diverting stoma decreases the leak rate, as well as the need for urgent reoperation [69]. When deciding on whether a patient would benefit from a defunctioning stoma, our approach has been to try to estimate a patient's risk of leak considering the risk factors as temporary (modifiable) or permanent (non-modifiable). In the presence of several modifiable factors, the subsequent stoma closure would be expected to have a significantly lower risk of leak than the anastomosis being protected. However, when the factors causing concern for an increased risk of anastomotic leak are non-modifiable, a diverting stoma for anything other than high-risk distal rectal anastomoses is likely not helpful, as there will still be a risk of leak at the time of loop stoma closure. In those situations, if the risk of leak is felt to be sufficiently high, consideration should be given to a permanent stoma.

Risk Evaluation and Informed Consent

Prior to obtaining informed consent, the patient and the surgeon must have a clear discussion of the risks and benefits of the surgery. This discussion may take place at the time of the first visit prior to signing consent if the patient is healthy or of moderate risk. In the case of a high-risk patient, the discussion should occur after the medical evaluation is complete and all risk reduction strategies have been put into place. At this time, the surgeon can evaluate the overall patient risk profile including patient, procedural, and anesthetic risks and review these with the patient. Additional factors that must be considered include the present disease state, the potential for recurrent disease or symptoms, and the possibility of disease progression. It is extremely important that your patient has a clear understanding of the treatment, risks, and decisions that are being made. In situations of excessive risk, the surgical plan may have to be altered and compromised, or in some cases, a nonoperative approach may be appropriate.

Summary Pearls

Perioperative risk assessment is an essential part of sound surgical decision making. As the surgeon, you must perform a basic screening examination to assess your patient's overall health and fitness for surgery and obtain appropriate consultation when required. With a thorough understanding of their underlying health issues, interventions (where possible) to optimize their overall condition can be undertaken. Ultimately, it is your responsibility not only to ensure that each patient has their procedure selected to effectively treat the disease process in question but also to perform the procedure as safely as possible to minimize perioperative morbidity and mortality.

References

1. Fleisher LA, Beckman JA, Brown KA, et al. ACC/AHA 2007 guidelines on perioperative cardiovascular evaluation and care for noncardiac surgery: executive summary: a report of the American College of Cardiology/American Heart Association Task Force on Practice Guidelines (writing committee to revise the 2002 guidelines on perioperative cardiovascular evaluation for noncardiac surgery). J Am Coll Cardiol. 2007;50(17):1707–32. Erratum in: J Am Coll Cardiol. 2008;52(9):794–7.
2. Fleisher LA, Beckman JA, Brown KA, et al. ACC/AHA 2007 guidelines on perioperative cardiovascular evaluation and care for noncardiac surgery: a report of the American College of Cardiology/American Heart Association Task Force on Practice Guidelines (writing committee to revise the 2002 guidelines on perioperative cardiovascular evaluation for noncardiac surgery). Circulation. 2007;116(17):e418–99. Erratum in: Circulation. 2008;117(5):e154. Circulation. 2008;118(9):e143–4.
3. Reynolds TM, National Institute for Health and Clinical Excellence; Clinical Science Reviews Committee of the Association for Clinical Biochemistry. National Institute for Health and Clinical Excellence guidelines on preoperative tests: the use of routine preoperative tests for elective surgery. Ann Clin Biochem. 2006; 43(Pt 1):13–6.
4. Green CJ, Maxwell R, Verne J, Martin RM, Blazeby JM. The influence of NICE guidance on the uptake of laparoscopic surgery for colorectal cancer. J Public Health (Oxf). 2009;31(4):541–5.
5. Dewan SK, Zheng SB, Xia SJ. Preoperative geriatric assessment: comprehensive, multidisciplinary and proactive. Eur J Intern Med. 2012;23(6):487–94.
6. Lanier WL. A three-decade perspective on anesthesia safety. Am Surg. 2006;72(11):985–9.
7. Cohen MM, Duncan PG, Tate RB. Does anesthesia contribute to operative mortality? JAMA. 1988;260(19):2859–63.
8. Wolters U, Wolf T, Stutzer H, Schroder T. ASA classification and perioperative variables as predictors of postoperative outcome. Br J Anaesth. 1996;77(2):217–22.
9. Maurer SG, Chen AL, Hiebert R, et al. Comparison of outcomes of using spinal versus general anesthesia in total hip arthroplasty. Am J Orthop. 2007;36(7):E101–6.
10. Naesh O, Hindberg I, Friis J, Christiansen C. General versus regional anaesthesia and platelet aggregation in minor surgery. Eur J Anaesthesiol. 1994;11(3):169–73.
11. Parker SD, Breslow MJ, Frank SM, et al. Catecholamine and cortisol responses to lower extremity revascularization: correlation with outcome variables. Perioperative ischemia randomized anesthesia trial study group. Crit Care Med. 1995;23(12):1954–61.
12. Werawatganon T, Charuluxanun S. Patient controlled intravenous opioid analgesia versus continuous epidural analgesia for pain after intra-abdominal surgery. Cochrane Database Syst Rev. 2005;(1): CD004088.
13. Harvey S, Young D, Brampton W, et al. Pulmonary artery catheters for adult patients in intensive care. Cochrane Database Syst Rev. 2006;(3):CD003408.

14. Sandham JD, Hull RD, Brant RF, et al. A randomized controlled trial of the use of pulmonary-artery catheters in high-risk surgical patients. N Engl J Med. 2003;348(1):5–14.
15. Catena E, Mele D. Role of intraoperative transesophageal echocardiography in patients undergoing noncardiac surgery. J Cardiovasc Med (Hagerstown). 2008;9(10):993–1003.
16. Finlayson EV, Birkmeyer JD. Operative mortality with elective surgery in older adults. Eff Clin Pract. 2001;4(4):172–7. Erratum in: Eff Clin Pract. 2001; 4(5):235.
17. Linn BS, Linn MW, Wallen N. Evaluation of results of surgical procedures in the elderly. Ann Surg. 1982;195(1):90–6.
18. Smetana GW, Lawrence VA, Cornell JE, American College of Physicians. Preoperative pulmonary risk stratification for noncardiothoracic surgery: systematic review for the American College of Physicians. Ann Intern Med. 2006;144(8):581–95.
19. Lubin MF. Is age a risk factor for surgery? Med Clin North Am. 1993;77(2):327–33.
20. Turrentine FE, Wang H, Simpson VB, Jones RS. Surgical risk factors, morbidity, and mortality in elderly patients. J Am Coll Surg. 2006;203(6):865–77.
21. Pelavski AD, de Miguel M, Lacasta A, Rochera MI, Roca M. Anaemia and transfusion in nonagenarians undergoing emergency, non-traumatic surgery: a prospective observational study. Transfus Med. 2013;23(4):238–44. doi:10.1111/tme.12011.
22. Hosking MP, Warner MA, Lobdell CM, Offord KP, Melton 3rd LJ. Outcomes of surgery in patients 90 years of age and older. JAMA. 1989;261(13):1909–15.
23. Fleisher LA, American College of Cardiology/American Heart Association. Cardiac risk stratification for noncardiac surgery: update from the American College of Cardiology/American Heart Association 2007 guidelines. Cleve Clin J Med. 2009;76 Suppl 4:S9–15.
24. Fleischmann KE, Beckman JA, Buller CE, et al. 2009 ACCF/AHA focused update on perioperative beta blockade: a report of the American College of Cardiology Foundation/American Heart Association Task Force on Practice Guidelines. Circulation. 2009;120(21):2123–51.
25. Reilly Jr JJ. Preoperative and postoperative care of standard and high risk surgical patients. Hematol Oncol Clin North Am. 1997;11(3):449–59.
26. Wilson RJ, Davies S, Yates D, et al. Impaired functional capacity is associated with all-cause mortality after major elective intra-abdominal surgery. Br J Anaesth. 2010;105(3):297–303.
27. Bradley KA, Rubinsky AD, Sun H, et al. Alcohol screening and risk of postoperative complications in male VA patients undergoing major non-cardiac surgery. J Gen Intern Med. 2011;26(2):162–9.
28. Tønnesen H, Nielsen PR, Lauritzen JB, Møller AM. Smoking and alcohol intervention before surgery: evidence for best practice. Br J Anaesth. 2009;102(3):297–306.
29. Jones R, Nyawo B, Jamieson S, Clark S. Current smoking predicts increased operative mortality and morbidity after cardiac surgery in the elderly. Interact Cardiovasc Thorac Surg. 2011;12(3):449–53.
30. Mills E, Eyawo O, Lockhart I, Kelly S, Wu P, Ebbert JO. Smoking cessation reduces postoperative complications: a systematic review and meta-analysis. Am J Med. 2011;124(2):144–54.e8.
31. Ang-Lee MK, Moss J, Yuan CS. Herbal medicines and perioperative care. JAMA. 2001;286(2):208–16.
32. Kaplan EB, Sheiner LB, Boeckmann AJ, et al. The usefulness of preoperative laboratory screening. JAMA. 1985;253(24):3576–81.
33. Narr BJ, Hansen TR, Warner MA. Preoperative laboratory screening in healthy Mayo patients: cost-effective elimination of tests and unchanged outcomes. Mayo Clin Proc. 1991;66(2):155–9.
34. Narr BJ, Warner ME, Schroeder DR, Warner MA. Outcomes of patients with no laboratory assessment before anesthesia and a surgical procedure. Mayo Clin Proc. 1997;72(6):505–9.
35. Benarroch-Gampel J, Sheffield KM, Duncan CB, et al. Preoperative laboratory testing in patients undergoing elective low-risk ambulatory surgery. Ann Surg. 2012;256(3):518–28.
36. Smetana GW, Macpherson DS. The case against routine preoperative laboratory testing. Med Clin North Am. 2003;87(1):7–40.
37. Causey MW, Maykel JA, Hatch Q, Miller S, Steele SR. Identifying risk factors for renal failure and myocardial infarction following colorectal surgery. J Surg Res. 2011;170(1):32–7.
38. Goldman L, Caldera DL, Nussbaum SR, et al. Multifactorial index of cardiac risk in noncardiac surgical procedures. N Engl J Med. 1977;297(16):845–50.
39. Owens WD, Felts JA, Spitznagel Jr EL. ASA physical status classifications: a study of consistency of ratings. Anesthesiology. 1978;49:239–43.
40. Lee TH, Marcantonio ER, Mangione CM, et al. Derivation and prospective validation of a simple index for prediction of cardiac risk of major noncardiac surgery. Circulation. 1999;100(10):1043–9.
41. Devereaux PJ, Goldman L, Cook DJ, Gilbert K, Leslie K, Guyatt GH. Perioperative cardiac events in patients undergoing noncardiac surgery: a review of the magnitude of the problem, the pathophysiology of the events and methods to estimate and communicate risk. Can Med Assoc J. 2005;173(6):627–34.
42. Devereaux PJ, Goldman L, Yusuf S, Gilbert K, Leslie K, Guyatt GH. Surveillance and prevention of major perioperative ischemic cardiac events in patients undergoing noncardiac surgery: a review. Can Med Assoc J. 2005;173(7):779–88.
43. Gupta PK, Gupta H, Sundaram A, et al. Development and validation of a risk calculator for prediction of cardiac risk after surgery. Circulation. 2011;124(4):381–7.
44. Surgical cardiac risk calculator. Available online at: http://www.surgicalriskcalculator.com/miorcardiacarrest. Accessed June 2013.
45. POISE Study Group, Devereaux PJ, Yang H, Yusuf S, Guyatt G, Leslie K, Villar JC, Xavier D, Chrolavicius S, Greenspan L, Pogue J, Pais P, Liu L, Xu S, Málaga G, Avezum A, Chan M, Montori VM, Jacka M, Choi P. Effects of extended-release metoprolol succinate in patients undergoing non-cardiac surgery (POISE trial): a randomised controlled trial. Lancet. 2008;371(9627):1839–47.
46. Dunkelgrun M, Boersma E, Schouten O, Koopman-van Gemert AW, van Poorten F, Bax JJ, Thomson IR, Poldermans D, Dutch Echocardiographic Cardiac Risk Evaluation Applying Stress Echocardiography Study Group. Bisoprolol and fluvastatin for the reduction of perioperative cardiac mortality and myocardial infarction in intermediate-risk patients undergoing noncardiovascular surgery: a randomized controlled trial (DECREASE-IV). Ann Surg. 2009;249(6):921–6.
47. Hall JC, Tarala RA, Hall JL, Mander J. A multivariate analysis of the risk of pulmonary complications after laparotomy. Chest. 1991;99(4):923–7.
48. Memtsoudis S, Liu SS, Ma Y, et al. Perioperative pulmonary outcomes in patients with sleep apnea after noncardiac surgery. Anesth Analg. 2011;112(1):113–21.
49. Lai HC, Lai HC, Wang KY, et al. Severe pulmonary hypertension complicates postoperative outcome of noncardiac surgery. Br J Anaesth. 2007;99(2):184–90.
50. Brooks-Brunn JA. Predictors of postoperative pulmonary complications following abdominal surgery. Chest. 1997;111(3):564–71.
51. McAlister FA, Khan NA, Straus SE, et al. Accuracy of the preoperative assessment in predicting pulmonary risk after nonthoracic surgery. Am J Respir Crit Care Med. 2003;167(5):741–4.
52. Schwenk W, Haase O, Neudecker J, Müller JM. Short term benefits for laparoscopic colorectal resection. Cochrane Database Syst Rev. 2005;(3):CD003145.
53. Qaseem A, Snow V, Fittermna N, et al. Risk assessment for and strategies to reduce perioperative pulmonary complications for

patients undergoing noncardiothoracic surgery: a guideline from the American College of Physicians. Ann Intern Med. 2006; 144(8):575–80.
54. US Department of Health and Human Services. 2011 National Institute of Diabetes and Digestive and Kidney Diseases (NIDDK), National Institutes of Health (NIH) annual report. Available at: http://kidney.niddk.nih.gov/kudiseases/pubs/kustats/#4. Accessed June 2013.
55. Canadian Association of Radiologists. 2011 consensus guidelines for the prevention of contrast induced nephropathy. Available at: http://www.car.ca/uploads/standards%20guidelines/20110617_en_prevention_cin.pdf. Accessed June 2013.
56. Drolet S, Maclean AR, Myers RP, Shaheen AA, Dixon E, Buie WD. Morbidity and mortality following colorectal surgery in patients with end-stage renal failure: a population-based study. Dis Colon Rectum. 2010;53(11):1508–16.
57. Cooley EK, McPhee JT, Simons JP, Sweeney WB, Tseng JF, Alavi K. Colorectal neoplasia screening before age 50? Current epidemiologic trends in the United States. Dis Colon Rectum. 2009;52(2):222–9.
58. Ata A, Valerian BT, Lee EC, Bestle SL, Elmendorf SL, Stain SC. The effect of diabetes mellitus on surgical site infections after colorectal and noncolorectal general surgical operations. Am Surg. 2010;76(7):697–702.
59. Mansour A, Watson W, Shayani V, Pickleman J. Abdominal operations in patients with cirrhosis: still a major surgical challenge. Surgery. 1997;122(4):730–5.
60. Kamath PS, Wiesner RH, Malinchoc M, et al. A model to predict survival in patients with end-stage liver disease. Hepatology. 2001;33(2):464–70.
61. MELD Score. Available at: http://www.mayoclinic.org/meld/mayomodel9.html. Accessed June 2013.
62. Hedrick TL, Sawyer RG, Friel CM, Stukenborg GJ. A method for estimating the risk of surgical site infection in patients with abdominal colorectal procedures. Dis Colon Rectum. 2013;56(5):627–37.
63. Cima R, Dankbar E, Lovely J, Pendlimari R, Aronhalt K, Nehring S, Hyke R, Tyndale D, Rogers J, Quast L, Colorectal Surgical Site Infection Reduction Team. Colorectal surgery surgical site infection reduction program: a national surgical quality improvement program – driven multidisciplinary single-institution experience. J Am Coll Surg. 2013;216(1):23–33.
64. Webster J, Osborne S. Preoperative bathing or showering with skin antiseptics to prevent surgical site infection. Cochrane Database Syst Rev. 2012;(9):CD004985.
65. Reid K, Pockney P, Draganic B, Smith SR. Barrier wound protection decreases surgical site infection in open elective colorectal surgery: a randomized clinical trial. Dis Colon Rectum. 2010;53(10):1374–80.
66. Hawn MT, Vick CC, Richman J, Holman W, Deierhoi RJ, Graham LA, Henderson WG, Itani KM. Surgical site infection prevention: time to move beyond the surgical care improvement program. Ann Surg. 2011;254(3):494–9.
67. Kao LS, Millas SG, Pedroza C, Tyson JE, Lally KP. Should perioperative supplemental oxygen be routinely recommended for surgery patients? A Bayesian meta-analysis. Ann Surg. 2012;256(6):894–901.
68. Reinke CE, Showalter S, Mahmoud NN, Kelz RR. Comparison of anastomotic leak rate after colorectal surgery using different databases. Dis Colon Rectum. 2013;56(5):638–44.
69. Montedori A, Cirocchi R, Farinella E, Sciannameo F, Abraha I. Covering ileo- or colostomy in anterior resection for rectal carcinoma. Cochrane Database Syst Rev. 2010;(5):CD006878.
70. American Society of Anesthesiologists (ASA) website: http://www.asahq.org/Home/For-Members/Clinical-Information/ASA-Physical-Status-Classification-System.

Perioperative Nutrition Support in Colorectal Surgery

3

Justin A. Maykel

Key Points

- In the year 2014, malnutrition remains prevalent yet under recognized in surgical patients.
- The timely and appropriate delivery of nutritional support to malnourished patients decreases postoperative complications, shortens hospital length of stay, and may decrease postoperative mortality.
- While the enteral route is preferred when feasible, total parenteral nutrition is safe and provides equivalent benefit when delivered appropriately.
- Perioperative feeding of malnourished patients appears to be the most efficacious approach but can be difficult to coordinate and deliver.

With proper use of total parenteral nutrition when necessary and use of the gastrointestinal tract when possible, malnutrition need no longer add to the morbidity and mortality of surgical patients.

Josef E. Fischer
AJS, 1980

Introduction

In the early 1970s, the widespread prevalence of protein-calorie malnutrition in hospitalized patients was defined [1, 2] and recognized to have a major influence on clinical outcome, specifically patient morbidity and mortality [3]. Subsequently, there have been extraordinary advances in the fields of surgical nutrition and metabolism. Today, invasive nutritional therapies are commonly employed in hospitalized patients and virtually universal in the critically ill. Enteral access techniques and specialized formulas have revolutionized the ability to use the GI tract to support the metabolic responses to systemic injury, inflammation, and infection. Central venous access techniques and technologic advances in total parenteral nutrition (TPN) components and compounding make it possible to provide nutritional and metabolic support when the enteral route is inaccessible or functionally inadequate. In the field of colorectal surgery, we are commonly faced with challenging patients who are malnourished due to advanced malignancies or inflammatory bowel disease that result in intestinal blockages, intestinal fistulas, poor absorptive capacity, and large volume losses from the GI tract. The literature continues to evaluate the role for nutritional support in both chronic disease and acute illness, delivered via the enteral and parental routes, and in the preoperative and postoperative settings; yet, there are few studies that concentrate exclusively on colorectal disease and colorectal patients. Additionally there is marked heterogeneity involving study design, patient populations under investigation (degree of malnutrition, disease process, etc.), and feeding protocols. Using published studies and personal experience, I will attempt to give the reader an understanding of the overreaching concepts while detailing those scenarios most commonly encountered by the practicing surgeon.

Prevalence and Impact of Malnutrition

Key Concept: While the overall prevalence of malnutrition is high, it remains woefully unrecognized and unaddressed in many of the highest at-risk patients. Poor nutritional status directly correlates with worse outcomes.

Specifically looking at patients undergoing gastrointestinal surgery, the prevalence of malnutrition can be as high as 50 % [4]; yet, it remains unrecognized in upwards of 50 % of patients who are at considerable nutritional risk [5], reflecting

J.A. Maykel, MD
Division of Colorectal Surgery, Department of Surgery,
UMass Memorial Medical Center,
University of Massachusetts Medical School,
Worcester, MA, USA
e-mail: justin.maykel@umassmemorial.org

S.R. Steele et al. (eds.), *Complexities in Colorectal Surgery*,
DOI 10.1007/978-1-4614-9022-7_3, © Springer Science+Business Media New York 2014

a generalized lack of appreciation and understanding of the extent and importance of the problem. Additionally, the degree of malnutrition worsens during the course of hospital admission, particularly after 16 days, highlighting the importance of ongoing assessment and appropriate intervention [6]. This may be due to illness or inadequate consumption of delivered hospital food [7]. Nutritional risk tends to be a reflection of the patient's overall health and, in oncology, has correlated with the primary tumor site (i.e., worse with esophageal), higher Eastern Cooperative Oncology Group score (range 0–5), and the presence of anorexia or fatigue [8]. Such nutritional risk is associated with increased postoperative complications, longer length of stay, and higher mortality following elective surgery [9] and is particularly pronounced in patient with colorectal cancer [10].

Patient Assessment

Key Concept: Although several instruments are available to help assess nutritional status, nothing is more effective than specific findings on routine history and physical examination.

The initiation of invasive nutritional support should be based on a comprehensive, up-front nutritional assessment. Several objective options exist and have been studied over time including body composition analysis (bioelectrical impedance, displacement, exchange of labeled ions, total body counters, magnetic resonance imaging, and computed tomography), anthropomorphic measurements (creatinine height index, triceps skinfold thickness, arm muscle circumference), biochemical measurements (serum proteins, nitrogen balance, protein breakdown, measurements of immunologic function), and indirect calorimetry. The vast majority of these studies are of historical significance and are rarely used currently outside of investigative studies.

Practically speaking, the evaluation of the potentially malnourished patient begins with the history and physical examination. Most patients will complain of some degree of intolerance of oral intake as a result of poor appetite, nausea, abdominal bloating, abdominal pain, and weakness. Symptoms may be exacerbated by drug side effects and interactions as well as the hypermetabolic state often seen with advanced cancers and inflammatory conditions. Patients will relate a recent weight loss, typically over a 1- to 3-month time period. On physical examination, you will find the patient appearing thin, pale, and weak with muscle wasting and loose skin. These variables can be objectified using grading systems such as the relatively intuitive Subjective Global Assessment (SGA) to classify patients as well nourished, moderately malnourished, or severely malnourished [11]. The SGA utilizes five features of the history (weight loss over 6 months, dietary intake change, gastrointestinal symptoms, functional capacity, and the impact of disease on nutritional requirements) and four features of the clinical exam (loss of subcutaneous fat, muscle wasting, ankle edema, sacral edema, ascites) to elicit a SGA rank based on subjective weighting. Any practitioner should be able to use such an intuitive system to assess patients with ease and with a high degree of inter-rater agreement [12]. Similarly, the Nutritional Risk Index (NRI) uses weight loss and serum albumin to calculate a score which can classify a patient's nutritional status, NRI = (1.489 × serum albumin, g/L) + (41.7 × current weight/usual weight) with the usual weight defined as the stable weight 6 months or more before illness. The nuances of other screening tools such as the nutritional risk screening (NRS) 2002 and Reilly's NRS remain controversial regarding predictive ability and clinical utility. It is important to note that while a patient may appear obese on exam or by BMI, depletion of protein stores can still render them malnourished.

Albumin

Key Concept: Trending albumin over time (i.e., weeks) may be beneficial, but in the acute setting albumin levels have several physiological-based limitations.

Serum albumin level has been considered the "classic test" which reflects overall nutritional status, with serum concentration of <3.0 g/dL defining the malnourished state. However, in real practice, its utility and reliability is limited. This is a very important point to be stressed. As a serum protein, levels fluctuate for many reasons, including production alterations in the catabolic or anabolic states, external losses, or redistribution between the various fluid compartments of the body [13]. As such, a low value may reflect either decreased synthesis or increased degradation. What is well known is that albumin levels fall precipitously in the setting of metabolic stress and sepsis. During the acute phase response, certain proteins (such as IL1, TNF, and CRP) increase to help facilitate the immune response to eliminate microbes, control tissue damage, and initiate the repair process. Albumin is a serum protein that *decreases* during the acute phase response, apparently serving as "metabolic compensator" and helping to minimize transport of nutrients to microbes. When patients are fluid overloaded with increased extravascular space, albumin shifts from the intravascular fluid into the interstitium where it is diluted and degraded. Other short turnover proteins such as prealbumin, transferrin, and retinol-binding protein have similar limitations as nutritional markers as a result of variable half-lives and response to dietary intake and renal/liver dysfunction, although all of these proteins can be useful when followed as trends over time. Such trending can be particularly helpful when patients are receiving apparently adequate nutrition, but the serum albumin level remains low or even falls over time. This should prompt a comprehensive investigation looking for a source of infection that is preventing the patient from recovering from a catabolic state. This may be due to an obscure infection such as an undiscovered intra-abdominal abscess, persisting bacteremia, or inadequately treated colitis. In a recent review, higher baseline serum albumin was found to predict improved survival for patients with cancer of the gastrointestinal tract; however, causality has not been shown as preoperative intravenous infusion has not been shown to impact overall mortality [14].

When discussing the nutritional state of a patient, the standard question heard is: "What is the albumin or prealbumin level?" You should not let the discussion end there. Rather follow with these questions: "What is the patient's hydration status? Is the patient acutely ill? Is there an ongoing infection? Has the patient lost weight over the preceding 3 months?" If the patient is coming to the office from home, in the well-hydrated state without active infection, then a low serum albumin can be reflective of their overall nutritional state. In any other situation, it is an unreliable predictor of nutrition when taken out of context alone and more likely represents a reflection of overall illness severity. When a patient is acutely ill or even healthy but involved in a major trauma, you should expect (and predictably will find) albumin levels of <3.0 g/dL. While low serum albumin is widely recognized as a risk factor for postoperative morbidity, it remains generally undetermined if this correlation is a reflection of overall systemic illness, nutritional status, or a combination of both.

Nitrogen Balance

Key Concept: Nitrogen balance is calculated easily and can provide insight into the patient's catabolic (or anabolic) state to help guide feeding regimens or prompt additional evaluation for occult sources of ongoing sepsis.

The change in total body protein can be assessed by estimating nitrogen balance, as 16 % of protein is nitrogen and almost all body nitrogen is in protein. The calculation of nitrogen balance can be useful, particularly in patients who require prolonged nutritional support due to intestinal failure or those who do not appear to be responding to adequate protein and calorie administration. In the clinical setting, nitrogen balance is calculated by determining the total nitrogen intake and the total losses via urinary, skin, and gastrointestinal losses. An accurate 24-h urine collection and total protein intake are the only necessary data points:

Intake – loss (urine 90 %, stool 5 %, integument 5 %)

[*Protein intake* (g)/6.25] – *urinary urea* (g) – 2 (stool and skin) – 2 (non-urea nitrogen)

While a positive value is indicative of an anabolic state, a negative value represents a persisting state of catabolism.

Table 3.1 Common baseline markers of malnutrition

BMI <18 kg/m^2
Weight loss >10 %
Low SGA score
Nonstressed state serum albumin <3.0 g/dL

This can be as a result of underfeeding or, commonly, due to a persisting source of stress such as inadequately treated infection or persisting low-grade sepsis. With comparisons over time (i.e., week to week), a failure to convert to an anabolic state may prompt manipulation of feeding formulation or delivery mode or may even prompt further investigation of ongoing sepsis (similar to a persisting low albumin level).

In the critical care setting, indirect calorimetry, utilizing the metabolic cart, can be very useful to determine energy expenditure, the potential of overfeeding, and the relative contribution/utilization of protein, carbohydrates, and fat to overall metabolism. This data is commonly obtained and interpreted by an experience critical care team helping to care for critically ill patients in partnership with the colorectal surgeon.

Cancer Cachexia

Similar to the stress response, it is worth mentioning the cancer cachexia syndrome as it is prevalent and associated with reduced physical function, tolerance of treatment, and survival [15]. This is reflective of the patient's physical appearance. This was defined as a multifactorial syndrome with an ongoing loss of skeletal muscle mass (with or without loss of fat mass) that cannot be fully reversed by conventional nutritional support and leads to progressive functional impairment. Its pathophysiology is characterized by a negative protein and energy balance driven by a variable combination of reduced food intake and abnormal metabolism that is driven by proinflammatory cytokines including interleukin (IL)-1, (IL)-6, and tumor necrosis factor (TNF)-α. There is evidence that "chronic inflammation" as a result of low-grade tumor-induced activation of the host immune system shares several characteristics with the "acute phase response" to injury (Table 3.1).

Initiation of Nutritional Support

Key Concept: Although relatively healthy patients may safely wait several days prior to initiation of therapy, at-risk patients or those with moderate insults achieve optimal outcomes with early implementation of nutritional support.

For the well or mildly malnourished patient with an ongoing moderate systemic inflammatory response, initiating invasive feeding 5–7 days, or even more conservatively 7–10 days, after a period of fasting (if oral intake has not resumed) is a reasonable and well-accepted guideline. These principles reflect evidence that up to 10 days of routine fluid and electrolyte therapy can be tolerated without clinical harm in this circumstance [16]. Those with a poor premorbid nutritional status (i.e., more than 10 % weight loss or BMI less than 18 kg/m^2) and superimposed illness are not as able to mount an adequate inflammatory response, which primarily impairs wound healing and immune function. This nutritionally related impairment of protein synthetic capacity increases susceptibility to infectious complications and organ failure. It is therefore important not to delay nutritional therapy and to intervene within the first several days. Although it has been shown to be more effective to feed moderately malnourished individuals for 7 days prior to an elective major operative procedure [17], present day reality is that preoperative or early post-injury feeding is generally not the rule. This practice needs to be reconsidered. For those with the most severe injuries which increase resting energy expenditure by 50 % or more, such as multiple trauma, major burns, closed head injury, and severe sepsis, all of which commonly result in lean tissue losses of 600–900 g/day without feeding, early feeding is essential. In this group of patients, even in the absence of pre-illness weight loss (rarely encountered by the colorectal surgeon), adjuvant nutritional therapy should be started soon after the acute resuscitation and metabolic issues are resolved. In this setting, early feeding may diminish the intensity of the systemic inflammatory response [18, 19], which could be an important factor in improved clinical outcome. Those patients who fall in between these extremes are the most challenging with regard to delivery choice and timing, and hopefully this chapter will better arm the reader regarding the role and benefits of nutritional support.

Nutritional Options: Enteral and Parenteral

Key Concept: *Nutritional supplementation has a storied history that encompasses several unique attempts to help patients improve their status*.

The goals of nutritional provision should be to provide adequate protein (at least 1 g/kg/day and optimally 1.5 g/kg/day) and energy (at least 1,000 kcal/day and optimally 25 kcal/kg/day) along with all essential nutrients, so as to allow optimal protein synthesis for the support of the immune system, wound healing, and vital organ function. Fortunately, there are two available options, enteral and parenteral nutrition, to reach these goals in essentially all patients.

The administration of supplemental enteral nutrition dates back hundreds of years. The ancient Egyptians provided support with enemas of wine, milk, whey, wheat, and barley. In 1790, Hunter created an orogastric tube made of a whalebone probe covered with eel skin attached to a bladder pump. After an assassination attempt in 1881, President Garfield was kept alive for 79 days with every 4-h rectal infusions of peptonized beef, broth, and whiskey. Furthermore, in 1918, Anderson placed the first nasojejunal feeding tube.

The ability to provide intravenous nutrition support came from revolutionary work done at the University of Pennsylvania in the 1960s. In 1962, Rhoads began infusing high volume peripheral solutions followed by diuretics. In 1966, Dudrick, Vars, and Rhoads documented their ability to support normal growth and development of beagle puppies with TPN. Finally in 1968, Dudrick and Wilmore demonstrated that they were able to safely support growth and development of infant fed entirely by TPN. This milestone revolutionized the nutritional support of surgical patients and has had a transformational impact on perioperative morbidity and mortality that continues to this day.

Enteral Feeding

Key Concept: *Although the dictum "Whenever possible, feed the gut" is likely accurate, there is very little data in human studies to back up its superiority over the parenteral route*.

It is commonly stated that the administration of enteral nutrition is "more physiologic" and its absence results in gut mucosal atrophy and increased intestinal permeability, predisposing to bacterial translocation and increased rates of septic complications [20]. Experimental evidence confirms that mucosal atrophy occurs with short-term bowel rest in animals [21], but human studies to date do not support these findings. Remaining NPO over a short time course (up to 1 month) has no substantial effect on mucosal architecture [22], while chronic starvation and malnutrition in humans do result in changes in villous architecture [23].

Several investigators have looked at the potential clinical benefits attributable to enteral feeding. There exists a large cohort of animal studies showing that functional stimulation of the GI tract resulting in the release of hormonal, biliary, and pancreatic secretions prevents mucosal atrophy [24]. Enteral nutrients also improve intestinal blood flow, increase the systemic and local immune response, increase the secretion of IgA, and increase the production of trophic hormones. Although these findings become considerably more vague when humans are studied and clinical outcomes are evaluated, there is strong suggestive evidence for benefit of early feeding, particularly enteral, in the most critically ill [18, 19].

In 1997, Reynolds et al. sought to answer the question if early enteral feeding after major upper GI surgery modulates gut barrier function and decreases the risk of major infectious complications compared with bowel rest and parenteral nutrition [25]. According to previous studies, TPN had been associated with an exaggerated acute phase and metabolic response after injury or endotoxin challenge, a response that could be attenuated by enteral nutrition [26]. The investigators prospectively randomized 67 surgical patients to either 7 days of TPN or enteral feeding via operative jejunostomy tubes. They showed that there was no clinical benefit attributable to the enteral route of nutrient administration when compared to the parenteral route. Furthermore, intestinal permeability was equally increased postoperatively in both groups (measured by lactose-mannitol ratios and serum anti-endotoxin core antibodies), but the degree was not influenced by the provision of enteral or parenteral nutrition. In addition, the magnitude of surgery-induced changes in the acute phase reactants, albumin and C-reactive protein, were not different between groups. Their results revealed that major surgery does profoundly influence gut barrier function, but there was no evidence that enteral nutrition modulated gut barrier function or that septic morbidity was altered.

Early Enteral Feeding Versus NPO

Key Concept: Early enteral feeding is likely not harmful, though has questionable evidence-based benefit compared to NPO for otherwise healthy patients undergoing surgery. Some data exists citing improved outcomes to early enteral feeding in the critically ill.

If there does not appear to be a significant difference in the stress response and clinical outcome between enterally and parenterally fed patients, then is there a difference between patients fed enterally and those fed not at all? This question was studied in an extremely convincing article conducted by Heslin et al. from the Memorial Sloan-Kettering Cancer Center [16]. The authors prospectively randomized 195 patients undergoing surgery for major upper gastrointestinal cancer. The enterally fed group was administered an immune-enhancing diet via a jejunostomy tube, begun on POD #1 and advanced to a goal of 25 kcal/kg. The control group was administered intravenous crystalloid solutions. It is important to note that the patients studied in this trial were not malnourished, with mean preoperative weight loss of only 6 % and initial serum albumin concentration of 4.0 g/dL. The results revealed no significant differences in postoperative complications, hospital stay, or mortality. The authors concluded that there is no benefit to early enteral feeding in postoperative general surgical patients who are not malnourished at baseline.

A meta-analysis [27] looked at the 11 prospective randomized controlled trials comparing the practice of early enteral feeding to maintaining patients NPO after *elective gastrointestinal surgery*. Their analysis of 837 patients concluded that (1) there is no clear advantage to keeping patients NPO after elective GI surgery and (2) early feeding *may* be of benefit in decreasing infections and shortening postoperative length of stay. A closer evaluation of their pooled data revealed that the mean length of hospital stay was only reduced by 0.84 days. Although there was an increase in "any type of infection," when considered individually, there was no difference in the incidence of anastomotic dehiscence, wound infections, pneumonia, intra-abdominal abscess, or mortality. Today early enteral feeding is a key component to enhanced recovery after surgery (ERAS) programs routinely used following colon resection surgery.

In 2001, Marik and Zaloga performed another meta-analysis, this time looking at the 15 randomized controlled trials that compared early with delayed enteral nutrition in *critically ill* surgical patients [28]. A total of 753 patients were analyzed: early enteral nutrition was associated with a significantly lower incidence of infections (RR reduction 0.45) and reduced length of hospital stay (2.2 days). There were no differences in noninfectious complications or mortality. The authors concluded that their pooled data supports the practice of early initiation of enteral feeding but that their conclusion should be interpreted with caution because of the heterogeneity between studies.

In summary, it has been sufficiently demonstrated that the provision of nutrients is important to both support the immune system and heal surgical wounds. Investigators have further studied the route, timing, and metabolic response of nutritional support. Reasonable conclusions based on the studies quoted above would be that:

1. There is no benefit from the immediate administration of enteral nutrition to patients who undergo routine general surgical procedures but are well nourished at baseline.
2. When patients are either malnourished or in the post-injury stressed state, there is no obvious harm (and there may be a clinical benefit) to the initiation of immediate enteral feeding, particularly in the more critically ill patient.
3. The specific clinical benefits of a more aggressive approach have yet to be confirmed and will likely require better powered future studies which focus on particular subsets of patients.

Enteral Shortcomings

Key Concept: The benefit of enteral feeding may be hindered by an inability to tolerate feeds with either a nasojejunal or nasogastric route.

While there appears to be support in the literature for early enteral nutrition, most especially with immune-enhancing formulas, the majority of studies are handicapped by the high prevalence of gastrointestinal intolerance leading to inadequate tube feed administration. In fact, several studies have shown that patients who rely on enteral feeding alone are underfed. In 1995, Heyland et al. enrolled 99 consecutive ICU patients and recorded the initiating time and tolerance of tube feeds [29]. They found that approximately one half of critically ill, hypermetabolic ICU patients were intolerant of enteral feeding due to gastrointestinal dysfunction. Subsequently, in 2001, De Jonghe followed 51 consecutive ICU patients for the first 14 days of nutritional delivery [30]. The investigators discovered inadequate routine delivery of enteral nutrition, with more than half of the study patients receiving <70 % of their nutritional goals. On further inspection, the etiology was multifactorial, equally distributed among the following: digestive intolerance (high gastric residual >200 cc, constipation, diarrhea, abdominal distention, vomiting, and regurgitation), airway management issues, and discontinuation for diagnostic procedures.

To address this well-defined problem of enteral feeding intolerance and resultant inadequate nutrition delivery, multiple studies have been performed to evaluate whether a potential change in clinical practice may improve outcome. When providing enteral nutrition, the decision to feed into the stomach or into the small bowel has been both a point of debate and of substantial clinical investigation. One approach has been to determine if there is a noticeable clinical difference when delivering enteral formulas into the stomach, into the duodenum, or into the jejunum. When discussing "transpyloric" or "postpyloric" feeding, most investigators distinguish between delivering nutrients (1) into some portion of the duodenum or (2) beyond the ligament of Treitz, into the proximal jejunum. The hypothesis has been that in bypassing the region of potential gastroduodenal dysmotility, nutrients directly infused into the jejunum would improve tolerance while decreasing the potential for feeding complications such as aspiration (Fig. 3.1).

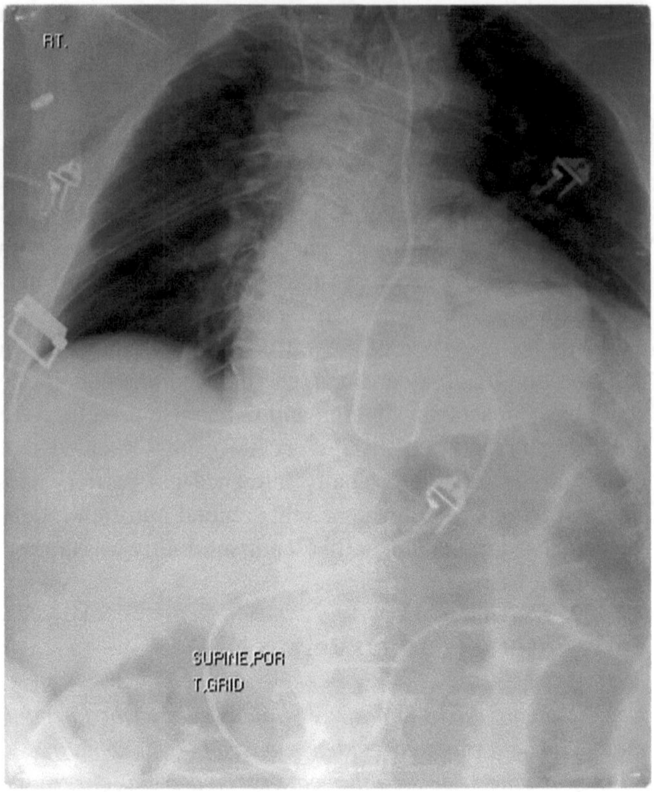

Fig. 3.1 Postpyloric positioning of nasoenteric feeding tube

Aspiration

When investigators have prospectively compared nasogastric to nasoduodenal feeding in principally medical ICU patients, there has been no evidence for decreased rates of aspiration [31] or of aspiration pneumonia [32–34]. Similar findings have been noted when comparing nasogastric to nasojejunal feeding [35–37]. This is likely due to the lower esophageal sphincter being stented open by any tube, regardless of where its tip is positioned.

Esparza et al conducted a trial in 2001 which randomized 54 ICU patients to either gastric or transpyloric feeding [31]. All feeds were tagged with technetium 99m-radiolabeled sulfur colloid, and the pulmonary secretions or lungs were scanned on a daily basis to determine whether aspiration had occurred. There was a nonsignificant difference in aspiration between the gastric and transpylorically fed patients (7 % vs. 13 %). These findings suggest that regurgitation of postpylorically delivered feeds exists secondary to retrograde peristalsis but does not result in an increase in actual aspiration or in clinically definable pneumonia.

Feeding Tolerance

Key Concept: Nasogastric and nasojejunal routes have similar rates of feeding tolerance.

The medications that have been employed as prokinetic agents include antidopaminergic agents (i.e., metoclopramide), serotonergic agents (i.e., cisapride), and motilin receptor agonists (i.e., erythromycin). While there is some support for a role in the setting of gastroparesis, these agents have been proven useless in impacting the degree or duration small bowel or colonic ileus [38]. In addition to lack of efficacy, administration of many of these agents results in unacceptable side effects. Cisapride is no longer available due to cardiac arrhythmias and risk of sudden death. The practicing surgeon commonly adds such agents with a hope of stimulating GI functional recovery, often understanding the lack of benefit while under recognizing the potential risks. These agents should not be used at present, as we await new formulations with more reliable and predictable results. Alvimopan is a peripheral μ antagonist that may prophylactically prevent postoperative ileus but must be initiated prior to narcotic administration.

Regarding the issue of feeding tolerance, several studies do reveal significantly greater nutrient delivery when feeding beyond the pylorus [32, 34] while others do not [33, 35–37]. This difference appears to be primarily related to the practice of holding feeds for high gastric residuals, the most frequent gastrointestinal complication associated with enteral feeding leading to decreased nutritional intake [39]. When a more aggressive feeding protocol is followed, nasogastrically fed patients, despite having higher gastric residual volumes, receive equivalent amounts of enteral nutrition to those fed nasojejunally [35].

One of the earliest studies that evaluated the potential difference between intragastric and jejunal feedings was performed in 1992 by Montecalvo et al. [40]. They prospectively randomized 38 ICU patients to receive feeds through either gastric or endoscopically placed jejunal tubes. Those patients fed by the jejunal route received a significantly higher proportion of their goal caloric intake (46.9 % vs. 61 %, $p<.05$) but had equal rates of pneumonia (0 % vs. 10 %, $p=\text{NS}$).

In 2002, Davies et al. performed a prospective, randomized trial to evaluate the potential benefits of nasojejunal (NJ) feeding compared to nasogastric (NG) feeding [35]. By feeding directly into the jejunum, the authors hypothesized that the patients would be more tolerant of enteral nutrition. The study distinguished between criteria for "ceasing" tube feeds and criteria for declaring a patient "intolerant" of feeds. Instead of using the traditional cutoff range for high gastric residual volumes (150–200 cc), the authors continued feeds until a residual measured >250 cc beyond the previous residual measurement. They also commenced feeds at a rate of 20 cc/h and aggressively advanced by 20 cc every 4 h. Patients were only declared "intolerant" when, over a 48-h period, (1) feeds were stopped four times due to one of their predefined complications or (2) a total gastric residual volumes of 2,000 cc was reached. By these criteria, 4/31 patients in the NJ group were intolerant, although all 31 were eventually tolerant of enteral feeds after a holding period. A total of 11/35 patients in the NG group were intolerant. Of the 11 who were intolerant, 10 were eventually tolerant, either by NG or NJ feeding. Only 1 patient went on to TPN.

Although the authors did demonstrate a significant difference in gastric residual volumes (incidence 32 % vs. 74 %), there was no difference in feeding tolerance. Once feeding was initiated, there was no difference between the groups with regard to the volume delivered at 24 and 48 h or the time to reach target rate. Also, there were no differences in clinical complications such as bleeding, pneumonia, sepsis, SIRS, or mortality. It should be noted that there was a 1-day delay in initiating enteral feeding in the NJ group. This was directly attributable to a scheduling delay required to arrange endoscopy by the gastroenterologist for tube placement. The endoscopic placement of jejunal tubes does appear to be technically feasible (98 % success rate) and safe but is the effort and expense worth the trouble? As the enteral feeding tubes were inadvertently removed in approximately one-third of the patients, tube dislodgment remains a major problem and is likely a major factor in reaching goal nutrition. NG tubes can be replaced at the bedside, but NJ tubes replacement typically requires repeat endoscopy or radiologic assistance.

Although NJ feeding results in reduced gastric residual volumes, this feeding method does not consistently improve feeding tolerance. It can be helpful in certain subsets of patients, suggesting that NJ feeding can be an alternative to TPN in the patient proven or likely to be intolerant to NG feeding. This is an important finding. Its applicability to populations with higher likelihood of gastrointestinal intolerance such as postoperative patients or those with severe pancreatitis or closed head injury will require further study before implementation as a standard for all patients.

Enteral Complications

Key Concept: Though perhaps not as well publicized, enteral feeding has its own unique set of potential complications surgeons should be aware of.

One of the arguments used in support of enteral over parenteral feeding revolves around the morbidity associated with central venous line placement and maintenance. In fact, enteral feeding practices can often lead to unique adverse effects of their own such as high gastric residuals leading to reflux, emesis and aspiration, abdominal distention, diarrhea, constipation, and rarely mesenteric ischemia. Mechanical complications include misplacement (endobronchial, intrapulmonary, and transesophageal), dislodgement, or malfunction from luminal blockage. Finally, enteral feeding (particularly of ICU patients) is regularly discontinued for both diagnostic and interventional procedures, often resulting in patient underfeeding (Fig. 3.2).

The above complications become particularly important when one attempts to bypass the physiologic brake of gastroduodenal dysmotility by placing a postpyloric feeding tube. There is a very small but substantial risk of mesenteric ischemia associated with jejunal feeding (estimated at 1 in 1,359), which is most likely to occur in patients showing signs of abdominal pain, distention, increased NG drainage, or intestinal ileus [41]. Given this uncommon but serious potential complication with NJ feeding, protocols to avoid high-risk patients such as hypotensive patients receiving pressor agents or those with significant abdominal pain seem appropriate, since its low incidence renders this complication outside the ability to study clinically. Fortunately, feeding-related small bowel necrosis is not encountered by most surgeons or intensivists, but this complication carries a significant mortality (86 %).

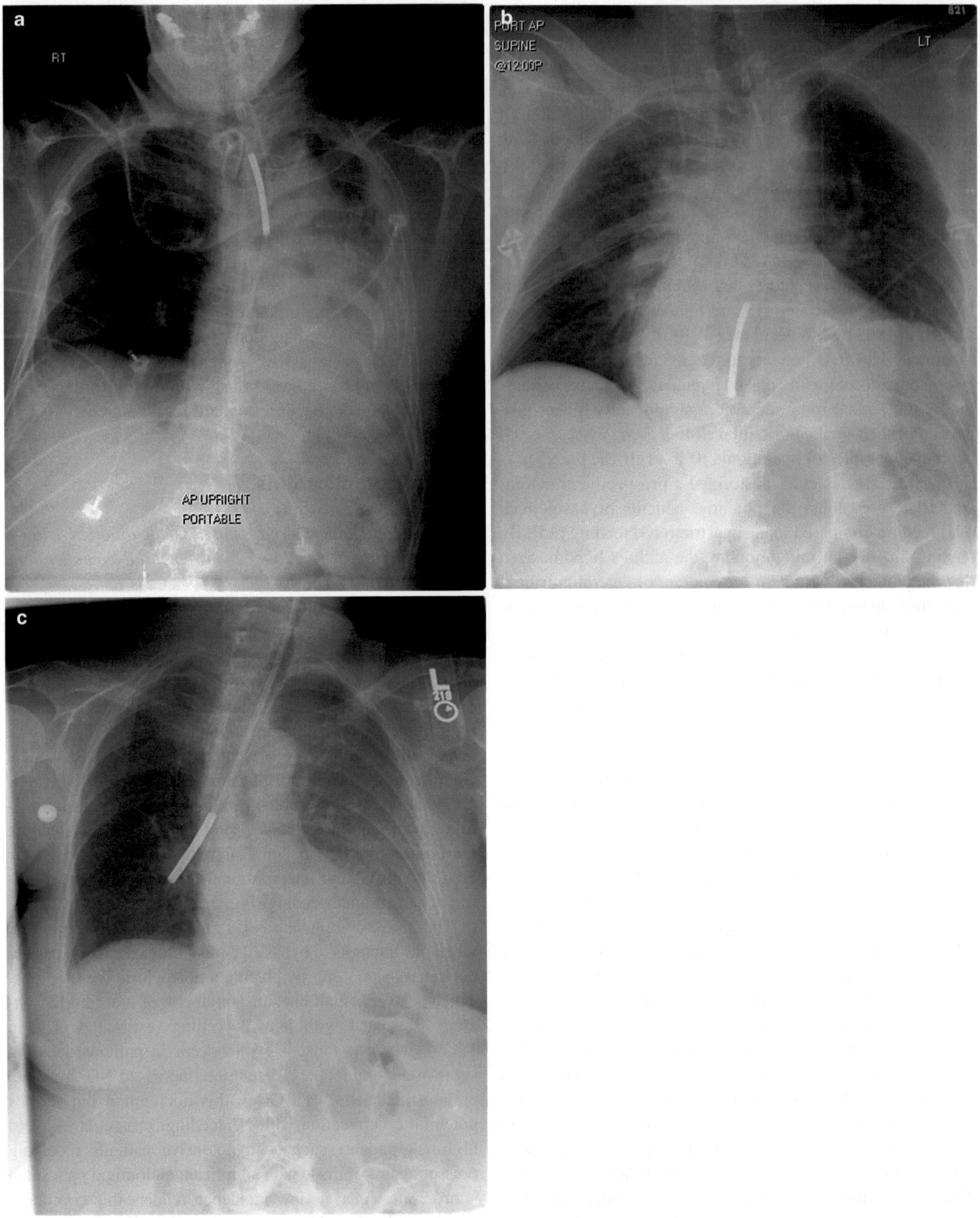

Fig. 3.2 Malpositioned nasoenteric feeding tubes, highlighting the importance of verifying tip location prior to initiation of feeds. (**a**) Coiled tip in proximal esophagus (**b**). Tip in mid-esophagus (**c**). Tip in right mainstem bronchus

Total Parenteral Nutrition

Key Concept: Underlying problems with the available literature regarding perioperative TPN use make widespread reliable conclusions difficult. Surgeons should be aware of proper formulation and practice guidelines, as well as the potential complications that can arise with the use of TPN.

Unfortunately, the literature that evaluates the role for parenteral support is typically old, employing outdated practices and generally of low quality due to heterogeneous patient populations, variable study designs, and excessive feeding protocols. Early studies and subsequent meta-analyses have revealed conflicting results.

Von Meyenfeldt et al. published one of the earliest randomized controlled trials evaluating the impact of preoperative TPN on postoperative morbidity [42]. The authors randomized 50 patients to 10 days of preoperative TPN and 50 patients to 10 days of preoperative enteral nutrition. These patients were compared to a group of 50 malnourished control patients. The investigators observed a significant decrease in postoperative complications in patients who administered preoperative nutrition and were high risk (>10 % weight loss and >500 cc blood loss) ($p<0.05$).

In 1997, an expert committee reviewed all published studies evaluating the use of TPN in the perioperative setting [43]. When delivered preoperatively, TPN appeared to decrease the risk of postoperative complications by 10 %, yet no difference in mortality was noted. When delivered postoperatively, TPN was found to increase postoperative complications by 10 %, again with no mortality difference. Even at the time the authors recognized that the type and quantity of nutrients delivered were suboptimal and calories were given in excess of metabolic needs, potentially impacting outcomes.

In 2000, Bozzetti et al. looked at the role of perioperative TPN in malnourished gastrointestinal cancer patients. 90 patients with gastric or colorectal tumors and >10 % weight loss were randomized to 10 days of preoperative and 9 days of postoperative nutrition vs. control group [44]. The TPN group suffered fewer postoperative complications 37 % vs. 57 % ($p=0.03$) and fewer deaths (0 vs. 5, $p=0.05$.). Even though the patients were overfed at >35 kcal/kg, the overall and infectious complications were fewer, likely as a result of appropriate selection of highest risk, malnourished patients.

Complications

Catheter

The placement of a central venous catheter is necessary for the initiation of total parenteral nutrition. The hyperosmolar solution must be delivered into the large diameter, high-flow vena cava to prevent phlebitis seen when delivered into the peripheral veins. A PICC line is currently the most common form of access, supplanting the triple lumen placed at the internal jugular or subclavian location. While considered safer with less risk of pneumothorax or injury to the chest vessels, PICC placement is not benign and can still be complicated by misplacement, dislodgment, cardiac arrhythmias, thrombosis, and infection. Long-term tunneled lines may be more resistant to infection, though are more invasive with their own set of complications. All catheters are at risk for infection, and this is a direct consequence of local care and access technique. Thrombosis can complicate lines in the upper extremities due to intraluminal thrombus or fibrin clot at the catheter tip. If a catheter-related thrombosis is diagnosed, the catheter should be removed and the patient systemically anticoagulated. Less common complications include pneumothorax, vascular injury, air embolism, thoracic duct injury, brachial plexus injury, and catheter erosion.

Metabolic

TPN should be considered a compounded medication and therefore requires an understanding of its components and risks of administration. While some institutions have "standardized" formulas or even nutrition support teams to guide the prescription process, many surgeons are tasked with writing a customized solution on a daily basis. Inappropriate formulation can result in electrolyte abnormalities (commonly including potassium and magnesium) as well as acid–base disturbances. Excess calcium or phosphorus can lead to precipitation. Excess water can cause hyponatremia. One of the most important issues related to TPN administration surrounds glycemic control. Excessive dextrose administration, particularly to a diabetic patient or those on steroids, can iatrogenically create a state of hyperglycemia with significant impact of patient morbidity.

How to Write TPN

Key Concept: Matching the TPN formulation with the individual patient's needs is an obvious, yet understated (and underperformed), critical aspect to better outcomes.

This review of potential complications of TPN prompts a review of a safe way to initiate and advance TPN. While each institution varies regarding TPN formula options and compounding process, this review will highlight some of the salient points that help the practitioner prescribe TPN in a systematic and safe fashion (Table 3.2).

Enteral Versus Parenteral

Key Concept: When given properly and avoiding hyperglycemia, both the enteral and parenteral routes can adequately provide ideal nutritional supplementation with similar outcomes.

Table 3.2 Systematic approach to the safe and appropriate prescription of TPN (*may vary based on institution's products and protocols*)

Initial calculations

1. Determine the "feeding weight":

Calculate ideal body weight (IBW)

Men: 106 lb for 1st 5 ft and 6 lb for each inch thereafter

Women: 100 lb for the 1st 5 ft and 5 lb for each inch thereafter

Compare to actual body weight (ABW) or usual body weight (UBW)

If a big discrepancy, calculate adjusted feeding weight

If patient is underweight, generally use IBW

If patient is obese (>120 % IBW), then add 25 % of the difference between the ABW and IBW to the IBW

Amputations

IBW less 6 % for BKA

IBW less 9 % for AKA

Using the example of a 70 kg person ("feeding weight"):

2. Calculate *GOAL* nutritional support. *Usually*

(a) Protein: 1.5 g/kg/day ($1.5 \times 70 = 105$ g)

(b) Kilocalories: 25 kcal/kg/day ($25 \times 70 = 1{,}750$ kcal)

3. Determine the components of the GOAL TPN admixture (no lipids/2:1)

(a) Start with total *kilocalories*

1,750 kcal

(b) Calculate how much of total kcal will come from goal *protein*

$105\ \text{g} \times 4\ \text{kcal/g} = 420$ kcal

(c) Subtract this amount of calories from the goal/total

$1{,}750 - 420 = 1{,}330$ kcal.

(d) Make up the difference with *dextrose*

$1{,}330\ \text{kcal} \div 3.4\ \text{kcal/g} = 390$ g dextrose

4. Determine the components of the GOAL TPN admixture (with lipids/3:1)

(a) Start with total *kilocalories*

1,750 kcal

(b) Calculate 20 % (or 30 %) of the total calories, and provide this as *lipids*

$1{,}750 \times 0.2 = 350$ kcal

$350\ \text{kcal} \div 9\ \text{kcal/g} = 38$ g (may round off to 35 g lipids (so lipids actually provide 315 kcal))

(c) Determine how much of total kcal will come from *protein*

$105\ \text{g} \times 4\ \text{kcal/g} = 420$ kcal

(d) Subtract the protein and fat calories from the total and administer the remaining calories as *dextrose*

$1{,}750 - 315 - 420 = 1{,}015$ kcal

$1{,}015 \div 3.4\ \text{kcal/g} = 300$ g dextrose

5. Final *volume* (*maximally* concentrated)

(a) Amino acids (10 % stock solution)	105 g = 1,050 cc
(b) Dextrose (70 % stock solution)	300 g = 430 cc
(c) Lipids (20 % stock solution)	35 g = 175 cc
	= 1,655 cc total

How to advance TPN safely

1. Day#1 "Starter Formula": 1,000 cc/70gAA/150 g dextrose

Not much thought necessary as a start

Typically will test glucose tolerance, without significant hyperglycemia

2. If tolerated (blood sugars <150 mg/dL), advance to day#2 formula:

1,000 cc/70gAA/210 g dextrose

Can also advance to goal protein safely if eager to move forward

3. If tolerated, advance protein to goal and then dextrose by 50 g/day (if hyperglycemia or diabetes) or 100 g/day until reach goal

4. Insulin administration:

(a) Rule

Cover dextrose in TPN with insulin in TPN (or SQ sliding scale)

Cover dextrose in tube feeds with sliding scale or NPH

(b) Typically it is safe to put 10 units in TPN for everybody

Table 3.2 (continued)

(c) Add up previous day's sliding scale and add 2/3 of total to what is already in the current bag	
(d) If advancing dextrose amount, increase insulin *proportionally*	
(e) If hyperglycemic, do not advance dextrose until blood sugars are controlled (under 120–150 mg/dL)	
(f) If difficult to control blood sugars because of insulin resistance, be quick to switch to an insulin drip, especially in the SICU	
Electrolytes	
1. Na: depends on volume status and losses	
2. K: depends on urine output and losses	
Typical urine: 20 or 40 mEq/L if on Lasix	
3. Cl: maximize if metabolic alkalosis	
4. Acetate: maximize if metabolic acidosis	
5. Ca: RDA 10 mEq/day	
6. Mg: RDA 10 mEq/day	
7. Phos: RDA 30–40 mmol/day	
Routine upon starting TPN (day #1)	
1. Start aggressive insulin sliding scale and QID BS checks for goal BS under 120 mg/dL	
2. Check triglyceride level	
Lipids contraindicated if >400 mg/dL	
3. If on heparin, may add to TPN bag (6,000 units in TPN = 5,000 units SC BID)	
4. If on Zantac, may add to bag (150 mg/day if normal renal function)	
5. If on Reglan, may add to bag (40 mg/day if normal renal function)	
6. Remember to reverse the above when stopping TPN	
Some things to remember	
1. Ca/phos solubility curve (can get chart from Pharmacy)	
2. Lipid concentration must be at least 2 % (20 g/L)	
3. If lipids in bag, total Ca and Mg sum must be ≤20 mEq/L	
4. There is a minimum required volume for solubility, so use these two formulas to see if the macronutrients fit:	
Standard AA	(AA × 7) + D + (L × 3.5) must be ≤ 70
If branched-chain AA	(AA × 11) + D + (L × 3.5) ≤ 70
5. If using BCAA, maximum of 100 g/day	
6. HCl cannot be added if lipids in bag	
7. Remember kilocalories *outside* of TPN:	
(a) Propofol is in a 10 % lipid emulsion, so you get 1 kcal/cc of propofol	
(b) D5W for meds and treatment of hypernatremia	
(c) Patients on CVVH(D) often have D5 solutions as return fluid	
(d) Patients on peritoneal dialysis	
(e) Protein/calories from concurrent enteral feeds	
8. Other potential additives:	
Hydrochloric acid (HCl). Not compatible with lipids	
Supplemental zinc (for open wounds, decubitus ulcers, or diarrhea)	
Typically 10 mg/day	

The literature over the past decades is replete with clinical trials comparing enteral and parenteral nutrition. Some conclude that parenteral feeding is equivalent to enteral feeding [45–47] while others conclude that enteral feeding is better than parenteral feeding [48–50]. Absent a clear consensus, post hoc analysis does reveal a common flaw in many of the studies purporting an advantage to enteral feeding. GI tolerance limits the total volume of solution that can be provided to critically ill patients to about 1,500 cc/day. When study goals are set at 35 kcal/kg/day, this can only be consistently attained when parenteral nutrition is delivered through a central venous catheter. This dichotomy commonly sets up a situation where enterally fed patients receive substantially less energy than parenterally fed subjects. On the other hand, providing parenteral nutrition at 35 kcal/kg/day or greater produces hyperglycemia in the majority of patients [51]. Hyperglycemia clearly induces immunosuppression, resulting in an increased risk of postoperative complications and adverse outcomes [52]. Van Den Berghe showed that in critically ill patients, all of who were adequately fed (approximately 25 kcal/kg/day either enterally or parenterally), intensive insulin therapy aiming for euglycemia reduced bloodstream infections by 46 % and overall mortality by 42 % [53]. There was no difference in outcome for those fed exclusively enterally, exclusively parenterally, or with combined feeding with adequate control of blood glucose. This finding underscores the fact that studies must properly compare feeding protocols that maintain equal glycemic control and provide equivalent intakes of protein and calories for *both* routes.

Since the 1991 Veteran's Affairs study evaluating the efficacy of preoperative TPN identified an increased infection risk in certain subgroups of patients [54], there has been a general recommendation favoring the use of enteral nutrition over total parenteral nutrition. Closer examination of that study reveals that it was actually a study of overfeeding in the TPN group marked by resultant hyperglycemia. The total energy intake of the TPN group was 46 kcal/kg/day (2,944 kcal/day) while the ad libitum group consumed 20 kcal/kg/day (1,280 kcal/day). Energy expenditure in such postoperative patients would be estimated to be 25 kcal/kg/day [55]. With this degree of feeding-induced hyperglycemia, the immunosuppressive effects would be great enough to negate any potential benefit to preoperative feeding, with the exception of the subgroup, which was severely malnourished. This was, in fact, exactly and not surprisingly what was found.

More recent studies that provide patients with roughly equivalent amounts of nutrients at modest levels demonstrate that there is essentially no clinical difference between enteral and parenteral nutrition [47, 56]. For example, Braga et al. designed a prospective RCT to evaluate the potential clinical, metabolic, and economic advantages of enteral nutrition over parenteral nutrition [46]. Two hundred and fifty-seven surgical patients were randomized to receive early postoperative TPN or early postoperative TEN via a jejunal feeding tube. Mean energy intakes were equal between groups (1,632 ± 281 kcal TPN vs. 1,522 ± 317 kcal TEN), and there was no difference in rate of hyperglycemia (defined as serum glucose >200 mg/dL) (9.1 % TPN vs. 4.7 % TEN). Although enteral nutrition was found to improve gut oxygenation (as assessed by cecal microprobe), there was no difference in infectious complication rates, noninfectious complication rates, length of hospital stay, mortality, or in nutritional, inflammatory, or immunologic variables.

Most recently, Wu et al published a prospective randomized controlled trial evaluating the use of perioperative artificial nutrition in malnourished gastrointestinal cancer (stomach, colon, and rectum) patients [57]. Four hundred and sixty-seven elective patients who were moderately to severely malnourished surgical by SGA were assigned to 7 days of preoperative and 7 days of postoperative parenteral or enteral nutrition vs. a simple control group. Patients were fed appropriately with 25 kcal/kg/day. Complications occurred in 18 % of patients receiving nutrition and 34 % of control patients ($p = 0.012$), and postoperative stay was longer in the control group (23 days vs. 12 days, $p = 0.0001$). A mortality difference was also seen comparing study and control patients (2.1 % vs. 6.0 %, $p = 0.003$). This study shows not only the overall impact of nutritional support but highlights the importance of providing the appropriate quantity via the most appropriate route over an adequate duration. Patients who were unable to tolerate enteral nutrition were fed with TPN, and combination regimens were utilized as well. There was no difference in septic complications seen comparing enteral and parentally fed patients (13 % vs. 16 %, $p = 0.36$).

Therefore, in the year 2014, it appears irrefutable that, when delivered appropriately, both forms of nutritional support can be expected to improve organ function, immune competence, and wound healing in appropriately selected patients [22].

Perioperative Management

Key Concept: Despite limited high-level evidence, preoperative nutrition through either the enteral or parenteral route is likely beneficial, especially in the malnourished patient. Additional benefits may be seen with immune-modulated formulas.

In colorectal surgery, patients who present in the malnourished state do so as a consequence of the underlying disease process, which affects the gastrointestinal tract. Inflammatory bowel disease, intestinal obstruction, large tumors, fistulizing diseases, and patients with diarrhea are often unable to sustain themselves orally due to a poor appetite or resultant abdominal bloating and pain. This limits the ability to intervene preoperatively, particularly when considering utilizing the enteral route. Oral nutritional supplements that provide defined quantities of protein, calories, and vitamins can be offered and encouraged in almost every setting but obstruction. These have been shown to improve postoperative outcomes. Appetite stimulants such as Megace can help those patients with poor appetite but are unlikely to augment intake of these patients who are functionally obstructed. Nasogastric tubes, nasojejunal tubes, and gastrostomy tubes can be inserted and utilized. As most patients are deficient, an oral multivitamin/mineral supplement should be recommended for 2 weeks before surgery at 300–400 % the recommended daily values [58].

Unfortunately, the use of preoperative enteral nutrition has not been well studied in either the well-nourished or malnourished GI surgery patient populations. A recent Cochrane review [59] highlights this paucity of evidence and the reality that many of the studies are outdated—with only two trials evaluating the administration of enteral nutrition (years 1992 and 2009) including only 120 participants and a high risk of bias. Neither study showed any difference in primary outcomes. The three studies that evaluated preoperative parenteral nutrition (years 1982, 1988, and 1992) showed a significant reduction in postoperative complications, predominantly in malnourished patients.

Immunonutrition

Major injury, whether traumatic or surgery induced, results in significant metabolic and immunologic sequelae which influence patient recovery. Specific "immune-modulating" substances such as arginine, glutamine, nucleotides, and omega-3 fatty acids/fish oil have been shown to modulate the host response, resulting in improved immune function. The clinical trials evaluating the efficacy of these formulas have supported an improved postoperative clinical course when patients are compared to those receiving standard enteral formulas [60–62] and provide the only available studies evaluating preoperative feeding.

In 1992, Daly et al. were the first to study the clinical effects of early enteral feeding with immune-enhancing diets by prospectively randomizing 85 patients undergoing surgery for upper gastrointestinal malignancies to either a standard or experimental (Impact) enteral diet [63]. Postoperative nutrition was delivered via a jejunostomy tube, starting on POD#1 and continuing until POD#7. The two groups were well matched and received equivalent volumes of tube feeds (1,421 vs. 1,285 kcal/day). The patients who were administered the immune-modulating diet experienced a significant improvement in both postoperative wound healing and infectious complications, along with a shorter length of hospital stay. The only flaw in this study was that the patients were fed isocalorically but not isonitrogenously (15.6 vs. 9.0 g of Nitrogen per day), leaving the possibility that their findings may be partially explained by differential protein administration, although this is unlikely.

A recent meta-analysis consisting of 21 randomized controlled trials including 2,730 patients reviewed the literature evaluating immunonutrition following major elective gastrointestinal surgery [64]. Immunonutrition decreased overall complications when delivered before surgery (OR 0.48 CI 0.34–0.69), before and after surgery (OR 0.39 CI 0.28–0.54), and after surgery (OR 0.46 CI 0.25–0.84). In the end there were fewer infectious complications and shorter hospital length of stay but no influence on mortality. The heterogeneity of the studies made it difficult to comment to the specific role of malnutrition on outcomes. What does appear clear is that if it is possible to give immune-modifying nutrition support early in the course of illness and to give it in rather large amounts, its benefits are more easily detected.

Braga et al. similarly showed quite convincingly that the administration of an immune-enhancing diet perioperatively resulted in a significant clinical benefit [65]. They randomized 206 candidates for elective surgery to treat malignancies of the colon, rectum, stomach, or pancreas to receive either an immune-enhancing formula (Impact) or a control enteral formula (isonitrogenous, isocaloric). Patients were administered 1 l per day for 7 days preoperatively followed by jejunal infusions of the same formulas postoperatively, starting 6 h after operation and continued until postoperative day 7. The perioperative group experienced significantly fewer postoperative infections (14 % vs. 30 %) and a shorter hospital length of stay (11.1 days vs. 12.9 days). These findings were consistent, regardless of the baseline nutritional status, and the authors concluded that the perioperative supplementation of immunonutrition provided metabolic and immunologic advantages that may be related to the ability to attain adequate levels before the surgical insult. Because of the preoperative feeding protocol, the formula intake was not limited by postoperative gastrointestinal intolerance.

Total Parenteral Nutrition

The challenge with initiating TPN preoperatively deals with the complexities of coordination. To safely and properly initiate TPN, a patient needs to be monitored for glycemic control, volume tolerance, and electrolyte abnormalities, particularly when severely malnourished due to the risk of developing the refeeding syndrome (development of electrolyte abnormalities, volume overload, and congestive heart failure). Advancement of TPN from an initial formula to goal formula often takes several days following placement of a central venous line. It is nearly impossible to accomplish this safely on an outpatient basis, yet it can be a challenge to obtain insurance approval for hospital admission. Fortunately most patients who are moderately to severely malnourished (representing the population to theoretically benefit most from this approach) are commonly dealing with other medical issues that warrant hospital admissions, such as bowel instruction, failure to thrive, or severe diarrhea with dehydration. While admitted, the surgeon can take advantage of this opportunity to obtain central venous access and initiate parental nutrition. Once goal formula has been reached and other medical issues stabilized, the patient can be transitioned to a subacute care center or home with nursing support. Oftentimes the nutrition can be cycled to free the patient and provide a "break" during the daytime hours. Once the TPN has been started, there is less dependence on the patient's oral intake for nutritional support, and oral intake can be considered a supplement to the protein and calories being reliably delivered intravenously.

Postoperative Management

Key Concept: *Nutritional support is not required in the immediate resuscitative period following major surgery; however, it should be initiated shortly thereafter by whatever route is more feasible.*

During the immediate postoperative period, intravenous nutritional support should be held. The body is recovering from a major stress (surgery) and the stress response induces a period of hyperglycemia and insulin resistance. The focus should be on fluid resuscitation with standardized isotonic solutions as opposed to hyperosmolar hyperglycemic solutions that are compounded in a variety of formulations. Once the "metabolic response to injury" has resolved and oral intake had resumed, the surgeon can commonly readvance the diet and avoid the reinitiating of TPN all together. For those patients who are less likely to support themselves with oral intake, TPN should be restarted on postoperative day #3. The preoperative goal formula can often be restarted. For those patients who received a gastrostomy tube or jejunostomy tube at the time of surgery, tube feeds can be started and advanced unless a postoperative ileus develops. The relatively immediate initiation of enteral feeding after surgery fits well into established enhanced recovery after surgery (ERAS) protocols that are commonly followed by colorectal surgeons, but one must be careful not to push early oral intake too aggressively for those patients who have been chronically obstructed.

A particular challenge arises when it is time to discharge the patient yet they remain dependent on TPN. It is often advantageous to begin cycling the TPN prior to discharge. This provides the surgeon with an opportunity to monitor the patient's response to increased TPN volume delivered per hour, with its potential impact on glycemic control and volume tolerance. In addition, cycling provides the patient a period of time disconnected from the pump for physical therapy or activities of daily life. Though it remains a commonly held misperception, there is no evidence to suggest that there is any appetite suppression during TPN infusion, so this should not have an impact on oral food interest or intake.

The outpatient prescription of TPN typically becomes the responsibility of the discharging physician. This can be challenging for both inexperienced surgeons and for patients with complex medical issues including heart failure, renal dysfunction, or high volume losses from the GI tract. Some institutions have home TPN services, others rely on expertise from home infusions pharmacists or dieticians, while others may have a local expert to provide consultation. Regardless, the surgeons should be aware that patients must be followed very closely as outpatients with regular blood work and manipulation of the TPN formulas dependent on oral intake and changes in coverall clinical status.

Summary/Pearls

The field of surgical nutrition is complicated and remains incompletely studied, resulting in a widespread lack of command of the topic. Unfortunately this general lack of focused training coupled with a lack of quality evidence handicaps the surgeon's ability to consistently consider the importance, recognize the prevalence, and initiate appropriate perioperative nutritional intervention. Nutrition can provide a powerful adjunct to the care provided to your patients, particularly those at high risk. By simply remembering these important points and understanding where to find supportive resources at your institution, you will lead the effort towards improving the overall care of your patients:

1. Albumin is generally an unreliable marker of overall nutritional status and more likely reflects overall severity of illness.
2. Extensive animal studies have shown that early enteral feeding after injury provides both physiologic and immunologic benefits.
3. Although one would intuitively assume that enteral feeding is the more "physiologic" route of nutrition administration, these findings have not been well verified in humans.
4. The numerous studies that compare early to delayed enteral feeding in general surgical and critically ill patients appear to ascribe a small benefit to early postoperative or post-injury feeding in particular patient subsets. Inherent harm does not appear to result from its administration.
5. More recent studies that use immediate immune-modulating formulas, result in decreased infectious complications and shorter length of hospital stay, particularly when a minimal volume is infused (approximating 800 cc/day or 30 cc/h).
6. It appears that *peri*operative supplementation with immunonutrition is the most successful means of improving patient outcome, in both well and malnourished patients.
7. Enteral feeding is severely limited by gastrointestinal intolerance, commonly leading to inadequate nutrition administration and the underfeeding of critically ill, hypermetabolic patients.
8. Promotility agents have been inconsistently helpful in improving GI tolerance.
9. The use of postpyloric feeding tubes, when studied in prospective, randomized trials, provides no benefit to decreasing the incidence of pulmonary aspiration. There is conflicting evidence whether this practice improves feeding tolerance, and this advantage may be limited to specific patient populations.
10. It appears that the practices of preoperative supplementation, more aggressive postoperative feeding protocols, and/or more diligent avoidance or minimization of unnecessary postoperative feeding disruptions would close the gap between what is prescribed and what is delivered. These measures appear more reasonable and more cost-effective than trying to obtain and maintain postpyloric access.
11. Balancing minimal potential risk with potential future benefit/need, always consider placement of a gastrostomy

tube, jejunostomy tube, or both at the conclusion of every operation.

12. When delivered isonitrogenously and isocalorically, coupled with fastidious serum glucose control, there no longer appears to exist a difference in patient outcome when administered enteral or parenteral nutrition.
13. When patients have declared themselves intermittently or completely intolerant of enteral feeding, supplement or supplant their feeding goals with TPN.
14. Patients who are malnourished benefit from perioperative nutritional support using TPN, enteral feeding, or immunonutrition resulting in an approximately 25 % decreased complication rate.

References

1. Bistrian BR, Blackburn GL, Vitale J, Cochran D, Naylor J. Prevalence of malnutrition in general medical patients. JAMA. 1976;235(15):1567–70.
2. Bistrian BR, Blackburn GL, Hallowell E, Heddle R. Protein status of general surgical patients. JAMA. 1974;230(6):858–60.
3. Mullen JL, Gertner MH, Buzby GP, Goodhart GL, Rosato EF. Implications of malnutrition in the surgical patient. Arch Surg. 1979;114(2):121–5.
4. Schiesser M, Kirchhoff P, Muller MK, Schafer M, Clavien PA. The correlation of nutrition risk index, nutrition risk score, and bioimpedance analysis with postoperative complications in patients undergoing gastrointestinal surgery. Surgery. 2009;145(5):519–26.
5. McWhirter JP, Pennington CR. Incidence and recognition of malnutrition in hospital. BMJ. 1994;308(6934):945–8.
6. Kyle UG, Schneider SM, Pirlich M, Lochs H, Hebuterne X, Pichard C. Does nutritional risk, as assessed by Nutritional Risk Index, increase during hospital stay? A multinational population-based study. Clin Nutr. 2005;24(4):516–24.
7. Dupertuis YM, Kossovsky MP, Kyle UG, Raguso CA, Genton L, Pichard C. Food intake in 1707 hospitalised patients: a prospective comprehensive hospital survey. Clin Nutr. 2003;22(2):115–23.
8. Bozzetti F, Mariani L, Lo Vullo S, Amerio ML, Biffi R, Caccialanza G, et al. The nutritional risk in oncology: a study of 1,453 cancer outpatients. Support Care Cancer. 2012;20(8):1919–28.
9. Sorensen J, Kondrup J, Prokopowicz J, Schiesser M, Krahenbuhl L, Meier R, et al. EuroOOPS: an international, multicentre study to implement nutritional risk screening and evaluate clinical outcome. Clin Nutr. 2008;27(3):340–9.
10. Schwegler I, von Holzen A, Gutzwiller JP, Schlumpf R, Muhlebach S, Stanga Z. Nutritional risk is a clinical predictor of postoperative mortality and morbidity in surgery for colorectal cancer. Br J Surg. 2010;97(1):92–7.
11. Baker JP, Detsky AS, Wesson DE, Wolman SL, Stewart S, Whitewell J, et al. Nutritional assessment: a comparison of clinical judgement and objective measurements. N Engl J Med. 1982; 306(16):969–72.
12. Detsky AS, McLaughlin JR, Baker JP, Johnston N, Whittaker S, Mendelson RA, et al. What is subjective global assessment of nutritional status? JPEN J Parenter Enteral Nutr. 1987;11(1):8–13.
13. Doweiko JP, Nompleggi DJ. The role of albumin in human physiology and pathophysiology, part III: albumin and disease states. JPEN J Parenter Enteral Nutr. 1991;15(4):476–83.
14. Gupta D, Lis CG. Pretreatment serum albumin as a predictor of cancer survival: a systematic review of the epidemiological literature. Nutr J. 2010;9:69.
15. Fearon K, Strasser F, Anker SD, Bosaeus I, Bruera E, Fainsinger RL, et al. Definition and classification of cancer cachexia: an international consensus. Lancet Oncol. 2011;12(5):489–95.
16. Heslin MJ, Latkany L, Leung D, Brooks AD, Hochwald SN, Pisters PW, et al. A prospective, randomized trial of early enteral feeding after resection of upper gastrointestinal malignancy. Ann Surg. 1997;226(4):567–77; discussion 577–80.
17. Muller JM, Brenner U, Dienst C, Pichlmaier H. Preoperative parenteral feeding in patients with gastrointestinal carcinoma. Lancet. 1982;1(8263):68–71.
18. Taylor SJ, Fettes SB, Jewkes C, Nelson RJ. Prospective, randomized, controlled trial to determine the effect of early enhanced enteral nutrition on clinical outcome in mechanically ventilated patients suffering head injury. Crit Care Med. 1999;27(11): 2525–31.
19. Windsor AC, Kanwar S, Li AG, Barnes E, Guthrie JA, Spark JI, et al. Compared with parenteral nutrition, enteral feeding attenuates the acute phase response and improves disease severity in acute pancreatitis. Gut. 1998;42(3):431–5.
20. Alverdy JC, Aoys E, Moss GS. Total parenteral nutrition promotes bacterial translocation from the gut. Surgery. 1988;104(2):185–90.
21. Hughes CA, Prince A, Dowling RH. Speed of change in pancreatic mass and in intestinal bacteriology of parenterally fed rats. Clin Sci (Lond). 1980;59(5):329–36.
22. Sedman PC, MacFie J, Palmer MD, Mitchell CJ, Sagar PM. Preoperative total parenteral nutrition is not associated with mucosal atrophy or bacterial translocation in humans. Br J Surg. 1995;82(12):1663–7.
23. Pironi L, Paganelli GM, Miglioli M, Biasco G, Santucci R, Ruggeri E, et al. Morphologic and cytoproliferative patterns of duodenal mucosa in two patients after long-term total parenteral nutrition: changes with oral refeeding and relation to intestinal resection. JPEN J Parenter Enteral Nutr. 1994;18(4):351–4.
24. Carr CS, Ling KD, Boulos P, Singer M. Randomised trial of safety and efficacy of immediate postoperative enteral feeding in patients undergoing gastrointestinal resection. BMJ. 1996;312(7035): 869–71.
25. Reynolds JV, Kanwar S, Welsh FK, Windsor AC, Murchan P, Barclay GR, et al. 1997 Harry M. Vars Research Award. Does the route of feeding modify gut barrier function and clinical outcome in patients after major upper gastrointestinal surgery? JPEN J Parenter Enteral Nutr. 1997;21(4):196–201.
26. Fong YM, Marano MA, Barber A, He W, Moldawer LL, Bushman ED, et al. Total parenteral nutrition and bowel rest modify the metabolic response to endotoxin in humans. Ann Surg. 1989;210(4):449–56; discussion 456–7.
27. Lewis SJ, Egger M, Sylvester PA, Thomas S. Early enteral feeding versus "nil by mouth" after gastrointestinal surgery: systematic review and meta-analysis of controlled trials. BMJ. 2001;323 (7316):773–6.
28. Marik PE, Zaloga GP. Early enteral nutrition in acutely ill patients: a systematic review. Crit Care Med. 2001;29(12):2264–70.
29. Heyland D, Cook DJ, Winder B, Brylowski L, Van deMark H, Guyatt G. Enteral nutrition in the critically ill patient: a prospective survey. Crit Care Med. 1995;23(6):1055–60.
30. De Jonghe B, Appere-De-Vechi C, Fournier M, Tran B, Merrer J, Melchior JC, et al. A prospective survey of nutritional support practices in intensive care unit patients: what is prescribed? What is delivered? Crit Care Med. 2001;29(1):8–12.
31. Esparza J, Boivin MA, Hartshorne MF, Levy H. Equal aspiration rates in gastrically and transpylorically fed critically ill patients. Intensive Care Med. 2001;27(4):660–4.
32. Kearns PJ, Chin D, Mueller L, Wallace K, Jensen WA, Kirsch CM. The incidence of ventilator-associated pneumonia and success in nutrient delivery with gastric versus small intestinal feeding: a randomized clinical trial. Crit Care Med. 2000;28(6):1742–6.

33. Strong RM, Condon SC, Solinger MR, Namihas BN, Ito-Wong LA, Leuty JE. Equal aspiration rates from postpylorus and intragastric-placed small-bore nasoenteric feeding tubes: a randomized, prospective study. JPEN J Parenter Enteral Nutr. 1992;16(1):59–63.
34. Kortbeek JB, Haigh PI, Doig C. Duodenal versus gastric feeding in ventilated blunt trauma patients: a randomized controlled trial. J Trauma. 1999;46(6):992–6; discussion 996–8.
35. Davies AR, Froomes PR, French CJ, Bellomo R, Gutteridge GA, Nyulasi I, et al. Randomized comparison of nasojejunal and nasogastric feeding in critically ill patients. Crit Care Med. 2002; 30(3):586–90.
36. Neumann DA, DeLegge MH. Gastric versus small-bowel tube feeding in the intensive care unit: a prospective comparison of efficacy. Crit Care Med. 2002;30(7):1436–8.
37. Montejo JC, Grau T, Acosta J, Ruiz-Santana S, Planas M, Garcia-De-Lorenzo A, et al. Multicenter, prospective, randomized, single-blind study comparing the efficacy and gastrointestinal complications of early jejunal feeding with early gastric feeding in critically ill patients. Crit Care Med. 2002;30(4):796–800.
38. Karamanolis G, Tack J. Promotility medications – now and in the future. Dig Dis. 2006;24(3–4):297–307.
39. Montejo JC. Enteral nutrition-related gastrointestinal complications in critically ill patients: a multicenter study. The Nutritional and Metabolic Working Group of the Spanish Society of Intensive Care Medicine and Coronary Units. Crit Care Med. 1999;27(8):1447–53.
40. Montecalvo MA, Steger KA, Farber HW, Smith BF, Dennis RC, Fitzpatrick GF, et al. Nutritional outcome and pneumonia in critical care patients randomized to gastric versus jejunal tube feedings. The Critical Care Research Team. Crit Care Med. 1992;20(10): 1377–87.
41. Schunn CD, Daly JM. Small bowel necrosis associated with postoperative jejunal tube feeding. J Am Coll Surg. 1995;180(4): 410–6.
42. Von Meyenfeldt MF, Meijerink WJ, Rouflart MM, Builmaassen MT, Soeters PB. Perioperative nutritional support: a randomised clinical trial. Clin Nutr. 1992;11(4):180–6.
43. Klein S, Kinney J, Jeejeebhoy K, Alpers D, Hellerstein M, Murray M, et al. Nutrition support in clinical practice: review of published data and recommendations for future research directions. Clin Nutr. 1997;16(4):193–218.
44. Bozzetti F, Gavazzi C, Miceli R, Rossi N, Mariani L, Cozzaglio L, et al. Perioperative total parenteral nutrition in malnourished, gastrointestinal cancer patients: a randomized, clinical trial. JPEN J Parenter Enteral Nutr. 2000;24(1):7–14.
45. Adams S, Dellinger EP, Wertz MJ, Oreskovich MR, Simonowitz D, Johansen K. Enteral versus parenteral nutritional support following laparotomy for trauma: a randomized prospective trial. J Trauma. 1986;26(10):882–91.
46. Braga M, Gianotti L, Gentilini O, Parisi V, Salis C, Di Carlo V. Early postoperative enteral nutrition improves gut oxygenation and reduces costs compared with total parenteral nutrition. Crit Care Med. 2001;29(2):242–8.
47. Pacelli F, Bossola M, Papa V, Malerba M, Modesti C, Sgadari A, et al. Enteral vs parenteral nutrition after major abdominal surgery: an even match. Arch Surg. 2001;136(8):933–6.
48. Kudsk KA, Croce MA, Fabian TC, Minard G, Tolley EA, Poret HA, et al. Enteral versus parenteral feeding. Effects on septic morbidity after blunt and penetrating abdominal trauma. Ann Surg. 1992;215(5):503–11; discussion 511–3.
49. Moore FA, Moore EE, Jones TN, McCroskey BL, Peterson VM. TEN versus TPN following major abdominal trauma – reduced septic morbidity. J Trauma. 1989;29(7):916–22; discussion 922–3.
50. Moore FA, Feliciano DV, Andrassy RJ, McArdle AH, Booth FV, Morgenstein-Wagner TB, et al. Early enteral feeding, compared with parenteral, reduces postoperative septic complications. The results of a meta-analysis. Ann Surg. 1992;216(2):172–83.
51. Rosmarin DK, Wardlaw GM, Mirtallo J. Hyperglycemia associated with high, continuous infusion rates of total parenteral nutrition dextrose. Nutr Clin Pract. 1996;11(4):151–6.
52. McCowen KC, Malhotra A, Bistrian BR. Stress-induced hyperglycemia. Crit Care Clin. 2001;17(1):107–24.
53. van den Berghe G, Wouters P, Weekers F, Verwaest C, Bruyninckx F, Schetz M, et al. Intensive insulin therapy in critically ill patients. N Engl J Med. 2001;345(19):1359–67.
54. The Veterans Affairs Total Parenteral Nutrition Cooperative Study Group. Perioperative total parenteral nutrition in surgical patients. N Engl J Med. 1991;325(8):525–32.
55. Hunter DC, Jaksic T, Lewis D, Benotti PN, Blackburn GL, Bistrian BR. Resting energy expenditure in the critically ill: estimations versus measurement. Br J Surg. 1988;75(9):875–8.
56. Woodcock NP, Zeigler D, Palmer MD, Buckley P, Mitchell CJ, MacFie J. Enteral versus parenteral nutrition: a pragmatic study. Nutrition. 2001;17(1):1–12.
57. Wu GH, Liu ZH, Wu ZH, Wu ZG. Perioperative artificial nutrition in malnourished gastrointestinal cancer patients. World J Gastroenterol. 2006;12(15):2441–4.
58. Stohs SJ, Dudrick SJ. Nutritional supplements in the surgical patient. Surg Clin North Am. 2011;91(4):933–44, x.
59. Burden S, Todd C, Hill J, Lal S. Pre-operative nutrition support in patients undergoing gastrointestinal surgery. Cochrane Database Syst Rev. 2012;(11):CD008879.
60. Heys SD, Walker LG, Smith I, Eremin O. Enteral nutritional supplementation with key nutrients in patients with critical illness and cancer: a meta-analysis of randomized controlled clinical trials. Ann Surg. 1999;229(4):467–77.
61. Beale RJ, Bryg DJ, Bihari DJ. Immunonutrition in the critically ill: a systematic review of clinical outcome. Crit Care Med. 1999; 27(12):2799–805.
62. Heyland DK, Novak F, Drover JW, Jain M, Su X, Suchner U. Should immunonutrition become routine in critically ill patients? A systematic review of the evidence. JAMA. 2001;286(8):944–53.
63. Daly JM, Lieberman MD, Goldfine J, Shou J, Weintraub F, Rosato EF, et al. Enteral nutrition with supplemental arginine, RNA, and omega-3 fatty acids in patients after operation: immunologic, metabolic, and clinical outcome. Surgery. 1992;112(1):56–67.
64. Cerantola Y, Hubner M, Grass F, Demartines N, Schafer M. Immunonutrition in gastrointestinal surgery. Br J Surg. 2011;98(1):37–48.
65. Braga M, Gianotti L, Radaelli G, Vignali A, Mari G, Gentilini O, et al. Perioperative immunonutrition in patients undergoing cancer surgery: results of a randomized double-blind phase 3 trial. Arch Surg. 1999;134(4):428–33.

Part II
The Abdomen

Diverticulitis: Beyond the Basics

4

Patricia L. Roberts

Key Points

- The recommendations for surgery for uncomplicated and complicated diverticular disease have changed in the last decade.
- Triggering factors for an initial attack of diverticulitis and risk factors for subsequent attacks are not well defined.
- Recommendations for sigmoid resection after recurrent attacks of diverticulitis should take into account the severity and frequency of attacks.
- The optimal operation for purulent peritonitis is not defined, and the role of laparoscopic lavage is evolving.
- Minimally invasive techniques have an increasing role in the treatment of uncomplicated and complicated diverticular disease.

Introduction

Diverticulitis is the 5th most costly gastrointestinal disease in the United States and accounts for approximately 298,000 admissions per year, resulting in 1.5 million inpatient days per year [1]. In addition, over one-third of colectomies and colostomies are performed for a primary indication of diverticular disease [2]. Our understanding of the disease and recommendations for treatment has changed markedly in the last decade, and this chapter reviews some of the current controversies and guidelines for management of diverticulitis.

Indications for Surgery

Key Concept: The decision to recommend elective surgery should be individualized to each patient and should consider the risks of operative therapy, the overall medical condition of the patient, and other factors such as the effects on lifestyle (professional and personal) imposed by recurrent attacks, inability to exclude carcinoma, severity of the attacks, as well as chronic or lingering symptoms that may constitute "smoldering" disease.

Until recently, the recommendations for surgery were quite straightforward. A number of societies recommended elective resection after two attacks of uncomplicated diverticulitis and after one attack of complicated diverticulitis [3–6]. Diverticulitis in young patients (generally defined as under the age of 50 years old) was felt to have a more virulent course, and resection was recommended after one attack of diverticulitis [5]. A number of decision analyses, systematic reviews, and other publications have challenged our conventional wisdom about recommendations for surgery for diverticulitis and have suggested that it is safe to wait until the third or fourth attack of diverticulitis before considering resection [7, 8]. Furthermore, it has been suggested that there is no data to support resection after a second attack of diverticulitis and that it is essentially time to review of teaching for diverticulitis [9, 10]. The American Society of Colon and Rectal Surgeons' practice parameters have been modified stating that the "number of attacks is not an overriding factor" in recommending surgery [11]. The Association of Coloproctology of Great Britain and Ireland recommended that the "decision to perform an elective resection should be made on an individual basis after the assessment of the particular circumstances of the patient" [12].

Overall, it is widely quoted that of all individuals with diverticulosis, only approximately 10–25 % will develop

P.L. Roberts, MD
Division of Surgery, Department of Colon and Rectal Surgery, Lahey Clinic, Tufts University School of Medicine,
41 Mall Rd., Burlington, MA 01805, USA
e-mail: patricia.l.roberts@lahey.org

Electronic supplementary material The online version of this chapter (doi: 10.1007/978-1-4614-9022-7_4) contains supplementary material, which is available to authorized users. Videos can also be accessed at http://www.springerimages.com/videos/978-1-4614-9021-0.

S.R. Steele et al. (eds.), *Complexities in Colorectal Surgery*,
DOI 10.1007/978-1-4614-9022-7_4, © Springer Science+Business Media New York 2014

diverticulitis. After one attack of diverticulitis, approximately 30 % of patients will have another attack of diverticulitis. After a second attack of diverticulitis, over 50 % of patients will have another attack of diverticulitis. In reviewing the literature, there appears to be little scientific basis for these recommendations.

The indications for surgery for diverticulitis are broadly divided into indications for surgery for uncomplicated and for complicated diverticulitis, the latter being associated with fistula, abscess, obstruction, or perforation. Diverticular bleeding is associated with diverticulosis and not diverticulitis.

Indications for Surgery: Uncomplicated Diverticulitis

Key Concept: Performing an elective sigmoid colectomy after recovery from uncomplicated acute diverticulitis should be individualized based on several patient- and disease-specific variables, though no longer should focus on the number of attacks or the age of the patient alone.

In considering the recommendations for surgery for attacks of uncomplicated diverticulitis, one needs to consider the risk of subsequent attacks of diverticulitis, the severity of recurrent attacks of diverticulitis, the risk that one of the subsequent attacks will be associated with the need for emergency surgery and a colostomy, and the risk of developing complicated diverticulitis.

Risk of Subsequent Attacks of Diverticulitis After Recovery from Uncomplicated Diverticulitis

Although we frequently quote a risk of developing diverticulitis or 10–25 % in the presence of diverticulosis, there is no population-based data assessing this risk. After recovery from an attack of diverticulitis, we frequently quote a 30 % chance of developing another attack of diverticulitis. There is considerable variation based on the definition of an attack of diverticulitis and the length of time of follow-up. Parks, who followed 521 patients with 99.6 % follow-up, has been frequently cited and quoted as recommending resection after the second attack because of the morbidity of subsequent attacks [13]. Careful analysis of his patient cohorts shows that of the 317 patients treated medically, only 78 (24.6 %) had a subsequent attack, 12 (3.8 %) had a third attack, and only 5 (1.6 %) had a fourth attack [8]. In this series of patients, if surgery were performed after a second attack of diverticulitis, as has been conventionally recommended, 17 readmissions would have been prevented at a cost of 61 presumed unnecessary operations. Another cohort of 366 patients admitted over a 10-year period revealed a recurrence rate of 22 % [14]. In this group of patients, surgery performed after the second attack would have prevented 29 recurrent attacks by performing 57 operations, of which 28 would *not* have been necessary. The authors subsequently updated their series and stated that there was no data to support resection after the second attack of diverticulitis [15]. An additional study of 2,551 patients who were initially treated successfully medically for diverticulitis (with a mean follow-up of 9 years) resulted in only 13 % of patients with recurrent attacks and only 7 % of patients who required colectomy [16]. A conservative policy for managing acute sigmoid diverticulitis was found to be safe in the short and long term in a prospectively followed cohort of 232 patients from 1990 to 2004 [17]. Thus, several studies have suggested that the majority of patients who recover from an episode of diverticulitis have no further attacks. Evaluation of inpatients may be associated with a higher risk of diverticulitis, presumably since such patients, compared to outpatients, would be expected to have more severe diverticulitis. We have found a 36 % recurrence rate in 672 patients, the majority of whom were treated as inpatients [18]. The risk of recurrent diverticulitis appears to vary markedly, and patients with more severe disease most likely have a higher recurrence rate. Further investigations should focus on groups of patients at the highest risk for development of recurrent diverticulitis. The most recent practice parameters of the American Society of Colon and Rectal Surgeons suggest that the number of attacks of uncomplicated diverticulitis is "not necessarily the overriding factor in defining the appropriateness of surgery" [11].

Risk of Developing Complicated Diverticulitis After Recovery from an Attack of Uncomplicated Diverticulitis

The clinical course of diverticulitis appears to be determined by the first attack. Thus, patients who present with uncomplicated diverticulitis do not necessarily progress to have subsequent attacks of complicated diverticulitis [19, 20]. Chautems and colleagues found that 25 % of patients who recovered from uncomplicated diverticulitis had recurrent diverticulitis; none of these patients had subsequent attacks of complicated diverticulitis [19]. Eglinton and colleagues found a recurrence rate of 18.8 % overall in 502 patients but only a 5 % complicated recurrence rate [21]. In a study of 672 patients, we have found a 36 % rate of recurrent diverticulitis, but only 3.9 % of patients who had uncomplicated diverticulitis presented with a recurrent attack of complicated diverticulitis [18]. A study from the Mayo Clinic found that patients who had multiple attacks of diverticulitis had a lower risk of subsequently developing complicated diverticulitis [22].

Risk of Developing Free Perforation/Risk of Requiring Emergency Surgery and Stoma After Recovery from an Episode of Uncomplicated Diverticulitis

Patients have frequently been counseled to have an elective sigmoid resection after recovery from diverticulitis to avoid requiring an emergency resection and possible stoma with a subsequent attack. However, a number of studies have shown that the most severe attack of diverticulitis tends to be the first attack and an emergency stoma and/or urgent Hartmann resection is rarely required. A population-based study reviewed 25,058 patients with diverticulitis from 1987 to 2001. Emergency operation was required by 19.6 % of patients on the initial attack. Of those patients who recovered after an initial attack of diverticulitis without undergoing an operation, only 5.5 % required a subsequent emergency operation (7 % of young patients) [23]. Similarly, a systematic review of 85 papers showed that after recovery from one attack of diverticulitis, the risk of urgent Hartmann resection was 1 in 2,000 patient years of follow-up [9]. A subset of patients including those who are immunosuppressed and have chronic renal failure or collagen vascular disease are, however, 5 times more likely to have perforation after recovery from a single attack of diverticulitis, and therefore, resection should be considered in this subset of patients [24].

Smoldering Versus Discrete Attacks of Diverticulitis

Although there has been a great deal of focus on the number of attacks of diverticulitis a patient may have, patients who have a number of attacks in a short span of time more likely actually have smoldering diverticulitis, where a single attack of diverticulitis does not totally resolve with medical treatment. Elington and colleagues examined 502 patients with diverticulitis and noted a 35 % incidence of recurrent attacks of diverticulitis; the majority of recurrences occurred within 1 year of the index attack [21]. Boostrom and colleagues have suggested that the category of uncomplicated diverticulitis should be further refined into three categories including atypical, chronic/smoldering, and acute uncomplicated diverticulitis [25]. In a review of 907 consecutive patients who underwent sigmoid resection for diverticular disease, 82 % had acute resolving diverticulitis, 10 % had chronic or smoldering diverticulitis, and 8 % had atypical diverticulitis.

Severity of Disease and Indications for Surgery

The widespread use of CT scanning as the initial imaging modality in patients with suspected diverticulitis (in addition to history and physical examination) has allowed for a more thorough assessment and grading of the severity of disease. CT findings in diverticulitis include the presence of diverticula, pericolic inflammation, colonic wall thickening, and the presence of abscesses or fistula. The findings which correlate with severe disease include the presence of abscess, extraluminal air, and extraluminal contrast [26], while findings associated with mild disease include localized sigmoid wall thickening and inflammation of the pericolic fat. The presence of any of the severe findings on CT scan predicts a poor outcome and the likelihood of recurrent disease and the need for surgical intervention [19, 26]. In a study of 312 patients who underwent CT scanning for evaluation of acute left colonic diverticulitis, the finding of abscess and pockets of extraintestinal gas 5 mm in diameter or larger correlated with unfavorable outcome of nonoperative treatment [27].

We have noted that patients with a longer segment of disease (>5 cm) are more likely to have recurrent attacks of diverticulitis and have used this as one parameter in advising patients to have sigmoid resection after multiple attacks of diverticulitis [18]. We have also developed a scoring system for those patients who are less likely to resolve on conservative measures and require resection [28]. The scoring system is a point system that determines the risk of surgery within 90 days. The points are given for abscess >4 cm (2 points), pericolic free air (2 points), segment greater than 5 cm (2 points), pericolic abscess (5 points), and distant free air (7 points). Patients with 0–4 points have a less than 25 % risk of surgery in 90 days, patients with 5–9 points have a 25–50 % risk of surgery, and patients with >9 points have over a 50 % risk of requiring surgery with 90 days of presentation.

Other Considerations in Recommending Resection

Other patient-related factors are involved in the recommendations for surgery. I have found that patients who travel frequently particularly to areas with limited access to medical care often wish to have an elective laparoscopic sigmoid resection rather than risk another attack of diverticulitis in a remote area.

Risk of Recurrent Diverticulitis After Resection

Although patients may have persistent gastrointestinal symptoms following sigmoid resection for diverticulitis, the risk of recurrent diverticulitis is fairly small. Two studies have examined the risk of recurrent diverticulitis after sigmoid resection and have had similar conclusions. Benn and colleagues reviewed 501 patients who underwent sigmoid resection for diverticular disease at the Mayo Clinic. In 321 patients, the anastomosis was performed to the distal sigmoid colon, and 12.5 % of patients had recurrent diverticulitis, whereas 180 patients who had an anastomosis to the proximal rectum had only a 6.7 % incidence of recurrent diverticulitis [29]. The level of anastomosis was a significant risk factor for the development of recurrent diverticulitis. A subsequent study of 236 patients who were followed for 67 months had a similar conclusion that the level of anastomosis was the only predictor of recurrence, and patients with a colosigmoid versus a colorectal anastomosis had a four times higher rate of recurrence [30]. Of note, inflammation was found at the proximal resection margin in 30 patients (14 %), and there has been little focus on the proximal resection margin other than a recommendation to use "soft, pliable bowel." It has been suggested that limited resections have a greater tendency to develop recurrent symptoms, prompting the ACPGBI to suggest that the sigmoid flexure should be routinely mobilized in patients undergoing resection for diverticulitis [12, 30]. On the other hand, we have reviewed the NSQIP database and have noted a higher operative time and a higher rate of wound infection in patients who have undergone splenic flexure mobilization [31].

Young Patients and Diverticulitis

The prior recommendations of recommending resection after a single attack of diverticulitis in a young patient (defined as under the age of 50 years old) have also been reexamined. From a historical standpoint, diverticulitis in younger patients was previously felt to be more virulent, more likely to be associated with complications, and more likely to require resection [32, 33]. All series have consistently shown a striking male predominance in young patients with diverticulitis in contrast to older series, which have a slight female predominance [34]. Earlier series have shown a high rate of resection in this patient population [35]. Unfortunately, these series occurred prior to the use of CT scanning, and many patients were misdiagnosed and felt to have appendicitis. At laparotomy, diverticulitis was encountered and resection performed. Currently, there is no consensus on whether younger patients are at greater risk for complications or recurrent diverticulitis. Because of a longer life span, younger patients are certainly at greater risk for a higher cumulative recurrence. Yet, the clinical course of acute uncomplicated diverticulitis in young patients is similar to older patients, and therefore, resection is generally not required after the first attack of diverticulitis [36]. However, increasing numbers of young patients with diverticulitis are being seen, and a cohort of younger patients appears to have more severe disease. We recently reviewed 932 patients treated with diverticulitis who all underwent CT scan to establish a diagnosis. There were 243 patients (26 %) who were 50 years old or younger. Young patients were more likely to present with severe disease on CT scan (22 vs. 12 %) and more likely to have evidence of extraluminal air (22.4 % vs. 13.15, $P=0.014$) [37]. Further analysis from the state of California has shown that the increase in the number of sigmoid colectomies and hospitalizations for diverticulitis was due to an increasing number of young patients with the disease [38]. However, when simply considering uncomplicated disease, age, independent of other factors, should not be a major determinant in the decision for selecting elective operative versus nonoperative management following resolution of acute diverticulitis.

Laparoscopy and Indications for Surgery

Key Concept: *A laparoscopic approach is preferred over an open approach, when possible.*

Should the shift from open to laparoscopic colectomy change the indications for surgery for diverticulitis? The increase in the number of cholecystectomies performed since the adoption of laparoscopic techniques suggests that the indications for surgery in that setting may have changed. A laparoscopic resection that is associated with less pain, a quicker recovery, decreased length of stay, potentially less adhesions, and improved quality of life may be preferable to patients than having recurrent attacks of uncomplicated diverticulitis. While the safety and feasibility of laparoscopic colectomy are well established, as there is an increasing amount of data showing improved outcomes with a laparoscopic versus open technique, these results may make surgeons recommend resection more frequently, and the improved outcomes may make surgery a preferable option to patients. Data from the National Surgical Quality Improvement Project (NSQIP) has shown a lower incidence of surgical site infection (SSI) and sepsis after laparoscopic ($n=3{,}502$) versus open sigmoid resection ($n=3{,}468$) [39]. A randomized trial of open versus laparoscopic sigmoid resection showed a 30 % decrease in postoperative ileus and in length of hospital stay. The Sigma trial showed laparoscopic resection took longer but was associated with less blood loss, less pain, improved quality of life as measured by the SF 36, and less major complications [40]. All of these data combined suggest that changes in practice patterns may reflect more of an "end justifies the means" approach to recommending resection.

Nonoperative Management and Non-resective Treatment

Key Concept: *While the hallmark of diverticulitis therapy involves antibiotics, a select group of patients may benefit from supportive therapy alone including aminosalicylates and no requirement of antibiotic therapy.*

The mainstay of treatment for patients with acute diverticulitis has been antibiotics. Patients with severe symptoms and an inability to tolerate po are treated as inpatients with bowel rest, intravenous fluids, and broad-spectrum antibiotics. There are a number of antibiotic regimens used, though in each case the antimicrobial therapy is aimed at treating bowel flora. A systematic review has noted wide variation in the choice of antibiotics, duration of treatment, and the route of administration for diverticulitis [41]. Outpatients are treated with oral antibiotics and instructed on symptoms of worsening disease (worsening pain, high fever, inability to tolerate po fluids) in order to return for evaluation. Failure of outpatient therapy has been associated with the findings of fluid on CT scan and with female sex [42].

The role of antibiotics for uncomplicated disease has been questioned, and several studies have shown equivalent results without antibiotics. A retrospective review looked at 311 patients with diverticulitis treated as inpatients. There were 118 patients treated with antibiotics and 193 patients treated without antibiotics. Of those treated with antibiotics, 3 % required surgery, while 4 % of those who were initially treated without antibiotics were subsequently administered antibiotics. The rate of development of future events was the same in both groups [43].

The use of 5-ASA products has also been suggested for the treatment of diverticulitis, particularly in those patients who have inflammatory changes around the orifice of diverticulum—termed segmental colitis associated with diverticulitis or peridiverticulitis. Six randomized trials using 5-ASA products have enrolled a total of 818 patients [44]. The trials are heterogenous but have suggested improved outcomes for patients with uncomplicated diverticulitis treated with 5-ASA products. These medications may have a role in patients with smoldering diverticulitis who have residual inflammation but no obvious infectious focus.

My Recommendations for Elective Resection in the Setting of Uncomplicated Disease

Although the data supports a more conservative approach to uncomplicated diverticulitis, in my practice, I continue to see increasing numbers of patients at a young age with recurrent attacks of diverticulitis over a short span of time. While diverticulitis was an uncommon disease in patients under 50 years of age, close to 30 % of the patients who undergo sigmoid resection for diverticulitis at Lahey are under 50 years old. A number of these patients have severe diverticulitis with a long segment of disease and associated pericolic air or abscess. In such patients, especially with ongoing attacks of diverticulitis in a short time span, these bouts have a significant impact on quality of life and the ability to work and go about daily activities. Many otherwise fit patients prefer to undergo a single-stage laparoscopic sigmoid resection than face the prospect of recurrent attacks of diverticulitis. Conversely, it is important for patients to realize that the risk of free perforation and the need for an emergency stoma are quite low after recovery from an attack of uncomplicated diverticulitis; many patients are relieved to hear this and are subsequently less likely to proceed with surgery.

I take a more conservative approach for patients who have had multiple attacks of diagnosis at infrequent intervals. For instance, I generally do not recommend resection for a patient who presents with an attack of uncomplicated diverticulitis whose prior attacks were decades ago (and generally not confirmed by objective findings). I am also reluctant to recommend resection for patients with prominent irritable bowel symptoms and minimal inflammatory changes on CT scan.

Complicated Diverticulitis

Key Concept: Unlike uncomplicated disease, surgical resection of the colon is more common urgently or following recovery from an episode of complicated diverticulitis associated with abscess, fistula, obstruction, or perforation.

Complicated diverticulitis includes patients with associated abscess, fistula, obstruction, and perforation and is further subcategorized as acute complicated diverticulitis and chronic complicated diverticulitis. A large number of patients with complicated diverticulitis ultimately undergo sigmoid resection, and the goal of treating such patients is to optimize the patient condition and to ultimately convert an urgent or emergent process into an elective procedure, if possible. Complicated diverticulitis may be subdivided in chronic complicated diverticulitis (such as diverticular fistula and stricture) and acute complicated diverticulitis (such as abscess and perforation).

Diverticular Fistulas

Key Concept: Most diverticular fistulas require surgical resection of the involved colonic segment with interposition of healthy tissue between the anastomosis and adjacent organ to avoid fistula recurrence.

Fistulas associated with diverticulitis may occur to any adjacent organ and include colovesical, colovaginal, colouterine, coloenteric, and colocutaneous fistulas. Many patients with diverticular fistulas present with relatively few abdominal symptoms, presumably because the septic process has necessitated to an adjacent organ. It is common for such patients to present to another specialist initially such as urologists for a colovesical fistula with recurrent urinary tract infections or gynecologists for colovaginal fistulas with air or stool through the vagina.

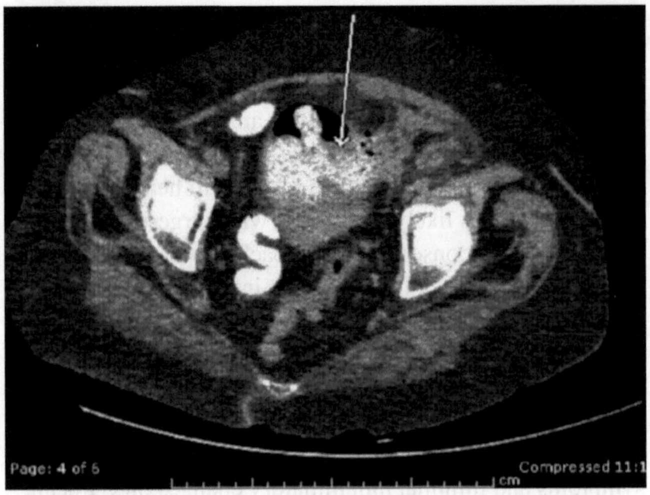

Fig. 4.1 Coronal image shows a colovaginal fistula (*arrow*) in a woman who has previously had a hysterectomy

The most common fistula is a colovesical fistula. Common signs and symptoms of colovesical fistula include pneumaturia, fecaluria, and polymicrobial urinary tract infections. Patients may not even have a history of an attack of diverticulitis. The fistula is suspected on clinical history, and the best objective test is a CT scan, where the presence of air in the bladder in the absence of prior instrumentation is indicative of a fistula. Cystoscopy and cystogram may also be utilized, demonstrating a cherry red spot or localized inflammation, but are less sensitive for detecting fistulas. Colonoscopy is useful to determine the etiology of the fistula and exclude a perforated colon cancer, which may present in a similar fashion. The majority of patients with a colovesical fistula may undergo a single-stage laparoscopic sigmoid resection where the fistula is pinched off, omentum (if available) is used to interpose between the bladder and the anastomosis, and a Foley catheter is left in place for drainage. I do not routinely use ureteral stents for chronic fistulas, but often use them for acute fistulas associated with an inflammatory phlegmon. In the latter case, stent placement facilitates identification of the ureters, which can be difficult and tedious with a significant phlegmon. My preference is to perform a cystogram prior to Foley catheter removal, but this study may be omitted in patients with a small fistula.

Colovaginal fistulas occur almost exclusively in patients who have undergone a prior hysterectomy. Presenting signs and symptoms include vaginal discharge and air per vagina. CT scan shows air in the vagina and may show the fistula tract (Fig. 4.1). Limited barium or Gastrografin studies can also be helpful in delineating the fistula tract. The majority of women undergo sigmoid resection, though elderly, debilitated patients with minimal symptoms may decline surgery. Once again, colonoscopy is useful to exclude a perforated colon cancer that may present with similar signs and symptoms. A similar operative approach is utilized to that of colovesical fistulas, pinching off the fistula and using omentum to interpose between the vagina and the anastomosis.

Colocutaneous fistulas rarely occur de novo and are generally associated with a leak from a prior anastomosis or with a prior percutaneous drain. In a large series of colocutaneous fistulas, leaving sigmoid colon distal to an anastomosis (i.e., not resecting the entire sigmoid colon) was a risk factor for the development of a fistula [45].

Diverticular Stricture

Key Concept: Symptomatic diverticular strictures should be resected; mucosal evaluation to exclude other diagnoses such as malignancy, IBD, or ischemia should be performed.

Strictures or partial obstruction may also occur in association with multiple attacks of diverticulitis. Many patients do not present with a complete large bowel obstruction but rather with progressive constipation and obstructive symptoms. Once again, endoscopic visualization of the mucosa is helpful to exclude other diagnoses such as colon cancer, a stricture resulting from ischemic colitis or from inflammatory bowel disease. Colonic stenting can be considered for patients with large bowel obstruction from diverticulitis with an aim toward stabilizing the patient, decompressing the bowel, and ultimately performing a single-stage sigmoid resection. Our success rate is poor for stenting diverticular disease and much better for stenting for obstructing cancer.

Diverticular Abscess

Key Concept: Image-guided percutaneous drainage is usually the most appropriate treatment for patients with large diverticular abscesses and does not necessarily require subsequent surgical resection.

Diverticulitis may be associated with an abscess in a small percent of cases. Approximately 10 % of patients hospitalized for diverticulitis at the Lahey Clinic have an associated abscess. Data from the Nationwide Inpatient Sample, the largest all-payer database of discharged patients in the country, shows that the incidence of diverticular abscess has increased from 5.9 % in 1995 to 9.6 % in 2005 [46]. The increasing numbers of patients with diverticular abscess may be related to the widespread and increasing usage of CT scanning for the initial diagnosis of diverticulitis. A number of staging systems have been utilized, but most commonly the Hinchey classification (with modifications thereof) is utilized. Stage 0 = mild clinical diverticulitis; stage 1a = confined pericolic inflammation/phlegmon; stage 1b = pericolic abscess; stage II = pelvic, intra-abdominal, or retrocolic abscess; stage III = purulent peritonitis; and stage IV = fecal peritonitis [47]. Many small abscesses (defined as those <4 cm) may be treated with antibiotics with successful

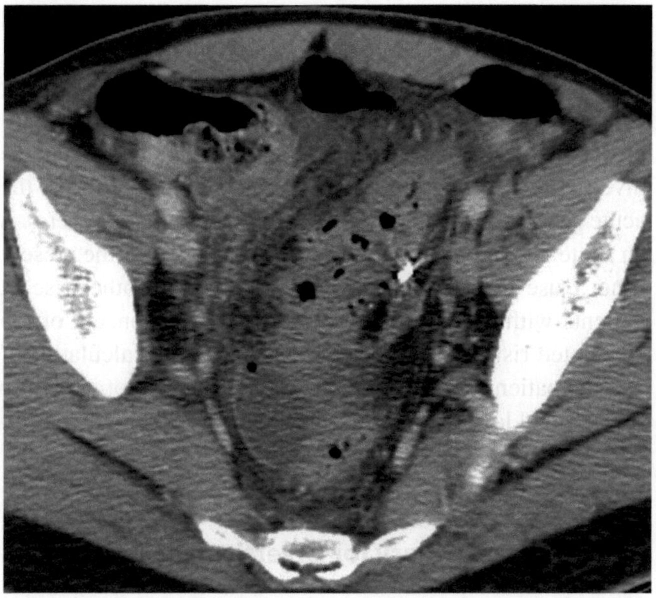

Fig. 4.2 Pelvic abscess (Hinchey II) with foci of free air

resolution and do not require percutaneous drainage or repetitive CT scans (especially if the patient is clinically responding with decrease in pain, fever, and leukocytosis) (Fig. 4.2) [48]. Combined series have shown that initial treatment with antibiotics (with or without percutaneous drainage) is successful in 30–56 % of patients [49]. Percutaneous drainage was initially used as a bridge to surgery; patients underwent drainage, sepsis resolved, and surgery was then performed electively [50]. Currently, percutaneous drainage is also used as definitive therapy, and some patients may not have further symptoms following successful resolution of the abscess. The decision to perform subsequent resection may therefore be made on an individual basis, recognizing patients with abscess have more severe diverticulitis and are more likely to require surgery. In rare cases, laparoscopic drainage may be performed if there is no radiologic window to drain an abscess (Video 4.1). The location of the abscess has been shown to help determine the clinical course, as those patients with more distant abscesses (i.e., Hinchey stage II) are more likely to require resection than patients with pericolic abscess. In a cohort of 465 patients, 73 patients (17 %) had an abscess, of which 45 patients had a pericolic abscess and 28 patients had a pelvic abscess. A larger number of patients with pelvic abscess (71 %) required surgery compared to those with pericolic abscess (51 %) [51].

Perforated Diverticulitis with Purulent or Feculent Peritonitis

Key Concept: The traditional therapy of mandatory colonic resection with or without diversion for perforated diverticulitis continues to evolve with the development of improved imaging, antibiotic success, endoscopic techniques, and implementation of laparoscopic lavage.

The optimal treatment for perforated diverticulitis and associated peritonitis continues to evolve. Options include Hartmann resection, sigmoid resection with primary anastomosis (in selected patients), sigmoid resection and primary anastomosis with proximal diversion, on-table lavage with primary anastomosis, and laparoscopic lavage without resection. Hartmann resection remains one of the most common operations performed for perforated diverticulitis but has a number of drawbacks. Approximately 30 % of patients never undergo reversal of the stoma [52, 53]. In addition, the operation has considerable morbidity and a reported mortality of up to 18.8 % [54]. Over the years, a number of other options have been advocated. Fibrin glue with suture repair and omental patching of the perforation has been reported [55]. Two studies (both underpowered) looked at the role of defunctioning the diseased segment with suture of the perforation and proximal diversion versus resection and had different conclusions [56, 57]. The role of on-table lavage in approaching patients with colonic emergencies has largely fallen out of favor since the need for bowel preparation has been challenged by a number of reviews [58]. A systematic review of 569 cases in 50 studies suggested that primary anastomosis with or without diversion was "safe in certain patients with peritonitis" but noted a mortality of 9.9 % and an anastomotic leak rate of 13.9 % [54].

In approaching the patient with perforated diverticulitis, it is important to distinguish between patients who have evidence of peritonitis on physical examination and those patients who have CT findings consistent with perforation but no objective findings of toxicity. While many surgeons trained in the 1970s or 1980s were taught that the finding of free air on a chest x-ray or KUB was an absolute indication for surgery, the findings of free air on CT imaging do not necessarily translate into similar recommendations. Dharmarajan and coworkers evaluated CT findings of perforated diverticulitis and devised a grading system based on the amount and location of abnormal air, which may assist with clinical decision-making [59]. While a grading system is a useful adjunct, I personally rely more heavily on the clinical status of the patient and base my initial strategy on the physical examination findings more than the CT findings alone.

There has recently been a renewed interest in the role of laparoscopic lavage without resection for patients with perforated diverticulitis and associated purulent peritonitis. In 1996, O'Sullivan and colleagues reported 8 patients with perforated diverticulitis and purulent peritonitis who underwent a laparoscopic lavage [60]. No resection of the sigmoid colon was performed, and patients were subsequently treated with intravenous antibiotics. At a follow-up of 12–48 months, no patient required subsequent resection, and no patient required an emergent colostomy. Based on these initial encouraging results, a prospective multi-institutional trial was subsequently performed of 100 patients with perforated diverticulitis who underwent laparoscopic lavage [61]. The median age was 62.5 years, and patients were followed for 36 months. The procedure was performed with an umbilical, suprapubic, and right lower quadrant ports, and patients were lavaged with 4 l of fluid or lavaged until the returns were clear. Eight out of the 100 patients were noted to have fecal peritonitis and were converted to an open procedure and underwent resection and stoma. Of the 92 patients who were managed with laparoscopic lavage, no patient required subsequent resection for diverticulitis at a median follow-up of 36 months. There was an overall 4 % morbidity and 3 % mortality rate for the cohort. Two patients developed a pelvic abscess and required drainage, while 2 patients presented with a subsequent attack of diverticulitis. The authors concluded that laparoscopic lavage was a reasonable alternative with low mortality and low morbidity, particularly when compared with Hartmann resection. Furthermore, they suggested that elective resection, even in this group of patients who presented with perforation, was probably unnecessary and that readmission was uncommon.

Currently, the role of laparoscopic lavage continues to evolve in the treatment of patients with perforated diverticulitis and associated purulent peritonitis. A number of additional small series have been reported, including a recent review article evaluating 12 nonrandomized studies encompassing 301 patients with a mean age of 57 years [62]. Although the majority of patients in these combined series had Hinchey III classification (i.e., purulent peritonitis), 25 % of patients had Hinchey II disease. In the Myers series, 25 % of patients also had Hinchey II disease, suggesting that some of these patients could potentially have been treated with bowel rest and antibiotics alone, along with subsequent percutaneous drainage for those patients developing abscesses [61]. In this combined series, the conversion rate was 4.9 %, while the mean complication rate was 18.9 % and mortality was 0.25 %. Subsequent resection was performed in 51 % of patients, and the majority of the resections were laparoscopic. In the future, we need to identify those patients who may optimally be treated by lavage. Further classification of the degree of peritonitis either by the Mannheim peritonitis index or the peritonitis severity score may help to further define the optimal candidate for lavage. Similarly, the need for subsequent resection has not been defined. In the Afshar series, the majority of patients who underwent elective resection did so because of surgeon preference [62]. It goes without saying that colonoscopic evaluation of the colon is important in patients to exclude a diagnosis of perforated colon cancer.

A number of guidelines have been refined to include a statement on lavage. The European Association for Endoscopic Surgery consensus statement of laparoscopy for abdominal emergencies states that "colon resection remains the gold standard, but laparoscopic lavage and drainage may be considered in some selected patients" [16]. The Association of Coloproctology of Great Britain and Ireland states that "laparoscopic lavage may play a role in some patients with acute diverticulitis. Whilst this is an alternative to resection in the acute setting for some patients, it is not certain whether it is an acute alternative to delayed resection" [12]. At the present time, I use laparoscopic lavage selectively in otherwise fit patients with perforated diverticulitis. In the concept of the calculated risk, we as the surgeons "make the calculations," and the patients "incur the potential risk." I do not generally recommend lavage to unstable patients or those with a number of other associated comorbidities.

Reoperative Surgery for Diverticular Disease

Key Concept: Reoperative surgery entails unique technical and decision-making challenges that need to be considered both prior to and at the time of surgery to optimize outcomes.

Reoperation for complicated diverticular disease occurs for two main reasons: as a planned procedure to restore intestinal continuity after resection, stoma, and Hartmann closure of the rectum and as an unplanned procedure to treat complications or unanticipated events after initial resection and primary anastomosis. The latter occurrence is mainly due to anastomotic leakage but may occur from fistula, abscess, or stricture at the anastomosis. This section discusses considerations prior to reoperative surgery including anatomy, timing of reoperation, anatomic considerations, preoperative preparation, conduct of the operation, and outcome.

Reoperative Surgery After Hartmann Resection

The Hartmann resection was first described by Henri Hartmann for the treatment of rectal cancer in which he described two patients presenting with obstruction in whom he resected the tumor and closed the "superior part of the rectum and left it in the peritoneum without disturbing the pelvic floor" [63]. The procedure quickly became the procedure of choice for the majority of patients who underwent emergency surgery for perforated diverticulitis in the second half of the twentieth century, replacing the three-stage procedure of initial colostomy, subsequent resection, and finally colostomy takedown that was advocated by Lockhart-Mummery [64, 65]. Of note, Hartmann believed that reversal of the Hartmann procedure should not be attempted. Currently, Hartmann takedown still has significant morbidity and mortality and a relatively low reversal rate. Unfortunately, the risk of needing to return to the operating room for a repeat stoma remains high.

Timing

After Hartmann resection for perforated diverticulitis, most patients are eager to proceed as soon as possible with reversal of the colostomy. In contrast to patients who may be chronically ill with inflammatory bowel disease for years prior to resection, these patients often had never been ill before and had never anticipated leaving the hospital with a stoma after treatment for diverticulitis. Surgery for Hartmann reversal may be undertaken early (<3 months from initial surgery) or late (>3 months from initial surgery). There are advocates of each approach [66–70]. Proceeding with Hartmann takedown close to the time of initial surgery has several disadvantages, predominantly due to adhesions and the acute inflammatory response after initial surgery which may lead to a difficult dissection, potential enterotomies, and difficulty with identification of the Hartmann stump. While waiting for at least 3 months will presumably allow the patient sufficient time to heal and facilitate identification of the Hartmann stump, waiting longer may make identification of the stump more difficult secondary to fibrosis. The two approaches (waiting less than 3 months vs. greater than 3 months) have not been assessed in a randomized trial. My approach has been to wait for 3 months prior to Hartmann takedown. Waiting for this time period ideally reduces the difficulty and potential complications from adhesions.

Preoperative Preparation

General preoperative assessment of the patient should routinely be performed. Nutritional status is optimized. Cardiopulmonary disease is identified and evaluated. Reoperative pelvic surgery is associated with a high risk of thromboembolic complications, and patients are administered appropriate prophylaxis. Although increasing evidence suggests that mechanical bowel preparation is not necessary, I believe that it is preferable in reoperative surgery to minimize spillage in case the bowel is entered. Preoperative intravenous antibiotics are administered, although there is little evidence to support additional dosing.

Preoperative Imaging

For patients >50 years old who have not had prior colonic evaluation, a colonoscopy or barium enema should be performed. Prior to planning Hartmann takedown, my preference is to perform a barium enema through the stoma and a Gastrografin enema through the rectum. The Gastrografin enema is particularly useful as it gives an assessment of the length and configuration of the rectal segment and gives an assessment of any residual sigmoid colon and/or diverticula (Fig. 4.3). Many patients have undergone the initial resection by another surgeon; at times, because of intraoperative factors, a substantial amount of sigmoid colon is left in place. The road map of the specific anatomy is better determined by a Gastrografin study than by a flexible sigmoidoscopy, although both can be performed. These procedures are also helpful to evacuate retained fecal residue. Scybala retained in the rectum from the original Hartmann resection should be evacuated at this time or with distal rectal washout at the time of surgery to facilitate placement of a sizer and subsequently the EEA stapler. Even with a washout at the time of colostomy takedown, this may be difficult to accomplish.

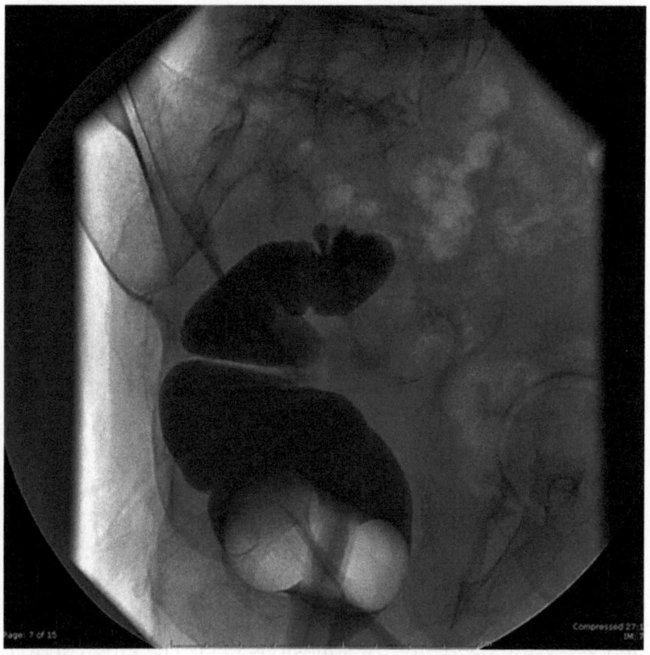

Fig. 4.3 Gastrografin enema shows residual sigmoid colon and diverticula

Intraoperative Considerations

Patient Positioning

Anticipate a long procedure and pad the patient's bony prominences accordingly. The patient may be placed in lithotomy position in Lloyd Davies, Allen, or Yellowfin stirrups. Care should be taken to avoid pressure on the peroneal nerves and the hips. Overall, my preferred position is aimed to have symmetric hip extension, knee flexion, and thigh abduction. Extreme hip extension beyond 60° can occasionally lead to femoral nerve palsies if a self-retaining retractor is positioned against the extended extremity. The perineum should be hanging slightly over the table to ensure easy passage of the EEA stapler. Rectal washout can be performed and a mushroom catheter left in the rectum if desired to facilitate identification of the Hartmann pouch. A proctoscope and/or sizer may also be used intraoperatively to identify the pouch. The vagina should also be included in the prep. Alternatively, my preference is to position the patient supine on a split leg table with the legs abducted. The split leg table avoids potential difficulties with long-standing lithotomy position including nerve injuries and compartment syndrome. Once again, care must be taken to ensure that the patient is positioned far enough down on the table that access to the anus (to pass the EEA stapler) can be achieved. A beanbag with the arms tucked at the sides can be helpful to ensure the patient does not slip cephalad on the table, especially when in steep Trendelenburg position.

Approach to the Procedure

The procedure may be undertaken by a laparoscopic or open approach. Adhesions encountered from previous surgery or prior infection may make a laparoscopic approach impossible. The extent and degree of adhesions may be difficult to predict; on occasion much less severe adhesions are encountered than anticipated, and the procedure progresses quite smoothly. Alternatively, with extensive adhesions, bowel injury may occur when attempting to enter the peritoneal cavity. A reasonable approach is the use of a "peek port" which entails entering the abdomen through a small incision and assessing the degree of adhesions [71]. The laparoscopic equipment is not opened until the feasibility of a laparoscopic hand-assisted approach is determined. Alternatively, a port can also be placed away from the site of the previous surgery to assess the degree of adhesions and the feasibility of a straight laparoscopic approach.

Exposure and Lighting

The importance of having adequate exposure and lighting cannot be overestimated with reoperative surgery. If an open approach is used, the incision should extend to the symphysis pubis. Cephalad extension of the midline incision may be needed if splenic flexure mobilization is needed. Operating between the patient's legs provides optimal visualization of the splenic flexure as does rotation of the table to a left-side-up position.

Adequate OR lighting, a headlight, and/or lighted pelvic retractors are helpful. A self-retaining retractor with bladder blade is also used. Straight blade (Wylie renal vein or St. Mark's) and curved (Deaver) retractors are available, with the former being more helpful for deep pelvic dissection, which is on occasion necessary to free up the Hartmann stump. Care must be taken to avoid placing these retractors on the drapes and causing a fire.

Initial Dissection

The initial dissection is focused on lysing all small bowel adhesions in the pelvis to be able to identify the Hartmann pouch. Ultimately, in the majority of cases, all small bowel adhesions from the ligament of Treitz to the ileocecal valve are lysed to be able to mobilize the colostomy and bring the proximal colon down to the pelvis without tension. The pelvic dissection associated with a prior Hartmann resection may be challenging secondary to dense adhesions and the inability to distinguish a plane suitable for dissection. It is advisable to lyse the filmy small bowel adhesions first and then attack the more difficult adhesions. With few exceptions, there are small bowel and/or omental adhesions to the top of the Hartmann pouch. Dense adhesions often occur to the top of the Hartmann pouch, and encountering staple material is an indication of proximity to this structure. If extremely dense adhesions are encountered, hydrodissection or infiltration of the fused area with saline with a small-gauge needle may be helpful [72]. The appendix can also be drawn down into the pelvis toward the Hartmann and may occasionally lead the surgeon to believe he or she has encountered the right ureter. The left ovary and tube, in particular, may be fused with the top of the Hartmann pouch. Bleeding from the pelvic wall may often occur from entering the fallopian tubes or a branch of the ovarian vessels.

The ureters should be identified, and the surgeon should be aware that they may be in an unanticipated position, particularly drawn in more medially, after prior surgery. Ureteral stents may be used in selected cases with prior severe pelvic sepsis or unclear anatomy. Stents do not prevent ureteral injury but facilitate the recognition of such injury. I selectively use stents in patients with hydronephrosis or a large amount of retroperitoneal inflammation. The vagina may be adherent to the rectum and dissection facilitated by placing a finger in the vagina to identify the proper planes.

The colostomy is mobilized by incising the mucocutaneous junction and trying to preserve all the mesenteric attachments. Injection with saline or local anesthetic around the mucocutaneous junction circumferentially may facilitate dissection. The stoma is resected and fresh bowel used for the intended anastomosis. Once the stoma is mobilized, the surgeon can generally assess whether there is adequate length for a tension-free anastomosis. Additional length is facilitated by a number of maneuvers including division of the lateral colonic attachments, takedown of the splenic flexure, division of the inferior mesenteric artery at the takeoff of the aorta, and division of the inferior mesenteric vein at the inferior border of the pancreas. Alternatively, further length can be achieved by mobilizing the rectum further distally and essentially bringing the Hartmann pouch up to the proximal bowel. Once complete mobilization of the proximal colon is performed and adhesiolysis is completed, the small bowel and colon can be packed into the upper abdomen.

Identification and Mobilization of the Hartmann Pouch

Once the small bowel is mobilized, the top of the Hartmann pouch can be identified. Some surgeons mark the top of the pouch with long suture material to facilitate identification. I have not found this to be helpful and have found that insertion of a proctoscope or flexible sigmoidoscope facilitates identification of the Hartmann pouch. The staple line of the Hartmann is identified, and the length of the pouch is usually longer than anticipated, even if it is located below the pelvic brim. If the staple line is adherent to the presacral fascia, it is generally safe to commence the dissection in the posterior midline, thus avoiding the ureters and the iliac vessels. It is not uncommon for the superior rectal artery to be left intact, and placing a Babcock clamp on the end of the Hartmann pouch and applying cephalad traction facilitate identification of the mesentery and straightening of the rectum. My practice is to mobilize and dissect out the Hartmann pouch at least to the mid- to proximal rectum. This is generally necessary to "straighten out the rectum," which often times has a concertina-like configuration following Hartmann resection. If this is not done, it is often difficult to guide the EEA stapler per anum to the top of the Hartmann pouch. Once the Hartmann pouch is mobilized, a small sizer is placed per rectum to ensure that this passes easily to the area of the intended anastomosis. In those patients who have had significant sepsis or in those who have had a long-standing Hartmann pouch, further mobilization may be needed. We have found that in women further dissection is often needed in the anterior cul-de-sac as the mid-rectum tends to angulate and adhere to the uterus. Despite further mobilization, some patients may still have a fairly fibrotic pelvis (in which the rectum is intrinsically normal but the surrounding tissues are fibrotic enough that it is impossible to pass a sizer). In this case, an EEA-stapled anastomosis may not be feasible and a handsewn anastomosis preferable. The top of the intended site of anastomosis is then re-resected and the integrity of the rectum tested by filling the pelvis with saline and insufflating the Hartmann pouch.

Performing the Anastomosis

I prefer using the EEA stapler to perform anastomosis after Hartmann resection. The anvil is placed in the proximal bowel. A handsewn purse string is placed, or a purse-string device may be used. A sizer is used to guide through the rectum to the top of the re-resected Hartmann pouch. Occasionally, it is difficult to introduce the stapler into the anus, and Khoury and Opelka have reported placement of a Faensler or Chelsea-Eaton anoscope with gradual dilatation of the sphincter and placement of the stapler shaft through the anoscope [73]. The EEA stapler is guided through with the trocar exiting at the top of the Hartmann pouch, the anvil is snugged up and secured, and the stapler is fired. The instrument is generally removed easily, and the tissue rings are inspected for thickness and integrity. The anastomosis is then tested by occluding the bowel proximally and introducing air through a proctoscope or a flexible sigmoidoscope [74].

Alternatives

There is no one single technique to perform an anastomosis after Hartmann takedown, and some ingenuity and employing other techniques may be necessary. The stapler may not pass up to the top of the rectum because of fibrosis and contraction, particularly if the patient has been diverted for many years. In this case, there are several alternatives. One option is to perform a handsewn anastomosis. Another option is to introduce the stapler and bring the trocar through the anterior rectal wall, thus performing an end of colon to side of rectum anastomosis [73]. Further options include employing a double purse-string technique in which a purse string is placed in the proximal colon and the distal end (rectum). The stapler is still introduced through the anus. A final technique employs a single purse string in the rectum and placing the stapler through the side of the proximal colon and completing the anastomosis by transecting the end of the colon with a TA stapler.

Abdominal Wall Closure

Following completion of the anastomosis, the abdomen is irrigated and the incision closed. A mass closure technique is superior to layered closure. A continuous abdominal wall closure is associated with a lower risk of abdominal wound dehiscence. Furthermore, a meta-analysis of six randomized controlled trials found that the risk of incisional hernia formation was significantly less with a continuous compared with an interrupted closure (regardless of the suture type used) [75]. The use of resorbable versus non-resorbable sutures results in no difference in dehiscence rates, but higher rates of persistent sinus formation and chronic wound problems occurred with non-resorbable sutures. Optimal primary wound closure is with a mass closure continuous technique with resorbable sutures placed at an interval of 1 cm apart and 1 cm back on the fascia [76]. Laparoscopic techniques minimize incision length and wound trauma and may be associated with less wound complications.

Reoperation for Sepsis and Anastomotic Complications After Hartmann Takedown

Key Concept: *Identification of anastomotic leak through testing is an integral part of left-sided anastomosis. For those experiencing a leak requiring operative intervention, deciding between proximal diversion alone and resection and diversion depends on the patient's clinical manifestations and the intraoperative findings.*

Anastomotic leak is among the most serious potential complications after Hartmann takedown (Fig. 4.4). The lack of a standardized definition precludes comparison among units and even a precise incidence of this complication. We have used the United Kingdom (UK) working party definition of leakage of gastrointestinal contents or contrast from a surgically constructed anastomosis [77]. In our unit, we have reviewed 998 left-sided colorectal anastomoses and have noted a clinical leak rate of 4.8 % [74]. Air leak testing was performed intraoperatively in 825 left colon anastomoses.

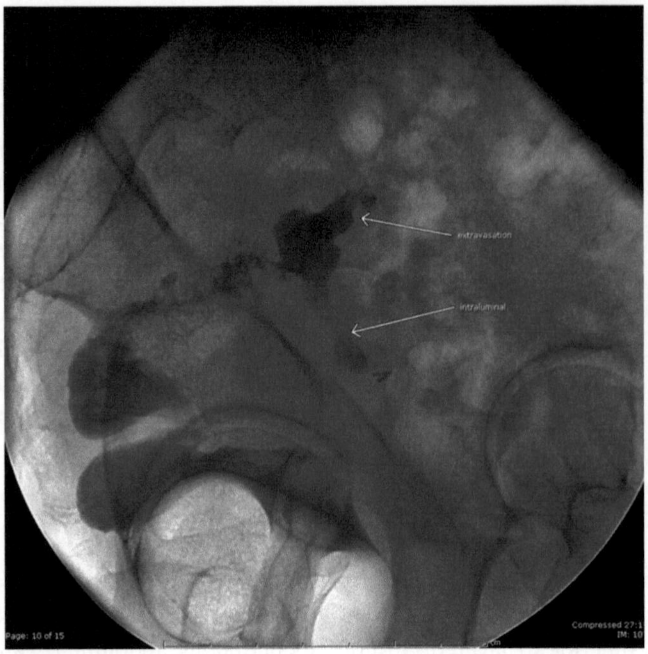

Fig. 4.4 Gastrografin enema shows a leak at the top of the Hartmann pouch with extravasation (*arrow*) and intraluminal contrast (*arrow*) into small bowel

A clinical leak was noted in 7.7 % of anastomosis with a positive air leak test compared with 3.8 % of anastomosis with a negative air leak test and 8.1 % of all untested anastomoses ($P<0.3$). The data suggest that air leak testing should be performed in all such anastomosis to allow the surgeon to detect and repair a leak at the time of initial procedure.

Management of anastomotic leak depends on the clinical manifestations of the leak and the overall condition of the patient. Anastomotic dehiscence may manifest as peritonitis, a colocutaneous fistula, an associated abscess, or even be relatively asymptomatic. For those patients with generalized peritonitis, urgent exploration is performed after fluid resuscitation and intravenous antibiotics. Stoma site marking is ideally done preoperatively. Placement in lithotomy position or on a split leg table is helpful in case sigmoidoscopy is needed. The two main intraoperative considerations are to leave the anastomosis in place and to divert proximally or to resect the anastomosis and perform a colostomy. In patients with total anastomotic dehiscence, a large defect, or concerns about the viability of the anastomosis, resection of the anastomosis is advisable. The distal end is stapled or handsewn, and the proximal colon brought out as a colostomy. Unfortunately, a substantial number of these patients will never undergo colostomy closure.

In selected cases of a small defect and a relatively stable patient, the anastomosis may be left in place and diverted proximally with either a colostomy or ileostomy. A recent meta-analysis suggested that an ileostomy was associated with less stoma-related complications and a lower incidence of abdominal wall hernias [78]. A concern of such an approach is leaving a large column of stool, which may then leak through the anastomosis resulting in ongoing pelvic sepsis. If a diverting ileostomy is performed, lavaging the distal bowel or endoscopically evacuating the distal bowel should be considered. An ileostomy may be associated with a high incidence of dehydration and the need for readmission, especially in elderly patients [79].

Chronic sepsis or anastomotic leak may also manifest as a colocutaneous fistula. A major risk factor for the development of a colocutaneous fistula is the anastomosis to the distal sigmoid colon and not the proximal rectum [45]. While selected cases may heal with good nutritional support and a tincture of time, re-resection of the anastomosis is needed for persistent fistulas.

Reoperation for Recurrent Diverticulitis

Key Concept: Re-resection of the prior anastomosis with special attention to the distal and proximal margins, along with ensuring a tension-free anastomosis, is paramount to improving outcomes for reoperative diverticular disease.

Recurrent diverticulitis following sigmoid resection is uncommon. In the patient presenting with abdominal pain following resection for diverticulitis, a thorough investigation should be undertaken to exclude other causes of abdominal pain including inflammatory bowel disease, irritable bowel syndrome, gynecologic disease, adhesive disease, and infectious complications from the initial resection. Recurrent diverticulitis should also be distinguished from poorly characterized pain following resection. A recent study of 325 patients who underwent either laparoscopic or open sigmoid resection for diverticulitis noted that 20 % of patients had ongoing functional symptoms [80]. Munson and colleagues found that 27.2 % of patients following resection for diverticular disease continued to have pain [81]. The most common risk factor associated with recurrent diverticulitis is failure to perform a colorectal anastomosis and performing a colocolic anastomosis with retained distal sigmoid colon as the proximal section margin (Fig. 4.3). Although diverticulitis may only involve a portion of the sigmoid colon, it is important to resect the sigmoid colon and perform resection to the proximal rectum. The rectum is identified at the level at which the tenia fan out, which is usually at the sacral promontory. In the presence of prior inflammation, this spot may not be readily apparent, in which case the level of the bowel just below the sacral promontory is a reasonable landmark. The proximal resection margin is less well established. While it is not necessary to resect all proximal diverticula, the anastomosis should be performed in soft pliable bowel. In the evaluation of the patient with recurrent diverticulitis, it is helpful to obtain prior records, including the pathology report and operative note, to ensure that the diagnosis was indeed diverticulitis and to review specific operative details.

Ureteral stents may be considered especially if the original operation was difficult, associated with unclear anatomy, or associated with postoperative pelvic sepsis or anastomotic complications. The patient should be prepared for the possibility of a temporary stoma, especially if the anastomosis is low. Adequate mobilization of the colon is key, and splenic flexure mobilization is necessary. If these various maneuvers do not result in sufficient mobility and allow a tension-free anastomosis, the middle colic vessels on occasion require division with blood supply of the residual colon based on the right and/or ileocolic vessels. Additional approaches such as bringing the right colon through a window in the mesentery or resecting further and bringing the hepatic flexure down to the rectum may be needed [82, 83].

The prior anastomosis may also be densely adherent to the presacral fascia. The presacral fascia is a condensation of the parietal endopelvic fascia, and it is important to get into the right plane; otherwise, massive pelvic bleeding may occur from the avalvular presacral veins which communicate with the basivertebral veins [84]. The sympathetic pelvic nerves run caudad and lateral over the presacral fascia to join the pelvic plexus laterally and are at risk for damage if the plane is not developed and exposed correctly. Depending on the difficulty of the pelvic dissection and the level of the anastomosis, fecal diversion may be necessary.

Reoperative surgery, in general, is challenging, and reoperative surgery for diverticulitis, specifically, is no exception. No one approach can be employed to guarantee success, and the surgeon must have a number of approaches and techniques in his or her armamentarium to ensure optimal patient outcome.

Conclusion

Our understanding and treatment of diverticulitis continue to evolve. Recent trends have shown increased use of laparoscopic techniques both for elective and emergency surgeries and a trend to primary anastomosis for both elective and urgent operations [85]. Although the literature supports a more conservative approach to patients with uncomplicated diverticulitis, there has been a dramatic increase in the frequency of elective surgical resection for diverticulitis by 38 %. The increase in elective surgical resection is nine times greater than the increase in urgent surgical resection, suggesting that clinical practice does not mirror the current recommendations.

Future investigations should focus on the identifying risk factors for recurrent diverticulitis and optimally identify those patients who require early surgical intervention. Ultimately increased understanding of this common disease will help physicians and surgeons in the prevention and treatment of diverticulitis.

Summary Pearls

Diverticulitis is one of the most common gastrointestinal diseases. The trend over the last decade has been toward a greater understanding of the disease that will ultimately result in a more "personalized" approach to the patient. I believe that we will ultimately be able to delineate the natural history of diverticular disease and predict the clinical course of disease for an individual patient. In the meantime, you should have a thorough understanding of all the factors involved when deciding on a management strategy to ensure optimal outcomes.

References

1. Available at http://hcup.ahrq.gov. Accessed 15 Dec 2012.
2. Salem L, Anaya DA, Flum DR. Temporal changes in the management of diverticulitis. J Surg Res. 2004;124(2):318–23.
3. Stollman NH, Raskin JB. Diagnosis and management of diverticular disease of the colon in adults. Ad hoc practice parameters committee of the American College of Gastroenterology. Am J Gastroenterol. 1999;94:3110–21.
4. Wong WD, Wexner SD, Lowry A, et al. Practice parameters for the treatment of sigmoid diverticulitis–supporting documentation. The Standards Task Force. The American Society of Colon and Rectal Surgeons. Dis Colon Rectum. 2000;43:290–7.
5. Surgical treatment of diverticulitis. Patient care committee of the Society for Surgery of the Alimentary Tract (SSAT). J Gastrointestinal Surg. 1999;3:212–13.
6. Kohler L, Sauerland L, Neugebauer E. Diagnosis and treatment of diverticular disease: results of a consensus development conference. The Scientific Committee of the European Association for Endoscopic Surgery. Surg Endosc. 1999;13:430–6.
7. Salem L, Veenstra D, Sullivan SD, et al. the timing of elective colectomy in diverticulitis: a decision analysis. J Am Coll Surg. 2004; 199:904–12.
8. Richards FJ, Hammitt JK. Timing of prophylactic surgery in prevention of diverticulitis recurrence: a cost effectiveness analysis. Dig Dis Sci. 2002;57(9):1903–8.
9. Janes S, Meagher A, Frizelle FA. Elective surgery after acute diverticulitis. Br J Surg. 2005;92(2):133–42.
10. Chapman J, Davies M, Wolff B, et al. Complicated diverticulitis: is it time to rethink the rules? Ann Surg. 2005;242:576–81; discussion 581–3.
11. Rafferty J, Shellito P, Hyman NH, Buie WD, Standards committee of American Society of Colon and Rectal Surgeons. Practice parameters for sigmoid diverticulitis. Dis Colon Rectum. 2006; 49(7):939–44.
12. Fozard JB, Armitage NC, Schofield JB, Jones OM, Association of Coloproctology of Great Britain and Ireland. ACPGBI position statement on elective resection for diverticulitis. Colorectal Dis. 2011;13 Suppl 3:1–11.
13. Parks TG. Natural history of diverticular disease of the colon: a review of 521 cases. BMJ. 1969;4:639–45.
14. Makela J, Vuolio S, Kiviniemi H, et al. Natural history of diverticular disease; when to operate? Dis Colon Rectum. 1998;41:1523–8.
15. Makela JT, Kiviniemi HO, Laitinen ST. Spectrum of disease and outcome among patients with acute diverticulitis. Dig Surg. 2010;27(3):190–6.
16. Broderick-Villa G, Burchette FJ, Collin JC, Abbas MA, et al. Hospitalization for acute diverticulitis does not mandate routine elective colectomy. Arch Surg. 2005;140:576–81.

17. Shaikh S, Kurkowski ZH. Outcome of a conservative policy for managing acute sigmoid diverticulitis. Br J Surg. 2007;94:876–9.
18. Hall JF, Roberts PL, Ricciardi R, Read T, Scheirey C, Wald C, et al. Long-term follow-up after an initial episode of diverticulitis: what are the predictors of recurrence? Dis Colon Rectum. 2011;54(3):283–8.
19. Chautems RC, Ambrosetti P, Ludwig A, et al. Long term follow-up after the first acute episode of sigmoid diverticulitis; is surgery mandatory? A prospective study of 118 patients. Dis Colon Rectum. 2002;49:939–44.
20. Haglund U, Hellberg R, Johnson C, et al. Complicated diverticular disease of the sigmoid colon. An Analysis of short and long term outcome in 293 patients. Ann Chir Gynaecol. 1970;68:41–6.
21. Eglinton T, Nguyen T, Raniga S, Dixon L, Dobbs B, Frizelle FA. Patterns of recurrence in patients with acute diverticulitis. Br J Surg. 2010;97(6):952–7.
22. Chapman JR, Dozois EJ, Wolff BG, Gullerud RE, Larson DR. Diverticulitis; a progressive disease? Do multiple recurrences predict less favorable outcomes? Ann Surg. 2006;243(6):876–80; discussion 880–3.
23. Anaya DA, Flum DR. Risk of emergency colectomy and colostomy in patients with diverticular disease. Arch Surg. 2005;140(7):681–5.
24. Klarenbeek BR, Samuels M, van der Wal MA, van der Peet DL, Meijerink WF, Cuesta MA. Indications for elective sigmoid resection in diverticular disease. Ann Surg. 2010;251(4):670–4.
25. Boostrom SY, Wolff BG, Cima RR, Merchea A, Dozois EJ, Larson DW. Uncomplicated diverticulitis, more complicated than we thought. J Gastrointest Surg. 2012;16:1744–9.
26. Ambrosetti P, Grossholz M, Becker C, Terrier F, Morel P. Computed tomography in acute left colonic diverticulitis. Br J Surg. 1997;84:532–4.
27. Poletti PA, Platon A, Rutschmann O, Kinkel K, Nyikus V, Ghiorghui S, Morel P, et al. Acute left colonic diverticulitis; can CT findings be used to predict recurrence? Am J Roentgenol. 2004;182(5):1159065.
28. Hall JF, Roberts PL, Ricciardi R, Read TE, Marcello PW, Schoetz DJ. The Lahey Score; a simple score to predict the need for early surgical intervention for diverticulitis. In: Presented at the American College of Surgeons, 2012.
29. Benn PL, Wolff BG, Ilstrup DM. Level of anastomosis and recurrent colonic diverticulitis. Am J Surg. 1986;151:269–71.
30. Thaler K, Baig MK, Berho M, et al. Determinants of recurrence after sigmoid resection for uncomplicated diverticulitis. Dis Colon Rectum. 2003;46(3):385–8.
31. Carlson RM, Roberts PL, Hall JF, Marcello PW, Read TE, Ricciardi R. Is routine splenic flexure mobilization during anterior resection always necessary. In: Presented at the American Society of Colon and Rectal Surgeons Annual meeting, San Antonio, 2012.
32. Schauer PR, Ramos R, Ghiatas AA, et al. Virulent diverticular disease in young obese men. Am J Surg. 1992;164:443–6.
33. Ouriel K, Schwartz SI. Diverticular disease in the young patients. Surg Gynecol Obstet. 1983;16:1–5.
34. Acousta JA, Grebene ML, Doberneck RC, et al. Colonic diverticular disease in patients 40 years old or younger. Am Surg. 1992;58:605–7.
35. Janes S, Meagher A, Faragher IG, Shedda S, Frizelle FA. The place of elective surgery following acute diverticulitis in young patients: when is surgery indicated? An analysis of the literature. Dis Colon Rectum. 2009;52(5):1008–16.
36. Vignati PV, Welch JP, Cohen JL. Long-term management of diverticulitis in young patients. Dis Colon Rectum. 1995;38:627–9.
37. Hall JF, Roberts PL, Ricciardi R, Marcello PW, Scheirey C, Wald C, et al. Colonic diverticulitis: does age predict severity of disease on CT imaging. Dis Colon Rectum. 2010;53(2):121–5.
38. Etzioni DA, Cannom RR, Ault GT, Beart Jr RW, Kaiser AM. Diverticulitis in California from 1995 to 2006; increased rates of treatment for younger patients. Am Surg. 2009;75(10):981–5.
39. Russ AJ, Obma KL, Rajamanickam V, Wan Y, Heise CP, Foley EF, et al. Laparoscopy improves short-term outcomes after surgery for diverticular disease. Gastroenterology. 2010;138(7):2267–74.
40. Klarenbeek BR, Veenhof A, Bergamaschi R, van der Peet DL, van den Broek WT, de Lange ES, et al. Laparoscopic sigmoid resection for diverticulitis decreases major morbidity rates: a randomized control trial; short term results of the Sigma Trial. Ann Surg. 2009;249(1):39–44.
41. Ridgway PF, Latif A, Shabbir J, Ofriokuma F, Hurley MJ, Evoy D, et al. Randomized controlled trial of oral vs intravenous therapy for the clinically diagnosed acute uncomplicated diverticulitis. Colorectal Dis. 2009;11(9):941–6.
42. Etzioni DA, Chiu VY, Cannom RR, Burchette RJ, Haigh PI, Abbas MA. Outpatient treatment of acute diverticulitis and predictors of failure. Dis Colon Rectum. 2010;53(6):861–5.
43. Hjern F, Josephson T, Altman D, Holmstrom B, Mellgren A, Pollack J, et al. Conservative treatment of acute colonic diverticulitis; are antibiotics always mandatory? Scan J Gastroenterol. 2007;42(1):41–7.
44. Gatta L, Vakil N, Vaira D, Pilotto A, Curlo M, Comparato G, Leandro G, et al. Efficacy of 5-ASA in the treatment of colonic diverticular disease. J Clin Gastroenerol. 2010;44(2):113–6.
45. Fazio VW, Church JM, Jagelman DG. Colocutaneous fistulas complicated diverticulitis. Dis Colon Rectum. 1987;30(2):89–94.
46. Ricciardi R, Baxter NN, Read TE, Marcello PW, Hall J, Roberts PL. Is the decline in the surgical treatment for diverticulitis associated with an increase in complicated diverticulitis? Dis Colon Rectum. 2009;52(9):1558–63.
47. Hinchey EJ, Schaal PG, Richards GK. Treatment of perforated diverticular disease of the colon. Adv Surg. 1978;12:85–109.
48. Siewert B, Tye G, Kruskal J, et al. Impact of CT-guided drainage in the treatment of diverticular abscess: size matters. AJR Am J Roentgenol. 2006;186:680–6.
49. Soumain S, Thomas S, Mohan PP, Khan N, Khan Z, Raju T. Management of Hinchey II diverticulitis. World J Gastroenterol. 2008;14(47):7163–9.
50. Saini S, Mueller PR, Wittenberg J, Butch RJ, Rodkey GV, Welch CE. Percutaneous drainage of diverticular abscess. An adjunct to surgical therapy. Arch Surg. 1986;121(4):475–8.
51. Ambrosetti P, Chautems R, Soravia C, et al. Long-term outcome of mesocolic and pelvic diverticular abscesses: a prospective study of 73 cases. Dis Colon Rectum. 2005;48:787–91.
52. Seetharam S, Paige J, Horgan PG. Impact of socioeconomic deprivation and primary pathology on rate of reversal of Hartmann's procedure. Am J Surg. 2003;186:154–7.
53. Maggard MA, Zingmond D, O'Connell JB, Ko CY. What proportion of patients with an ostomy (for diverticulitis) get reversed? Am Surg. 2004;70(10):928–31.
54. Salem L, Flum DR. Primary anastomosis or Hartmann's procedures for patients with diverticular peritonitis? A Systematic review. Dis Colon Rectum. 2004;47:1953–64.
55. Karoui M, Champault A, Pautrat K, Valleur P, Cherqui D, Champault G. Laparoscopic peritoneal lavage or primary anastomosis with defunctioning stoma for Hinchey 3 complicated diverticulitis: results of a comparative study. Dis Colon Rectum. 2009;52(4):609–15.
56. Krukowski ZH, Matheson NA. Emergency surgery for diverticular disease complicated by generalized and faecal peritonitis; a review. Br J Surg. 1984;71(12):921–7.
57. Zeitoun G, Laurent A, Rouffet F, Hay J, Fingerhut A, Paquet J, Pellon G, et al. Multicentre, randomized clinical trial of primary versus secondary sigmoid resection in generalized peritonitis complicating sigmoid diverticulitis. Br J Surg. 2000;87(10):1366–74.
58. Slim K, Vicaut E, Launay-Savary MV, et al. Updated systemic review and meta-analysis of randomized clinical trials on the role of mechanical bowel preparation before colorectal surgery. Ann Surg. 2009;249(2):203–9.

59. Dharmarajan S, Hunt SR, Birnbaum EH, Fleshman JW, Mutch MG. The efficacy of nonoperative management of acute complicated diverticulitis. Dis Colon Rectum. 2011;54(6):663–71.
60. O'Sullivan GC, Murphy D, O'Brien MG, Ireland A. Laparoscopic management of generalized peritonitis due to perforated colonic diverticula. Am J Surg. 1996;171(4):432–4.
61. Myers E, Hurley M, O'Sullivan GC, Kavanagh D, Wilson I, Winter DC. Laparoscopic peritoneal lavage for generalized peritonitis due to perforated diverticulitis. Br J Surg. 2008;95(1):97–101.
62. Afshar S, Kurer MA. Laparoscopic peritoneal lavage for perforated sigmoid diverticulitis. Colorectal Dis. 2012;14920:135–42.
63. Hartmann H. Nouveau procede d'ablation des cancers de la partie terminale du colon pelvien. Congres Francais de Chirugia. 1923;30:2241. Cited by: Corman ML. Classic articles in colonic and rectal surgery. Dis Colon Rectum. 1984;27:273.
64. Lockhart-Mummery JP. Late results in diverticulitis. Lancet. 1938;2:1401–2.
65. Smithwick RH. Experiences with surgical management of diverticulitis of sigmoid. Ann Surg. 1942;15:969–85.
66. Albarran SA, Shimoens C, Van de Winkel N, et al. Restoration of digestive continuity after Hartmann's procedure: ASA score is a predictive factor for risk of postoperative complications. Acta Chir Belg. 2009;109:714–9.
67. Khan AL, Ah-See AK, Crofts TJ, et al. Reversal of Hartmann's colostomy. J R Coll Surg Edinb. 1994;39:239–42.
68. Keck JO, Collopy BT, Ryan PJ, et al. Reversal of Hartmann's procedure: effect of timing and technique on ease and safety. Dis Colon Rectum. 1994;37:243–8.
69. Fleming FJ, Gillen P. Reversal of Hartmann's procedure following acute diverticulitis: is timing everything? Int J Colorectal Dis. 2009;24:1219–25.
70. Salem L, Anaya DA, Roberts KE, et al. Hartmann's colectomy and reversal in diverticulitis: a population-level assessment. Dis Colon Rectum. 2005;48:988–95.
71. Read TE, Salgado J, Ferraro D, et al. "Peek port": a novel approach for avoiding conversion in laparoscopic colectomy. Surg Endosc. 2009;23(3):477–81.
72. Worsey MJ, Fazio VW. Reoperative Pelvic Surgery. In: Yeo CJ, Dempsey DT, Klein AS, Pemberton JH, Peters JH, editors. Shackelford's Surgery of the Alimentary Tract. 6th ed. Philadelphia: Saunders/Elsevier; 2007. p. 2409–18.
73. Khoury DA, Opelka FG. Anoscopic-assisted insertion of end-to-end anastomosing staplers. Dis Colon Rectum. 1995;38:533–4.
74. Ricciardi R, Roberts PL, Marcello PW, Hall JF, Read TE, Schoetz DJ. Anastomotic leak testing after colorectal resection: what are the data? Arch Surg. 2009;144(5):407–11.
75. Hodgson NC. The search for an ideal method of abdominal fascial closure: a meta-analysis. Ann Surg. 2000;231(3):436–42.
76. Ceydeli A, Rucinski J, Wise L. Finding the best abdominal closure: an evidence-based review of the literature. Curr Surg. 2005;62(2):220–5.
77. Bruce J, Krukowski ZH, Al-Khairy G, Russell EM, Park KG. Systematic review of the definition and measurement of anastomotic leak after gastrointestinal surgery. Br J Surg. 2001;88(9):1157–68.
78. Tilney HS, Sains PS, Lovegrove RE, et al. Comparison of outcomes following ileostomy versus colostomy for defunctioning colorectal anastomoses. World J Surg. 2007;31:1141–5.
79. Hayden DM, Pinzon MC, Francescatti AB, Edquist SC, Malczewski MR, Jolley JM. Hospital readmission for fluid and electrolyte abnormalities following ileostomy construction. Preventable or unpredictable. J Gastrointest Surg. 2013;17:298–303. Epub 2012 Nov 29.
80. Levack MM, Savitt LF, Berger DL, Shellito PC, Hodin RA, Rattner DW, et al. Sigmoidectomy syndrome? Patients' perspectives on the functional outcomes following surgery for diverticulitis. Dis Colon Rectum. 2012;55(1):10–7.
81. Munson KD, Hensien MA, Jacob LN, et al. Diverticulitis-a comprehensive follow-up. Dis Colon Rectum. 1996;39:318–22.
82. Le TH, Gathright Jr JB. Reconstitution of intestinal continuity after extended left colectomy. Dis Colon Rectum. 1993;36:197–8.
83. Beck DE. Intraoperative anastomotic challenges. In: Whitlow CB, Beck DE, Margolin DA, Hicks TC, Timmcke AE, editors. Improved outcomes in colon and Rectal Surgery. London: Informa Healthcare; 2010. p. 33–55.
84. Qinyao W, Wejiin S, Youren Z, et al. New concepts in severe presacral hemorrhage during proctectomy. Arch Surg. 1985;120:1013–20.
85. Masoomi H, Buchberg BS, Magno C, Mills SD, Stamos MJ. Trends in diverticulitis management in the United States from 2002 to 2007. Arch Surg. 2011;146(4):400–6.

Carcinomatosis: Cytoreduction and Heated Intraperitoneal Chemotherapy (HIPEC) Versus Palliation

5

Björn L.D.M. Brücher, Avital Itzhak, Anton Bilchik, Aviram Nissan, and Alexander Stojadinovic

Abbreviations

BMI	Body mass index
CC score	Completeness of cytoreduction score
CDSS	Clinical decision support systems
CRC	Colorectal cancer
CRS	Cytoreductive surgery
CT	Computed tomography
CTR-1	Copper transport protein-1
DPAM	Disseminated peritoneal adenomucinosis
EPIC	Early postoperative IP chemotherapy
HIPEC	Hyperthermic intraperitoneal Chemotherapy
ICU	Intensive care unit
IV	Intravenous
NCCTG	North Central Cancer Treatment Group
OR	Operating room
PC	Peritoneal carcinomatosis
PCI	Peritoneal cancer index
PSM	Peritoneal surface malignancy
QOL	Quality of life
RCT	Randomized controlled trial
TPN	Total parenteral nutrition

B.L.D.M. Brücher, MD, PhD, FRCS (Engl), FACS (✉)
Department of Surgery, Bon Secours Cancer Institute,
Richmond, VA, USA

INCORE = International Consortium of Research of the Theodor-Billroth-Academy®, Richmond, VA, Germany-Israel-Serbia-USA
e-mail: b-bruecher@gmx.de

A. Itzhak, MD, FACS
Department of Surgery, Bon Secours Cancer Institute,
Richmond, VA, USA

Uniformed Services University of the Health
Sciences, Bethesda, MD, USA

A. Bilchik, MD, PhD, FACS
Department of Surgery, John Wayne Cancer
Institute, Santa Monica, CA, USA

A. Nissan, MD, FACS
Department of Surgery, Hadassah-Hebrew University,
Jerusalem, Israel

United States Military Cancer Institute, Bethesda, MD, USA

A. Stojadinovic, MD, FACS
Department of Surgery, Bon Secours Cancer Institute,
Richmond, VA, USA

Uniformed Services University of the Health
Sciences, Bethesda, MD, USA

United States Military Cancer Institute, Bethesda, MD, USA

Contributing Author Declaration
We certify that all individuals who qualify as authors have been listed; each author has participated in one or more of the following areas: conception and design of this work, the acquisition and/or analysis of data, the writing and/or critical revision of the document, and supervision of this cooperative research effort. All contributing authors approve of the submission of this version of the manuscript and assert that the document represents valid work. If information derived from another source was used in this manuscript, we obtained all necessary approvals to use it and made appropriate acknowledgements in the document. All contributing authors take public responsibility for this work.

Disclaimer
The views expressed in this manuscript are those of the authors and do not reflect the official policy of the Department of the Army, the Department of Defense, or the US Government.

S.R. Steele et al. (eds.), *Complexities in Colorectal Surgery*,
DOI 10.1007/978-1-4614-9022-7_5, © Springer Science+Business Media New York 2014

Key Points

- Tumor biology is an extremely important, yet difficult to quantify, factor for overall outcomes.
- Proper patient selection is the key to cytoreductive surgery and HIPEC.
- Understand not only good candidates but also patients with contraindications based on preoperative staging, as they will not derive any benefit.
- Select patients with peritoneal surface malignancy can be cured.
- Cytoreductive surgery and HIPEC is challenging and has the potential for increased morbidity.
- A multimodality approach includes lifelong surveillance and the potential for repeated treatments.

Background, Basics, and Rationale

General Aspects, Epidemiology

Key Concept: *Cytoreductive surgery and heated intraperitoneal chemotherapy prolongs survival in carefully selected patients in whom complete resection of all grossly apparent disease can be attained (completeness of cytoreduction score 0/1).*

It remains controversial if patients suffering from PSM of CRC origin should be treated by a time-, labor-, and cost-intensive multimodal interdisciplinary therapeutic approach using CRS + HIPEC, or if palliative treatment remains the standard of practice. In this chapter, we try to provide a broad overview of the multifaceted considerations in order to provide a critical assessment of this controversial matter and provide guiding principles as to how best to implement such an approach.

As people worldwide grow older, common afflictions increase in incidence—coronary heart diseases, diabetes mellitus, dementia, and cancer. One of every four deaths in the USA is due to cancer [1], and cancer is the leading cause of death among Hispanics in the USA [2]. A total of 1,638,910 new cancer cases and 577,190 deaths from cancer were projected to occur in the USA in 2012 alone [1]. Of these, ~150,000 patients are diagnosed with CRC and nearly 50,000 die from this disease each year [1]. More pertinent to the present discussion, approximately 8,000 patients in the USA are diagnosed with synchronous PSM of colorectal cancer origin annually [3, 4]. An overview of disease-specific consideration in PSM is shown in Table 5.1.

Peritoneal surface malignancy of CRC origin is a frequent manifestation in the natural history of the disease, and it is associated with marked deterioration in quality of life (QOL) and very poor prognosis. Peritoneal disease spread continues to be a common mode of disease progression for intra-abdominal malignancies. Eight percent of patients with CRC have synchronous peritoneal spread of disease at time of primary resection, and up to 25 % of patients with recurrent CRC have disease confined to the peritoneal cavity [3]. In about 30 % of patients with CRC, PSM is the main reason for disease-specific mortality [9]. On the positive side, ~50 % of patients who develop PSM from CRC may have curative treatment by an R0-resection.

Confinement of disease to a limited extent of the peritoneal surface in the absence of systemic spread of disease has served as the basis for surgical eradication of disease through aggressive CRS + HIPEC. Survival during the time when patients with PSM from CRC had been treated by systemic therapy alone, typically 5-FU, was limited to approximately 6 months (range 5–7 months) [9, 10]. Among patients who suffered from PSM due to CRC and had simultaneous malignant bowel obstruction, the survival was even worse—limited to 3 months [11]. Based on recent experience, however, a paradigm shift has occurred.

Change of Paradigm

Key Concept: *The results that can be obtained with cytoreduction and heated intraperitoneal chemotherapy for resectable peritoneal surface malignancy of colorectal cancer origin are similar to hepatic resection for resectable colorectal cancer metastasis, with 5-year overall survival of ~45 %.*

A clear change of paradigm occurred slowly within the past 50 years, in part due to the increasing recognition that PSM is a regional disease once limited to a compartment—the abdomen. It was not, as once thought, a systemic disease for which only palliative intervention was indicated [3]. It was not until the 1980s that the generally held fatalistic view

Table 5.1 Disease-specific considerations in PSM

Primary tumor	Incidence (%)	Disease-specific considerations in PSM	Reference
CRC	30	Cause of disease-specific mortality in 30 %	Esquivel et al. [40]
Small bowel	40	Synchronous PSM at time of diagnosis in 50 %	Brücher et al. [6]
Stomach (pT3/4)	50	Synchronous PSM in 50 % at time of first surgical exploration	Xu et al. [7]
Ovarian	75	Synchronous PSM at time of diagnosis in 50 %	Armstrong et al. [8]

CRC colorectal carcinoma, *pT3/4* locally advanced tumor categories, *PSM* peritoneal surface malignancy of PC gave way to a new way of thinking with regard to treatment options and treatment-specific prognosis; such options expanded beyond purely palliative and/or best supportive therapy. During the 1990s, pioneering surgeons such as Paul Sugarbaker and Francois Gilly were the principal driving forces that moved away from that fatalistic approach toward a curative treatment approach by using CRC + HIPEC in carefully selected patients that could benefit from such an aggressive treatment intervention [3, 4, 12–16]. Disease once limited to bleak outcomes of 3–6 month median survival with therapy could, in selected cases, be treated aggressively with CRS + HIPEC and have strikingly improved outcomes [9, 10]. In fact, patients undergoing complete resection of PSM from CRC followed by HIPEC could attain median survival of 21–40 months, while patients with pseudomyxoma peritonei were reported to have 20-year survival of up to 70 % [17]. However, these results clearly depended on the extent of peritoneal surface tumor burden and completeness of cytoreduction [18]. The curative treatment approach in PC is a demanding and complex interdisciplinary procedure in which surgeons, anesthetists, oncologists, gastroenterologists, dieticians, physical and occupational therapists, psychologists, and case managers, among others, should be equally involved in the patient-centered, integrative, team approach to cancer care. It must be emphasized that CRS, HIPEC, and systemic therapy are not competitive therapies, and this can be recognized by the fact that in France this therapeutic paradigm has already incorporated into French Guidelines for standards of practice [19]. In 2012, Germany integrated this approach into national treatment guidelines as a therapeutic option [20]. Surgical oncologists caring for patients with PC need a wide range of training and experience that extends well beyond the technical aspects of surgical care and includes understanding of the biology of disease, assessment of the extent of disease, careful patient selection, administration of HIPEC, and related anesthetic and safety considerations, as well as postoperative interventions for secondary surgical events. Understanding of the fundamentals of peritoneal surface disease-specific anatomy and embryology is essential.

Anatomy and Embryology

Key Concept: *The pelvic–peritoneal partition serves as the anatomic basis for the delivery of dose-dense heated intraperitoneal chemotherapy.*

A detailed description of the ultrastructure of the peritoneum was published by Baron in 1941 [21] and reviewed recently by us [20]. The distinct histological structure of the peritoneum is evident in a special type of vascular anatomy and also its specific function. The peritoneum consists of a single-cell layer of mesothelial cells, with a basal membrane beneath it along with five layers of connective tissue (interstitial cells and a matrix of collagen, hyaline, and proteoglycans), with a total thickness of 90 μm [3, 22]. As it also contains other cellular elements such as pericytes, parenchymal cells, and blood capillary vessels, the peritoneum is often referred to as the "peritoneal membrane." The functions of the peritoneum include maintenance of the mobility of intra-abdominal organs relative to the abdominal wall. This is achieved through a lubricant secreted by the peritoneal membrane consisting of glycosaminoglycans and phospholipids. The membrane further fulfills an important function in defense against intra-abdominal infections. It is also thought that the peritoneum represents the principal barrier and initial line of defense against dissemination of malignant cells and establishment of peritoneal carcinomatosis [23]. This view is supported by research, which has shown that intraperitoneal injection of aggressive tumor cell lines leads to a corresponding increase in tumor cell activity in the peritoneal membrane [3]. The interaction between its single layer of mesothelial cells together with associated blood capillaries and surrounding interstitial matrix contributes to this line of defense [24]. In fact, the peritoneal membrane is regarded as an organ itself [3] and its surface area approximates 7,500 cm^2 and is in direct contact with all intra-abdominal organs.

At the end of the third week of gestation, the intraembryonic mesoderm divides bilaterally into the mesoderm, the intermediate mesoderm, and the lateral plate. In the lateral plate, a mesothelial cell layer divides into the parietal and visceral mesoderm. The parietal mesoderm, which lines the intraembryonic celomic cavity, becomes the parietal peritoneum, the parietal pleura, and the pericardium. From the visceral mesodermal layer, the visceral peritoneum, visceral pleura, and epicardium develop. The dorsal mesentery, to which the intestinal tube is attached, represents the junction between the parietal and visceral peritoneum. Understanding this embryology and anatomical relationship is important in the technical execution of cytoreduction [3]. It is also important to recognize that there is practically never any tumor penetration into the underlying organ structures (e.g., kidney, spleen) in cases of PC. This is probably due to the peritoneum's embryologically delineated barrier function.

Classification and Types of Growth of PC

Key Concept: *Irrespective of the growth pattern of peritoneal surface malignancy, the predominant factor-determining outcome is the ability to achieve complete cytoreduction.*

Peritoneal surface malignancy can be subdivided into primary and secondary forms [3]. Primary PSM consists of invasion by a mesothelioma or pseudomyxoma peritonei—both extremely rare tumor entities. Secondary PC originates most commonly from gastrointestinal tumors [25–27] or urogenital tumors [28]. Other forms of secondary PC involve less common primary epithelial malignancies such as malignant melanoma or breast carcinoma. There are important differences between growth types in peritoneal carcinomatosis pertaining to involvement of the bowel, supporting mesentery, and its critical vascular structures; these are important to consider when estimating likelihood of achieving complete cytoreduction with CRS, particularly when there is substantial involvement of the mesenteric pedicle, or root of the mesentery (Fig. 5.1), [3].

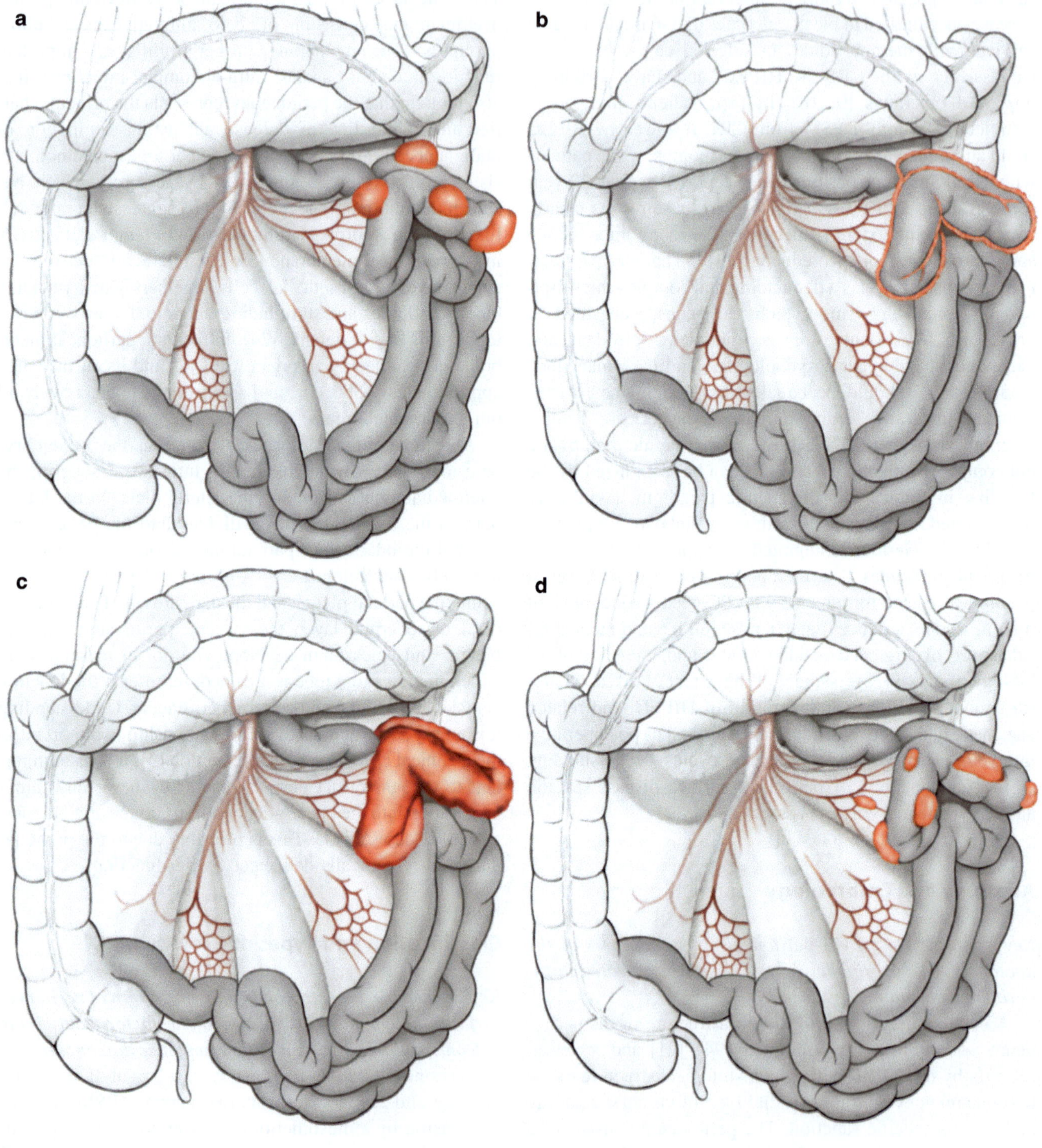

Fig. 5.1 (a–e) Growth patterns in peritoneal carcinomatosis on the small bowel (Modified from Brücher et al. [3])

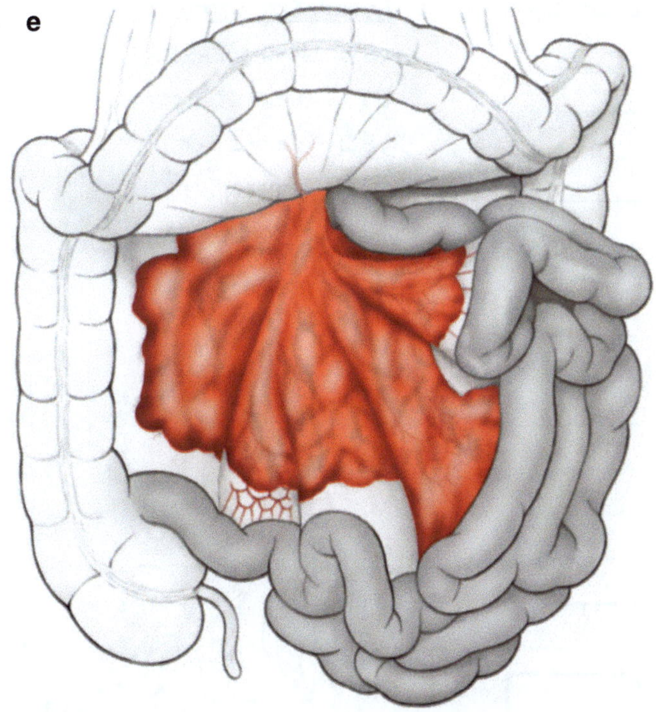

Fig. 5.1 (continued)

History and Rationale for Intraperitoneal Drug Therapy

Key Concept: Heated intraperitoneal chemotherapy is indicated for treatment of non-visible or <1 mm peritoneal surface tumor deposits.

The history of intraperitoneal drug therapy was reported recently [20]. The earliest report mentioned in the literature about the use of intraperitoneal "drug therapy" was by the English surgeon, Christopher Warrick in 1744 [29]. The Belgium surgeon, WP Ceelen, together with a US colleague, MF Flessner, reported on the biophysics of intraperitoneal therapy [30] that Warrick injected into the peritoneal cavity, a mixture of "Bristol" water and "claret," a Bordeaux wine, in the female, Jane Roman, who suffered from malignant ascites. The cytotoxic nitrogen mustard, which had been in use during World War II, was investigated in the 1950s in clinical trials for the purpose of intraperitoneal therapy [31]. In 1978, Dedrick reported about the pharmacokinetics of intraperitoneal drug delivery, distribution, and clearance given the peritoneal–plasma partition. This anatomical barrier provides the fundamental rationale for intraperitoneal drug delivery, such that a much higher drug concentration can be used than administered systemically, because peritoneal drug clearance is much slower than plasma clearance [32]. Intraperitoneal drug delivery has been proven to be efficient and effective in patients with minimal ("infra-millimetric") or microscopic residual disease following cytoreductive surgery [30]. Hence, cytoreductive surgery

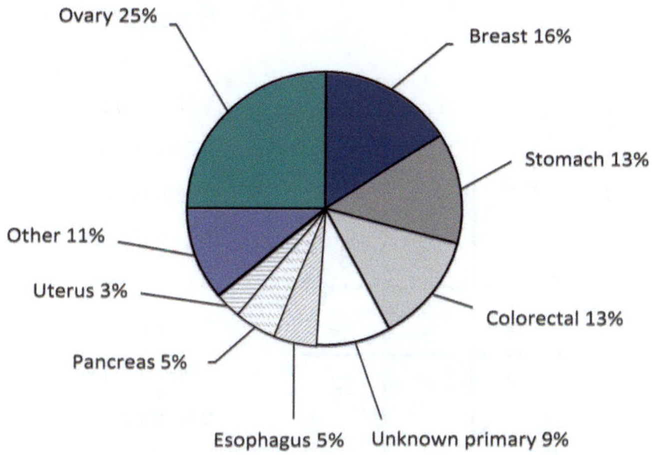

Fig. 5.2 Primary etiology of malignant ascites (Modified from: Avantunde and Parson [33])

is intended to clear visible peritoneal surface disease, while HIPEC is indicated for treatment of non-visible or <1 mm peritoneal tumor deposits, as intraperitoneal chemotherapy penetrates only a millimeter in depth during HIPEC. The reason why intraperitoneal therapy emerged early in the history of regional therapy seems to be related to the challenge of alleviating symptomatic malignant ascites. There are various epithelial malignancies that may lead to symptomatic ascites; these are shown in Fig. 5.2 [33]. Malignant ascites reflects a symptom of peritoneal carcinomatosis, and it indicates the presence of malignant cells within the peritoneal cavity. The biodynamic effects of intraperitoneal drug administration were shown to be dependent on a number of key variables, such as diffusion and convection (dependent on molecular weight of the agent administered), and interstitial fluid pressure; malignant tumors characteristically have elevated interstitial fluid pressure, which serves as a barrier for connective drug transport. Flessner et al. showed that the structure of the peritoneal intracellular matrix is the major source of resistance to macromolecular drug transport [34]. The tumor penetration distance measured experimentally ranges from a few cell layers (generally <1 mm) to a maximum of 3–5 mm [30]. Active and passive transport across the cell membrane leads to better and somewhat worse intracellular drug concentration, and the mode of transport influences the efficacy of regional drug application. Additionally, in the case of cisplatin, the copper transport protein-1(CTR1) regulates uptake in human cancer cells [35]. Additionally, preclinical models have shown that hypotonic carrier fluids lower interstitial fluid pressure and increase intraperitoneal pressure, leading to enhanced peritoneal drug penetration [30].

Peritoneal Cancer Index (PCI)

Key Concept: A key quantitative prognostic index is the peritoneal cancer index (PCI). Cytoreductive surgery should not be

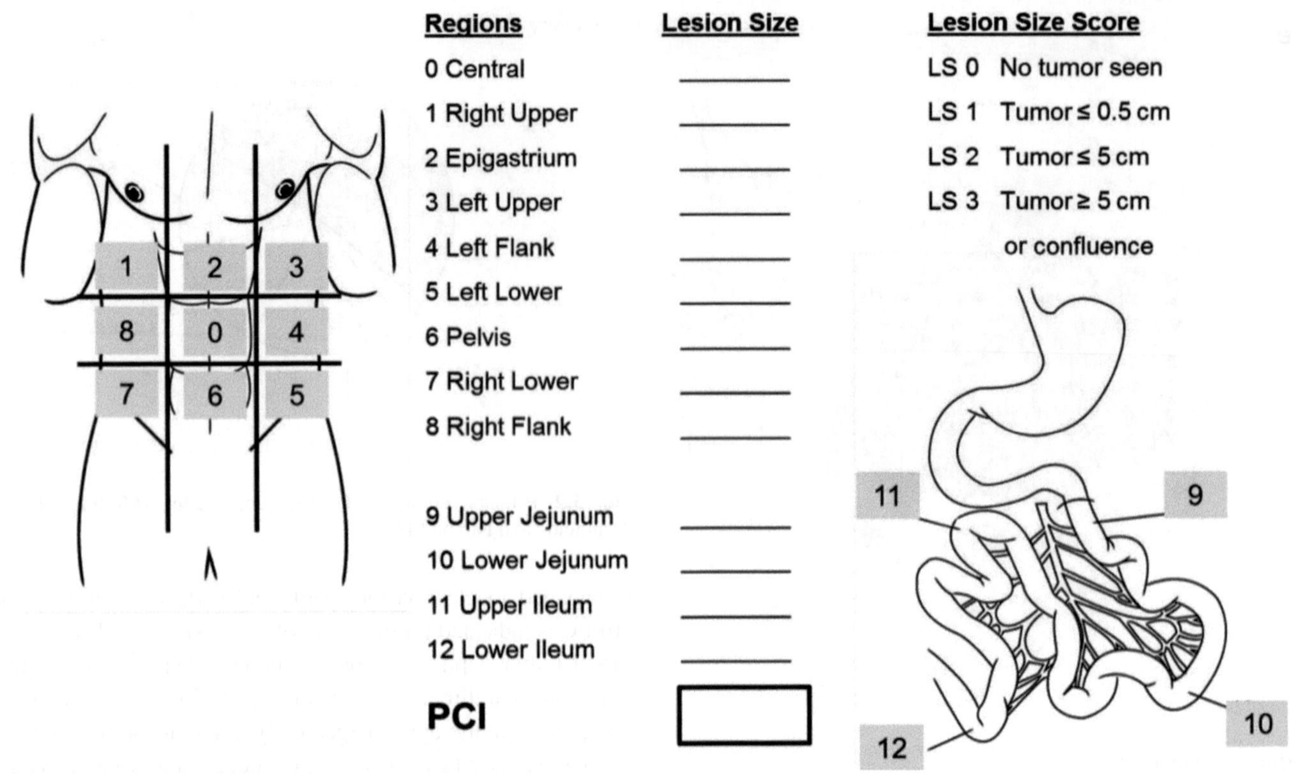

Fig. 5.3 The peritoneal cancer index (*PCI*) (Modified from: modified according Jacquet and Sugarbaker [37])

undertaken with curative in patients with PCI ≥20, as the results of CRS + HIPEC are not different than systemic therapy alone.

Presurgical extent of disease evaluation should provide reliable information about the tumor location, the extent of peritoneal tumor burden, and distribution and extent of the disease so that diligent patient selection can be carried out [3]. Studies on the preoperative clinical staging of PC have shown that the reliability of computed tomography (CT) for predicting the stage of the disease is somewhat limited [36]. As reviewed earlier [3], various scoring systems are currently in use for the assessment of peritoneal surface disease burden:

- Sugarbaker's peritoneal cancer index (PCI) [37] (Fig. 5.3)
- Verwaal's N score [38]
- Gilly's classification [16]
- P score [39]

The PCI [37] is well established, currently in use at the major PSM centers worldwide (Fig. 5.3), and was confirmed as the preferred scoring system by a consensus conference held in Milan in 2006 [40]. Sugarbaker divides the abdominal compartment into nine regions (Regions 0 through 9), and the small bowel separately into four regions (Regions 10 through 13). After exploring the abdomen, all single regions are assigned a score corresponding to the greatest possible extent of tumor involvement by size of the largest peritoneal surface lesion within that region (lesion size from 0, no tumor seen, to 3, tumor >5 cm). Out of this, the maximum possible number of points in the PCI is thus 39, and the lowest is 0. Sugarbaker's analyses revealed that patients with a PCI score of less than 20 have a reasonable likelihood of complete cytoreduction, thereby prognosis (in comparison with the previous approach of palliative chemotherapy alone and/or best supportive care) that may be favorably impacted by CRS + HIPEC. A challenge for the future will be reliable pre-therapeutic (before surgical exploration) prediction of tumor involvement of the small bowel and/or mesentery, as this represents one of the major limiting factors for the ability to achieve complete cytoreduction with CRS. The Society of Surgical Oncology has published surgical selection criteria for patients with PSM in 2006 [40].

Residual Tumor Classification (Completeness of Cytoreduction, CC Score)

Key Concept: Another key prognostic indicator is completeness of cytoreduction (CC) score. The goal is to attain complete removal of all grossly evident disease (CC0) or to leave behind only a few minute deposits of peritoneal surface tumor that can be treated effectively with HIPEC (CC1). Therefore, complete CRS implies both CC0 and CC1. The only way in which the patient can achieve long-term benefit is through having complete cytoreduction (CC0/1).

The major basis for prognosis in surgical oncology is completeness of resection, obtaining complete clearance of

Table 5.2 Completeness of cytoreduction (CC) score

CC 0	No residual tumor (= R0 resection) (en bloc resection)
CC 1	<0.25 cm residual tumor tissue (complete cytoreduction)
CC 2	0.25–2.5 cm residual tumor tissue (incomplete cytoreduction with moderate residual tumor proportion)
CC 3	>2.5 cm residual tumor tissue (incomplete cytoreduction with high residual tumor proportion)

Modified from Sugarbaker [41]

grossly apparent disease. This is usually determined by the R-classification (residual tumor classification). CRS is also based on the target criteria used in surgical oncology—achieving complete macroscopic and microscopic freedom from tumor (R0 resection). It is difficult to communicate in terms of R0 resection after multivisceral resection in the context of CRS. Therefore, the classification of "completeness of cytoreduction," so-called CC classification [41], was developed and also affirmed at the 2006 consensus conference in Milan (Table 5.2) [40]. In patients with mucinous pseudomyxoma peritonei who undergo CRS + HIPEC, the R0 resection referred to elsewhere in the gastrointestinal tract is equivalent to CC 0 (no residual tumor) and CC1 status (<0.25 cm residual tumor tissue),whereas in invasive gastrointestinal tumors such as CRC and/or gastric carcinomas, R0 resection is only equivalent to CC 0 status. Completeness of resection is of paramount importance for patients with PC, and it has been clearly shown that patients with CC 0/CC 1 resections have a significantly improved survival period than those who do not [41–44]. In fact, there is no indication for CRS/HIPEC treatment in the setting of incomplete cytoreduction (CC2/3). Therefore, the CC classification is important not only in patient selection for CRS (only those in whom CC 0/1 status can be achieved should undergo attempted CRS) but also in estimating oncological outcome of CRS for a given CC score, which has been shown to be of significant prognostic value, serving as a surrogate marker for disease-free and overall survival after CRS for patients with PSM due to CRC [45, 46].

HIPEC: Technique, Rationale, and Drugs

Key Concept: *The strategic rationale for HIPEC includes increased chemotherapeutic agent concentration/dose at the intended site of action, increased cytotoxic effect of the administered intraperitoneal agent, reduced systemic absorption and toxicity of the chemotherapeutic, homogeneous distribution of intraperitoneal chemotherapy, and direct antitumor effect of hyperthermia.*

Hyperthermic intraperitoneal chemotherapy (HIPEC) can be carried out as an open ("coliseum") or closed procedure [3]. The coliseum technique allows manual distribution of the perfusate during HIPEC that is extremely important for certain anatomical regions. The principle is that the abdomen is initially filled with a carrier solution (dialysis or Ringer's solution). The carrier solution is then passed through the HIPEC machine to heat it. Once a steady-state temperature of minimum of 42 °C has been reached (optimally a mean temperature of 43–44 °C), the chemotherapeutic agent is added and HIPEC starts. The intra-abdominal temperature is measured every minute, and patient-specific temperatures (bladder, head, esophageal, and/or rectal temperature probe temperature assessed by the anesthetist) are also closely monitored and recorded. After 30–90 min of HIPEC, the carrier solution is drained along with the chemotherapeutic agent, and the abdomen is lavaged with approximately 8–10 L of Ringer's solution. Both the perfusate and lavage solutions must be disposed of as potentially hazardous waste material. Locoregional (intraperitoneal) administration of chemotherapy increases the local concentration of the chemotherapeutic agent at the site of action, the peritoneal surface. This reduces the systemic toxicity of the treatment, but at the expense of potentially increased postoperative morbidity related to the surgical procedure [47]. Some institutions create the anastomosis before and some after the administration of HIPEC. One animal study showed that anastomotic insufficiency is more likely to occur when systemic 5-fluorouracil (5-FU) treatment is carried out around the time of HIPEC than when locoregional chemotherapy is used alone [48]. Another study in a rat model showed that HIPEC consistently resulted in delayed healing of colonic anastomosis [49], raising the question whether technical modifications (e.g., proximal diversion) are indicated in the setting of HIPEC.

In HIPEC, the carrier solution (dialysis or Ringer's solution) is initially heated to a temperature of 43 °C, with instillation of the chemotherapeutic agent only being carried out afterwards. The chemotherapeutic agent is circulated in the peritoneal cavity administered for 30–90 min, depending on the preference of the peritoneal carcinomatosis center concerned and the agent being utilized. When HIPEC has been completed at a mean temperature of 43–44 °C, the abdomen may be lavaged. Postoperatively, the patient is monitored in an intensive care unit. It is important to note that cisplatin-containing substances in particular can also have direct cardiotoxic effects. As a result of the large wound surface, it is possible for *cis*-diaminedichloroplatinum (CDDP) to be washed into the bloodstream, leading to cardiotoxicity, for which care in a monitored setting following operation is imperative.

At present, the agents used in HIPEC are mainly mitomycin C, cisplatin (CDDP), oxaliplatin, and doxorubicin. Intraperitoneal administration of chemotherapeutic agent achieves high response rates in patients with peritoneal carcinomatosis, as the peritoneum–plasma barrier makes it possible to administer high doses of the drug [50]. On the basis of analyses conducted during peritoneal dialysis, Dedrick et al.

Table 5.3 Rationale for hyperthermic delivery of intraperitoneal chemotherapy immediately after colorectal surgery

Increased penetration of the chemotherapeutic agent into tissue
Increased cytotoxic effect
Cytotoxic effect of hyperthermia itself
Reduced systemic toxicity of administered agent at higher concentrations
Direct treatment of free intraperitoneal tumor cells

Modified from Brücher et al. [3]

showed in 1978 that the peritoneal permeability of hydrophilic cancer drugs is lower than the known plasma clearance of the same agents [32]. The chemotherapeutic drugs mitomycin C, cisplatin, and/or oxaliplatin are the agents of choice for HIPEC. These drugs have a relatively high molecular weight (mitomycin C, 334 Da; cisplatin, 300 Da; oxaliplatin, 397 Da). Due to reduced permeability into the plasma through the peritoneal barrier, they consequently have lower systemic concentrations and thus lower associated toxicity [51, 52]. The challenge when interpreting the international literature is that there are also centers in which systemic chemotherapy is administered simultaneously with heated agents delivered into the peritoneal cavity [3]. Another important variable aside from the type (open versus closed technique) and duration (30, 60, 90 min) of HIPEC is the temperature at which the chemotherapy is delivered into the peritoneal cavity (generally >41.5 °C). Hyperthermia above 41 °C alone produces a direct antitumor effect. However, tumor cells react through upregulation of heat shock proteins, which may be able to produce some thermal tolerance [53]. This cytotoxic effect has been demonstrated only for drugs containing platinum [54] and for mitomycin C [55]. It is also important to recognize that hyperthermia itself has deeper tissue effects [56]. The rationale for hyperthermic delivery of intraperitoneal chemotherapy immediately after CRS is summarized in Table 5.3 [3]. Deeper tissue effects of HIPEC are discussed in the following section.

Multimodal Therapy in Peritoneal Carcinomatosis

Key Concept: Multimodality therapy consisting of cytoreductive surgery + HIPEC in patients with CRC peritoneal carcinomatosis is superior over systemic therapy alone.

Published randomized phase III trials in PSM and CRC had been recently reviewed in detail [4]. In this and another recent review addressing the application of the second look operation [20], it was emphasized that systemic multidrug chemotherapy alone has not altered significantly the natural history and/or prognosis of patients with PSM and CRC. First-line 5-fluorouracil-based regimens (5-FU/leucovorin (LV) including oxaliplatin (FOLFOX) and irinotecan (IFL, FOLFIRI) with or without targeted monoclnal antibody therapy using bevacizumab (IFL/bevacizumab) or cetuximab (Erbitux) have increased response rates to a range of 25–55 % and median overall survival rates from 12 to 24 months compared to the benchmark regimen applied as the standard of practice over the past 40 years (5-FU or 5-FU/LV) [57–65]. A retrospective pooled analysis of over 2,000 study subjects enrolled in the North Central Cancer Treatment Group (NCCTG) Phase III Trials N9741 and N9841 demonstrated a median survival of 12.7 months in patients with peritoneal spread of CRC [66]. Treatment-adjusted analysis showed that patients with PSM and CRC have worse survival compared to patients with advanced CRC and distant metastases without PSM ($p = 0.0006$). Oncological outcome in patients with PSM of CRC origin treated by second line 5-FU + leucovorin + oxaliplatin (FOLFOX) was not significantly improved. Progression-free survival was ~6 months. This is in contradistinction to reported median survival rates between 19 and 63 months in experienced centers using CRS + HIPEC to treat limited PSM of CRC origin (that can be completely resected), underscoring the advantage of this multimodality therapeutic approach [19, 67–69]. Although FOLFOX was found to be superior to irinotecan + 5-FU/leucovorin (IFL) and irinotecan + oxaliplatin (IROX) as first-line therapy in the pooled analysis of the NCCTG trials by Franko et al., no survival benefit was apparent with second line use [66]. Systemic multidrug chemotherapy has not altered the natural history of peritoneal carcinomatosis as patients suffer disease progression and functional deterioration due to visceral obstruction, malignant ascites, and cancer cachexia over a limited median survival [4].

The multimodality therapy approach, using systemic chemotherapy plus aggressive CRS and HIPEC, has shown clearly promising results. The randomized controlled trial (RCT) of Verwaal et al. demonstrated a statistically significant survival advantage for this therapeutic approach [67, 68]. This was an RCT comparing CRS + HIPEC versus 5-FU-based systemic chemotherapy, which demonstrated a significant OS benefit with median survival of 22 months versus 12 months and 2-year survival of 44 % versus 22 %, respectively [67, 68]. *The study also determined that ~5 patients must undergo CRS + HIPEC for one patient to experience survival advantage at 3 years.*

Other studies have shown that patients with PC from CRC treated with chemotherapy alone have a median survival of 5–19 months, whereas those treated with CRS + HIPEC for early PC from CRC have reported median survival in the range of 48–63 months and 5-year survival of ~50 % following complete cytoreduction and HIPEC [4]. This data represents significant progress over the past 20 years for what was once thought to be a preterminal condition for which only palliative intervention was previously considered. It is also important to recognize what data is

Table 5.4 Unanswered questions in the multimodal treatment approach for peritoneal surface malignancy (PSM)

Chemotherapy preoperatively (neoadjuvant setting) followed by CRS + HIPEC versus
CRS + HIPEC alone versus
CRS + HIPEC + intraoperative systemic chemotherapy versus
CRS + HIPEC followed by postoperative chemotherapy (adjuvant setting) versus
Taking all 4 aspects into account: neoadjuvant + CRS + HIPEC + intraoperative chemotherapy + plus adjuvant chemotherapy

CRS cytoreductive surgery, *HIPEC* heated intraperitoneal chemotherapy

needed in order to further advance and optimize this multimodality treatment approach for PC of CRC origin. This is summarized in Table 5.4. One particular interesting consideration is that of neoadjuvant systemic therapy. Response to neoadjuvant therapy can provide important insights into the biology of disease, tumor response to treatment, and surgical decision making in terms of likelihood of achieving complete cytoreduction. Future clinical trials are likely to address this important unanswered question pertaining to the role of neoadjuvant therapy as part of multimodality treatment in PC from CRC [70].

Patient selection is critical in terms of maximizing oncological benefit of multimodality treatment, with the critical determinant being likelihood of achieving complete cytoreduction (CC 0/1). Clinical decision support systems (CDSS) based on specific clinical, pathological, biomarker, and patient data will ultimately facilitate risk stratification, further enable patient selection for CRS + HIPEC, optimize selection of high-risk patients for PC to undergo second look laparotomy, and individualize multimodality therapy in patients with PSM in CRC [71]. One major problem in patients with PSM of CRC origin is that approximately 50 % will have recurrence of disease after treatment [72, 73], which serves as the fundamental basis for performing a second look operation.

Second Look Concept

Key Concept: *Second look laparotomy*: *…a new plan for early intervention in patients with high risk for local-regional recurrence after primary colon cancer surgery…The high incidence of prolonged survival in this group of patients with early definitive intervention supports the concept of maximal benefit in patients with minimal disease.*

– Paul A. Sugarbaker

We have recently reviewed this in detail and will summarize the key points here [20]. Completeness of cytoreduction (CC0/1) and limited peritoneal surface disease (PCI <20) are associated with improved survival following CRS/HIPEC. Importantly, not only is survival improved after CRS + HIPEC for limited PC but also operative morbidity and mortality is significantly reduced because surgery is less extensive. Early peritoneal carcinomatosis is undetectable by conventional imaging or through the use of biomarkers; therein lays the challenge. Second look laparotomy followed by CRS + HIPEC data could only be generated thus far because some groups have performed the so-called second look laparotomy to identify patients that could potentially benefit from second CRS + HIPEC at a time when none of the patients had clinical or radiographic evidence of recurrent PSM [74–76]. The rationale for performing second look laparotomy (generally not laparoscopy, as this modality cannot expose all relevant planes of dissection to ascertain presence of and magnitude of PC) is to identify PSM of CRC origin early in the natural history of the disease in patients at high risk of having disease recurrence. The goal is to identify at-risk patients when tumor volume is below an important clinically detectable threshold, recognizing that completeness of cytoreduction is more readily attained when peritoneal surface disease is of limited extent (PCI <20), where the oncological impact of CRS + HIPEC conducted with curative intent is greatest [37]. As pointed out before [20], the concept of second look operation in cancer is over 60 years old, was probably established in 1948, and first described by Wangensteen in 1949 [5, 77, 78]. Different groups studied the "second look approach" in different tumor types for various indications: cancer staging, palliative treatment in cancer recurrence, and other non-cancer-related diseases, such as mesenteric artery occlusion and in postoperative complication algorithms [5, 27, 72–105]. Esquivel and Sugarbaker investigated a large number of patients with PSM of appendiceal origin during a 12-year period [5, 74]. Out of 321 patients, 98 patients (31 %) underwent second look procedure followed by CRS + HIPEC. The overall 5-year survival rate in these 98 of 321 patients was 74 % compared to 68 % in the remaining 223 of 321 patients. These data clearly show that there is a subpopulation of patients that may benefit from follow-up second look laparotomy and CRS + HIPEC. On the other hand, symptomatic patients, who present with bowel obstruction as a symptom or have a large amount of tumor (PCI >20), have significantly worse survival; hence, patients with a high amount of tumor load have questionable benefit from either second look laparotomy or CRS + HIPEC. In fact, there is no overall survival benefit when CRS is undertaken for patients with PCI exceeding 20 [37]. Maggiori et al. investigated 41 patients with PSM of CRC origin who underwent second look operation and who had no clinical or radiomorphological sign of recurrence at the time of second look. Over half of the patients (23/41, 56 %) underwent subsequent CRS + HIPEC [76]. The reported 5-year overall survival rate was 90 % and 5-year disease-free survival, 44 %. An important finding in this study was that early peritoneal surface recurrence of

CRC could be identified absent clinical or radiomorphological signs of disease at a time in its natural history when the oncological benefit of CRS + HIPEC could be maximized. Importantly at-risk asymptomatic patients can be diagnosed with PSM over 50 % of the time. Sugarbaker focused on clinical parameters to identify these at-risk patient in an effort to improve selection and provide clinical decision support to the surgical oncology community; he published suggestions for guidelines for second look operation [72, 73] The major aim of second look operation is to achieve complete tumor resection (R0 resection, CC 0/1 resection). The limited extent of PC that may be identified during the second look in asymptomatic patients lends itself to completeness of tumor resection, estimation of prognosis, and positively impacting patient outcomes through multimodality therapy, CRS + HIPEC. Therefore, patients with limited local–regional recurrence may have more benefit compared to possibly symptomatic patients with a high tumor burden, PCI. Recently, a group of experts in PSM suggested decision support algorithms for patients presenting for the first time with CRC and for those with recurrent CRC or already scheduled for programmed second look operation, which are discussed in the following section. Patients considered at risk for peritoneal carcinomatosis that may benefit from second look laparotomy include patients with perforated primary tumors (iatrogenic or spontaneous), completely resected synchronous limited PC at initial operation, synchronous ovarian metastases, and possibly T4 lesions that required adjacent organ resection and emergency presentation for obstructing/bleeding lesions that underwent surgery.

Decision Making/Preoperative Work-up

Indications and Interdisciplinary Tumor Board

Key Concept: An important element in patient selection for CRS + HIPEC is careful evaluation of the diagnosis and stage of disease as well as resectability of the peritoneal surface malignancy and operability of the patient; the findings of diagnostic testing must be reviewed by an interdisciplinary tumor board in order to arrive at an individualized plan of care.

A patient-centered, integrated, comprehensive, and evidence-based team approach is a "must" in individual cancer therapy. This individualized care approach to patients afflicted by cancer demands that each patient is carefully evaluated, and the findings of diagnostic testing reviewed collectively by a team that in the venue of an interdisciplinary tumor board arrive at an individualized plan of care. All prior patient reports of any treatment intervention, histopathological review, laboratory parameter dynamics during multimodal treatment, and radiomorphological imaging are mandatory elements requiring review by the team prior to treatment recommendations, which must take into account available best level evidence. In addition to such team members as surgical, medical, and radiation oncologists, radiologists, geneticists, pathologists, psychologists, rehabilitation specialists, nurses, as well as students should be involved as part of the interdisciplinary tumor board. An example of an interdisciplinary tumor board structure is shown in Fig. 5.4. Interactions with external stakeholders in academia, administration, and government are shown.

The indications for CRS + HIPEC in patients with PSM have been reviewed by several authors [27, 96] and are shown in Table 5.5 [96]. Factors to consider in patient selection for CRS + HIPEC include disease-free interval; extra-abdominal metastases; extent of liver metastases; histology of the primary tumor; local–regional tumor burden (PCI); expected completeness of cytoreduction (CC0/1); patient age, comorbidity, and performance status; carcinomatosis-related complications (SBO, ascites); and prior systemic therapy (toxicity, resistance). A recent expert review of CRS + HIPEC for CRC [20] suggested two clinical decision support algorithms for patients presenting with a diagnosis of CRC (Fig. 5.5) and those who present with CRC recurrence or are already planned for programmed second look laparotomy (Fig. 5.6).

Contraindications

Key Concepts: Contraindications to CRS + HIPEC include but are not limited to patient with inability to tolerate the operation (poor performance status), PCI >19, prohibitive medical comorbidities, extra-abdominal metastases, massive retroperitoneal tumor involvement and/or root of mesentery invasion, extensive small bowel disease, >3 liver metastases, and aggressive biology (high grade, signet ring cell).

These can be divided into absolute and relative contraindications [3] (Table 5.6). CRS + HIPEC can only provide survival benefit in patients having good performance status, limited peritoneal surface disease, and those in whom complete cytoreduction is highly likely. Thus, cytoreductive surgery and HIPEC should not be pursued in patients with poor performance status (Karnofsky <70), weight loss ≥10 %, unremitting pain; carcinomatosis-related morbidity (ascites, SBO involving >1 SB segment); prohibitive medical comorbidities (cardiac, pulmonary, renal, hepatic, florid infection); extra-abdominal metastases; massive retroperitoneal involvement or root of mesentery invasion by tumor; extensive small bowel disease (high risk of short-bowel syndrome if resected); unresectable peritoneal disease (PCI ≥20); or aggressive biology (high-grade, signet ring). It is important to note that liver (≤3) metastases and peritoneal disease progression while on chemotherapy are not contraindications for CRS + HIPEC so long as complete cytoreduction can be

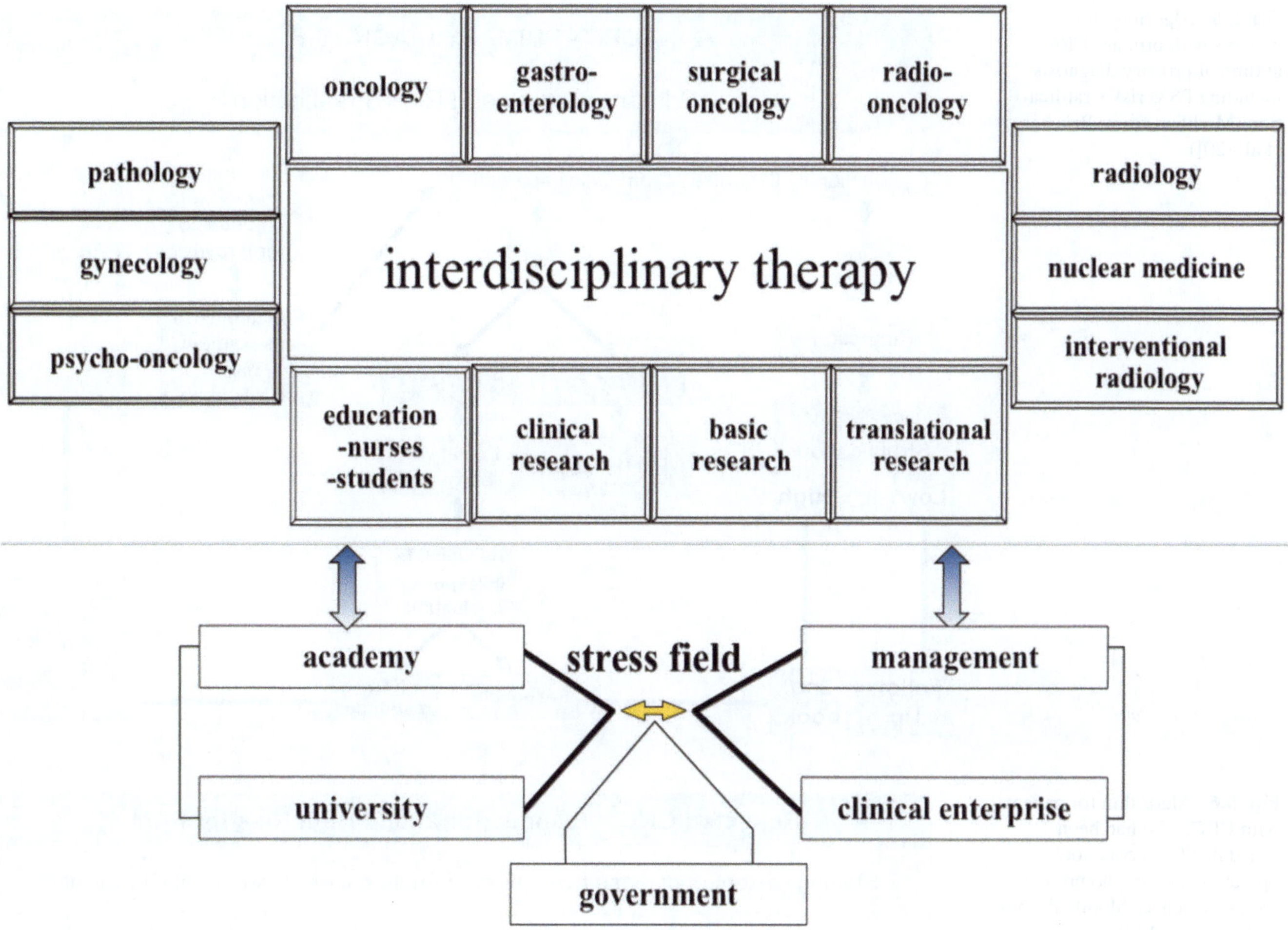

Fig. 5.4 Interdisciplinary tumor board including interactions with academia, administration, and government

Table 5.5 Indications for cytoreductive surgery (CRS) and hyperthermic intraperitoneal chemotherapy (HIPEC)

PSM	Indications
Primary peritoneal neoplasms	Diffuse malignant peritoneal mesothelioma (epitheloid type)
	Well-differentiated peritoneal mesothelioma
	Multicystic peritoneal mesothelioma
	Papillary serous primary peritoneal mesothelioma
	Primary peritoneal adenocarcinoma
Secondary peritoneal neoplasms	Gastrointestinal carcinoma (appendix carcinoma, CRC, small bowel carcinoma, gastric carcinoma, pancreas carcinoma)
	Gynecological/urogenital tumors (e.g., epithelial ovarian cancer)
	Other rare primary tumors with potential peritoneal metastasis (e.g., malignant melanoma, breast cancer, cervix carcinoma, bladder carcinoma)

Modified from Brücher [96]
PSM peritoneal surface malignancy, *CRC* colorectal carcinoma

achieved. CRS is contraindicated in patients with PCI >19, as median survival is no different after CRS/HIPEC than that obtained with systemic therapy alone (~18 months). These decisions in selecting patients for CRS + HIPEC with curative intent are best made in centers of excellence with multidisciplinary teams devoted to the care of patients with PSM.

Quantitative Prognostic Factors (QPIs)

Key Concept: *Cross-sectional and functional imaging with CT and CT/positron emission tomography [PET]) is the first-choice diagnostic test in the work-up of peritoneal carcinomatosis*; *however, these modalities often underestimate*

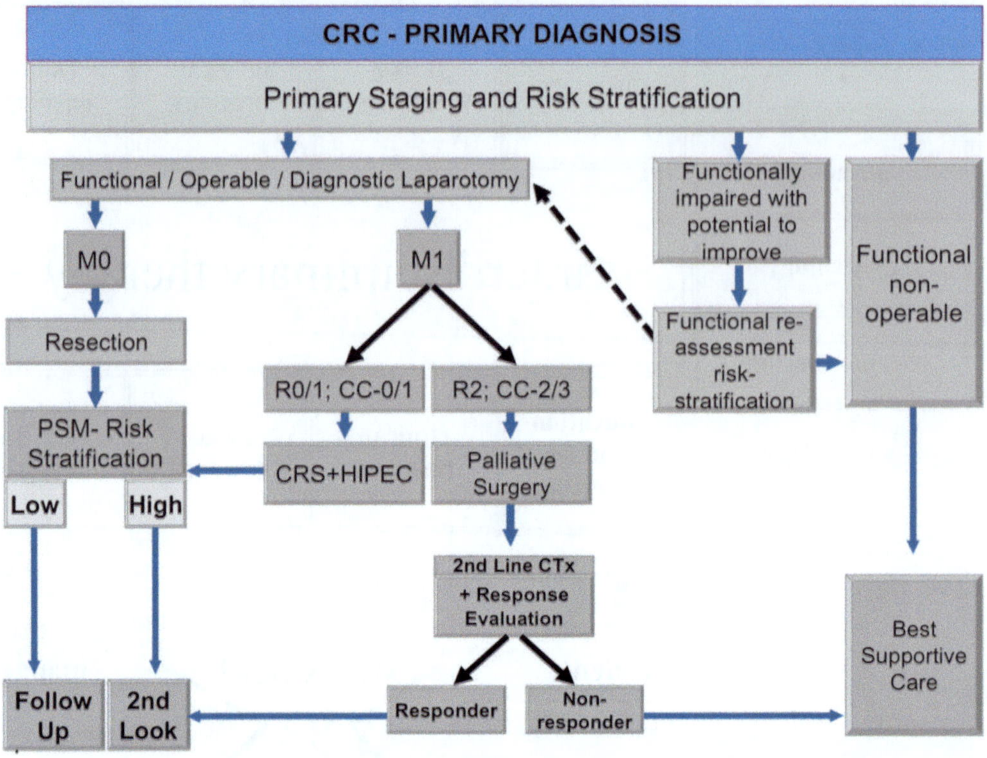

Fig. 5.5 Algorithm for patients with primary CRC at time of primary diagnosis including PSM risk stratification (Modified from: Brücher et al. [20])

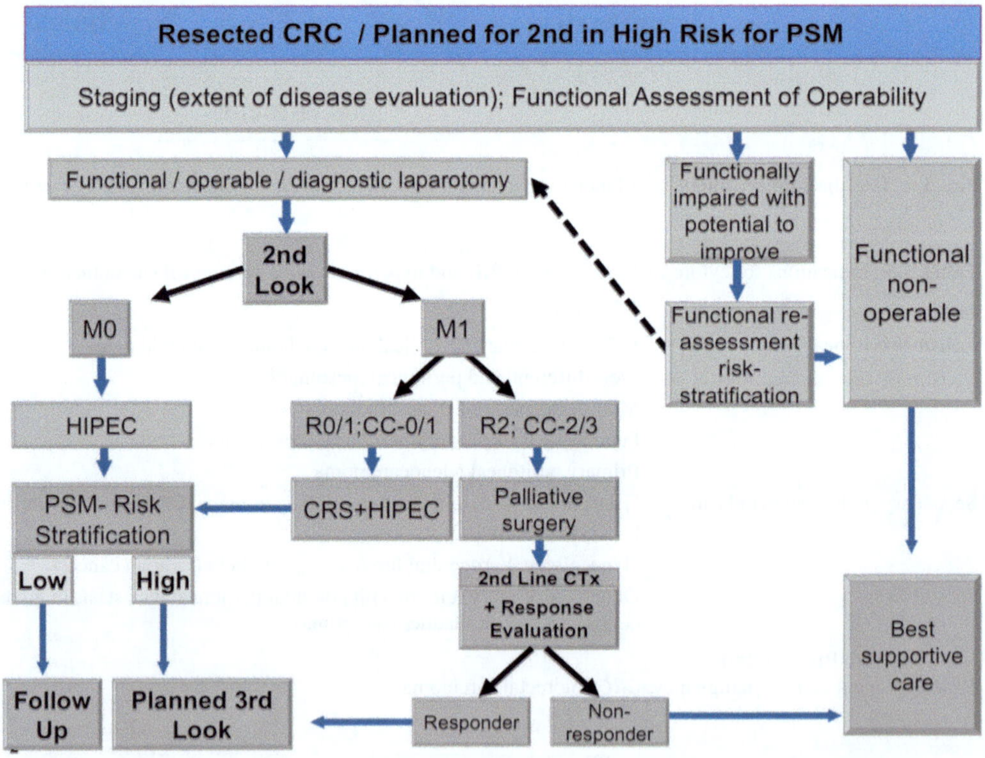

Fig. 5.6 Algorithm for patients with CRC, who had been scheduled for second look operation and/or who present with recurrence (Modified from Brücher et al. [20])

preoperative PCI necessitating laparoscopic or open laparotomy staging of extent of disease in order to determine likelihood of CC0/1.

Clinically very important are quantitative prognostic indicators (QPIs) [3], although the quality of the evidence supporting their use in clinical practice varies from one tumor entity to another and high-level published evidence is sometimes lacking. No data are available on tumor markers as qualitative prognostic markers in PSM. With regard to histopathology, the only available data show that patients

Table 5.6 Absolute and relative contraindications to cytoreductive surgery (CRS) and hyperthermic intraperitoneal chemotherapy (HIPEC)

Absolute contraindications
Massive involvement of the retroperitoneum
Invasion of the mesenteric pedicle
Massive small-bowel involvement (that would result in a short bowel after radical resection)
Unresectable intra-abdominal and/or extra-abdominal metastases
Incurable second malignancy
Karnofsky index <70
Relative contraindications
High body mass index
Cardiac contraindication
Hepatic contraindication
Renal contraindication
Florid infection
Acute ileus

Modified from Brücher et al. [3]

with poorer differentiation (high-grade, signet ring cell) have worse prognosis than those with well/moderately differentiated cancers. The value of preoperative cross-sectional imaging (CT, MRI) appears to be limited to patients with mucinous PSM. Our own research on the use of preoperative ^{18}F-fluorodeoxyglucose-positron emission tomography and computed tomography (FDG-PET/CT) scanning in comparison with the intraoperative PCI score shows that it has prognostic value [36]. The Sugarbaker PCI score ($P<0.0001$) and CC score ($P<0.001$) are both clinically relevant prognostic factors in PSM of CRC origin [41].

Ethical Considerations

Key Concept: We must do our best to inform our patients and to enhance their comprehension about their disease and prognosis; most importantly to communicate to them our best estimate of likelihood of cure of their disease.

Independent of the underlying cancer leading to PSM, our society has a kind of Zeitgeist: that peritoneal carcinomatosis means "death soon." This follows decades of therapeutic nihilism for this stage of cancer. Treatment of patients who suffer from peritoneal carcinomatosis is a burden for both patient and provider, for it is a formidable problem and the treatment is extensive in nature and burdensome itself. This was, is, and always will be a situation that tests our forbearance, our resolve, and at times our faith, as we are often confronted at times with malignancy and intervene at the crossroads of potentially curative and palliative treatment in the face of incompletely defined tumor biology. Combating PSM means being aware about areas of potential ethical conflict: informed consent, treatment refusal, treatment waiver, decision-making ability, capacity to consent, truth at the bedside, truth in the OR, the ICU, confidentiality, research on patients, termination of life-sustaining measures, preserving hope while communicating the actual implications of clinical findings, among others. Dealing with the diagnosis of PSM means to be aware that we must often confront life-limiting challenges. The philosopher *Epikur* (341–270 ante Christi) stated "Ars moriendi ars vivendi" meaning *the art of dying is the art of living*. This refers to the process of how to die well and can lead one to conclude that terms such as palliative care, supportive care, or terminal care are second rate and inconsistent with that ethos. Ethics has as one of its main tenets that humans have the freedom to decide. It has been shown that patients with advanced malignancy are willing to accept high-risk interventions and toxic treatments for a slight (even 1 %) chance of cancer cure; at the same time, most patients would not accept such therapy without cure, even if it may significantly increase anticipated survival [97]. A recent study of patients participating in the Cancer Care Outcomes Research and Surveillance (CanCORS) study found that over 80 % of those with CRC did not report understanding that chemotherapy was unlikely to cure their cancer. The authors concluded that "many patients receiving chemotherapy for incurable cancers may not understand that chemotherapy is unlikely to be curative, which could compromise their ability to make informed treatment decisions that are consonant with their preferences" [97]. It is our ethical obligation as human beings and physicians to do our best to inform our patients and to enhance their comprehension about their disease, even if the patient's satisfaction with the health-care provider and or system is negatively impacted.

Intraoperative Work-up

Cytoreductive Surgery: Logistics, Strategy, and Technique

Key Concepts: High-voltage electrosurgery is utilized for cytoreduction of peritoneal surface malignancy, thereby generating a significant amount of smoke during the procedure which necessitates the use of proper operating room ventilation and a smoke evacuator system used continuously over the surgical field. Heated intraperitoneal chemotherapy is safe for the surgical team and operating room personnel as chemotherapy exposure is negligible, particularly with adherence to universal precautions, and environmental/individual protective measures.

Cytoreductive surgery is a major operation including multiple visceral resections and stripping of peritoneal surfaces. Complex surgical maneuvers such as liver mobilization or full exploration of the omental bursa including the upper recess (the area between the right crura of the diaphragm, liver, and vena cava) and the foramen of Winslow are mandatory to establish CC-0/1 [98]. Therefore, even in the face of limited peritoneal surface disease, cytoreduction is considered a complex abdominal operation and requires a dedicated team and adherence to a comprehensive, standardized preoperative preparation protocol. The HIPEC procedure puts the operating room (OR) and intensive care unit (ICU) personnel within unfamiliar territory at outside their proverbial "comfort zone." Even in high-volume cancer centers, handling and delivering cytotoxic agents is not a routine in most ORs. Therefore, careful planning and detailed preparation, transport, administration, disposal, and safety protocols should be followed in order to avoid errors risking the patient or OR staff.

Preoperative planning is conducted in two levels. The first level is oncological and the second level is technical.

Oncological Planning

Oncological planning was outlined before ("Indications") and includes:

(a) Indication for surgery (disease type, disease status, PCI)
(b) Lack of contraindications (extraperitoneal disease, PCI >20, >3 liver metastases, poor performance status)
(c) Surgical history (prior surgical procedures for PSM or resection of primary tumor)
(d) Oncological history (date of diagnosis, age at diagnosis, stage at primary diagnosis, prior treatments delivered, and response evaluation)

In most centers this is done in a tumor board setting and discussed by a multidisciplinary team. In patients that are found to be eligible for CRS + HIPEC, the HIPEC protocol is decided upon and the patient is then scheduled for surgery.

Technical Planning

This is done by a dedicated team including surgical oncologist, anesthesiologist, ICU specialist, medical oncology, OR nurse, nutrition nurse, stoma nurse, pharmacy, and perfusionist.

The procedure is planned according to the following parameters:

Surgical Planning

Type of Disease

Diseases such as disseminated peritoneal adenomucinosis (DPAM) or benign cystic mesothelioma tend to adhere to organs and not to penetrate into the tissue; therefore, they require less visceral resections and result in less surgical trauma and consequent operative morbidity. Other diseases such as serous papillary adenocarcinoma of the ovary or adenocarcinoma of the colon are more likely to penetrate into organs and tissues and as a result require more visceral resections, and the extent of surgical trauma and attendant morbidity are higher [99].

Extent and Location of Disease

The complexity of the procedure, its success, and the rate of postoperative complications are highly correlated with extent of disease as measured by PCI [100]. Volume of disease and location of disease require careful consideration for detailed surgical and anesthetic planning as they may impact postoperative course and recovery. For example, large volume of disease located between the right lobe of the liver and right diaphragm requires liver mobilization and retraction that may result in periods of low blood pressure as a result of vena caval compression. Full stripping of the diaphragm requires the insertion of a chest drain in order to avoid postoperative pleural effusions. Another example is tumor in the abdominal wall. Disease recurrence in surgical scars is common in patients with PSM [101]. When abdominal wall tumor masses exist, careful surgical planning of abdominal wall resection and reconstruction is required.

Approach to "Critical Lesions"

Lesions that are located in places that may have a significant impact on the course or outcome of surgery are defined as "critical lesions." It is important to distinguish between lesions that will prevent surgery (as part of exclusion criteria or contraindications to surgery) and "critical lesions." In surgical planning, lesions located in the following areas should be considered critical:

1. *Liver hilum*: Dissection of the liver hilum is time-consuming and may be associated with increased risk of hemorrhage.
2. *Upper recess of lesser sac*: Resection of lesions located in this area is technically demanding. Various solutions exist including full mobilization of the liver off the retrohepatic vena cava and approach from the right side, distal control in the mediastinum by creating a window in the diaphragm and more.
3. *Third portion of the duodenum or lesions invading the head of the pancreas*: Careful assessment of such lesions should be conducted in order to avoid dissection that will eventually lead to pancreaticoduodenectomy.
4. *Pancreatic capsule and hilum of spleen*: Such lesions may lead to pancreatic injury and fistula formation.
5. *Retroperitoneum*: Although retroperitoneal disease is a contraindication for CRS + HIPEC, in many cases, the peritoneal planes were violated by previous surgery, and as a result, peritoneal disease invades the retroperitoneum. In such cases, if complete cytoreduction is achievable, the prognosis of the patients is expected to be the same as disease limited to the abdomen/peritoneal cavity. However, in such patients, ureteral or vascular involvement should be carefully assessed and adequate measures taken including ureteral stenting, planning of ureteral resection and reimplantation, and the possibility of vascular encasement or involvement requiring vascular procedures.
6. *Pelvic sidewall*: Much like the retroperitoneum, the pelvic sidewall is rarely invaded by tumor deposits in surgery naive patients. However, following pelvic surgery, ureteral

Table 5.7 Suggestions for hyperthermic intraperitoneal chemotherapy (HIPEC) + early postoperative intraperitoneal chemotherapy (EPIC) – EPIC protocols in adenocarcinoma of the appendix (including pseudomyxoma peritonei) and the colon

(a) Adenocarcinoma of the appendix (including pseudomyxoma peritonei)		
Agent	Mitomycin C	
Dose	15 mg/m^2	At time 0
Second dose	5 mg/m^2	At 45 min
Perfusion duration	90 min	
Inflow temp.	44 °C	
(b) Adenocarcinoma of the colon (Protocol #1)		
Agent 1	i.v. 5-flourouracil	10 min before perfusion
Dose	400 mg/m^2	
	i.v. leucovorin	60 min before perfusion
Dose	20 mg/m^2	
Agent 2	Mitomycin C	
Dose	15 mg/m^2	At time 0
Second dose	5 mg/m^2	At 45 min
Perfusion duration	90 min	
Inflow temp.	44 °C	
(c) Adenocarcinoma of the colon (Protocol #2)		
Agent 1	i.v. 5-flourouracil	10 min before perfusion
Dose	400 mg/m^2	
	i.v. leucovorin	60 min before perfusion
Dose	20 mg/m^2	
Agent 2	Oxaliplatin	(In D5W)
Dose	460 mg/m^2	At time 0
Perfusion duration	60 min	
Inflow temp.	44 °C	

or vascular involvement should be carefully assessed and the adequate measures taken including ureteral stenting, planning of ureteral resection and reimplantation, and the possibility of vascular encasement or involvement requiring vascular procedures.

Abdominal Wall Assessment

Abdominal wall assessment is important for surgical planning. Not only the presence, but the location and size of tumor deposits in the abdominal wall, as well as the location of previous scars including trocar sites and drain sites should be taken into consideration and excised; prior midline scar excision includes umbilicus excision. Hernias, either incisional or inguinal-femoral, may harbor tumor deposits and should be recognized and later, during surgery, addressed in a fashion that hernia sacs are completely excised and hernia defects repaired. It is not only important for the prevention of postoperative wound dehiscence, but also for those who use closed perfusion technique for HIPEC, it is important to close all incisions in a way that the chemotherapy cannot leak during perfusion. Therefore, careful history and review of operative reports, physical examination, and detailed review of all cross-sectional imaging is essential for abdominal wall assessment.

Approach to Liver Metastasis

If up to three liver metastases are present, then according to the PSOG consensus statement, the patient is eligible for CRS + HIPEC. In such cases, it is important to carefully calculate the volume of the remaining liver since a "small for size" liver will not only be the result of previous chemotherapy delivered but may also be a result of HIPEC. Intraoperative ultrasound is used to define the location of the liver lesions and to rule out additional lesions missed by the cross-sectional imaging, which can occur in up to 15–20 % of cases that would lead to reconsideration of the intended operation.

For the surgical evaluation high-resolution CT can provide sufficient data, in most cases PET-CT will provide the data required for surgical planning combined with its more important role, to rule out extraperitoneal disease. In selected cases, MRI or MR angiogram (MRA) is required. Staging laparoscopy is used routinely by some, but in most centers, it is used for selected cases both for exclusion of patients and for better operative planning [102].

HIPEC Planning

Most centers use closed HIPEC and some use early postoperative IP chemotherapy (EPIC) protocols (see Table 5.7a–c for suggested protocols in adenocarcinoma of the appendix

Table 5.8 Preoperative testing for cytoreductive surgery (CRS) and hyperthermic intraperitoneal chemotherapy (HIPEC)

Test	Author group	International survey	Comments
CBC	All patients	100 %	
Chemistry	All patients	100 %	Including LFT and RFT
PT–PTT	All patients	100 %	
Blood type and cross	All patients	100 %	
EKG	Age >40 years	93 %	
Chest X-ray	Age >40 years	Not reported	
PFT	Age >40 years	28 %	Asthma or heavy smoker at all ages
Carotid duplex	Age >40 years	Not reported	
Echocardiogram	Age >40 years	24 %	Patients exposed to cardiotoxic agents at any age
Stress test for thallium dipyridamole	Age >40 years	Not reported	Patients exposed to cardiotoxic agents at any age

Modified from Bell et al. [103]
LFT liver function tests, *RFT* renal function tests, *PFT* pulmonary function tests

including pseudomyxoma peritonei and the colon). However, each patient should undergo individual assessment by the CRS/HIPEC team including validation of weight and height, calculation of body surface area, and careful evaluation of:

(a) Prior chemotherapy regimens delivered with special attention to response and toxicity.
(b) Renal, liver, and cardiac function that may necessitate dose modifications.
(c) Dose adjustments should be made for age and comorbid conditions.

After the appropriate protocol is decided upon by the medical and surgical oncologists and all dose modifications are made, the pharmacist, perfusionist, anesthesiologist, and ICU specialist are all informed about the HIPEC ± EPIC protocols to be used. In our practice, the final cytotoxic prescription is written by the medical oncologist and the orders in the patient's chart are signed by the surgical oncologist.

Anesthesia Planning

Preoperative planning of anesthesia is no different than in every major surgical procedure. By careful history and physical examination, the anesthesiologist can define the operative risk using the ASA classification. Because of the duration of the procedure, the major surgical trauma, and the delivery of chemotherapy, additional tests are routinely applied in most centers. Bell et al. from the Basingstoke group reviewed the perioperative management of patients in medical centers experienced in CRS + HIPEC [103]: anesthesiologists in 41 centers were asked to participate in a web-based questionnaire—the data was completed by 29 centers with a cumulative experience in almost 8,500 patients. In Table 5.8, we summarized the preoperative testing conducted in our center and combined it with the findings of the Basingstoke group's international survey.

Patients with large volume pseudomyxoma peritonei may have elevated abdominal pressure resulting in reduced functional residual lung capacity leading to a difficulty in ventilation and may also have low venous return to the heart leading to drop in blood pressure during induction of anesthesia or during surgery. Therefore, they all should undergo maximal cardiac and respiratory evaluation before surgery regardless of age.

Nutritional Planning

The general underlying working hypothesis is that all patients undergoing CRS + HIPEC are malnourished. Therefore, nutritional evaluation is conducted to record the level of malnourishment. History and physical examination are the most important. Recent weight loss as percentage of current body weight is essential. Body mass index (BMI), serum albumin, and prealbumin are of less importance unless albumin or prealbumin are very low. In such cases, preoperative nutritional support is recommended. Total parenteral nutrition (TPN) is selectively used by most centers until caloric requirements can be met via the enteral route. In our practice, dedicated central venous access line (PICC line) for TPN is inserted routinely, and TPN is used in all patients until oral diet resumed.

Stoma Planning

All patients are evaluated by a stoma nurse. Detailed education is the initial step followed by physical examination and marking (with the patient in the upright position is the best location for both ileostomy and colostomy). It is of great importance to choose the location of the stoma away from old surgical scars or port sites to be resected during operation.

Perioperative Antibiotic Prophylaxis

All patients undergoing cytoreduction and HIPEC must be covered by IV broad-spectrum antibiotics. In our practice a second-generation cephalosporin + metronidazole are given with induction of anesthesia (30 min before skin incision), re-dosed intraoperatively, and given for up to 5 days if HIPEC is administered. This protocol is modified in cases of allergies or in case of in-hospital infection with bacteria resistant to one of the antibiotic drugs, with resistance documented within the past 6 months.

Venous Thromboembolism Prophylaxis

Subcutaneous low molecular heparin is administrated starting 12 h before surgery until 30 days post-discharge from the hospital.

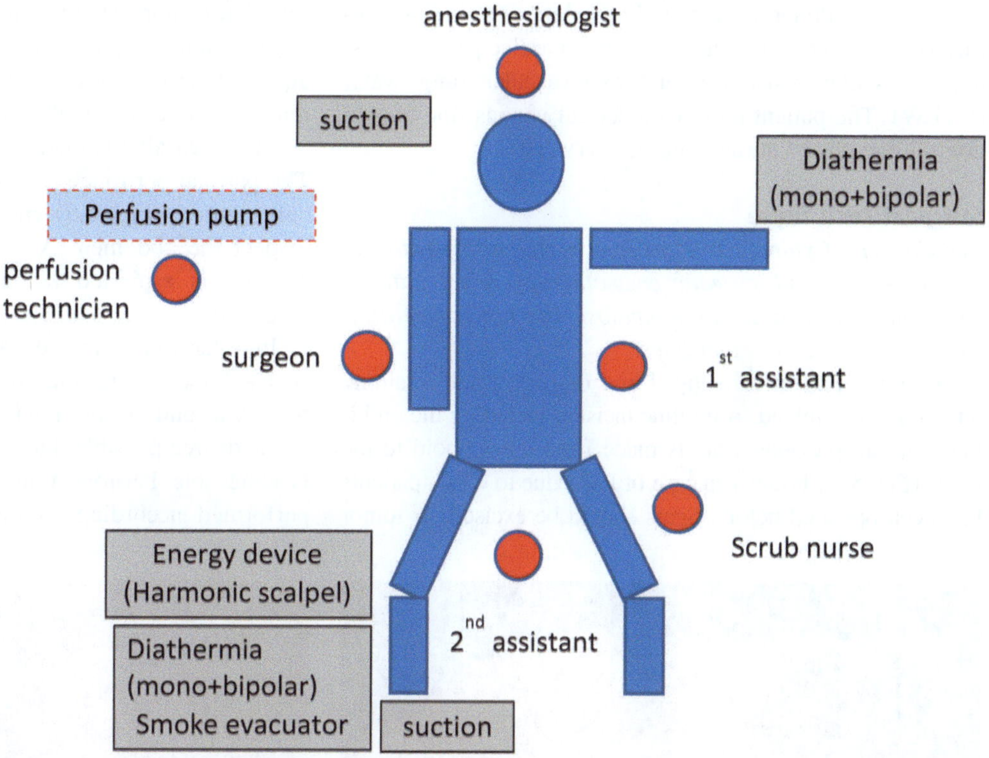

Fig. 5.7 Patient positioning for CRS + HIPEC

Mechanical Bowel Preparation

Patients with PSM undergoing CRS + HIPEC are prone to infections due to multifactorial immunosuppression. Therefore, unlike many patients undergoing colonic resections, patients before CRS should undergo bowel preparation. Mechanical bowel preparation combined with oral neomycin and metronidazole is practiced by most centers.

Skin Preparation

In several centers, mainly in Europe, the patient is washed by several antiseptic solutions and following shower is dressed with a paper-sterile gown.

Operating Room

In many centers combined general and thoracic epidural are used. After the insertion of the epidural catheter and induction of anesthesia, the following invasive monitoring lines are inserted:

- Arterial line
- High-flow central line
- Femoral and jugular lines for PiCCO® monitoring
- Esophageal thermometer
- Urinary bladder thermometer

The patient is positioned on a temperature control device (CritiCool® Systems, MTRE™, Mennen Medical Corp, Feasterville-Trevose, PA, USA). The patient is wrapped by a blanket containing fluid at a certain temperature set by the operator. By multi-temperature sensing, the temperature of the patient is managed at a level set by the anesthesiologist. During the HIPEC procedure, the device is used to cool the patient achieving a fixed temperature of 37 °C for the entire procedure. By using this microprocessor-controlled temperature management unit, using feedback from the patient's core and skin temperature sensors, the proprietary control algorithm responds by modifying water temperature such that patient target temperature will be achieved precisely.

Induction of Anesthesia and Monitoring

In most patients, induction of anesthesia is no different than for any other major abdominal operation. However, in patients with pseudomyxoma peritonei or large intra-abdominal tumor masses, large quantity of mucin or ascites, rapid sequence intubation is recommended due to increased risk of aspiration. Another important consideration in such patients is decreased venous return to the heart due to inferior vena caval compression resulting in a sudden drop in blood pressure [104].

Following induction of general endotracheal anesthesia and multiple line placements, the patient is positioned in the lithotomy position (Fig. 5.7). Intermittent compression stockings are applied to the lower extremities of all patients and activated from entrance to the operating room until the fifth postoperative day. Positioning, padding points of pressure, and securing location of lines and devices are carefully confirmed before the patient is draped.

Hemodynamic monitoring during the procedure is essential. Some centers use advanced hemodynamic monitoring such as LIDCO® (LidcoLtD, Cambridge, UK) [105] or NICOM® (Cheeta Medical™, Tel Aviv, Israel) [106] with less invasive nature or the pulse-induced contour cardiac output (PiCCO®, Philips Healthcare, Andover, MA, USA). This is a device that quantifies several parameters, including continuous (pulse contour) cardiac output, cardiac preload, systemic vascular resistance, and extravascular lung water (EVLW). The patient requires a central venous line and an arterial line placed in the femoral artery [107].

Surgical Technique

Key Concept: *Cytoreductive surgery, heated intraperitoneal chemotherapy, and systemic chemotherapy select patients with colorectal cancer carcinomatosis are not competitive, rather complementary therapies.*

After the patient is prepped and draped, a self-retaining retractor is assembled. A midline incision including the umbilicus and all previous scars is made from the xiphoid to the pubis (Fig. 5.8). Usually in case of PSM due to CRC, patients had been operated before. Scars should be excised, as tumor cells can be implanted within those. If a patient had a former median midline laparotomy from the xiphoid to the pubis, the umbilicus needs to be excised also. The completion of the laparotomy is done later to allow a complete abdominal exposure.

The linea alba is opened keeping the peritoneum intact. The parietal peritoneum is then stripped down to the paracolic gutters (Fig. 5.9) and a small window is created to inspect the abdomen. Adhesions are lysed and mucin, if present, is aspirated using a large-caliber suction tube (Fig. 5.10).

In order to have the best available exposure, large masses such as bulky ovarian metastasis or omental cake are removed first. A second exploration is then made in order to be certain to the degree possible that complete cytoreduction (CC 0/1) is achievable. Peritonectomy procedures (Table 5.9) are then performed according to the methods described by P.H.

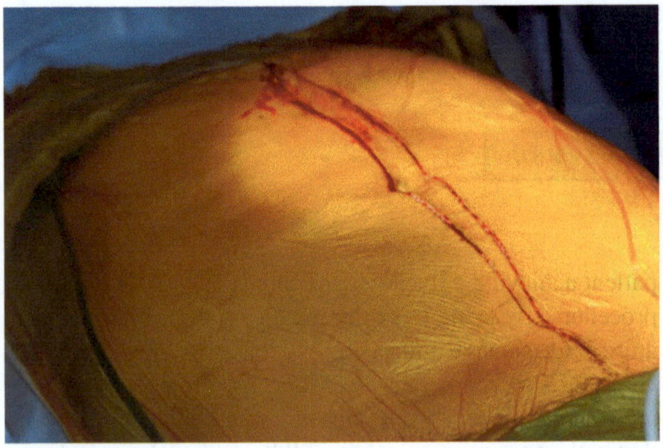

Fig. 5.8 Midline abdominal incision

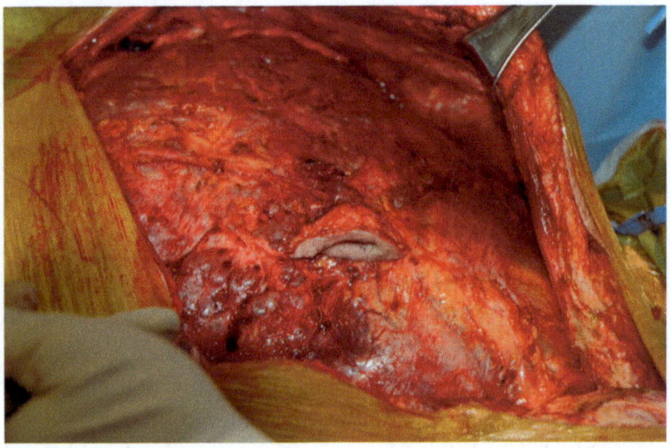

Fig. 5.9 Extraperitoneal dissection to the paracolic gutters

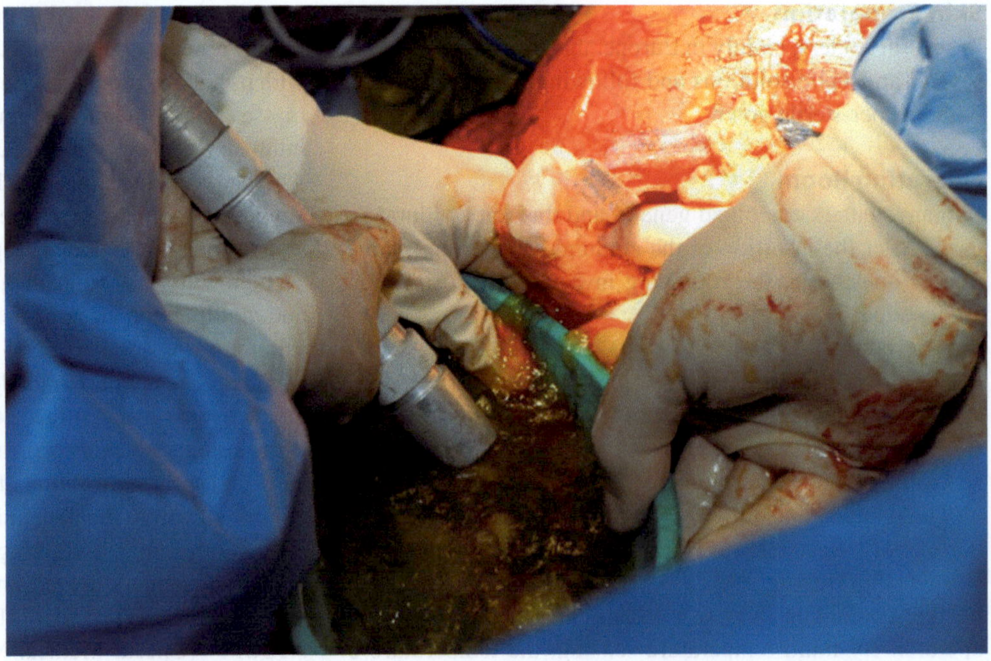

Fig. 5.10 Aspiration of mucin using a large-caliber suction tube

Table 5.9 Surgical resections in peritoneal surface malignancies (PSM) differentiated into parietal and visceral procedures (when possible)

Parietal peritoneal stripping of the anterior abdominal wall including surgical scars
Parietal left subphrenic (diaphragmatic) peritonectomy (± splenectomy)
Parietal right subphrenic (diaphragmatic) peritonectomy
Visceral peritoneal dissection at the falciform ligament at the round ligament of the liver and the Glisson's capsule
Visceral peritoneal dissection of the Ligamentum Terres including opening the hepatic bridge between right and left liver lobe at the umbilical fissure
Parietal left middle abdominal parietal stripping including paracolic gutter
Parietal right middle abdominal parietal stripping including paracolic gutter
Parietal peritonectomy of Morison' pouch
Omentectomy (greater omentum) with resection of the gastrocolic ligament
Omentectomy (minor omentum) ± cholecystectomy, dissection of the hepatoduodenal ligament and/or dissection of the infradiaphragmatic retro-hepatic caval area
Visceral peritoneal stripping of the bladder
Multivisceral resection of stomach, small bowel, colon (ascending, transverse, descending, or sigmoid colon), rectum, uterus, ovary, and/or vagina

Modified from Brücher et al. [3]

Sugarbaker and anastomoses completed prior to HIPEC per surgeon preference [108].

Cytoreductive surgery in PSM does not mean complete routine stripping of the peritoneal wall; it means to resect the tumor-involved areas only. Due to former operations, any adhesions have to be cleared, the liver as well as the mesenteric root has to be mobilized completely, and areas of potential pitfalls have to be cleared as well such as the retro-hepatic caval area, hepatoduodenal ligament, umbilical fissure, etc. as indicated. After completion of adhesiolysis, the parietal peritonectomy can be performed in parts: ventral wall, left and right upper quadrant, as well as middle right and left abdominal peritoneum and pelvis. Sugarbaker described 6 peritonectomy procedures:

1. Total anterior parietal peritonectomy
2. Greater omentectomy [with or without splenectomy]
3. Right subphrenic peritonectomy
4. Left subphrenic peritonectomy
5. Pelvic peritonectomy
6. Lesser omentectomy with or without cholecystectomy

The parietal peritonectomy procedures usually do not require blood replacement. Afterwards, additional visceral required cytoreductive surgical procedures can be performed. It remains the choice of the surgeon whether to perform anastomosis before or after HIPEC. We suggest a double-sutured hand anastomosis. In the case of a high-risk low rectal anastomosis, it might be necessary to perform a fecal diversion or a defunctioning stoma. This stoma can be closed within 3 months after postoperative recovery and prior to commencing further adjuvant chemotherapy, in case it is needed.

After the parietal peritonectomy and the necessary visceral resections, HIPEC is administered. For the coliseum technique, the ventral wall is sutured onto the retractor system and lifted up. Afterwards, the drains (from the HIPEC machine to the patient and those from the patient to the machine) are inserted. After the HIPEC is completed with all the necessary documentation of patient temperatures, the abdomen is usually washed out with 8–10 L of saline. A summary of the possible surgical resections in PSM differentiated into parietal and visceral procedures (when possible) is shown in Table 5.9.

Perioperative Chemotherapy

Preparation for perfusion should start 2 h before estimated time of perfusion. Urine output should be measured every 15 min with a minimum requirement of 25 mL in 15 min. Urine output may be increased by using low dose furosemide or by a drip of dopamine at a low diuretic dose. The patient's temperature should be maintained between 35 and 37 °C. Using a standard heating device may create a challenge to keeping the temperature in this range; on the other hand, use of a multisensor temperature control device with both warming and cooling capabilities makes temperature-keeping a lot easier.

In centers that use concomitant systemic 5-FU and leucovorin, intravenous (IV) folinic acid (leucovorin) is administrated 1 h before IV administration of 5-flourouracil. Following the administration of IV 5-flourouracil, the patient is connected to the perfusion device and perfusion with 0.9 % NaCl is commenced (we use the closed method). Platinum compounds such as cisplatinum or oxaliplatinum are best preserved in D5W solution, but in the short-term (30–60 min) delivery of these compounds in the HIPEC setting, the amount of the degradation of the drug in 0.9 % NaCl is minimal. If perfusion is conducted using D5W, hyponatremia should be prevented by intravenous administration of 0.9 % NaCl solution.

Temperature is measured by five probes (Fig. 5.11):

(a) Patient esophageal probe
(b) Patient bladder probe (tissue heating probe)
(c) Device (heat exchanger)
(d) Inflow
(e) Outflow

Average temperature is calculated as $T_{\text{inflow}} + T_{\text{outflow}}/2$

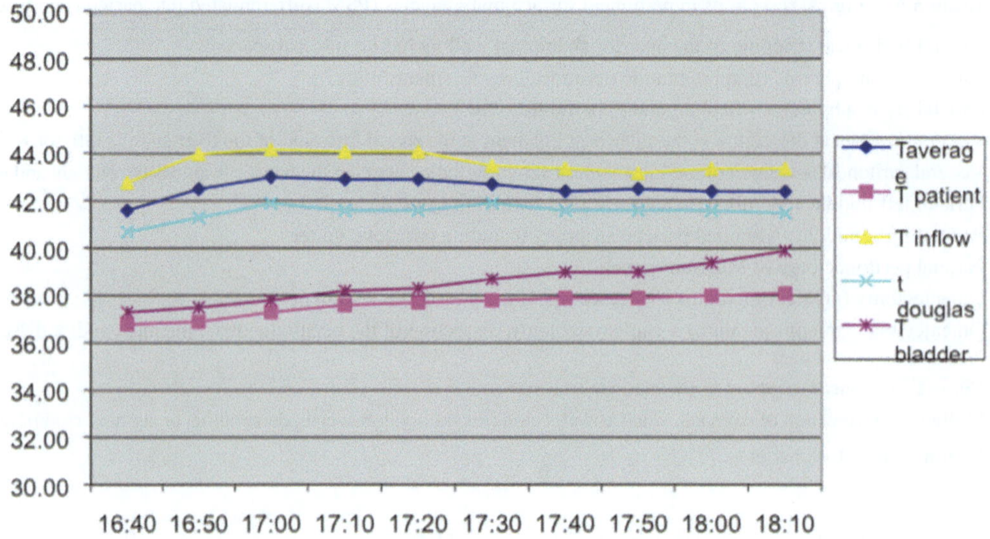

Fig. 5.11 Five-probe temperature monitoring output

Once inflow temperature of 44 °C and average temperature is above 41 °C, chemotherapy is added to the reservoir and HIPEC commences. All team members present in the operating theater are dressed with eye protection, masks, waterproof gowns, and non-permeable gloves in accordance with institutional safety standards [109, 110].

In the closed technique, it is advised to measure intra-abdominal pressure by a catheter introduced into the peritoneal cavity before closure connected to a transducer and a monitor. Intra-abdominal pressure should not exceed 25 mmHg.

At this point antiemetics are administrated in order to prevent postoperative nausea and vomiting.

At the end of the HIPEC procedure, all waste is disposed into special containers designated for cytotoxic disposal and marked accordingly.

The patient is transferred to the ICU where cytotoxic isolation of all secretions is maintained for additional 72 h.

Early Postoperative Intraperitoneal Chemotherapy (EPIC)

Administration of EPIC is done in most centers in the ICU or in step-down units. Delivery of EPIC can be performed either through the HIPEC inflow and outflow tubes left at the time of surgery or through a peritoneal port inserted at the time of surgery. EPIC protocols vary between institutions; though in most cases, 5-day protocols incorporating an agent such as 5-flourouracil are different then when the cytotoxic agents perfused during HIPEC are selected.

Complete CRS Not Achievable: What Now?

The completeness of cytoreduction is classified according to the CC score [41] and CC 0/1 is the goal of CRS. If it is clear that a CC 0/1 resection cannot be achieved, then there is certainly no role for HIPEC. The outcome of CC 2/3 resection for PSM of CRC origin, in terms of overall survival, is no different than with systemic therapy alone. Hence, no major cytoreductive procedure should be undertaken. If visceral obstruction is present, a stoma should be avoided if possible and bypass operation should be considered. Any kind of additional operation, particularly splenectomy, cholecystectomy, or other multivisceral operation is not indicated when complete cytoreduction cannot be attained. If there is diffuse gastric involvement by tumor, a percutaneous gastrostomy tube should be considered along with jejunostomy feeding tube placement.

Postoperative Considerations

Key Concept: Cytoreductive surgery and HIPEC requires an experienced and dedicated team within a center of excellence committed to the care of patients with peritoneal surface malignancy. In the best of hands, operative morbidity (Grade 3 and 4) and mortality are ~30 and 3 %, respectively.

Morbidity and Mortality

Key Concept: The goal is to identify patients with peritoneal carcinomatosis early in the course of their disease, as postoperative morbidity and mortality are significantly lower when the extent of peritoneal disease is low, because operation is less extensive on this basis. CRS + HIPEC is a very complex surgical endeavor with a steep learning curve (~150 cases for attaining acceptable competence including adequate radicality of resection and acceptable operative morbidity and mortality). These complex operations should

Table 5.10 Complications that can occur after cytoreductive surgery (CRS) and hyperthermic intraperitoneal chemotherapy (HIPEC) in patients with peritoneal surface malignancy (PSM) [115–117]

Metachronous peritoneal carcinomatosis ($P=0.009$)
Peritoneal carcinomatosis index ≥13 ($P=0.012$)
Five or more affected regions ($P=0.04$)
Incomplete initial cytoreductive surgery ($P=0.035$)
Blood transfusion requirements due to intraoperative blood loss ($P=0.28$)
Three or more anastomoses ($P=0.018$)

be conducted in dedicated centers of excellence with adequate experience in CRS+HIPEC.

According to the literature, the postoperative morbidity rates ranges from 14 to 40 % [38, 111–115]. The major concern in the postoperative morbidity of patients after CRS+HIPEC is that it is substantially different from the familiar morbidity/mortality associated with other so-called traditional surgical procedures. Pain as one of the major signs of perioperative morbidity typically does not occur after peritonectomy when complications develop. Patients with complications are usually identified clinically due to fatigue, failure to progress, fever, tachycardia, or leukocytosis or thrombocytosis. Simultaneous pancytopenia occurring after HIPEC may aggravate the situation even more. A heightened awareness and index of suspicion as well as aggressive postoperative diagnostic approach are absolutely necessary, because the central symptom of potential postoperative morbidity "pain" is seldom reported after peritonectomy.

Cytoreductive surgery with HIPEC is associated with high morbidity and mortality in the range 0–12 % (Table 5.10). The high morbidity and mortality are related to the extent of surgery, the effects of perioperative chemotherapy, effects of hyperthermia, and to the impaired immune response of patients with metastatic disease and prior systemic chemotherapy. In a recent publication, Glehen et al. [118] presented data from 25 French-speaking institutions reporting morbidity and mortality after 1,344 cytoreductive surgery and HIPEC procedures or early EPIC conducted in 1,290 patients with peritoneal carcinomatosis from non-gynecologic malignancies. They found Grades 3 and 4 complications in 403 patients (34 %) with reoperation rate of 14 %, enterocutaneous fistula in 10 %, bleeding in 8 %, intra-abdominal abscess in 7 %, and sever neutropenia in 13 % of patients. The mean hospital stay was 24 ± 17 days. They identified three significant risk factors for complication: age, extent of disease (PCI), and institution (low volume). A report from an international registry of 506 patients reported a mortality of 4 % and severe morbidity of 23 %, with GI fistula occurring in 8 % [119]. Another recent report of 2,298 patients treated at 16 high-volume centers with CRS+HIPEC for pseudomyxoma peritonei [120] cited treatment-related mortality in 2 % and major operative complications in 24 %.

There are many reports of complications associated with CRS+HIPEC, with some variability of the major morbidity between 20–40 % and mortality of 0–12 %. This variability stems from the different definitions of major complications, lack of uniform reporting system for surgical complications, variability in patients, disease types, and individual center's volume and expertise [45, 100, 116, 121–132]. Like in any other complex surgical technique, there is a learning curve [133]. Learning and assimilating a new technology is a complex process; therefore, there are two learning curves to consider: a surgeon's learning curve and an institution's learning curve—reaching a plateau after 100–140 cases within a single center [134]. Learning curve and the rate of morbidity and mortality associated with it can be significantly reduced in a new HIPEC program with close mentorship of a high-volume center as was shown by the Milan group [135–137].

Complication Management and Patient Follow-Up

Since the morbidity of CRS+HIPEC is high, in order to reduce mortality, several topics should be addressed before initiating a HIPEC program:

1. Nursing staff acquainted with complex gastrointestinal surgery that may alert the surgeon of any clinical deterioration in a timely manner.
2. Mid-high level residents (postgraduate year 3–5) or available staff on call that can address any clinical issue early on.
3. Availability of a high-quality invasive radiology service.
4. Availability of an operating theater for emergency 24 h a day, 7 days a week.
5. Availability of ICU beds for readmission of the patient with major complication if needed.

Most complications are related to the operative procedure and should be addressed the same way surgical complications are addressed in every patient following abdominal surgery. In addition, most common complications associated with HIPEC include paralytic ileus related not only to the surgical procedure but also to the impact of heat on the enteric nervous system [138], neutropenia associated with systemic absorption of some of the HIPEC agents with bone marrow suppression ability, and hepatotoxicity of some agents such as mitomycin C or oxaliplatinum [123]. Renal failure is a known adverse event of cisplatinum and can be prevented by perioperative administration of IV sodium thiosulfate. Wound necrosis and infection may be associated with cytotoxic effect of the HIPEC or EPIC agents. Many of the abdominal wall closures require synthetic or biological graft placement, and there is only scarce data regarding the impact of cytotoxic agents on these materials [139].

Pearls and Practical Tips in Peritoneal Cytoreductive Surgery

1. Low lithotomy position is preferred for CRS.
2. Strong suction apparatus is necessary to control the spoke resulting from high-energy cautery used for cytoreduction.
3. The preferred anastomotic technique is hand-sewn anastomosis in two layers. We recommend outer layer with 3.0 sutures (PDS or Vicryl) and internal layer with 4.0 PDS.
4. Generally, chromic sutures are not used for anastomosis. The best results in our experimental and clinical experience are attained with PDS or Prolene suture. Some groups use Vicryl for the outer layer of the double-sutured anastomosis.
5. Do not use anti-adhesive barriers around an anastomosis if cytoreductive surgery includes an anastomosis.
6. We use 10 L of water irrigation after HIPEC to reduce postoperative intra-abdominal infection.
7. We recommend against irrigating the peritoneal cavity with saline after HIPEC. Patients receiving peritoneal irrigation with saline following oxaliplatin/HIPEC tend to get hyponatremic after the operation. What's more, the oxaliplatin will precipitate in saline, whereas it is diluted in D5W.
8. Major hepatobiliary or pancreatic resections, though generally regarded as contraindications to cytoreductive surgery, can be safely undertaken in selected cases when all grossly apparent disease can be cleared (CC0/1) surgically.
9. If major liver resection is undertaken with cytoreductive surgery, early liver dysfunction is common, but liver failure is uncommon in patients with normal preoperative liver function.
10. If we perform a major liver resection during CRS, we place topical hemostatic over the cut surface and then leave a moist lap pad against the cut surface during the HIPEC because of the negative pressure exerted by the outgoing tube, which can generate bleeding from the liver surface.
11. We are especially mindful of this bleeding risk and pay close attention to the appearance of the peritoneal fluid return early in the course of HIPEC for signs of liver hemorrhage.
12. Prior to major liver resection, it is our practice to administer vitamin C, 1.0 g twice daily, for at least a week prior to operation.
13. Furthermore, we continue intravenous vitamin C postoperatively, including zinc and multivitamin supplementation in an effort to improve surgical wound healing.
14. In patients that receive intraoperative chemotherapy, we administer prophylactic antibiotics for 5 days following operation.
15. Patients are kept on strict contact precautions until the leukopenia and thrombocytopenia commonly encountered after perioperative chemotherapy resolves.
16. The critical parameter in assessing the impact of cytoreductive surgery and patient prognosis is postoperative PCI.
17. Cytoreductive surgery is complex and places a significant burden on both the patient and the surgeon. If it is possible to render the patient free of all grossly apparent disease (CC0/1), then all reasonable efforts should be undertaken to that end.
18. Even in the presence of extensive miliary disease with 1–2 mm lesions implanted throughout the peritoneal cavity, we endeavor to take the time it takes to meticulously remove all apparent disease, one lesion at a time using low voltage argon beam coagulator with short bursts. Furthermore, we gently scrape to the lesion from the bowel with the back of a scalpel, and if needed place one or two seromuscular stitches at the ablated site to reduce the risk of consequent fistula formation.
19. Some groups of experts prefer performing selective peritonectomy and some a complete peritonectomy (including peritoneum with and without grossly evident tumor implants) at time of cytoreductive surgery.
20. It is our practice to resect the ovaries, greater omentum, and lesser omentum-hepatogastric ligament during cytoreductive surgery.
21. We prefer to perform cytoreduction before the HIPEC and to complete the reconstruction/anastomoses after the HIPEC. Bowel edema with 30 min of oxaliplatin/HIPEC does not appear to be clinically significant. This is different if groups perform 90 min of HIPEC.
22. Prior to anastomosis following HIPEC, we trim back the bowel edges to get rid of any potential malignant cells along the stapled edge that were exposed to HIPEC.
23. For prolonged cytoreductive cases (>8 h), we keep patients intubated on mechanical ventilation overnight in the ICU.
24. For patients requiring subtotal colectomy, we prefer to retain the cecum and preserve the ileocecal valve whenever possible, as fluid and electrolyte management for the next 1 year while on systemic chemotherapy is so much simpler than in cases where the ileocecal valve is resected. In cases where the cecum appears diseased, we make every effort to ablate as much of the disease as possible and bring most of the cecum outside the abdomen as a matured stoma, leaving the ileocecal valve within the peritoneal cavity.
25. As we plan a second look laparotomy within 1 year following CRS/HIPEC in all our patients, we prefer anastomosis when colectomy is performed.
26. If in the course of peritoneal stripping off the hemidiaphragm, we breach the diaphragm and identify it only after the HIPEC, we then insert a small chest tube to treat the inevitable effusion that ensues.

27. Our suture of choice for diaphragmatic repair is Prolene monofilament.
28. Great care must be taken when performing peritoneal stripping in the region of the pericardium so as to avoid a breach of that membrane.
29. If one can avoid splenectomy during the course of CRS, then one should. In cases where splenectomy is anticipated, vaccination is administered prior to operation.
30. If resection of the pancreas is required during CRS for clearance of all apparent disease, then we leave peripancreatic drains to closed, low-pressure suction.

Funding This work is supported by the Henry M. Jackson Foundation for the Advancement of Military Medicine, INCORE, International Consortium of Research Excellence of the Theodor-Billroth-Academy [TBA®], Germany-Israel-USA and the US Military Cancer Institute.

Acknowledgement The authors are grateful to Tiffany Felix for her editorial assistance with this collaborative effort.

References

1. Siegel R, Naishadham D, Jemal A. Cancer statistics 2012. CA Cancer J Clin. 2012;62(1):10–29. doi:10.3322/caac.20138. Epub 2012 Jan 4.
2. Siegel R, Naishadam D, Jemal A. Cancer statistics for Hispanics/Latinos 2012. CA Cancer J Clin. 2012;62(5):2883–98. doi:10.3322/caa.21153.
3. Brücher BLDM, Piso P, Verwaal V, Esquivel J, Derraco M, Yonemura Y, Gonzalez-Moreno S, Pelz J, Königsrainer A, Ströhlein M, Levine EA, Morris D, Bartlett D, Glehen O, Garofalo A, Nissan A. Peritoneal carcinomatosis: cytoreductive surgery and HIPEC–overview and basics. Cancer Invest. 2012;30(3):209–24.
4. Itzhak A, Brücher BLDM, Nissan A, Stojadinovic A. Randomized clinical trials for colorectal cancer peritoneal surface malignancy. Surg Clin North Am. 2012;21:665–88.
5. Griffen Jr WO, Gilbertsen VA, Wangensteen OH. The second look operation for abdominal malignancies 1948–1963. Natl Cancer Inst Monogr. 1964;15:267–76.
6. Brücher BLDM, Roder JD, Fink U, Stein HJ, Busch R, Siewert JR. Prognostic factors in resected primary small bowel tumors. Digestive Surgery. 1998;15:42–51.
7. Xu DZ, Zhan YQ, Sun XW, Cao SM, Geng QR. Meta-analysis of intraperitoneal chemotherapy for gastric cancer. W J Gastroenterol. 2004;15(10):2727–30.
8. Armstrong DK, Bundy B, Wenzel L, Huang HQ, Baergen R, Lele S, Copeland LJ, Walker JL, Burger RA. Gynecologic Oncology Group. Intraperitoneal cisplatin and paclitaxel in ovarian cancer. N Engl J Med. 2006;354(1):34–43.
9. Jayne DG, Fook S, Loi C, Seow-Choen F. Peritoneal carcinomatosis from colorectal cancer. Br J Surg. 2002;89(12):1545–50.
10. Chu DZ, Lang NP, Thompson C, et al. Pertoneal carcinomatosis in nongynecological malignancy: a prospective study of prognostic factors. Cancer. 1989;63:364–7.
11. Blair SL, Chu DZ, Schwarz RE. Outcome of palliative operations for malignant bowel obstruction in patients with peritoneal carcinomatosis from nongynecological cancer. Ann Surg Oncol. 2001;8:632–7.
12. Sugarbaker PH, Gianola FJ, Speyer JC, Wesley R, Barofsky I, Meyers CE. Prospective randomized trial of intravenous versus intraperitoneal 5-fluorouracil in patients with advanced colon and rectal cancer. Surgery. 1985;98(3):414–22.
13. Sugarbaker PH, Gianola FJ, Speyer JC, Wesley R, Barofsky I, Myers CE. Prospective randomized trial of intravenous versus intraperitoneal 5-FU in patients with advanced colon and rectal cancer. Semin Oncol. 1985;12(3 Suppl 4):1–11.
14. Gilly F, Carry PY, Sayag AC, Braillon GB, Volloch AA, Panteix GG, James IM, Chatelard PA. Treatment of peritoneal carcinomatosis by intraperitoneal chemot-hyperthermia with Mtomycin C. Initial experience. Ann Chir. 1990;44(7):545–51.
15. Gilly FN, Beaujard A, Glehen O, Grandclement E, Caillot JL, Francois Y, Sadeghi-Looyeh B, Gueugniaud PY, Garbit F, Benoit M, Bienvenu J, Vignal J. Peritonectomy combined with intraperitoneal chemohyperthermia in abdominal cancer with peritoneal carcinomatosis: phaseI-II study. Anticancer Res. 1999;19(3B): 2317–21.
16. Gilly FN, Carry PY, Sayag AC, Brachet A, Panteix G, Salle B, Bienvenu J, Burgard G, Guibert B, Banssillon V, Braillon G. Regional chemotherapy and intraoperative hyperthermia for digestivecancerswithperitonealcarcinomatosis. Hepatogastroenterology. 1994;41:124–9.
17. Sugarbaker PH. New standard of care for appendiceal epithelial malignancies and pseudomyxomaperitonei syndrome. Lancet Oncol. 2006;7:69–76.
18. Sadeghi B, Arvieux C, Glehen O, Beaujard AC, Rivoire M, Baulieux J, Fontaumard E, Brachet A, Caillot JL, Faure JL, Porcheron J, Peix JL, Francois Y, Vignal J, Gilly FN. Peritoneal carcinomatosis from non-gynecologic malignancies: results of the EVOCAPE 1 multicentric prospective study. Cancer. 2000;88(2): 358–63.
19. Elias D, GIlly F, Boutitie F, Quenet F, Bereder JM, Manavelt B, Lorimier G, Dube P, Glehen O. Peritoneal carcinomatosis treated with surgery and perioperative intraperitoneal chemotherapy: retrospective analysis of 523 patients from a multicentric French study. J Clin Oncol. 2010;28(1):63–8.
20. Brücher BLDM, Stojadinovic A, Bilchik A, Nissan A, Avital I. Identifying patient at risk of peritoneal surface malignancy of colorectal cancer origin. The role of 2nd look laparotomy. J Cancer. 2013;4:262–9.
21. Baron MA. Structure of the intestinal peritoneum in man. Am J Anat. 1941;69:439–97.
22. Flessner M, Henegar J, Bigler S, Genous L. Is the peritoneum a significant transport barrier in peritoneal dialysis. Perit Dial Int. 2003;23:542–9.
23. Sugarbaker PH. Peritoneum as the first line of defense in carcinomatosis. J Surg Oncol. 2007;95:93–6.
24. Stelin G, Rippe B. A phenomenological interpretation of the variation in dialysate volume with dwell time in CAPD. Kidney Int. 1990;38:465–72.
25. Sugarbaker PH, Schellinx ME, Chang D, Koslowe P, von Meyerfeldt M. Peritoneal carcinomatosis from adenocarcinoma of the colon. World J Surg. 1996;5:585–91.
26. Yonemura Y, Bandou E, Kawamura T, Endou Y, Sasaki T. Quantitative prognostic indicators of peritoneal dissemination of gastric cancer. Eur J Surg Oncol. 2006;32:602–6.
27. Gonzalez-Moreno S, Ortega-Perez G, Gonzalez-Bayon L. Indications and patient selection for cytoreductive surgery and perioperative intraperitoneal chemotherapy. J Surg Oncol. 2009;100: 287–92.
28. Rufián S, Muñoz-Casares FC, Briceño J, Diaz CJ, Rubio MJ, Ortega R, Ciria R, Morillo M, Aranda E, Muntane J, Pera C. Radical surgery–peritonectomy and intraoperative intraperitoneal chemotherapy for the treatment of peritoneal carcinomatosis in recurrent or primary ovarian cancer. J Surg Oncol. 2006;94: 316–24.

29. Warrick C. An improvement on the practice of tapping; whereby that operation instead of a relief of symptoms, becomes an absolute cure for an ascites, exemplified in the case of Jane Roman; and recommended to the consideration of the Royal Society, by Christopher Warrick, of Turo, Surgeon. Philos Trans R Soc Lond B Biol Sci. 1744;43:12–9.
30. Ceelen WP, Flessner MF. Intraperitoneal therapy for peritoneal tumors: biophysics and clinical evidence. Nat Rev Clin Oncol. 2010;7:108–15.
31. Weisberger AS, Levine B, Storaasli JP. Use of nitrogen mustard in treatment of serous effusions of neoplastic origin. J Am Med Assoc. 1955;159:1704–7.
32. Dedrick RL, Myers CE, Bungay PM, De Vita VT. Pharmacokinetic rationale for peritoneal drug administration in the treatment of ovarian cancer. Cancer Treat Rep. 1978;62:1–11.
33. Avantunde AA, Parson SL. Pattern and prognostic factors in patients with malignant ascites: a retrospective study. Ann Oncol. 2007;18(5):945–9.
34. Flessner M, Choi J, Credit K, Deverkadra R, Henderson K. Resistance of tumor interstitial pressure to the penetration intraperitoneally delivered antibodies into metastatic ovarian tumors. Clin Cancer Res. 2005;11:3117–25.
35. Holzer AK, Samimi G, Katano K, Naerdemann W, Lin X, Safaei R, Howell SB. The cooper influx transporter human cooper transport protein 1 regulates the uptake in human ovarian carcinoma cells. Mol Pharmacol. 2004;66(4):817–23.
36. Pfannenberg C, Konigsrainer I, Aschoff P, Öksüz M, Zieker D, Beckert S, Symons S, Nieselt K, Glatzle J, Brücher BLDM, Claussen CD, Konigsrainer A. 18F-FDG-PET/CT to select patients with peritoneal carcinomatosis for cytoreductive surgery and hyperthermic intraperitoneal chemotherapy. Ann Surg Oncol. 2009;16(5):1295–303.
37. Jacquet P, Sugarbaker PH. Current methodologies for clinical assessment of patients with peritoneal carcinomatosis. J Exp Clin Cancer Res. 1996;15:49–58.
38. Verwaal VJ, Van Tinteren H, Van Ruth S, Zoetmulder FAN. Predicting the survival of patients with peritoneal carcinomatosis of colorectal origin treated by aggressive cytoreduction and hyperthermic intraperitoneal chemotherapy. Br J Surg. 2004;91:739–46.
39. Kajitani T, Japanese Research Society for Gastric Cancer. The general rules for the gastric cancer study in surgery and pathology. Part I. Clinical classification. Jpn J Surg. 1981;11:127–39.
40. Esquivel J, Sticca R, Sugarbaker P, Levine E, Yan TD, Alexander R, Baratti D, Bartlett D, Barone R, Barrios P, Bieligk S, Bretcha-Boix P, Chang CK, Chu F, Chu Q, Daniel S, de Bree E, Deraco M, Dominguez-Parra L, Elias D, Flynn R, Foster J, Garofalo A, Gilly FN, Glehen O, Gomez-Portilla A, Gonzalez-Bayon L, Gonzalez-Moreno S, Goodman M, Gushchin V, Hanna N, Hartmann J, Harrison L, Hoefer R, Kane J, Kecmanovic D, Kelley S, Kuhn J, LaMont J, Lange J, Li B, Loggie B, Mahteme H, Mann G, Martin R, Misih RA, Moran B, Morris D, Onate-Ocana L, Petrelli N, Philippe G, Pingpank J, Pitroff A, Piso P, Quinones M, Riley L, Rutstein L, Saha S, Alrawi S, Sardi A, Schneebaum S, Shen P, Shibata D, Spellman J, Stojadinovic A, Stewart J, Torres-Melero J, Tuttle T, Verwaal V, Villar J, Wilkinson N, Younan R, Zeh H, Zoetmulder F, Sebbag G. Cytoreductive surgery and hyperthermic intraperitoneal chemotherapy in the management of peritoneal surface malignancies of colonic origin: a consensus statement. Society of Surgical Oncology. Ann Surg Oncol. 2007;14:128–33.
41. Sugarbaker PH. Peritonectomy procedures. Surg Oncol Clin N Am. 2003;12:703–27.
42. Sugarbaker PH. Successful management of microscopic residual disease in large bowel cancer. Cancer Chemother Pharmacol. 1999;43(Suppl):S15–25.
43. Sugarbaker PH, Chang D. Results of treatment of 385 patients with peritoneal surface spread of appendiceal malignancy. Ann Surg Oncol. 1999;6:727–31.
44. Glehen O, Cotte E, Kusamura S, Deraco M, Baratti D, Passot G, Beaujard AC, Noel GF. Hyperthermic intraperitoneal chemotherapy: nomenclature and modalities of perfusion. J Surg Oncol. 2008;98:242–6.
45. Chua TC, Yan TD, Saxena A, Morris DL. Should the treatment of peritoneal carcinomatosis by cytoreductive surgery and hyperthermic intraperitoneal chemotherapy still be regarded as a high morbid procedure ? Ann Surg. 2009;249:900–7.
46. Gonzalez-Moreno S, Kusamura S, Baratti D, Deraco M. Postoperative residual disease evaluation in the locoreginal treatment of peritoneal surface malignancy. J Surg Oncol. 2008;98: 237–41.
47. Sugarbaker PH. Observations concerning cancer spread within the peritoneal cavity and concepts supporting an ordered pathophysiology. In: Sugarbaker PH, editor. Peritoneal carcinomatosis: principles of management. Boston: Kluwer; 1996. p. 79–100.
48. Ozel L, Ozel MS, Toros AB, Kara M, Ozkan KS, Tellioglu G, Krand O, Koyuturk M, Berber I. Effect of early preoperative 5-fluorouracil on the integrity of colonic anastomoses in rats. World J Gastroenterol. 2009;15(33):4156–62.
49. Pelz JO, Doerfer J, Decker M, Dimmler A, Hohenberger W, Meyer T. Hyperthermic intraperitoneal chemoperfusion (HIPEC) decrease wound strength of colonic anastomosis in a rat model. Int J Colorectal Dis. 2007;22:941–7.
50. Van der Speeten K, Stuart OA, Sugarbaker PH. Using pharmacologic data to plan clinical treatments for patients with peritoneal surface malignancy. Curr Drug Discov Technol. 2009;6:72–81.
51. Sugarbaker PH, Graves T, DeBruijn EA, Cunliffe WJ, Mullins RE, Hull WE, Oliff L, Schlag P. Rationale for early postoperative intraperitoneal chemotherapy (EPIC) in patients with advanced gastrointestinal cancer. Cancer Res. 1990;50:5790–4.
52. Sugarbaker PH, Mora JT, Carmignani P, Stuart OA, Yoo D. Update on chemotherapeutic agents utilized for perioperative intraperitoneal chemotherapy. Oncologist. 2005;10:112–22.
53. Lepock JR. How do cells respond to their thermal environment? Int J Hyperthermia. 2005;21:681–7.
54. Kusumoto T, Holden SA, Teicher BA. Hyperthermia and platinum complexes: time between treatments and synergy in vitro and in vivo. Int J Hyperthermia. 1995;11:575–86.
55. Barlogie B, Corry PM, Drewinko B. In vitro thermochemotherapy of human colon cancer cells with *cis*-dichlorodiammineplatinum (II) and mitomycin C. Cancer Res. 1980;40:1165–8.
56. Jacquet P, Averbach A, Stuart OA, Chang D, Sugarbaker PH. Hyperthermic intraperitoneal doxorubicin: pharmacokinetics, metabolism, and tissue distribution in a rat model. Cancer Chemother Pharmacol. 1998;41:147–54.
57. Saltz LB, Cox JV, Blanke C, et al. Irinotecan plus fluorouracil and leucovorin for metastatic colorectal cancer. Irinotecan Study Group. N Engl J Med. 2000;343(13):905–14.
58. Douillard JY, Cunningham D, Roth AD, et al. Irinotecan combined with fluorouracil compared with fluorouracil alone as first-line treatment for metastatic colorectal cancer: a multicentre randomised trial. Lancet. 2000;355(9209):1041–7.
59. Giacchetti S, Perpoint B, Zidani R, et al. Phase III multicenter randomized trial of oxaliplatin added to chronomodulated fluorouracil-leucovorin as first-line treatment of metastatic colorectal cancer. J Clin Oncol. 2000;18(1):136–47.
60. Rothenberg ML, Oza AM, Bigelow RH, et al. Superiority of oxaliplatin and fluorouracil-leucovorin compared with either therapy alone in patients with progressive colorectal cancer after irinotecan and fluorouracil-leucovorin: interim results of a phase III trial. J Clin Oncol. 2003;21(11):2059–69.
61. Goldberg RM, Sargent DJ, Morton RF, et al. A randomized controlled trial of fluorouracil plus leucovorin, irinotecan, and oxaliplatin combinations in patients with previously untreated metastatic colorectal cancer. J Clin Oncol. 2004;22(1):23–30.

62. Tournigand C, Andre T, Achille E, et al. FOLFIRI followed by FOLFOX6 or the reverse sequence in advanced colorectal cancer: a randomized GERCOR study. J Clin Oncol. 2004;22(2):229–37.
63. Hurwitz H, Fehrenbacher L, Novotny W, et al. Bevacizumab plus irinotecan, fluorouracil, and leucovorin for metastatic colorectal cancer. N Engl J Med. 2004;350(23):2335–42.
64. Colucci G, Gebbia V, Paoletti G, et al. Phase III randomized trial of FOLFIRI versus FOLFOX4 in the treatment of advanced colorectal cancer: a multicenter study of the Gruppo Oncologico Dell'Italia Meridionale. J Clin Oncol. 2005;23(22):4866–75.
65. Goldberg RM, Sargent DJ, Morton RF, et al. Randomized controlled trial of reduced-dose bolus fluorouracil plus leucovorin and irinotecan or infused fluorouracil plus leucovorin and oxaliplatin in patients with previously untreated metastatic colorectal cancer: a North American Intergroup Trial. J Clin Oncol. 2006;24(21):3347–53.
66. Franko J, Shi Q, Goldman CD, Pockaj BA, Nelson GD, Goldberg RM, Pitot HC, Grothey A, Alberts SR, Sargent DJ. Treatment of colorectal peritoneal carcinomatosis with systemic chemotherapy: a pooled analysis of North Central Cancer Treatment Group Phase III Trials N971 and N9841. J Clin Oncol. 2012;30:263–76.
67. Verwaal V, Ruth S, Bree E, et al. Randomized trial of cytoreduction and hyperthermic intraperitoneal chemotherapy versus systemic chemotherapy and palliative surgery in patients with peritoneal carcinomatosis of colorectal cancer. J Clin Oncol. 2003;21:3737–43.
68. Verwaal VJ, van Ruth S, Witkamp A, Boot H, van Slooten G, Zoetmulder FA. Long-term survival of peritoneal carcinomatosis of colorectal origin. Ann Surg Oncol. 2005;12(1):65–71.
69. Glehen O, Kwiatkowski F, Sugarbaker PH, Elias D, Levine EA, De Simone M, Barone R, Yonemura Y, Caaliere F, Quente F, Gutman M, Tentes AA, Lorimier G, Bernard JL, Bereder JM, Porcheron J, Gomez-Portilla A, Shen P, Deraco M, Rat P. Cytoreductive surgery combined with perioperative intraperitoneal chemotherapy for the management of peritoneal carcinomatosis from colorectal cancer: a multi-institutional study. J Clin Oncol. 2004;22(16):3284–92.
70. Brücher BL, Bilchik A, Nissan A, Avital I, Stojadinovic A. Tumor response criteria: are they appropriate? Future Oncol. 2012;8(8): 903–6.
71. Stojadinovic A, Bilchik A, Smith D, Eberhardt JS, Ward EB, Nissan A, Johnson EK, Protic M, Peoples GE, Avital I, Steele SR. Clinical decision support and individualized prediction of survival in colon cancer: bayesian belief network model. Ann Surg Oncol. 2013;20:161–74.
72. Sugarbaker PH. Revised guidelines for second-look surgery in patients with colon and rectal cancer. Clin Transl Oncol. 2010;12(9): 621–8.
73. Sugarbaker P. Second-look surgery for colorectal cancer: revised selection factors and new treatment options for greater success. Int J Surg Oncol. 2011;2011:915078. Epub 2010 Dec 5.
74. Esquivel J, Sugarbaker PH. Second-look surgery in patients with peritoneal dissemination from appendiceal malignancy: analysis of prognostic factors in 98 patients. Ann Surg. 2001;234(2):198–205.
75. Elias D, Honoré C, Dumont F, Ducreux M, Boige V, Malka D, Burtin P, Dromain C, Goéré D. Results of systematic second-look surgery plus HIPEC in asymptomatic patients presenting a high risk of developing colorectal peritoneal carcinomatosis. Ann Surg. 2011;254(2):289–93.
76. Maggiori L, Elias D. Curative treatment of colorectal peritoneal carcinomatosis: current status and future trends. Eur J Surg Oncol. 2010;36(7):599–603.
77. Wangensteen OH. Cancer of the colon and rectum; with special reference to earlier recognition of alimentary tract malignancy; secondary delayed re-entry of the abdomen in patients exhibiting lymph node involvement; subtotal primary excision of the colon; operation in obstruction. Wis Med J. 1949;48:591–7.
78. Wangensteen OH, Lewis FJ, Tongen LA. The second look in cancer surgery: a patient with colic cancer and involve lymph nodes negative on the sixth look. J Lancet. 1951;71(8):303–7.
79. Bleday R, Steele Jr G. Second-look surgery for recurrent colorectal carcinoma: is it worthwhile? Semin Surg Oncol. 1991;7(3):171–6.
80. Bucci L, Benassai G, Santoro GA. Second look in colorectal surgery. Dis Colon Rectum. 1994;37(2 Suppl):S123–6.
81. Elias D, Goéré D, Di Pietrantonio D, Boige V, Malka D, Kohneh-Shahri N, Dromain C, Ducreux M. Results of systematic second-look surgery in patients at high risk of developing colorectal peritoneal carcinomatosis. Ann Surg. 2008;247(3):445–50.
82. Gilbertsen VA, Wangensteen OH. A summary of thirteen years' experience with the second look program. Surg Gynecol Obstet. 1962;114:438–42.
83. Grotz RL, Pemberton JH. Second look surgery–a shell game? Am J Gastroenterol. 1992;87(6):804–5.
84. Lefevre JH, Elias DM. Cytoreductive surgery plus intraperitoneal chemohyperthermia in patients with colorectal cancer at high risk for local-regional recurrence. Cancer J. 2009;15(3):200–3.
85. Martin Jr EW, James KK, Hurtubise PE, Catalano P, Minton JP. The use of CEA as an early indicator for gastrointestinal tumor recurrence and second-look procedures. Cancer. 1977;39(2):440–6.
86. Martin Jr EW, Carey LC. Second-look surgery for colorectal cancer. The second time around. Ann Surg. 1991;214(3):321–5; discussion 326–7.
87. Minton JP, Hoehn JL, Gerber DM, Horsley JS, Connolly DP, Salwan F, Fletcher WS, Cruz Jr AB, Gatchell FG, Oviedo M, et al. Results of a 400-patient carcinoembryonic antigen second-look colorectal cancer study. Cancer. 1985;55(6):1284–90.
88. Osteen RT, Guyton S, Steele Jr G, Wilson RE. Maligant intestinal obstruction. Surgery. 1980;87:611–5.
89. Portilla AG, Sugarbaker PH, Chang D. Second-look surgery after cytoreduction and intraperitoneal chemotherapy for peritoneal carcinomatosis from colorectal cancer: analysis of prognostic features. World J Surg. 1999;23(1):23–9.
90. Ripley RT, Davis JL, Kemp CD, Steinberg SM, Toomey MA, Itzhak A. Prospective randomized trial evaluating mandatory second look surgery with HIPEC and CRS vs. standard of care in patients at high risk of developing colorectal peritoneal metastases. Trials. 2010;11:62.
91. Rittgers RA, Steele Jr G, Zamcheck N, Loewenstein MS, Sugarbaker PH, Mayer RJ, Lokich JJ, Maltz J, Wilso RE. Transient carcinoembryonic antigen (CEA) elevations following resection of colorectal cancer: a limitation in the use of serial CEA levels as an indicator for second-look surgery. J Natl Cancer Inst. 1978;61(2):315–8.
92. Santoro BT, Griffen Jr WO, Wangensteen C. The second look procedure in the management of ovarian malignancies and pseudomyxoma peritonei. Surgery. 1961;50:354–8.
93. Spears H, Petrelli NJ, Herrera L, MItelman A. Treatment of bowel obstruction after operation for colorectal carcinoma. Am J Surg. 1998;155:383–6.
94. Walsh HPJ, Schofield PF. Is laparotomy for small bowel obstruction justified in patients with previously treated malignancy? Br J Surg. 1984;71:933–5.
95. Zivanovic O, Barakat RR, Sabbatini PJ, Brown CL, Konner JA, Aghajanian CA, Abu-Rustum NR, Levine DA. Prognostic factors for patients with stage IV epithelial ovarian cancer receiving intraperitoneal chemotherapy after second-look assessment: results of long-term follow-up. Cancer. 2008;112(12):2690–7.
96. Brücher BLDM, Königsrainer A. Peritonealcarcinose. Chirurgische Allgemeine Zeitung. 2010;11(1):17–31.
97. Weeks JC, Catalano PJ, Cronin A, Finkelman MD, Mack JW, Keating NL, Schrag D. Patients' expectations about effects of chemotherapy for advanced cancer. N Engl J Med. 2012;367(17): 1616–25.

98. Sugarbaker PH. Peritonectomy procedures. Ann Surg. 1995;221(1): 29–42.
99. Helm CW, Bristow RE, Kusamura S, Baratti D, Deraco M. Hyperthermic intraperitoneal chemotherapy with and without cytoreductive surgery for epithelial ovarian cancer. J Surg Oncol. 2008;98(4):283–90.
100. Casado-Adam A, Alderman R, Stuart OA, Chang D, Sugarbaker PH. Gastrointestinal complications in 147 consecutive patients with peritoneal surface malignancy treated by cytoreductive surgery and perioperative intraperitoneal chemotherapy. Int J Surg Oncol. 2011;2011:468698. Epub 2011 Oct 16.
101. Koea JB, Lanouette N, Paty PB, Guillem JG, Cohen AM. Abdominal wall recurrence after colorectal resection for cancer. Dis Colon Rectum. 2000;43(5):628–32.
102. Valle M, Federici O, Garofalo A. Patient selection for cytoreductive surgery and hyperthermic intraperitoneal chemotherapy, and role of laparoscopy in diagnosis, staging, and treatment. Surg Oncol Clin N Am. 2012;21(4):515–31.
103. Bell JC, Rylah BG, Chambers RW, Peet H, Mohamed F, Moran BJ. Perioperative management of patients undergoing cytoreductive surgery combined with heated intraperitoneal chemotherapy for peritoneal surface malignancy: a multi-institutional experience. Ann Surg Oncol. 2012;19:4244–51.
104. Raspe C, Piso P, Wiesenack C, Bucher M. Anesthetic management in patients undergoing hyperthermic chemotherapy. Curr Opin Anaesthesiol. 2012;25(3):348–55.
105. Pearse R, Dawson D, Fawcett J, Rhodes A, Grounds RM, Bennett ED. Early goal-directed therapy after major surgery reduces complications and duration of hospital stay. A randomised, controlled trial. Crit Care. 2005;9(6):687–93.
106. Raval NY, Squara P, Cleman M, Yalamanchili K, Winklmaier M, Burkhoff D. Multicenter evaluation of noninvasive cardiac output measurement by bioreactance technique. J Clin Monit Comput. 2008;22(2):113–9.
107. Montenij LJ, de Waal EE, Buhre WF. Arterial waveform analysis in anesthesia and critical care. Curr Opin Anaesthesiol. 2011;24(6): 651–6.
108. Sugarbaker PH. Peritonectomy procedures. Ann Surg. 1995;221(1): 29–42.
109. Wallemacq PE, Capron A, Vanbinst R, Boeckmans E, Gillard J, Favier B. Permeability of 13 different gloves to 13 cytotoxic agents under controlled dynamic conditions. Am J Health Syst Pharm. 2006;63(6):547–56.
110. Peters BG. Technical considerations in the preparation and dispensing of chemotherapy. Top Hosp Pharm Manage. 1995;14(4):78–88.
111. Stephens AD, Alderman R, Chang D, Edwards GD, Esquivel J, Sebbag G, Steves MA, Sugarbaker PH. Morbidity and mortality analysis of 200 treatments with cytoreductive surgery and hyperthermic intraoperative intraperitoneal chemotherapy using coliseum technique. Ann Surg Oncol. 1999;6:790–6.
112. Saxena A, Yan TD, Morris DL. A critical evaluation of risk factors for complications after cytoreductive surgery and perioperative intraperitoneal chemotherapy for colorectal peritoneal carcinomatosis. World J Surg. 2010;34:70–8.
113. Saxena A, Chua TC, Yan TD, Morris DL. Postoperative pancreatic fistula after cytoreductive surgery and perioperative intraperitoneal chemotherapy: incidence, risk, factors, management and clinical sequelae. Ann Surg Oncol. 2010;17(5):1302–10.
114. Kerscher AG, Mallalieu J, Pitroff A, Kerscher F, Esquivel J. Morbidity and mortality of 109 consecutive cytoreductive procedures with hyperthermic intraperitoneal chemotherapy (HIPEC) performed at a community hospital. World J Surg. 2010;34:62–9.
115. Glehen O, Osinsky D, Cotte E, Kwiatkowski F, Freyer G, Isaac S, Trillet-Lenoir V, Sayag-Beaujard AC, Francois Y, Vignal J, Gilly FN. Intraperitoneal chemohyperthermia using a closed abdominal procedure and cytoreductive surgery for the treatment of peritoneal carcinomatosis: morbidity and mortality analysis of 216 consecutive procedures. Ann Surg Oncol. 2003;10(8):863–9.
116. Franko J, Gusani NJ, Holtzman MP, Ahrendt SA, Jones HL, Zeh 3rd HJ, Bartlett DL. Multivisceral resection does not affect morbidity and survival after cytoreductive surgery and chemoperfusion for carcinomatosis from colorectal cancer. Ann Surg Oncol. 2008;15(11):3065–72.
117. Kusamura S, Younan R, Baratti D, Costanzo P, Favaro M, Gavazzci C, Deraco M. Cytoreductive surgery followed by intraperitoneal hyperthermic perfusion: analysis of morbidity and mortality in 209 peritoneal surface malignancies treated with closed abdomen technique. Cancer. 2006;106(5):1144–53.
118. Glehen O, Gilly FN, Boutitie F, Bereder JM, Quenet F, Sideris L, Mansvelt B, Lorimier G, Msika S, Elias D, French Surgical Association. Toward curative treatment of peritoneal carcinomatosis from nonovarian origin by cytoreductive surgery combined with perioperative intraperitoneal chemotherapy: a multi-institutional study of 1,290 patients. Cancer. 2010;116(24):5608–18.
119. Glehen O, Kwiatkowski F, Sugarbaker PH, Elias D, Levine EA, De Simone M, Barone R, Yonemura Y, Cavaliere F, Quenet F, Gutman M, Tentes AA, Lorimier G, Bernard JL, Bereder JM, Porcheron J, Gomez-Portilla A, Shen P, Deraco M, Rat P. Cytoreductive surgery combined with perioperative intraperitoneal chemotherapy for the management of peritoneal carcinomatosis from colorectal cancer: a multi-institutional study. J Clin Oncol. 2004;22(16):3284–92.
120. Chua TC, Moran BJ, Sugarbaker PH, Levine EA, Glehen O, Gilly FN, Baratti D, Deraco M, Elias D, Sardi A, Liauw W, Yan TD, Barrios P, Gómez Portilla A, de Hingh IH, Ceelen WP, Pelz JO, Piso P, González-Moreno S, Van Der Speeten K, Morris DL. Early- and long-term outcome data of patients with pseudomyxoma peritonei from appendiceal origin treated by a strategy of cytoreductive surgery and hyperthermic intraperitoneal chemotherapy. J Clin Oncol. 2012;30(20):2449–56.
121. McConnell YJ, Mack LA, Francis WP, Ho T, Temple WJ. HIPEC+EPIC versus HIPEC-alone: differences in major complications following cytoreduction surgery for peritoneal malignancy. J Surg Oncol. 2013;107:591–6. doi:10.1002/jso.23276.
122. Preti V, Chang D, Sugarbaker PH. Pulmonary complications following cytoreductive surgery and perioperative chemotherapy in 147 consecutive patients. Gastroenterol Res Pract. 2012;2012:635314. Epub 2012 Aug 13.
123. Di Miceli D, Alfieri S, Caprino P, Menghi R, Quero G, Cina C, Pericoli Ridolfini M, Doglietto GB. Complications related to hyperthermia during hyperthermic intraoperative intraperitoneal chemotherapy (HIPEC) treatment. Do they exist? Eur Rev Med Pharmacol Sci. 2012;16(6):737–42.
124. Glockzin G, von Breitenbuch P, Schlitt HJ, Piso P. Treatment-related morbidity and toxicity of CRS and oxaliplatin-based HIPEC compared to a mitomycin and doxorubicin-based HIPEC protocol in patients with peritoneal carcinomatosis: a matched-pair analysis. J Surg Oncol. 2013;107:574–8. doi:10.1002/jso.23228.
125. Baratti D, Kusamura S, Mingrone E, Balestra MR, Laterza B, Deraco M. Identification of a subgroup of patients at highest risk for complications after surgical cytoreduction and hyperthermic intraperitoneal chemotherapy. Ann Surg. 2012;256(2):334–41.
126. Baratti D, Kusamura S, Laterza B, Balestra MR, Deraco M. Early and long-term postoperative management following cytoreductive surgery and hyperthermic intraperitoneal chemotherapy. World J Gastrointest Oncol. 2010;2(1):36–43.
127. Dovern E, de Hingh IH, Verwaal VJ, van Driel WJ, Nienhuijs SW. Hyperthermic intraperitoneal chemotherapy added to the treatment of ovarian cancer. A review of achieved results and complications. Eur J Gynaecol Oncol. 2010;31(3):256–61.
128. Roviello F, Pinto E, Corso G, Pedrazzani C, Caruso S, Filippeschi M, Petrioli R, Marsili S, Mazzei MA, Marrelli D. Safety and potential benefit of hyperthermic intraperitoneal chemotherapy

(HIPEC) in peritoneal carcinomatosis from primary or recurrent ovarian cancer. J Surg Oncol. 2010;102(6):663–70.
129. Kerscher AG, Mallalieu J, Pitroff A, Kerscher F, Esquivel J. Morbidity and mortality of 109 consecutive cytoreductive procedures with hyperthermic intraperitoneal chemotherapy (HIPEC) performed at a community hospital. World J Surg. 2010;34(1):62–9.
130. Jaehne J. Cytoreductive procedures-strategies to reduce postoperative morbidity and management of surgical complications with special emphasis on anastomotic leaks. J Surg Oncol. 2009;100(4):302–5.
131. Glockzin G, Schlitt HJ, Piso P. Peritoneal carcinomatosis: patients selection, perioperative complications and quality of life related to cytoreductive surgery and hyperthermic intraperitoneal chemotherapy. World J Surg Oncol. 2009;7:5.
132. Younan R, Kusamura S, Baratti D, Cloutier AS, Deraco M. Morbidity, toxicity, and mortality classification systems in the local regional treatment of peritoneal surface malignancy. J Surg Oncol. 2008;98(4):253–7.
133. Mohamed F, Moran BJ. Morbidity and mortality with cytoreductive surgery and intraperitoneal chemotherapy: the importance of a learning curve. Cancer J. 2009;15(3):196–9.
134. Chua TC, Yan TD, Smigielski ME, Zhu KJ, Ng KM, Zhao J, Morris DL. Long-term survival in patients with pseudomyxoma peritonei treated with cytoreductive surgery and perioperative intraperitoneal chemotherapy: 10 years of experience from a single institution. Ann Surg Oncol. 2009;16(7):1903–11.
135. Kusamura S, Baratti D, Hutanu I, Rossi P, Deraco M. The importance of the learning curve and surveillance of surgical performance in peritoneal surface malignancy programs. Surg Oncol Clin N Am. 2012;21(4):559–76.
136. Kusamura S, Baratti D, Virzì S, Bonomi S, Iusco DR, Grassi A, Hutanu I, Deraco M. Learning curve for cytoreductive surgery and hyperthermic intraperitoneal chemotherapy in peritoneal surface malignancies: analysis of two centres. J Surg Oncol. 2013;107:312–9. doi:10.1002/jso.23231.
137. Kusamura S, Baratti D, Deraco M. Multidimensional analysis of the learning curve for cytoreductive surgery and hyperthermic intraperitoneal chemotherapy in peritoneal surface malignancies. Ann Surg. 2012;255(2):348–56.
138. Burke S, Abu-Wasel B, Eid A, Nissan A, Hanani M. Differential effect of hyperthermia on nerves and smooth muscle of the mouse ileum. J Surg Oncol. 2011;103(1):92–100.
139. Boutros C, Somasundar P, Espat NJ. Early results on the use of biomaterials as adjuvant to abdominal wall closure following cytoreduction and hyperthermic intraperitoneal chemotherapy. World J Surg Oncol. 2010;8:72.

Metastatic Colorectal Cancer

6

Steven Mills and Michael J. Stamos

Key Points

- Given the various treatment options for a patient with Stage 4 colorectal cancer, it is strongly recommended to employ a multidisciplinary team approach.
- An aggressive, yet realistic, approach to treatment of a patient with metastatic colorectal cancer can result in a cure for selected patients.
- Taking a stepwise approach to treatment of metastatic colorectal cancer is recommended to attempt to increase survival.
- Surgeons treating patients with metastatic colorectal cancer need to be aware of various palliative surgical and nonsurgical options.

Introduction

Despite availability of an effective screening tool, colorectal cancer remains a common and deadly cancer. Of the estimated 143,000 new cases of colorectal cancer predicted for 2012 [1], around 28,000 (20 %) will present as Stage 4, meaning presence of metastatic disease at the time of diagnosis. The most common sites of metastatic disease for colon and rectal cancer are the liver followed by the lungs. The presentation of metastatic disease (either at initial presentation or as a subsequent recurrence) and pattern (single site vs. multiple site) can present treatment dilemmas for physicians. There is also a wide range of metastatic cancer load among patients with Stage 4 colorectal cancer, further complicating the picture (Fig. 6.1); as such, what to do for the patient with a single liver metastasis will often be very different from the patient with multiple liver metastases or multiple sites of metastatic spread. Further, one must individualize the treatment plan based upon the patient's goal for therapy and the overall condition of the patient. Whereas management for early-stage primary cancers can often be fairly straightforward, in treating the patient with metastatic disease, a multidisciplinary approach is often needed to determine the appropriate use of preoperative chemotherapy or radiation therapy, whether to proceed with initial curative or palliative operation or other procedures, postoperative adjuvant therapy, and the involvement of a palliative care team. Though much of the following can be extrapolated to the patient with recurrent disease, this chapter will focus on patients presenting with Stage 4 disease.

Multidisciplinary Approach

Key Concept: A multidisciplinary tumor board to review the specifics of each individual patient's case provides a great opportunity to determine the ideal treatment plan and optimize outcomes.

A multidisciplinary approach to treatments of all types of cancer has long been advocated [2]. Given that many different modalities may be utilized in the treatment of Stage 4 colorectal cancer, a multidisciplinary approach is strongly recommended. The various disciplines can include surgery (including colorectal surgery, hepatobiliary surgery, thoracic surgery), medical oncology, radiation oncology, palliative care, radiology, and pathology. Through a thorough discussion of the patient's overall condition and symptoms, the goals of care and potential curative versus palliative intent of treatment can be made. Many centers employ a tumor board conference where an individual case can be presented to representatives from each of the above specialties. A review of the patient's history, relevant radiologic studies, pathology, and general medical condition can be made followed by discussion and input from all members of the team. This will allow for understanding of the condition of the patient, any

S. Mills, MD (✉) • M.J. Stamos, MD
Department of Surgery, University of California, Irvine,
333 City Blvd. West, Suite 700, Orange, CA 92868, USA
e-mail: sdmills@uci.edu; mstamos@uci.edu

S.R. Steele et al. (eds.), *Complexities in Colorectal Surgery*,
DOI 10.1007/978-1-4614-9022-7_6, © Springer Science+Business Media New York 2014

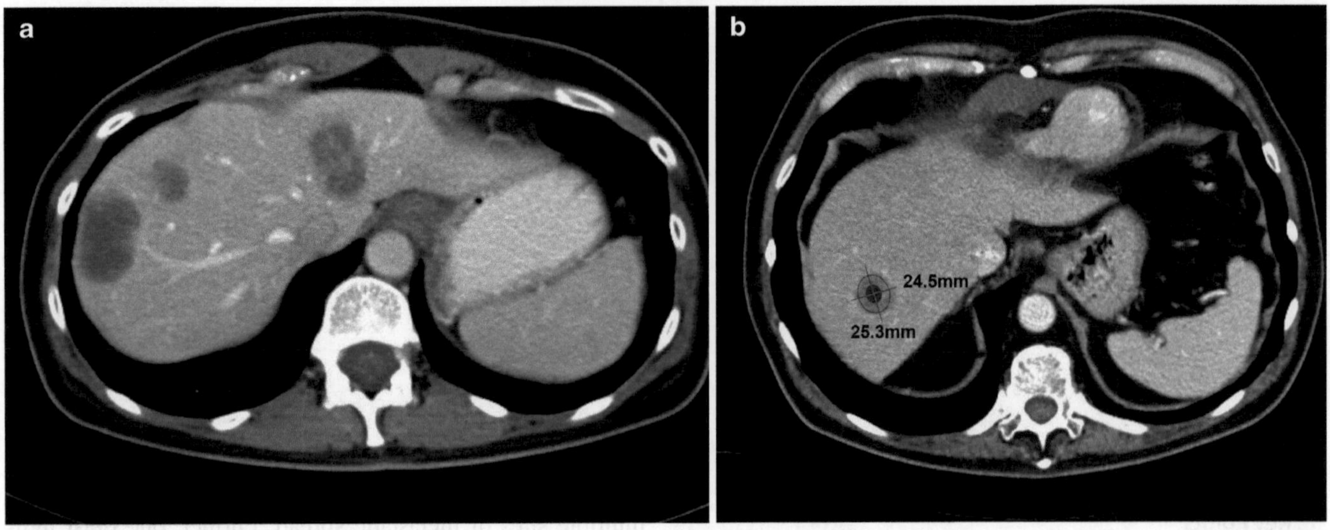

Fig. 6.1 CT scan images of two patients presenting with metastatic involvement of the liver. Image (**a**) represents a 47-year-old woman with rectal cancer and multiple, bilobar liver lesions. Image (**b**) represents a 54-year-old man with rectosigmoid cancer and a single site of metastatic disease in the liver. Both patients have been treated with a multidisciplinary approach and are currently free of disease

prior treatments, as well as an explanation of goals of care. An honest discussion of the realistic expectations and prognosis of the patient can occur as well. Finally, the team can formulate a plan to include inclusion/exclusion of each therapeutic modality as well as discuss and plan for timing of each of the included treatments. This up-front communication will assure that all members of a patient's treatment team are "on the same page." An additional by-product of this is that the patient may further benefit from this communication by frequently precluding the need for multiple initial consults, thereby saving the patient time and energy.

Often, the questions raised at the multidisciplinary meeting revolve around timing of chemotherapy and/or radiation and the role of surgical resection. Occasionally, the oncologists and surgeons disagree as to the expectations of therapy, appropriate timing of the various therapeutic options, or when care is futile. It is not always clear which opinion is most appropriate for the patient, especially with very complex cases that cannot easily be compared to a specific trial or literature search for guidance. In cases where there are strongly held opinions that are divergent, it should be recommended to the patient to obtain a second opinion, most often from both medical oncology as well as another experienced surgeon.

Evolution of Care

Key Concept: Improvements in chemotherapeutics have allowed longer survival and an evolving role for resection following response to therapy.

In the past, many patients presenting with Stage 4 disease were started on chemotherapy (5-FU and leucovorin), and there was often felt to be a limited role for any operation. As chemotherapeutics have evolved over the last two decades (with the addition of oxaliplatin, irinotecan, cetuximab, bevacizumab, and others), patients are living longer (median survival up to 24 months or more) than ever before [3, 4], and an ever-increasing number of patients have a realistic chance of cure. As we continue to better understand the biology of colorectal cancers and the role for various adjuvant therapies, outcomes will continue to improve. A significant number of patients with initially surgically incurable disease burden are currently being treated aggressively with what has become neoadjuvant chemotherapy to the point that surgical options for cure are once again entertained. An example of this would be a patient presenting with extensive liver metastases to the point that curative resection is not feasible. After several rounds of chemotherapy, the tumor burden in the liver is reduced to the point that curative intent treatment is possible.

The Food and Drug Administration (FDA) has recently approved two new chemotherapy agents for the treatment of metastatic disease. Aflibercept (commercial name Zaltrap™, also known as VEGF Trap) is a fusion protein which binds all forms of vascular endothelial growth factor-A (VEGF-A), as well as VEGF-B, and placental growth factor (PIGF). The VELOUR study was a multinational, randomized, double-blind trial comparing FOLFIRI in combination with either Zaltrap™ or placebo. The study randomized 1,226 patients who previously had been treated with an oxaliplatin-based regimen. The addition of Zaltrap™ to the FOLFIRI regimen significantly improved both overall survival (13.5 vs. 12.1 months) and progression-free survival (6.9 vs. 4.7 months) [5].

The FDA also recently approved regorafenib (commercial name Stivarga™), an oral multi-kinase inhibitor which targets angiogenic, stromal, and oncogenic receptor tyrosine kinases. The CORRECT study enrolled 760 individuals whose disease had progressed during or within 3 months following the last administration of approved standard therapies. Median overall survival for regorafenib was 6.4 months, compared with 5.0 months for those who received placebo [6]. While modest improvements in survival with these additional agents may not significantly change practice patterns, they represent other options for patients with previously recalcitrant disease.

The past two decades have not only seen an improvement in available chemotherapeutic agents, but we have also seen an improvement in the understanding of the role of liver resection for metastatic lesions as well as the enhanced utilization of ablative techniques (e.g., radiofrequency ablation). Indications for operation have broadened, while contraindications have loosened as the operations have become safer and more common (see below—Liver Metastases).

Indications for Operation

Key Concept: Clear communication with the patient and their family is critical to discuss the goals and realistic expectations of an operation in the setting of metastatic disease.

There are two general goals of an operation: curative and palliative. More to the point, when discussing the indication for operation in patients with colorectal cancer, the goal is generally either to attempt a cure (curative) or to relieve a specific symptom (palliative). The specific indication for a patient set to undergo palliative operation will depend upon the symptom/complaint to be alleviated, such as to relieve an obstruction. It is important that during preoperative discussions and evaluation, the surgeon clearly identifies the goal of an operation with the patient and family members. A realistic discussion of prognosis is important in order for the patient to understand any proposed procedure and to have realistic expectations of the operation as well as the postoperative course.

Of the roughly 20 % of patients that present with Stage 4 disease, there is a substantial subset that has a realistic chance of being treated and cured, for example, a patient with colon cancer and unilobar liver metastases. There are multiple options for treatment of this patient in terms of order of therapy. In general, the patient will benefit from chemotherapy and surgical resection of both the primary as well as the liver for cure. Again, a strong recommendation for multidisciplinary planning is made. Traditionally, these patients underwent colon resection followed by liver resection (or occasionally synchronously) followed by systemic chemotherapy. Recently, many experts have recommended taking a "liver first" approach to these patients and perhaps proceed with systemic chemotherapy to establish an effective regimen, followed by liver resection [7]. The colon resection may also occur at the same operation, or, alternatively, they may be performed in a staged setting. We generally base that decision upon the condition of the patient, the extent and difficulty of the liver and colonic resections, and how well/easily the liver resection goes. For staged operations, some patients will benefit from further systemic chemotherapy between the procedures [8]. Alternatively, the patient could undergo the second resection prior to resumption of systemic chemotherapy. Our bias is to base recommendations for treatment on the patient's symptoms and response to therapy. Colonic lesions that virtually "melt away" are left to further rounds of chemotherapy (Fig. 6.2), whereas significant bleeding or nearly obstructive lesions typically warrant consideration for resection followed by completion chemotherapy.

Unfortunately, some patients will present with Stage 4 disease for which cure is not realistic. Determining which symptoms can be surgically palliated is a very difficult process. A patient may have vague symptoms and be found to have metastatic disease, but determining cause and effect for a specific symptom, and thereby determining the possibility of surgical palliation, can be challenging. Bowel obstruction may be a more intuitive predicament as CT scanning can often show the site of obstruction, in the case of malignant obstruction, a mass at the transition point (Fig. 6.3). The question becomes what to do about the obstruction. Options would include surgical resection, an intraluminal colonic stent, chemotherapy, or hospice, with or without placement of a gastrostomy tube to vent the GI tract. Each of these choices depends heavily on the extent of the disease and the condition and wishes of the patient. Obviously a relatively young patient with extensive disease but otherwise good reserve is often treated very differently from an octogenarian with CHF and chronic renal failure that may have a small amount of bleeding and isolated otherwise potentially resectable metastases. In general, a malignant bowel obstruction is a very serious and ominous occurrence. Historically, surgical procedures for these patients have been fraught with complications and an in-hospital mortality of 21–28 % [9, 10].

In the case of suspected malignant bowel obstruction, each patient's ability to undergo a major resection must be independently evaluated. Further, it is useful to determine what, if any, therapeutic options remain for the postoperative period (e.g., chemotherapy or radiation therapy). For patients with large bowel obstruction, we prefer endoscopic stenting when feasible and possible, at least initially. For patients with malignant small bowel obstruction, we generally will attempt one surgical exploration (laparoscopic when possible) for decompression via resection, internal bypass, or diversion. For a patient who is not suitable for exploration, or who is highly suspected to be inoperable based on imaging or prior attempts at relieving obstructions, a decompressive "venting" gastrostomy tube (percutaneous, endoscopic, or surgical) is often beneficial.

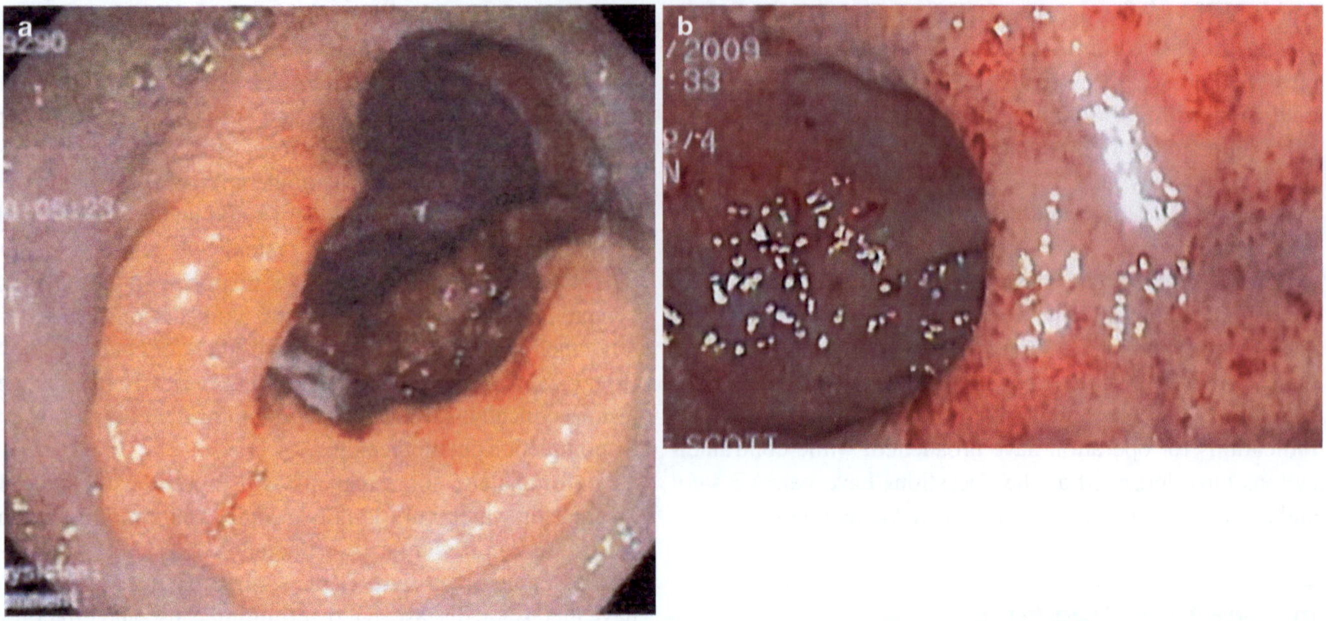

Fig. 6.2 Endoscopic view pre- (**a**) and post- (**b**) chemoradiation therapy demonstrating complete regression of the tumor (Courtesy of Scott R. Steele MD)

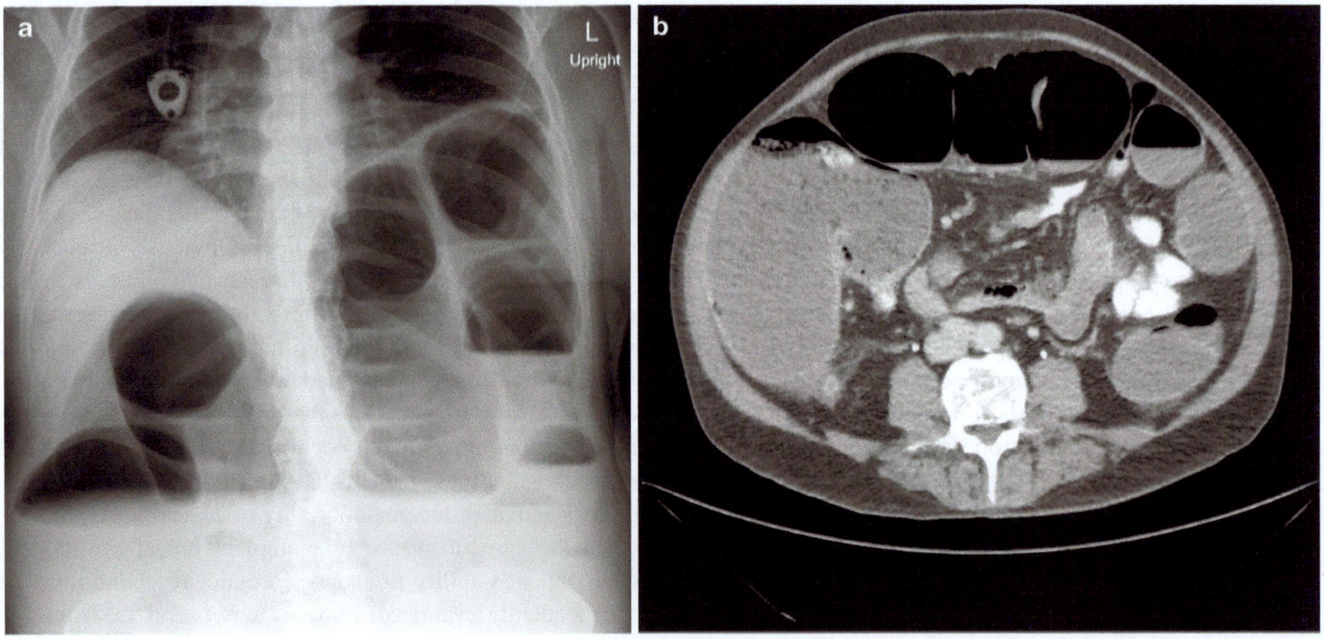

Fig. 6.3 Imaging of a malignant colon obstruction. Image (**a**) is plain film of distal colon obstruction, while Image (**b**) represents the corresponding CT scan image

Should I Biopsy the Metastasis?

Key Concept: Unless otherwise directed by a multidisciplinary panel to guide therapy, metastatic disease in the setting of a known CRC does not require biopsy.

National Comprehensive Cancer Network (NCCN) guidelines recommend that every patient with a diagnosis of colon or rectal cancer should undergo, among other things, a CT scan of the chest, abdomen, and pelvis to evaluate for evidence of metastatic disease [11]. When abnormalities are found on these studies suggestive of metastases, a decision must be made regarding whether or not a biopsy of a metastatic site needs to be performed. CT findings can be quite suggestive of metastatic disease, and in the patient with a diagnosis of colorectal cancer, these findings alone are often adequate for initiation of treatment. In some cases,

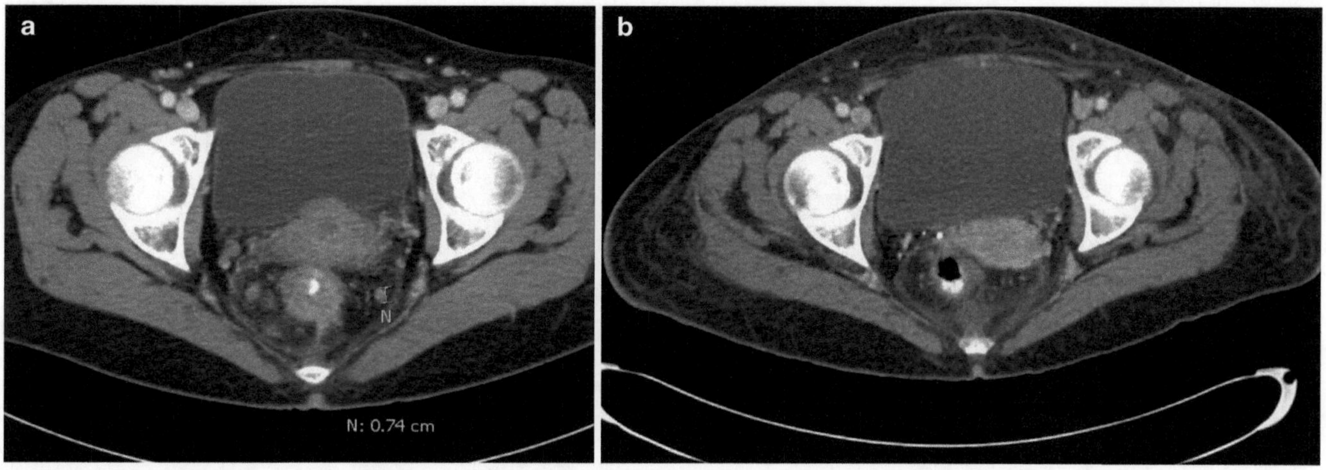

Fig. 6.4 CT Images pre- (**a**) and post- (**b**) chemoradiation therapy demonstrating tumor and lymph node regression

the addition of positron emission testing (PET) may further substantiate the need for systemic treatment, though the routine use of PET scan for every patient with a new diagnosis of colon or rectal cancer is not recommended by the NCCN [11]. In cases where there is some question about the diagnosis and the course of action would be altered if metastatic disease were confirmed, biopsy should be considered. We would generally recommend image-guided percutaneous needle biopsy where appropriate. However, for a patient with a known colorectal malignancy and CT findings strongly suggestive of malignant disease (and especially if the lesions are also PET-avid), routine biopsy is not necessary and may be harmful in terms of complications (e.g., bleeding) or tumor seeding.

What Should I Do with the Primary Lesion in the Patient with Extensive Disease?

Key Concept: While some evidence suggests improvement in outcomes with resection of the primary site, this has not been substantiated. Focus on the response to treatment and degree of symptoms.

Considering the primary tumor in the setting of metastatic disease, there has not been a clear consensus as to what, if anything, should be done. A recent review has suggested that there is a survival advantage to resection of the primary tumor [12]. They did note, however, that selection bias could in part be used to explain the advantage and, therefore, recommended further, prospective, studies. A subsequent Cochrane Review concluded that resection of the primary tumor is not associated with a survival benefit nor does it consistently result in a decrease in the tumor-related complications [13]. They felt that given the lack of strong evidence to recommend either for or against resection of the primary tumor, further clinical trials are warranted. In our practice (excepting for near obstruction), we will initiate chemotherapy and evaluate for the response to therapy. If the patient has a favorable or nearly complete clinical response (especially if the metastatic sites respond), we will reevaluate for resectability (Fig. 6.4). If imaging demonstrates resectable disease in a good surgical candidate, we will proceed with attempted resection of both sites. We have also come across the occasional case where there is a complete clinical response without any disease activity on PET (i.e., regression of all lesions) and have resected the primary site (Fig. 6.5). Ensuring the lesion is marked prior to chemotherapy (i.e., India ink tattoo, clip) has proved to be beneficial in this situation. Finally, for patients who continue to have progression, we must monitor for evidence of impending obstruction and be prepared to act accordingly.

What Treatment Modality Should Come First?

Key Concept: The extent of the disease, primary symptoms, and ability of the patient to tolerate various options should be discussed among the multidisciplinary census to determine a unified treatment plan.

Decisions about the order of various treatments (chemotherapy, operation, stenting, radiation therapy in cases of rectal cancer) will depend upon the sites and extent of metastatic disease as well as symptoms—especially obstruction or impending obstruction of the primary lesion. Again, multidisciplinary discussions are highly recommended. For patients without evidence of obstruction, and isolated liver or lung metastases, up-front chemotherapy would generally be started, with operation reserved for the metastases and primary lesion after several rounds of chemotherapy, assuming that the lesions are responding. Subsequently, the surgical resection(s) can be undertaken, either in one operation or in staged procedures. The decision is much more difficult for

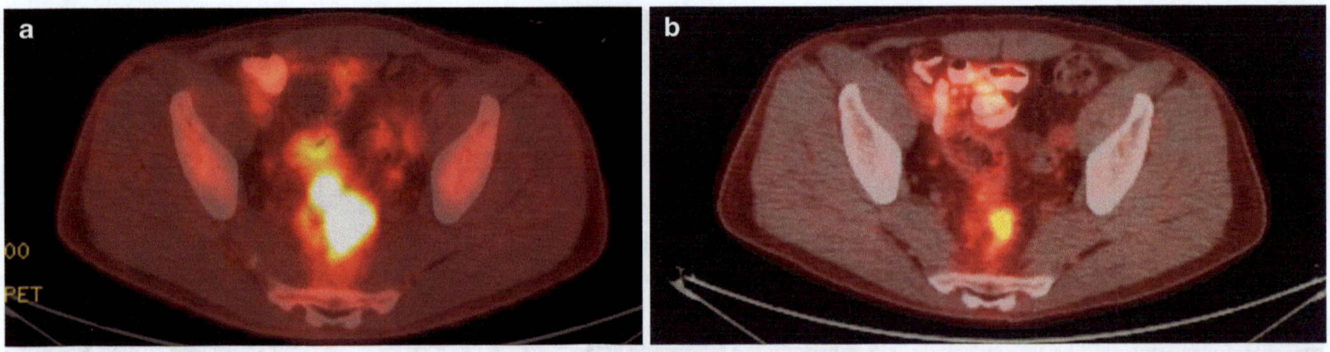

Fig. 6.5 Pre- (**a**) and post- (**b**) chemoradiation PET-CT images demonstrating absence of PET-positive activity on follow-up imaging

patients with multisite metastatic disease. In the past, these patients were generally felt to be incurable, with the possible exception of an isolated pulmonary metastasis in concert with limited liver metastases. Currently, multisite metastases, including select patients with peritoneal spread, can be considered for aggressive curative intent treatment, but generally only if they show response to up-front chemotherapy.

For surgeons, it is important to take into consideration the specific chemotherapeutic agents the oncologists are planning to use. This is especially important with the increasing use of bevacizumab, as it has been linked to bowel perforations. There has therefore been some concern about treating metastatic disease with systemic chemotherapy and bevacizumab, while the primary tumor remains within the colon. However, McCahill and colleagues demonstrated that the use of mFOLFOX6 plus bevacizumab did not result in an increased rate of complications associated to the primary tumor [14]. When an operation is planned for a patient on bevacizumab, it is recommended to wait 6 weeks following the last dose of bevacizumab prior to operating if possible, in order to decrease surgical complications that may be attributed to the antiangiogenic effects of bevacizumab [15]. For all other chemotherapeutic agents, we typically delay any operation at least 4 weeks (6–8 weeks for bevacizumab) when feasible, but one must weigh the risks of operating with chemotherapeutics circulating versus continued symptoms or progression during the delay.

The Obstructed Patient: What Now?

Key Concept: Several methods exist to deal with an impending obstruction and are at least in part predicated on the symptoms and location of the lesion.

For patients with a colon or rectal obstruction/near obstruction, the first step of treatment is generally to relieve the obstruction. In broad terms this can be performed in three fashions: resection of the primary lesion, diversion via a proximal stoma, or utilizing an intraluminal stent. Most

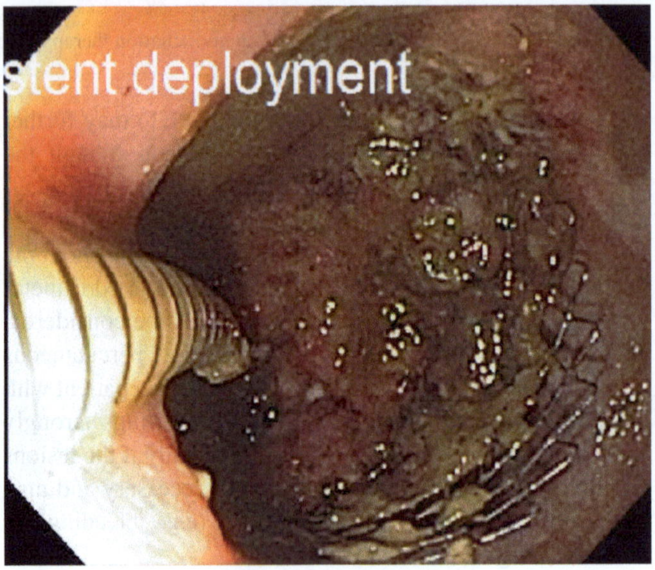

Fig. 6.6 Endoscopic placement of colonic stent

patients, when faced with these options, would choose to avoid a stoma and would therefore prefer an attempt at intraluminal stenting. Assuming that the lesion is not too low within the rectum and that the obstruction can be technically stented, there is a high technical success rate for placement of a stent [16–18]. The most recent series show both technical success and clinical success over 90 % of the time (Fig. 6.6). There is relatively low incidence of related morbidity, with migration, and tumor ingrowth being the most common (Fig. 6.7). Fortunately, perforation is uncommon although Manes et al. did note that the rate of perforation was considerably higher in patients receiving bevacizumab [17].

For distal rectal lesions, there may not be enough space for placement of a stent. The distal end of the stent needs to be above the pelvic floor (levator muscles) to avoid patient discomfort from the stent (Fig. 6.8). When there is no sufficient room for placement of a stent, diversion (proximal stoma) or primary resection may be needed, depending on the degree of obstruction. Occasionally, laser recanalization

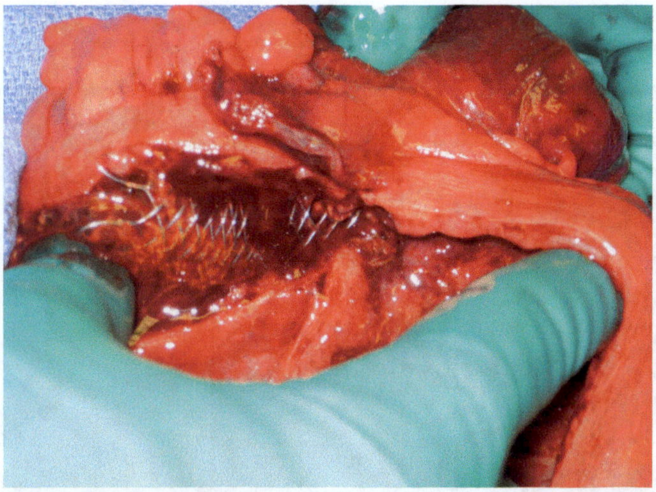

Fig. 6.7 Colonic stent perforation

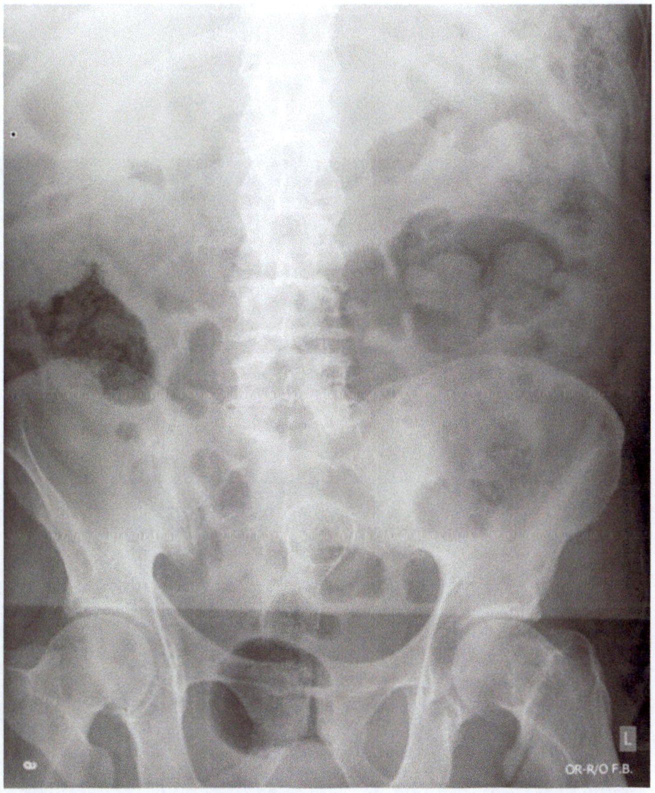

Fig. 6.8 Radiograph showing endorectal stent in place to relieve obstruction

can be effective in avoiding need for a stoma. Given that most such patients are candidates for pelvic irradiation prior to operation, we generally observe these patients closely during the first couple of weeks of radiation as long as they do not have evidence of complete obstruction, or we divert them with a laparoscopic sigmoid colostomy. Alternatively, for a patient with widespread metastatic disease, there may not be a primary role for pelvic radiation. As the goal of radiation is usually to decrease the rates of local (pelvic) recurrence, the patient with extensive, widespread metastases may not realize this potential benefit, and often the delay in full systemic chemotherapy may not be warranted. If the metastatic disease respond to the up-front chemotherapy, there may be a subsequent role for palliative pelvic radiation or for preoperative radiation (e.g., prior to attempt at cure).

When systemic chemotherapy is chosen as the initial approach, in some circumstances, the primary tumor shrinks considerably or even responds completely. What is the role for resection of the colon or rectum in this circumstance, and is there still a need/role for radiation in the case of a mid or low rectal cancer? Is there an indication to remove the primary source in the setting of metastatic disease? The answers to these questions are complex and need to be approached on a patient-specific basis. Sometimes these decisions are easy, such as for a patient whose primary tumor shrinks, but less significant treatment effect on the metastatic disease is observed, or who develops further metastatic disease despite ongoing chemotherapy. In these cases, there is very little, if any, role for resection of the primary tumor. However, as stated before, in a patient who has response of their liver/pulmonary disease or has disease that is resectable after up-front chemotherapy, there may well be a role in resecting the primary site of disease, especially in cases where the goal of operation is cure. Finally, there is occasionally a patient who would benefit from a palliative resection, especially in a situation where perineal pain from sphincter invasion has occurred or where the primary tumor continues to cause obstructive symptoms which are disabling.

Specific Sites of Disease

Liver

Key Concept: Metastatic disease to the liver is increasingly resected (or otherwise treated), even with bilobar involvement, based on the degree of functioning parenchyma that will remain after resection.

Colorectal cancer, when it metastasizes, most commonly spreads to the liver, followed by the lungs. Years ago, it was felt that any liver metastasis was a death sentence. However, limited resection for solitary liver metastases was initially shown to be safe and feasible, and an apparent oncologic benefit was demonstrated. Over time, indications expanded to include multiple metastases. With continued improvement, more aggressive therapy has been undertaken to treat patients, even with fairly high tumor burden at presentation (Fig. 6.9). The current paradigm in specialized and experienced programs centers around the amount of residual healthy liver remaining as the main determining factor in treating patients with liver metastases via resection. The other factor of importance remains the presence of extrahepatic disease.

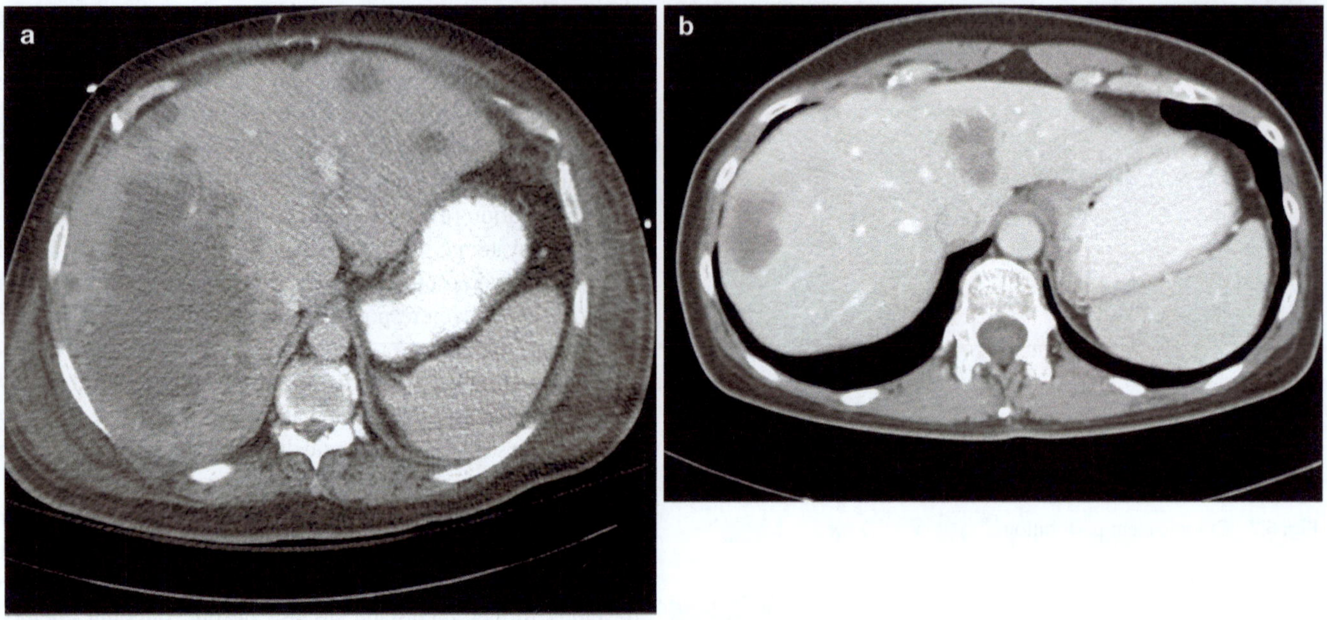

Fig. 6.9 (**a**, **b**) CT scan images of two patients with varying amounts of bilobar liver disease

As mentioned earlier, even some patients who would have been deemed unresectable (not potentially curable) due to inadequate normal liver have been able to be downsized to the point that they are candidates for potentially curative operation. Progressing from the traditional view that metastatic disease represented a death sentence, more than three decades of data argue against that view. With hepatectomy, select patients with colorectal cancer metastasized to the liver can realize 5-year disease-free survival of 28–58 % [19–25].

The data support treatment of a patient with liver metastases, but prior to embarking on operative therapy, one must understand the keys to liver resection. Certainly, achieving a negative margin is among the most important factors. More than a decade ago, Scheele demonstrated that a negative margin (R0 resection) had a vastly superior median survival (44 months) compared to those with R1 or R2 margins (14 months) [26]. The ability to achieve a negative margin, along with improved adjuvant therapy, has led surgeons to broaden indications for hepatectomy. As mentioned above, the most common limiting factor in liver resective surgery is the ability to have adequate functioning liver remaining postoperatively. It is generally felt that adequate liver remnant can be defined as 20 % of initial volume, as long as the remaining liver is normal.

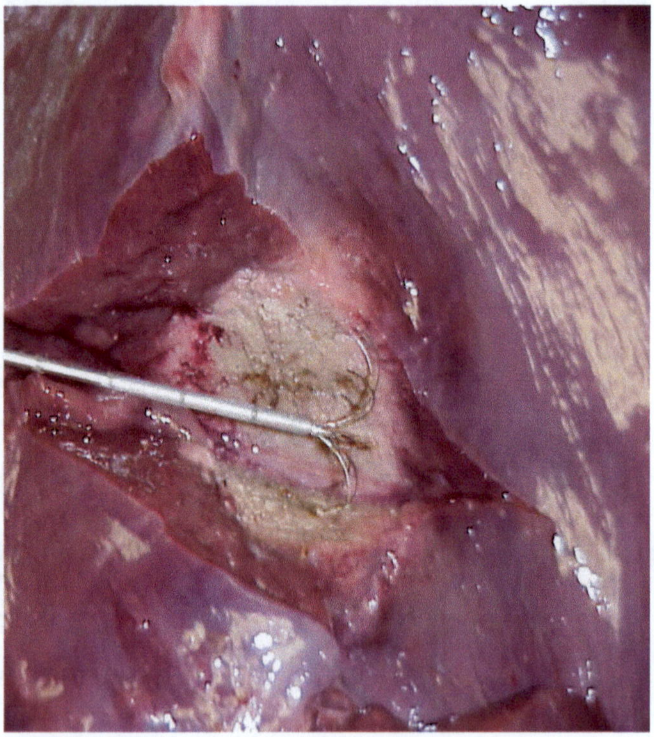

Fig. 6.10 Evaluation image of RFA probe in place in the liver (Courtesy of David Imagawa, MD)

There have also been several technological advancements in the past decade for treating liver metastases. Although surgical resection remains the "gold standard," alternative techniques to treat liver metastases, such as radiofrequency ablation (RFA) (Fig. 6.10), cryotherapy, irreversible electroporation, microwave ablation, selective internal radiation therapy (SIRT), and chemoembolization, are being increasingly utilized either as primary treatment or in conjunction with liver resection—especially in the setting of bilobar disease. RFA (the most commonly performed ablation method in the USA of those listed) can be performed percutaneously, laparoscopically, or in an open fashion.

After localization of the metastatic lesion, the RFA probe is inserted (under image guidance) and then activated. The tumor is heated, causing coagulation necrosis. Given that the effect is heat based, vessels located near tumors may act as a "heat-sink," potentially explaining the somewhat higher recurrence rate seen with RFA compared to resection. However, reasonable results have been obtained in multiple studies [27–30]. Further studies have been advocated [31].

Lung

Key Concept: Lung lesions are normally treated with chemotherapy primarily. Resection is typically reserved for those patients able to tolerate a pulmonary resection with isolated metastases.

Distal rectal cancers, by virtue of the systemic (rather than portal) venous drainage, are more likely to first spread to the lungs compared to other primary sites. However, given that isolated pulmonary metastases are not as commonly encountered as liver metastases, data supporting resection are not as compelling. That said, there are studies supporting resection of pulmonary metastases, with results surprisingly similar to outcomes for hepatic metastasectomy. For example, Pfannschmidt et al. [32, 33] twice reviewed the literature regarding pulmonary metastasectomy for colorectal metastases and noted that although there were no randomized trials to evaluate, the retrospective data demonstrated an improved survival rate for the highly selected group of patients who underwent pulmonary metastasectomy. Another large review in 2010 was less convinced [34]. After reviewing the data, the authors felt that any connection between increased survival and lung resection was unfounded due to a lack of sufficiently good data and that a randomized trial was warranted. With these issues in mind, we approach each patient with isolated pulmonary metastases on an individual basis. If, after full staging, the patient still appears to have only isolated lung metastases and the primary lesion is resectable, we will usually treat with up-front systemic chemotherapy and then resect the lung lesions first (or resect the primary lesion simultaneously as able) if response is seen. If the patient does well and continues to have no other evidence for disease, we will then tackle the primary lesion either before or after the addition of further systemic chemotherapy. If, on the other hand, the patient is found to be unresectable in the thorax or has other sites of disease, continuation of systemic chemotherapy, as indicated, is routine.

Peritoneal Metastases

Key Concept: Peritoneal carcinomatosis represents "drop" metastases that may be approached with combination therapy in rare instances. The ability to select proper patients (i.e., healthy, low PCI score) and achieve a complete cytoreduction is imperative.

Carcinomatosis is a dreaded pattern of spread of colorectal cancer (Fig. 6.11). Unfortunately, up to 15 % of patients may present with carcinomatosis at the time of initial diagnosis and an even higher rate of carcinomatosis exists with patients who have recurrent disease [35, 36]. Though traditionally felt to be incurable, carcinomatosis can be treated, and in some cases, a cure can be achieved, through the use of cytoreductive surgery, peritoneal stripping, and intraperitoneal chemotherapy. There are two general methods of delivering the chemotherapy, intraoperative hyperthermic intraperitoneal chemotherapy (HIPEC) (Fig. 6.12) and early postoperative intraperitoneal chemotherapy (EPIC). The use of cytoreductive surgery and intraperitoneal chemotherapy for colorectal carcinomatosis is based upon the practice championed by Sugarbaker for treating pseudomyxoma peritonei [37]. An intraoperative staging system (PCI) is employed describing the extent of carcinomatosis on a scale of 1–39 [38]. For patients with otherwise surgically treatable disease, HIPEC should be considered as long as a complete cytoreduction is possible [39–41]. Outcomes are best for patients with PCI below 20 at time of exploration and in whom a complete/near complete cytoreduction is possible [42].

Ovary

Key Concept: Only involved ovaries should be resected, and prophylactic oophorectomy is typically not warranted.

The ovaries can become involved in women with advanced colorectal cancer. A recent review of 180 cases of colorectal cancer in women demonstrated an overall prevalence of colorectal cancer metastasis to the ovary of 2.7 %, but fewer than half that number were isolated metastases to the ovary [43]. In the past, it was routine for women to undergo concomitant bilateral oophorectomy with resection of the primary colorectal lesion. Currently, only ovaries that are involved via direct extension or which are morphologically involved should be removed, when feasible, but prophylactic oophorectomy is not generally recommended except for suspected/known cases of Lynch syndrome [44].

Brain

Key Concept: Only in rare instances are brain metastases addressed and normally as a palliative measure.

Limited data exist on brain metastases, and isolated brain metastases are extremely rare. Sundermeyer et al. [45] demonstrated that only 3 % of patients with colorectal cancer develop brain metastases. They develop more commonly in

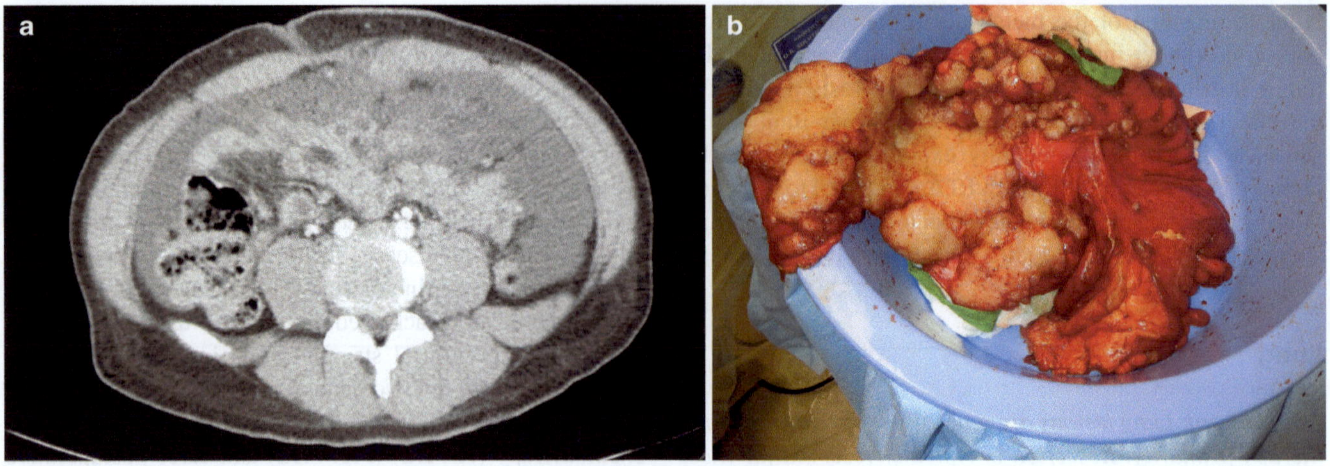

Fig. 6.11 Carcinomatosis leading to bowel obstruction. Image (**a**) demonstrates CT scan findings of extensive carcinomatosis. Image (**b**) (Courtesy of Alessio Pigazzi, MD) represents surgical specimen of large debulking procedure

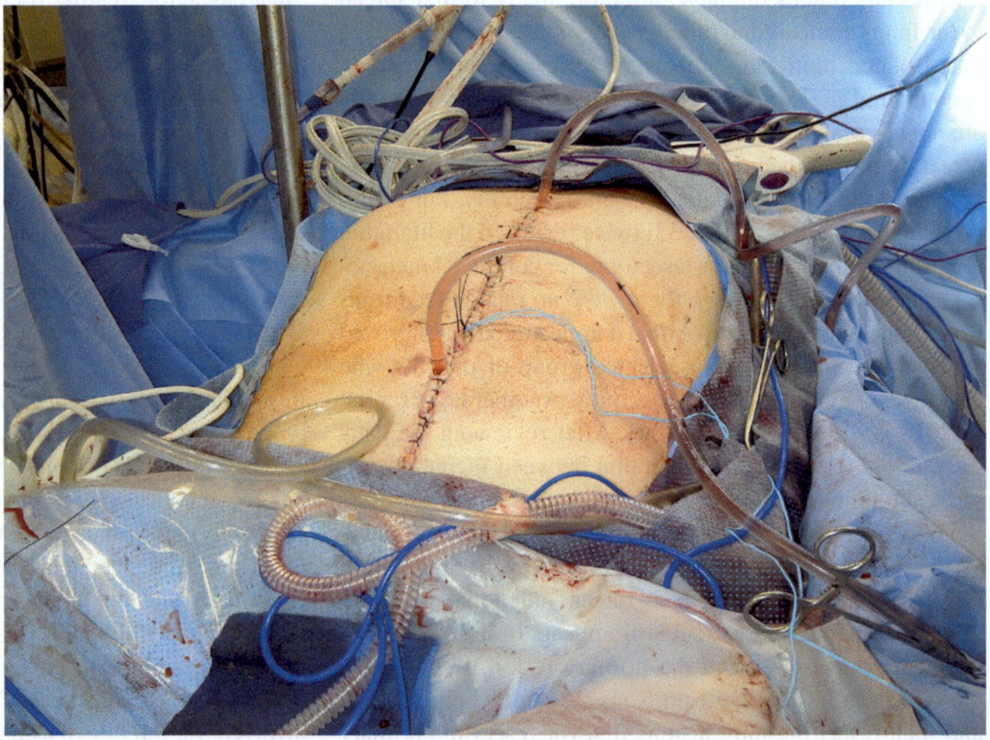

Fig. 6.12 Intraoperative photograph of patient undergoing HIPEC, with catheters in place (Courtesy of Alessio Pigazzi, MD)

patients who already have pulmonary metastases. Treatment is almost always palliative and therefore should be dictated by symptoms.

Controversial Points

Age of Patient: Should we treat patients differently based upon their age?

Is there a difference between the Stage 4 patient who is 48 years old versus the patient who is 84? That is, should a patient be treated differently based primarily upon age alone, or should we look at something else to determine how aggressive to be, such as comorbidities (ASA) and patient/family desires? There is no specific literature to guide decision making for elderly patients with Stage 4 colorectal cancer; however, there is some related information regarding elderly patients undergoing colon cancer treatment that can be extrapolated. In terms of treating the elderly, age alone should not be a reason to exclude a patient from colon resection or even from systemic chemotherapy [46]. It has been shown that when chemotherapy is appropriately given for Stage 3 patients, despite being older, it is generally well tolerated with even fewer adverse reactions than younger patients and improves overall survival. Older patients receiving chemotherapy have also been reported to have similar disease-specific survival as their younger counterparts. Yet, this data was for Stage 3 patients, not Stage 4, and one must take a realistic approach to treating the elderly with metastatic disease. In this more advanced stage, we simply go back to one initial point regarding treatment indications: the surgeon must evaluate and discuss with the patient and their family about maintaining *realistic* goals of care and the possibility of futility.

As a patient presents for consideration of resection—any patient, regardless of age—they arrive with expectations and desires. Some may have met with other physicians (surgeons or otherwise) and may have already been told what to expect to hear from you (rightly or wrongly). When a patient arrives with set expectations, it is critical to have an open, honest, and clear discussion about potential outcomes and various options that are reasonable. Though their expectations and yours may not be initially aligned, it is imperative that you leave that meeting united prior to proceeding. Any other way forward is a setup for failure.

The Patient with a "Near Obstruction"

As stated briefly earlier, not infrequently a patient will present with an impending obstruction. The endoscopist may or may not have been able to traverse the lesion with the scope, and the patient may have varying degrees of symptoms associated with obstruction. When these patients also have metastatic disease on work up, we generally commence with systemic chemotherapy. The question of whether or not the primary "near-obstructing" lesion needs to be addressed first can be a complicated situation. The surgeon must consider whether or not the patient is having significant symptoms of obstruction (smaller stools, difficulty with BM, loose bowel movements, obstipation, bloating, etc.) or "simply" a non-traversable lesion on endoscopy. For patients suffering from symptoms of obstruction (even partial), we would generally attempt to place an intraluminal stent. Resection and proximal diversion are also options, although you have to weigh the risks of each of these against other options in light of the patient (and their overall clinical state) sitting in front of you. For patients with questionable or intermittent obstructive symptoms, in general, if it is possible to pass a colonoscope through the lesion, it is not likely to cause an imminent obstruction, especially if the patient is being treated with an effective chemotherapeutic regimen. For these patients we will continue (or initiate) chemotherapy.

A more difficult situation is when, occasionally, a patient develops an obstruction during chemotherapy. Often these patients are not ideal candidates for surgical intervention given the systemic effects of chemotherapy and possibly of any biologic therapy concurrently employed. When this occurs, our first choice would be intraluminal stent placement. Given the high technical and clinical success rates that we previously highlighted, this typically provides adequate relief of the obstruction. However, if diversion is required, we would always recommend creating a loop stoma or mucous fistula to avoid a closed-loop obstruction and possible perforation. This is generally obtained via an "end-loop" colostomy [47], which we generally perform laparoscopically (Fig. 6.13). We create the stoma by stapling off the distal segment and then opening a corner of the defunctionalized limb at the inferior aspect of the colostomy, thereby allowing for the use of a normal colostomy appliance but allowing for decompression of the distal, obstructed limb.

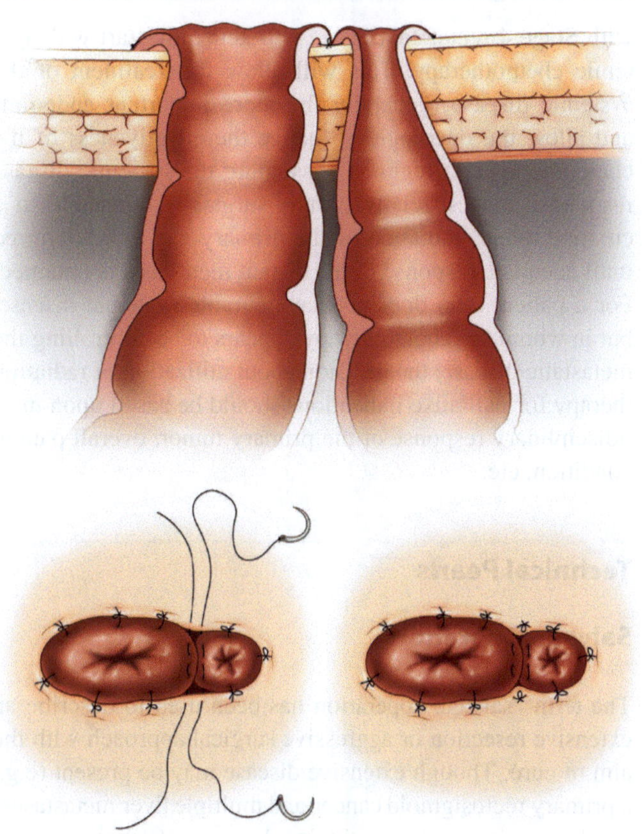

Fig. 6.13 End-loop stoma with distal defunctionalized bowel matured through the same incision

Role of Radiation for Rectal Cancer in Patients with Stage 4 Disease

Key Concept: Radiation plays a secondary role in patients with metastatic disease and often for primary palliation of symptoms.

When treating patients with resectable rectal cancer, the use of radiation in the "neoadjuvant" setting is primary to decrease the risk of locoregional recurrence. For a patient with Stage 4 rectal cancer, we will generally start with systemic chemotherapy. This will allow for treatment of the systemic disease (generally the more important endpoint) and allow the oncologist to gauge the effectiveness of the chemotherapeutic regimen. Assuming the systemic disease responds, and especially if it is surgically amenable to a curative intent, radiation of the primary would be deferred until adequate response of the distant metastasis is obtained. For a patient who does not have curable systemic disease, but in whom the chemotherapy appears to be controlling the metastatic disease, the decision about utilization of radiation therapy for palliative indications should be based upon multidisciplinary response of the primary tumor, overall patient condition, etc.

Technical Pearls

Salvage Operation

The term "salvage" operation has been used to describe an extensive resection or aggressive surgical approach with the aim of cure. Though extensive disease may be present (e.g., a primary rectosigmoid cancer and multiple liver metastases) or a large primary tumor with involvement of other organs or the abdominal wall, an attempt is planned for an aggressive surgical approach (salvage) with the hope of providing a curative (R0) operation. Prior to any attempt at salvage, an in-depth discussion should be had with the patient. A clear discussion of goals and possible operative scenarios (such as what the patient's wishes are for various potential operative discoveries) is necessary. The patient should generally be given a bowel preparation, when feasible.

Prior to any pelvic exenteration or liver resection surgery, we strongly recommend first performing diagnostic laparoscopy to look for carcinomatosis. If carcinomatosis is encountered, one should calculate the peritoneal cancer index (PCI) [38] to determine if the patient would be a candidate for cytoreductive surgery (see above), although this is rarely done in the presence of significant metastatic disease.

If the decision is made to proceed with resection, one should first start with adequate exposure. As most of these cases are performed through a full laparotomy incision, the use of an abdominal wall retractor (such as a Bookwalter, Omni, or other retractor system) is essential. In certain situations, as determined by the surgeon's experience, skill-set, and needs of the procedure, a laparoscopic or robotic approach may be feasible. Regardless of approach, we recommend that mobilization be the first step. Prior to committing to resection by performing any step that cannot be undone (i.e., to "burn a bridge"—to divide the bowel or devascularize a segment), the surgeon should attempt either to assure that there is nothing precluding the completion of the operation or to assure a safe way out of the procedure (e.g., the ability to create a stoma). Once the resection is complete, reconstruction is performed.

For extensive pelvic procedures, procedures in reoperative fields, or if ureter involvement is suspected, one should consider the preoperative placement of ureteral catheters. They may aid in identification of the ureter even in a situation where they are obscured or displaced by tumor or scar. Further, in the event of ureteral injury, they can help to identify the injury (visualization of the catheter).

Palliative Care

Some patients are not appropriate for curative treatment. The question of when to decide to "back off" can be very difficult for both the patient and the surgeon. As questions about futility of care, palliation, and/or hospice arise, involvement of a palliative care team would be worthwhile. Adding their input will aid the patient and family member in decision making regarding myriad end-of-life issues. Some patients may benefit from placement of a venting gastrostomy tube (percutaneous or laparoscopic assisted) to palliate the effects of bowel obstruction.

Summary Pearls

The management of Stage 4 colorectal cancer is complex. Given the multimodal therapy options, a multidisciplinary team approach should be used, primarily a medical oncologist, radiation oncologist (in the case of rectal cancer), and a surgeon. With the recent advancements of all aspects of cancer treatment, patients with metastatic disease are living longer, and we are extending indications and options for curative intent. When you are treating a patient with metastatic disease, take a stepwise approach, and treat each of the various sites of disease. This will allow you to convert some patients to a potentially curable state. You must be willing to be aggressive with indications and treatment when appropriate, but also be realistic. Discussions with the patient and family are important, and you should be open and genuine. Surgical and nonsurgical options for palliation are available and should be utilized as indicated. As a surgeon who treats colorectal cancer, you should be familiar with all of the various options and treatment scenarios.

References

1. Siegel R, Naishadham D, Jemal A. Cancer statistics, 2012. CA Cancer J Clin. 2012;62(1):10–29.
2. Ko C, Chaudhry S. The need for a multidisciplinary approach to cancer care. J Surg Res. 2002;105(1):53–7.
3. Fuchs CS, Marshall J, Barrueco J. Randomized, controlled trial of irinotecan plus infusional, bolus, or oral fluoropyrimidines in

first-line treatment of metastatic colorectal cancer: updated results from the BICC-C study. J Clin Oncol. 2008;26(4):689–90.
4. Hochster HS, Hart LL, Ramanathan RK, Childs BH, Hainsworth JD, Cohn AL, et al. Safety and efficacy of oxaliplatin and fluoropyrimidine regimens with or without bevacizumab as first-line treatment of metastatic colorectal cancer: results of the TREE Study. J Clin Oncol. 2008;26(21):3523–9.
5. Gaya A, Tse V. A preclinical and clinical review of aflibercept for the management of cancer. Cancer Treat Rev. 2012;38(5):484–93.
6. Grothey A. Results of a phase III randomized, double-blind, placebo-controlled, multicenter trial (CORRECT) of regorafenib plus best supportive care (BSC) versus placebo plus BSC in patients (pts) with metastatic colorectal cancer (mCRC) who have progressed after standard therapies. In: Gastrointestinal cancers symposium of the American Society of Clinical Oncology, San Framcisco, CA, USA, 21 Jan 2012.
7. Nordlinger B, Sorbye H, Glimelius B, Poston GJ, Schlag PM, Rougier P, et al. Perioperative chemotherapy with FOLFOX4 and surgery versus surgery alone for resectable liver metastases from colorectal cancer (EORTC Intergroup trial 40983): a randomized controlled trial. Lancet. 2008;371(9617):1007–16.
8. Sorbye H, Mauer M, Gruenberger T, Glimelius B, Poston GJ, Schlag PM, et al. Predictive factors for the benefit of perioperative FOLFOX for resectable liver metastasis in colorectal cancer patients (EORTC Intergroup Trial 40983). Ann Surg. 2012;255(3):534–9.
9. Mucha P. Small intestine obstruction. Surg Clin North Am. 1987;67:597–620.
10. Butler JA, Cameron BL, Morrow M, Kahng K, Tom J. Small bowel obstruction in patients with a prior history of cancer. Am J Surg. 1991;162:624–8.
11. NCCN Colon Cancer Guidelines (version 1.2013). National Comprehensive Cancer Network. 2013. Available at http://www.nccn.org/professionals/physician_gls/f_guidelines.asp#colon. Accessed Feb 2013.
12. Venderbosch S, de Wilt JH, Teerenstra S, Loosveld OH, van Bochove A, Sinnige HA, et al. Prognostic value of resection of primary tumor in patients with stage IV colorectal cancer: retrospective analysis of two randomized studies and a review of the literature. Ann Surg Oncol. 2011;18(12):3252–60.
13. Cirocchi R, Trastulli S, Abraha I, Vettoretto N, Boselli C, Montedori A, et al. Non-resection versus resection for an asymptomatic primary tumour in patients with unresectable stage IV colorectal cancer. Cochrane Database Syst Rev. 2012;(8):CD008997.
14. McCahill LE, Yothers G, Sharif S, Petrelli NJ, Lai LL, Bechar N, et al. Primary mFOLFOX6 plus bevacizumab without resection of the primary tumor for patients presenting with surgically unresectable metastatic colon cancer and an intact asymptomatic colon cancer: definitive analysis of NSABP trial C-10. J Clin Oncol. 2012;30(26):3223–8.
15. Hompes D, Ruers T. Review: incidence and clinical significance of Bevacizumab-related non-surgical and surgical serious adverse events in metastatic colorectal cancer. Eur J Surg Oncol. 2011;37(9):737–46.
16. Law WL, Choi HK, Lee YM, Chu KW. Palliation for advanced malignant colorectal obstruction by self-expanding metallic stents: prospective evaluation of outcomes. Dis Colon Rectum. 2004;47(1):39–43.
17. Manes G, de Bellis M, Fuccio L, Repici A, Masci E, Ardizzone S, et al. Endoscopic palliation in patients with incurable malignant colorectal obstruction by means of self-expanding metal stent: analysis of results and predictors of outcomes in a large multicenter series. Arch Surg. 2011;146(10):1157–62.
18. Lamazza A, Fiori E, Scillaci A, Demasi E, Pontone S, Sterpetti AV. Self-expandable metallic stents in patients with stage IV obstructing colorectal cancer. World J Surg. 2012;36(12):2931–6.
19. Scheele J, Stangl T, Altendorf-Hofmann A. Hepatic metastases from colorectal carcinoma: impact of surgical resection on the natural history. Br J Surg. 1990;77:1241–6.
20. Scheele J, Stangl R, Atlendorf-Hofmann A, Paul M. Resection of colorectal liver metastases. World J Surg. 1995;19(1):59–71.
21. Nordlinger B, Guiguet M, Vaillant JC, Valladur P, Boudjema K, Bachellier P, et al. Surgical resection of colorectal carcinoma metastases to the liver. A prognostic scoring system to improve case selection, based on 1568 patients. Cancer. 1996;77:1254–62.
22. Choti MA, Sitzmann JV, Tiburi ME, Sumetchotimetha W, Rangsin R, Schulck RD, et al. Trends in ling-term survival following liver resection for hepatic colorectal metastases. Ann Surg. 2002;235(2):759–66.
23. Fernandez FG, Drebin JA, Linchan DC, Dehdashti F, Siegel BA, Strasberg SM. Five year survival after resection of hepatic metastases from colorectal cancer in patients screened by positron emission tomography with F-18 fluorodeoxyglucose (FDG-PET). Ann Surg. 2004;240(3):438–47.
24. Pawlik TM, Scoggins CR, Zorzi D, Abdalla EK, Andres A, Eng C, et al. Effect of surgical margin status on survival and site of recurrence after hepatic resection from colorectal metastases. Ann Surg. 2005;241(5):715–22.
25. Tomlinson JS, Jarnagin WR, DeMatteo RP, Fong Y, Kornprat P, Gonen M, et al. Actual 10-year survival after resection of colorectal liver metastases defines cure. J Clin Oncol. 2007;25(29):4575–80.
26. Scheele J, Altendorf-Hoffman A, Grube T, Hohenbreger W, Stangl R, Schmidt K. Resection of colorectal liver metastases. What prognostic factors determine patient selection? Chirurg. 2001;72(5):547–60.
27. Abdalla EK, Vauthey JN, Ellis LM, Ellis V, Pollock R, Broglio KR, et al. Recurrence and outcomes following hepatic resection, radiofrequency ablation, and combined resection/ablation for colorectal liver metastases. Ann Surg. 2004;239(6):818–25.
28. Sorensen SM, Mortensen FV, Nielsen DT. Radiofrequency ablation of colorectal liver metastases: long-term survival. Acta Radiol. 2007;48(3):253–8.
29. Siperstein AE, Berber E, Ballem N, Parikh RT. Survival after radiofrequency ablation of colorectal liver metastases: 10-year experience. Ann Surg. 2007;246(4):559–65.
30. Kennedy TJ, Cassera MA, Khajanchee YS, Diwan TS, Hammill CW, Hansen PD. Laparoscopic radiofrequency ablation for the management of colorectal liver metastases: 10-year experience. J Surg Oncol. 2013;107(4):324–8.
31. Cirocchi R, Trastulli S, Boselli C, Montedori A, Cavaliere D, Parisi A, et al. Radiofrequency ablation in the treatment of liver metastases from colorectal cancer. Cochrane Database Syst Rev. 2012;(6):CD006317.
32. Pfannschmidt J, Dienemann H, Hoffmann H. Surgical resection of pulmonary metastases from colorectal cancer: a systematic review of published series. Ann Thorac Surg. 2007;84(1):324–38.
33. Pfannschmidt J, Dienemann H, Hoffmann H. Reported outcome factors for pulmonary resection in metastatic colorectal cancer. J Thorac Oncol. 2010;5(6 Suppl 2):S172–8.
34. Fiorentino F, Hunt I, Teoh K, Treasure T, Utley M. Pulmonary metastasectomy in colorectal cancer: a systematic review and quantitative synthesis. J R Soc Med. 2010;103(2):60–6.
35. Sugarbaker PH, Cunliffe WJ, Belliveau J, de Brulin EA, Graves T, Mullins RE, et al. Rationale for integrating early postoperative intraperitoneal chemotherapy into the surgical treatment of gastrointestinal cancer. Semin Oncol. 1989;16(4 Suppl 6):83–97.
36. Dawson LE, Russell AH, Tong D, Wisbeck WM. Adenocarcinoma of the sigmoid colon: sites of initial dissemination and clinical patterns of recurrence following surgery alone. J Surg Oncol. 1983;22(2):95–9.
37. Sugarbaker PH, Zhu BW, Sese GB, Shmookler B. Peritoneal carcinomatosis from appendiceal cancer: results in 69 patients treated by cytoreductive surgery and intraperitoneal chemotherapy. Dis Colon Rectum. 1993;36(4):323–9.
38. Sugarbaker PH, Averbach AM, Jacquet P, Stuart OA, Stephens AD. Hyperthermic intraoperative intraperitoneal chemotherapy (HIIC) with mitomycin C. Surg Technol Int. 1996;5:245–9.

39. Verwaal VJ, van Ruth S, de Bree E, van Sloothen GW, van Tinteren H, Zoetmulder FA. Randomized trial of cytoreduction and hyperthermic intraperitoneal chemotherapy versus systemic chemotherapy and palliative surgery in patients with peritoneal carcinomatosis of colorectal cancer. J Clin Oncol. 2003;21(20):3737–43.
40. Elias D, Glehen O, Pocard M, Quenet F, Goere D, Arvieux C, et al. A comparative study of complete cytoreductive surgery plus intraperitoneal chemotherapy to treat peritoneal dissemination from colon, rectum, small bowel, and nonpseudomyxoma appendix. Ann Surg. 2010;251(5):896–901.
41. Elias D, Lefevre JH, Chevalier J, Brouquet A, Marchal F, Classe JM, et al. Complete cytoreductive surgery plus intraperitoneal chemohyperthermia with oxaliplatin for peritoneal carcinomatosis of colorectal origin. J Clin Oncol. 2009;27(5):681–5.
42. Van Sweringen HL, Hanseman DJ, Ahmad SA, Edwards MJ, Sussman JJ. Predictors of survival in patients with high-grade peritoneal metastases undergoing cytoreductive surgery and hyperthermic intraperitoneal chemotherapy. Surgery. 2012;152(4):617–24.
43. Omranipour R, Abasahi A. Ovarian metastases in colorectal cancer. Int J Gynecol Cancer. 2009;19(9):1524–8.
44. Chang GJ, Kaiser AM, Mills S, Rafferty JF, Buie WD, Standards Practice Task Force of the American Society of Colon and Rectal Surgeons. Practice parameters for the management of colon cancer. Dis Colon Rectum. 2012;55(8):831–43.
45. Sundermeyer ML, Meropol NJ, Rogatko A, Wang H, Cohen SJ. Changing patterns of bone and brain metastases in patients with colorectal cancer. Clin Colorectal Cancer. 2005;5(2):108–13.
46. Audisio RA, Papamichael D. Treatment of colorectal cancer in older patients. Nat Rev Gastroenterol Hepatol. 2012;9(12):716–25.
47. Prasad ML, Pearl RK, Abcarian H. End-loop colostomy. Surg Gynecol Obstet. 1984;158(4):380–2.

Enterocutaneous Fistulas

7

Willem A. Bemelman and Marja A. Boermeester

Key Points

- The management of enterocutaneous fistulas should be performed according to SNAP (Sepsis, Nutrition, Anatomy, Procedure).
- Timing of reconstructive surgery should be at least 6 months after the last surgery.
- Patients dependent on parenteral nutrition or with metabolic issues require an abdominal reconstruction, if their risk profile is acceptable.
- Abdominal wall reconstruction is essential for successful fistula closure.

Initial Evaluation

The general principle of management of enterocutaneous fistula can be summarized in the acronym SNAP, which represents Sepsis, Nutrition, Anatomy, Procedure.

1. Sepsis
   - Remove cause and control sepsis.
   - Drain abscess cavities.
   - Wound care and skin protection.
2. Nutrition
   - Control fluid and electrolyte intake (restriction depends on fistula output).
   - Total parenteral nutrition/enteral nutrition.
3. Anatomy
   - CT: define abscess cavities.
   - Inside-to-outside contrast video radiography or MR enteroclysis (determine upstream absorption length).
   - Completion of road map as preoperative work-up (MR, colonography, fistulogram).
4. Procedure

Controlling Sepsis

Key Concept: *Initial focus should be on source control, resuscitation, and early antibiotics to reverse the septic process.*

The treatment of abdominal sepsis in the acute setting is characterized by preservation or restoration of organ function to provide adequate perfusion and oxygenation. A rapid sequence in treatment steps involves resuscitation, antimicrobial therapy, and surgery. Resuscitation comprises all measures taken to sustain adequate perfusion and oxygenation. Adequate resuscitation in the first 6 h of a septic shock improves mortality rate significantly [1]. Early administration of antibiotic therapy is of great importance. With every delay of 30 min after the diagnosis, mortality rate increases with an odds ratio of 1.021 (95 % CI 1.003–1.038) [2]. Early administration of antibiotics gives a 33 % relative risk reduction of mortality in patients with bacteremia admitted to the intensive care unit [3]. Empiric antimicrobial therapy should be aimed at expected strains, while there is no preference for one of the various available empiric antibiotic regimes [4]. When culture results and their susceptibility become available, the antibiotic regime should be reviewed once more and, if necessary, adapted. Colonization and infection with yeast and fungi is common in ICU patients, especially with *Candida* spp. [5] A meta-analysis has shown that antifungal prophylaxis is useful in reducing yeast infections in severely ill patients with either a single-drug antifungal prophylaxis (odds ratio 0.54, 95 % CI 0.39–0.75) or with selective bowel decontamination (odds ratio 0.29, 95 % CI 0.18–0.45) [6].

W.A. Bemelman, MD, PhD (✉) • M.A. Boermeester, MD, PhD
Department of Surgery, Academic Medical Center,
University of Amsterdam, Meibergdreef 9,
Amsterdam 1105 AZ, The Netherlands
e-mail: w.a.bemelman@amc.uva.nl; m.a.boermeester@amc.uva.nl

S.R. Steele et al. (eds.), *Complexities in Colorectal Surgery*,
DOI 10.1007/978-1-4614-9022-7_7, © Springer Science+Business Media New York 2014

To prevent one yeast infection, 20 patients have to be treated with single-drug prophylaxis, or 18 patients have to be treated with selective bowel decontamination. Furthermore, mortality rates are lower with antifungal prophylaxis with a combined odds ratio (single-drug or selective bowel decontamination regimes) of 0.23 (95 % CI 0.09–0.60) [6].

Surgery remains the cornerstone for the treatment of peritonitis where elimination of the infectious focus (source control) and prevention of an ongoing infection are key features. This can comprise not only surgical intervention, but also additional measures such as a radiological intervention or the removal of an infected catheter [7]. The underlying condition and the anatomical site causing secondary peritonitis dictate which procedure is most appropriate. Specific surgical techniques used for each condition are not discussed here, as the variety of underlying causes would call for an extensive description, which is beyond the scope of this chapter. Effort must be made to achieve complete source control in the early phase of the disease and in a single surgical procedure. Source control is of greater importance than restoration of normal function and/or anatomy [8]. Rinsing of the abdominal cavity with saline, or even antibiotics, or antiseptic agents in case of an intra-abdominal infection is a common practice in surgery. To the surprise of many, none of the intra-abdominally used solutions have any proven positive effect on the outcome of secondary peritonitis [9], whereas rinsing can damage mesothelial cells which play a key role in the immune reaction [10]. Therefore, the proverb "the solution to pollution is dilution" seems a dogma to divert from. Elimination of the infectious focus makes drain placement unnecessary and potentially harmful. Drain placement in general should be reserved for percutaneous drainage of fluid collections that develop during the postoperative course. In some cases a monitor drain can be useful, such as after primary closure of a duodenal perforation. Just as important, whenever possible, closure of the abdominal cavity (by fascial closure) is important to prevent fluid losses, fistula formation, and permanent abdominal hernia.

Despite adequate source control during the initial emergency laparotomy, a re-laparotomy may sometimes be necessary depending on the patient's clinical course. In general, only in the setting of clinical deterioration or insufficient improvement in the first few days will a re-laparotomy be performed. This is called the "on-demand" strategy. There are several reasons to prefer the on-demand strategy above the planned re-laparotomy strategy. A meta-analysis of observational studies showed a nonsignificant lower mortality implementing the on-demand strategy (combined odds ratio 0.70, 95 % CI 0.27–1.80) [11]. In 2007 the only randomized trial comparing the on-demand and planned strategies was published (RELAP trial) [12]. For this trial, 510 patients with secondary peritonitis were registered, of which more than half were excluded because of an APACHE-II score ≤10. Two hundred and thirty-two patients were included (116 on-demand and 116 planned re-laparotomy). A nonsignificant lower mortality was found in the on-demand group compared with the planned re-laparotomy group (29 % versus 36 %, $p = 0.22$). Even for the most severely ill patients with an APACHE-II score >20, this pattern was observed (Fig. 7.1). This important finding argues against the dogma that the most severely ill patient in particular benefits from the planned re-laparotomy strategy. While sounding

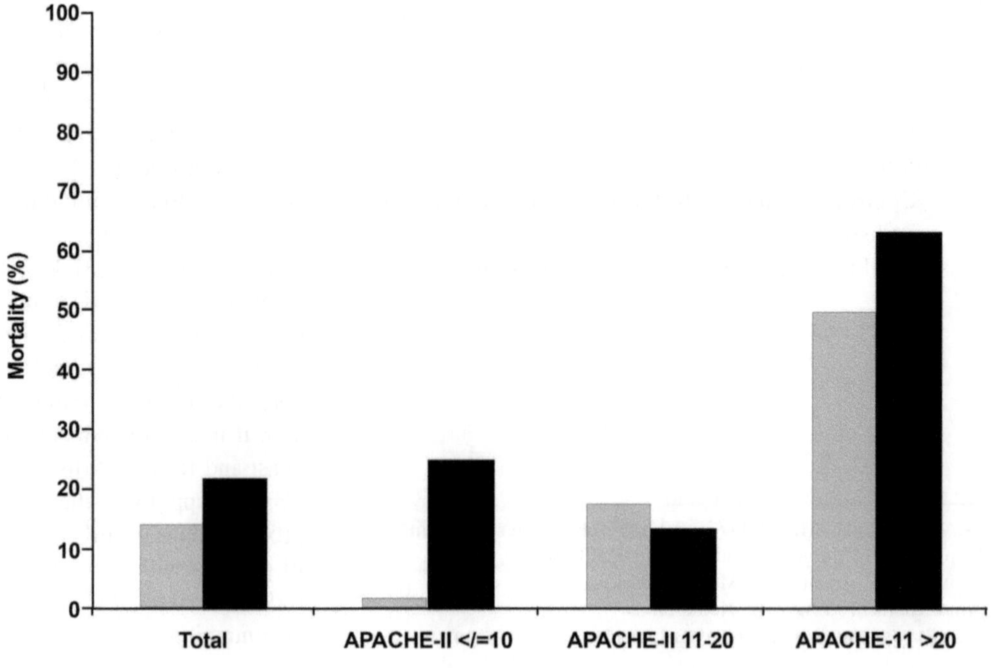

Fig. 7.1 Mortality of secondary peritonitis patients, divided based on the severity of disease expressed by the APACHE-II score. Two surgical strategies were compared per category, re-laparotomy on-demand (□) and planned re-laparotomy (■). A total of 510 patients were registered; patients with an APACHE-II score >10 were randomized in two strata (11–20 and >20) between on-demand and planned re-laparotomy strategy

oversimplified, only the patients that "need" to return to the operating room are those that should be reexplored. Additionally the on-demand strategy significantly decreases healthcare utilization, resulting in a cost reduction of USD 23,000 per patient [13]. Patients treated with the on-demand strategy are admitted shorter to the ICU and hospital. Less repeat laparotomies are performed in the on-demand group and 113 versus 233 in the planned re-laparotomy group. Furthermore, the rate of unnecessary re-laparotomies was significantly lower in the on-demand group compared with the planned re-laparotomy group (31 % versus 66 %, $p < 0.001$).

The acute phase of abdominal sepsis may at some point lead to the development of an enterocutaneous fistula or even several fistulas. Factors that contribute to this unfortunate course of disease are:

- Ongoing peritonitis, in particular when combined with multiple laparotomies within a short period of time
- A bowel anastomosis *in situ*
- Open abdomen
- Inadequate drainage of intra-abdominal abscesses or infected fluid collections
- Synthetic meshes in contaminated environment used as bridging or inlay and meshes of whatever material when positioned as an inlay

When an enterocutaneous fistula has developed, it is important to verify whether there is an ongoing intra-abdominal infection. Certainly in the case of a fistula that has a tract from intestine to abdominal wall, remaining abscesses of infected fluid collections have devastating effects. Imaging work-up in this situation should be performed by contrast-enhanced computed tomography (CT). Intravenous contrast is needed in a septic patient, even when renal function is compromised, since an inadequate diagnosis is in the end more harmful than the risk of increased renal insufficiency related to use of contrast. Use of oral contrast that can be applied via the nasogastric tube can enhance CT accuracy in specific cases, although the gain in diagnostic accuracy is limited. Therefore, paralytic ileus that frequently accompanies abdominal sepsis—hampering enteral contrast work-up—should not delay CT imaging.

Thus far, reliable CT accuracy data come from patients suspected of having secondary peritonitis after elective abdominal surgery. The positive predictive value of CT to detect an abdominal source of sepsis (ruling in) is 71 % (95 % CI 57–83 %), leaving a margin of error. However, the negative predictive value for an abdominal source of sepsis (ruling out) is 15 % (95 % CI 6–32 %) making it a reliable modality [14]. In contrast, there are no data on the accuracy of CT after an initial operation for peritonitis and none in the setting of an open abdomen. For fistulas in an open abdomen setting, without any tract, imaging of the fistula is a less pressing matter initially. Harm has been done with early aggressive attempts at closing the fistula, and spontaneous closure of open abdomen fistulas is anecdotal. It is more important to focus on sepsis control.

Overall, antibiotics are usually not indicated merely because of fistulas. Use of antibiotics after the initial event of abdominal sepsis should be reserved for ongoing or new-onset peritonitis or during (percutaneous) drainage in a septic patient, preferably based on previous culture results and resistance pattern.

Managing Patient Expectations and the Importance of "Patience"

Key Concept: Surgeons need to avoid the temptation to rush patients back to the operating room for an attempt to close the enterocutaneous fistula. Explaining the usual extended timeline to the patient and family will be helpful to controlling emotions and managing expectations.

Fistulas usually develop after multiple laparotomies, in an open abdomen, and days after the initial septic event. As a rule of thumb, re-laparotomy for a fistula more than 7–10 days and less than 6 months after previous laparotomy, after multiple recent re-laparotomies, or in case of an open abdomen, is not advised. This means that, in general, the moment intestinal fluid is seen coming out of the laparotomy wound (after fascial closure), a drain, an old drain opening, or the open abdomen, surgery is not an option at that time. This should be made clear to the patient, family, and other involved doctors such as intensivists. Although tempting, any additional surgery in the first phase of a fistula to treat this fistula is a futile attempt and should be avoided. Remember that "early fistula surgery is for the surgeon not for the patient; we surgeons need to be patient."

Initial fistula management comprises restoring and monitoring of fluid and electrolyte balance, adequate nutrition, and wound care. Apart from CT in case of clinical suspicion of ongoing infection, no imaging of the fistula tract is needed or desirable. The only exception to this rule is leakage or fistulas from the proximal gastrointestinal tract, such as from a surgically closed duodenal perforation or biliary leakage such as leakage from a hepaticojejunostomy or after cholecystectomy. In these cases a percutaneous transhepatic catheter (PTC) drainage is very effective, and after cholecystectomy endoscopic retrograde cholangiography (ERC) and stenting may provide source control.

Wound management should focus on skin protection, using modern wound management systems, which collect fistula fluid and at the same time allow granulation and (near) closure of the wound. Figure 7.2 shows an example of inadequate wound management in the presence of a fistula. Other ways to protect the skin are reduction of fistula production and fluid composition (see section "Rehabilitation phase").

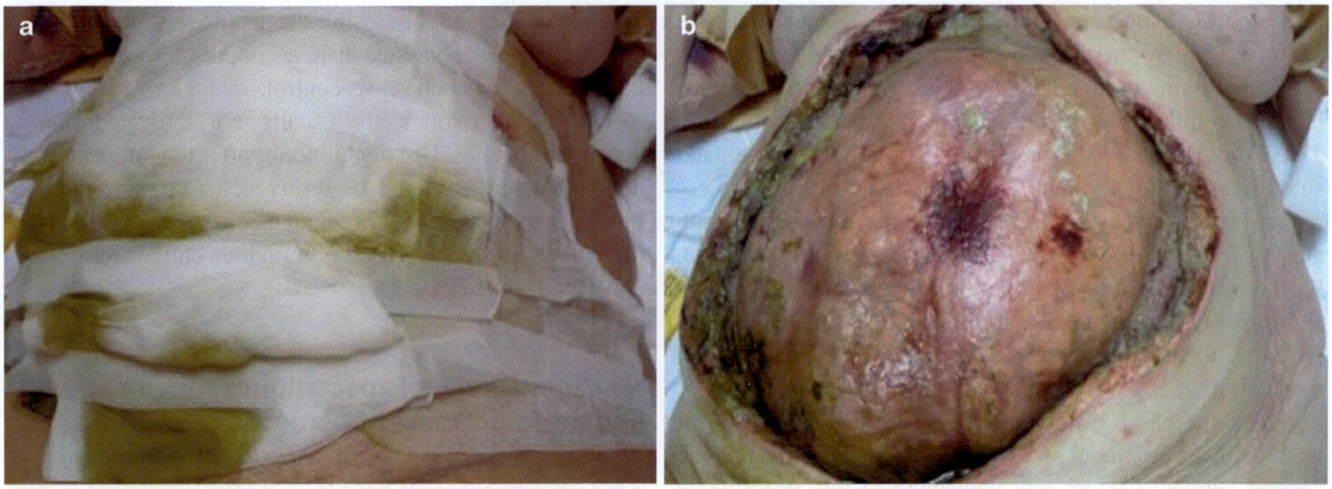

Fig. 7.2 Inadequate wound management of fistula in open abdomen

Evaluation of the Fistula

Defining the Anatomy

Key Concept: *In the phase II stabilization period, in absence of ongoing sepsis, defining the fistula anatomy can be performed with the aid of a small bowel contrast studies, CT, or preferably, MR enteroclysis.*

During phase I (≤2 days after its presentation) of enterocutaneous fistula management, focus is on its diagnosis and evaluation of coexisting ongoing peritonitis, as has been described in the previous paragraph. The diagnosis of a fistula can be relatively simple if evident bowel content is seen in wound or drain or open abdomen. Usually we can deduce the most likely cause of this leakage, i.e., anastomotic leakage, leakage from a primary closed duodenal perforation, leakage from an oversewn iatrogenic bowel injury, bile leakage, and open rectum stump. In most cases we can only have a fair guess toward the origin of the fistula. During phase I, this is typically all the information required to determine an action plan, as the radiological evaluation is predominantly a CT directed at the detection of a coexisting ongoing infection as an underlying cause of the fistula or as a mechanism that prohibits fistula closure. The old practice of instilling methylene blue via a gastric tube is not very informative and should be abandoned in an era of modern imaging.

During phase II, the stabilization phase (≤10–14 days), focus is on fluid, metabolic and electrolyte balance, adequate nutrition, and wound care. Percutaneous drainage of an intra-abdominal abscess may still play a role in this phase. When untreated infections or non-drained abscesses are no longer an issue, it is time to have a more exact location of the fistula. This is done by "inside-to-outside" contrast imaging and not by fistulogram ("outside-to-inside" contrast imaging). Manipulation in the fistula is not helpful for accurate localization and likely to disturb any potential for spontaneous closure. A fistulogram with water-soluble contrast no longer is considered the "gold standard" for examining a fistula. Inside-to-outside contrast imaging can comprise small bowel contrast radiography with contrast administered via a post-pyloric tube or by mouth, or MR enteroclysis, if the patient's condition allows. The advantage of MR enteroclysis is that it provides a clear image of the fistula tract as well as the surrounding tissues and any abscess cavity connected to the fistula tract. For initial imaging of a proximal fistula during phase II, contrast radiography usually suffices. In this phase (1) the length of the intestinal tract proximal to the (first) fistula and (2) the length of the fistula tract from intestine to abdominal wall/"outside world" are the primary information needed to determine whether (a) enteral feeding is of any use with respect to absorption length and (b) enteral feeding is feasible with respect to location (e.g., duodenal leak versus fistula of the ileum) and chances of spontaneous closure (e.g., long fistula tract versus fistula in open abdomen). For ICU patients these modalities can be replaced by enteral and intravenous contrast-enhanced CT, but visualization of the fistula anatomy and origin is less clear. For suspicion of a fistula of colonic origin, enteral and intravenous contrast-enhanced CT may be helpful or more feasible and sensitive in this stage than contrast radiography of the colon.

Endoscopy can also be helpful in determining the origin of the disease that caused the fistula, but it is not a particularly helpful or necessary study to reveal a fistula. Biopsy samples could be useful if inflammatory bowel disease, radiation enteritis, or malignancy is suspected. In specific cases with a very proximal, (e.g., esophageal) or very distal (e.g., rectal) origin of a fistula, endoscopy may be useful because of the possibility of endoscopic therapy. Nevertheless, endoscopy should not be considered as a first-step diagnostic tool. Examples of endoscopic fistula therapy are bridging stents in the esophagus or transrectal endoscopic drainage or local vacuum sponge treatment. For gastric and duodenal fistulas, contrast imaging is preferred over endoscopy, as endoscopic fistula therapy does not play a major role in these locations.

Nutritional Support

Key Concept: Adequate nutritional support through both the enteral or parenteral route is paramount for both an attempt of spontaneous closure as well as preparation for operative intervention, if required.

Intestinal failure due to an enterocutaneous fistula is caused by a functional short bowel syndrome. In this situation, the absolute bowel length may be adequate; however, the absorption capacity is only relevant in the intestine proximal from the fistula. The small bowel distal from the fistula is, for all practical purposes, defunctionalized. Therefore, intestinal failure typically presents as malabsorption leading to intractable diarrhea (or output), dehydration (secondary to high-output losses), malnutrition, and weight loss. Total parenteral nutrition (TPN) is the mainstay of therapy for patients with intestinal failure and in particular for those with high-output fistulas, distal obstruction, and ongoing sepsis. TPN maintains good nutritional status and control of fluid, calorie, nitrogen, and electrolyte intake. Moreover, output reduction by TPN reduces wound care problems and risk of dehydration. TPN reduces the maximal secretory capacity of the gastrointestinal tract by 30–50 %. Malnutrition is often a silent, but significant, cause of morbidity and mortality in patients with enterocutaneous fistulas. An additional great advantage of TPN is that it is independent of fistula anatomy.

While the practice of TPN for enterocutaneous fistula has been adopted widely, even for high-output fistulas, additional enteral feeding is beneficial. The primary role of nutritional support, whether enteral or parenteral, is the prevention of malnutrition. Randomized trials investigating outcomes in patients kept "nil by mouth" have not been performed. In fact, it has never been proven that fistula closure rates improve dramatically with TPN compared to enteral nutrition. The concept of "bowel rest" has been based largely on the observation of output reduction, yet output reduction has never been proven to be related to fistula closure [15].

When comparing the oral and intravenous routes, the advantages of enteral nutrition include avoidance of catheter-related complications (sepsis, thrombosis), trophic effect on bowel mucosa, support of immunological and barrier functions of the gut, reduced risk of bacterial translocation, and stimulation of bowel adaptation. Enteral nutrition should be used whenever possible, to some extent, although high-output small bowel fistulas as a rule require supplemental parenteral nutrition to prevent malnutrition and manage output.

Fistuloclysis (i.e., feeding distal to the fistula) is believed to prevent atrophy of the small intestine distal to an enterocutaneous fistula and is performed by placing a feeding catheter into the fistula opening. Some surgeons also believe that subsequent reconstructive surgery is made technically easier, though that statement has never been substantiated. Provided there is more than 75 cm of healthy small intestine available downstream for absorption distal to the fistula opening [16], fistuloclysis makes theoretical sense from a nutritional standpoint and may indeed prevent mucosal atrophy. However, in clinical practice, the enormous effort to provide this fistula feeding often does not outweigh its disadvantages, such as additional wound care difficulties, decreased mobilization of the patient, relatively limited contribution to overall nutrient demand (e.g., feeding the distal ileum has limited nutrient absorption), and unpredictable absorption of nutrients. Therefore, the practitioner must consider the reality that distal feeding does not provide adequate, predictable, and balanced nutrition, whereas TPN combined with proximal enteral feeding does.

Postoperative Nutrition

Key Concept: Intravenous nutrition requirements continue even after definitive surgery due to problems with absorption until adaptation is complete.

It is important to remember that after fistula surgery the downstream part of the intestine has limited function for a prolonged period of time. Although some enteral nutrition is still possible and preferable, resorption of enteral nutrients is not optimal until after the postoperative adaptation phase with intestinal mucosal restoration. Therefore, postoperative TPN is essential to ensure adequate nutrient intake without the pressure of enteral intake to fulfill this need.

Rehabilitation Phase

How to Control Fistula Output and Role of Adjunctive Medications

Key Concept: Several classes of medications are available and often required to reduce fistula output.

The standard regimen to reduce fistula output, if needed, is the use of high-dose antidiarrheals in a combination of loperamide, codeine, and proton pump inhibitors (PPIs). Loperamide acts in the gastrointestinal tract on both cholinergic and noncholinergic mechanisms, thereby decreasing the activity of both longitudinal and circular muscles. Codeine sulfate is an opioid analgesic with weak analgesic properties. Yet its "side effects" include an ability to decrease gastric, biliary, and pancreatic secretions; cause a reduction in motility; and are associated with an increase in tone in the gastric antrum and the duodenum. Digestion in the small intestine is delayed, and propulsive contractions are decreased. Codeine can cause a spasm of the sphincter of Oddi, thereby increasing biliary tract pressure. PPIs are lipophilic weak bases that cross the parietal cell membrane and enter the acidic parietal cell canaliculus. In this acidic environment, the PPI becomes protonated, producing the activated sulfenamide form of the drug that binds covalently with the H^+/K^+ ATPase enzyme that results in irreversible inhibition of acid secretion by the proton pump. PPIs pantoprazole, esomeprazole, and rabeprazole were more effective in increasing gastric pH and decreasing gastric volume than omeprazole [17]. It is our general practice, after a short period observing natural behavior of the fistula, to start with loperamide, a PPI, and codeine.

Cholestyramine can be added to this regimen, in particular when corrosive action of fistula output creates a wound care problem. Cholestyramine is a chloride salt of a strongly basic non-digestible anion-exchange resin used as a bile salt sequestrant. It binds to bile acids in the intestine to form an insoluble complex, which is excreted in the feces.

It should be especially noted that bulk-forming laxatives are not part of the standard regimen of medical treatment of high-output fistulas. These agents absorb water and cause a softening of stool mass. In addition, the bulk-forming laxatives cause an enlargement of the stools that stimulates propulsive movements in the GI tract and encourages the passage of intestinal contents.

Somatostatin analogues inhibit the release of gastrin, cholecystokinin, secretin, motilin, and other gastrointestinal hormones. This results in a decreased secretion of bicarbonate, water, and pancreatic enzymes into the intestine and an increased water and electrolyte absorption, thereby reducing the intestinal fluid volume. Moreover, analogues relax intestinal smooth muscle, which increases the intestinal capacity. For somatostatin and somatostatin analogues such as octreotide, there is no equivocal evidence that closure rate is improved. In a recent meta-analysis that included randomized trials comparing somatostatin or one of its analogues with control treatment, closure rates are improved by the somatostatin analogues octreotide (5 trials) and lanreotide (1 trial) (RR 1.36 (95 % CI 1.12–1.63); $I^2=47$ %) [18]. This effect is dominated by the results of the two largest trials comprising 192 of 307 pooled patients and including not only 114 small bowel fistulas, but as much as 101 pancreatic and gastric fistulas. The pooled effect of somatostatin is hampered by heterogeneous results ($I^2=84$ %). There is conflicting evidence about its capacity, on top of standard regimen, to reduce output and time to spontaneous closure. We primarily use somatostatin in the setting of high-output fistula despite adequate loperamide, PPIs, and codeine causing fluid and electrolyte disturbances and wound care problems.

Creative Ways for Wound Care

Key Concept: Due to the nature of these wounds, often you are required to think "outside of the box" for innovative solutions to control effluent and protect the skin.

Various solutions can be applied for wound management of high-output fistula. Wound management systems (Fig. 7.3) and negative pressure wound therapy (NPWT) systems with either foam (Fig. 7.4) or gauzes (Fig. 7.5) deliver excellent solutions. In general, wound care in patients with enterocutaneous fistula is tailor-made, and choices must be made per patient, depending on output, localization, abdominal shape, and skin folds. These include wound appliances that can be cut to shape, suction catheters, and adhesive paste dressings to build up or flatten irregularly shaped wounds. When available, often the incorporation of wound care or enterostomal therapist provides additional knowledge and experience that are invaluable to this aspect of care of ECF patients.

Dealing with Medications for Underlying Disease

Key Concept: While fistulas in the setting of active Crohn's disease may close with immunosuppressive therapy, in general the diseased section of bowel needs to be removed.

The presence of Crohn's disease, diverticulitis, cancer, or radiation enteritis in the segment of bowel related to the enterocutaneous fistula is a poor prognostic factor. As a rule of thumb, the fistula will never close as long as the diseased segment is in place. Most enterocutaneous fistulas in the setting of Crohn's disease are postoperative fistula due to a sealed anastomotic leak. Spontaneous fistula in Crohn's disease might close with medical therapy using anti-TNF agents. A systematic review Ford et al. indicated that the number needed to treat to obtain remission is one patient in eight for all anti-TNF agents and four for infliximab [19]. So, definite closure of the fistula is achieved only in some at the expense of expensive maintenance therapy. Surgical resection of the diseased segment is mostly required after optimization of the patient.

Fig. 7.3 Examples of tailor-made fistula wound care. (**a**) A deeper laying enterocutaneous fistula with a skin wall. (**b**) Solution for the (here shown) massive, painful skin erosion caused by fistula effluent (We thank Yvonne Lutgens, specialist nurse, Academic Medical Center (AMC), Amsterdam, for these pictures)

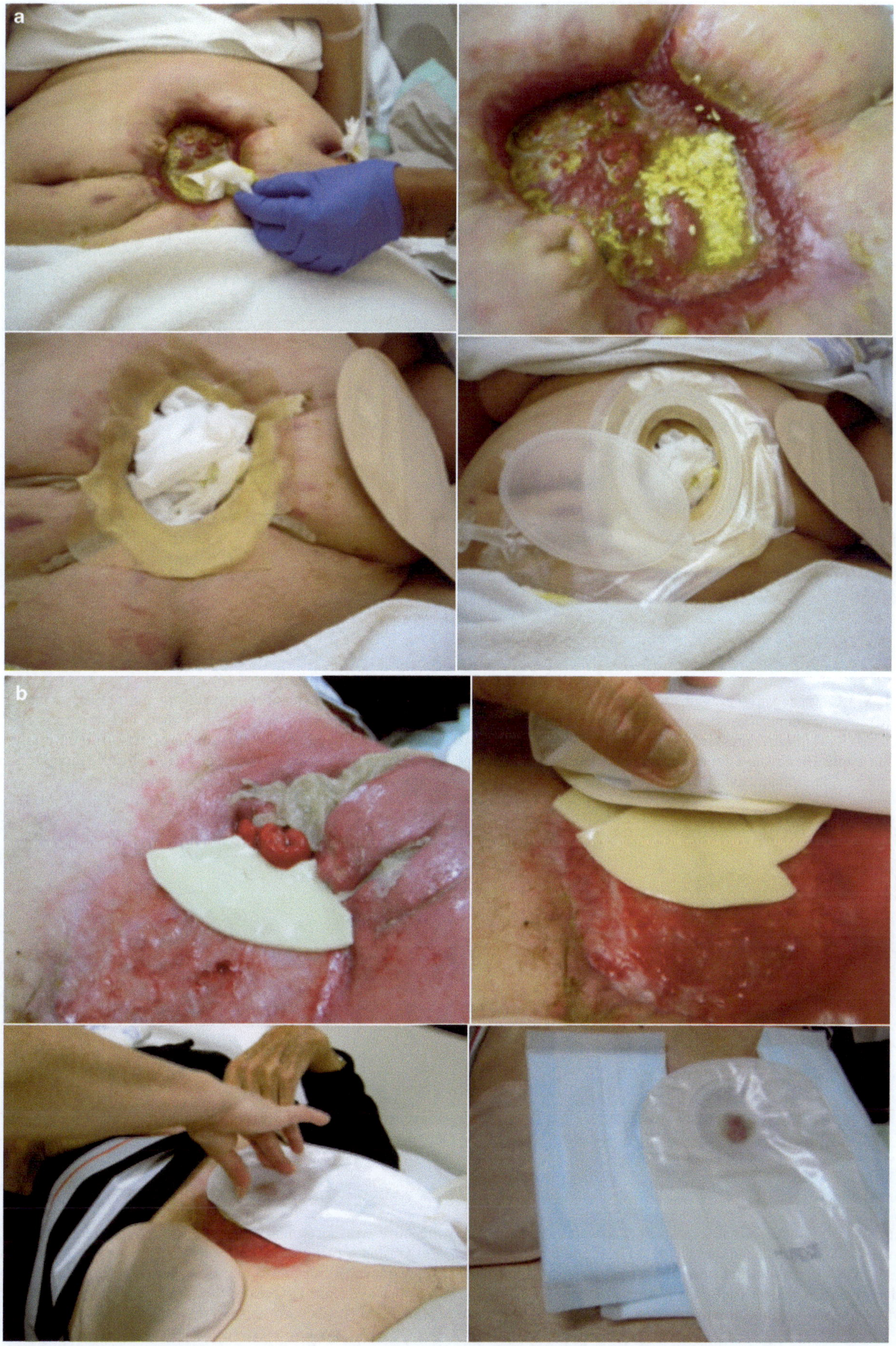

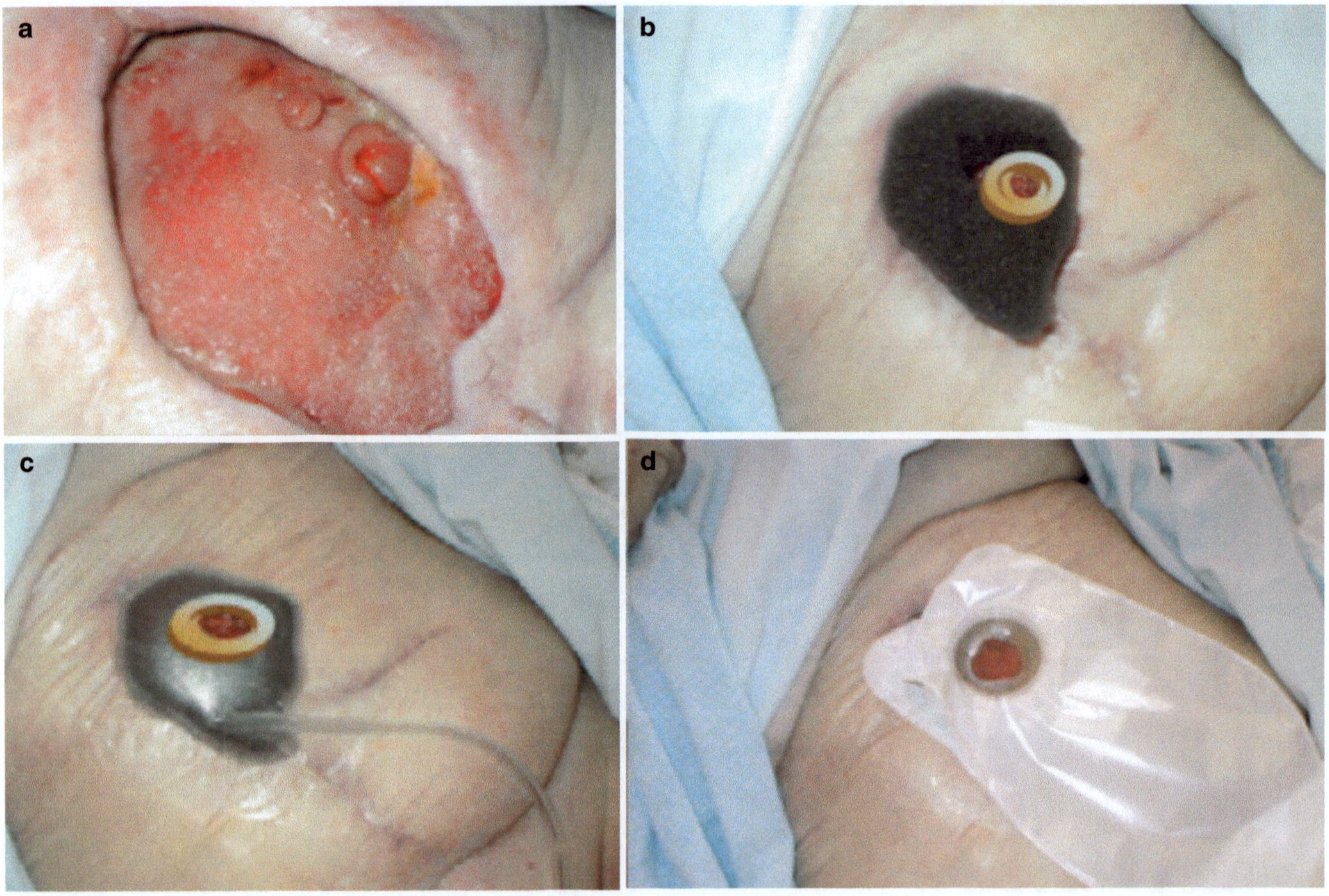

Fig. 7.4 V.A.C. ® negative pressure wound therapy to isolate the fistula. (**a**) View of granulating open abdomen with fistula. Wound care by V.A.C. ® (KCI) negative pressure wound therapy (NPWT) system to isolate the fistula. (**b**) Create a donut of petroleum gauze allowing for a clear 1 cm margin around fistula mouth. (**c**) Invert a stoma ring into a cone to sit inside donut with fistula mouth clearly visible. V.A.C.® GranuFoam™ Dressing to cover wound bed appropriately without overlapping donut. (**d**) Successful fistula isolation with stoma bag applied on top to collect secretions (We thank Chris Borsten, KCI Medical, Houten, the Netherlands, for these pictures)

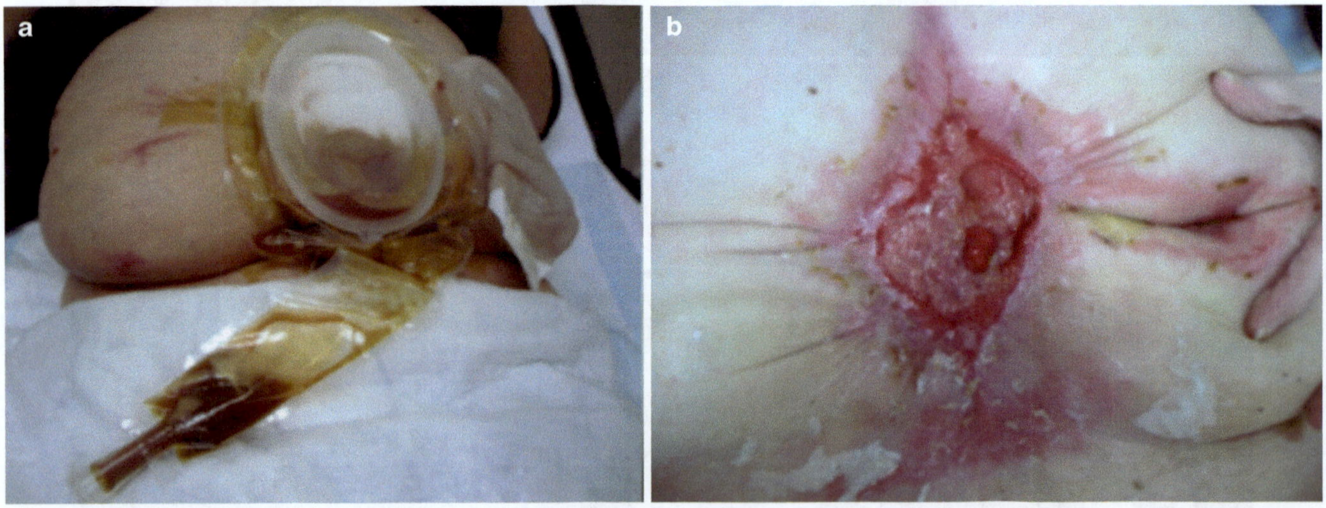

Fig. 7.5 Avance ® gauze negative pressure wound therapy to isolate the fistula. (**a**) Standard wound manager leaks in sitting position, twice a day. (**b**) View of granulating open abdomen with fistula and clear corrosive injury, on patient's left side a stoma is seen. (**c, d**) Wound care was changed to hydrocolloid with (Avance ®, Mölnlycke) gauze negative pressure wound therapy (NPWT) system to isolate the fistula. (**e**) On top a two-part stoma system. (**f**) 60 mmHg negative pressure on fistula environment, fistula itself is isolated from negative pressure (We thank Yvonne Lutgens, specialist nurse, Academic Medical Center (AMC), Amsterdam, for the photographs)

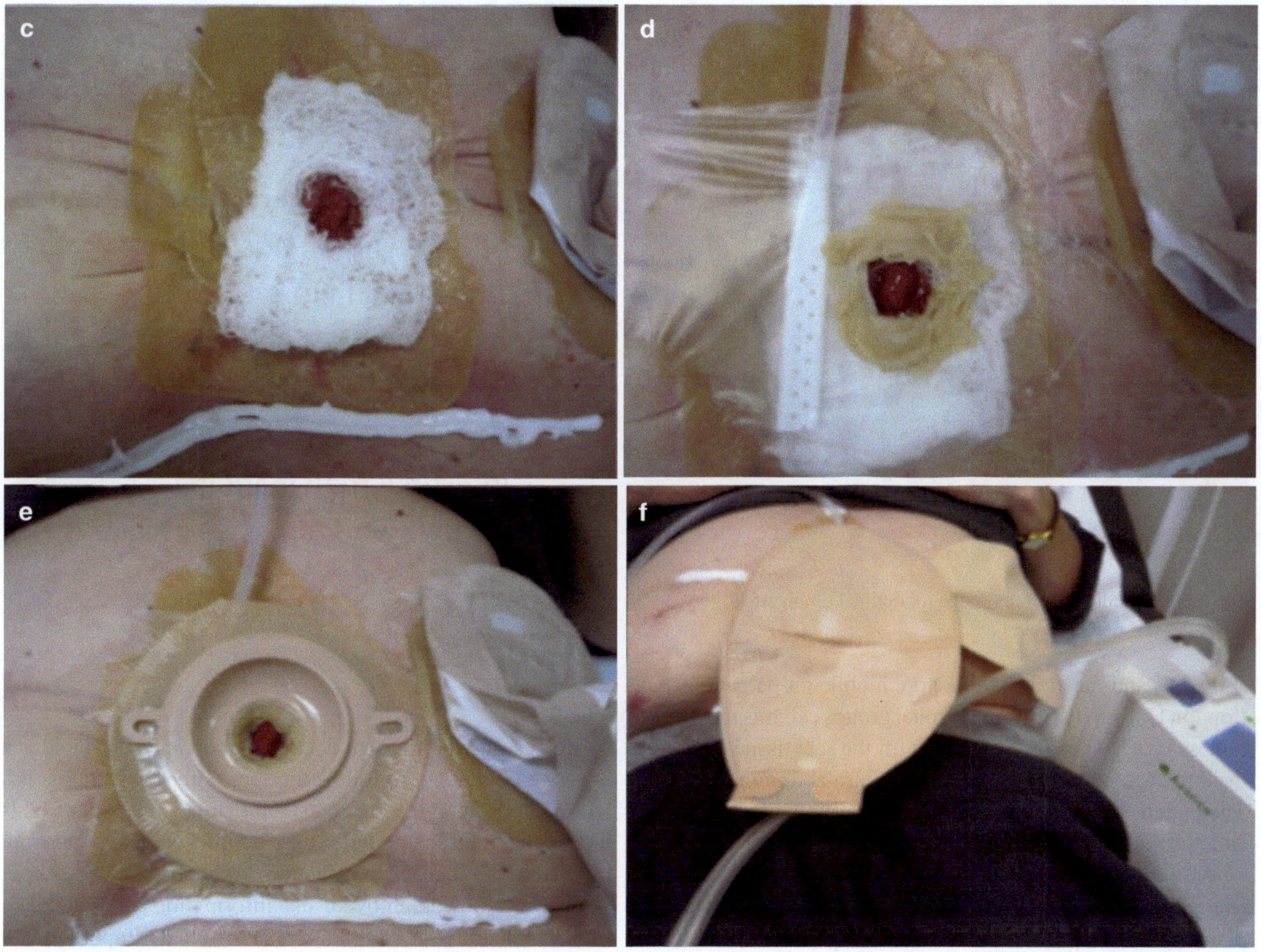

Fig. 7.5 (continued)

Surgical Evaluation

Spontaneous Closure or Not?

Key Concept: Spontaneous closure of an ECF is widely variable, with several underlying factors that help to predict a high or low likelihood.

Overall, a 7–70 % spontaneous closure rate is reported for ECF [15, 20, 21]. Of spontaneous closing enterocutaneous fistulas, the vast majority close within 4–12 weeks of conservative treatment [15]. In general, these fistulas are simple lateral fistulas arising from small bowel anastomotic leaks within otherwise normal bowel. Fistula closure is unlikely with foreign body, diseased bowel (radiation enteritis, malignancy, Crohn's disease), epithelialization of the fistula tract, a short fistula tract (<2 cm), distal obstruction, eversion of mucosa in the wound, sepsis, high output, malnutrition, unfavorable fistula site (stomach, duodenum, proximal jejunum, ileum), and complicated lateral fistula (from an infected segment or with surrounding infiltrate). Favorable fistula features are as follows: no underlying bowel disease, long fistula tract, no sepsis, low output, well nourished, and favorable fistula site (esophageal, duodenal stump, pancreaticobiliary, colon).

Timing of Operation

Key Concept: Waiting at least 6 months to operate on ECF is associated with better outcomes. During this time, full optimization and planning are crucial to overall success.

In general, the rule of thumb for timing of surgery of a recent enterocutaneous fistula is "not now!" Optimal timing of definitive surgical intervention is at least 6 months after the last laparotomy or last sign of ongoing intra-abdominal infection. Early surgery for enterocutaneous fistula is associated with more recurrent fistula [20, 22]. In addition, physical examination findings that suggest optimal timing include fistulas with mucocutaneous continuity should begin to protrude

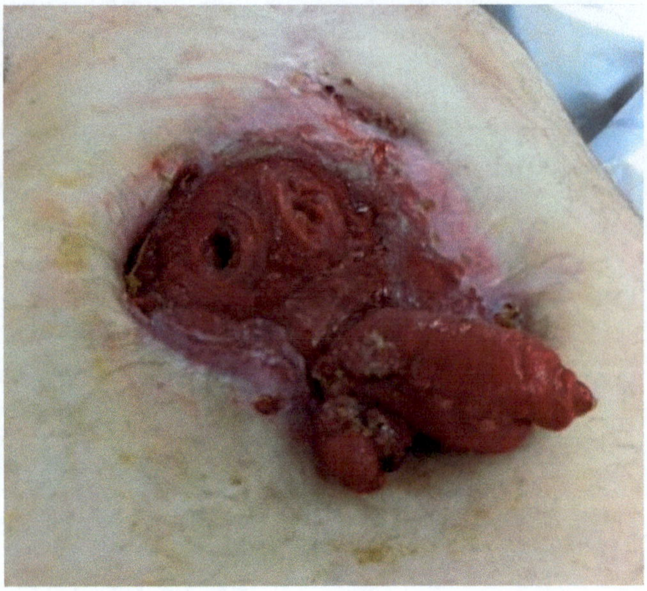

Fig. 7.6 Protruding fistula as a sign for optimal timing of surgery

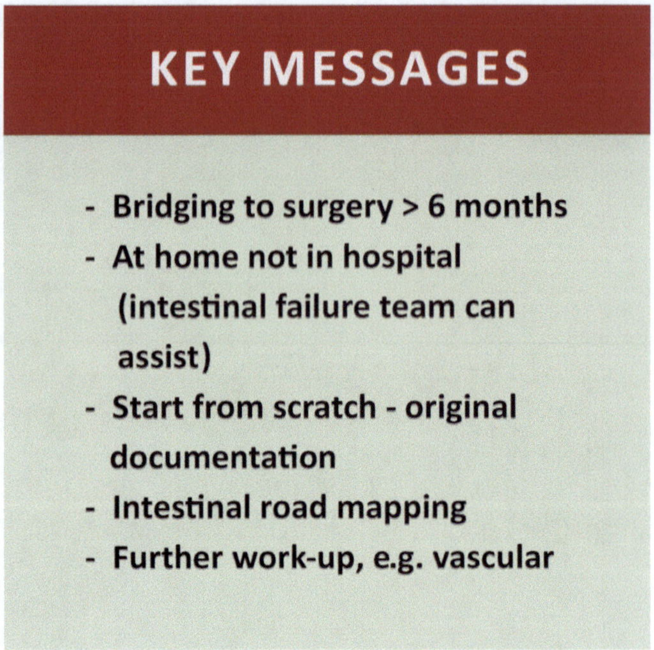

Fig. 7.7 Key messages of surgical work-up

(Fig. 7.6) and the abdomen is more mobile on palpation (the London University College Hospital groups call this the "wobbliness sign"). Classically you can lift the scar tissue covering the laparostomy from the underlying (intra-abdominal) bowel. The patient must be fully optimized conditionally, medically, and nutritionally prior to reconstructive surgery.

Also prior to surgery, a complete road map of the gastrointestinal tract is very helpful for guidance in operative strategy planning and to prevent preoperative surprises or oversights of additional fistula or downstream obstructions. Although complete adhesiolysis is an essential part of successful reconstructive surgery, in some cases part of the intestinal windings cannot be entangled—in particular in the pelvic region—without a too high risk of bowel lesions. A reliable road map of the intestinal tract reduces the risk that in those areas bowel obstructions are overseen. An ideal surgical work-up consists of small bowel contrast radiography with contrast administered via a post-pyloric tube (or by mouth in case of a very proximal fistula) or MR enteroclysis (presently the preferred imaging technique), colonography (if the colon may be reconnected in the intestinal tract), and a fistulogram (if MR enteroclysis does not provide a complete small bowel road map). Frequently bowel length is found to be different from what has been reported in medical records. Key messages of the surgical work-up are summarized in Fig. 7.7.

Reviewing the Prior Operative Notes: Does It Help?

Key Concept: Review of all the original reports provides insight into not only what you may encounter, but also helps avoid pitfalls and repetition of interpretation mistakes.

Reviewing of important documentation in its original form is very essential not to follow the same slippery path that has led to the development of intestinal fistulas in a patient. This means that a discharge letter may be informative, but cannot be the only source of information. Apart from clarity about segments of bowel removed, also information about the position and anatomy of anastomoses is extremely important.

For example, a 52-year-old female was referred to our intestinal failure clinic to evaluate surgical options given her short bowel. She had received daily TPN for 3 years at the time of her referral. According to her medical records, she had about 140 cm of small intestine left, ending on an enterostomy, and her colon had been removed. The length of the rectosigmoid stump was not mentioned explicitly. To evaluate reconstructive options, a MR enteroclysis was performed and a colonography (Fig. 7.8). Total intestinal length on imaging was estimated to be well over 200 cm and a complete colon was in situ. After surgical restoration of intestinal continuity and an adaptation period, TPN was no longer needed.

Techniques

Preoperative Preparation

Key Concept: Planning out all aspects of surgery, from the opening incision to the need for reconstruction of the abdominal wall at closure, will aid in minimizing complications and avoid surprises.

When approaching the complex abdomen, sufficient preoperative planning is of great importance. This involves an assess-

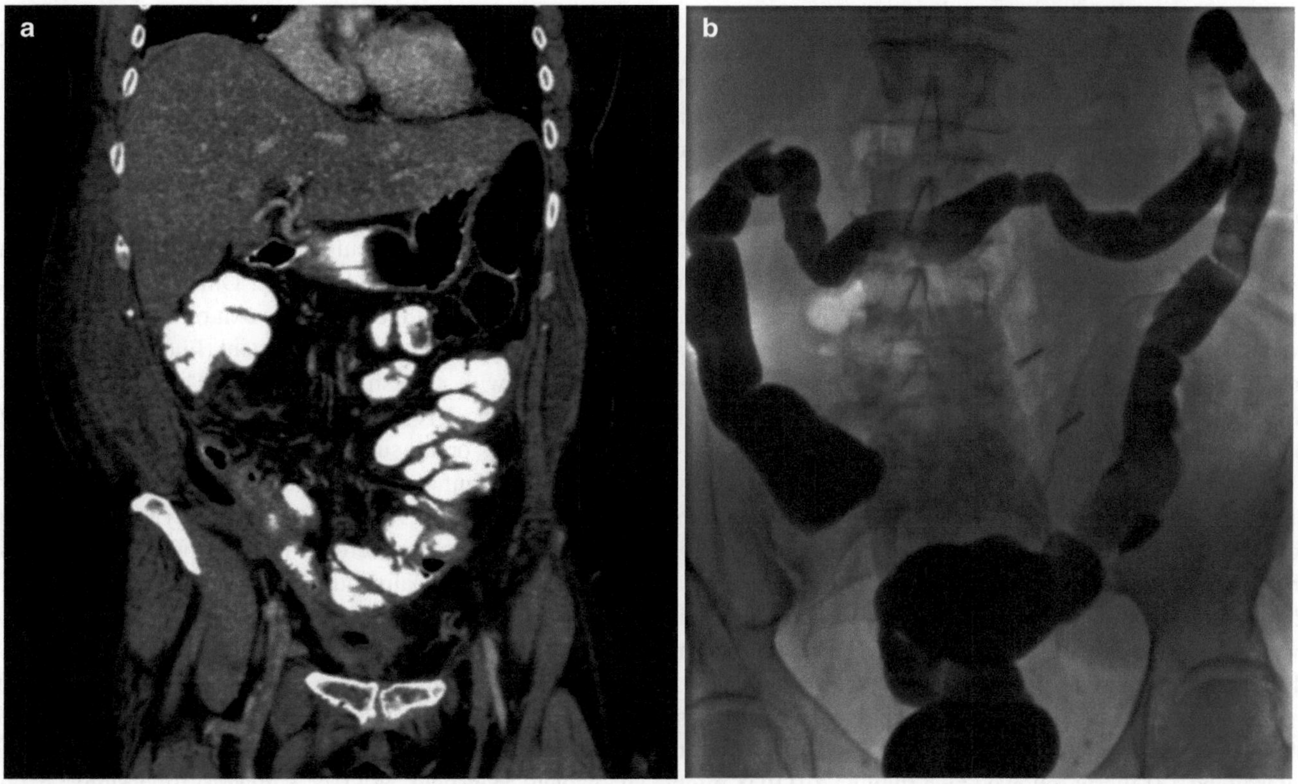

Fig. 7.8 MR entercolysis (**a**) and colonography (**b**) as part of a road map work-up of a short bowel patient, discovering much more bowel length than documented

ment of multiple different components of the surgery, including the ofttimes most important determination of where to start attempting to enter the abdomen safely. In addition, preoperative evaluation of the need of abdominal wall reconstruction helps in assessing the requirement of special meshes. Patients recovered from an abdominal disaster generally have an incisional hernia covered with either granulation tissue (plastron), a split skin, or subcutaneous fat with skin. CT or MR of the abdomen can tell you where there is a safe place to start entering the abdomen (i.e., where there is no bowel below the surface). If no safe place can be found, the abdomen can best be entered subxiphoidally in the upper midline, where most likely the liver or the stomach will be encountered first. In general, entering below the xyphoid is the best option for safe entry.

Imaging can also show you the separation of the rectal muscle indicating whether abdominal wall reconstruction is necessary. It helps to determine whether the abdominal wall can be closed using a component separation technique either with "reinforcement" with a mesh or whether the remaining defect even after extensive mobilization needs to be "bridged" by a biological mesh [23].

Surgical Approach

Key Concept: The tool kit of technical success comprises of meticulous technique, adhesiolysis under visual control of separate bowel loops, and covering repaired or re-anastomosed bowel parts with visceral peritoneum from healthy organs (i.e., omentum, small bowel, mesentery). Abdominal wall reconstruction and closure of the abdominal cavity is paramount.

The overlying skin is incised at the predetermined place. The abdominal cavity is carefully reached by pulling up the subcutaneous edges with Kocher or Ochsner clamps. Once inside, fascial edges are clamped and the skin is incised, excising the plastron (i.e., the remains of the open abdomen composed of granulation tissue and underlying bowel and omentum) step by step by detaching it from the underlying small bowel. This must be performed under visual control, identifying bowel loops stuck underneath before cutting the skin. Avoid incising the skin on the fingertip, because sometimes it is difficult to feel the presence of a collapsed atrophic small bowel loop with the finger. The plastron is excised including the fistula openings.

If an ostomy is present, and if it is planned to close or revise, the procedure can be initiated with dissecting the ostomy free from its position on the abdomen in order to find a safe entrance via the ostomy site. Adhesions should be lysed where this can be done easily. Leave the difficult part of adhesiolysis for later. If surrounding loops are lysed, the difficult part will become easier. Try to isolate one small bowel loop at a time, and use the antimesenteric site of the bowel to stay in the right plane (no fat there). Lyse bowel loops separately and not "en masse." Most often, the small bowel loops are stuck to the skin or plastron. If it is not safe to lyse the bowel from the plastron, one can leave parts of the plastron on the bowel as long as it has no skin.

Repair serosal defects immediately after lyses of the affected loop, or mark them with a suture for later repair. Later on during the procedure, these defects might be difficult to find or one might forget altogether, leading to further fistula or sepsis. We prefer to use a flexible monofilament like a PDS 4-0. This suture is the least traumatic to the friable bowel. Vicryl sutures are traumatic and resolve rapidly. Position the stitches seromuscularly; avoid full-thickness bites oversewing seromuscular defects. A serosal defect might become a transmural defect if the sutures are full thickness. If the anatomy is unclear, a full adhesiolysis might be necessary. Otherwise it is best to avoid unnecessary high-risk adhesiolysis.

Sometimes it is easier to find the right plane of adhesiolysis by turning the bowel loop around. The plane between the loops might be easier to identify from the back. Staying in the proper plane is of great importance to avoid serosal defects and bleeding. Use a pair of scissors with a blunt tip pushing and cutting the tissue forward rather than cutting through the tissue right away.

Pay particular attention to full-thickness lesions, as these should be repaired meticulously. Two-layer closure with interrupted 4-0 Vicryl followed by a running 4-0 PDS might be necessary. These repaired lesions must be covered with undamaged organs like omentum, small bowel, or colon to separate them from other repaired defects or anastomoses and the abdominal wall incision. Never leave the sutured defects exposed to the suture midline incision or a mesh.

The fistula opening in the bowel must be excised and closed, rather than simply oversewn, in order to prevent recurrent fistula. Usually a segmental resection with anastomosis is required [24]. An anastomosis needs to be covered by visceral peritoneum, whenever possible, and should not in any case be positioned adjacent to the laparotomy wound, which increases the risk of a recurrent fistula. A good place to "hide" an anastomosis of the small intestine is close to the mesocolon or covered by omentum. Also, other intestinal loops are ideal for covering an anastomosis. Full abdominal wall closure is essential to reduce the risk of recurrent fistulas or anastomotic leakage. In other words, an open abdomen does not combine with fistula repair, ever.

Abdominal Wall Reconstruction

Key Concept: Abdominal wall reconstruction is a regular aspect of managing ECF patients, and surgeons should be facile with or involve someone with experience and knowledge with these techniques.

Rarely, the abdominal wall can be closed without tension. Mostly, a one- or double-sided component separation technique must be applied to bring the rectal muscles together. Before suturing the wound edges, they must be cleaned of peritoneum and fatty tissue. These structures do not support the abdominal wall reconstruction and might become necrotic, giving rise to a higher chance of infection and dehiscence. Use a flexible, slowly absorbable, monofilament polydioxanone (PDS) 0 or PDS 1 with a circle taper (CT) or tapercut needle to avoid unnecessary large holes in the fascia. When tightening the sutures, they should be pulled in the direction of their exit of the tissue. Otherwise, holes in the fascia will be torn at the site of the exit of the sutures.

In many cases, either reinforcement (Fig. 7.9) or bridging (Fig. 7.10) with a mesh is necessary. The choice of mesh depends on the level of contamination, the location of the mesh (Fig. 7.9; onlay, sublay, or intraperitoneal), and whether it is used to reinforce or to bridge. Muscle (skin) flaps are rarely necessary and require the availability of a plastic surgeon. A considerable increase in the morbidity rate of the donor site of flap repairs must be anticipated, when required. Unfortunately, evidence is lacking which techniques and meshes are best used to close the abdominal defects [23].

Onlay reinforcement can be done using Vicryl meshes (temporary) in largely contaminated conditions or by using biologicals such as Strattice™ (LifeCell, Bridgewater, NJ), Permacol™ (Covidien, Mansfield, MA), or Surgisis® Biodesign™ (Cook Medical, Bloomington, IN). If a sublay reinforcement is possible, a lightweight polypropylene mesh is the most cost-effective solution. If the abdominal wall cannot be closed, the defect is best bridged by a (intraperitoneal) biological mesh. All bridging meshes must be fixed using full-thickness transmuscular/transfascial PDS (or Prolene) sutures with a circle taper needle placed at some distance from the mesh using them as tension wires to pull the mesh flat and tight. Excellent results have been documented in the RICH study, examining the use of Strattice™ non-cross-linked biomesh in challenging abdomens, i.e., contaminated ventral hernias [25]. It is of note that only 4 % of included patients also had fistulas.

The component separation technique is always accompanied by an extensive subcutaneous wound, where fluids can readily accumulate. Large suction drains are therefore advised on both sides of the abdomen. Complication rate of abdominal reconstructions is high, up to 90 % in some reports. Thankfully, the majority of the morbidity is caused by superficial wound infection that can be readily treated. Minimal invasive and endoscopic techniques have been described to perform the component separation technique to avoid the extensive subcutaneous wound and its associated morbidity [26–28].

Dealing with a Stoma

Key Concept: Having a plan for a new stoma or how to deal with the wound following takedown of a present one is paramount when considering reconstruction of the abdominal wall.

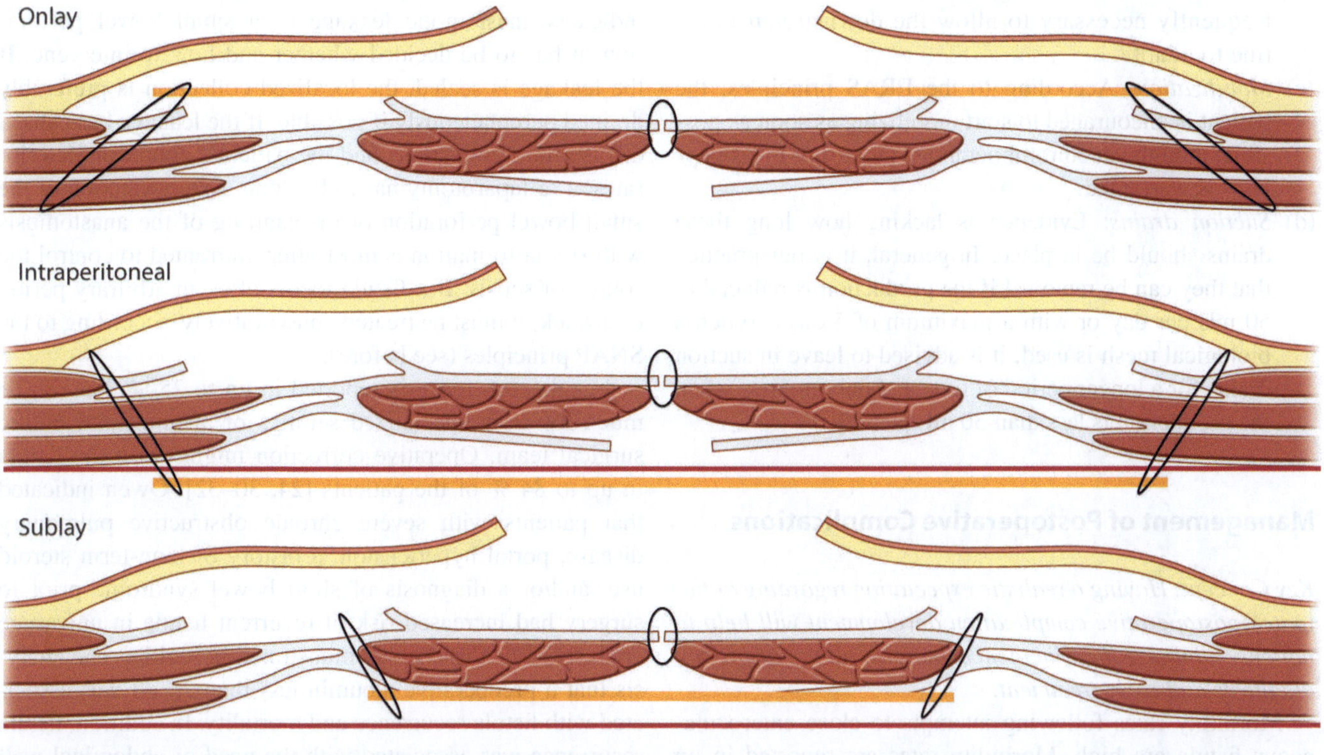

Fig. 7.9 Reinforcement with mesh after component separation technique in three different positions only, intraperitoneal and sublay. Full-thickness sutures fixate the mesh acting as tension wires

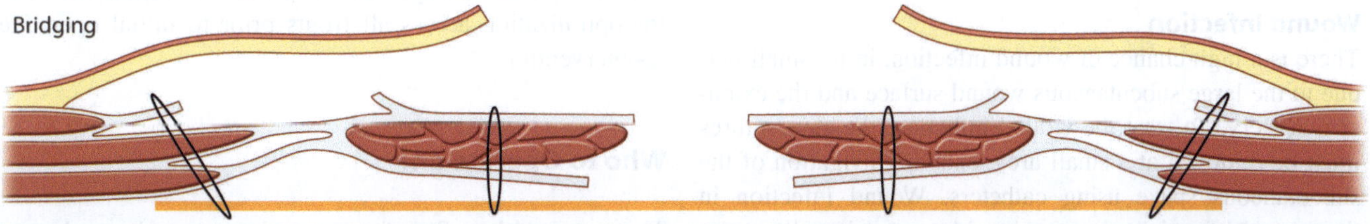

Fig. 7.10 The component separation technique has been insufficient to bring the abdominal wall together. The mesh is used to close the gap (bridging)

The objective of the abdominal reconstruction is to close all fistulas and ostomies and reconstruct the abdominal wall. Abdominal reconstruction is hindered by ostomies, although ostomies can traverse meshes if necessary. Primary surgery encompassing low anterior anastomoses or ileoanal anastomoses will mostly require a defunctioning ileostomy. In surgery for the complex abdomen, defunctioning of low anastomoses is therefore an absolute necessity.

Follow-up

Postoperative Management

Key Concept: *Having a pathway that involves plans for wound care, drain management, nutrition support, and physical therapy is crucial to minimizing complications.*

(a) *Antibiotics*: There is no evidence of any benefit of prolonged perioperative administration of antibiotics. A prophylactic schedule is advised (typically ≤24 h). Only in the case of gross contamination should a therapeutic schedule be given.

(b) *Feeding*: If given parenteral nutrition preoperatively, this should be continued until the patient is able to tolerate sufficient enteral feeding. According to the Enhanced Recovery After Surgery (ERAS) principles, the oral intake can be advanced as soon as tolerated [29]. Anticipating a higher chance of postoperative ileus due to extensive adhesiolysis, one might limit this to fluids and protein-enriched drinks in the first days after surgery. Importantly, the part of the intestine downstream from the fistula is atrophic and postoperatively has limited function for a prolonged period of time. A bridging period with TPN is frequently necessary to allow the downstream intestine to adapt.

(c) *Mobilization*: According to the ERAS principles, the patient is encouraged to start mobilizing as soon as possible, though venothromboembolic (VTE/DVT) prophylaxis is warranted.

(d) *Suction drains*: Evidence is lacking how long these drains should be in place. In general, it is our practice that they can be removed if the production is reduced to 50 mL per day or with a maximum of 5 days. When a biological mesh is used, it is advised to leave in suction drains for a longer period of time and only remove when the production is less than 30 mL per day.

Management of Postoperative Complications

Key Concept: *Having a realistic expectation regarding anticipated postoperative complication development will help to not only minimize their incidence, but also allow for prompt diagnosis and early treatment.*

Morbidity rates following attempts to close enterocutaneous fistula are high. Morbidity rates are reported in up to 90 % with 30-day mortalities in between 5 and 10 % [24, 30–33].

Wound Infection

There is a high chance of wound infection, in no small part due to the large subcutaneous wound surface and the extensive surgery. To treat the wound infection, the skin sutures must be removed at a small area, enabling irrigation of the subcutaneous space using catheters. Wound infection in these types of patients is not treated by removing all sutures because the skin may then become completely dehiscent, and the underlying abdominal wall reconstruction is rendered at risk.

Bleeding

Preferably, postoperative bleeding is managed conservatively. Large subcutaneous hematomas sometimes need to be evacuated surgically because of the high likelihood of infection and prolonged wound care. It is advised to approximate the skin after such drainage procedure and not to leave it wide open. Currently, adjuvant topical medications such as fibrin glue, thrombin-based gels, and powders have not proven to minimize bleeding complications.

Anastomotic Leakage and Recurrent Enterocutaneous Fistula

Key Concept: *Recurrent ECF is a possibility, especially with underlying risk factors, and surgeons should be aware of the signs of symptoms.*

If shortly after surgery to repair the fistula the patient deteriorates, imaging is imperative (preferably a CT). If imaging indicates anastomotic leakage or a small bowel perforation, it has to be decided whether and how to intervene. If the leakage is sealed, the localized collection is preferably drained percutaneously if possible. If the leakage has caused diffuse fluid collections and the patient's condition deteriorates, a re-laparotomy has to be done. Exteriorization of the small bowel perforation or dismantling of the anastomosis with stoma formation is most often warranted to control the source of sepsis. If a fistula recurs after an arbitrary period of a week, it must be treated conservatively, according to the SNAP principles (see before).

Fistula recurrence is reported in up to 25 %, but can be much lower in specialized settings of an intestinal failure surgical team. Operative correction might close the fistula in up to 84 % of the patients [24, 30–32]. Owen indicated that patients with severe chronic obstructive pulmonary disease, portal hypertension, a history of long-term steroid use, and/or a diagnosis of short bowel syndrome prior to surgery had increased risk of recurrent fistula in univariate analysis [30]. Visschers demonstrated in multivariate analysis that a preoperative albumin less than 25 g/l was associated with fistula recurrence and mortality. In addition, fistula recurrence was associated with the need of abdominal wall reconstruction [31]. Martinez concluded that independent predictors of recurrent fistula were a preoperative albumin <30 g/l and an age >55 [32]. This highlights the need for optimization across all fronts prior to initial operative re-intervention.

Who to Operate on?

The expected benefits of an operation must always be out weighed against the risks. The decision to operate depends on the (biological) age of the patient, comorbidities, the extent of the required reconstruction, and the motivation of the patient. High-risk patients with small-output fistula that can be treated with a stoma bag should not undergo an operation. Patients depending on parenteral nutrition or with metabolic issues require an abdominal reconstruction if the risk is acceptable. There is no rule of thumb which patient to operate. This decision should be made together with the patient. While factors such as a BMI of less than 20 and a totally dependent functional status are associated with a high 1-year mortality [30], it is ultimately your surgical judgment that plays the primary role for determining who should and should not get an operation.

Summary Pearls

Unfortunately, the development of enterocutaneous fistulas remains an untoward possibility for patients undergoing laparotomy. Once identified, adhering to the general principles of SNAP (Sepsis, Nutrition, Anatomy, Procedure) will help guide your management while minimizing subsequent morbidity and mortality. You should avoid the urge to re-intervene within 6 months for fistula closure and instead discuss a realistic timeline with patients and their families. Full attention should then be on the optimization of the patient's overall health (bridging to surgery with a specialized team), while planning out the surgery from preoperative complete road mapping, via initial incision to working through exactly how you will get the abdomen closed. Despite the multitude of challenges, success lies in the details of preoperative work-up and surgery itself and taking time to think completing through the various situations that will arise along the way.

References

1. Dellinger RP, Levy MM, Carlet JM, et al. Surviving Sepsis Campaign: international guidelines for management of severe sepsis and septic shock: 2008. Crit Care Med. 2008;36:296–327.
2. Barie PS, Hydo LJ, Shou J, et al. Influence of antibiotic therapy on mortality of critical surgical illness caused or complicated by infection. Surg Infect (Larchmt). 2005;6:41–54.
3. Ibrahim EH, Sherman G, Ward S, et al. The influence of inadequate antimicrobial treatment of bloodstream infections on patient outcomes in the ICU setting. Chest. 2000;118:146–55.
4. Wong PF, Gilliam AD, Kumar S, et al. Antibiotic regimens for secondary peritonitis of gastrointestinal origin in adults. Cochrane Database Syst Rev. 2005;(2):CD004539.
5. Hedderwick SA, Lyons MJ, Liu M, et al. Epidemiology of yeast colonization in the intensive care unit. Eur J Clin Microbiol Infect Dis. 2000;19:663–70.
6. van Till JWO, van Ruler O, Lamme B, et al. Single-drug therapy or selective decontamination of the digestive tract as antifungal prophylaxis in critically ill patients: a systematic review. Crit Care. 2007;11:R126.
7. Jimenez MF, Marshall JC. Source control in the management of sepsis. Intensive Care Med. 2001;27 Suppl 1:S49–62.
8. Boermeester MA. Surgical approaches to peritonitis. Br J Surg. 2007;94:1317–8.
9. Schein M. Surgical management of intra-abdominal infection: is there any evidence? Langenbecks Arch Surg. 2002;387:1–7.
10. van Westreenen M, Mul FJ, Pronk A, et al. Influence of peroperative lavage solutions on peritoneal defence mechanisms in vitro. Eur J Surg. 1999;165:1066–71.
11. Lamme B, Boermeester MA, Reitsma JB, et al. Meta-analysis of relaparotomy for secondary peritonitis. Br J Surg. 2002;89:1516–24.
12. van Ruler O, Mahler CW, Boer KR, et al. Comparison of on-demand vs planned relaparotomy strategy in patients with severe peritonitis: a randomized trial. JAMA. 2007;298:865–72.
13. Opmeer BC, Boer KR, van Ruler O, et al. Costs of relaparotomy on-demand versus planned relaparotomy in patients with severe peritonitis: an economic evaluation within a randomized controlled trial. Crit Care. 2010;14:R97.
14. Go HL, Baarslag HJ, Vermeulen H, et al. A comparative study to validate the use of ultrasonography and computed tomography in patients with post-operative intra-abdominal sepsis. Eur J Radiol. 2005;54:383–7.
15. Lloyd DAJ, Gabe SM, Windsor ACJ. Nutrition and management of enterocutaneous fistula. Br J Surg. 2006;93:1045–55.
16. Kaushal M, Carlson GL. Management of enterocutaneous fistulas. Clin Colon Rectal Surg. 2004;17:79–88.
17. Gursoy O, Memiş D, Sut N. Effect of proton pump inhibitors on gastric juice volume, gastric pH and gastric intramucosal pH in critically ill patients: a randomized, double-blind, placebo-controlled study. Clin Drug Investig. 2008;28:777–82.
18. Rahbour G, Siddiqui MR, Ullah MR, Gabe SM, Warusavitarne J, Vaizey CJ. A meta-analysis of outcomes following use of somatostatin and its analogues for the management of enterocutaneous fistulas. Ann Surg. 2012;256:946–54.
19. Ford AC, Sandborn WJ, Khan KJ, Hanauer SB, Talley NJ, Moayyedi P. Efficacy of biological therapies in inflammatory bowel disease: systematic review and meta-analysis. Am J Gastroenterol. 2011;106(4):644–59.
20. Hollington P, Mawdsley J, Lim W, Gabe SM, Forbes A, Windsor AJ. An 11-year experience of enterocutaneous fistula. Br J Surg. 2004;91:1646–51.
21. Datta V, Engledow A, Chan S, Forbes A, Cohen CR, Windsor A. The management of enterocutaneous fistula in a regional unit in the United Kingdom: a prospective study. Dis Colon Rectum. 2010;53:192–9.
22. Lynch AC, Delaney CP, Senagore AJ, Connor JT, Remzi FH, Fazio VW. Clinical outcome and factors predictive of recurrence after enterocutaneous fistula surgery. Ann Surg. 2004;240:825–31.
23. Ghazi B, Deigni O, Yezhelyev M, Losken A. Current options in the management of complex abdominal wall defects. Ann Plast Surg. 2011;66:488–92.
24. Lynch AC, Delaney CP, Senagore AJ, Connor JT, Remzi FH, Fazio VW. Clinical outcome and factors predictive of recurrence after enterocutaneous fistula surgery. J Gastrointest Surg. 2012;16:156–63; discussion 163–4.
25. Itani KM, Rosen M, Vargo D, Awad SS, Denoto 3rd G, Butler CE, RICH Study Group. Prospective study of single-stage repair of contaminated hernias using a biologic porcine tissue matrix: the RICH Study. Surgery. 2012;152(3):498–505.
26. Ko JH, Wang EC, Salvay DM, Paul BC, Dumanian GA. Abdominal wall reconstruction: lessons learned from 200 "components separation" procedures. Arch Surg. 2009;144:1047–55.
27. Ghali S, Turza KC, Baumann DP, Butler CE. Minimally invasive component separation results in fewer wound-healing complications than open component separation for large ventral hernia repairs. J Am Coll Surg. 2012;214:981–9.
28. Tong WM, Hope W, Overby DW, Hultman CS. Comparison of outcome after mesh-only repair, laparoscopic component separation, and open component separation. Ann Plast Surg. 2011;66:551–6.
29. Kehlet H, Wilmore DW. Multimodal strategies to improve surgical outcome. Am J Surg. 2002;183(6):630–41.
30. Owen RM, Love TP, Perez SD, Srinivasan JK, Sharma J, Pollock JD, Haack CI, Sweeney JF, Galloway JR. Definitive surgical treatment of enterocutaneous fistula: outcomes of a 23-year experience. Arch Surg. 2012;15:1–9.
31. Visschers RG, Olde Damink SW, Winkens B, Soeters PB, van Gemert WG. Treatment strategies in 135 consecutive patients with enterocutaneous fistulas. World J Surg. 2008;32:445–53.
32. Martinez JL, Luque-de-León E, Ballinas-Oseguera G, Mendez JD, Juárez-Oropeza MA, Román-Ramos R. Factors predictive of recurrence and mortality after surgical repair of enterocutaneous fistula. J Gastrointest Surg. 2012;16:156–64.
33. Wind J, van Koperen PJ, Slors JF, Bemelman WA. Single-stage closure of enterocutaneous fistula and stomas in the presence of large abdominal wall defects using the components separation technique. Am J Surg. 2009;197(1):24–9.

Enteroatmospheric Fistula

8

Eric Keith Johnson

Key Points

- Enteroatmospheric fistulas (EAF) are different than enterocutaneous fistulas.
- Control of the EAF effluent is a primary initial focus.
- Prevention is the key, with closure of the abdomen by an assortment of techniques.
- Nutritional optimization is key to both initial patient stabilization and preparation for eventual surgical management.
- Extensive abdominal wall reconstruction is often required. Familiarity with several reconstructive techniques and strategies is crucial for optimal outcomes.

Introduction

Patient morbidity can result from technical errors, or it can simply be an unavoidable outcome related to a disease process and its surgical management. Some postoperative complications "come with the territory"—such as a possible wound infection or anastomotic leak in the setting of colectomy. On the other hand, enteroatmospheric fistula (EAF) is a complex and highly morbid complication, and one that is extremely painful and difficult for the patient, surgeon, nurse, and family alike. Occurrence of an EAF was a rare event as recently as 30 years ago and was often followed quickly by mortality due to sepsis, electrolyte imbalance, and malnutrition.

E.K. Johnson, MD, FACS, FASCRS
Department of Surgery, Madigan Healthcare System, Uniformed Services University of the Health Sciences, 9040a Fitzsimmons Dr, Fort Lewis, Tacoma, WA 98431, USA
e-mail: doktrj@gmail.com

Modern surgical and critical care of the most complex disease processes has ironically led to both an increase in the incidence of this complication and an improved ability to care for those afflicted with this malady. While enterocutaneous fistula (ECF) was not uncommon in "the old days," it is a different disease process from EAF in several aspects. There is clearly an overlap in the way these entities are addressed, yet there are also distinct differences in terms of nutritional, medical, wound, and surgical management needs. The purpose of the chapter will be to highlight these differences and outline various strategies to assist in improving the care of these most complicated of patients.

History: The Evolving Concept of EAF

Key Concept: *EAF has always been around, but changes in surgery including the open abdomen have led to this being a more common occurrence.*

EAF was an unusual occurrence prior to 1980. Changes in the way we surgically manage those with severe intra-abdominal sepsis and multiple traumatic injuries, even in the setting of hemodynamic instability, as well as the recognition of the entity of abdominal compartment syndrome, have led to an increase in the incidence of EAF. Many of our surgical mentors tell tales of being taught to close the abdomen at all costs after the completion of a laparotomy. An improved understanding of perioperative physiology has led to the option of managing specific patients using an "open abdomen" technique, referred to by some as laparostomy. Each of the previous scenarios has in common the potential necessity of a laparostomy wound or open abdomen.

In the early 1980s, publications began to describe the use of this planned open technique. The earliest reports depict its use in the treatment of severe abdominal sepsis [1–5]. A later report, credited as the first to describe damage control laparotomy, involves the use of an abbreviated laparotomy and packing technique in patients developing coagulopathy during surgery [6]. While these authors did not leave the

S.R. Steele et al. (eds.), *Complexities in Colorectal Surgery*,
DOI 10.1007/978-1-4614-9022-7_8, © Springer Science+Business Media New York 2014

abdomen open, they did set the tone for the development of the modern concept of damage control surgery, which includes this component [7]. Theoretical concerns over the negative physiological effects of intra-abdominal hypertension led to bench and animal research that validated the open abdomen concept [8]. Subsequently, there was a rise in the use of a decompressive laparotomy in patients demonstrating end-organ dysfunction in the face of elevated uncontrollable intra-abdominal pressure. Once again, the common denominator involved an abdominal wall left purposely open.

As with many new developments in surgical care, initial reports of success did not necessarily list the associated negative outcomes. With 20–30 years of experience with this sort of management strategy, it is now well demonstrated that the most common acute complication resulting from the open abdomen is EAF, with the most common chronic complication being incisional hernia [9]. EAF is currently reported to occur in up to 25 % of patients managed with an open abdomen [10].

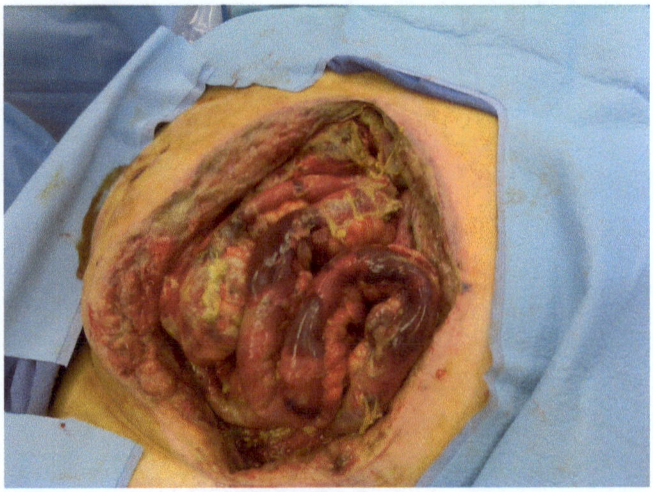

Fig. 8.1 Patient with intra-abdominal sepsis and gut ischemia. While there is no EAF present, they are a prime candidate for this complication

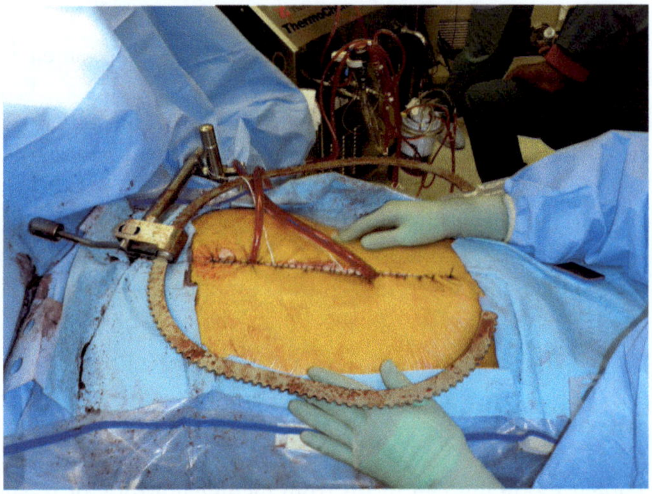

Fig. 8.2 Patient undergoing cytoreduction and HIPEC. These patients are at high risk for dehiscence and subsequent exposure of intra-abdominal viscera

Clinical Presentation and Defining Goals

Key Concept: EAF presents with effluent into the wound. This is most common in patients with exposed bowel. Adhering to the tenets of patient stabilization, anatomic definition, skin protection, nutritional repletion, and eventual definitive reconstruction helps optimize outcomes.

Unlike many postsurgical complications, EAF typically becomes quite obvious when it occurs. One common situation is in a patient being managed with an open abdomen for at least several days. Despite the best efforts to ensure that exposed bowel is kept moist and that trauma to the viscera is avoided, a small erosion occurs in a segment of hollow viscera leading to drainage of intestinal content into the wound (for purposes of this chapter, we will group enteroatmospheric and coloatmospheric fistulas under the label EAF). If the patient is fortunate, the fistula output is low and located in a shallow wound where the output is easier to control (i.e., ECF). Unfortunately, most often this is not the case. Any attempt to perform simple suture closure of the bowel is ill advised as it will almost always fail and result in a larger opening in the bowel wall.

EAF occurs most commonly in the setting of an open abdomen related to trauma and damage control laparotomy, decompressive laparotomy in the setting of high intra-abdominal pressure (IAP), or elective surgery "gone wrong" with a resulting anastomotic leak or missed enterotomy. They also develop in patients who present with an acute abdominal septic process (Fig. 8.1), in those in which we are unable to achieve abdominal closure at the completion of laparotomy secondary to bowel edema and in those with large fascial dehiscences where remaining fascial quality prohibits effective abdominal wall closure resulting in the open abdomen. Modern procedures such as hyperthermic intraperitoneal chemotherapy used to treat peritoneal surface malignancy similarly lend themselves to this sort of complication (Fig. 8.2) [11, 12].

Once an EAF occurs, the patient and surgeon must embark upon what is typically a long journey toward healing. This healing/management process can be arbitrarily broken down into phases of treatment, as has been cited by many authors [13, 14]. Regardless of the specifics of any particular management scheme, they all tend to be based on a few sound tenets: recognition and stabilization, anatomic definition/decision planning, and definitive surgery, if needed [14]. The early phase is characterized first by determining if an EAF is present, followed by early fluid and electrolyte resuscitation, and control of any remaining septic focus. The latter remains an important distinction with EAF patients, where this is often not an issue, as opposed to those with an enterocutaneous fistula. Also in the initial phase, focus is on control of fistula output, protection of surrounding skin, and early nutritional support. The intermediate phase involves defining the fistula anatomy, securing durable access for nutritional support, and planning for the potential of spontaneous closure vs. committing to the long process of definitive surgical management. The late or final phase in management is made up of definitive surgical therapy to close the EAF, reconstruction of the abdominal wall defect that almost always accompanies this process, and prevention of complications related to the closure itself. The remainder of the chapter will address the abovementioned issues with specific attention dedicated to several areas of controversy surrounding the management of EAF.

Prevention

It is important to stress that the best approach to an EAF is to prevent its occurrence altogether (Fig. 8.3). While this disastrous event may be unavoidable, there are factors that increase its risk. Initially it was felt that development of an EAF was increased in patients with an open abdomen for reasons other than trauma; however, a recent report showed this not to be true [15]. Undoubtedly, every attempt should be made to close the open abdomen as soon as possible. While we obviously lack randomized data proving that increased duration of bowel exposure to the outside environment results in an increased rate of EAF formation, this is clearly the consensus [16, 17]. A report published in 2005 reviewing complications experienced in 344 damage control laparotomies showed a higher rate of complications, including EAF, if the abdomen was left open longer than 8 days [18].

Problem: The Fascia Won't Close Initially, Now What?

Key Concept: *Overlying closure through a variety of techniques is the best way to help prevent EAF formation.*

The reality of the situation is that the surgeon cannot simply choose a convenient time to close the abdomen. Typically one has to wait for resolution of visceral edema so that fascial closure can be achieved without leading to intra-abdominal hypertension. There are several reported techniques to potentially reduce the rate of EAF formation in the abdomen left open, and there are also several methods reported to decrease time to closure in these patients. Schecter and colleagues advocate covering the viscera with a non-adherent drape, and performing a skin only closure as an intermediate when fascial re-approximation is not possible [19]. While this seems intuitive, it is based more on expert opinion than any data and may actually result in repetitive trauma to the skin if multiple reoperations are required prior to definitive closure. There are certainly potentially better systems in use today that may hasten fascial closure (Figs. 8.4, 8.5, 8.6, and 8.7).

The planned ventral hernia (PVH) approach utilizes absorbable polyglactin mesh to create a fascial bridge,

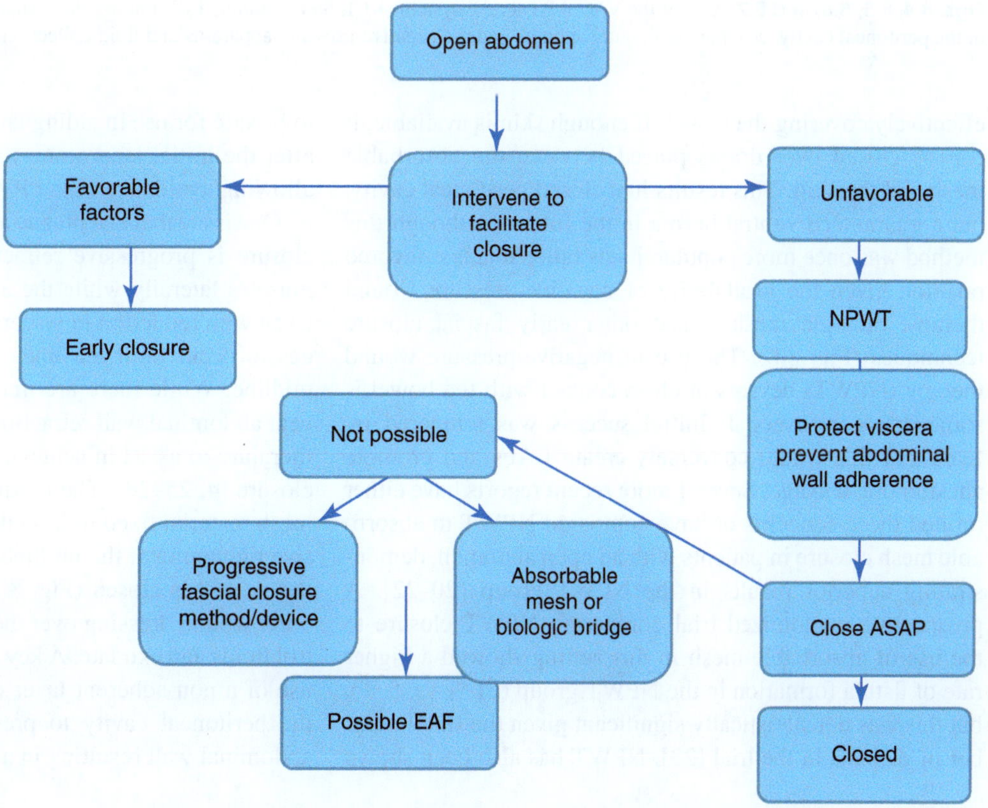

Fig. 8.3 A suggested management scheme for the open abdomen with focus on prevention of EAF. *ASAP* as soon as possible, *EAF* enteroatmospheric fistula, *NPWT* negative-pressure wound therapy

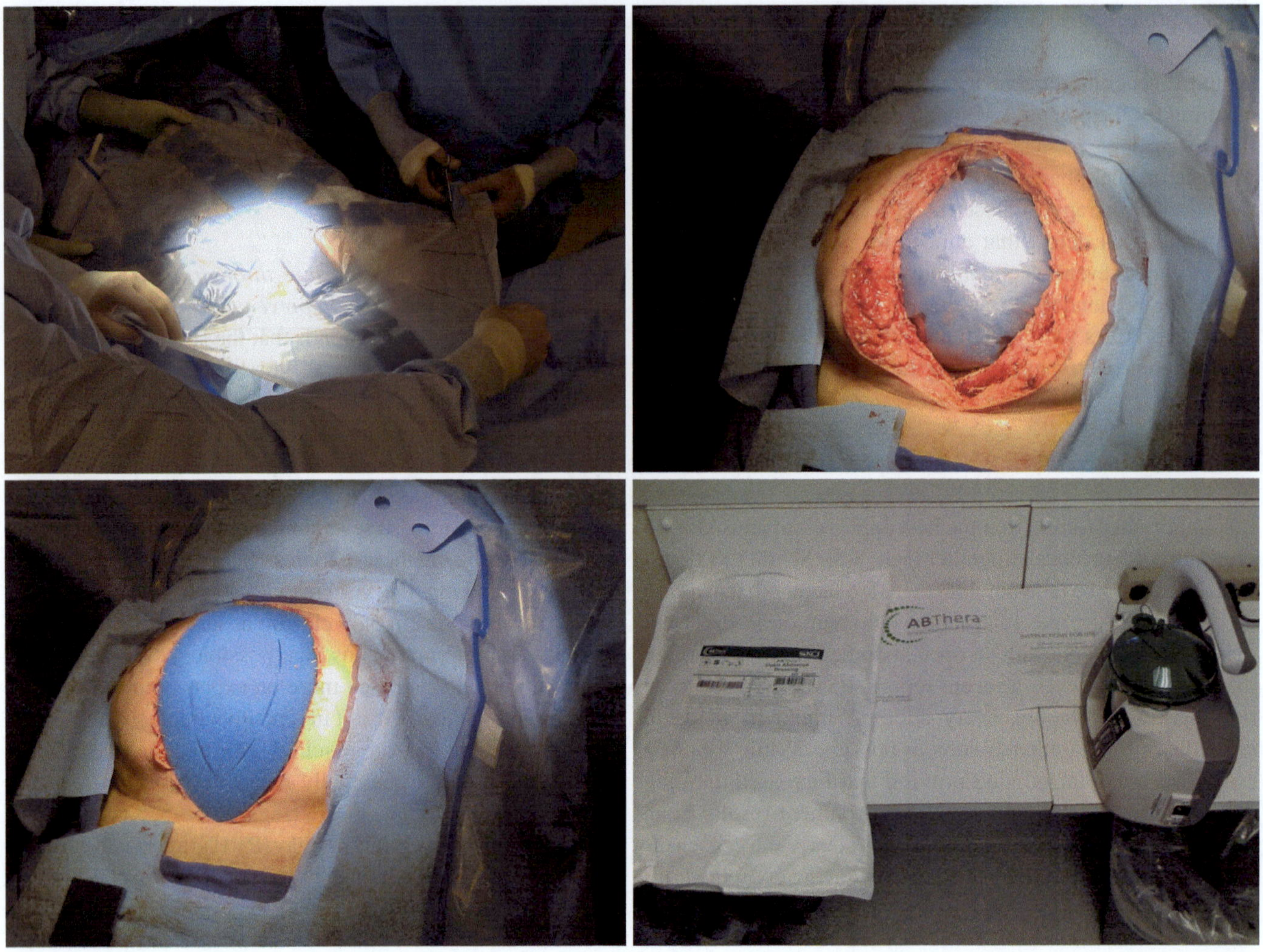

Figs. 8.4, 8.5, 8.6, and 8.7 Use of the VAC ABThera™ system (KCI, San Antonio, TX). Photos show sizing of the protective drape, placement in the peritoneal cavity, coverage with outer sponge, and the negative-pressure apparatus and fluid collection chamber

effectively covering the bowel. If enough skin is available, it can be closed over drains placed between the absorbable mesh and the skin. This results in a closed peritoneal cavity, but a guaranteed ventral hernia in the future. Although this method was once more popular, it has fallen to a less favored position given the availability of negative-pressure wound therapy, biologic meshes, and other early fascial closure techniques (Fig. 8.8). The use of negative-pressure wound therapy (NPWT) devices in close contact with the bowel is somewhat controversial. Initial success was tempered by fears that this would conversely create EAFs and promote anastomotic leakage. Several more recent reports have either refuted these concerns or have compared NPWT to absorbable mesh closure in patients with an open abdomen, demonstrating superior results in the NPWT group [20–22]. A prospective randomized trial comparing NPWT closure to the use of absorbable mesh in this setting showed a higher rate of fistula formation in the NPWT group (21 % vs. 5 %), but this was not statistically significant given the small number of patients in the trial [23]. NPWT has also been shown to be safe for use in aiding late fascial closure (up to a month after the initial laparotomy) with a low rate of fistulization, allowing avoidance of the PVH approach altogether [24].

One issue that can plague any effort to achieve early fascial closure is progressive retraction of the rectus and oblique muscles laterally while the abdomen is left open (Fig. 8.9). Even with reduction in visceral edema, this retraction continues to occur until the linea alba is re-approximated in the midline. While there are many techniques available to prevent abdominal wall retraction, some have been shown in the literature to assist in achieving early (faster) abdominal wall closure [4, 25–28]. The uniting factor involves some type of mesh material fixed to fascial edges, combined with progressive tightening at the midline as visceral edema resolves and the wound is closed (Fig. 8.10). NPWT is employed as an outer wound dressing over the top of the mesh bridge to control fluids and exudate. A key aspect of these techniques is the use of a non-adherent layer or sheet over the viscera inside the peritoneal cavity to prevent adhesions to the anterior abdominal wall resulting in a frozen abdomen.

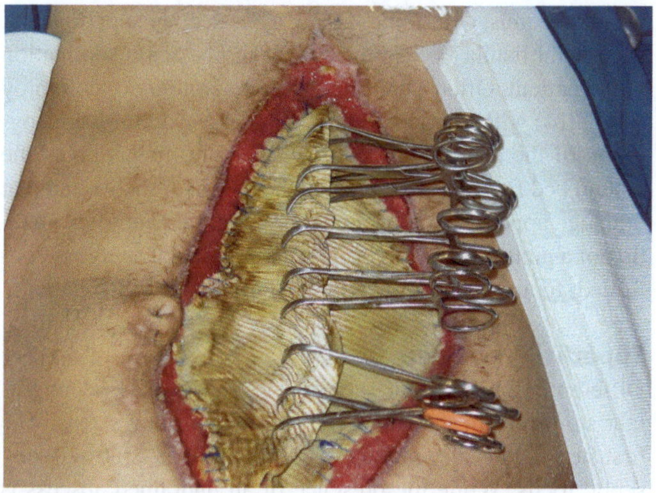

Fig. 8.8 Combat casualty managed with an open abdomen employing coverage of the viscera with PTFE mesh sewn to the fascial edges with progressive tightening at the midline as edema resolves. This is the so-called EDAC (early definitive abdominal closure) technique utilized at Walter Reed Army Medical Center

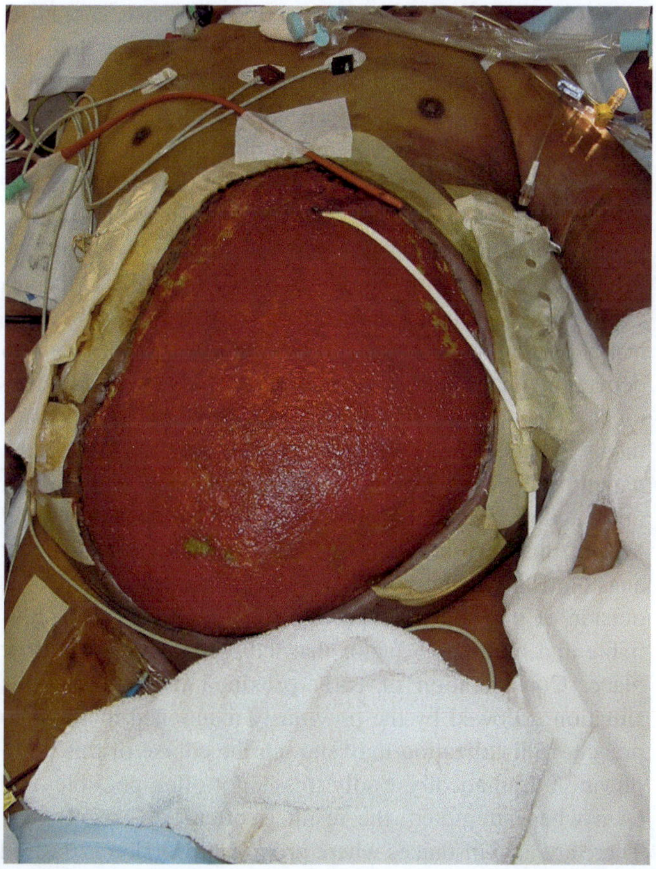

Fig. 8.9 A patient managed with an open abdomen after a repair of a ruptured abdominal aortic aneurysm. This patient was managed in the pre-NPWT days, and the viscera are covered with a healthy bed of granulation tissue. A Foley catheter has been placed in the stomach for feeding purposes

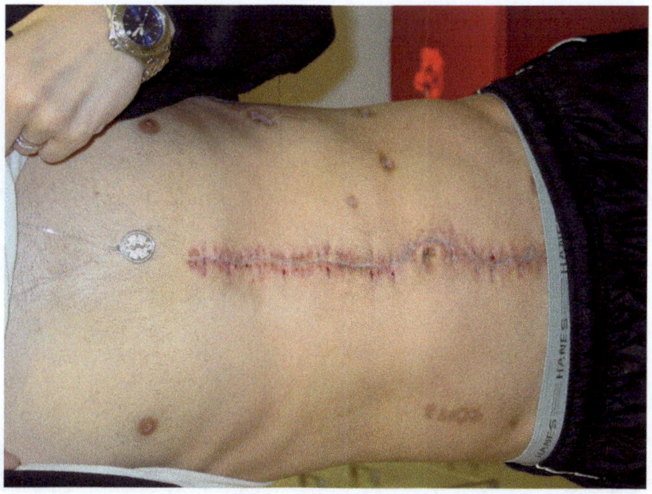

Fig. 8.10 EDAC patient after closure of the fascia primarily at the midline

In cases where several days have passed and early closure seems impractical, one may choose to use biologic mesh bridges to achieve fascial "closure" with either skin re-approximation over drains or NPWT over top of the biologic graft (Fig. 8.11). While this has been shown to result in a high rate of incisional hernia formation [29, 30], it achieves the goal of skin closure over the viscera and has been shown to result in a low rate of bowel fistulization [31]. While some believe that placement of a biologic bridge results almost universally in an incisional hernia over the long term, others have shown that this complication can be minimized (33 % vs. 83 %) if skin closure over the biologic bridge can be achieved immediately [32]. Follow-up in this particular study was short (9 months), limiting the generalizability of the conclusions. Early closure using a variation of the component separation technique (CST) can be performed and has been shown to potentially eliminate the risk of fistulization [33]. However, one must consider the risk of eliminating future options for abdominal wall reconstruction should CST failure occur. The first effort with CST is usually the best and potentially the only chance to achieve a desirable result.

An Ounce of Prevention

Key Concept: Avoiding serosal tears in dressing changes and early nutritional support in the open abdomen setting helps reduce EAF formation.

It is imperative that an experienced member of the surgical team be present during dressing changes for the patient with an open laparotomy wound. This can ensure the avoidance of trauma to the underlying viscera as well as early recognition of areas of deserosalization that are likely precursors of an EAF. Girard reported securing of human acellular dermal matrix (HADM) sheets to areas of intestinal deserosalization with fibrin glue [34]. This was performed in two patients felt to be at risk for EAF, which

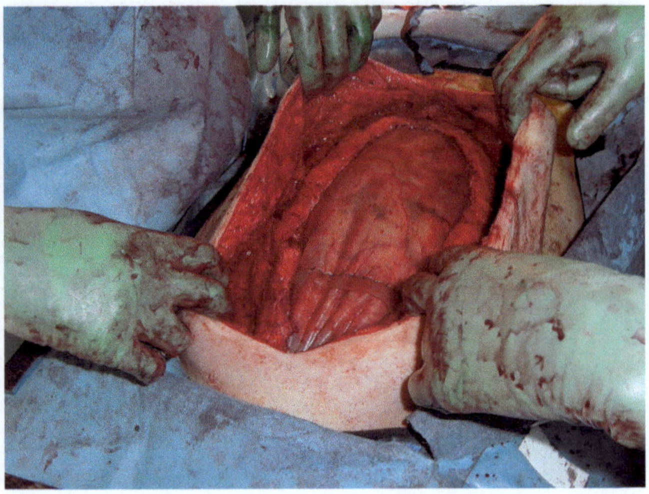

Fig. 8.11 A large fascial diastasis that has been bridged with a biologic mesh. While this is not optimal in terms of hernia repair, it may be an acceptable option to obtain visceral coverage

ultimately did not occur in either. The use of this method has also been reported to be successful in closing small EAFs [35, 36].

While nutritional optimization is central to the care of a patient with a gastrointestinal fistula, it is almost as important in the prevention of an EAF. A patient with an open abdomen is in an extreme catabolic state with increased nutritional requirements. The benefits of enteral nutrition over parenteral nutrition are well established in surgical patients, and the use of early (less than or equal to 4 days after laparotomy) enteral nutrition has been shown to result in a statistically significant reduction in the rate of EAF formation, as well as a faster time to abdominal closure [37]. While no single strategy will prevent EAF in every patient managed with an open abdomen, the above mentioned tools may be tailored into the care for these patients to minimize the risk of this devastating complication.

Problem: So You Have an EAF (The Early Phase)

Key Concept: In the early phase, the goals are to categorize the EAF as superficial or deep to help define an uncontrolled infection, followed by implementation of sepsis control, nutritional therapy, and skin protection measures. Success (or failure) with each of these components has an interrelated effect on optimizing the others.

Diagnosis

Unfortunately, despite our best preventive efforts, some patients will develop an enteroatmospheric fistula (Fig. 8.12). Recognition of this complication is not typically difficult, as one will appreciate either stool or bilious material draining from the open wound (Fig. 8.13). Once these signs are recognized, one must determine if the EAF is deep or superficial. A superficial fistula is easy to see during physical examination of the patient. Often a clearly visible enterotomy or colotomy (Fig. 8.14) will be noted, but in many cases, definitive recognition of the source may be more difficult. Irrigation of the wound bed followed by focus on the region of the wound that drainage appears to emanate from will often lead to localization of a pinhole enterotomy. Once a superficial source is confirmed, focus can turn to early supportive care of the patient.

Superficial vs. Deep

Differentiation between superficial or deep EAF is important simply from the standpoint of uncontrolled sepsis. The first step in the early phase after recognition is control of any septic focus. While the presence of an undrained abscess is uncommon in the patient with an EAF, it is more common in an individual with a deep fistula source. The typical scenario is an anastomotic leakage in a patient being managed with an open abdomen. If the site of anastomosis lies deep within the peritoneal cavity, undrained collections may be present despite the fact that some drainage is noted in the open wound. Computed tomographic scanning is the best method to demonstrate any intraperitoneal collection needing attention. A patient showing systemic signs of sepsis should be treated with broad-spectrum antibiotics and undergo drainage of any septic collection. In some cases this can be performed percutaneously using CT guidance; however, in others this is not possible due to lack of an intervening safe window of passage for needle and drain. It is this group of individuals that may require early reoperation simply for control of sepsis.

In a small but fortunate subset of these individuals, the problem of EAF may be addressed definitively at the re-exploration through resection of the leaking segment of bowel with reanastomosis, proximal diversion, or both depending on the individual setting and sound surgical judgment. When considering the decision to perform an anastomosis in this setting, we must account for the fact that the patient will likely continue to require management with an open abdomen and that they initially developed the EAF/leak in this very environment. The expectation that a new anastomosis will heal in a worse environment is unlikely, outside of the rare event of discovering an isolated identifiable and modifiable factor that led to the leak in the first place. Consideration of early proximal diversion in this situation followed by the previously mentioned methods to prevent re-fistulization may shorten the course of this complication dramatically. Sadly this is not often possible, and even when attempted, the result is often EAF recurrence. There are also instances where proximal diversion is desired but impossible due to mesenteric foreshortening and bowel immobility. In cases such as this, the only option available may be to widely drain a leak with multiple closed suction or sump-type drains. Elimination of oral/enteral intake may be required to achieve effective control of drainage.

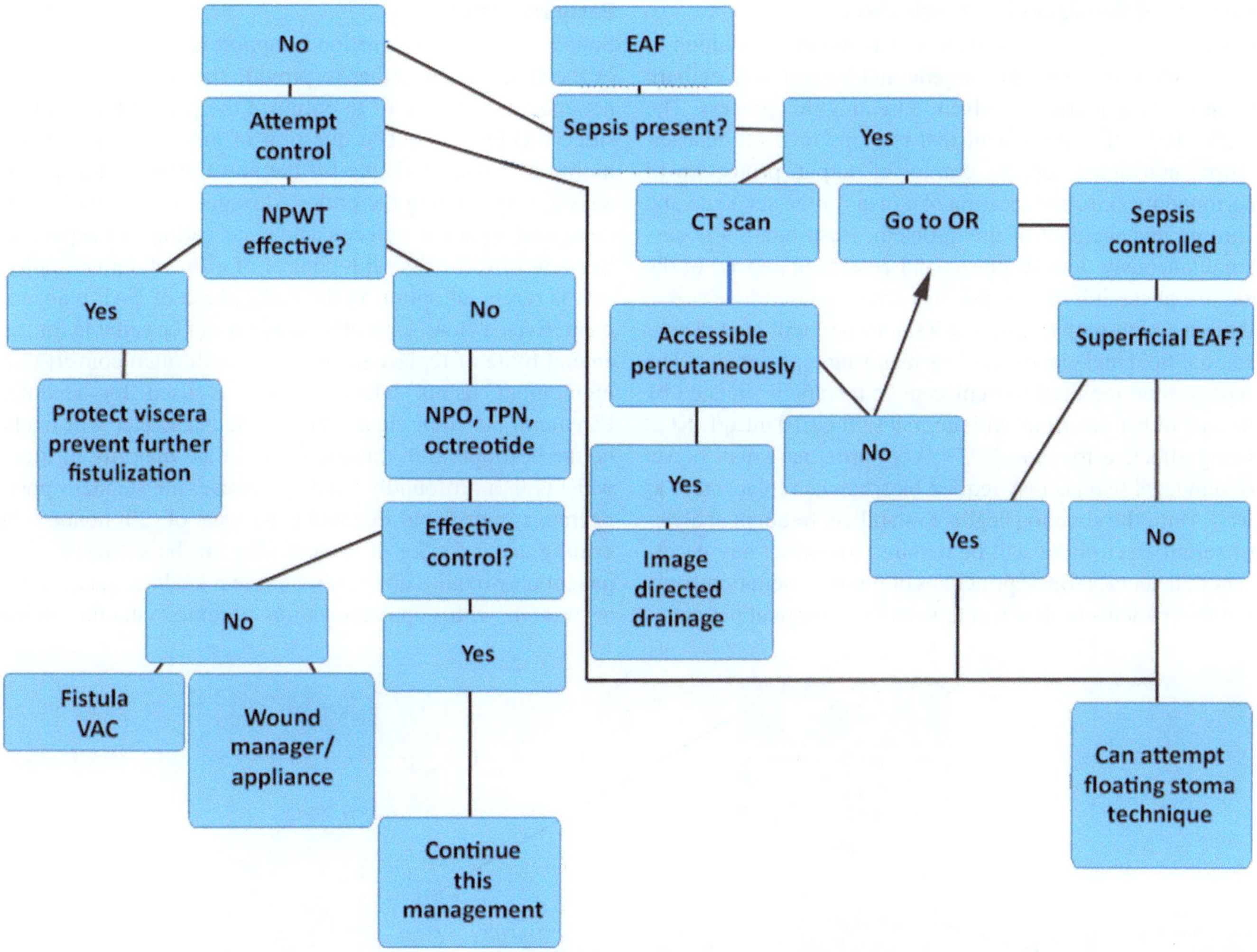

Fig. 8.12 Algorithm depicting methods useful in managing an enteroatmospheric fistula after it is initially discovered. *EAF* enteroatmospheric fistula, *NPWT* negative-pressure wound therapy, *OR* operating room, *NPO* nothing per os, *TPN* total parenteral nutrition, *VAC* vacuum-assisted closure device

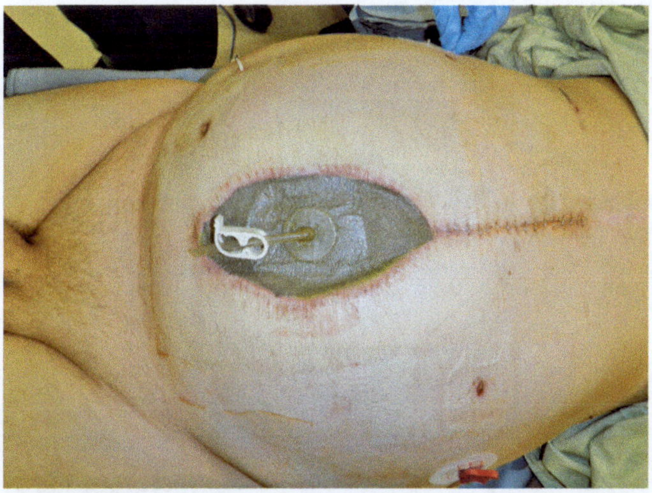

Fig. 8.13 Image showing a NPWT system that has been overwhelmed by a high-output EAF. This dressing was placed less than 1 day prior to this photo

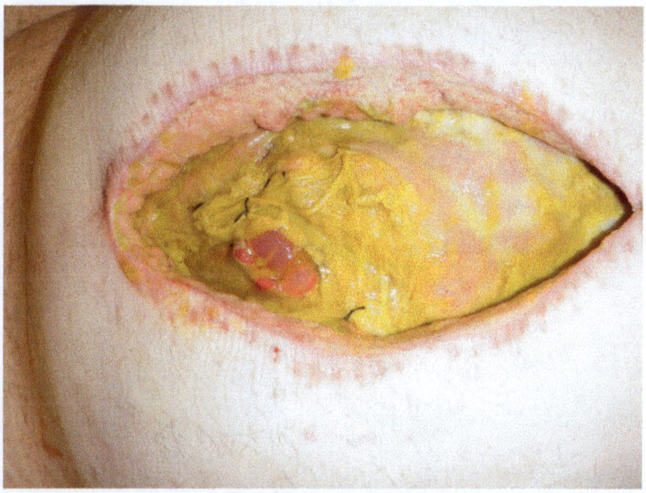

Fig. 8.14 A superficial coloatmospheric fistula

Control of Sepsis and Resuscitation

Once it is recognized that there will be no rapid solution to the problem of EAF, the surgeon and patient will embark upon the long journey involved in treating this process. The early phase of management that remains involves resuscitation, nutritional support, control of output, protection of surrounding skin, and creation of a plan for the subacute and chronic management of this problem. Resuscitation occurs simultaneously with diagnosis and control of sepsis. In the earliest phase, it is often sepsis that drives resuscitative needs, though a high-output fistula (>500 mL/day) will lead to substantial fluid and electrolyte loss requiring replacement. The type of fluid required for replacement therapy is dictated by the site of fistula origin, with normal saline + 10 mEq/L KCL being effective for most EAFs. Very proximal small bowel or duodenal fistulas may require bicarbonate replacement as well. Until the situation begins to stabilize, frequent analysis of serum electrolytes will be required to correct any necessary deficiencies. Basic principles of fluid resuscitation apply to these patients as they would to any postsurgical patient.

Early Nutrition

Sound and effective nutritional support is central to the care of the EAF patient either to provide the highest chance of nonoperative closure or to optimize the patient for eventual surgery (Fig. 8.15). The question of enteral vs. parenteral nutrition is always simple for the nutritionist—with enteral almost always being the preferred route—but is much more complex for patient, surgeon, and nurse caring for the patient. Because of difficulty with control of effluent, enteral nutrition is rarely an option in the early phase of EAF management. Even a "low"-output fistula may not be suitable for the enteral route of replacement, as they will often convert to a high-output fistula when the gut is used for feeding. Parenteral nutrition via a central venous catheter will likely be the best option in this phase. With the majority of these patients in a profoundly catabolic phase, the standard postoperative nutritional recommendations of 20 nonprotein kcal/kg and 1.5 g/kg of protein may not be sufficient. The patient may require up to 30 nonprotein kcal/kg and 2.5 g/kg of protein with supplementation of zinc, vitamins, trace

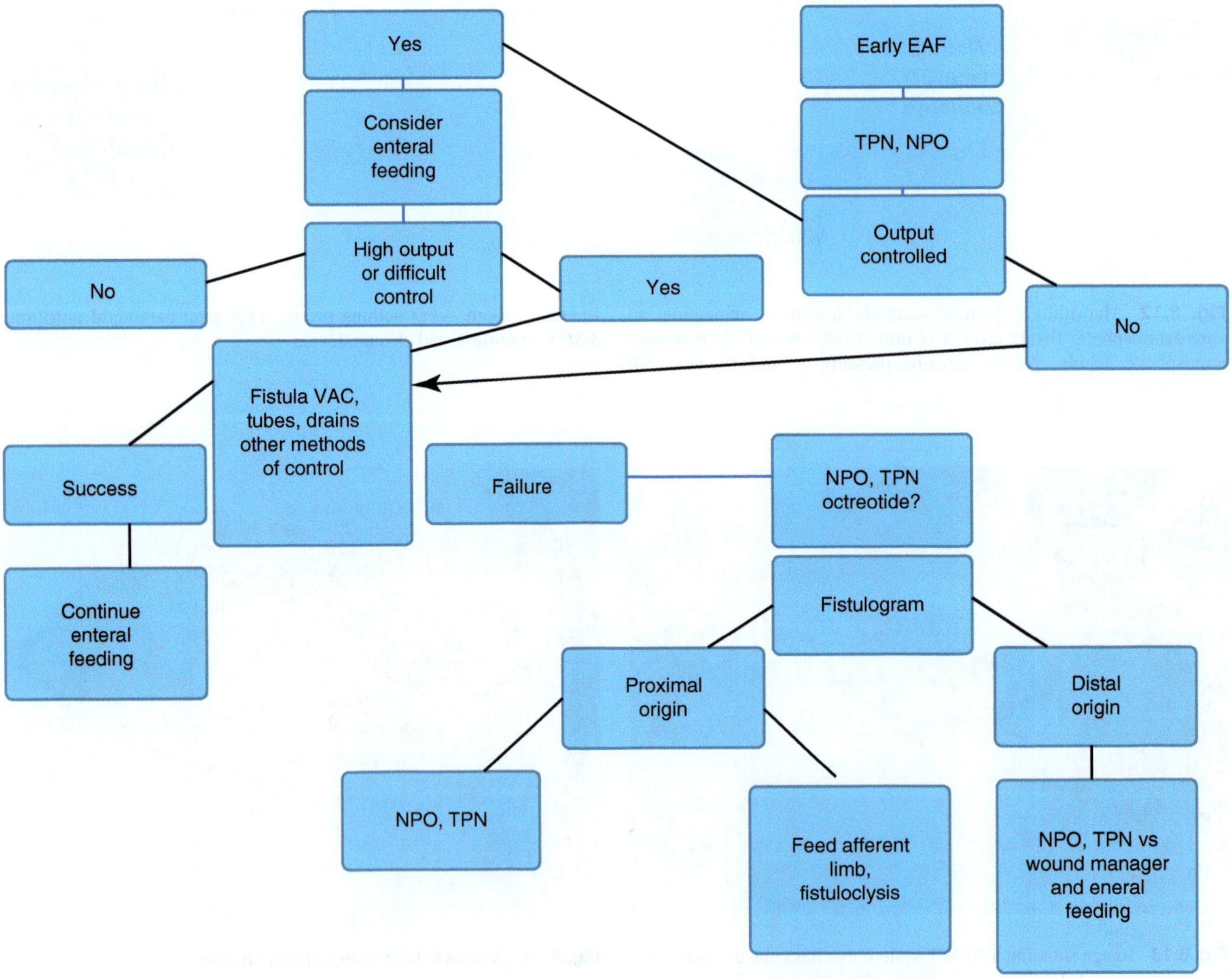

Fig. 8.15 Algorithm illustrating a feeding strategy to be used early after discovery of an EAF. *EAF* enteroatmospheric fistula, *NPO* nothing per os, *TPN* total parenteral nutrition, *VAC* vacuum-assisted closure device

elements, and five to ten times the standard recommendation of vitamin C [13]. Additional copper, folic acid, and vitamin B12 are often also needed [38].

Assessment of nutritional adequacy should also begin in the early phase with twice weekly measurements of serum prealbumin. The serum C-reactive protein level is also often helpful in determining whether or not the patient remains in the acute inflammatory phase or has ongoing sepsis. No matter how much nutritional support is provided, it is difficult to make measurable gains in the nutritional status of an actively septic individual. This again illustrates the importance of sepsis control in optimizing a patient's chance to heal an EAF nonoperatively or at least provide favorable conditions for a future required surgical procedure.

Effluent Control and Skin Protection

It is worth repeating that the poorly controlled EAF is a nightmare for the patient and everyone involved in their care. It is a source of embarrassment and discomfort for the patient, frustration for the surgeon, and results in the consumption of a tremendous amount of nursing and disposable medical resources. Early control of EAF output is therefore critical, as contact between the skin and drainage will result in significant skin damage that may limit options for subsequent control. A sound first step is to stop any and all oral intake. Bowel rest will likely not eliminate EAF output, but will significantly reduce the quantity. Use of a nasogastric tube on intermittent suction may also aid in reducing the quantity of effluent. In the majority of cases, the use of NPWT will have already been employed, and simple continuation of this will be all that is needed to obtain early effluent control. EAFs that result in higher effluent output will often overwhelm NPWT systems resulting in the requirement for dressing changes on a daily basis or even more frequently. This again can overwhelm both manpower and resources requiring advanced methods of control (Figs. 8.16, 8.17, and 8.18). The involvement of an enterostomal therapist or experienced wound care team cannot be overemphasized [39]. If the patient is being cared for in a facility without these resources, transfer to a higher level of care should certainly be considered.

There are several available options for skin protection using any of a variety of topical skin barriers. Again, the enterostomal therapist/wound care team will be familiar with the available options, and use of these materials should be employed early. Advanced method of effluent management as well as pharmacologic adjuncts to the management of EAF will be discussed in the next section.

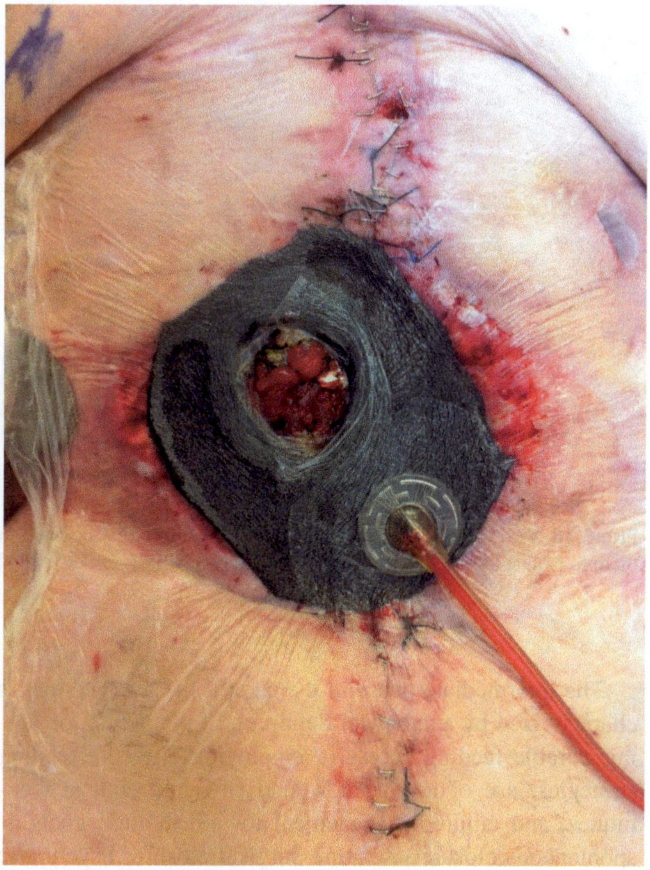

Fig. 8.16 The "fistula VAC." The EAF has been isolated from the rest of the wound bed allowing the benefits of NPWT while controlling effluent using and ostomy appliance

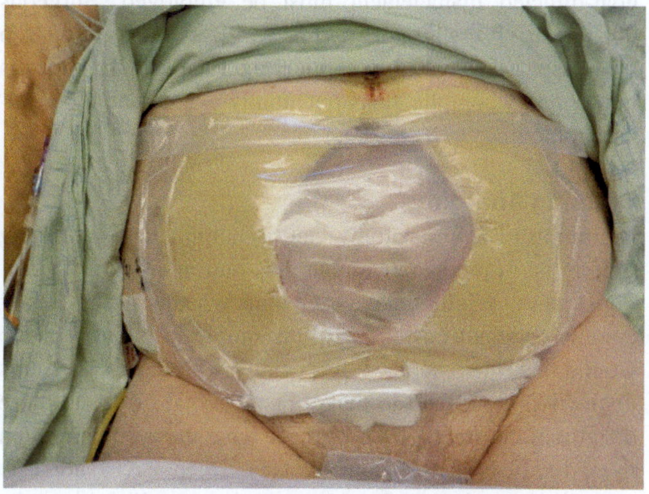

Fig. 8.17 Use of a large custom fit wound appliance. This technique is useful when NPWT fails to adequately control fistula effluent

Intermediate Phase

Key Concept: *Once the patient has stabilized, the focus shifts to using enteral nutrition, defining the fistula anatomy, identifying potential sources hindering EAF resolution, and mobilization or discharge of the patient through advanced wound protection. This may allow the EAF to close spontaneously or prepare the patient for surgery.*

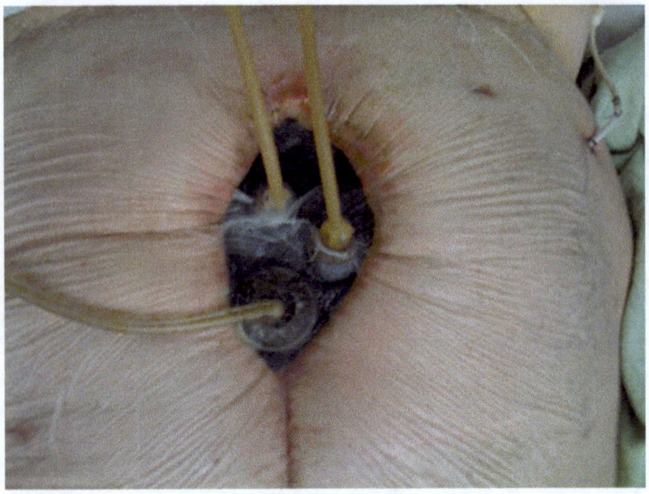

Fig. 8.18 Use of baby bottle nipples with Malecot drains inserted in them to isolate two EAFs from the wound bed so NPWT could be used

The intermediate phase in the care of the EAF patient is characterized by anatomical definition of the fistula, obtaining durable feeding access or employing alternate feeding strategies, use of advanced wound care and control techniques, and tailored management toward defined goals of spontaneous closure vs. future surgical closure. Psychiatric and social support of the individual with EAF cannot be overstated. It is this phase of management where the patient, their family, and nursing will apply pressure to the surgeon in hope of a quick fix. Unfortunately, there is no easy way out of this complication, and patience with well-defined goal-directed management must be employed. Surgeons must resist pressure to attempt surgical intervention too soon, as the error of early surgical intervention often results in secondary complications potentially worse than the original problem.

Defining Anatomy

Definition of EAF anatomy can be helpful in determining prognosis, in preoperative planning, and in creating a feeding strategy. While it may be obvious whether an EAF is of colonic or small bowel origin on simple inspection of the wound bed, in some cases (especially with deep EAF), this distinction is difficult to make. Fistulas that originate more distally in the small bowel or those from the colon are often more likely to close spontaneously. Deep EAFs are also more likely to close, as long as sepsis is controlled, given the length of the fistula tract. While these statements are difficult to support directly with evidence, one can extrapolate from evidence that reveals lower spontaneous closure rates in fistulas with proximal origin or high output [40]. There is also some evidence to suggest that ECFs that have developed in trauma patients may be more likely to close than in others; however, it is unknown if this association applies to those with an EAF [41]. Knowledge of the likelihood of spontaneous closure will affect the goal-directed management plan as well as provide reasonable expectations for the patient and others involved in their care. Site of origin may also directly impact upon the decision to feed enterally or parenterally.

We are often required to perform some sort of radiographic study to make a definitive determination of the site of fistula origin. There are several options available to the surgeon for this purpose. The fistulogram is the classic study to assist in this purpose. Performance of a fistulogram involves intubation of the fistula tract from the outside using various tubing or catheter devices that will facilitate direct contrast instillation into the tract. A scout radiograph should be obtained prior to any contrast administration. This will assist in visualizing any clips or anastomotic staples in the area of question that may be related to the process of fistulization. Contrast should be administered gently under low pressure while visualizing the area of interest using fluoroscopy. The use of a balloon tipped catheter inflated with low pressure may assist in maintaining intraluminal contrast thereby improving the image. A well-performed fistulogram of a deep EAF will define the tract, its length, the origin, and any associated abscess cavity. Fistulograms performed on superficial EAFs may assist in determination of how proximal or distal the origin of the fistula is in the GI tract. Water-soluble contrast should be used when performing these studies. While barium tends to provide greater detail, water-soluble contrast material works well and alleviates the risk of peritonitis related to barium extravasation in some circumstances. Any barium retained in the GI tract tends to form concretions that can be very difficult to clear and may hinder further radiographic evaluations. As a general rule, barium is simply best avoided in these patients. A fistulogram may also aid in the identification of distal obstruction as well as adjacent or associated foreign bodies—both factors that will tend to preclude spontaneous fistula closure. Alternatively, a small bowel follow-through after ingestion of oral water-soluble contrast may also be helpful in identifying the discussed findings.

Computed tomography scanning is probably the most useful modality for imaging a patient with an EAF to determine if there are other associated intraperitoneal abnormalities. When oral and IV contrast are used, one may in fact achieve direct visualization of the origin of the EAF, as well as information related to tract length, associated abscess, adjacent inflammation, presence and relation of foreign body, and any potential distal obstruction. Cross-sectional imaging with CT also provides the obvious advantage of facilitating percutaneous drainage of intra-abdominal fluid collections. MRI and ultrasound examination may also be helpful in select circumstances but are less frequently employed methods of imaging in these patients.

Nutrition

As mentioned, the purpose of imaging is to define the situation anatomically such that an intervention can be undertaken to improve outcome, if possible. Intervention may be direct, as in the case of abscess drainage, or indirect such as implementation of an enteral feeding plan based on anatomy. In cases where fistulas are located distally, it may be possible to provide all nutritional intake by mouth without substantially increasing fistula output to a level where control becomes difficult. In cases where the fistula origin is very proximal, enteral feeding can often be achieved via a tube inserted into the efferent portion of the tract. The majority of intestinal absorptive surface can be utilized, and high volume biliopancreatic secretions can be re-fed into the distal bowel [13]. Some patients will simply not be candidates for enteral nutrition (although it should always be the first choice) and will require extended administration of total parenteral nutrition (TPN). These individuals will require durable central venous access in some form. Line sepsis and TPN-associated liver disease remain major morbidities in those who require this form of nutritional therapy. While debatable, when fistula anatomy is favorable for a higher likelihood of spontaneous closure, some physicians prefer the parenteral route alone in order to keep effluent output low. If spontaneous closure seems unlikely, which is often the case, feeding enterally may be the best way to boost nutritional status in preparation for future surgery.

Effluent Control and Skin Protection

In the intermediate phase, control of fistula effluent remains extremely difficult. As patients regain strength, simple mobilization and, eventually, life beyond the hospital become a reality. This poses challenges to the effluent control aspect of care. In order to re-feed biliopancreatic secretions, they must be effectively controlled and collected. While possible through use of nasogastric tubes and NPWT systems, this is a much more difficult task in practice. High-output EAFs will tend to overwhelm NPWT systems requiring extremely frequent dressing changes and resulting in high cost. For those without as much experience in dealing with this situation, it should be highlighted that an EAF that arises in the setting of the open abdomen often actually gets worse before it starts to get better (Figs. 8.19, 8.20, 8.21, and 8.22). Control of effluent and protection of surrounding skin present a true challenge in this period. Poor control of gastrointestinal secretions will lead to a frustrated patient and nursing staff.

Aggressive effort toward the above goals is warranted immediately and may require considerable thought. Several authors have developed methods and systems, simply out of need, to address these concerns [42–48]. Creation of a "floating stoma" has even been reported and may be useful in specific circumstances [49]. All of these methods address a few simple ideas: "dam off" the EAF from surrounding bowel or granulation tissue, provide NPWT to surrounding tissues to assist with healing and exudate control, protect the surrounding skin to assist with dressing adherence and use in future surgery, and prevention of trauma to underlying viscera to eliminate the potential for additional EAF formation (Figs. 8.23, 8.24, 8.25, and 8.26). Any system that can address all of these concerns will be effective, but none specifically designed for the purpose of EAF control has been marketed. It therefore requires considerable effort from the care team to design a custom device for a particular patient and to ensure its effective use on a daily basis. This is where a competent enterostomal therapist or wound care team is worth their weight in gold.

In cases where effluent control is simply impossible with NPWT-based wound care systems, the only remaining option may be the use of what amounts to a large stoma appliance or wound manager (Fig. 8.27) [48]. These devices can be custom cut to the size and shape of the open wound and function much like a standard ostomy appliance. They come in a variety of sizes and are marketed by at least two companies currently. If the surrounding skin is in good shape, a watertight seal can be maintained with effective collection of effluent in a large pouch. Despite continued contact with gastrointestinal secretions, granulation tissue will somewhat surprisingly continue to form over the underlying viscera, and the wound will contract over time (Figs. 8.28, 8.29, 8.30, 8.31, and 8.32). The wound appliance should be replaced with a fresh one as needed or ideally every 4–5 days, much like an ostomy appliance is managed. As a general rule, changes should be as infrequent as possible to limit trauma to the underlying skin.

Pharmacologic Therapy

Key Concept: Several pharmacological agents including octreotide, somatostatin, acid-reducing medications, and antimotility drugs aid in decreasing EAF effluent volume and ultimately help in EAF control, volume and electrolyte abnormalities, wound care, and closure.

Ultimately, the goal remains for either spontaneous EAF closure, provision of an acceptable wound bed for performance of split-thickness skin grafting (STSG), or optimization of the overall situation in preparation for future surgery. Optimal control of fistula output is key to achieving these goals but, as stated, can often be difficult in execution. In this case, pharmacologic adjuncts assist in reduction of fistula output and aid in EAF effluent control. The most widely utilized and studied adjunct is octreotide. Octreotide is the long-acting synthetic analogue of somatostatin, a naturally occurring hormone that reduces gastrointestinal, biliary, and pancreatic secretions while increasing intestinal electrolyte and water absorption [50]. These effects are understandably beneficial in the patient with an EAF. Though often not stated, the drug also has the potentially negative effects of

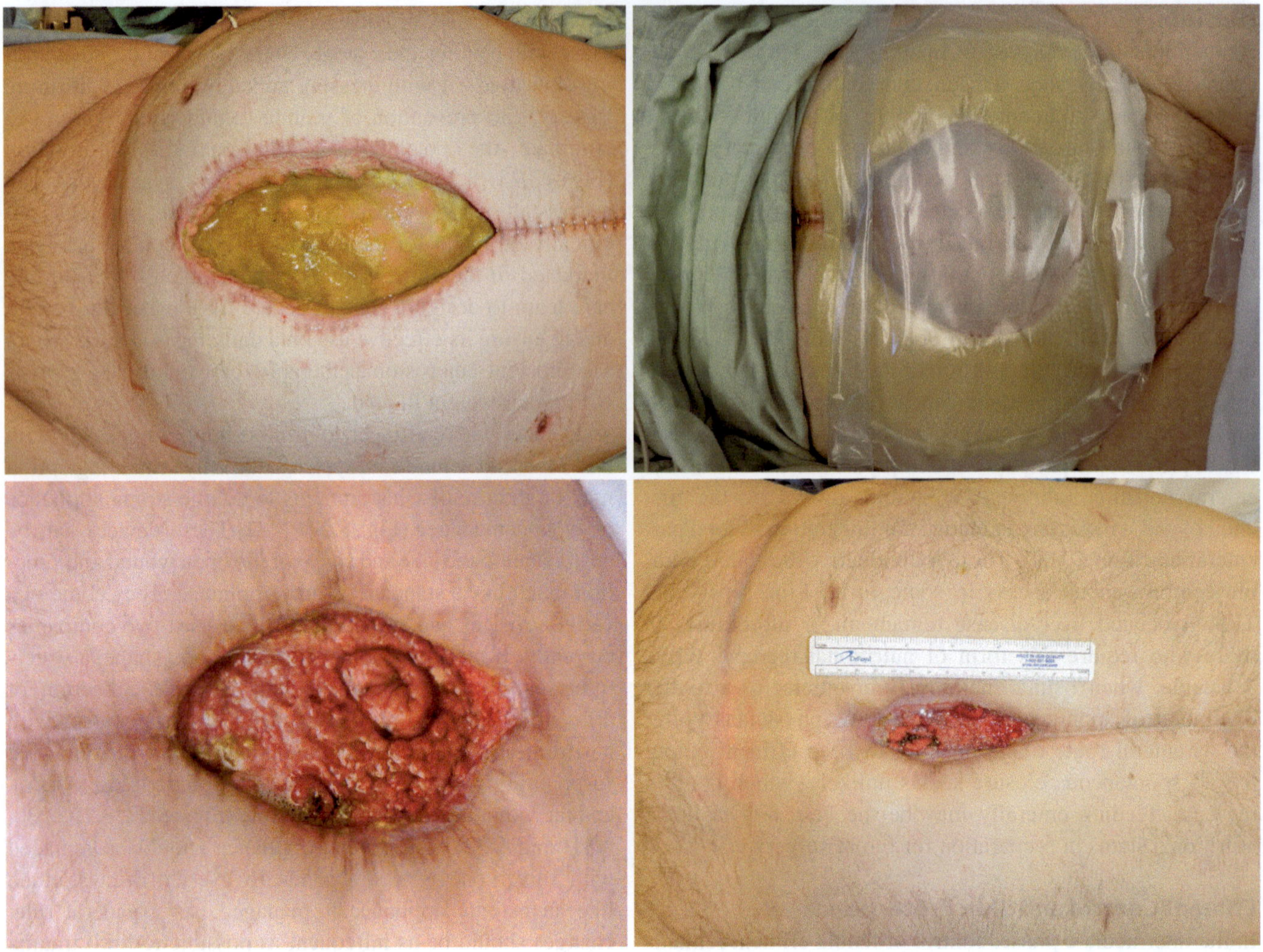

Figs. 8.19, 8.20, 8.21, and 8.22 This series of images shows an EAF patient as they progress through the phases of management. The first image shows a large poorly controlled EAF associated with a wound that actually gets wider initially and is controlled with a wound appliance. Over time the wound bed granulates and contracts ultimately leaving the patient with a very small open wound with two mature fistulas

decreasing the release of growth hormone and thyroid stimulating hormone [51].

The role of octreotide in the management of EAF has not been specifically investigated; however, numerous studies of the drug's use in patients with enterocutaneous fistulas exist [50, 52–61]. Claims that octreotide and somatostatin reduce fistula output and result in a higher rate of spontaneous fistula closure are controversial. A 2011 meta-analysis of the role of these drugs in patients with enterocutaneous fistulas concluded that both drugs shorten the time to fistula closure, but only somatostatin improved the rate of spontaneous closure [52]. There are several analyses that show a reduction in fistula output with the use of these medications [55–57, 59, 61], while others show questionable or no benefit [50, 53, 60]. A single center study of 60 ECF patients showed no benefit to the use of octreotide, though did show an increase in septic and thrombotic complications in those in which the drug was used [58]. Another randomized controlled trial of the use of these drugs in 2004 showed that both somatostatin and octreotide reduced time to ECF closure as well as overall hospital costs [54]. Given the mixed nature of reports in the literature, the use of these pharmacologic adjuncts should be individualized in EAF patients, keeping in mind the potential negative effects and complications associated with their use. Drugs such as proton-pump inhibitors and histamine-2 receptor blockers have been shown to be beneficial in patients with short-gut syndrome [62]. The benefit is at least in part related to a reduction in upper gastrointestinal secretions. While most EAF patients will be receiving one of these drugs given the nature of their disease, there may be a benefit,

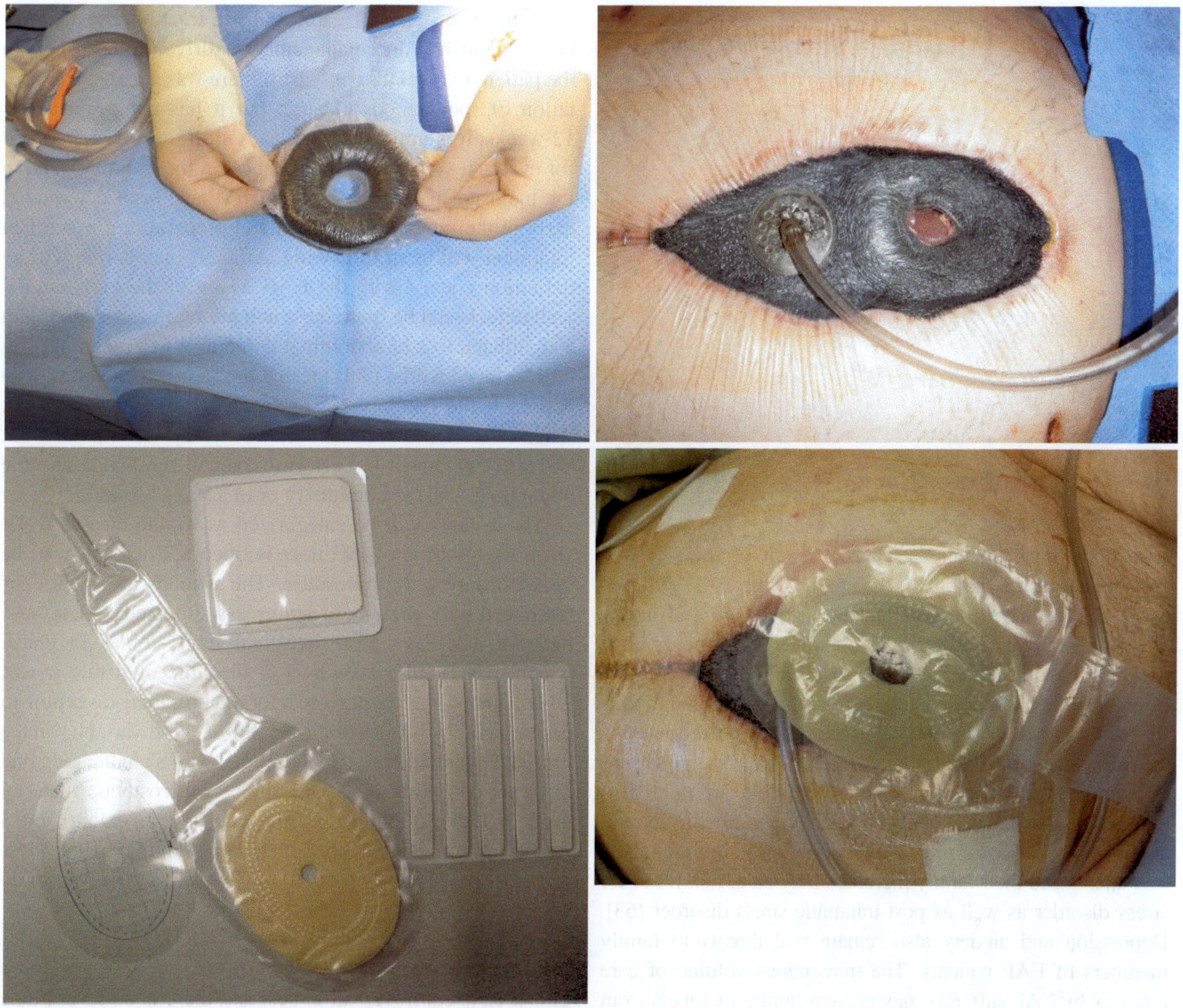

Figs. 8.23, 8.24, 8.25, and 8.26 This series of images depicts construction of a "fistula VAC." A "donut" is constructed out of sponge and nonporous drape. This is utilized to dam off the EAF from the surrounding wound. Stoma paste and powder can be used to facilitate this. The remaining wound bed is covered with sponge and drape. A fistula appliance is placed over the EAF to control effluent

although unproven, in reducing EAF output. Patients with more distal fistulas may benefit from the use of loperamide to control effluent, although there is no data to support this drug's use for this purpose.

Psychiatric Implications of EAF

Key Concept: *The psychiatric toll on both the patient and surgeon is tremendous. Open discussion between all parties, including airing of frustrations, anger, or concerns, is beneficial. Managing expectations and the involvement of mental health specialists can aid in this process.*

Dealing with an EAF presents numerous challenges to the patient and their family. There are significant psychiatric implications associated with this disease process. Unfortunately, EAF is a problem with no rapid solution. In the best cases a fistula may close nonoperatively after a significant amount of time (i.e., months) and intensive care management. Patient activity is typically severely limited during the early and intermediate phases of disease. Difficulties with effluent control can prevent a patient from ambulating any significant distance and may completely eliminate the ability to perform normal activities of daily living. Problems

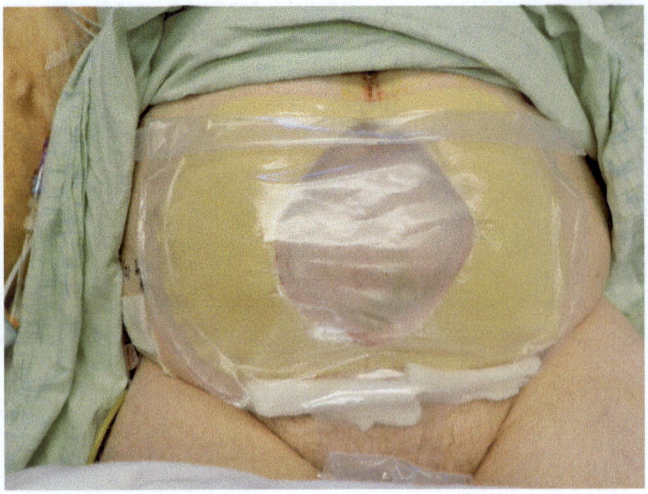

Fig. 8.27 Wound appliance in place

with body image occur as a direct result of the physical appearance of the abdomen, the smell of the EAF effluent, and the potential or actual leakage around wound appliances that can be devastating for a patient's psyche. Even if a patient becomes stable enough to leave the hospital, they often become homebound and reclusive, with limited mobility, while they await spontaneous closure or corrective surgery. Because of this, patients and family will often pressure the surgical team for a quick solution. While no published data addresses the issue in EAF patients specifically, depression is clearly a major problem faced by these individuals.

Patients and their family members may be at risk for acute stress disorder as well as post-traumatic stress disorder [63]. Depression and anxiety also remain real threats to family members of EAF patients. The tremendous volume of care required by EAF sufferers may prevent family members from keeping normal work schedules and often can result in the need for family members to completely change their daily life to provide support to a loved one. Awareness of the psychological impact of this disease on patient and family is critical for the surgeon. Referral for psychiatric care will often be required. Most importantly, the surgeon must not allow pressure from the family or patient to have a negative impact on the long-term plan of care. Rushing to the operating room to solve a "perceived" problem may result in worsening of the "real" problem as well as the potential of burned bridges for the future.

Late/Chronic Phase

Key Concept: *Failure of spontaneous closure leads to a period of preparation prior to surgical intervention. This process lasts several months and is dictated by the individual's nutritional, overall health, and overlying skin and EAF status. Optimization of these factors and extensive planning that includes both the reestablishment of gastrointestinal tract continuity and abdominal wall reconstruction is required.*

In the late phase of care, realistic treatment goals have been established and management is driven to best prepare the patient to meet these goals. If there was a realistic expectation of spontaneous closure, but it has not occurred by 12 weeks, it is unlikely to occur. A shift toward preparation for eventual surgery is probably best in these individuals. In the majority of EAF cases, this will have been determined early in the intermediate phase and preparation for surgical treatment will be in full swing. An incisional hernia will by definition coexist with the EAF. Many of these abdominal wall defects can be quite large and are often associated with a significant loss of abdominal domain. When planning, you will be faced with a multifaceted problem: when and how to approach the fistula, how to repair the associated hernia, whether or not to reconstruct a functional abdominal wall, and whether or not to perform repair of the fistula and the abdominal wall concomitantly or in a staged fashion.

These cases will be categorized as wound classes II–IV since the gastrointestinal tract is open and will have to be violated during the procedure. The wounds are often contaminated with bacteria or are grossly infected. Often these patients will have gastrointestinal tract stomas in place, which may require takedown at the time of fistula repair, while others may require temporary proximal diversion to protect a high-risk anastomosis. All of these variables make the decision to address the abdominal wall a challenging one in terms of timing of repair, choice of prosthetic material used in reconstruction, and the decision to embark on a staged vs. non-staged approach. From this, two major questions always lurk: when do you re-operate and on whom do you attempt surgery?

Timing of Surgery

This area is controversial at best and there is no level I data to support any specific period of delay prior to an attempt at closure of an EAF or abdominal wall reconstruction. Most experienced surgeons would agree that a period of *at least* 3 months after the initial laparotomy or fistula formation would be advised before any attempt at operative repair. This allows time for intra-abdominal adhesions to soften, for inflammatory processes to resolve, and reduces risk of iatrogenic bowel injury during the reparative procedure. In patients who have had split-thickness skin grafting directly over bowel, definitive surgery is routinely deferred until the graft is no longer adherent to the underlying viscera. This can be determined with a simple "pinch" test (Fig. 8.33) by pinching the skin graft between the index finger and thumb to see if it lifts freely from the intestine underneath. In general, this takes longer than 3 months and can take up to a year before conditions are ideal for proceeding with surgery.

Various authors have reported delays that range between 2 and 929 days from initial temporary abdominal closure to attempted definitive reconstruction [64–67], with mean times

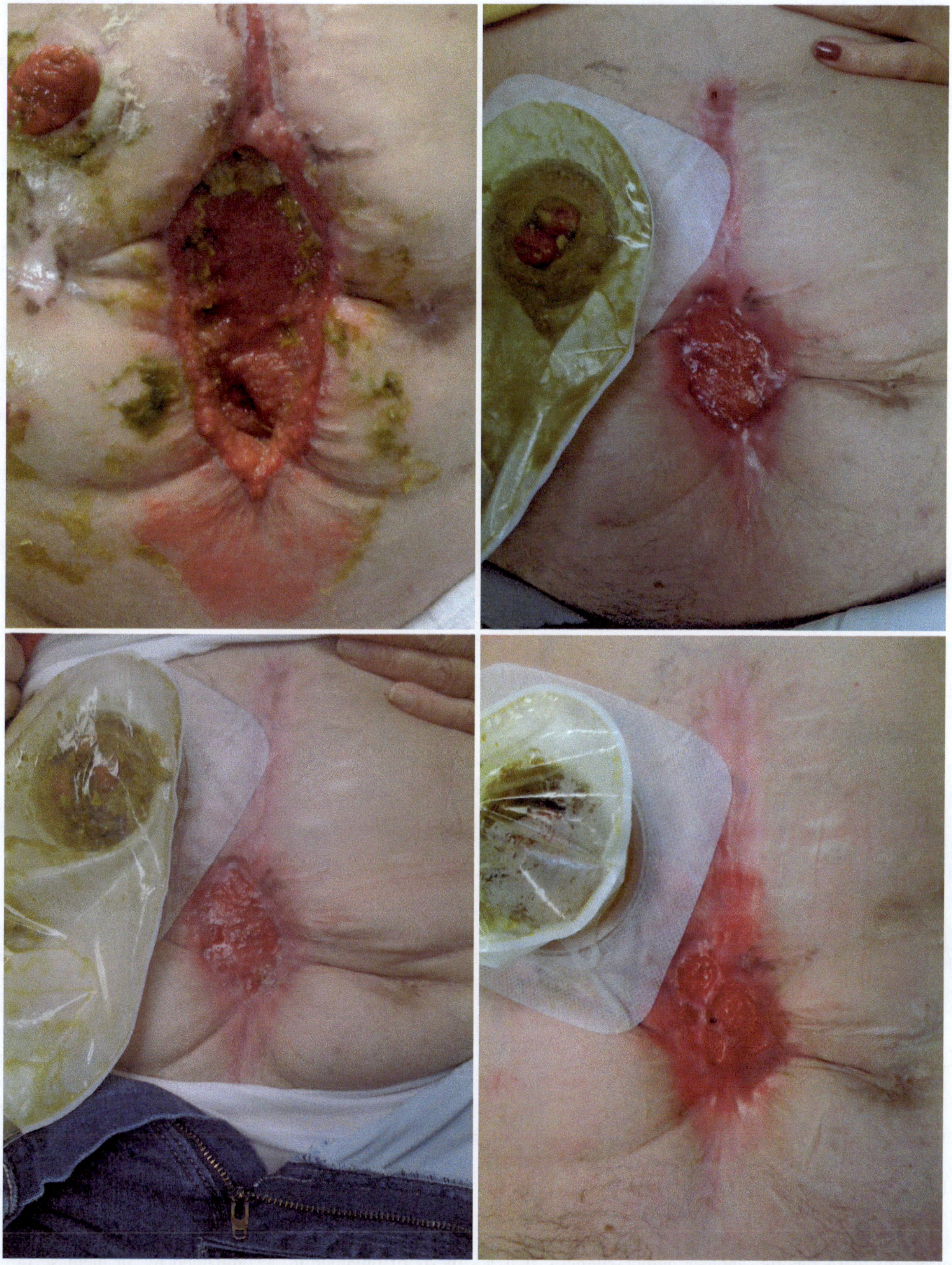

Figs. 8.28, 8.29, 8.30, 8.31, and 8.32 This series of images shows a poorly controlled deep EAF with resulting skin irritation and an adjacent loop ileostomy. This individual was managed with a wound appliance, and despite chronic contact of the wound bed with fistula effluent, the wound contracted nicely over time with resultant spontaneous closure of the deep EAF. The ostomy was taken down and the patient did well

Figs. 8.28, 8.29, 8.30, 8.31, and 8.32 (continued)

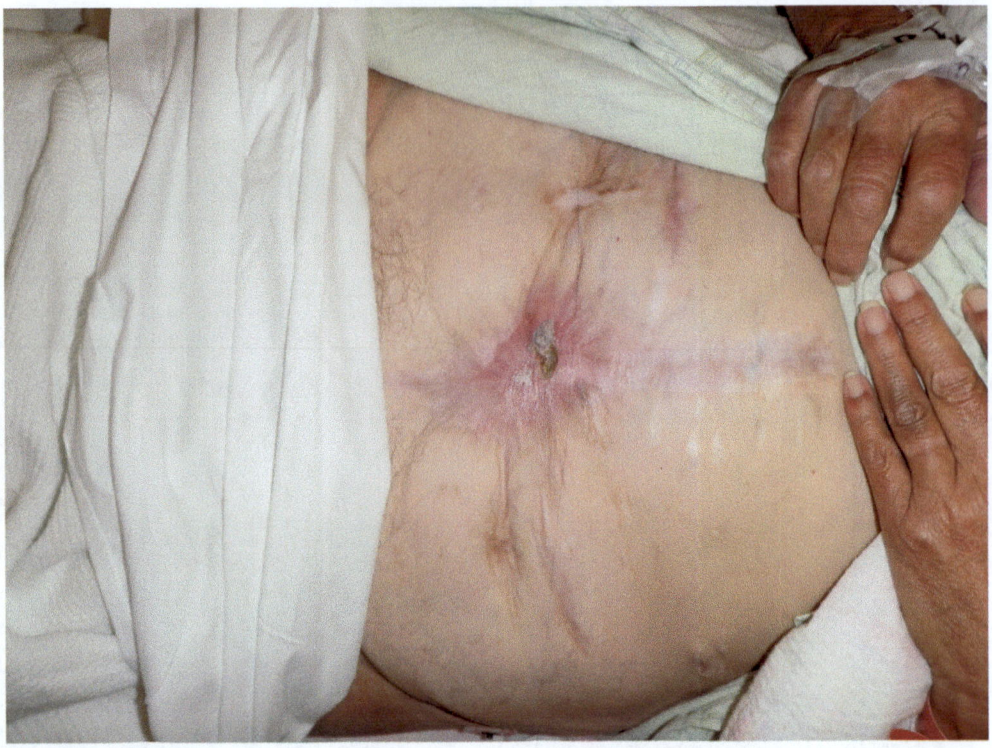

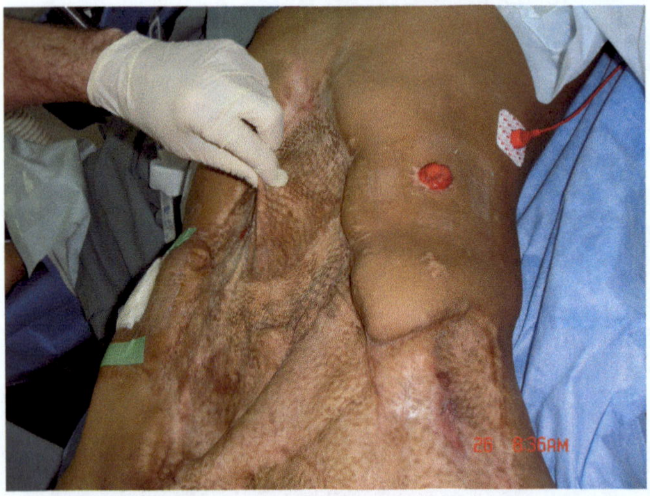

Fig. 8.33 The "pinch" test that can be done to assess readiness for reconstructive surgery

to attempted reconstruction of 311 days [65], 184 days [66], and 585 days [67]. Due to the retrospective nature of these studies, it is difficult to relate the success of a reconstructive effort with the timing of surgery. What is clear, though, is that a waiting period of 6 months or longer is common. Contrary to these reports, another author suggests that a delay of longer than 12 months may be associated with increased loss of domain, thereby making a tension-free repair more difficult leading to an increased recurrence [64]. It must be noted that these studies included many patients that did not have EAFs and simply required abdominal wall reconstruction after management with a planned ventral hernia strategy after an open abdomen. Regardless, any reconstructive attempt must be well planned, and the optimal timing will be intimately related to resolution of inflammation, softening of the surrounding tissues, improvement in nutritional status, and overall fitness of the patient. Surgical judgment based on these multiple factors is likely the key to success.

Optimization: Preparation for Surgery

Optimization of these factors prior to surgery can be achieved through utilization of an appropriate delay, aggressive nutritional strategy, overall medical and physical re-conditioning, and detailed planning. No matter what nutritional strategy is employed, the patient's overall nutritional status should be assessed. This is likely best accomplished through the measurement of serum prealbumin levels, albumin and protein levels. It is best to see a sustained achievement of normal levels to ensure adequate nutritional status over time. Any sudden decrease in the serum level of prealbumin should be followed by measurement of serum C-reactive protein (CRP), as any secondary infection or inflammatory process will lead to an acute phase response with a decrease in synthesis of prealbumin accompanied by an increase in CRP. Sometimes this may be an early sign of line sepsis, pneumonia, or recurrent intra-abdominal abscess and should prompt further investigation and avoidance of any extensive surgical procedure. Any reconstructive procedure performed on a malnourished patient is doomed to failure. This may be the single most important factor to optimize prior to surgery.

Medical and physical optimization will require support from a multidisciplinary team of providers including internists, medical subspecialists, physical therapists, and social workers. Diligent preparation in these areas will ease recovery from major reconstructive procedures and must be emphasized. Detailed planning for reconstruction starts first with obtaining an abdominopelvic CT scan utilizing IV and enteral contrast. Imaging will assist in defining areas of potential ongoing inflammation and obstruction, as well as provide detailed information about abdominal wall musculature and its relation to underlying structures. The distance of rectus diastasis can be accurately measured, and a safe site of entry can potentially be chosen. This information will assist the surgeon in determining potential sizes and types of reinforcing materials that will have to be on hand and may in fact determine the best approach to abdominal wall closure and reconstruction.

Staged vs. Non-staged Approaches

Key Concept: One or more extensive operations may be required to achieve EAF and abdominal wall closure. Planning for this involves setting well-defined goals, communicating these with the patient and their family, avoidance of overaggressive surgery, and knowledge of "bail-out" strategies.

As previously stated, an individual that has been patiently awaiting corrective surgery for an EAF will often push their surgeon to achieve a quick single-stage solution to their problem. The prospect of undergoing two or more major surgical procedures to correct all existing problems may not be palatable to patient or family. Advocates of a single-stage approach to this problem cite this advantage, as well as a potential decrease in overall morbidity by avoiding multiple procedures. A second approach to the problems of gastrointestinal tract fistulae and coexisting abdominal wall defects is to handle these issues remotely from one another at separate surgeries in order to improve the outcomes associated with the abdominal wall reconstruction.

When using complex reconstructive techniques such as component separation, [68] (Fig. 8.34) or flaps, the first attempt will be the easiest and most likely to achieve success. Proponents of the staged procedure cite several advantages. Given the contaminated nature of these cases performed in patients with fistulae and/or intestinal stomas, infectious complications may be decreased, as well as improving overall closure rates, and decreasing the rates of recurrent hernia by performing the abdominal wall reconstruction after the EAF has been addressed. Aside from the risk of infection, the nutritional status of these patients may be far superior after repair of their fistula and complete reliance on enteral feeding utilizing the entire GI tract.

There are no prospective studies that have randomized patients to a staged vs. non-staged approach to these problems. There are several small retrospective analyses of patients that required surgical management of both fistulae (not all EAF) and large abdominal wall defects, some of which took a staged approach [66] and some of which did not [69, 70]. One retrospective review of 19 patients with high-output EAFs associated with large abdominal wall defects revealed a 31.5 % re-fistulization rate after the initial procedure performed to repair the digestive tract fistula [66]. The investigators used a staged approach to abdominal wall reconstruction employing the use of flap procedures, but unfortunately did not report the results of the reconstruction in their manuscript. It is certainly reasonable to assume that the cases where re-fistulization occurred would have likely failed any abdominal wall reconstructive attempt had the procedures been performed concomitantly.

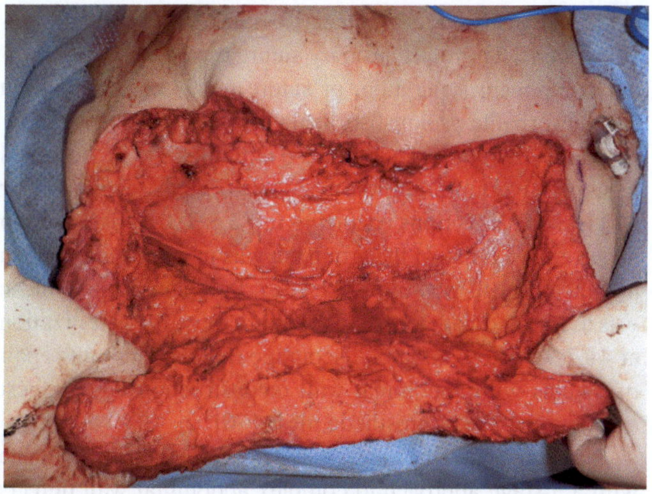

Fig. 8.34 A unilateral traditional "Ramirez" component separation. Unilateral fascial release may be all that is needed in some cases to get approximation of the rectus fascia at the midline

A retrospective study of 32 patients that had either intestinal stomas or enterocutaneous fistulae in the presence of large abdominal wall defects who subsequently underwent single-stage closure of the gastrointestinal tract and their abdominal wall defect using a component separation technique reported a 28 % rate of wound complications, 21 % recurrence of hernia, and 26 % recurrence of fistulae with a median follow-up of 20 months [69]. The authors concluded that the rates of hernia recurrence and re-fistulization were acceptable, although the definition of acceptable is certainly open for debate. Because of the difficulty associated with the care of these patients, the United Kingdom has established specialized intestinal failure units to assist in, and potentially improve the care of these difficult cases [70]. The standard management in one of these units has been to perform repair of the fistula with concomitant abdominal wall closure/reconstruction after initial optimization of the patient's overall condition—focusing mainly on nutritional support and control of sepsis. Sixty-one patients underwent 63 operations to close digestive tract fistulae associated with open abdominal wounds. They used primary suture repair, with and without component separation, or suture repair in combination with absorbable or nonabsorbable prosthetic mesh to reconstruct the abdominal wall in these individuals. The observed postoperative mortality rate was 4.8 %, with respiratory or surgical site infections occurring in 82.5 %. Re-fistulization occurred in 11.1 % of the group but was more common when prosthetic mesh was used (24.1 %). Porcine collagen mesh was associated with a particularly high rate of re-fistulization at 41.7 %. These authors discourage the concomitant repair of fistulas with abdominal wall reconstruction and suggest avoiding the use of prosthetic mesh [70].

Jernigan and colleagues [64] reviewed their experience with a 3-stage approach to complex abdominal wall defects in 274 patients over 8 years. They did not specifically address individuals with fistulae, but all patients were critically ill and were managed with open abdomens. Their management scheme was as follows: stage 1, absorbable mesh insertion for temporary closure (with mesh pleating and delayed closure if edema resolved within 3–5 days); stage 2, mesh removal after 2–3 weeks and formation of a planned ventral hernia through placement of a split-thickness skin graft over granulation tissue or a full-thickness skin closure over viscera; and stage 3, definitive abdominal wall reconstruction after 6–12 months using the modified component separation technique. Of note, 39 % of the patients died during stage 1 secondary to shock. Of the 166 patients who lived and had absorbable mesh placed, 22 % underwent delayed fascial closure. In the stage 2 group, there were nine deaths from multisystem organ failure, with 96 % of the remaining 120 patients having a skin graft placed over the viscera. A total of 14 fistulae occurred (8 % of survivors). To date, 73 of the 120 have undergone definitive abdominal wall reconstruction with no deaths and a 5 % rate of recurrent hernia at a mean follow-up of 24 months. This large, retrospective study demonstrates nicely how a well thought-out and staged reconstructive plan can result in low mortality with good long-term results. Application of these results to the patient with an EAF must be done cautiously, however, as these patients were not analyzed separately as a specific group.

Abdominal Wall Reconstruction (AWR)

Key Concept: Reconstruction of the abdominal wall may be the most difficult aspect of the case, fraught with high complication rates. Expertise is crucial to successful results and may require a multidisciplinary approach along with use of mesh, flap, or tissue transfer techniques.

Reconstruction of the abdominal wall can be a complex and high-risk procedure. When performing definitive surgery for EAF, one immediate goal is to obtain closure of the abdomen over the visceral repair (Fig. 8.35). Exposure of bowel to the environment is one factor that likely led to formation of an EAF to begin with and must be avoided at this stage at all costs. The approach to closure of the abdominal wall will be dictated in part by the decision to stage the repair or not. There is no ideal technique or simple approach to AWR. Component separation techniques (CST) and flap reconstructions tend to be technically demanding and can be associated with an increased incidence of wound problems depending on the approach used; however, they can provide a functional abdominal wall reconstruction. Simple mesh underlay closure of fascial defects will result in an acceptable hernia repair, but often leaves the patient with a large area of laxity on the anterior abdominal wall. The lack of a functional anterior abdominal wall may limit their physical activity in the future, and the finished appearance may be cosmetically inferior. It is important to consider a patient's functional status and expectations when determining which approach to use for abdominal wall reconstruction and hernia repair (Figs. 8.36 and 8.37).

The CST originally popularized by Ramirez in 1990 [68] involves separating the rectus muscle from the posterior rectus sheath and the external oblique muscle from the internal oblique, thereby resulting in medial advancement of approximately 5 cm at the epigastrium, 10 cm at the waistline, and 3 cm in the suprapubic region unilaterally (Fig. 8.38). This can be coupled with mesh reinforcement and restores a dynamic and functional abdominal wall. There are several reports in the literature on the success of CST in the management of large ventral hernias, revealing rates of hernia recurrence from 6 to 52 % [68, 71–83]. It may seem intuitive, but it is worth stating that larger hernia defects are more likely to recur and they are more likely to require mesh-bridging techniques whether or not CST is used. Ideally, CST is used to facilitate full re-approximation of the rectus complex in the midline with some sort of mesh buttress. Some defects are so large that bridging will still be required even after performance of component separation. One can expect higher recurrence rates in these scenarios.

A randomized comparison of CST to prosthetic mesh closure with an expanded PTFE patch in 39 patients [78] showed that wound complications were more frequent in the prosthetic group and 38 % of the patients closed with mesh required its removal later because of infectious complications. Recurrent hernia was noted in 52 % of those undergoing CST and in 36 % of those with prosthetic repair. While it is difficult to draw definitive conclusions from this small study, the two methods were statistically equivalent in this group. Several minor modifications of the CST technique have been reported in the literature with varying success rates [74, 75, 81, 84]. All of these reports involved either single cases or very small groups of patients. More recently there has been a surge of interest in the use of the posterior CST, [81] likely related to the ability to exploit the retro-rectus space for placement of mesh reinforcement. Many of those who were major proponents of the classic anterior CST have shifted to the posterior approach.

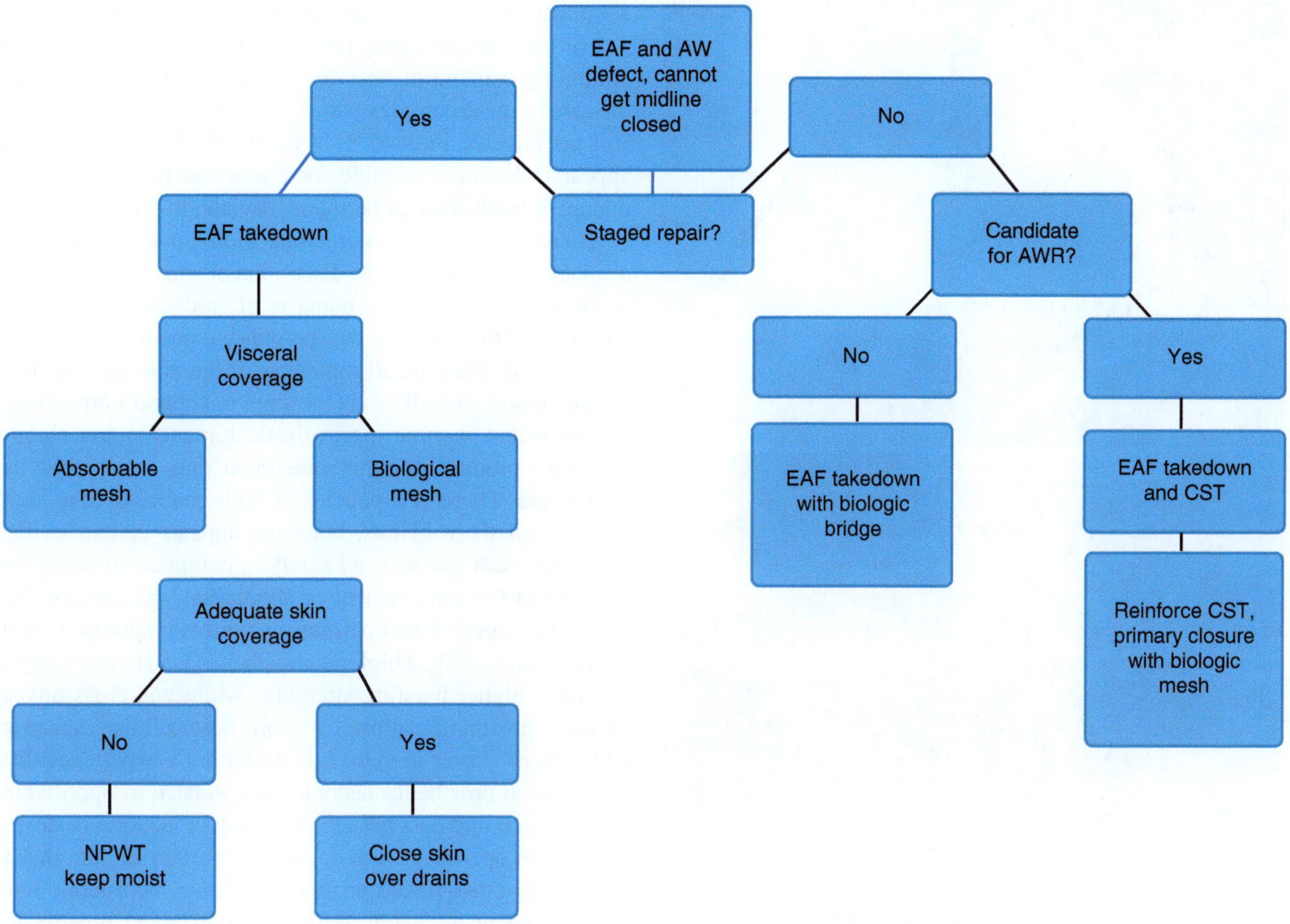

Fig. 8.35 Algorithm illustrating a strategy for abdominal wall reconstruction in EAF patients. *EAF* enteroatmospheric fistula, *AW* abdominal wall, *AWR* abdominal wall reconstruction, *CST* component separation technique, *NPWT* negative-pressure wound therapy

Utilization of CST may assist in AWR by increasing abdominal domain. Comparisons of preoperative and post operative CT scans of the abdomen and pelvis after CST repair of large abdominal wall hernias with associated loss of domain have shown significant increases in the intra-abdominal volume without any significant change in diaphragmatic height [85]. It may be possible to restore lost domain without the unfavorable result of pulmonary compromise secondary to a loss of thoracic volume.

One of the major criticisms of the anterior CST approach is the large bilateral skin flaps that result from the dissection necessary for exposure during the procedure. Flap complications comprise the majority of wound occurrences noted with this procedure. Several approaches have been devised to avoid the seroma and potential infections that can be common. The use of fibrin sealant has been shown to reduce seroma and wound infection rates in patients undergoing traditional anterior CST [82]. Placing numerous "quilting" mattress sutures has been described to eliminate dead space with the potential decrease in seroma formation but has not been studied prospectively. Rosen et al. [83] described the use of a laparoscopic component separation technique in seven patients that altogether eliminates the large flaps created using the open technique. The technique is similar to that used in TEPP laparoscopic inguinal hernia repair. Release of Scarpa's fascia should also be performed with this approach, although care must be taken not to divide the linea semilunaris itself. After performance of the CST portion of the case laparoscopically, the midline may be reconstructed using either a laparoscopic or open approach—a requirement in all EAF patients treated with a single-stage procedure. Short-term follow-up of patients treated with this technique has shown acceptable outcomes. Laparoscopic CST has been shown to be inferior with regard to mobility in a porcine model, as it yielded only 86 % of the medial mobilization of the rectus that was achieved with the open technique [86]. In cadaveric testing the two have been shown to be equivalent [87]. Another minimally invasive method of achieving a lateral release has been described by creating small tunnels from the midline incision instead of large flaps [88]. While this technique is approached through a large midline incision, it avoids the creation of large flaps with their attendant

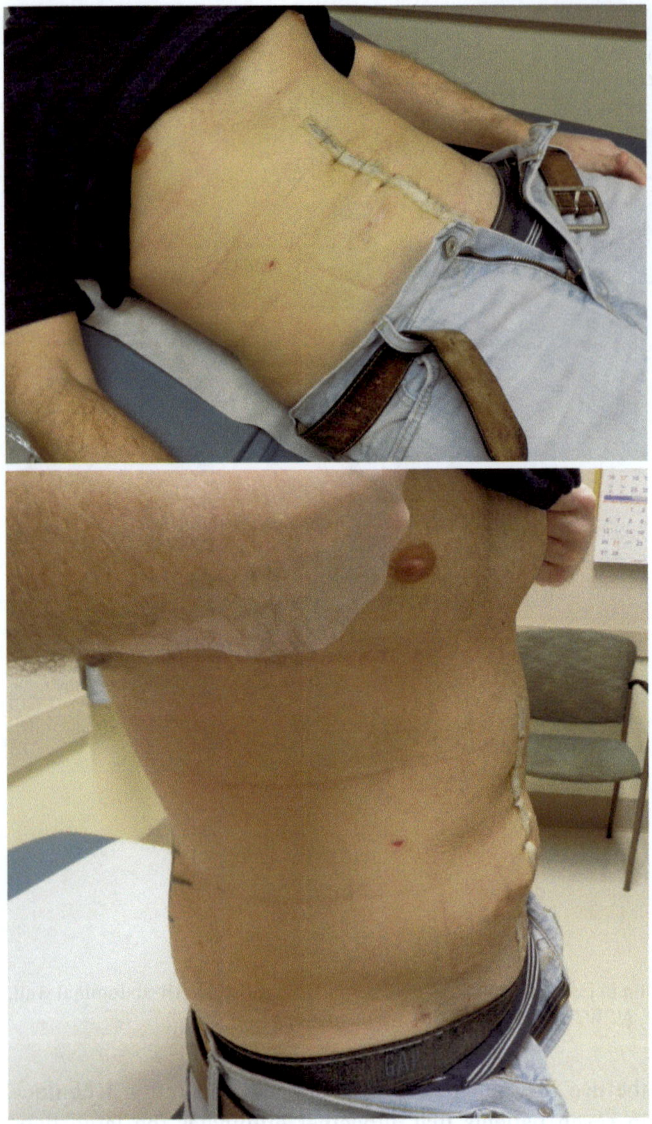

Figs. 8.36 and 8.37 These images show a young patient after a functional abdominal wall reconstruction. Note the obvious positioning of the rectus back in the midline as well as his ability to perform a sit-up

wound morbidity, potentially making it ideal in the case of single-stage repair of EAF. Laparoscopic and other minimally invasive approaches to component separation are relatively new, and to date, no randomized comparisons of these techniques with traditional techniques have been undertaken.

Biologic or Synthetic Mesh

Key Concept: Choice of mesh involves factors ranging from the risk of infection, strength and durability to incorporation, to personal preference. Regardless of choice, primary myofascial apposition along with the mesh vs. using a mesh "bridge" results in decreased hernia formation.

AWR performed at the time of EAF repair will occur in a contaminated or potentially grossly infected environment. This precludes the placement of a permanent prosthetic or alloplastic mesh as a bridge or reinforcement secondary to risk of infection requiring prosthetic removal. The advent of biologic prosthetic meshes has provided one more tool for the care of these complex patients. While these materials can still get infected in 0–40 % of cases [29, 30, 89–106], they appear to be more suitable for placement in contaminated operative fields than do permanent synthetic prosthetics.

There are currently numerous biologic mesh products available on the market, the discussion of which is beyond the scope of this chapter. The majority of products are collagen-based, and this collagen can be either cross-linked or non-cross-linked. They are all somewhat different in the way they are processed, and all products claim to support normal host fibroblast and vascular ingrowth. Each manufacturer claims that their product is either integrated into or replaced by host tissue. There is a paucity of high-quality data to support any of these claims, but what appears certain is that these materials can be used safely in complicated scenarios to assist in the achievement of abdominal wall closure and visceral coverage when permanent synthetic options cannot be used. Cross-linked biologic prosthetics tend to be stronger and have higher bursting strengths, while non-cross-linked biologic prosthetics allow for more host cellular ingrowth and "resorb" faster in vivo. It is the author's experience that cross-linked prosthetics become encapsulated as opposed to incorporated into host tissues. This may or may not be desirable to the operating surgeon. It is important to note that a completely cross-linked prosthetic will not incorporate into host tissues at all, while partially cross-linked prosthetics will incorporate to some degree.

The majority of data available for biologic mesh use in AWR involves three products: AlloDerm® (LifeCell Corporation, Branchburg, NJ) [29, 30, 96–106], Surgisis® (Cook Biotech, West Lafayette, IN) [93–95], and Permacol™ (Covidien Surgical, Mansfield, MA) [89–92]. AlloDerm studies included between 10 and 144 patients revealing hernia recurrence rates between 0 and 100 % with variable follow-up. There is unfortunately a fair amount of heterogeneity in the approach to reconstruction within each study, making it difficult to draw definitive conclusion from the data. Reports of Permacol™ use include between 1 and 28 patients with hernia recurrence rates of 0–15 % with variable length of follow-up [89–92]. Several studies on the use of Surgisis® to repair both ventral and inguinal hernia defects in contaminated environments have been published [93–95]. These studies have included between 20 and 53 patients with mean follow-up periods of 14–19 months and showed hernia recurrence rates of 0–30 %. All ventral repairs completed in these studies were performed using a fascial-bridging technique. One study of the use of a non-cross-linked porcine dermal scaffold in the abdominal wall reconstruction of 16 patients reported a 7 % hernia recurrence rate after 16.5 months of follow-up [105]. Importantly, the majority of these patients

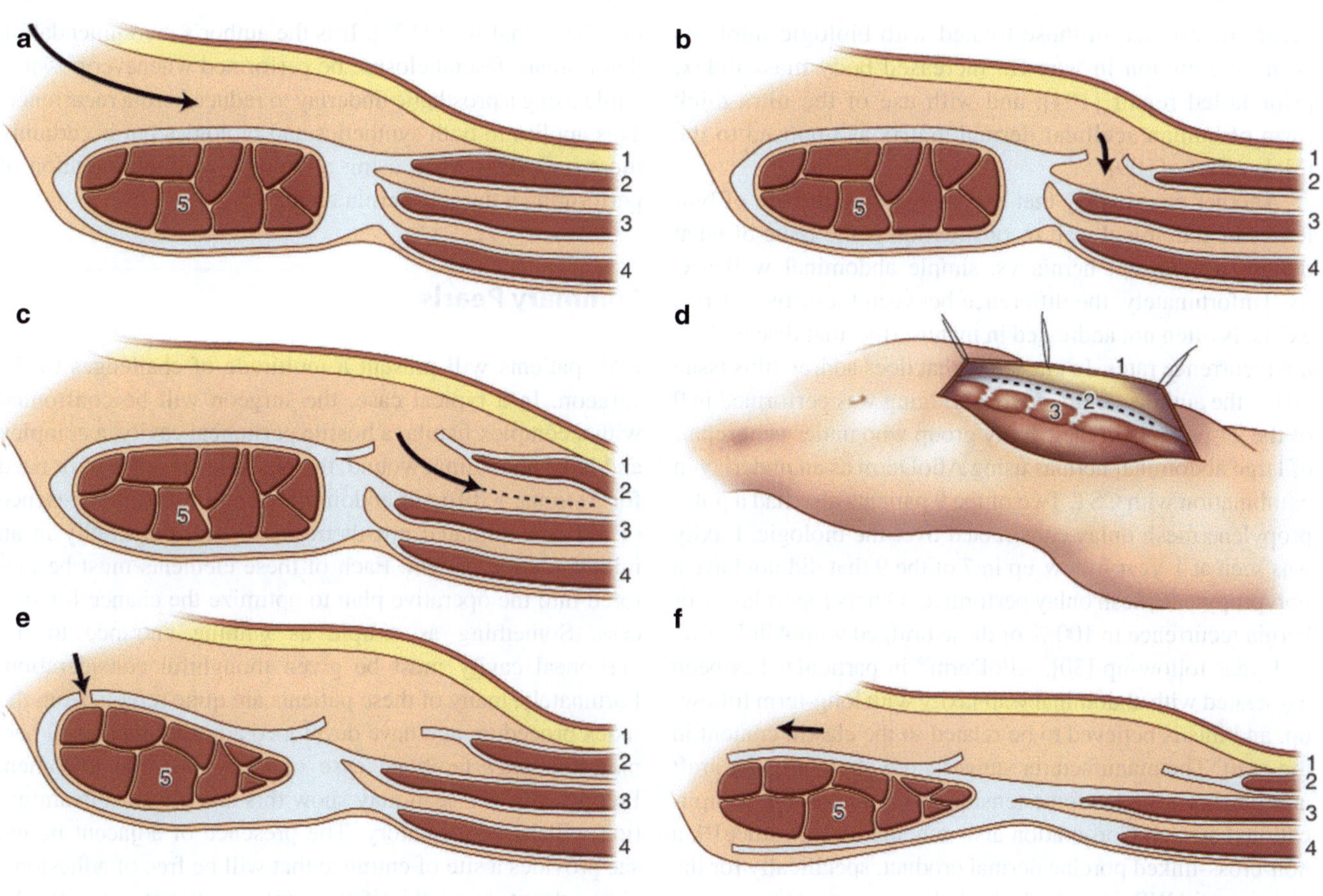

Fig. 8.38 These drawings depict the anatomy of the rectus and oblique muscles on one side of the anterior abdominal wall. The traditional "Ramirez" anterior component separation is shown. Release of the external oblique is performed and the space between the external and internal obliques is developed out to the flank. The posterior rectus fascia is also released. *Arrows* indicate the direction of dissection, (**a–f**) indicate the order of dissection, *1–4* indicate the layers of the abdominal wall and muscles

underwent CST, and they achieved complete apposition and closure of the rectus muscles in 88 %. The porcine matrix was used as a reinforcing underlay in the majority of these patients but was used as a bridge graft in those where rectus apposition could not be achieved. The only recurrence was noted in a patient who was "bridged" (Fig. 8.39).

There is some controversy as to whether or not bridging a fascial defect with a biologic prosthetic is an adequate hernia repair. A retrospective review of 11 patients that had large complex hernias bridged with human acellular dermal matrix found an 80 % hernia recurrence rate at a mean follow-up of 24 months and a cost of $5,100 per patient [29]. The manuscript title asserts that bridging with a biologic may simply result in an expensive hernia sac. Another study showed that a biologic mesh-reinforced primary repair (involving CST in most) had only a 20 % recurrence, while 80 % of patients who were bridged with the same biologic mesh-reinforced primary repair had hernia recurrence [96]. The obvious confounder in this study is that patients who were bridged had larger defects that were more likely to recur in any case. Comparison of biologic reinforcement of CST with historical controls

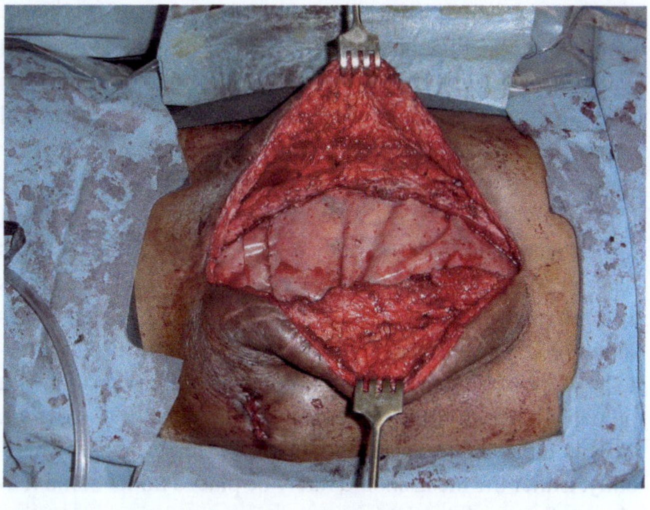

Fig. 8.39 A bridge repair with a biologic mesh

who were not reinforced shows a decreased recurrence rate in hernias that did not require bridging [97]. There have been other reports that surgical site infection is more common with larger biologic implants [103] and that hernia recurrence in those treated with biologic implants is more common in women, increased body mass index, prior failed repair [104], and with use of the ultra-thick form of human acellular dermal matrix as opposed to the thick variety [100].

Another controversy that exists regarding the use of biologics in abdominal wall reconstruction is the issue of what defines a recurrent hernia vs. simple abdominal wall laxity. Unfortunately, the difference between these two, if one exists, is often not addressed in manuscripts that discuss hernia recurrence rates. In one study that does address this issue [101], the authors comment that bridging was performed in 9 of the 27 patients in their study group who underwent repair of large abdominal hernias using AlloDerm as an underlay in combination with CST. Two of the 9 patients also had a polypropylene mesh onlay constructed over the biologic. Laxity was seen at 1-year follow-up in 7 of the 9 that did not have a polypropylene mesh onlay performed. Others report laxity or hernia recurrence in 100 % of those bridged with AlloDerm® at 1 year follow-up [30]. AlloDerm® in particular has been associated with abdominal wall laxity with long-term follow-up, and this is believed to be related to the elastin content in the graft. The manufacturer suggests pre-stretching the graft and placing it under some tension to minimize this complication. LifeCell Corporation also now markets Strattice™, a non-cross-linked porcine dermal product, specifically for the purpose of AWR given its lack of elastin content.

In the situation of a staged abdominal wall reconstruction in a patient that has previously undergone EAF repair with simple visceral coverage, a synthetic prosthetic mesh may be appropriate to use (for a clean wound class I). The issue of bridging vs. complete myofascial re-approximation is pertinent in the select patient population with complex abdominal wall defects. While the idea of tension-free hernia repair has made its way from use in the inguinal region to use in ventral hernia repair; it may be that this concept is fundamentally flawed. It is obvious that bringing a patient's fascia together in the midline under extreme tension increases the risk of failure; however, a certain amount of tension on a repair is desired. When surgeons place a piece of prosthetic mesh as an underlay to bridge a fascial defect, a degree of tension is intentionally placed upon the underlay mesh to fascia interface. A prosthetic placed with no tension at all results in a palpable bulge or soft spot at the location of the fascial defect. This is undesirable to patients both physically and cosmetically. Either the mesh should likely be placed under some tension to flatten abdominal contour or a component separation should be performed to achieve complete myofascial approximation and a functional abdominal wall reconstruction. This issue is controversial and is not strongly supported by data; however, a 2005 review of 188 patients with large abdominal hernias showed a recurrence rate of 31 % in patients treated with a fascial-bridging synthetic prosthetic vs. 9 % in those that had complete restoration of myofascial continuity of the abdominal wall [106]. It is the author's recommendation that primary fascial closure be performed whenever possible while using a prosthetic underlay to reduce hernia recurrence. This applies to both synthetics and biologics but is certainly more important when using a biologic with the intention of performing a durable hernia repair.

Summary Pearls

EAF patients will present a multitude of challenges to the surgeon. In a typical case, the surgeon will be confronted with a complex fistula, a hostile peritoneal cavity, a complex and large abdominal wound, the possible presence of or need for a stoma, a difficult abdominal contour, and the presence of old contaminated prosthetic mesh—all potentially in an initially septic patient. Each of these elements must be factored into the operative plan to optimize the chance for success. Something as simple as gaining entrance to the peritoneal cavity must be given thoughtful consideration. Fortunately, many of these patients are quite remote from the index procedure and have developed adjacent incisional hernias that may facilitate ease of entry into the abdomen. Preoperative CT scan may show this and physical examination will be confirmatory. The presence of adjacent hernia sac provides a site of entrance that will be free of adhesions. Take advantage of this if it is present. If not, one may be forced to enter in the midline where dense adhesions between the bowel and anterior abdominal wall will create difficulty and potentially enterotomies. Lateral entry into the abdomen should be avoided as it may limit the options for CST during the reconstructive portion of the procedure.

Performing a complete adhesiolysis during laparotomy is tempting and can certainly be achieved in some circumstances. Yet, if there are no signs of bowel obstruction either clinically or radiographically, it is likely best to limit adhesiolysis to areas of necessity. The risk of enterotomy is high, and the likelihood of re-fistulization increases with every enterotomy created. Fistulas should be resected and the remaining bowel re-anastomosed. The temptation to free an area of fistulized bowel followed by primary closure should be reserved for situations where it is the only possibility. These repairs tend to break down and are discouraged.

The patient with an ostomy presents an additional challenge. The surgeon must first consider if the stoma should be closed or left in place. The length of remaining bowel, continence status, presence of a parastomal hernia, and potential for the need to perform a high-risk distal anastomosis must all be considered. If the need for a stoma remains, it is easiest to leave the existing stoma in place. If AWR is performed at the time of EAF closure, it is likely that the abdominal wall contour will change to some degree. A stoma site that was prime preoperatively may be completely unsuitable after AWR. This is especially important with high-output stomas and

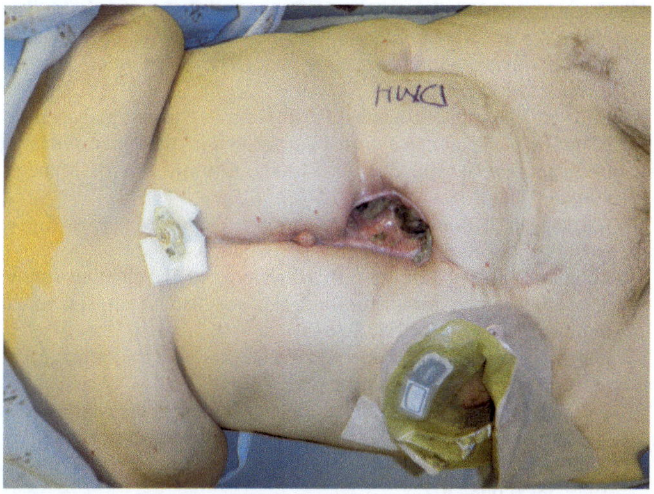

Fig. 8.40 A patient previously operated upon where "incorporated" polypropylene mesh was left in place. She suffered midline wound breakdown and bowel fistulization through the mesh. Ultimately this mesh was excised and she underwent AWR with a good result

ileostomies. If this situation is encountered, the best course of action is to re-site the stoma. You won't have the luxury of selecting an appropriate site preoperatively, so familiarity with the concepts of selecting an optimal stoma site is critical. The stoma can be delivered through a keyhole in any mesh used as reinforcement, and should be located through the rectus muscle. Parastomal hernias can be repaired using the Sugarbaker technique or can also be addressed via relocation of the stoma and primary closure with mesh reinforcement. High-risk or distal colorectal/coloanal anastomoses should be covered with a proximal stoma. You have one good shot at helping these patients, and clinical sequelae of a leaking anastomosis will destroy any chance of success. If any previous mesh is encountered during the procedure, remove it completely (Fig. 8.40). The old adage that "incorporated mesh" is fine to leave behind is a terrible pitfall. While controversial, it is this author's opinion that leaving old and potentially infected mesh behind is a recipe for failure.

Finally, often in the profession of surgery, true wisdom involves knowing when to say when. There are some EAF patients that, despite our best efforts and intentions, simply cannot be helped with surgery. Unfortunately there is no surgical "crystal ball" that will allow us to reliably make this assessment. Though it may sound obvious, these procedures are extremely stressful on the patient, and those in poor medical condition with severe cardiopulmonary disease may not tolerate this stress. Some patients will learn to live harmoniously with an EAF over time. In some, the fistula simply becomes a poorly sited stoma that can be effectively controlled with an appliance and wound care products. An elderly patient with significant comorbidities and a well-controlled EAF may be best left alone. Give this considerable thought and ensure adequate counseling of the patient prior to making the commitment to surgical repair.

References

1. Duff JH, Moffat J. Abdominal sepsis managed by leaving abdomen open. Surgery. 1981;90(4):774–8.
2. Maetani S, Tobe T. Open peritoneal drainage as effective treatment of advanced peritonitis. Surgery. 1981;90(5):804–9.
3. Mughal MM, Bancewicz J, Irving MH. 'Laparostomy': a technique for management of intractable intra-abdominal sepsis. Br J Surg. 1986;73(4):253–9.
4. Hedderich GS, Wexler MJ, McLean AP, Meakins JL. The septic abdomen: open management with Marlex mesh with a zipper. Surgery. 1986;99(4):399–408.
5. Ivatury RR, Nallathambi M, Rohman M, Stahl WM. Open management of the posttraumatic septic abdomen. Am Surg. 1990;56(9): 548–52.
6. Stone HH, Strom PR, Mullins RJ. Management of the major coagulopathy with onset during laparotomy. Ann Surg. 1983; 197(5):532–5.
7. Burch JM, Ortiz VB, Richardson RJ, Martin RR, Mattox KL, Jordan GL. Abbreviated laparotomy and planned reoperation for critically injured patients. Ann Surg. 1992;215(5):476–84.
8. Barnes GE, Laine GA, Giam PY, Smith EE, Granger HJ. Cardiovascular responses to elevation of intra-abdominal hydrostatic pressure. Am J Physiol. 1985;248(2):R208–13.
9. Tremblay LN, Feliciano DV, Schmidt J, et al. Skin only or silo closure in the critically ill patient with an open abdomen. Am J Surg. 2001;182(6):670–5.
10. D'Hont M, Devriendt D, Van Rooy F, et al. Treatment of small-bowel fistulae in the open abdomen with topical negative-pressure therapy. Am J Surg. 2011;202(2):e20–4.
11. Pelz JOW, Doerfer J, Decker M, Dimmler A, Hohenberger W, Meyer T. Hyperthermic intraperitoneal chemoperfusion (HIPEC) decrease wound strength of colonic anastomosis in a rat model. Int J Colorectal Dis. 2007;22(8):941–7.
12. Boutros C, Somasundar P, Espat NJ. Early results on the use of biomaterials as adjuvant to abdominal wall closure following cytoreduction and hyperthermic intraperitoneal chemotherapy. World J Surg Oncol. 2010;72(8):1–7.
13. Polk TM, Schwab CW. Metabolic and nutritional support of the enterocutaneous fistula patient: a three-phase approach. World J Surg. 2012;36(3):524–33.
14. Schecter WP. Management of enterocutaneous fistulas. Surg Clin North Am. 2011;91(3):481–91.
15. Kritayakirana K, Maggio PM, Brundage S, Purtill MA, Staudenmayer K, Spain DA. Outcomes and complications of open abdomen technique for managing non-trauma patients. J Emerg Trauma Shock. 2010;3(2):118–22.
16. Bjorck M, D'Amours SK, Hamilton AE. Closure of the open abdomen. Am Surg. 2011;77 suppl 1:S58–61.
17. Fabian TC. Damage control in trauma: laparotomy wound management acute to chronic. Surg Clin North Am. 2007;87(1):73–93.
18. Miller RS, Morris Jr JA, Diaz Jr JJ, Herring MB, May AK. Complications after 344 damage-control open celiotomies. J Trauma. 2005;59(6):1365–71.
19. Schecter WP, Ivatury RR, Rotondo MF, Hirshberg A. Open abdomen after trauma and abdominal sepsis: a strategy for management. J Am Coll Surg. 2006;203(3):390–6.
20. Prichayudh S, Sriussadaporn S, Samorn P, et al. Management of open abdomen with an absorbable mesh closure. Surg Today. 2011;41(1):72–8.
21. Stevens P. Vacuum-assisted closure of laparostomy wounds: a critical review of the literature. Int Wound J. 2009;6(4):259–66.
22. Shaikh IA, Ballard-Wilson A, Yalamarthi S, Amin AI. Use of topical negative pressure in assisted abdominal closure does not lead to high incidence of enteric fistulae. Colorectal Dis. 2010;12(9):931–4.
23. Bee TK, Croce MA, Maginotti LJ, et al. Temporary abdominal closure techniques: a prospective randomized trial comparing polyglactin

910 mesh and vacuum-assisted closure. J Trauma. 2008;65: 337–44.
24. Miller PR, Thompson JT, Faler BJ, Meredith JW, Chang MC. Late fascial closure in lieu of ventral hernia: the next step in open abdomen management. J Trauma. 2002;53(5):843–9.
25. Acosta S, Bjarnason T, Petersson U, et al. Multicentre prospective study of fascial closure rate after open abdomen with vacuum and mesh-mediated fascial traction. Br J Surg. 2011;98(5):735–43.
26. Koss W, Ho HC, Yu M, et al. Preventing loss of domain: a management strategy for closure of the "open abdomen" during the initial hospitalization. J Surg Educ. 2009;66(2):89–95.
27. Vertrees A, Greer L, Pickett C, et al. Modern management of complex open abdominal wounds of war: a 5-year experience. J Am Coll Surg. 2008;207(6):801–9.
28. Kafie FE, Tessier DJ, Williams RA, et al. Serial abdominal closure technique (the "SAC" procedure): a novel method for delayed closure of the abdominal wall. Am Surg. 2003;69(2):102–5.
29. Blatnik J, Jin J, Rosen M. Abdominal hernia repair with bridging acellular dermal matrix- an expensive hernia sac. Am J Surg. 2008;196:47–50.
30. De Moya M, Dunham M, Inaba K, et al. Long-term outcome of acellular dermal matrix when used for large traumatic open abdomen. J Trauma. 2008;65:349–53.
31. Scott BG, Welsh FJ, Pham HQ, et al. Early aggressive closure of the open abdomen. J Trauma. 2006;60(1):17–22.
32. Schuster R, Singh J, Safadi BY, Wren SM. The use of acellular dermal matrix for contaminated abdominal wall defects: wound status predicts success. Am J Surg. 2006;192(5):594–7.
33. Kushimoto S, Yamamoto Y, Aiboshi J, et al. Usefulness of the bilateral anterior rectus abdominis sheath turnover flap method for early fascial closure in patients requiring open abdominal management. World J Surg. 2007;31(1):2–8.
34. Girard S, Sideman M, Spain DA. A novel approach to the problem of intestinal fistulization arising in patients managed with open peritoneal cavities. Am J Surg. 2002;184(2):166–7.
35. Becker HP, Willms A, Schwab R. Small bowel fistulas and the open abdomen. Scand J Surg. 2007;96(4):263–71.
36. Jamshidi R, Schecter WP. Biological dressings for the management of enteric fistulas in the open abdomen: a preliminary report. Arch Surg. 2007;142(8):793–6.
37. Collier B, Guillamondegui O, Cotton B, et al. Feeding the open abdomen. J Parenter Enteral Nutr. 2007;31(5):410–5.
38. Evenson AR, Fischer JE. Current management of enterocutaneous fistula. J Gastrointest Surg. 2006;10(3):455–64.
39. Harris C, Shannon R. An innovative enterostomal therapy nurse model of community wound care delivery: a retrospective cost-effectiveness analysis. J Wound Ostomy Continence Nurs. 2008;35(2): 169–83.
40. Martinez JL, Luque-de-Leon E, Mier J, Blanco-Benevides R, Robledo F. Systematic management of postoperative enterocutaneous fistulas: factors related to outcomes. World J Surg. 2008;32(3):436–43.
41. Fischer PE, Fabian TC, Magnotti LJ, et al. A ten-year review of enterocutaneous fistulas after laparotomy for trauma. J Trauma. 2009;67(5):924–8.
42. Wright A, Wright M. Bedside management of an abdominal wound containing an enteroatmospheric fistula: a case report. Ostomy Wound Manage. 2011;57(1):28–32.
43. Ramsay PT, Mejia VA. Management of enteroatmospheric fistulae in the open abdomen. Am Surg. 2010;76(6):637–9.
44. Layton B, Dubose J, Nichols S, Connaughton J, Jones T, Pratt J. Pacifying the open abdomen with concomitant intestinal fistula: a novel approach. Am J Surg. 2010;199(4):e48–50.
45. Al-Khoury G, Kaufman D, Hirshberg A. Improved control of exposed fistula in the open abdomen. J Am Coll Surg. 2008;206(2): 397–8.
46. Goverman J, Yelon JA, Platz JJ, Singson RC, Turcinovic M. The "Fistula-VAC", a technique for management of enterocutaneous fistulae arising within the open abdomen: a report of 5 cases. J Trauma. 2006;60(2):428–31.
47. O'Brien B, Landis-Erdman J, Erwin-Toth P. Nursing management of multiple enterocutaneous fistulae located in the center of a large open abdominal wound: a case study. Ostomy Wound Manage. 1998;44(1):20–4.
48. Geoghegan J, Robert K. The Convatec Wound Manager: a new stoma appliance. Br J Clin Prac. 1990;44(12):750–1.
49. Subramanian MJ, Liscum KR, Hirshberg A. The floating stoma: a new technique for controlling exposed fistulae in abdominal trauma. J Trauma. 2002;53:386–8.
50. Dorta G. Role of octreotide and somatostatin in the treatment of intestinal fistulae. Digestion. 1999;60 suppl(2):53–6.
51. Battershill PE, Clissold SP. Octreotide: a review of its pharmacodynamic and pharmacokinetic properties, and therapeutic potential in conditions associated with excessive peptide secretion. Drugs. 1989;38(5):658–702.
52. Stevens P, Foulkes RE, Hartford-Benyon JS, Delicata RJ. Systematic review and meta-analysis of the role of somatostatin and its analogues in the treatment of enterocutaneous fistula. Eur J Gastroenterol Hepatol. 2011;23(10):912–22.
53. Draus Jr JM, Huss SA, Harty NJ, Cheadle WG, Larson GM. Enterocutaneous fistula: are treatments improving? Surgery. 2006;140(4):570–6.
54. Leandros E, Antonakis PT, Albanopoulos K, Dervenis C, Konstadoulakis MM. Somatostatin versus octreotide in the treatment of patients with gastrointestinal and pancreatic fistulas. Can J Gastroenterol. 2004;18(5):303–6.
55. Alivizatos V, Felekis D, Zorbalas A. Evaluation of the effectiveness of octreotide in the conservative treatment of postoperative enterocutaneous fistulas. Hepatogastroenterology. 2002;49(46):1010–2.
56. Hesse U, Ysebaert D, de Hemptinne B. Role of somatostatin-14 and its analogues in the management of gastrointestinal fistulae: clinical data. Gut. 2001;49 suppl 4:iv11–21.
57. Makhdoom ZA, Komar MJ, Still CD. Nutrition and enterocutaneous fistulas. J Clin Gastroenterol. 2000;31(3):195–204.
58. Alvarez C, McFadden DW, Reber HA. Complicated enterocutaneous fistulas: failure of octreotide to improve healing. World J Surg. 2000;24(5):533–7.
59. Paran H, Neufeld D, Kaplan O, Klausner J, Freund U. Octreotide for treatment of postoperative alimentary tract fistulas. World J Surg. 1995;19(3):430–3.
60. Sancho JJ, di Costanzo J, Nubiola P, et al. Randomized double-blind placebo-controlled trial of early octreotide in patients with postoperative enterocutaneous fistula. Br J Surg. 1995;82(5): 638–41.
61. Kocak S, Bumin C, Karayalcin K, Alacayir I, Aribal D. Treatment of external biliary, pancreatic, and intestinal fistulas with a somatostatin analogue. Dig Dis. 1994;12(1):62–8.
62. Tang SJ, Nieto JM, Jensen DM, Ohning GV, Pisegna JR. The novel use of an intravenous proton pump inhibitor in a patient with short bowel syndrome. J Clin Gastroenterol. 2002;34(1):62–3.
63. Hickman Jr RL, Douglas SL. Impact of chronic critical illness on the psychological outcomes of family members. AACN Adv Crit Care. 2010;21(1):80–91.
64. Jernigan TW, Fabian TC, Croce MA, et al. Staged management of giant abdominal wall defects. Ann Surg. 2003;238:349–57.
65. Joels CS, Vanderveer AS, Newcomb WL, et al. Abdominal wall reconstruction after temporary abdominal closure: a ten-year review. Surg Innov. 2006;13:223–30.
66. Dionigi G, Dionigi R, Rovera F, et al. Treatment of high output entero-cutaneous fistulae associated with large abdominal wall defects: single center experience. Int J Surg. 2008;6:51–6.

67. Rodriguez ED, Bluebond-Langner R, Silverman RP, et al. Abdominal wall reconstruction following severe loss of domain: The R Adams Cowley Shock Trauma Center algorithm. Plast Reconstr Surg. 2007;120:669–80.
68. Ramirez OM, Ruas E, Dellon L. "Components separation" method for closure of abdominal-wall defects: an anatomic and clinical study. Plast Reconstr Surg. 1990;86:519–26.
69. Wind J, van Koperen PJ, Slors FM, Bemelman WA. Single-stage closure of enterocutaneous fistula and stomas in the presence of large abdominal wall defects using the components separation technique. Am J Surg. 2009;197:24–9.
70. Connolly PT, Teubner A, Lees NP, Anderson ID, Scott NA, Carlson GL. Outcome of reconstructive surgery for intestinal fistula in the open abdomen. Ann Surg. 2008;247:440–4.
71. De Vries Reilingh TS, van Goor H, Charbon JA, et al. Repair of giant midline abdominal wall hernias: "components separation technique" versus prosthetic repair. World J Surg. 2007;31: 756–63.
72. Dragu A, Klein P, Unglaub F, et al. Tensiometry as a decision tool for abdominal wall reconstruction with component separation. World J Surg. 2009;33:1174–80.
73. Vargo D. Component separation in the management of the difficult abdominal wall. Am J Surg. 2004;188:633–7.
74. Shabatian H, Lee D, Abbas MA. Components separation: a solution to complex abdominal wall defects. Am Surg. 2008;74:912–6.
75. De Vries Reilingh TS, van Goor H, Rosman C, et al. "Components separation technique" for the repair of large abdominal wall hernias. J Am Coll Surg. 2003;196:32–7.
76. Howdieshell TR, Proctor CD, Sternberg E, Cué JI, Mondy JS, Hawkins ML. Temporary abdominal closure followed by definitive abdominal wall reconstruction of the open abdomen. Am J Surg. 2004;188:301–6.
77. Lowe JB, Lowe JB, Baty JD, Garza JR. Risks associated with "components separation" for closure of complex abdominal wall defects. Plast Reconstr Surg. 2003;111:1276–83.
78. Ewart CJ, Lankford AB, Gamboa MG. Successful closure of abdominal wall hernias using components separation technique. Ann Plast Surg. 2003;50:269–74.
79. Carbonell AM, Cobb WS, Chen SM. Posterior components separation during retromuscular hernia repair. Hernia. 2008;12: 359–62.
80. Ennis LS, Young JS, Gampper TJ, Drake DB. The "open-book" variation of component separation for repair of massive midline abdominal wall hernia. Am Surg. 2003;69:733–43.
81. Tobias AM, Low DW. The use of subfascial vicryl mesh buttress to aid in the closure of massive ventral hernias following damage-control laparotomy. Plast Reconstr Surg. 2003;112: 766–76.
82. Kingsnorth AN, Shahid MK, Valliattu AJ, Hadden RA, Porter CS. Open onlay mesh repair for major abdominal wall hernias with selective use of components separation and fibrin sealant. World J Surg. 2008;32:26–30.
83. Rosen MJ, Jin J, McGee MF, Williams C, Marks J, Ponsky JL. Laparoscopic component separation in the single-stage treatment of infected abdominal wall prosthetic removal. Hernia. 2007;11: 435–40.
84. Stark B, Strigård K. Definitive reconstruction of full-thickness abdominal wall defects initially treated with skin grafting of exposed intestines. Hernia. 2007;11:533–6.
85. Hadad I, Small W, Dumanian GA. Repair of massive ventral hernias with the separation of parts technique: reversal of the 'lost domain'. Am Surg. 2009;75:301–6.
86. Rosen MJ, Williams C, Jin J, et al. Laparoscopic versus open-component separation: a comparative analysis in a porcine model. Am J Surg. 2007;194:385–9.
87. Milburn ML, Shah PK, Friedman EB, et al. Laparoscopically assisted components separation technique for ventral incisional hernia repair. Hernia. 2007;11:157–61.
88. Maas SM, van Engeland M, Leeksma NG, Bleichrodt RP. A modification of the "components separation" technique for closure of abdominal wall defects in the presence of an enterostomy. J Am Coll Surg. 1999;189:138–40.
89. Liyanage SH, Purohit GS, Frye JNR, Giordano P. Anterior abdominal wall reconstruction with a Permacol implant. J Plast Reconstr Aesthet Surg. 2006;59:553–5.
90. Parker DM, Armstrong PJ, Frizzi JD, North JH. Porcine dermal collagen (Permacol) for abdominal wall reconstruction. Curr Surg. 2006;63:255–8.
91. Shaikh FM, Giri SK, Durrani S, Waldron D, Grace PA. Experience with porcine acellular dermal collagen implant in one-stage tension-free reconstruction of acute and chronic abdominal wall defects. World J Surg. 2007;31:1966–72.
92. Hsu PW, Salgado CJ, Kent K, et al. Evaluation of porcine dermal collagen (Permacol) used in abdominal wall reconstruction. J Plast Reconstr Aesthet Surg. 2009;62(11):1484–9.
93. Franklin ME, Gonzalez JJ, Glass JL. Use of porcine small intestinal submucosa as a prosthetic device for laparoscopic repair of hernias in contaminated fields: 2-year follow-up. Hernia. 2004;8:186–9.
94. Ueno T, Pickett LC, de la Fuente S, Lawson DC, Pappas TN. Clinical application of porcine small intestinal submucosa in the management of infected or potentially contaminated abdominal defects. J Gastrointest Surg. 2004;8:109–12.
95. Helton WS, Fisichella PM, Berger R, Horgan S, Espat NJ, Abcarian H. Short-term outcomes with small intestinal submucosa for ventral abdominal hernia. Arch Surg. 2005;140:549–62.
96. Jin H, Rosen MJ, Blatnik J, et al. Use of acellular dermal matrix for complicated ventral hernia repair: does technique affect outcomes? J Am Coll Surg. 2007;205:654–60.
97. Espinosa-de-los-Monteros A, de la Torre JI, Marrero I, Andrades P, Davis MR, Vasconez LO. Utilization of human cadaveric acellular dermis for abdominal hernia reconstruction. Ann Plast Surg. 2007;58:264–7.
98. Patton JH, Berry S, Kralovich KA. Use of human acellular dermal matrix in complex and contaminated abdominal wall reconstructions. Am J Surg. 2007;193:360–3.
99. Bellows CF, Albo D, Berger DH, Awad SS. Abdominal wall repair using human acellular dermis. Am J Surg. 2007;194:192–8.
100. Misra S, Raj PK, Tarr SM, Treat RC. Results of AlloDerm use in abdominal hernia repair. Hernia. 2008;12:247–50.
101. Bluebond-Langner R, Keifa ES, Mithani S, Bochicchio GV, Scalea T, Rodriguez ED. Recurrent abdominal laxity following interpositional human acellular dermal matrix. Ann Plast Surg. 2008;60:76–80.
102. Taner T, Cima RR, Larson WV, Dozios EJ, Pemberton JH, Wolff BG. Surgical treatment of complex enterocutaneous fistulas in IBD patients using human acellular dermal matrix. Inflamm Bowel Dis. 2009;15:1208–12.
103. Maurice SM, Skeete DA. Use of human acellular dermal matrix for abdominal wall reconstructions. Am J Surg. 2009;197:35–42.
104. Lin JH, Spoerke N, Deveney C, Martindale R. Reconstruction of complex abdominal wall hernias using acellular human dermal matrix: a single institution experience. Am J Surg. 2008; 197:599–603.
105. Pomahac B, Aflaki P. Use of a non-cross linked porcine dermal scaffold in abdominal wall reconstruction. Am J Surg. 2010; 199(1):22–7.
106. Espinosa-de-los-Monteros A, de la Torre JI, Ahumada LA, Person DW, Rosenberg LZ, Vasconez LO. Reconstruction of the abdominal wall for incisional hernia repair. Am J Surg. 2006;191: 173–7.

Technical Tips for Difficult Stomas

9

Alia Whitehead, Adrian Seah, and Peter Cataldo

Key Points

- Constructing a high-quality stoma will directly correlate to decreasing complications and improving your patient's quality of life.
- Proper stoma marking up front is the likely the single best thing you can do to help minimize complications.
- A stoma site above the umbilicus is often the "best" location in difficult situations to ensure adequate viability and length.
- Prior to constructing a stoma, always first ask yourself if one is needed at all.

Introduction

Key Concept: Intestinal stoma creation, though often seen as the minor component of a major abdominal operation, will have a significant and lasting impact on the patient.

Intestinal stomas are the surgical exteriorization of either small or large bowel to the anterior abdominal wall. The ultimate purpose when creating a diverting stoma is to prevent the fecal stream from reaching a distal segment of the distal small bowel or large intestine for the purpose of either treating or preventing a leak. Permanent stomas are required when the altered anatomy prohibits reestablishment of gastrointestinal continuity, the risks of undergoing another surgery are too prohibitive due to patient comorbidities, or the functional results of a reanastomosis would adversely impact quality of life. Regardless of the type of ostomy, living with a stoma can exact a tremendous psychological burden on patients and requires adjustments to routine activities of daily living. However, quality of life studies in individuals with stomas support the idea that ostomy function is directly correlated with patient satisfaction [1]. As a result, we must make a concerted effort to individualize treatment plans with the goal being to create a functioning and an appropriate stoma.

Successful ostomy creation requires significant planning and discussion. The process starts with understanding the patient's lifestyle, occupation, clothing preferences, bowel function, and any disabilities. The patient's abdomen must be carefully examined for skin folds and preexisting scars. This preoperative information will help create a healthy stoma in the correct site and using the correct segment of bowel. Unfortunately, even the best-planned stoma can still be difficult to construct. While most surgeons can readily make a "serviceable" stoma in an ideal patient, you need to have some tricks in your "bag" to help out with the tough cases, as well as making the good ones great. Our goal of this chapter is to review general techniques of stoma creation and to identify what factors exist that complicate stoma creation. In addition, we will discuss possible solutions and tips to overcome these challenges.

Preoperative Assessment

Key Concept: First, figure out if a stoma is required. If it is, enlist the help of an enterostomal therapist, when possible, and together as a team, ensure marking is in the ideal location for each individual person.

The easiest way to avoid a stoma complication is to avoid stoma formation altogether. While this may sound flippant, it

A. Whitehead, MD • A. Seah, MD
Department of Surgery, Fletcher Allen Health Center, University of Vermont, 111 Colchester Avenue, Burlington, VT 05401, USA
e-mail: alia.whitehead@vtmednet.org; adrian.seah@vtmednet.org

P. Cataldo, MD (✉)
Department of Surgery, Fletcher Allen Health Center, University of Vermont, 111 Colchester Avenue, Mailstop 320FL4, Burlington, VT 05401, USA
e-mail: peter.cataldo@vtmednet.org

S.R. Steele et al. (eds.), *Complexities in Colorectal Surgery*,
DOI 10.1007/978-1-4614-9022-7_9, © Springer Science+Business Media New York 2014

merits some thought. When planning for a temporary or permanent stoma, one should ask, "Will this stoma provide the best possible functional result for my patient in this situation?" In the case of the temporary stoma, "Am I creating the stoma that will lead to the simplest, safest future reversal?" In some cases, the slightly higher risk of a primary anastomosis may be preferable to a stoma that severely impacts a patient's lifestyle. While the discussion of whether or not an ostomy is always necessary in the emergent situation with unprepped bowel is beyond the scope of this chapter, it should be remembered and carefully considered before creating any stoma.

If the creation of an ostomy is unavoidable, careful preoperative preparation is essential. The importance of a thorough history and physical exam, even in the emergent setting, cannot be overemphasized. If performed properly, creation of a stoma in the emergent setting is not associated with increased postoperative morbidity [2]. Preoperative preparation begins with informed consent, especially in the emergency situation where a patient is likely to be completely unaware that he or she may need an ostomy. Ideally, each conversation will also include a careful social history that assesses disabilities, clothing styles, occupation, and living circumstances. For example, an ostomy in an elderly patient with visual impairment and arthritis might take away his or her ability to live independently. A stoma that sits under a patient's belt line will not only be uncomfortable and affect clothing choices but may be injured by contact with the belt [2]. It is also essential to evaluate the patient's bowel habits. A rectal resection and low pelvic anastomosis may render a marginally continent patient totally incontinent. In these situations, stoma formation could avoid an unpleasant and embarrassing operative result.

In an ideal situation, preoperative stoma preparation and site marking should be a collaborative effort among the surgeon, patient, and enterostomal (ET) therapist or nurse [2]. A study by Bass et al. showed that preoperative marking by an ET therapist reduced overall and early complications when compared to patients that were not marked preoperatively [3]. However, it is imperative that every surgeon is adept at selecting and marking the stoma site in the case that an ET therapist is not available. If possible, the site should be examined with the patient lying, sitting, and standing to confirm optimum placement. The site should be centered on an at least 2 in. flat area of healthy skin away from scars, skin creases, and bony prominences. The belt line and the apex of the convex curvature of the infraumbilical fold should be avoided. In the obese patient, it may be advantageous for both the surgeon and the patient to site the stoma in the supraumbilical area. Finally, it is essential that the stoma is visible to the patient. An obstructed view will inevitably lead to stoma neglect. Individuals with disabilities, such as spinal cord injury, should be marked in the position they spend most time to facilitate appliance fitting and care.

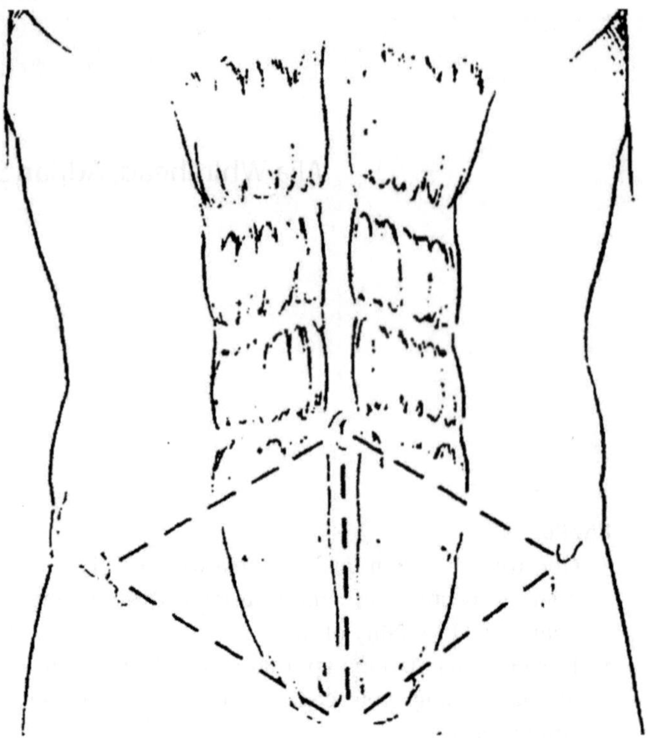

Fig. 9.1 The ostomy triangle (With permission from Cataldo and MacKeigan [4]. Copyright © 2004 by Marcel Dekker Inc. All rights reserved)

Marking should begin with identification of the "ostomy triangle" bounded by the anterior superior iliac spine, the pubic tubercle, and the umbilicus (Fig. 9.1). The stoma is placed at the center of this triangle, through the rectus muscle. Traditionally, an ileostomy is placed on the right and a colostomy on the left. However, if "conventional" placement will lead to stoma tension, the surgeon may need to choose an alternate site.

Prevention of Parastomal Hernias

Key Concept: Although parastomal hernias are a relatively common complication, several technical maneuvers including mesh use, tunneling, and proper sizing of the trephine can help minimize this complication from developing.

In addition to stoma location, stomal trephine size is also important and, if done improperly, can lead to complications. Too small of an opening can cause stoma ischemia, while too large an opening can lead to parastomal hernia. The incidence of symptomatic parastomal hernia is as high as 39 % for colostomies and 6 % for loop ileostomies [5]. When identified by computed tomography, the incidence of parastomal hernia with a colostomy may be as high as 78 % [6]. Up to one-third of these patients eventually require surgical repair due to pain, incarceration, obstruction, and poor appliance fitting [6].

One technique for hernia prevention is to mature the stoma through the extraperitoneal route. This has been done during end sigmoid colostomy creation after laparoscopic abdominoperineal resection with promising results [7]. The stomas that were created through the transperitoneal route developed more parastomal hernias within a shorter period of time when compared to the extraperitoneal route. A large meta-analysis of 1,071 patients also showed that extraperitoneal colostomy is associated with a lower rate of postoperative parastomal hernia as compared to intraperitoneal colostomy [8]. Again, this is only applicable to patients undergoing permanent colostomy. For this technique, an incision is made in the parietal peritoneum immediately lateral to the transected end of the descending colon. A tunnel is then made that extends through the retroperitoneal tissues into the deep surface of the anterior abdominal wall. This tunnel is then connected to the stoma site on the anterior abdominal wall. Finally, the bowel is passed through the tunnel [9].

When hernias do occur, mesh is often required to close or repair the defect. In an attempt to reduce the rate of hernias, surgeons began placing mesh prophylactically. Several small studies have shown promising results with prophylactic mesh placement [6]. Two randomized trials using a lightweight polypropylene mesh found significantly more parastomal hernias in the no mesh group (53.7 %) when compared with the mesh group (14.8 %; $P<0.001$) [6]. Additionally, the patients in the mesh group that did develop a hernia did not require surgical intervention as often. Mesh-related complications were rare. Most studies have looked at prosthetic mesh but biologic mesh has also been utilized prophylactically with similar results. However, the cost may be prohibitive [10]. The PREVENT trial, a multicenter randomized controlled study, is currently underway to determine if a retromuscular, preperitoneal monofilament polypropylene mesh at the stoma site can prevent parastomal hernias in patients receiving a permanent end colostomy without unacceptable complications [6].

The PREVENT trial uses a standardized technique for mesh placement [6]. First, the bowel intended for colostomy is stapled closed to minimize contamination. The trephine is created by excision of the skin oval at the preoperatively marked ostomy site without excising any subcutaneous tissue. After exposing the anterior rectus sheath, a cross-shaped incision is made in the fascia. The rectus abdominis muscle is split in the direction of the fibers. A retromuscular space is created and dissected to the lateral stomal border via the midline laparotomy. The posterior fascia/peritoneum is left undisturbed. Then a 10×10 cm piece of mesh, with a cross-shaped incision in the center to allow for passage of the colonic loop, is placed above the posterior rectus sheath. The lateral corners of the mesh are fixed with two absorbable monofilament sutures. The posterior fascia is opened over the trephine in the mesh, and the bowel gradually passed through. The running suture that closes the midline incision includes the medial border of the mesh and the peritoneum, thus preventing contact between the mesh and the viscera. Finally, the stoma is matured.

There are some opponents of prophylactic mesh placement, however, who say that it is too time-consuming and difficult to perform laparoscopically. One such group has proposed a stapled mesh stoma reinforcement technique, or SMART, to prevent parastomal hernias [11]. After excision of the skin and soft tissue cylinder, opening of the anterior rectus sheath, and splitting of the muscle, the posterior sheath/peritoneum is pierced with the tips of forceps used to grasp the anvil shaft of a circular stapling gun (28 mm) that was placed within the abdominal cavity. The anvil shaft is withdrawn through the posterior rectus sheath and exteriorized. The fully extended trocar of the gun, preloaded with a circular configured mesh 5 cm in diameter, is mated with the exteriorized anvil shaft. The gun is closed, fired, and removed, encompassing a disc of mesh, posterior rectus sheath, and peritoneum, leaving a precise reinforced stapled trephine. The outer mesh circumference is sutured to the anterior rectus sheath so it lines the trephine. The stoma is then fashioned in the usual way. If a prophylactic mesh is required, my preference is to use a square piece of mesh large enough to surround the stoma with a 2–3 cm ring of mesh in contact with the fascia. A cruciate incision is placed in the mesh. The mesh is placed deep to the anterior rectus sheath but superficial to the rectus muscle. The mesh is tacked to the anterior rectus fascia at the four corners. It is not sutured directly to the stoma. At this time there is conflicting evidence as to the benefit of prophylactic mesh in the prevention of parastomal hernias, and I do not use it universally.

End Ostomy Creation

Key Concept: Whether creating an end colostomy or ileostomy, the technique and principles are similar. The main difference will be how much the final stoma protrudes from the skin.

There are certain key aspects to creating an ideal end stoma. Among the principles:

1. Create a circular skin incision approximately 2.5 cm in diameter at the previously marked site and excise the skin.
2. Part the subcutaneous tissue with small retractors until the anterior rectus sheath is exposed. Do not excise this tissue.
3. Make a vertical incision in the anterior rectus sheath approximately 3 cm in length. At the midpoint of the incision, make a perpendicular 1 cm incision laterally. This will keep the stoma opening away from the midline incision.

4. Split the rectus abdominis muscle in the direction of its fibers.
5. Create a vertical incision in the posterior rectus sheath.
6. Deliver the previously divided bowel through the abdominal wall without twisting it. "Pushing" from within the abdominal cavity is preferred to "pulling" when exteriorizing the bowel.
7. Again confirm that the bowel is viable and not twisted.
8. For a colostomy, the colon should extend 2 cm above the skin surface. For an ileostomy, 5 cm of bowel should be pulled through. The matured colostomy should protrude 0.5–1 cm above the skin. The matured ileostomy should protrude 2–2.5 cm.
9. Excise the staple line at end of the bowel cleanly with a #10 scalpel blade. Ileostomies must be everted. Eversion of a colostomy is optional and should ideally be dictated by the stomal therapist who will be working with the patient long term. The abdominal incision should be closed before this step. However, if there is concern that the stoma is under too much tension or has questionable viability, the abdomen can be closed after maturation of the stoma.
10. Perform the enterocutaneous anastomosis with interrupted absorbable sutures that take full-thickness bites of the end of the colon and the subcuticular layer of the skin.
    (a) Colostomies may be matured flush or can be everted similar to ileostomies. For flush creation, full-thickness bites of the terminal end of the bowel are followed by corresponding dermal bites on the stoma trephine. Sutures through the skin may lead to "mucosal islands," or small growths of mucosa, in the skin surrounding the stoma and therefore should be avoided.
    (b) Ileostomy eversion is created by placing "triplicate" sutures. First, the suture is placed through the dermis, followed by a seromuscular bite 4–5 cm from the proximal to the end of the ileum. The final bite is passed full thickness through the cut end of the bowel. Three everting sutures, away from the mesentery, will often even the stoma effectively. Gaps can be closed with standard sutures between the triplicate sutures.

Loop Ileostomy Creation

Key Concept: While loop ileostomies are ideal for a temporary diversion, some will become permanent; therefore, it is imperative that you construct as best of a stoma as possible.

When simple fecal diversion is required, a loop ileostomy will allow for easier reversal. However, it is important to remember that a significant number of diverting stomas become permanent. Therefore, creating a stoma that functions well and is easily reversible can be, and often is, the difference between reversal and life with a permanent ostomy. The purpose of a diverting stoma is to prevent fecal material from reaching a distal portion of the bowel, either because of fear of anastomotic leak or to treat a leak or injury. Diverting stomas do not decrease the incidence of anastomotic leak, per se, but instead decrease the related morbidity [12, 13]. When treating pelvic infection from a colonic source or when planning diversion of a low pelvic anastomosis, the two options are transverse loop colostomy and loop ileostomy. While it is important to be aware of both techniques, the loop ileostomy is clearly the superior procedure [14]:

1. Identify an appropriate loop terminal ileum that will protrude easily at the stoma site. A segment at least 20 cm from the ileocecal junction will facilitate subsequent stoma reversal. Any closer to the cecum may make a stapled anastomosis at the time of reversal more difficult. It is also important to confirm and mark the distal bowel with a suture to ensure proper orientation.
2. Make a circular skin incision that is slightly larger than that required for an end stoma at the previously marked site and excise the skin.
3. Part the subcutaneous tissue with small retractors until the anterior rectus sheath is exposed. Do not excise this tissue.
4. Make a vertical incision in the anterior rectus sheath approximately 2 cm in length. At the midpoint of the incision, make a perpendicular 1 cm incision laterally. This will keep the stoma opening away from the midline incision.
5. Split the rectus abdominis muscle in the direction of its fibers.
6. Make a vertical incision in the posterior rectus sheath.
7. Deliver the bowel through the abdominal wall. This can be facilitated by placing a small Penrose drain through a defect created in the mesentery adjacent to the bowel wall. The Penrose can then be used as a handle to help deliver the bowel. If desired, the catheter can later be exchanged for the stoma bridge. Be careful in friable bowel, as a drain (or some prefer to use an umbilical tape) can inadvertently "saw" through the bowel with excessive tension.
8. Again, the Alexis Wound Protector will facilitate passage of the bowel through the subcutaneous tissue, especially in obese individuals.
9. Confirm that the bowel is viable and not twisted by using the previously placed suture in the distal segment (Fig. 9.2).
10. Transect 80 % of the circumference of the antimesenteric portion of the bowel wall just above where the distal end meets the skin between two Allis clamps (Fig. 9.3).
11. Peel back the edges of the bowel to reveal the two openings. Exchange the catheter for the stoma bridge if desired. The proximal limb should still protrude approximately 2.5 cm, but the distal limb can site flush to the skin.

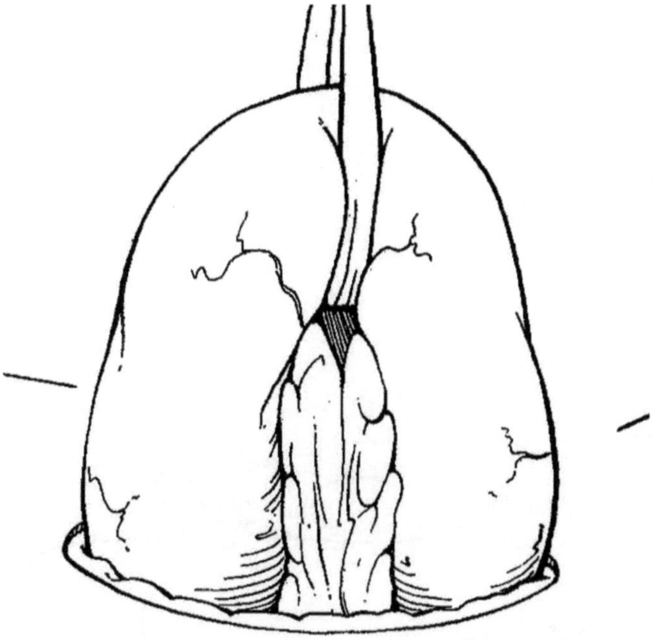

Fig. 9.2 Loop ileostomy creation. The ileum is elevated through stoma site with a Penrose drain. Care is taken to avoid twisting (With permission from Cataldo and MacKeigan [4]. Copyright © 2004 by Marcel Dekker Inc. All rights reserved)

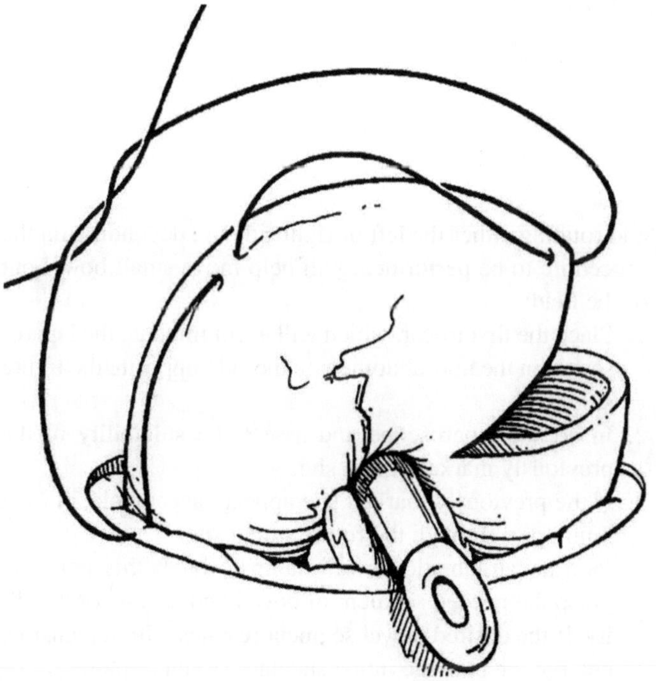

Fig. 9.3 Loop ileostomy creation. Eighty percent of the antimesenteric circumference is transected between Allis clamps (With permission from Cataldo and MacKeigan [4]. Copyright © 2004 by Marcel Dekker Inc. All rights reserved)

12. Perform the anastomosis with interrupted absorbable sutures that take full-thickness bites of the end of the bowel and the subcuticular layer of the skin. Small bites

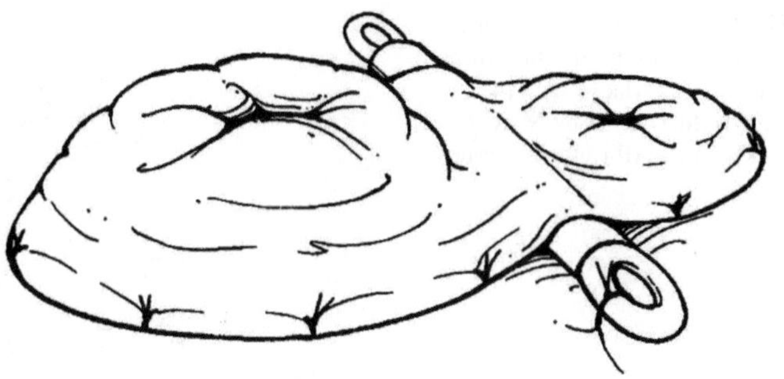

Fig. 9.4 Loop ileostomy creation. Proximal end of the ileum is everted with standard three-part sutures (With permission from Cataldo and MacKeigan [4]. Copyright © 2004 by Marcel Dekker Inc. All rights reserved)

are also taken of the seromuscular layer of the emerging colon at the level of the skin. It is best to mature the distal end without eversion using as little of the skin circumference as is practical. Evert the proximal end with standard three-part sutures on either side of the mesentery and the antimesenteric border (Fig. 9.4).

13. If using a bridge, remove it after 5 days. Of note, a bridge is rarely necessary.

End-Loop Stomas

Key Concept: By using an end-loop stoma that involves bringing the proximal and distal ends of the bowel out through the same trephine, you may be able to avoid a future laparotomy when restoring continuity at the appropriate time.

When creating a temporary stoma, it is always preferable, if possible, to bring the proximal and distal bowel loops through the same trephine in the abdominal wall. Among other advantages, this allows for stoma takedown without formal laparotomy. With standard loop stomas, this occurs by definition, but in other circumstances, it only occurs through proper technique and advanced planning. End-loop stomas can be created with remote intestinal segments following bowel resection. They consist of end-loop ileoileostomy, ileocolostomy, or colocolostomy. For example, it may be unsafe to perform a primary anastomosis after a right colectomy for trauma. An end-loop ileocolostomy is a viable alternative to an end ileostomy and long Hartmann's pouch, which would require a formal laparotomy for reversal in the future. Similar stomas can be performed following small bowel or left colon resections.

Whether using adjacent or remote intestinal segments, the technique for creating an end-loop stoma is similar. The stapled proximal end is passed through the preselected stoma site. Only the antimesenteric border of the stapled distal end is then advanced through the same trephine. The antimesenteric corner of the staple line is cut off, and the small open segment

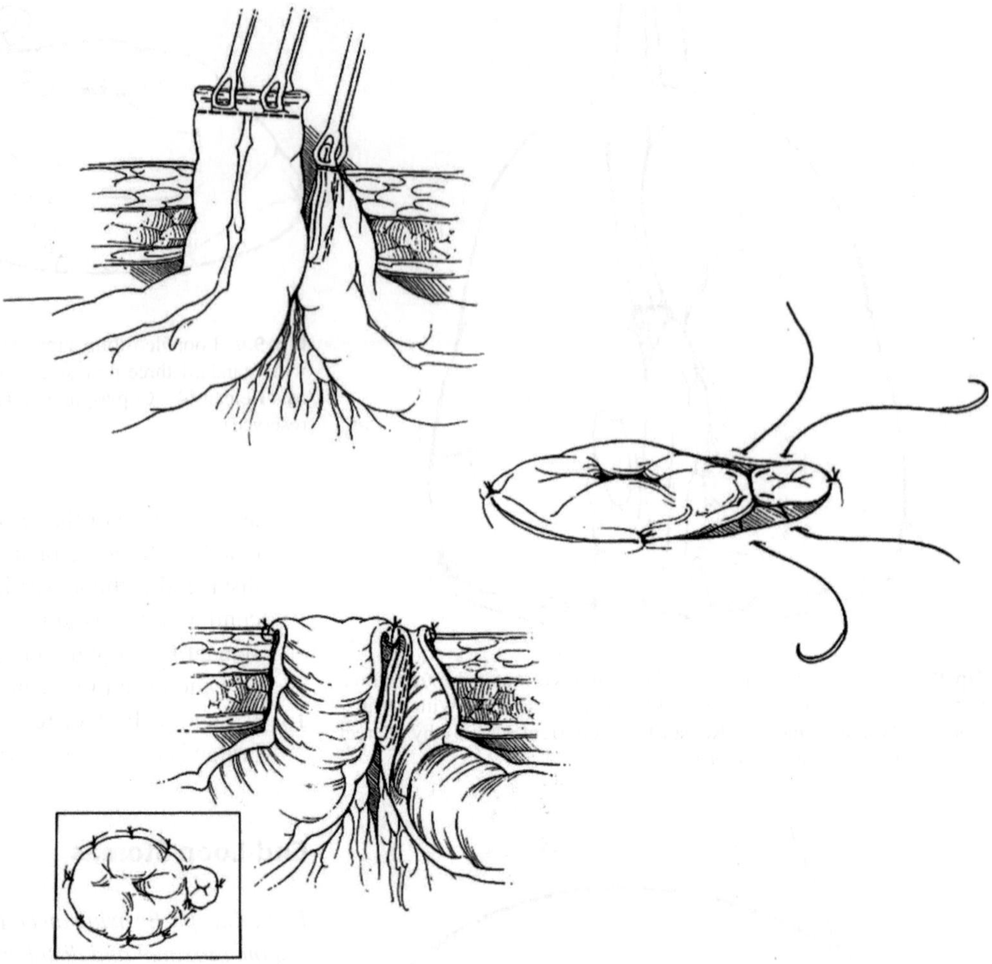

Fig. 9.5 End-loop colostomy creation (With permission from Cataldo and MacKeigan [4]. Copyright © 2004 by Marcel Dekker Inc. All rights reserved)

of the distal bowel is matured flush to the skin using as little of the stoma circumference as possible. The proximal end is then matured in the standard fashion. A small full-thickness stitch between the proximal and distal ends completes the procedure (Fig. 9.5). An end-loop sigmoid colostomy is an ideal stoma for distal fecal diversion for incontinence or in association with complex anorectal procedures.

Laparoscopic Ostomy Creation

Key Concept: A minimally invasive approach is an ideal alternative to either temporary or permanent diversion and can be performed through a single- or multi-port technique using similar principles as an open approach.

Fecal diversion for unresectable cancers or severe perineal disease or trauma is a fairly common procedure. Laparoscopic colostomy or ileostomy creation is an attractive alternative to a formal laparotomy, especially when ostomy creation is the sole purpose of the operation. As with any laparoscopic procedure, preoperative planning and patient positioning are key to success. Trendelenburg positioning and rotating either the left or right side up, depending on the procedure to be performed, will help move small bowel out of the field:

1. Place the first trocar, which will accommodate the laparoscope, in the mid-abdomen on the side opposite the future stoma.
2. Insert the laparoscope and assess the suitability of the previously marked stoma site.
3. If the previously marked site appears acceptable, place a 5 mm port through the future stoma site.
4. Pass an atraumatic bowel clamp through this port and grasp the needed segment of bowel and assess for mobility. If the desired bowel segment reaches without tension, enlarge the port site into a standard stoma trephine.
5. If the bowel requires mobilization, which is common in sigmoid colostomy creation, place an additional port and mobilize along the white line of Toldt.
6. Enlarge the fascial defect as needed and deliver the bowel through the stoma site without twisting. Prior to maturing the stoma, reestablish pneumoperitoneum and confirm proximal and distal orientation of the bowel.
7. Mature the stoma in the standard fashion.

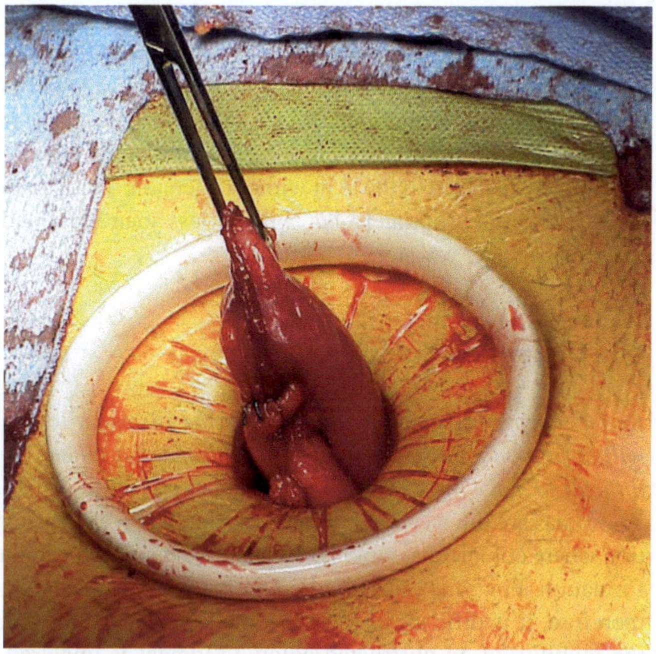

Fig. 9.6 An Alexis Wound Protector facilitates passage of bowel through the abdominal wall (With permission from Cataldo and MacKeigan [4]. Copyright © 2004 by Marcel Dekker Inc. All rights reserved)

The Obese Patient

Key Concept: Obesity presents multiple challenges with stoma creation such as ischemia and pouching complications. Several tricks can be used to facilitate a healthy viable stoma and help minimize wound complications.

Obesity can pose multiple challenges that range from siting a stoma to obtaining enough bowel length to span the subcutaneous tissue. Additionally, the mere process of bringing the bowel through the abdominal wall trephine can be difficult. Obesity is recognized as a risk factor for stoma complications, and obese patients are seven times more likely to suffer from stoma necrosis than nonobese patients [15]. Obese individuals have both a thick abdominal wall and a short, thick mesentery, making it quite difficult to construct a tension-free and well-vascularized stoma without trauma.

Fortunately, a few techniques have been described to assist the surgeon with these difficult patients. Horwood proposes the use of a surgical glove to reduce the trauma inflicted on the bowel and its blood supply as it passes through the trephine [16]. Meagher et al. use an Alexis Wound Protector in a similar fashion [17]. In addition, they feel that this technique allows the surgeon to make a smaller defect in the abdominal wall. We agree but argue that creation of any stoma, whether the patient is thin or obese, may benefit from the use of an Alexis Wound Protector (Fig. 9.6). When the abdominal wall is too thick to allow for a tension-free stoma, subcutaneous lipectomy may be an option [15]. In this instance, the subcutaneous fat is removed and the skin affixed to the fascia. Closed suction drainage helps to obliterate the dead space. Similarly, Klein et al. reported the removal of an elliptical segment of skin and subcutaneous tissue to facilitate the creation of a flat surface around the stoma [18].

While it is impossible to predict weight changes, you must remember that significant weight loss can draw the stoma caudally. If the original stoma was generously placed cephalad from any skin fold, this usually does not pose a problem. In those individuals where weight loss has caused stoma migration in to an anatomic fold, aside from conventional relocation via laparotomy with or without abdominoplasty, a panniculectomy can be performed [19]. For patients with smaller deformities, subcutaneous parastomal infiltration of porcine collagen may be a nonoperative option [20].

The Difficult Colostomy

Key Concept: Certain clinical situations often predict problems with constructing an ideal stoma. When confronted with these situations, use these tips as a checklist to make your life (and your stoma) easier.

The classic situation leading to a difficult colostomy creation occurs following emergency diverticular resection in an obese male with a shortened, thickened mesentery and a very thick abdominal wall. In this situation, creation of a well-perfused protruding colostomy can be very challenging. As previously mentioned, preoperative stoma site marking, particularly above the umbilicus, is invaluable. The well-mobilized descending colon will often protrude through the upper abdominal wall with less tension compared to the lower abdomen. In addition, there is often significantly less adipose tissue above the umbilicus. Finally, obese individuals manage the upper abdominal stomas better than the lower because of better visibility. The following tips will facilitate optimal stoma creation:

1. Determine if there is a safe alternative to colostomy creation. For example, resection and primary anastomosis with or without diverting ileostomy creation may be the better choice in some individuals.
2. Excise all inflamed colon.
3. The segment of colon used for the colostomy should be free of any inflamed tissue, thickening, or edema.
4. The left lateral peritoneal reflection should be taken down completely, leaving the left colon attached only to its midline mesentery.
5. Medial peritoneal attachments at the base of the colonic mesentery should be transected if further mobility is required.
6. Fully mobilize the splenic flexure.
7. If additional length is necessary, the inferior mesenteric artery can be ligated proximal to the take off of the left colic artery.

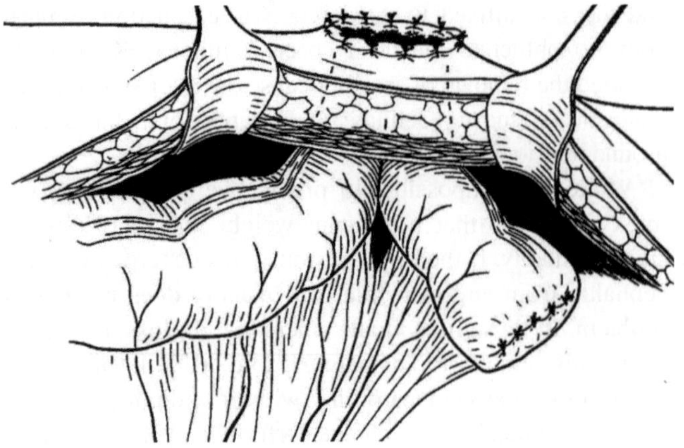

Fig. 9.7 Pseudo-loop colostomy

8. Create "windows" in the medial and lateral aspects of the mesocolon to increase length, similar to ileal-peritoneal windows when creating an ileal pouch-anal anastomosis.
9. The mesentery adjacent to the terminal left colon can be trimmed provided that a 1 cm segment of mesentery containing the marginal artery is left attached to the colonic wall.
10. An oversized abdominal trephine will often allow passage of a thick colonic mesentery, preventing venous congestion and subsequent stomal ischemia.
11. It cannot be stated enough that a stoma site above the umbilicus will decrease the thickness of the abdominal wall through which the colon must pass. Using this site will also decrease tension on the stoma since mobilized left colon reaches more easily to the abdominal wall above the umbilicus.
12. Placing an Alexis Wound Protector and rolling it in the standard fashion will increase the diameter of the trephine, decrease the thickness of the abdominal wall, and decrease friction between the bowel and the subcutaneous tissues. All of these factors will favor stoma creation. After the bowel is passed through the abdominal wall, the inner ring of the Alexis Wound Protector is transected and removed abdominally. The outer portion is removed around the stoma.
13. Any stoma where length or vascularity is tenuous should be matured prior to closure of the midline incision. This facilitates increased mobilization or selection of a different intestinal segment if stoma viability is in question.

Unfortunately, even utilizing each of these maneuvers may not produce a tension-free and viable stoma. In this case, it may be more appropriate to create an ileostomy. When even an ileostomy is not possible, a "pseudo-loop colostomy" can be created. Following the previously mentioned steps, a segment of colon several centimeters proximal to the stapled portion is selected (Fig. 9.7). An oversized trephine is created in the portion of the abdominal wall that results in the least colonic tension. Next, only the antimesenteric boarder of the previously selected colonic segment is passed through the abdominal wall. A small colostomy is made in the protruding bowel, and the antimesenteric boarder is primarily matured to the skin without eversion. This stoma will function appropriately but will be less than ideal and may require later revision.

The Distended Colon

Key Concept: Early decompression of the distended colon will correct many of the factors that will make it inherently difficult to make a good stoma with dilated bowel.

Stomas are often created in cases of a large bowel obstruction where colonic distention presents three barriers to stoma formation. First, the obstructed colon is by nature ischemic; therefore, it is difficult to assess stoma vascularity. Second, the mobility of an obstructed colonic segment is impaired, making it challenging to create a stoma that protrudes appropriately through the abdominal wall. Third, the dilated colon only passes through a large abdominal wall orifice, which can eventually lead to a parastomal hernia.

Decompression of the obstructed segment corrects all these difficulties. In extreme situations, this can be accomplished prior to passing the bowel through the abdominal wall. In this situation, it is also beneficial to mature the stoma prior to closing the abdominal incision. If possible, the colon is passed through the previously created stoma site. The staple line is resected and the bowel decompressed after protecting the operative field with towels. Once the bowel has been decompressed, it becomes more mobile and can be advanced further out of the abdomen. Its viability can then be reassessed. If the stoma's vascularity is adequate, it can be matured in the standard fashion. If not, the colon can be further mobilized with the abdomen still open, hopefully identifying a well-perfused segment that can be matured. This technique does increase the risk of intra-abdominal contamination but can be helpful in difficult situations.

The Difficult Ileostomy

Key Concept: Ileostomies can be as difficult to construct in certain patients as colostomies. Similar to a colostomy, you should be aware of several tips and tricks to ease the technical difficulty.

While creating a functioning ileostomy is generally not as challenging as a colostomy, the obese abdominal wall or a short, thickened mesentery can produce frustration. The following guidelines should prove beneficial:

1. As with a colostomy, consider supraumbilical placement.
2. Mobilization of the small bowel mesentery to the base of the duodenum, as done for an ileal pouch-anal anastomosis, often results in substantial mobility.
3. The ileocolic artery can nearly always be ligated at its origin without fear of subsequent ischemia.
4. An oversized abdominal wall trephine is beneficial in decreasing tension and improving perfusion in thickened bowel with short mesentery.
5. Although not ideal, a "noneverted" ileostomy can be created in an emergency situation.

Very rarely will these maneuvers not result in a viable ostomy. In this case a "pseudo-loop" technique can also be tried, substituting the ileum for colon (Fig. 9.7). The stoma will undoubtedly be difficult to manage for both the patient and the enterostomal therapy nurse and may require early takedown if it is temporary. If permanent, a revision is almost always necessary.

Unfortunately, challenging patients and situations will still arise in which the surgeon has to make sacrifices. It is not always possible to create the ideal stoma with the ideal bowel segment in the ideal location. In these situations, it is best to remember the real estate mantra "location, location, location." It is "better to create an ugly stoma in a good location, than to create a pretty stoma in a bad location."

The Compromised Stoma

Key Concept: Vascular insufficiency to a stoma can occur in many forms. While best to prevent this from occurrence, when it does, it is best to remember that the degree of ischemia predicts the natural repair process and the final anatomic result.

Despite best efforts, stomas with marginal viability are created and must be evaluated and managed in the perioperative period. Vascular compromise is the most serious early complication of stoma creation. The reported incidence of early stoma necrosis ranges from 2.3 to 17 %; I looked and don't have a good photo [2]. Ischemia can be mucosal, muscular, or full thickness. Any of these degrees of ischemia can be supra- or subfascial.

Stoma ischemia is often due to interruption of the segmental arterial supply to the exteriorized bowel segment. This can be avoided by two simple techniques. First, when possible, it is best to divide and complete preparation of the bowel before bringing it through the abdominal wall and maturing the stoma to allow for demarcation of any devitalized bowel. Second, you must remember how much mesentery can be removed from a segment of bowel without causing ischemia. For an end ileostomy, the mesentery can usually be detached from the bowel up to 5 cm without compromising the arterial blood supply [2]. If signs of ischemia appear after exteriorization of the bowel despite minimal devascularization, the tightness of the abdominal wall trephine should be evaluated.

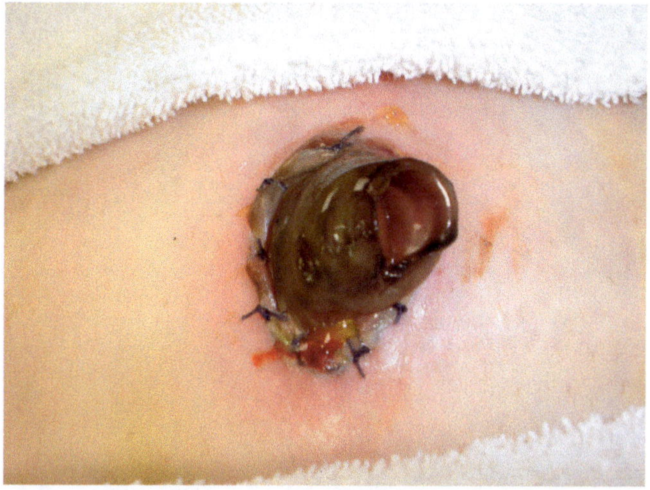

Fig. 9.8 Dusky stoma (Courtesy of Philip Y. Pearson, MD)

Vascular compromise of an end colostomy is generally secondary to division of collateral blood supply during mobilization. If high ligation of the inferior mesenteric artery is performed, every attempt should be made to preserve the ascending branch of the left colic artery [2]. Inadvertent division of the marginal artery or inadequate collateral circulation from the middle colic vessels can also cause bowel ischemia. Excessive trimming of epiploic fat or mesentery from the bowel should be avoided.

In general, mucosal ischemia will resolve without sequelae; muscular ischemia will result in fibrosis and stenosis. Suprafascial ischemia can be managed electively regardless of its degree, while full-thickness, subfascial ischemia must be treated urgently to avoid intra-abdominal fecal leakage and its consequences.

A simple, bedside test will help differentiate the different degrees and locations of intestinal ischemia. A lubricated blood collection tube is passed into the stoma orifice and illuminated with a penlight or an ophthalmoscope. If the mucosa is pink, no further evaluation is necessary as the ischemia will resolve on its own. If the mucosa appears dark below the fascial level, then the depth of ischemia must be assessed (Fig. 9.8). The stoma should be pricked with a needle; if right red bleeding appears, the muscle is well perfused and the ischemia is likely to resolve without issue. If muscular ischemia exists below the fascia, revision is mandatory. If it is suprafascial, stenosis is likely but does not always mandate urgent revision (Fig. 9.9). If the stoma is temporary, the stenosis can generally be managed until takedown is possible. If the stoma is permanent, revision is necessary. Depending on the patient's medical condition, it is often easier to perform revision sooner rather than later. If the viability of the stoma is still in question after test-tube examination, a pediatric proctoscope or flexible endoscope can be employed.

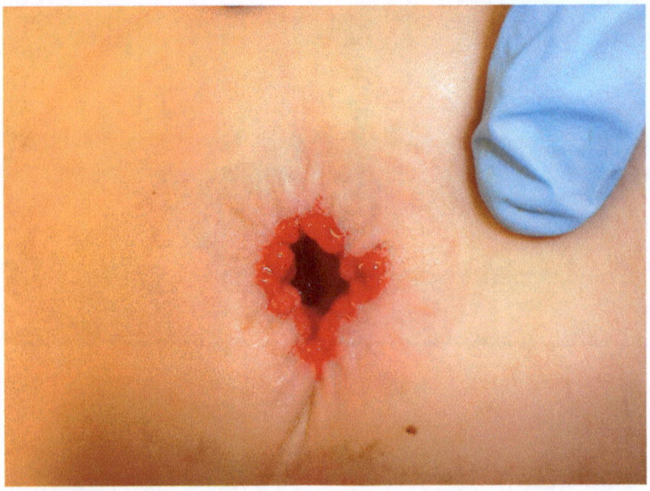

Fig. 9.9 Stenotic stoma (Courtesy of Philip Y. Pearson, MD)

Summary Pearls

Stoma creation is often the last component of a long and difficult operation and may seem trivial when compared with the essential portions of the surgery. Yet the stoma will undoubtedly have the largest impact on the patient's quality of life in the long term. A well-made and well-sited stoma will have minimal implications once the patient has adjusted to its presence. Alternatively, a difficult or complicated stoma will plague both the patient and the surgeon.

The easiest way to avoid a difficult stoma is to avoid stoma formation. When this is not possible, careful preoperative planning can help to avoid future complications. Both eventual stoma reversal, when appropriate, and long-term patient satisfaction should always be considered at the time of stoma creation, no matter how difficult and complex the procedure. Unfortunately, even a well-planned stoma can still cause problems. Prophylactic mesh placement may decrease the incidence of parastomal hernia. An experienced ET therapist can assist with many issues as they arise, but sometimes the only option is stoma revision.

References

1. McLeod RS, Lavery IC, Leatherman JR, Maryland PA, Fazio VW, Jagelman DG, Weakley FL. Factors affecting quality of life with a conventional ileostomy. World J Surg. 1986;10(3):474–80.
2. Kann BR. Early stomal complications. Clin Colon Rectal Surg. 2008;21:23–30.
3. Bass EM, Del Pino A, Tan A, Pearl RK, Orsay CP, Acarian H. Does preoperative stoma marking and education by the enterostomal therapist affect outcome? Dis Colon Rectum. 1997;40:440–2.
4. Cataldo P, MacKeigan JM, editors. Intestinal stomas: principles, techniques and management. 2nd ed. New York: Marcel Dekker; 2004.
5. Carne PWG, Robertson GM, Frizelle FA. Parastomal hernia. Br J Surg. 2003;90:784–93.
6. Brandsma HT, Hansson BM, Haan HV, Aufenacker TJ, Rosman C, Bleichrodt RP. PREVENTion of a parastomal hernia with a prosthetic mesh in patients undergoing permanent end-colostomy; the PREVENT-trial: study protocol for a multicenter randomized controlled trial. Trials. 2012;13(1):226.
7. Hamada M, Ozaki K, Muraoka G, Kawakita N, Nishioka Y. Permanent end-sigmoid colostomy through the extraperitoneal route prevents parastomal hernia after laparoscopic abdominoperineal resection. Dis Colon Rectum. 2012;55(9):963–9.
8. Lian L, Wu XR, He XS, Zou YF, Wu XJ, Lan P, et al. Extraperitoneal vs. intraperitoneal route for permanent colostomy: a meta-analysis of 1,071 patients. Int J Colorectal Dis. 2012;27(1):59–64.
9. Elliot-Smith A, Painter NS. Experiences with extraperitoneal colostomy and ileostomy. Gut. 1961;2:360–2.
10. Figel NA, Rostas JW, Ellis CN. Outcomes using a bioprosthetic mesh at the time of permanent stoma creation in preventing a parastomal hernia: a value analysis. Am J Surg. 2012;203(3):323–6.
11. Williams NS, Nair R, Bhan C. Stapled mesh stoma reinforcement technique (SMART) – a procedure to prevent parastomal herniation. Ann R Coll Surg Engl. 2011;93(2):169.
12. Mengual-Ballester M, García-Marín JA, Pellicer-Franco E, Guillén-Paredes MP, García-García ML, Cases-Baldó MJ, et al. Protective ileostomy: complications and mortality associated with its closure. Rev Esp Enferm Dig. 2012;104(7):350–4.
13. Shiomi A, Ito M, Saito N, Ohue M, Hirai T, Kubo Y, Moriya Y. Diverting stoma in rectal cancer surgery. A retrospective study of 329 patients from Japanese cancer centers. Int J Colorectal Dis. 2011;26(1):79–87.
14. Williams NS, Nasmyth DG, Jones D, Smith AH. De-functioning stomas: a prospective controlled trial comparing loop ileostomy with loop transverse colostomy. Br J Surg. 1986;73(7):566–70.
15. Meguid MM, McIvor A, Xenos L. Creation of a neoabdominal wall to facilitate emergency placement of a terminal ileostomy in a morbidly obese patient. Am J Surg. 1997;173(4):298–300.
16. Horwood J, Hay D. The 'glove cuff' technique for difficult stomas. Ann R Coll Surg Engl. 2009;91(5):438.
17. Meagher AP, Owen G, Gett R. Multimedia article. An improved technique for end stoma creation in obese patients. Dis Colon Rectum. 2009;52(3):531–3.
18. Klein FA, Herr HW, Sogani PC, Whitmore WF. Panniculectomy in conjunction with radical cystectomy in the obese patient. Surg Gynecol Obstet. 1983;156:31–3.
19. Zolfaghari S, Gauthier JC, Jarmuske MB, Boushey RP. Panniculectomy: an alternative approach to the revision of a difficult stoma. Colorectal Dis. 2011;13(7):176–7.
20. Arai Y, Okubo K. Correction of dermal contour defect with collagen injection: a simple management technique for difficult stoma care. J Urol. 1999;161:601–2.

Continent Ileostomy

10

Leif Hultén and Helge E. Myrvold

Key Points

- The continent ileostomy is a low-pressure reservoir capable of distension and holding capacity, allowing 3–4 evacuations/day.
- Stabilization of the nipple valve requires debulking of surrounding mesenteric fat tissues, four staple rows, anchoring of the pouch to the abdominal wall, and strict adherence to postoperative management routines to allow a gradual extension of the drainage period.
- Salvage procedures of nipple valve dysfunction include either rotating the reservoir and construction of a new nipple valve on the "former inlet" or construction of a new nipple valve on a transposed ileal segment.
- Dysplastic transformation in continent ileostomies is a rare phenomenon, and the risk of progression to cancer is small. Patients operated upon for familial polyposis are exceptions, as mucosal adenomas may develop. Regular endoscopic surveillance is mandatory.
- Persistent leakage after numerous nipple valve revisions, unsuccessful fistula operations, intractable pouchitis, and Crohn's disease are the common indications for excision.

L. Hultén, MD, PhD, FACS, ACGBI (Hon), ISUCRS (Hon), SICCR (Hon) (✉)
The Colorectal Unit, Department of Surgery, Sahlgrenska University Hospital SU/O, Göteborg 416 85, Sweden
e-mail: leif.hulten@surgery.gu.se

H.E. Myrvold, MD, PhD, SEC (Hon)
Department of Cancer Research and Molecular Medicine, Norwegian University of Science and Technology, Trondheim N-7491, Norway
e-mail: helge.myrvold@ntnu.no

The Continent Ileostomy: Complications, Their Management, and Its Place in the Future

Key Concept: Despite a relative decrease in its use, surgeons should be aware of how to interrogate a continent ileostomy and manage its potential complications.

Historical notes. The modern era of pouch surgery started with the introduction of the continent ileostomy in 1969 by Nils G. Kock. Originally Kock constructed a low-pressure reservoir by double folding a detubularized ileum segment to be used as a bladder substitute after total cystectomy. Subsequently he applied the same construction to create an intra-abdominal reservoir for collection and storage of intestinal effluent—the Kock pouch [1]. The construction was of a similar kind as that constructed by Tasker in the 1950s [2]. The intestine was split open, folded once, but instead of folding from side to side, according to the Tasker procedure, he folded the bowel from down upside or from upside down (Fig. 10.1). The motor activity is greatly reduced, resulting in virtually no pressure peaks up to a filling of ~300–400 ml. In the few first patients, the corner of the pouch was taken out through the abdominal wall as a conventional stoma in the belief that the rectus muscle might function as a closing mechanism. Leakage occurred frequently in this first series of patients, however, and several other techniques were put on trial subsequently in an attempt to improve continence. The "nipple valve", a short intussusception of the outlet segment, proved to be the most promising measure (Fig. 10.2).

In the 1970s and 1980s, the continent ileostomy gained popularity mainly in the USA and Canada, as well as in Europe—predominantly in Sweden, Norway, and Finland. Several modifications, such as the Barnett continent ileostomy and the T-pouch, have since evolved over the years. While the basic principle for the pouch construction is identical with the Kock pouch, the techniques used to achieve continence differ markedly.

Sir Alan Park used the ileal reservoir developed by Kock for endoanal anastomosis with preservation of the sphincter

S.R. Steele et al. (eds.), *Complexities in Colorectal Surgery*,
DOI 10.1007/978-1-4614-9022-7_10, © Springer Science+Business Media New York 2014

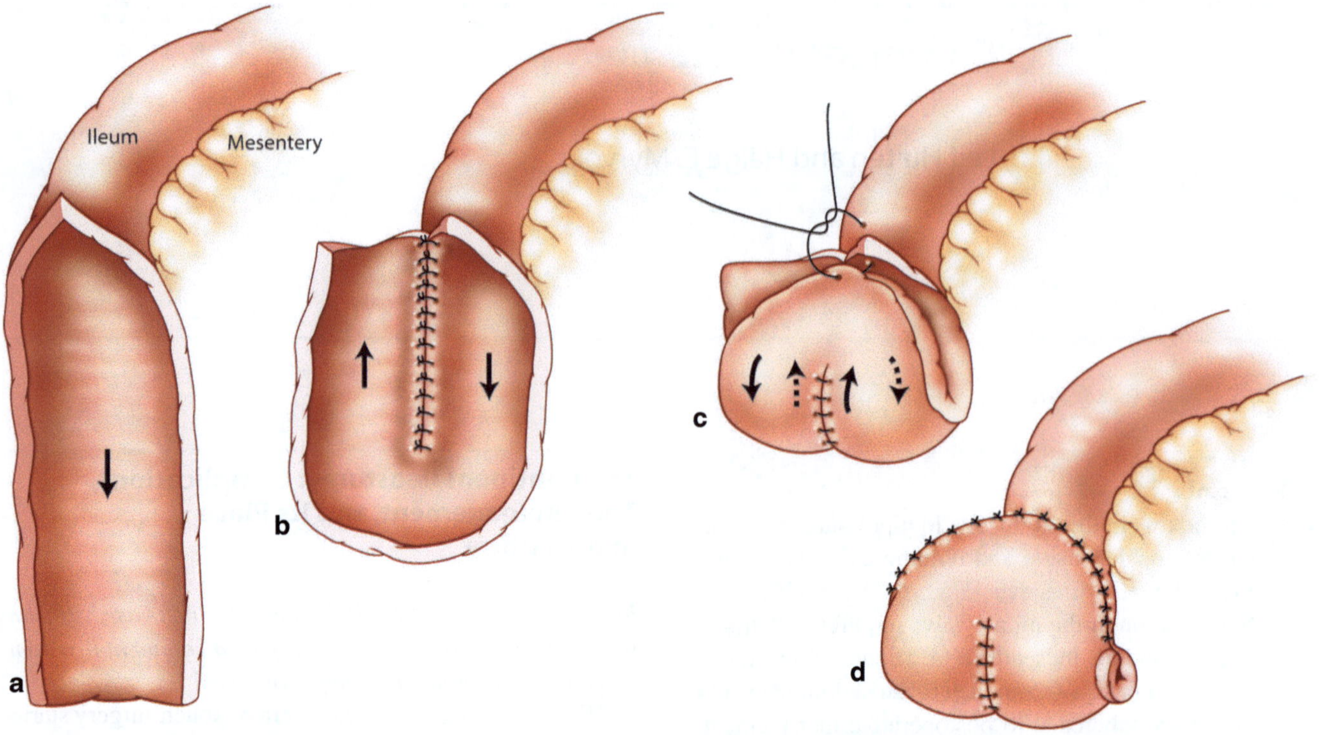

Fig. 10.1 The original procedure (**a**) Segment of terminal ileum (Arrow points to distal) (**b**) Folding of the bowel on itself and formation of the posterior wall. (**c**) Creation of the anterior wall of the pouch. (**d**) Completed pouch

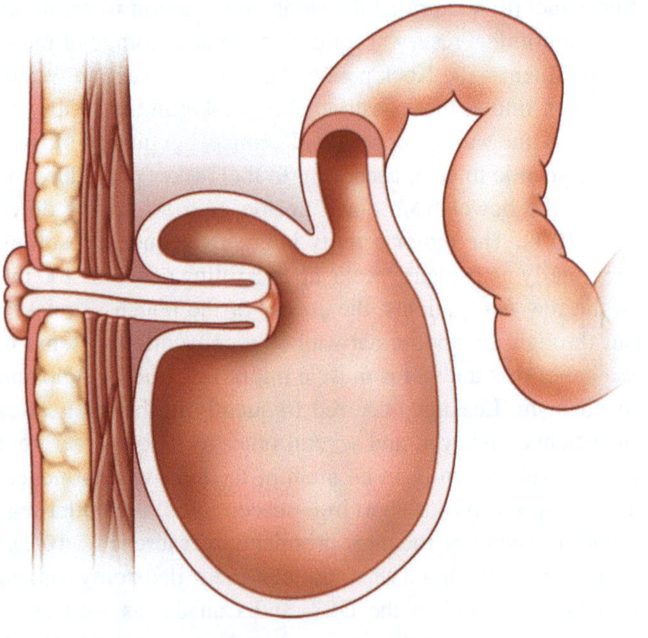

Fig. 10.2 The Kock reservoir with nipple valve

mechanism and published the first results on "restorative proctocolectomy" in 1978 [3]. This method is at present the preferred option worldwide for the surgical treatment of ulcerative colitis and familial adenomatous polyposis, and the demand for continent ileostomy is considerably reduced. However, the continent ileostomy continues to be routinely performed in a few specialized centres and other surgeons are often called upon to evaluate patients with troublesome continent ileostomies. The goals of this chapter are therefore to provide insight into the evaluation and management of potential complications associated with these pouches and allow surgeons to be more comfortable in caring for patients with continent ileostomies.

The Kock Pouch

Formation of the Ileal Pouch

Key Concept: Pouch construction uses terminal ileum for formation, with several different configurations.

The ileal pouch constructed according to the Kock original technique has proved to be an intestinal reservoir well designed to eliminate intraluminal pressure at filling and allowing to expand on distension. It has been convincingly demonstrated that the "double-folded" technique used offers a final pouch volume significantly larger than in pouches where the detubularized segment is folded side-to-side only [4, 5]. The reservoir will gradually reach a volume of 400–600 ml, a volume that will keep the number of evacuations to about three per day. For construction as suggested by Kock [6], 45 cm of the terminal ileum is sufficient—15 cm for the pouch outlet and nipple valve and 30 cm for the formation of the reservoir—while other authors [7], preferring a three-limb

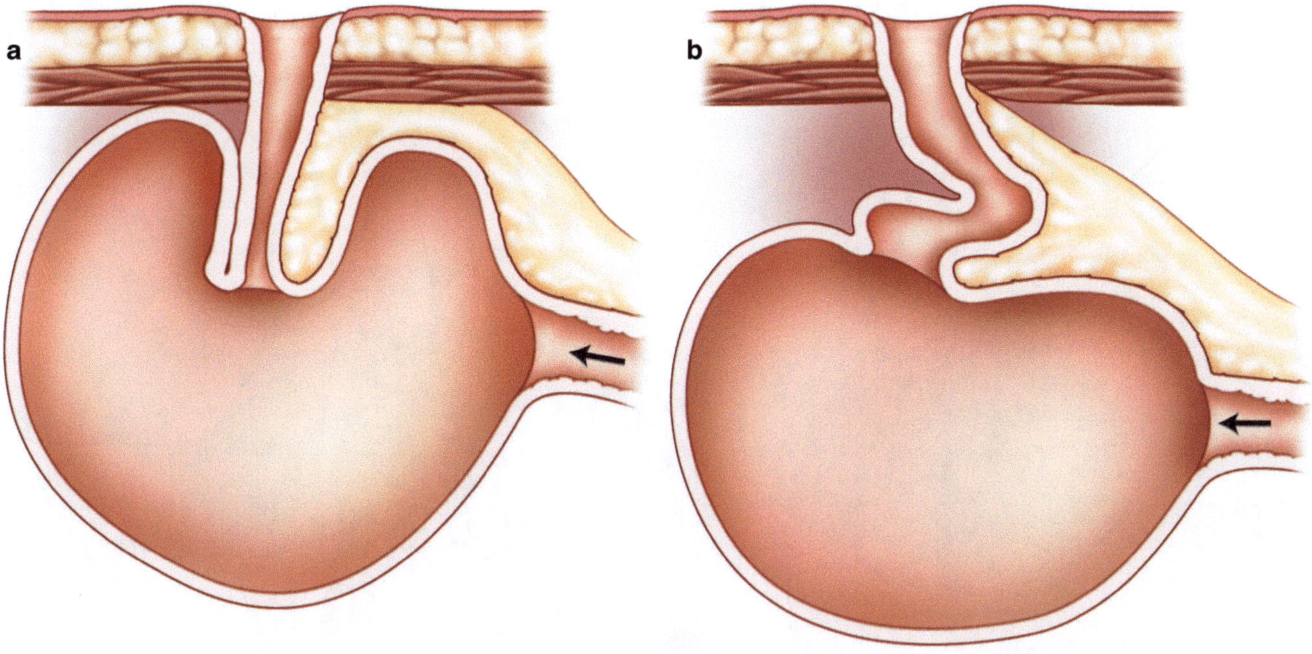

Fig. 10.3 Nipple valve sliding. (**a**) Arrow points to afferent limb. (**b**) The nipple valve has disappeared leading to intubation difficulties

ileal pouch, use a significantly longer segment of the terminal ileum for construction, though no improvement in function or in complication rate can be demonstrated.

Although the "nipple valve" was a promising technique to preserve continence, failures were common. When the reservoir distends, it stretches on the mesentery and puts stress on the valve. Over time, the valve may become reduced or finally disappear, leading to intubation difficulties and incontinence problems (Fig. 10.3). The method had to be changed several times over the years, until a stapling technique was introduced that ultimately has provided promising results. Nevertheless, the main problem in regard to the Kock pouch construction is the nipple valve construction, which remains "the Achilles heel" of the procedure to this day.

Formation of the Nipple Valve

Key Concept: While the nipple valve is the most difficult portion of the pouch construction, several technical points will minimize complications.

For a safe stabilization of the nipple valve, special attention and care should therefore be given to the following measures:

- Stripping of the peritoneal leaves and "defattening" of the nipple valve segment are important measures to reduce the bulk of tissue interposed in the intussusception (Fig. 10.4).
- The nipple valve should be stabilized by means of four staple rows: one staple row on each side of the mesentery, one on the antimesenteric side, and—to further prevent sliding and prolapse—one staple row anchoring the nipple valve to the wall of the reservoir (Fig. 10.5). To avoid necrosis of the tip of the nipple valve, removal of ten staples near the hinge of the stapling device is an important precaution.
- Moreover, a careful and correct construction of the exit conduit channel with firm anchoring of the reservoir to the abdominal wall is necessary.

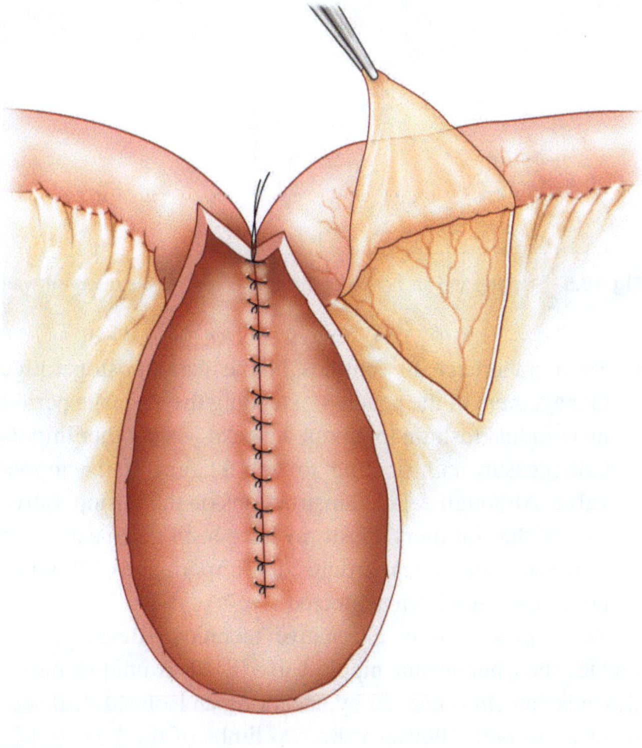

Fig. 10.4 Mesenteric stripping

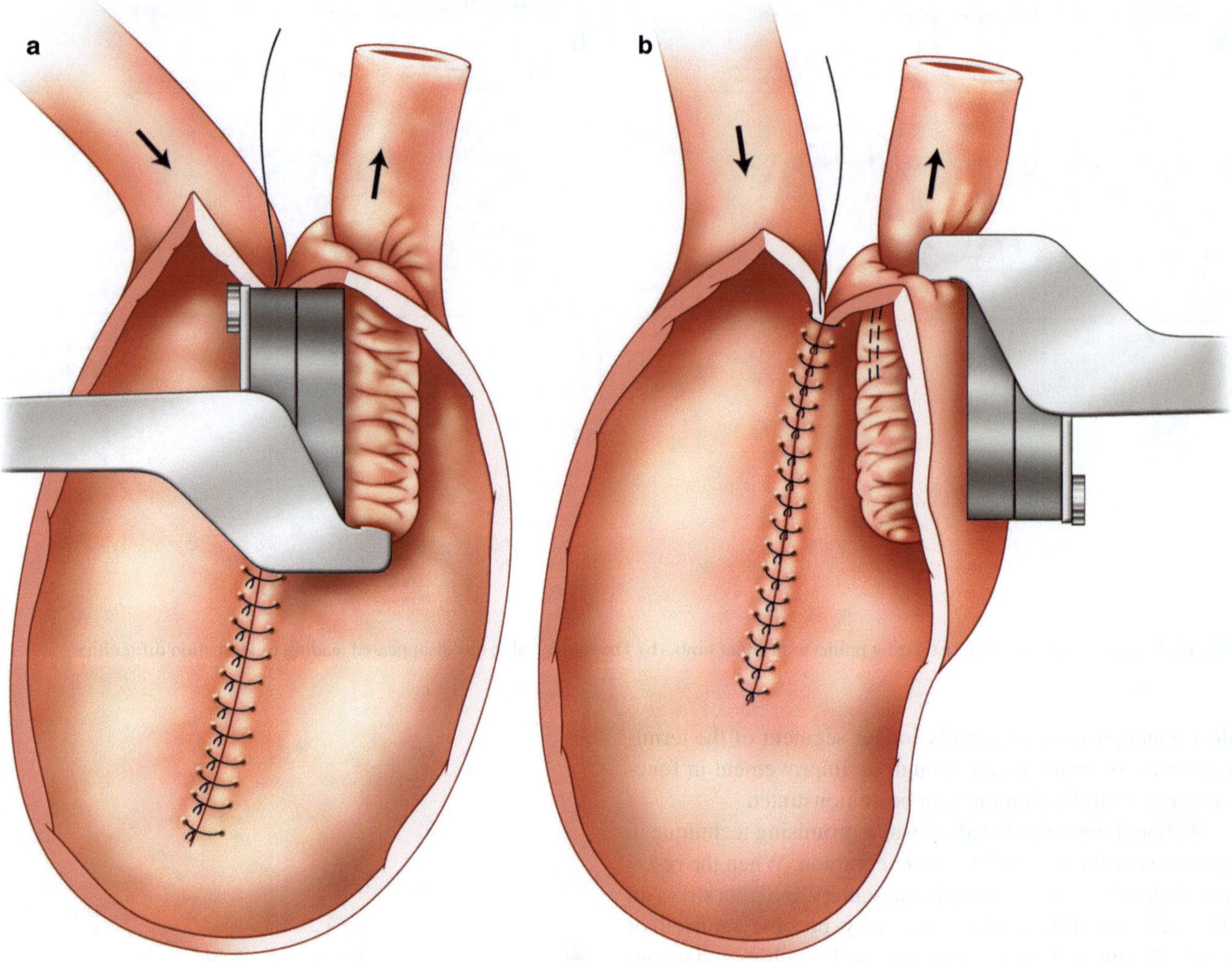

Fig. 10.5 Stapling and anchoring of the nipple valve to the reservoir wall. (**a**) Stapling of the nipple valve. (**b**)Anchoring the valve to the reservoir wall

- Strict adherence to routines in the early postoperative management of the pouch—extending the drainage period in a gradual fashion for about 4 weeks—is another important measure contributing to stabilization of the nipple valve. Although detailed instructions on the postoperative care of the continent ileostomy have been given extensive space in many recent articles, the importance of this last point has often been neglected.

The T-pouch is an alternative technique developed to replace the troublesome nipple valve [8, 9]. A unique antireflux mechanism is created by anchoring an isolated ileal segment as an outlet between the two limbs of the bowel "U", which will form the reservoir (Fig. 10.6). Results have been reported in a 10-year follow-up study [10], demonstrating an acceptable rate of complications and excellent functional results. Unfortunately, the technique is difficult and the procedure has yet to reach wide acceptance for faecal diversion.

The Barnett continent intestinal reservoir is another modification of the Kock pouch procedure. In this configuration, the afferent limb of the small bowel is used to construct the nipple valve and outlet. To improve continence, an intestinal segment with its lumen remaining in continuity with the pouch is wrapped as an intestinal collar around the base of the nipple valve, similar to a gastric fundoplication [11]. Collective results from five hospitals revealed similar complication rates and failures as with the traditional types of continent ileostomy commonly used [12, 13]. The procedure is complicated and the Barnett pouch has also not received general acceptance. The importance of this modification is still scientifically unproven.

Complications and Their Management

While there have been keen advocators for the continent ileostomy over the years, many surgeons have been reluctant to adopt the method considering the high postoperative morbidity—despite modifications in surgical technique and postoperative management.

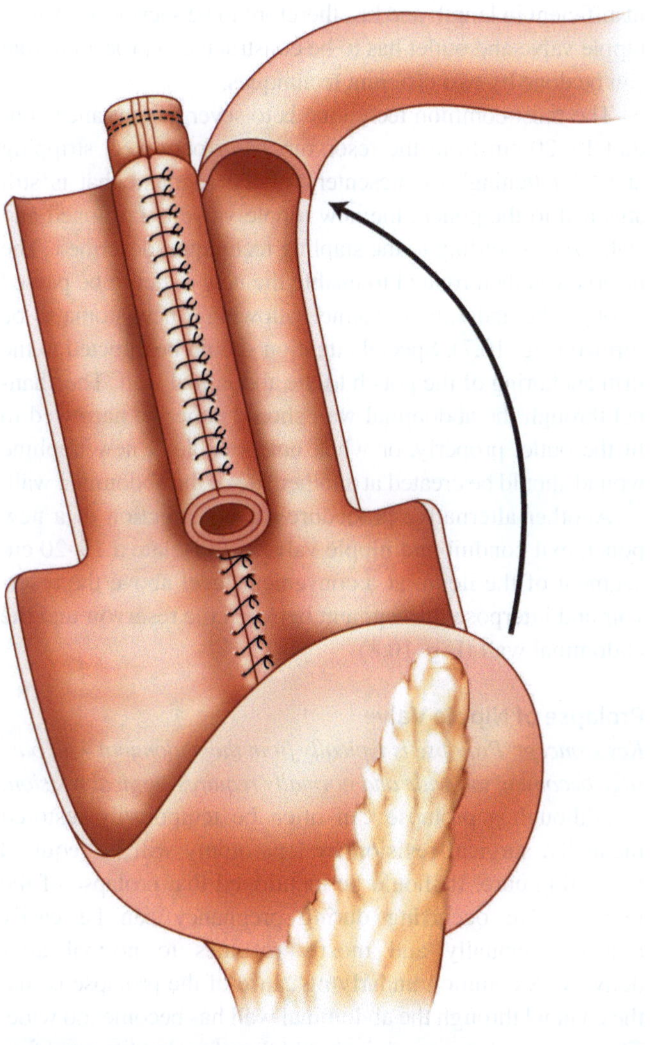

Fig. 10.6 The T-pouch

Early Complications

Key Concept: *Early complications with the continent ileostomy are similar to any other bowel surgery.*

With increasing experience on the part of surgeons, the early morbidity rate in terms of anastomotic leaks with peritonitis and/or intra-abdominal abscess, fistulas, and wound sepsis and dehiscence has been markedly reduced. Intestinal obstruction, local abscess, necrosis of the nipple valve, and fistula are reported to occur in about 10 %.

Late Complications

Key Concept: *Most of the complications developing later in the postoperative course are related to the nipple valve, and the success of the operation stands with the competence and stability of this intussusception.*

Late complications with pouch operations include those that are similar to any other bowel surgery, such as obstruction, stricture, and hernia. However, continent ileostomies have a unique set of late complications that are often related to the nipple valve including:

- Sliding and/or prolapse each render the pouch incontinent.
- Nipple valve slippage and stenosis are the most common causes of reoperation [14–17]. Overall revision rates range between 12.5 % [18] and 52 % [19].
- A fistula developing through the base of the nipple valve will also result in leakage of intestinal contents due to bypassing the valve. The complication seems to be an infrequent reason for reoperation however [14, 17].

The collective results imply that revisional surgery due to any of the above-mentioned defects has decreased from 40 to 50 % with the early techniques to about 20–25 % with the introduction of the currently most popular method of mesenteric stripping and stapling of the nipple valve. The need for reoperations has decreased significantly with increased experience of the surgical team to below 10 % [6, 18, 20, 21]. In concordance with the reduced rate of complications, surgical experience, and success of revisional surgery, the failure rate has decreased significantly and is currently reported between 4 and 10 % [6, 14, 17, 20–24], a failure rate which is comparable to that after restorative proctocolectomy [25–29].

Management of Complications

Key Concept: *The continent ileostomy is a demanding procedure with a high potential for complications, and special skill and experience are required for their recognition and management.*

Early Complications

- Local or diffuse peritonitis reflecting suture leakage or abscess require immediate and proper treatment. A local peritonitis with or without abscess should be drained. It is usually best to establish a loop ileostomy proximal to the affected area.
- A fistula either may heal spontaneously on this treatment or could be subject to revision by another operation 2 or 3 months later.
- Ischemic necrosis of the pouch outlet and/or the nipple valve may also occasionally develop in the early postoperative phase, a vascular complication mostly due to a faulty technique. Depending on its extension of the ischaemia, it may be successfully treated either conservatively by prolonged tube drainage of the pouch or, when more extensive as judged, by ileoscopy and be primarily managed by establishment of a defunctioning loop ileostomy. In both situations, revisional surgery may then be performed at a convenient time a few months later.

- Bleeding within the pouch during the first postoperative days is common, and the irrigation fluid will sometimes be heavily bloodstained. Profuse bleeding may sometimes occur, even after a careful suturing, with clots accumulating in the pouch blocking the draining catheter. Too little attention has been directed to the importance of the postoperative wide-bore (28Fr) catheter drainage. With strict irrigation routines and the use of a proper draining system, this complication should in most cases be possible to manage conservatively.

The importance of a defunctioning ileostomy for reducing the early morbidity rate, or at least minimizing the consequences of any complication developing during the early postoperative phase, may be controversial; however, such a safety measure should probably be recommended for the beginners before experience has been gained.

Late Complications

Key Concept: Despite surgical experience, improvements in technique, and strict routines in the postoperative care, sliding or prolapse of the nipple valve, or a nipple valve fistula, may develop resulting in incontinence and a need for surgical intervention.

Late complications typically manifest in predictable ways, and most involve problems with the nipple valve itself. In this section we will walk you through how to approach these often difficult situations.

Sliding of the Nipple Valve and Its Correction

Key Concept: Nipple valve sliding presents with problems with pouch intubation. While temporizing measures are possible, this most often requires formal operative revision.

Intubation difficulties of the reservoir and/or leakage of gas and faeces are symptoms indicating nipple valve sliding (Fig. 10.3). Confirmation of a defect valve can be done by using a flexible endoscope. In this context it should be mentioned that patients may sometimes present acutely with an over-distended reservoir due to inability to insert the catheter. The problem can be solved by using a small-size rigid sigmoidoscope (i.e. children's sigmoidoscope), by which it is possible to follow the typically angulated course into the reservoir under direct vision. An indwelling catheter can then be passed through the sigmoidoscope and left in place.

Revisional surgery through a formal laparotomy is required for reestablishment of continence in most cases, however. The surgical approach to be employed depends on the precise findings at laparotomy. The stoma and outlet is first dissected free and the reservoir mobilized into the wound. After opening the pouch, it may occasionally be possible to de-invaginate the intussusception simply by careful dissection and separation of layers of the nipple valve. Provided that the segment is sufficiently long, a nipple valve is reconstructed and fixed in position according to established technique. In most cases, however, the outlet segment is damaged by the dissection or insufficient in length and has therefore to be sacrificed. A new nipple valve and outlet has to be constructed, a procedure that can be done by two different techniques.

The most common technique is to sever the entrance conduit 15–20 cm from the reservoir. After peritoneal stripping and "defattening" of mesentery of the segment that is still attached to the pouch, the new nipple valve is fashioned and stabilized according to the stapling techniques described. The reservoir is then rotated to enable the new outlet to be passed through the abdominal channel, allowing a new stoma to be formed (Fig. 10.7). Special attention should be directed to the firm anchoring of the pouch to the abdominal wall. The channel through the abdominal wall should either be narrowed to fit the outlet properly, or when not possible, a new trephine wound should be created at another site of the abdominal wall.

Another alternative procedure for construction of a new pouch exit conduit and nipple valve is to isolate a 15–20 cm segment of the ileum at a convenient level above the reservoir and interpose the segment between the reservoir and the abdominal wall (Fig. 10.8).

Prolapse of Nipple Valve

Key Concept: Prolapse is typically from the abdominal wall passage becoming too wide and normally requires surgical revision.

Although a prolapse can often be temporarily restored manually, surgical revision by laparotomy will be required for lasting cure. It should be mentioned that prolapse of the nipple valve occurring during pregnancy can be easily reduced manually and mostly resumes to normal after delivery. A common underlying cause of the prolapse is that the channel through the abdominal wall has become too wide. The stoma and exit conduit should therefore be dissected free with complete mobilization of the reservoir. The channel should be narrowed by suturing the rectus muscle and the fascia, allowing the exit conduit to fit snugly. An alternative is to select another site for the ileostomy and create a new trephine wound through intact abdominal wall. Anchoring the nipple valve by stapling it to the wall of the reservoir has contributed greatly to prevent nipple valve dislocation (Fig. 10.5).

Parastomal Hernia

Parastomal hernia is rare but should be treated according to up-to-date techniques in the same way as any parastomal hernia. Because of the high recurrence rate after suture repair, the use of mesh in parastomal hernia repair is preferred [30].

Fistula Through the Nipple Valve

Key Concept: Internal fistulas are revised via laparotomy, and external fistulas are managed locally.

Fistulas may be external or internal bypassing the nipple valve (Fig. 10.9). The reported complication rate is about 25 % [17, 22], but reoperations may be successful [31]. The position of the fistula is mostly at the base of the nipple valve. Formerly silk sutures and/or synthetic material

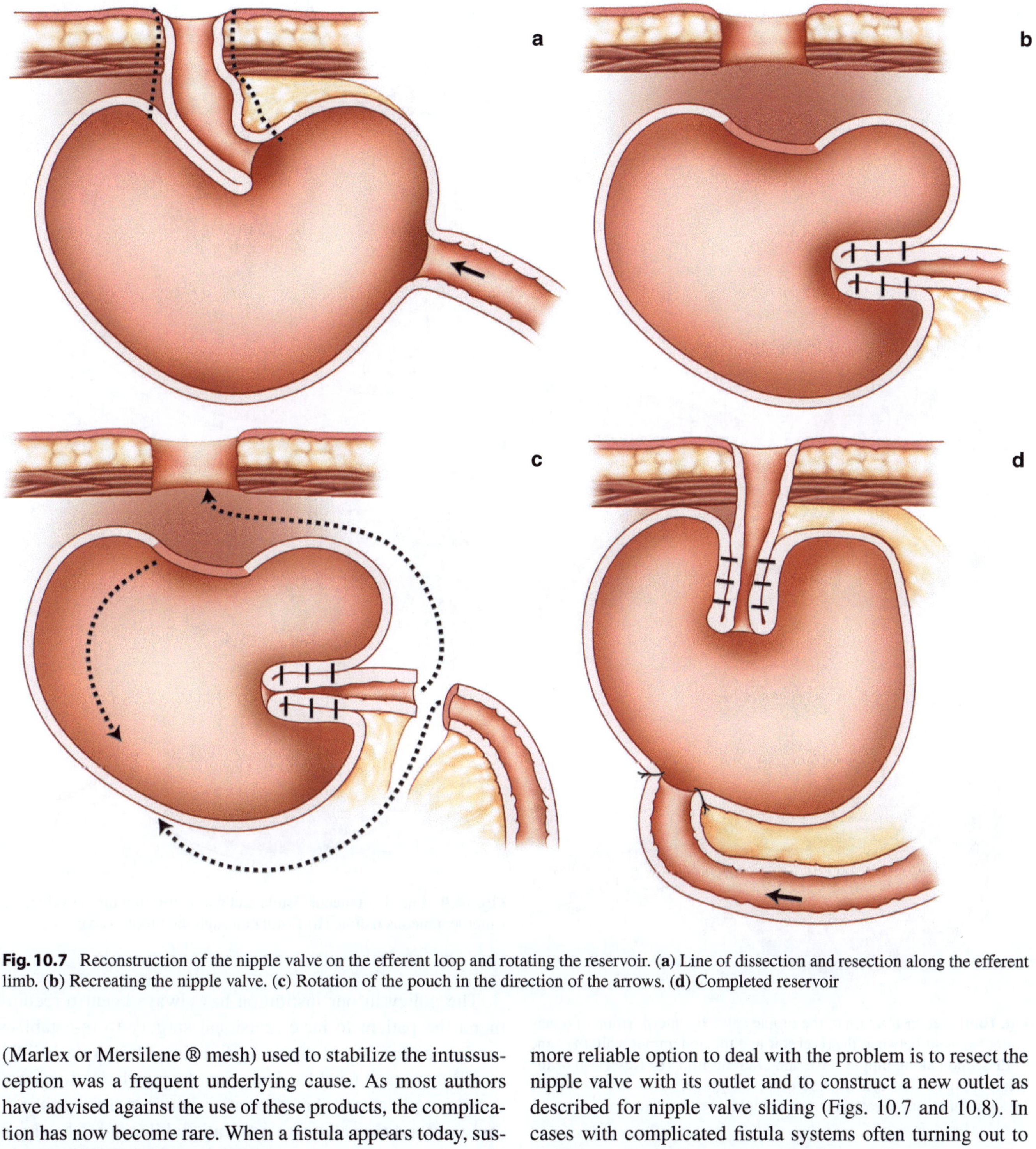

Fig. 10.7 Reconstruction of the nipple valve on the efferent loop and rotating the reservoir. (**a**) Line of dissection and resection along the efferent limb. (**b**) Recreating the nipple valve. (**c**) Rotation of the pouch in the direction of the arrows. (**d**) Completed reservoir

(Marlex or Mersilene ® mesh) used to stabilize the intussusception was a frequent underlying cause. As most authors have advised against the use of these products, the complication has now become rare. When a fistula appears today, suspicion of Crohn's disease arises.

While external fistulas should be best depicted by fistulography, internal fistulas are diagnosed by endoscopy. Repair of the external fistulas may be accomplished by local sutures after excision of its edges sometimes without a formal laparotomy. Internal fistulas through the nipple valve require laparotomy, however. Although desintussusception of the nipple valve and repair by excision of the fistula and reconstruction of the valve on the same intestinal segment may well be tried, such a repair is mostly unsuccessful. A more reliable option to deal with the problem is to resect the nipple valve with its outlet and to construct a new outlet as described for nipple valve sliding (Figs. 10.7 and 10.8). In cases with complicated fistula systems often turning out to be Crohn's disease, pouch excision and construction of a conventional ileostomy is often the best solution.

Miscellaneous

Perforation of the reservoir a very rare complication which might be caused by too vigorous insertion of the catheter or by penetration of a sharp food object such as a fishbone. The closure of a perforation—particularly when associated with peritonitis—should be protected by a defunctioning loop ileostomy. Volvulus of the reservoir has been reported, but

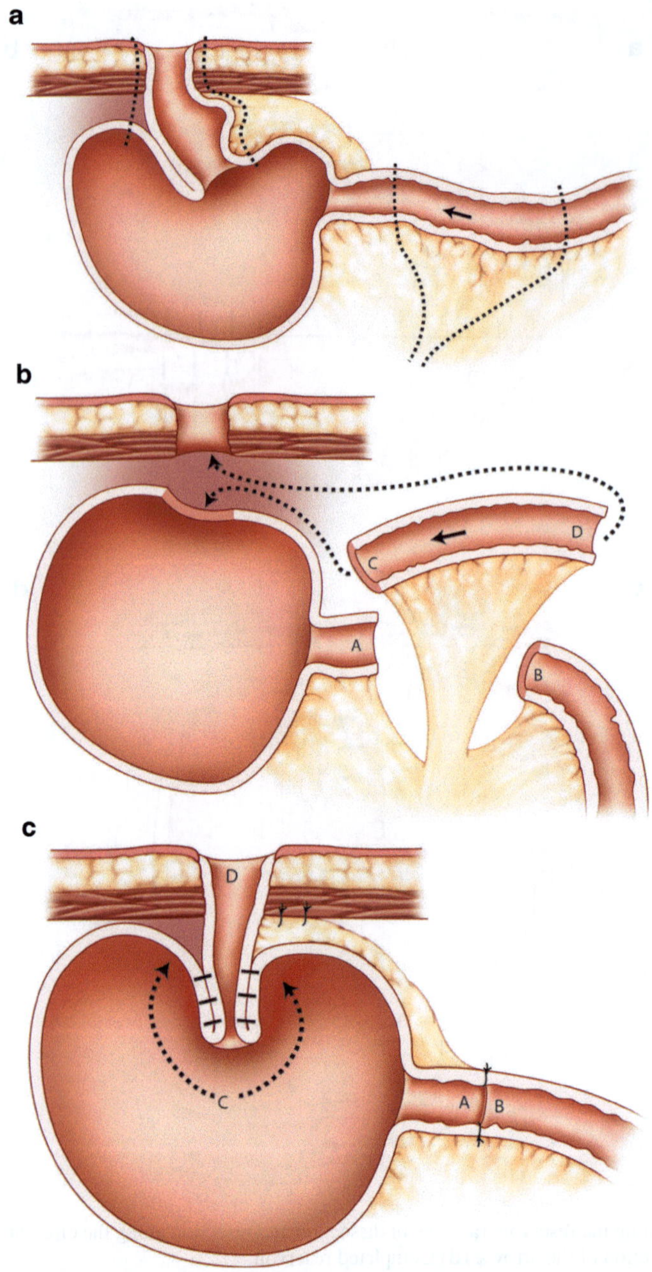

Fig. 10.8 Reconstruction of the nipple valve by interposition of a new outlet segment between the reservoir and the abdominal wall. (**a**) Line of dissection along nipple valve and afferent limb. (**b**) Resection of the original nipple and construction of new segment (C-D) for the nipple (arrows demonstrate rotation). (**c**) Completed reconstruction

should not occur if the fixation of the reservoir is performed according to current principles. Fibrosis of the tip of the nipple valve is another complication that may require dilatation and occasionally reconstruction. Skin stricture around the stoma is also common but is easily dealt with by local revision.

Recurrent Nipple Valve Complications

Key Concept: *Nipple valve dysfunction can be successfully revised, even after one or more previous revisions.*

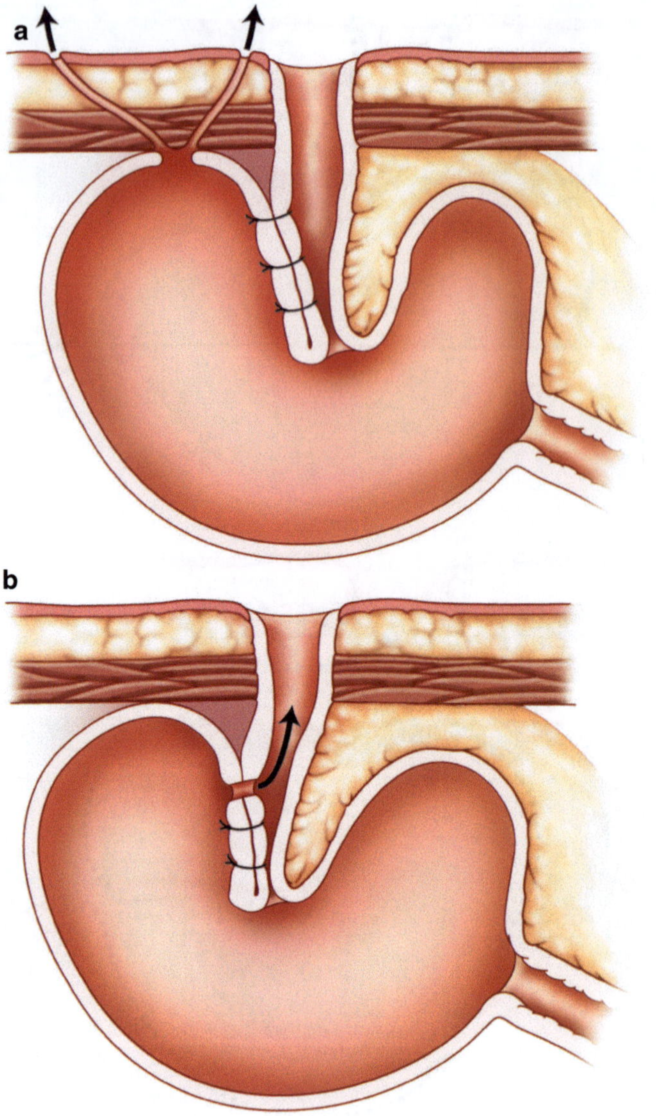

Fig. 10.9 Enterocutaneous fistula and fistula through nipple valve. (**a**) Enterocutaneous fistula. (**b**) Fistula through the nipple valve

The policy in our institution has always been to recommend the patient to have revisional surgery to re-establish continence in cases of nipple dysfunction. Only occasionally would there be a need for removing the pouch due to any of these complications. An association between the number of revisions and conversion to conventional ileostomy has been suggested, but has so far not been confirmed [15, 32, 33].

It must in this context be emphasized that surgical revision of nipple dysfunction, although requiring another laparotomy, is in fact not necessarily a major undertaking. Even if such a reconstruction is again followed by sliding or any other defect of the nipple valve function, a further operation for restoration of continence is mostly justified and will be successful eventually [34]. It appears also from our experience—amounting to 40–50 years clinical practice—that

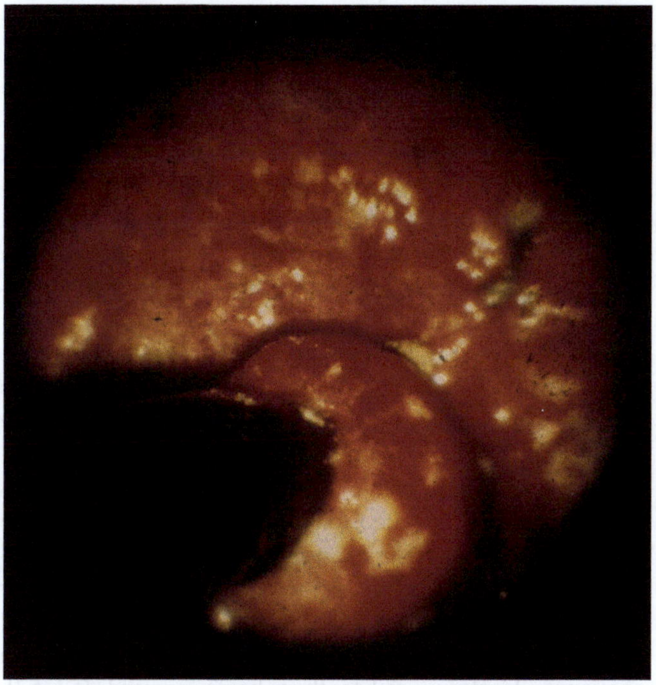

Fig. 10.10 Endoscopic view of acute pouchitis

once a patient has experienced the benefit of a continent ileostomy, such a patient usually insists on a further revision (even if it may be the third or fourth in order) and refuses to have the reservoir removed [35].

Ileitis (Pouchitis)

Key Concept: Similar to IPAA, continent ileostomies may develop pouchitis. Management is typically medical, though severe cases may require diversion or excision.

In patients with continent ileostomy, approximately one-third of the patients may experience episodes of pouchitis [14, 31, 33, 36]. The cause of this unspecific inflammatory reaction that sometimes develops in the reservoir and/or the afferent intestinal loop is still obscure [36, 37]. It may be mild or asymptomatic, apparent at endoscopy as reddened oedematous mucosa (Fig. 10.10). In more severe cases, the patients suffer from colicky abdominal pain and diarrhoea with liquid, bloodstained faeces. It is often readily reversed by oral antibiotics (metronidazole or ciprofloxacin), although continuous drainage may be required in severe cases. A loop ileostomy may occasionally be justified as an alternative measure, when other treatment has failed, and before removal of the pouch is decided. It has been suggested that the process is bacterial in origin. However, since the condition appears to be connected almost exclusively to patients operated upon for ulcerative colitis, and particularly to those suffering from primary sclerosing cholangitis, the reaction pattern is more likely to be inherent in the original disease. As compared to the other complications that can all be managed surgically, pouchitis is therefore considered a particularly distressing and ominous complication. When looked upon in a longer perspective, however, such fears appear to be unfounded. Although the overall failure rate of the Kock pouch may approach 10–15 %, pouchitis appears only occasionally to be the reason for pouch excision. Moreover, there is a general impression that the episodes of pouchitis become milder or may even disappear with the passage of time.

Epithelial Dysplasia and Cancer Risk

Key Concept: The development of dysplasia and cancer in the pouch is rare for most patients; however, adenomas in the setting of FAP are more common requiring surveillance.

Sporadic reports of dysplasia and occasional adenocarcinomas in the ileal pouch mucosa have been published [38], thus demonstrating the arrival of a further complication of the ileal pouch as another model of the multistep progression theory of cancer, taking normal mucosa through the stages of inflammation, dysplasia, and eventually carcinoma. Most reports suggest that dysplastic transformation in pelvic pouches is a rare phenomenon, and therefore, the risk of further progression to cancer should be small [39]. Others [40] claim the opposite view. Common to these studies is that the follow-up observation period is relatively short and casts doubts as to the reliability of these statements. The long-term results presented recently from a study on patients with a continent ileostomy are more reliable and reassuring. Considering an observation time of an average of 30 years and the comparatively large series of patients kept under close supervision, the incidence of mucosal dysplasia in the ileal pouch mucosa proved to be low, and no case of carcinoma or high-grade dysplasia was observed [41, 42]. Surveillance intervals should be left to the discretion of the provider.

Ileal Pouch Adenomas in Patients Operated for with Familial Adenomatous Polyposis (FAP)

The apparent ability of small bowel adenomas to develop many years after colectomy for familial polyposis may be a different problem in patients with a continent ileostomy [43–45]. Thus adenomas with the potential to progress to adenocarcinomas can develop even in the mucosa of the continent ileostomy. The risk of developing one or more adenomas over a 10-year period has been calculated to be about 35 %, and patients with adenomas appear also more likely to have duodenal and ampullary adenomas [46]. Regular endoscopic surveillance of FAP patients with a Kock pouch is therefore recommended at a frequency similar to that of upper gastrointestinal endoscopy. In general, most guidelines recommend every 3–5 years for upper endoscopy and every 1–2 years for IPAA patients.

Pouch Removal

Key Concept: Disease-specific, anatomic, and functional problems may occasionally lead to pouch excision.

Persistent leakage after numerous nipple valve revisions, unsuccessful fistula operations, intractable pouchitis, and Crohn's disease are the common indications for pouch removal. Removal rate is currently reported below 10 % [6, 14, 17, 20–24]. When the continent ileostomy fails, the pouch is usually excised and a conventional ileostomy established. Although a pouch constructed on a new ileal segment may well be possible, such a procedure is risky and usually not recommended as metabolic disturbances will inevitably occur and may lead to a short bowel syndrome eventually.

Criteria of Selection

Key Concept: Although the prevalence of continent ileostomies is decreasing, there remains well-defined cohort of patients for which this pouch may be useful.

The main indications for a continent ileostomy are ulcerative colitis and familiar polyposis, but the procedure has also been used in patients with multiple colorectal carcinomas, aganglionosis coli, coloanal incontinence, and severe constipation. In patients with Crohn's disease, the operation has been marred by a very high rate of immediate and late complications, and most surgeons therefore consider Crohn's disease a contraindication [47]. However, in highly selected cases (such as those undergoing proctocolectomy for Crohn's colitis without involvement of the distal ileum and disease-free for at least 5 years and still not accepting their conventional ileostomy), the procedure may still be justified and is often successful [48, 49]. In patients with familial adenomatous polyposis, the development of desmoids should be considered, as their occurrence will interfere with construction of a continent ileostomy.

Obese patients can often be a technical problem, as the mesenteric fat content may interfere with both the folding procedure and the valve construction. It is also often argued that the patient's manual skill will inevitably be reduced with ageing and might interfere with the evacuation routines, but in fact, these daily routines are less demanding than those used for the management of a conventional ileostomy. Provided that the patient is mentally fit, older age should therefore not be a contraindication to the Kock pouch.

Concluding Remarks

It appears reasonable to assume that anyone with a keen interest in colorectal surgery should be able to adopt the continent ileostomy technique in its present fashion and put it into practice with a good prospect of success. Complications will initially inevitably occur, requiring reintervention before the ideal functional stage is reached.

Experience and surgical skill are needed to improve the success rate, but competence is also required for proper management of the complications. A sufficiently large patient flow is of prime importance to achieve and maintain expertise in these respects, and the continent ileostomy should therefore be done in specialized surgical units where a team of surgeons must be prepared to accept a long-term commitment of these patients.

Since the advent of the pelvic pouch procedure, there are today even fewer advocates for the continent ileostomy. This is very unfortunate, as the technique has still a definite place in surgery [50]. There may be patients with a conventional ileostomy who may wish to undergo a conversion to a continent ileostomy due to ileostomy problems, or there may be patients who are considered unsuitable for a restorative proctocolectomy. Moreover, it appears that the excision rate for pelvic pouches increases with the passage of time [51, 52] and a failing pelvic pouch may be used for conversion to a continent ileostomy rather than being excised [53–57]. Therefore it is of our opinion that surgeons in specialty clinics offering patients a pelvic pouch should also be conversant and facile with the continent ileostomy technique.

The Continent Ileostomy: Its Place in the Future

Key Concept: In addition to primary construction following proctocolectomy, a continent ileostomy may be considered in carefully informed and strongly motivated patients with a failed ileal pouch-anal anastomosis.

The pelvic pouch procedure has become the chief method today for curative treatment of ulcerative colitis and familial polyposis. The failure rate after construction of a pelvic pouch in patients with ulcerative colitis (UC) varies. While Tulchinsky et al. [27] reported a failure rate of 9 % in 635 patients, with an average follow-up of 3 years, Korsgen and colleagues [58] reported a 19 % failure rate in 154 patients. Interestingly, most of the pouch failures seem to occur late postoperatively. Pelvic sepsis, poor function, pouchitis, and overlooked Crohn's disease (in that order) seem to be the main reasons for failures. The failure rate when calculated and expressed in crude figures is often unreliable, and actuarial methods should be a more correct statistical method to determine this cumulative risk. A life table calculation based on figures presented so far would imply that the cumulative risk for pelvic pouch failure in a UC patient is about 10–15 % over 10 years [14, 28, 59, 60] and 30–40 % in patients who develop septic complications [28, 52]. Time will tell, but the long-term results imply that the ileoanal pouch may not be the panacea it was initially thought to be.

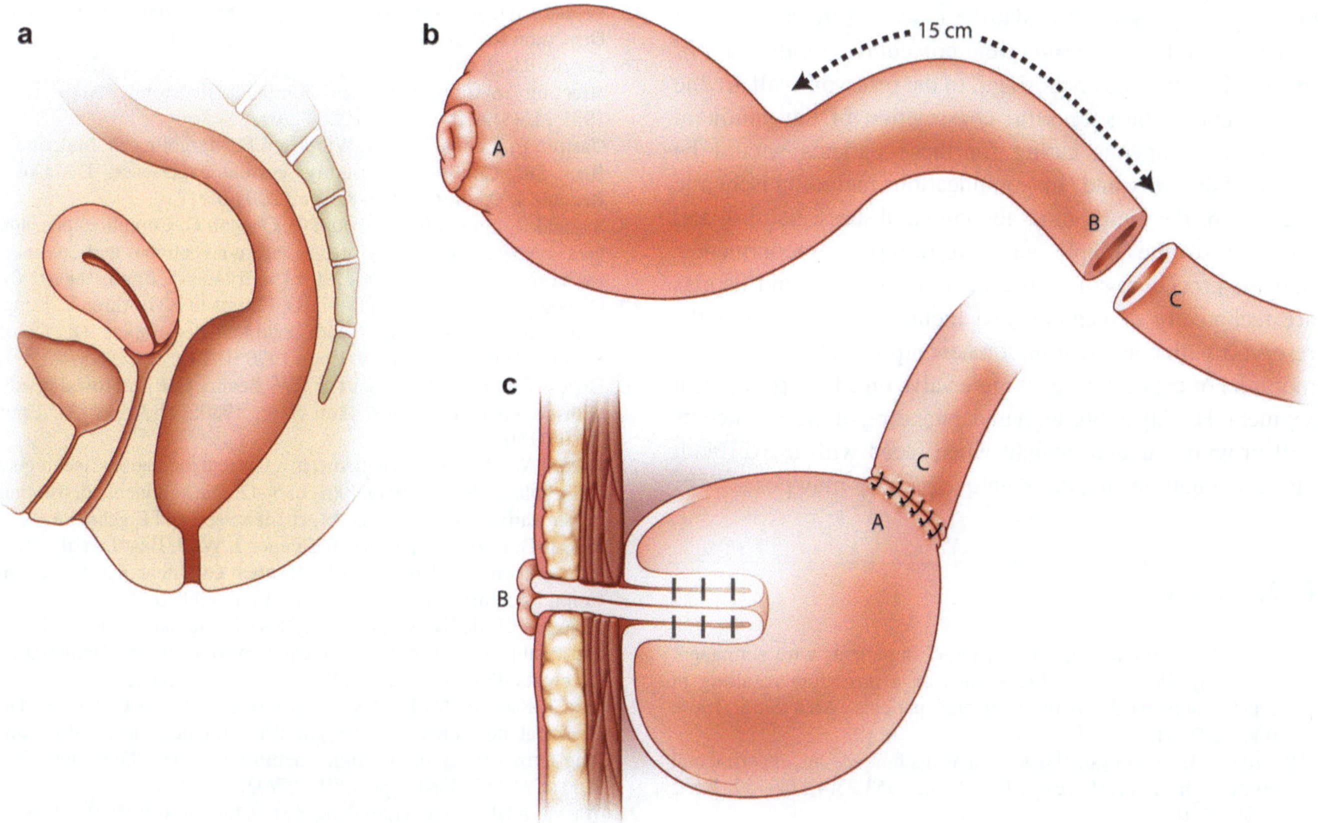

Fig. 10.11 Conversion of the failed pelvic pouch to continent ileostomy. (**a**) Cross-section of the pelvis with the failed pouch present. (**b**) Segment of bowel to be used to create the continent ileostomy with 15 cm needed for the nipple valve. (**c**) Completed continent ileostomy

There are three options that most readily come to mind for patients with a failing pelvic pouch: (1) it may simply be defunctionalized by a covering ileostomy, (2) revisional surgery may be done, and (3) the pouch may be excised. Clearly, the first option is mostly aimed to be just a temporary intervention. Refashioning of the pouch and/or the ileoanal anastomosis, which may well be tried, is often associated with an unsuccessful result. According to reports in the literature, pouch excision with construction of a conventional ileostomy appears to be the most common measure—even in specialized clinics. This is a very unfortunate decision, however, as such an operation will inevitably be associated with loss of a significant length of terminal ileum. Apart from the practical problems of a "high-flow" ileostomy, salt-water imbalance and malabsorbtion of bile acids and vitamin B12 will develop. Given the shortcomings of pouch excision or infinite diversion, conversion of a failed pouch to a continent ileostomy as suggested by Kusunoki et al. [53] and Hultén and associates [54, 56] should be a reasonable alternative. The terminal ileum is preserved and malabsorbtion consequences are avoided. For carefully informed and strongly motivated patients, conversion of the failed ileal pouch-anal anastomosis to a continent ileostomy should be recommended (Fig. 10.11). Recent reports [61, 62] from well-known colorectal centres confirm that such a conversion is a viable option with encouraging long-term results.

Apart from patients with a problematic conventional ileostomy and those unsuitable for a restorative proctocolectomy, candidates for a continent ileostomy are also the growing number of patients with a failed ileal pouch-anal anastomosis. It seems reasonable therefore to assume that there may well be a great revival of interest in the continent ileostomy technique in the future.

Summary Pearls

In summary, the low-pressure intestinal reservoir developed by N. G. Kock is the basis for modern pouch surgery, from continent ileostomy to ileal pouch-anal anastomosis, and remains a viable alternative for select patients to this day. Candidates for a continent ileostomy are patients with poorly functioning conventional ileostomy, patients with ulcerative colitis or familial adenomatous polyposis not suitable for restorative proctocolectomy, or patients with personal preference. A failed pelvic pouch or one that cannot be constructed during the operation can also be converted to a continent ileostomy. When performing the procedure, stabilization of the nipple valve and anchoring it to the reservoir wall are the key points in the successful construction of the continent ileostomy. Surgeons caring for these patients should be aware of the early and late complications including ischemic necrosis of the outlet, intra-abdominal abscess, fistulas, and slippage of the nipple valve resulting in incontinence. Salvage procedures of nipple valve dysfunction and fistulas are technically demanding and include either rotating the reservoir with construction of a new nipple valve on the former inlet or creating a new nipple valve on a transposed ileal segment. Having a thorough understanding of these concepts will provide valuable insight when faced with the difficult clinical situations that these unique patients may pose.

References

1. Kock NG. Intra-abdominal "reservoir" in patients with permanent ileostomy. Preliminary observations on a procedure resulting in fecal "continence" in five ileostomy patients. Arch Surg. 1969; 99(2):223–31.
2. Tasker JH. Ileo-cystoplasty: a new technique; an experimental study with report of a case. Br J Urol. 1953;25(4):349–57. Epub 1953/12/01.
3. Parks AG, Nocholls RJ. Proctectomy without ileostomy for ulcerative colitis. Br Med J. 1978;2:85–8.
4. Hulten L. [Capacity, motility and emptying of the ileal reservoir]. Ann Chir. 1993;47(10):1034–8. Epub 1993/01/01. Capacite, motilite et evacuation du reservoir ileal.
5. Kock NG, Hulten L, Myrvold HE. Ileoanal anastomosis with interposition of the ileal 'Kock pouch'. Preliminary results. Dis Colon Rectum. 1989;32(12):1050–4.
6. Kock NG, Brevinge H, Philipson BM, Ojerskog B. Continent ileostomy. The present technique and long term results. Ann Chir Gynaecol. 1986;75(2):63–70. Epub 1986/01/01.
7. Fazio VW, Tjandra JJ. Technique for nipple valve fixation to prevent valve slippage in continent ileostomy. Dis Colon Rectum. 1992;35(12):1177–9. Epub 1992/12/01.
8. Kaiser AM, Stein JP, Beart Jr RW. T-pouch: a new valve design for a continent ileostomy. Dis Colon Rectum. 2002;45(3):411–5. Epub 2002/06/18.
9. Skinner DG, Boyd SD, Lieskovsky G. An update on the Kock pouch for continent urinary diversion. Urol Clin North Am. 1987;14(4):789–95. Epub 1987/11/01.
10. Kaiser AM. T-pouch: results of the first 10 years with a nonintussuscepting continent ileostomy. Dis Colon Rectum. 2012;55(2): 155–62. Epub 2012/01/10.
11. Barnett WO. Current experiences with the continent intestinal reservoir. Surg Gynecol Obstet. 1989;168(1):1–5. Epub 1989/01/01.
12. Mullen P, Behrens D, Chalmers T, Berkey C, Paris M, Wynn M, et al. Barnett continent intestinal reservoir. Multicenter experience with an alternative to the Brooke ileostomy. Dis Colon Rectum. 1995;38(6):573–82. Epub 1995/06/01.
13. Behrens DT, Paris M, Luttrell JN. Conversion of failed ileal pouch-anal anastomosis to continent ileostomy. Dis Colon Rectum. 1999;42(4):490–5; discussion 5–6. Epub 1999/04/24.
14. Wasmuth HH, Svinsas M, Trano G, Rydning A, Endreseth BH, Wibe A, et al. Surgical load and long-term outcome for patients with Kock continent ileostomy. Colorectal Dis. 2007;9(8):713–7.
15. Lepisto AH, Jarvinen HJ. Durability of Kock continent ileostomy. Dis Colon Rectum. 2003;46(7):925–8. Epub 2003/07/09.
16. Dozois RR, Kelly KA, Ilstrup D, Beart Jr RW, Beahrs OH. Factors affecting revision rate after continent ileostomy. Arch Surg. 1981;116(5):610–3. Epub 1981/05/01.
17. Castillo E, Thomassie LM, Whitlow CB, Margolin DA, Malcolm J, Beck DE. Continent ileostomy: current experience. Dis Colon Rectum. 2005;48(6):1263–8. Epub 2005/06/17.
18. Sjodahl R, Lemon E, Nystrom PO, Olaison G. Complications, surgical revision and quality of life with conventional and continent ileostomy. Acta Chir Scand. 1990;156(5):403–7. Epub 1990/05/01.
19. Ojerskog B, Kock NG, Nilsson LO, Philipson BM, Ahren C. Long-term follow-up of patients with continent ileostomies. Dis Colon Rectum. 1990;33(3):184–9. Epub 1990/03/01.
20. Dozois RR, Kelly KA, Beart Jr RW, Beahrs OH. Improved results with continent ileostomy. Ann Surg. 1980;192(3):319–24. Epub 1980/09/01.
21. Ecker KW. [The continent ileostomy. Current indications, techniques and results]. Chirurg. 1999;70(6):635–42. Die kontinente Ileostomie. Gegenwartige Indikationen, Vorgehensweisen und Ergebnisse.
22. Nessar G, Fazio VW, Tekkis P, Connor J, Wu J, Bast J, et al. Long-term outcome and quality of life after continent ileostomy. Dis Colon Rectum. 2006;49(3):336–44. Epub 2006/02/02.
23. Hoekstra LT, de Zwart F, Guijt M, Bakx R, Gerhards MF. Morbidity and quality of life after continent ileostomy in the Netherlands. Colorectal Dis. 2009;11(7):719–25. Epub 2009/08/27.
24. Parc Y, Klouche M, Bennis M, Lefevre JH, Shields C, Tiret E. The continent ileostomy: an alternative to end ileostomy? Short and long-term results of a single institution series. Dig Liver Dis. 2011;43(10):779–83. Epub 2011/07/02.
25. Wasmuth HH, Trano G, Endreseth B, Rydning A, Wibe A, Myrvold HE. Long-term surgical load in patients with ileal pouch-anal anastomosis. Colorectal Dis. 2009;11(7):711–8. Epub 2009/08/27.
26. de Zeeuw S, Ali UA, Donders RA, Hueting WE, Keus F, van Laarhoven CJ. Update of complications and functional outcome of the ileo-pouch anal anastomosis: overview of evidence and meta-analysis of 96 observational studies. Int J Colorectal Dis. 2012;27(7):843–53. Epub 2012/01/10.
27. Tulchinsky H, Hawley PR, Nicholls J. Long-term failure after restorative proctocolectomy for ulcerative colitis. Ann Surg. 2003; 238(2):229–34.
28. Tekkis PP, Lovegrove RE, Tilney HS, Smith JJ, Sagar PM, Shorthouse AJ, et al. Long-term failure and function after restorative proctocolectomy – a multi-centre study of patients from the UK National Ileal Pouch Registry. Colorectal Dis. 2010;12(5): 433–41. Epub 2009/02/20.
29. Ikeuchi H, Uchino M, Matsuoka H, Bando T, Matsumoto T, Tomita N, et al. Surgery for ulcerative colitis in 1,000 patients. Int J Colorectal Dis. 2010;25(8):959–65. Epub 2010/03/11.
30. Hansson BM, Slater NJ, van der Velden AS, Groenewoud HM, Buyne OR, de Hingh IH, et al. Surgical techniques for parastomal hernia repair: a systematic review of the literature. Ann Surg. 2012;255(4):685–95. Epub 2012/03/16.
31. Fazio VW, Church JM. Complications and function of the continent ileostomy at the Cleveland Clinic. World J Surg. 1988;12(2):148–54. Epub 1988/04/01.
32. Lepisto A, Luukkonen P, Jarvinen HJ. Cumulative failure rate of ileal pouch-anal anastomosis and quality of life after failure. Dis Colon Rectum. 2002;45(10):1289–94.
33. Jarvinen HJ, Makitie A, Sivula A. Long-term results of continent ileostomy. Int J Colorectal Dis. 1986;1(1):40–3. Epub 1986/01/01.
34. Denoya PI, Schluender SJ, Bub DS, Gorfine SR, Bauer JJ. Delayed Kock pouch nipple valve failure: is revision indicated? Dis Colon Rectum. 2008;51(10):1544–7. Epub 2008/05/27.
35. Berndtsson IE, Lindholm E, Oresland T, Hulten L. Health-related quality of life and pouch function in continent ileostomy patients: a

30-year perspective. Dis Colon Rectum. 2004;47(12):2131–7. Epub 2005/01/20.
36. Svaninger G, Nordgren S, Oresland T, Hulten L. Incidence and characteristics of pouchitis in the Kock continent ileostomy and the pelvic pouch. Scand J Gastroenterol. 1993;28(8):695–700. Epub 1993/08/01.
37. Mahadevan U, Sandborn WJ. Diagnosis and management of pouchitis. Gastroenterology. 2003;124(6):1636–50. Epub 2003/05/23.
38. Cox CL, Butts DR, Roberts MP, Wessels RA, Bailey HR. Development of invasive adenocarcinoma in a long-standing Kock continent ileostomy: report of a case. Dis Colon Rectum. 1997;40(4):500–3. Epub 1997/04/01.
39. Sarigol S, Wyllie R, Gramlich T, Alexander F, Fazio V, Kay M, et al. Incidence of dysplasia in pelvic pouches in pediatric patients after ileal pouch-anal anastomosis for ulcerative colitis. J Pediatr Gastroenterol Nutr. 1999;28(4):429–34. Epub 1999/04/16.
40. Gullberg K, Stahlberg D, Liljeqvist L, Tribukait B, Reinholt FP, Veress B, et al. Neoplastic transformation of the pelvic pouch mucosa in patients with ulcerative colitis. Gastroenterology. 1997;112(5):1487–92. Epub 1997/05/01.
41. Duff SE, O'Dwyer ST, Hulten L, Willen R, Haboubi NY. Dysplasia in the ileoanal pouch. Colorectal Dis. 2002;4(6):420–9.
42. Hulten L, Willen R, Nilsson O, Safarani N, Haboubi N. Mucosal assessment for dysplasia and cancer in the ileal pouch mucosa in patients operated on for ulcerative colitis – a 30-year follow-up study. Dis Colon Rectum. 2002;45(4):448–52. Epub 2002/05/15.
43. Stryker SJ, Carney JA, Dozois RR. Multiple adenomatous polyps arising in a continent reservoir ileostomy. Int J Colorectal Dis. 1987;2(1):43–5. Epub 1987/02/01.
44. Parc YR, Olschwang S, Desaint B, Schmitt G, Parc RG, Tiret E. Familial adenomatous polyposis: prevalence of adenomas in the ileal pouch after restorative proctocolectomy. Ann Surg. 2001;233(3): 360–4. Epub 2001/02/27.
45. Church J. Ileoanal pouch neoplasia in familial adenomatous polyposis: an underestimated threat. Dis Colon Rectum. 2005;48(9): 1708–13. Epub 2005/06/07.
46. Alexander JR, Andrews JM, Buchi KN, Lee RG, Becker JM, Burt RW. High prevalence of adenomatous polyps of the duodenal papilla in familial adenomatous polyposis. Dig Dis Sci. 1989; 34(2):167–70. Epub 1989/02/01.
47. Mowat C, Cole A, Windsor A, Ahmad T, Arnott I, Driscoll R, et al. Guidelines for the management of inflammatory bowel disease in adults. Gut. 2011;60(5):571–607. Epub 2011/04/06.
48. de Oca J, Sanchez-Santos R, Rague JM, Biondo S, Pares D, Osorio A, et al. Long-term results of ileal pouch-anal anastomosis in Crohn's disease. Inflamm Bowel Dis. 2003;9(3):171–5. Epub 2003/06/07.
49. Bloom RJ, Larsen CP, Watt R, Oberhelman Jr HA. A reappraisal of the Kock continent ileostomy in patients with Crohn's disease. Surg Gynecol Obstet. 1986;162(2):105–8. Epub 1986/02/01.
50. Hulten L. Proctocolectomy and ileostomy to pouch surgery for ulcerative colitis. World J Surg. 1998;22(4):335–41. Epub 1998/04/02.
51. Setti Carraro P, Talbot IC, Nicholls RJ. Long term appraisal of the histological appearances of the ileal reservoir mucosa after restorative proctocolectomy for ulcerative colitis. Gut. 1994;35(12): 1721–7. Epub 1994/12/01.
52. Heuschen UA, Allemeyer EH, Hinz U, Lucas M, Herfarth C, Heuschen G. Outcome after septic complications in J pouch procedures. Br J Surg. 2002;89(2):194–200. Epub 2002/02/22.
53. Kusunoki M, Sakanoue Y, Shoji Y, Kusuhara K, Yamamura T, Utsunomiya J. Conversion of malfunctioning J pouch to Kock's pouch. Case report. Acta Chir Scand. 1990;156(2):179–81. Epub 1990/02/01.
54. Hulten L, Fasth S, Hallgren T, Oresland T. The failing pelvic pouch conversion to continent ileostomy. Int J Colorectal Dis. 1992;7(3):119–21. Epub 1992/09/01.
55. Behrens DT, Paris M, Luttrell J. Continent ileostomy can be offered as an option to patients who fail the ileal pouch-anal anastomosis (IPAA). Dis Colon Rectum. 1999;42(5):686.
56. Hulten L. Conversion of a pelvic pouch to a continent pouch (Kock pouch). Tech Coloproctol. 2001;5(3):192. Epub 2002/03/05.
57. Wasmuth HH, Trano G, Wibe A, Endreseth BH, Rydning A, Myrvold HE. Failed pelvic pouch substituted by continent ileostomy. Colorectal Dis. 2010;12(7 Online):e109–13. Epub 2009/04/04.
58. Keighley MR, Ogunbiyi OA, Korsgen S. Pitfalls and outcome in ileo-anal pouch surgery for ulcerative colitis. Neth J Med. 1997;50(2):S23–7. Epub 1997/02/01.
59. Setti-Carraro P, Ritchie JK, Wilkinson KH, Nicholls RJ, Hawley PR. The first 10 years' experience of restorative proctocolectomy for ulcerative colitis. Gut. 1994;35(8):1070–5.
60. Leowardi C, Hinz U, Tariverdian M, Kienle P, Herfarth C, Ulrich A, et al. Long-term outcome 10 years or more after restorative proctocolectomy and ileal pouch-anal anastomosis in patients with ulcerative colitis. Langenbecks Arch Surg. 2010;395(1):49–56. Epub 2009/03/13.
61. Lian L, Fazio VW, Remzi FH, Shen B, Dietz D, Kiran RP. Outcomes for patients undergoing continent ileostomy after a failed ileal pouch-anal anastomosis. Dis Colon Rectum. 2009;52(8):1409–14; discussion 4414–6. Epub 2009/07/21.
62. Wassmuth HH, Myrvold HE, Bengtsson J, Hulten L. Conversion of a failed pouch to a continent ileostomy: a controversy. Colorectal Dis. 2011;13(1):2–5. Epub 2010/12/25.

Part III

The Pelvis

Rectal Prolapse: Current Evaluation, Management, and Treatment of a Historically Recurring Disorder

11

Dana M. Hayden and Steven D. Wexner

Key Points

- Rectal prolapse is a surgical disorder for which there are a multitude of treatment options; however, conclusive evidence does not support any one operation as a panacea.
- Symptomology, comorbidities, and previous surgeries will guide the selection of the appropriate operation for prolapse.
- If a patient is medically fit, the transabdominal approach should be attempted for both initial and recurrent rectal prolapse, regardless of the initial operation.

Etiology and Epidemiology of Prolapse

Key Concept: Rectal prolapse affects both men and women and may be associated with constipation or fecal incontinence. Several anatomic conditions are commonly found with rectal prolapse.

Although an uncommon disorder, full-thickness rectal prolapse can drastically impair the quality of life. It was described as early as 1500 BC, depicting the protrusion of all layers of the rectum through the anal canal into the external environment (Fig. 11.1) [1]. Rectal prolapse can lead to several problems including fecal incontinence, obstructed defecation, bleeding, mucosal ulceration, mucous per rectum, and, rarely, bowel necrosis from strangulation [2, 3]. This disorder is more common in females, especially in the elderly population, although it affects both genders and patients of all ages, with an overall incidence of 4 per 1,000 [3]. Although prolapse is commonly thought to be associated with multiparty, one-third of females with rectal prolapse are nulliparous [4]. The peak incidence occurs in the seventh decade for women; interestingly for males with prolapse, it occurs at age 40 years or younger [4]. Although the exact etiology of prolapse remains unclear, it has been attributed to distal intussusception of the rectum and a combination of associated anatomic factors, including relaxation of the rectal suspensory ligaments, chronic straining, altered bowel transit, diastasis of the levator ani, increased width of the retrorectal space, an abnormally deep pouch of Douglas with an associated sliding hernia, and patulous anal sphincter [1, 4–6]. Surgical intervention is the only means of treatment; however, the type of operation still remains controversial, as illustrated by more than 100 different operations.

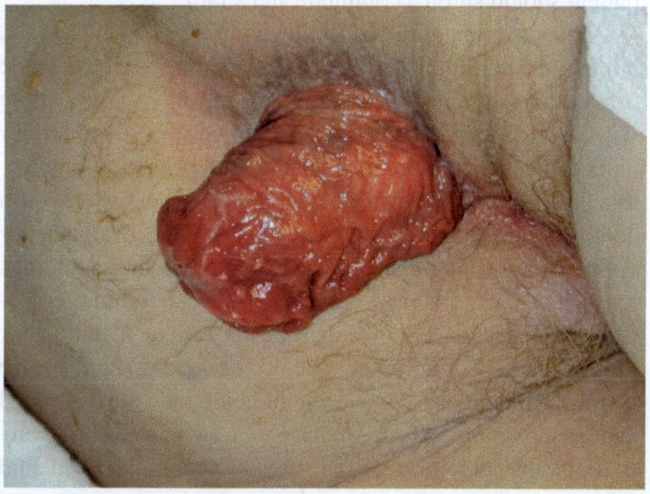

Fig. 11.1 Rectal prolapse

D.M. Hayden, MD, MPH
Department of General Surgery, Loyola University Medical Center, 2160 South First Avenue, Maywood, IL 60153, USA
e-mail: dhayden21@gmail.com

S.D. Wexner, MD, PhD (Hon), FACS, FRCS, FRCS(Ed) (✉)
Department of Colorectal Surgery, Cleveland Clinic Florida, 2950 Cleveland Clinic Blvd., Weston, FL 33331, USA
e-mail: wexners@ccf.org

S.R. Steele et al. (eds.), *Complexities in Colorectal Surgery*,
DOI 10.1007/978-1-4614-9022-7_11, © Springer Science+Business Media New York 2014

Evacuatory dysfunction frequently occurs with rectal prolapse and fecal incontinence has been found in approximately 50–75 % of patients with rectal prolapse [1, 4]. Several factors may contribute to this association: traumatic stretch of the sphincter complex by the protruding rectum or continuous stimulation of the rectoanal inhibitory reflex by the prolapse resulting in chronic low internal anal sphincter pressures and the presence of a direct conduit bypassing the sphincter mechanism [1, 4]. Interestingly, constipation is also a commonly associated feature of rectal prolapse, reported by 25–50 % of patients [4]. Although the mechanism is not clear, it appears to be related to difficulty with defecation due to an obstructing rectal intussusception, paradoxical puborectalis contraction, or colonic dysmotility [1, 4].

Diagnosis and Evaluation

Key Concept: Rectal prolapse is a clinical diagnosis. Underlying symptoms and risk factors should guide the evaluation.

History and physical examination are the key components to the diagnosis of full-thickness rectal prolapse. History and symptoms including persistent or spontaneous prolapse, prolapse with straining, and other symptoms including rectal pain, bleeding, mucous secretion, fecal incontinence, and constipation should be ascertained. Previous surgical history including colon resections or anorectal surgery and anorectal congenital anomalies repaired during childhood must be documented, as well as medical comorbidities. During the physical examination, reproduction of the prolapse with Valsalva should be performed; status of the anal sphincters, perineal descent, and associated pelvic organ prolapse should also be documented. If the prolapse is not reproduced in the lateral decubitus or prone positions in the office, the patient should sit on a commode and strain.

Adjunctive imaging and testing are not always necessary, but may be helpful. If the prolapse cannot be detected in the office, defecography should be performed. This procedure will also identify some associated pelvic floor disorders or defects that may require treatment as well [4]. A lifelong history of severe constipation should be investigated with colonic transit study and defecography to evaluate for colonic inertia or puborectalis dysfunction; these findings may change the planned operation (total abdominal colectomy with rectopexy) or aid in postoperative planning for biofeedback. Colonoscopy should be undertaken before operative intervention according to guidelines for colorectal cancer screening and surveillance as well as to exclude any findings that may change the surgical approach (incidental colon cancer or a tumor serving as lead point for rectal intussusception) [4]. Anorectal physiology testing may not be helpful since studies have shown that these tests do not reliably predict postoperative function after prolapse repair [4].

Types of Operative Repair

Key Concept: Understanding the risks, benefits, and technical details of the various approaches for rectal prolapse repair will aid in proper selection of operative repair and help optimize outcomes. In general, functional improvements for both constipation and fecal incontinence occur following both perineal and abdominal repair.

Perineal Operations

Key Concept: Perineal approaches are a second resort, normally to be used only in patients with medical comorbidities that prevent abdominal approaches. Your preferred choice is almost always to perform an Altemeier outside of mucosal or limited full-thickness prolapse where a Delorme may be useful.

Two main perineal operations are currently performed: the Altemeier (perineal rectosigmoidectomy) with or without levatorplasty and with or without colonic J pouch and the Delorme. Anal encirclement procedures, including the Thiersch operation, have for the most part been abandoned due to high complication rates (infection, erosion, breakage) and high recurrence rates [1]. The Delorme procedure, first described in 1900, is performed most commonly for mucosal prolapse or short full-thickness rectal prolapse [1, 4]. This operation involves circumferential mucosal sleeve resection of redundant mucosa with imbrication of the muscularis layer and then mucosal anastomosis [4]. The complete bowel wall is not resected. This perineal operation has been shown to improve incontinence when performed with or without a sphincteroplasty [1]. It may be technically more challenging than the Altemeier and has been reported to have higher recurrence rates as well [1]. Although complications are thought to occur less frequently than with the abdominal approach, urinary retention, infection, bleeding, and fecal impaction have been reported in 4–12 % [4]. Patients will usually have postoperative improvement of their fecal incontinence (25–70 %) and constipation (13–100 %); however, urgency and tenesmus may occur in a small percentage of patients [4].

Auffret in France first described perineal rectosigmoidectomy in 1882; a series of six cases were published by Mikulicz in 1889 [7]. Miles popularized the technique in 1933, although it was named after Altemeier, who described the technique with an associated levatorplasty in 1971, reporting a recurrence rate of only 2.8 % [2]. This operation involves transanal full-thickness resection of the rectum and sigmoid colon (Figs. 11.2 and 11.3). A coloanal anastomosis

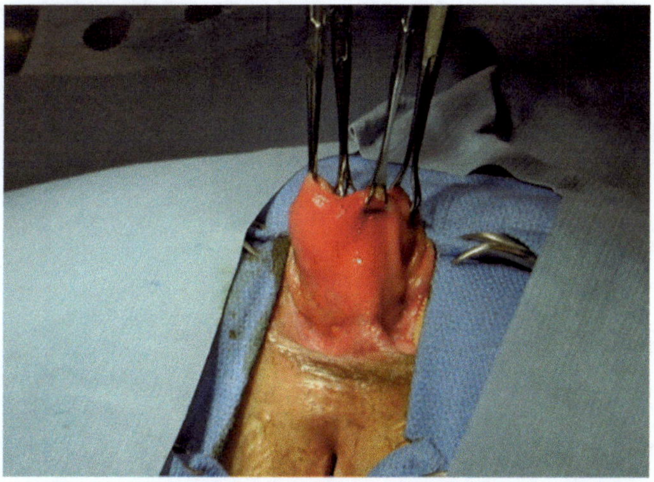

Fig. 11.2 Rectal prolapse during perineal repair

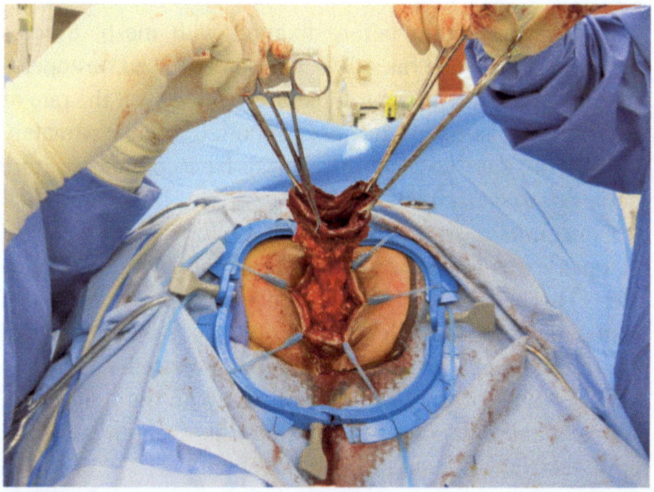

Fig. 11.3 Extraction of rectum and sigmoid during perineal proctosigmoidectomy

is then created with sutures or staples [4] (Fig. 11.4). Some surgeons reserve this perineal repair for older patients with comorbidities since major complications are reported to occur less often than after abdominal operations; the procedure can be performed without general anesthesia, and hospital stay is shorter [4]. Complications do occur, including pelvic bleeding, anastomotic leak, abscess, stricture, and bleeding from the anastomosis, but rates are typically less than 12 % [1, 4]. In addition, complications related to abdominal operations and pelvic dissection, such as sexual dysfunction, small bowel obstructions, wound infections, and incisional hernias, are avoided with the perineal approach [7]. Most studies show improvement in continence after perineal proctosigmoidectomy with levatorplasty similar to that seen after abdominal operations (20–90 %) [1]. Functional improvement in constipation is reported in a smaller number of series, with rates ranging from 61 to 100 %. The addition

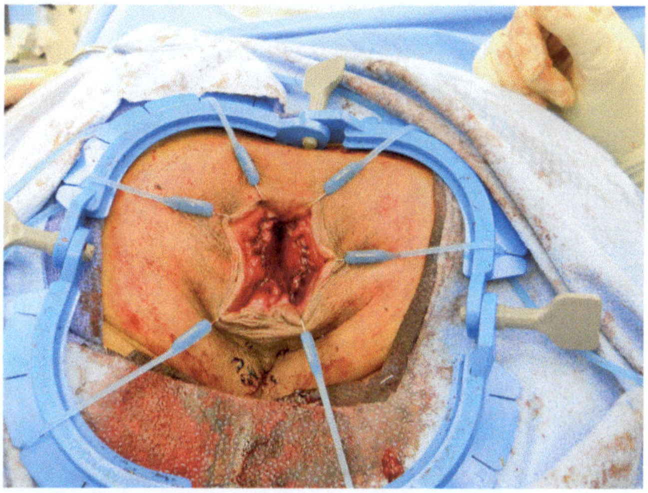

Fig. 11.4 Hand-sewn coloanal anastomosis during perineal proctosigmoidectomy

of the levatorplasty appears to decrease short-term recurrence rates and prolong the recurrence-free interval [1]. The addition of the colonic J pouch may also improve postoperative function. The senor author first described it and routinely employs it [8]. Some surgeons report low recurrence and morbidity rates with the perineal approach and advocate the Altemeier as the first-line treatment for patients of all ages.

Abdominal Operations

Key Concept: An abdominal operation, through either an open or minimally invasive approach, is the preferred operation for full-thickness rectal prolapse if the patient's risk profile permits. Regardless of the method chosen, adequate mobilization and fixation at the sacral promontory are required for optimal outcomes.

A variety of abdominal operations are performed to treat rectal prolapse based on the general principles of rectal mobilization and suspension of the rectum out of the pelvis. The operations vary by surgical technique (mobilization only, mobilization-rectopexy, mobilization-resection-rectopexy), means of access (laparoscopic or open) and method of fixation (suture or mesh) [9]. The extent of dissection, division of the lateral stalks, need for concomitant sigmoid resection, and method of rectal fixation are variable and remain points of controversy, as no single method has been shown to be more successful than the others and all have associated failures. Laparoscopy has been increasingly used for a variety of the prolapse repairs (including mesh or suture rectopexy and/or sigmoid resection) with similar recurrence and postoperative incontinence and constipation rates when compared to open surgery. Studies evaluating the laparoscopic approach indicate longer operative times but shorter hospital stays and lower overall costs [1].

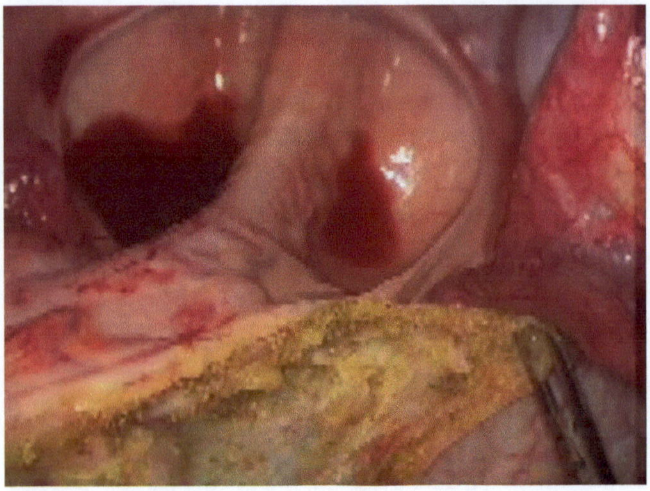

Fig. 11.5 Rectal mobilization during laparoscopic rectopexy

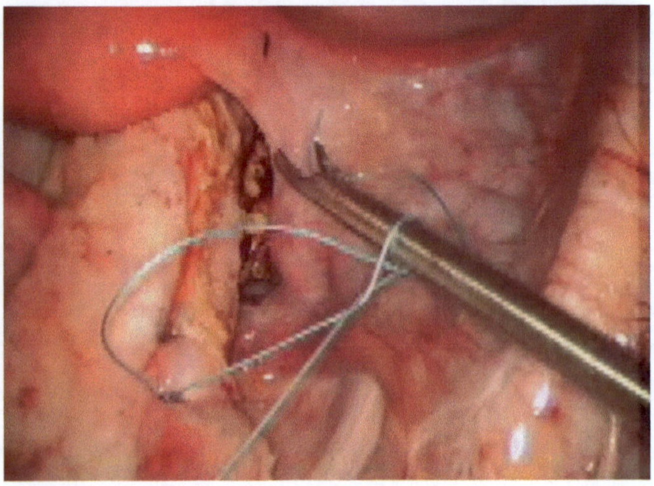

Fig. 11.6 Laparoscopic suture rectopexy

Mobilization of the rectum should extend caudally to the level of the pelvic floor musculature, specifically to the levator ani muscles, while the extent of lateral mobilization remains controversial (Fig. 11.5). In a small study performed by Speakman et al., division of the lateral stalks appeared to be associated with a high rate of postoperative constipation; however, division of the stalks was also found to be associated with decreased recurrence [1, 4]. Other studies have shown higher rates of constipation with stalk preservation [4]. Currently, most surgeons preserve the lateral stalks or may divide one lateral ligament.

The method of fixation of the rectum is also controversial, manifesting in the multitude of techniques available. Suture rectopexy is commonly performed with the advantage of avoiding the use of a prosthetic mesh, hopefully allowing good fixation with very little risk of infection or erosion, especially if a resection is performed concomitantly. Fixation with tacks has also been used. Rectopexy with mesh has been described with anterior or posterior placement [4]. The Ripstein repair and its variations involve placing a synthetic mesh around the mobilized rectum, attaching the mesh to the presacral fascia below the sacral promontory. Studies have shown low recurrence rates as well as improved incontinence in 20–60 % of patients [4]. Erosion and defecation problems have been noted with the anterior repair, and, accordingly, alternative approaches (attachment to the lateral mesorectum or variety of mesh types) have been used. The Wells mesh rectopexy originally used an Ivalon sponge (polyvinyl alcohol) with division of the lateral ligaments. The sponge is no longer used due to increased complications and postoperative constipation; however, this technique continues to be used with synthetic mesh [4]. Ventral mesh rectopexy (anterior mobilization of rectum) has also been described by D'Hoore et al., in order to decrease postoperative constipation. Orr-Loygue mesh rectopexy mobilizes both the anterior and posterior rectum before fixation with mesh. Studies show low recurrence rates (3.4 %) and decreased postoperative constipation with ventral rectopexy; however, the rate of new-onset constipation has been reported at approximately 14 % [4]. To date, no randomized trials have compared suture rectopexy to mesh fixation.

Concomitant sigmoid resection performed with suture rectopexy was first described by Frykman and Goldberg in 1969 [1]. The addition of the resection has decreased rates of postoperative constipation, but it does not appear to affect recurrence rates. The addition of a resection to the operation increases the potential risks associated with the transection of bowel and creation of an anastomosis, including anastomotic leak, abscess, and wound infection.

Laparoscopy and Rectal Prolapse Repair

Key Concept: A minimally invasive approach provides similar outcomes as open surgery, given experience and technical proficiency, and is increasingly being performed via laparoscopic and robotic means.

The first laparoscopic repair of rectal prolapse (rectopexy) was performed in 1992 [4]. Since that time, several studies have demonstrated that laparoscopy is safe and feasible for the treatment of prolapse (Figs. 11.6 and 11.7). Although these studies are small, they have shown similar recurrence and morbidity rates (4–8 % and 10–33 %, respectively) when compared to the open approach [4]. The benefits of laparoscopy have been reported in several studies. One small randomized trial by Solomon et al. found laparoscopy to be associated with less postoperative pain, faster return of bowel function, and shorter hospital stays, although operative times were longer [4, 10]. A meta-analysis performed in 2005 compared open to laparoscopic abdominal rectopexy [3]. This

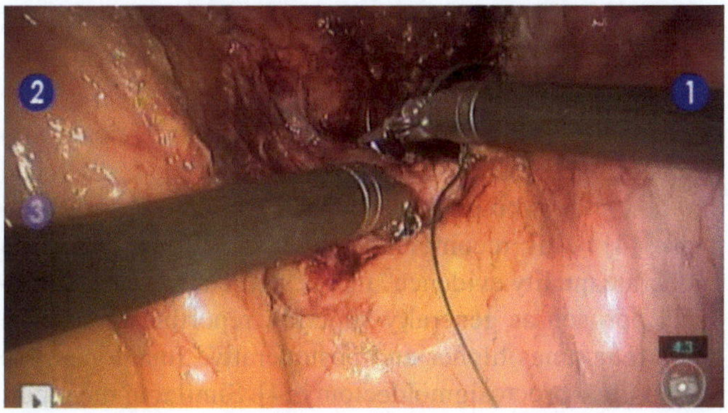

Fig. 11.7 Suture placement during robotically-assisted suture rectopexy

group found that operative time was longer for laparoscopy, but length of stay was shorter. However, overall recurrence was found to be similar between open and laparoscopic abdominal rectopexy with a mean follow-up time of 12–31 months for the included studies [3]. Byrne et al. investigated long-term functional outcomes between laparoscopic rectopexy and open and resection-rectopexy. They found that the recurrence rate remains low (7 % at 5 years and 11 % at 10 years follow-up) and that improvement of postoperative incontinence and constipation is similar when compared to the other operations; the majority of patients felt as if their constipation improved after surgery, and incontinence scores had improved [11]. The rate of wound complications also appeared to be lower in the laparoscopic group [4].

Robotic surgery has also been applied to the treatment of rectal prolapse (Fig. 11.7). There have been only a few series with small numbers reported. One small nonrandomized trial reported longer operating time and higher costs, but robotic-assisted mesh rectopexy was found to be safe and feasible [12]. Nonetheless, the visualization and ease of suturing during robotic surgery appears improved compared to conventional laparoscopy [4, 12]. Non-resectional rectopexy may be one of the better indications for robotic surgery as the procedure requires only a single docking of the robot and no incision is necessary for specimen retrieval. Moreover, unlike using laparoscopic instruments to suture the rectum to the anterior sacral fascia and periosteum, this step may potentially be reliably undertaken with the robotic platform.

Recurrence After Initial Repair

Key Concept: Recurrence rates increase with longer follow-up intervals and are typically higher with perineal procedures. An abdominal repair should be the initial approach when the patient's risk profile permits, while the type of procedure (i.e., rectopexy alone, mesh, resection) does not seem to influence recurrence rates.

Recurrence after initial prolapse repair has been reported to occur in 2–60 % of patients. These recurrence rates vary with type of approach, technique, preoperative anorectal and pelvic anatomy and function, and length of follow-up among other variables. Most studies have shown lower recurrence rates for abdominal repairs; whereas the reasons for this difference are not exactly clear, it is likely due to inadequate mobilization and resection of the rectum and sigmoid that results from lack of direct visualization during the perineal approach. Several studies have tried to identify predictors of recurrence. To date, there is very little conclusive evidence identifying specific risk factors. It is possible that rectal prolapse is just one symptom of overall pelvic floor dysfunction, which may recur if the overall pelvic environment is not changed.

Recurrence After Altemeier Procedure

Key Concept: The wide range of reported recurrence rates following an Altemeier are likely multifactorial and include technical variables (i.e., small resected segment, failure to enter the peritoneal cavity) and patient-driven factors (prior surgery, length of follow-up).

Several studies have examined the recurrence rates after perineal rectosigmoidectomy. In a literature review, the range of recurrence rates found for the Altemeier procedure was between 0 and 58 % [2]. In a study performed by Altomare et al., 17 (18 %) of 93 patients experienced complete recurrence after being followed for at least 12 months (median 41, 12–112). Six other patients had recurrence of mucosal prolapse only [2]. Of the 17 patients with full-thickness recurrence, repeat Altemeier was performed in 6, Delorme in 1, and Wells mesh rectopexy in 1; the 9 patients refused further surgery [2]. These authors found that only previous surgery for prolapse was associated with higher recurrence; other factors such as duration of follow-up, length of resected specimen, levatorplasty, age, sex, and severity of incontinence were not significantly associated [2]. At Washington University in St. Louis, Glasgow et al. found a recurrence rate of 8.5 % when 106 consecutive patients with full-thickness rectal prolapse had perineal proctectomy performed regardless of preoperative status (age, comorbidities, previous abdominal or anorectal surgery). In a study by Cirocco et al. published in 2010, 103 consecutive patients with full-thickness rectal prolapse were treated with perineal proctosigmoidectomy between 2000 and 2009. The authors reported that 61 % of patients had preoperative constipation; 94 % of these patients had improvement. Forty-seven percent had fecal incontinence, which improved in 85 % of patients following surgery [7]. This group found no recurrences with a mean follow-up of 43 months [7]. In their discussion, the authors allude to their lack of understanding regarding the historically high recurrence rates reported after perineal repair. Interestingly, in their literature review, cumulative recurrence rate was 37 % for studies performed before 1971 and only 10 % in reports published after 1971 [7]. The higher rates of recurrence were suspected to be due to poor surgical technique, especially in those cases where the mobilization failed to enter the peritoneal cavity.

Several studies have reported lower recurrence and improved outcomes after abdominal repair. Only one small randomized trial compared the perineal to transabdominal approach. Abdominal resection-rectopexy with pelvic floor repair was compared to perineal rectosigmoidectomy with pelvic floor repair in 20 elderly female patients with full-thickness rectal prolapse and fecal incontinence (10 patients in each arm) [13]. There were no recurrences following resection-rectopexy and only one after rectosigmoidectomy. Continence, frequency of defecation, maximal resting pressure, and compliance all appeared to improve more after resection-rectopexy versus perineal proctosigmoidectomy [13]. However, according to a Cochrane review by Bachoo et al. in 2000, which was updated by Tou et al. in 2008, no conclusive data indicate that the abdominal approach is superior to the perineal approach [14, 15]. This conclusion is likely due to the small number and size of randomized trials directly comparing both approaches. Perineal proctosigmoidectomy continues to constitute 50–60 % of operations conducted for rectal prolapse [15].

Recurrence After Abdominal Approach

Key Concept: Recurrence rates are similar among the various abdominal operations and in general are <10 % in single institutional studies, with larger series demonstrating higher rates at extended follow-up intervals.

In 2005, the Rectal Prolapse Recurrence Study Group evaluated recurrence of full-thickness rectal prolapse after abdominal operations [9]. They examined the individual pooled data for 643 patients. Overall recurrence was 1 %, 6 %, and almost 29 % at 1-, 5-, and 10-year follow-up, respectively, regardless of the method employed [9]. The surgical technique, means of access, and method of rectopexy all had no significant effect on recurrence [9]. Interestingly, the degree of complexity of the operation also did not influence recurrence (mobilization alone had similar recurrence compared to resection-rectopexy) [9]. Long-term recurrence rates were almost 30 % after 10 years, much higher than some proponents of the abdominal approach have reported in the short term.

In 2011, the Standards Practice Task Force of the American Society of Colon and Rectal Surgeons published practice parameters for rectal prolapse based on studies and trials performed between 1978 and 2010. Recommendations were formulated and graded on quality of evidence. This task force indicated that for patients who are acceptable surgical candidates, transabdominal rectal fixation should be the procedure of choice for rectal prolapse [4]. This recommendation was "strong, based on moderate quality evidence" that described the transabdominal approach as generally superior, reporting recurrence rates four times higher and postoperative function worse for perineal proctosigmoidectomy [4]. Similar to the report of Raftopoulos et al., this group noted that type of rectal fixation did not significantly influence recurrence. They noted recurrence after suture rectopexy to occur in 3–9 % of patients [4], reporting that worsening of preoperative constipation or new-onset constipation can occur with suture rectopexy [4]. This task force also indicated that the addition of resection to rectopexy was associated with lower recurrence and improved function for patients with preoperative constipation. Recurrence rates after resection-rectopexy were noted to be 2–5 %. However, complications were higher, likely due to associated anastomotic complications. It does appear that improvement of fecal incontinence after resection-rectopexy is less than seen without sigmoid colectomy [4].

Recurrence rates are also low for mesh rectopexy. Although higher morbidities did result from erosion or infection, recurrence was reported to be only 2.3–5 % [4]. A study performed at Cleveland Clinic by Hool et al. investigated recurrent rectal prolapse, management, and risk factors. They reported on 24 patients who were operated on for recurrent rectal prolapse out of 234 patients seen for prolapse from 1963 to 1993. Median time to recurrence was 2 years; however, 30 % occurred within 7 months of the initial operation [6]. The cause of recurrence was identified in 12 of the 24 patients; 11 were found to be associated with mesh used during the initial Ripstein repair (mesh pulled off from the rectum or sacrum, loose sling, misplacement or removal of mesh for pain) [6]. The majority of repairs for recurrent prolapse were performed transabdominally; only one patient had recurrence after the second repair (who also recurred after a third operation) [6].

Types of Operations for Recurrence

Key Concept: An abdominal repair should be the preferred approach, whenever possible, for recurrent prolapse patients. Any prior anastomosis should be resected when performing a second repair that involves a resection. You should exercise caution when considering early surgical intervention in patients with functional problems following abdominal prolapse repairs and rely instead on bowel regimen adjustments, bowel training, and time.

Rates of recurrence after prolapse repair have been reported between 10 and 20 %, regardless of the type of operation performed; rates as high as 30 % have been reported in some studies [1, 10]. It is unclear why recurrence rates are higher for perineal operations. Hypotheses include the ability to perform a complete rectal mobilization and fixation under direct visualization during abdominal operations and making more accurate decisions regarding resection and/or rectopexy [10]. Recurrences are considered either early (1–2 years), likely due to technical error, or late (>2 years), which may be due to patient-related factors. In a study of 78 patients with recurrent rectal prolapse, Steele et al. reported that 29 % of patients recurred in the first 7 months after the initial operation [10]. Overall re-recurrence occurred in 29 % of patients, significantly more after perineal repair for the recurrence versus an abdominal approach [10]. If a repair fails, evaluation including imaging for slow-transit constipation or puborectalis dysfunction, endoanal ultrasound, manometry, defecography, and colonoscopy should be performed depending on the associated features (constipation or incontinence). Comorbidities should also be investigated with cardiac and pulmonary testing when indicated because, if possible, repair of recurrent rectal prolapse should be attempted transabdominally. The reason for this is that secondary recurrence appears to be lower when compared to the perineal approach for recurrent prolapse [5, 10].

Fengler et al. examined the management of recurrent rectal prolapse. They identified 14 patients who underwent surgery for recurrence over a 10-year period. Most of these patients initially underwent perineal proctosigmoidectomy; however, surgeries for the recurrence included transabdominal and perineal approaches [16]. Although this study was small, no full-thickness prolapses were noted during the follow-up period (9–115 months) [16]. Pikarsky et al. evaluated the outcomes of 27 patients with repair of recurrent rectal prolapse versus 27 matched controls that underwent initial repair of rectal prolapse during the same time period. Perineal proctosigmoidectomy was the most commonly performed operation for recurrent prolapse, whereas perineal and transabdominal approaches were almost equivalently performed in the initial prolapse group [17]. Recurrence rates were not different between the recurrent and initial prolapse groups: 14.8 and 13.1 %, respectively [17]. The authors also found no differences in anorectal physiology testing, ultrasound, defecography, or concomitant anorectal pathology; thus, they could not identify other factors contributing to recurrence after prolapse surgery besides presumed technical errors [17].

If evaluation after recurrence reveals persistent or worsening constipation or a redundant sigmoid colon on imaging, resection is indicated regardless of the first operation. If constipation is persistent after non-resectional rectopexy, conservative measures including bowel retraining should be undertaken for a minimum of 6–12 months prior to consideration of a colectomy. Outside of the United States, sacral nerve stimulation might well be potentially indicated in this population but is currently unavailable for this indication in the United States. One must be very cautious when performing a sigmoid colectomy or subtotal colectomy after an initial non-resectional rectopexy, in particular if mesh has been used to stabilize the rectum either anteriorly or posteriorly. The risk of an infection is certainly of concern, and in addition, the amount of pelvic scarring may potentially increase the risk of pelvic bleeding and anastomotic difficulties. Moreover, if the initial anastomosis was performed at the 15-cm level, a more distal level of anastomosis might be required. One must be cautious about such an anastomosis especially if the patient has decreased sphincter tone and/or if a subtotal rather than a sigmoid colectomy is being considered, as postoperative diarrhea (or incontinence) may be extremely debilitating.

If a second resection is planned, removal of the previous anastomosis is important to prevent ischemia with resultant mucosal sloughing, anastomotic dehiscence, or stricture may occur [1, 16]. Fengler et al. noted mucosa sloughing after perineal proctosigmoidectomy was performed for recurrent prolapse after the initial operation was an anterior resection. They indicated that unless resection of the previous anastomosis is conducted, resection for the recurrence should be avoided [16]. The authors also noted that if the initial surgery was an Altemeier procedure, the anastomosis will likely prolapse; thus, repeat perineal proctosigmoidectomy should incorporate resection of the previous anastomosis, decreasing the likelihood of ischemia or anastomotic complications after the recurrent prolapse repair [16]. An attempt to preserve the superior hemorrhoidal artery during a resection-rectopexy should be made if a perineal proctosigmoidectomy was performed for the initial prolapse [1]. In the study by Steele et al., only two patients developed a stricture postoperatively. The authors partly attributed this low incidence to the preservation of the superior hemorrhoidal vascular supply when resection-rectopexy was performed after perineal proctosigmoidectomy [10].

Outcomes after repair of recurrent prolapse have been examined in only a few small studies. Recurrence rates have been shown to be equivalent to those after the initial surgery, regardless of the approach. There is also not much evidence evaluating incontinence or constipation after repair of recurrent prolapse. In a small study of 14 patients who underwent surgery for recurrent prolapse over a 10-year period, three patients were incontinent initially, and they remained incontinent even after successful repair of the recurrent prolapse [16]. It is the preference of the senior author to preserve the inferior mesenteric and superior rectal vessels during all abdominal resection-rectopexy procedures.

The discussion of laparoscopy and recurrent rectal prolapse is extremely limited. Tsugawa et al. published a case report in 2002. They used laparoscopic rectopexy safely in two patients, without complications or recurrence noted in a 2-year follow-up [18].

Our Treatment Preferences for Rectal Prolapse

Initial Rectal Prolapse

Key Concept: We prefer a laparoscopic abdominal approach, when feasible. Based on symptoms and subsequent work-up for significant constipation, this may involve a resection-rectopexy (when absent) or subtotal colectomy (when present).

If the patient is unfit for a transabdominal operation, then we would discuss with the patient the alternative transperineal options. If a transabdominal operation is planned and the patient has constipation, a colonic transit study should be undertaken to insure that a subtotal colectomy with ileorectal or ileosigmoid anastomosis is not potentially advisable. In addition, cinedefecography and/or water-soluble contrast enema testing may reveal a significantly redundant sigmoid colon that usually mitigates for concomitant sigmoid colectomy. Our preference is generally for a resection-rectopexy unless the patient has profound incontinence and limited sigmoid redundancy. The reason for a resection-rectopexy is to avoid the problems with constipation after non-resectional rectopexy that are likely to occur in this setting.

The procedure will preferentially be performed in a laparoscopic manner with a camera in an infraumbilical port and the two working ports in the right upper quadrant and right lower quadrant, respectively. We routinely employ ureteric catheters in patients in whom significant adhesions and/or fibrosis is expected. This operation is the only one in which we deliberately do not mobilize the splenic flexure as we wish to have a tension-free anastomosis without redundancy. Due to the inevitable redundancy of the left colon, splenic flexure mobilization is generally unnecessary. It is useful to try to avoid redundancy, and in fact, the sigmoid colectomy is performed to avoid redundancy. Therefore, routine splenic flexure mobilization in this scenario seems counterproductive.

In addition, we deliberately do not divide either the inferior mesenteric artery/vein or the superior rectal artery/vein. After full left colonic mobilization, the presacral space is entered, and a dissection as for a total mesorectal excision is undertaken to the level of the levator muscles. The mobilization proceeds with visual, digital, and flexible sigmoidoscopic assessment if necessary. Lateral dissection definitely decreases recurrence rates, although it very well may induce constipation. However, the concomitant performance of a sigmoid colectomy with the rectopexy should balance this potential problem. Therefore, the combination of resection and rectopexy with division of the lateral stalks would seem to offer the best combination of good outcomes – including simultaneously minimizing both recurrence rates and postoperative constipation.

After full mobilization, irrigation, and verification of meticulous hemostasis, a short suprapubic or short Pfannenstiel incision is made. The rectopexy is then generally undertaken utilizing two 0-Prolene sutures through each lateral stalk including the periosteum in a horizontal U-stitch. The three to four rectopexy sutures are tagged but not tied. The points of resection of the descending-sigmoid junction and the rectosigmoid junction are then divided. It is important that the superiormost rectopexy sutures are not in immediate proximity to the anastomosis to hopefully avoid any acute angulation of that anastomosis. The left colonic and sigmoidal vessels are divided with an energy source along the bowel wall in order to carefully preserve the superior rectal and inferior mesenteric vessels to insure optimal collateral blood supply. Division of these vessels has unfortunately been associated with rectal necrosis. A standard circular end-to-end anastomosis is performed between the descending colon and the rectum. The standard air insufflation test is undertaken using flexible endoscopic guidance, after which the rectopexy sutures are carefully secured. It is important to insure that the posterior aspects of the lateral stalks are tied flush against the periosteum and that there are no gaps through which small bowel might slip and become injured by the rectopexy sutures. After the sutures are secured, the air testing is again repeated with flexible sigmoidoscopy to also insure that the rectal lumen has not been compromised or narrowed. Ultimately a 19-mm suction drain is placed through a stab wound and left in the presacral space, and the abdomen is closed. An incision of greater than 7 cm is seldom necessary, except in obese patients.

We do not like to use mesh because of the risk of infection. Moreover, having operated on many patients in whom prolapse has recurred after mesh placement, it is only with great trepidation that we would perform anastomosis in the vicinity of the mesh. Moreover, excision of the mesh is often impossible without rectal resection, which then brings about the scenario of a low pelvic anastomosis. Sutures through the lateral stalks incorporating the anterior periosteum and presacral fascia should be sufficient to stabilize the rectum without need for introducing mesh.

Perineal Proctosigmoidectomy

Key Concept: Perineal approaches are used only for a select group of patients. Balancing adequate removal of redundant bowel with avoiding tension at the anastomosis is key to successful outcomes.

Once again, we prefer this operation for frail elderly patients and for patients with significant comorbidity, as well as for patients who have had prior failed perineal rectosigmoidectomy. In instances of circumferential mucosal prolapse or minimal circumferential full-thickness prolapse after failed perineal rectosigmoidectomy, a Delorme procedure could be considered. It is important as part of the Delorme procedure to ensure imbrications of the muscle prior to creating an anastomosis.

We perform this perineal operation with the patient in prone position, under general anesthesia or with an epidural or local with sedation. We use a handheld energy device for division of the mesorectum and mesentery. We slowly extract the rectum and sigmoid until there is resistance, carefully making sure that there is hemostasis and that no bleeding vessels retract into the anal canal. Once resistance is felt, the colon is manipulated to be sure that there is no more redundant sigmoid left. Although the entire redundancy should be extracted, there should be no tension on the coloanal anastomosis. The few tricks to try to decrease the rate of anastomotic leak include leaving enough laxity under the mesocolon to comfortably lift it from the recto-peritoneum, placing the anastomosis far enough cephalad to the rectopexy sutures to prevent acute angulation with obstruction, and preservation of the inferior mesenteric and superior rectal vessels. We also prefer to create a 6×6 to 8×8 cm colonic J pouch whenever possible.

Before the anastomosis is created, the levatorplasty is usually performed. With simple sutures, if possible the anterior and posterior levator muscles are plicated, ensuring that their outlet is narrowed without placing too much tension on the proximal colon that is about to be anastomosed to the anoderm. In general, it is much easier to plicate the anterior levator muscles although this approach is the converse of the Parks' posterior anal repair. Approximately 1–2 fingerbreadths left between the levatorplasty and the colon should be adequate. The levatorplasty may help decrease incontinence as well as provide more support to prevent recurrence. We hand sew our anastomoses with interrupted 3-0 Vicryl sutures; however, a transanal stapler can be used to create the anastomosis. A circular stapled anastomosis is performed in a manner akin to a PPH™ (Ethicon Endo-Surgery, Cincinnati, OH) procedure in that two circumferential purse strings can be used – one in the descending colon or colonic J-pouch and the other in the anoderm. In instances in which a stapled anastomosis is to be undertaken, sufficient redundancy must exist and in addition minimal size discrepancy. Furthermore, the initial incision should be at least 2 cm above the dentate line so that the anastomosis is not at or potentially even below the dentate line.

Incarcerated Rectal Prolapse

Perineal proctosigmoidectomy is the treatment of choice for incarcerated rectal prolapse, regardless of the patient's health. The operation is performed in standard fashion, making sure that the entire ischemic portion of the rectum and sigmoid is resected.

Concomitant Pelvic Prolapse

Key Concept: A complete evaluation for other pelvic floor disorders should be performed, as a multidisciplinary approach may be required to repair all defects.

It is the responsibility of the colorectal surgeon to ask about associated gynecological and urological symptoms when patients present with prolapse. During the physical examination, perineal descent or uterine, vaginal, or bladder prolapse may be noted. These patients are best managed with a multidisciplinary approach with consultation with urogynecology, and they should have a thorough evaluation including defecography, transvaginal and transrectal ultrasound, or urodynamic testing depending on the patient's presentation. Defecography is undertaken in cases of internal prolapse. I have not found any additional information to be gained from defecography in patients with visible circumferential full-thickness rectal prolapse.

Combined procedures are reasonable and usually preferred by the patient, although the surgical approach must be discussed initially in order to avoid placing mesh in the pelvis if a sigmoid resection is planned.

Recurrent Rectal Prolapse

Key Concept: In the setting of recurrent prolapse, a thorough history and physical examination will guide the need for adjuvant studies. When possible, a transabdominal repair should be your initial choice.

If a patient has recurrent full-thickness rectal prolapse, evaluation is guided by the patient's symptoms. If the patient has constipation that continued or worsened after the initial operation, a colonic transit study and defecography should be conducted to evaluate for potential colonic inertia or obstructed defecation syndrome. If the patient is incontinent, endoanal ultrasound, manometry, and physiologic testing should be performed. The positive findings may have contributed to failure of the initial repair and may change our next steps in management. It is reasonable to recommend biofeedback first if pelvic floor dysfunction is present before repairing the recurrent prolapse or postoperatively once the patient recovers. This method may help manage the patient's expectations after surgery.

Regardless of the initial repair, we recommend a transabdominal repair if the patient is medically fit. The selection of the operation is determined based on the previous repair and the patient's current symptoms. If the patient has no constipation and no evidence of sigmoid redundancy, we perform a suture rectopexy, regardless of whether the patient had a previous perineal repair or abdominal approach with or without resection. If constipation is also present, we add a resection, including the previous anastomosis if resection was performed initially. We again attempt to preserve the superior hemorrhoidal artery if resection is planned. Suture rectopexy without resection should not result in ischemia regardless of the previous repair.

If the patient had a previous perineal proctosigmoidectomy and is at excessive risk for a transabdominal operation, we perform a repeat perineal operation. If the previous anastomosis

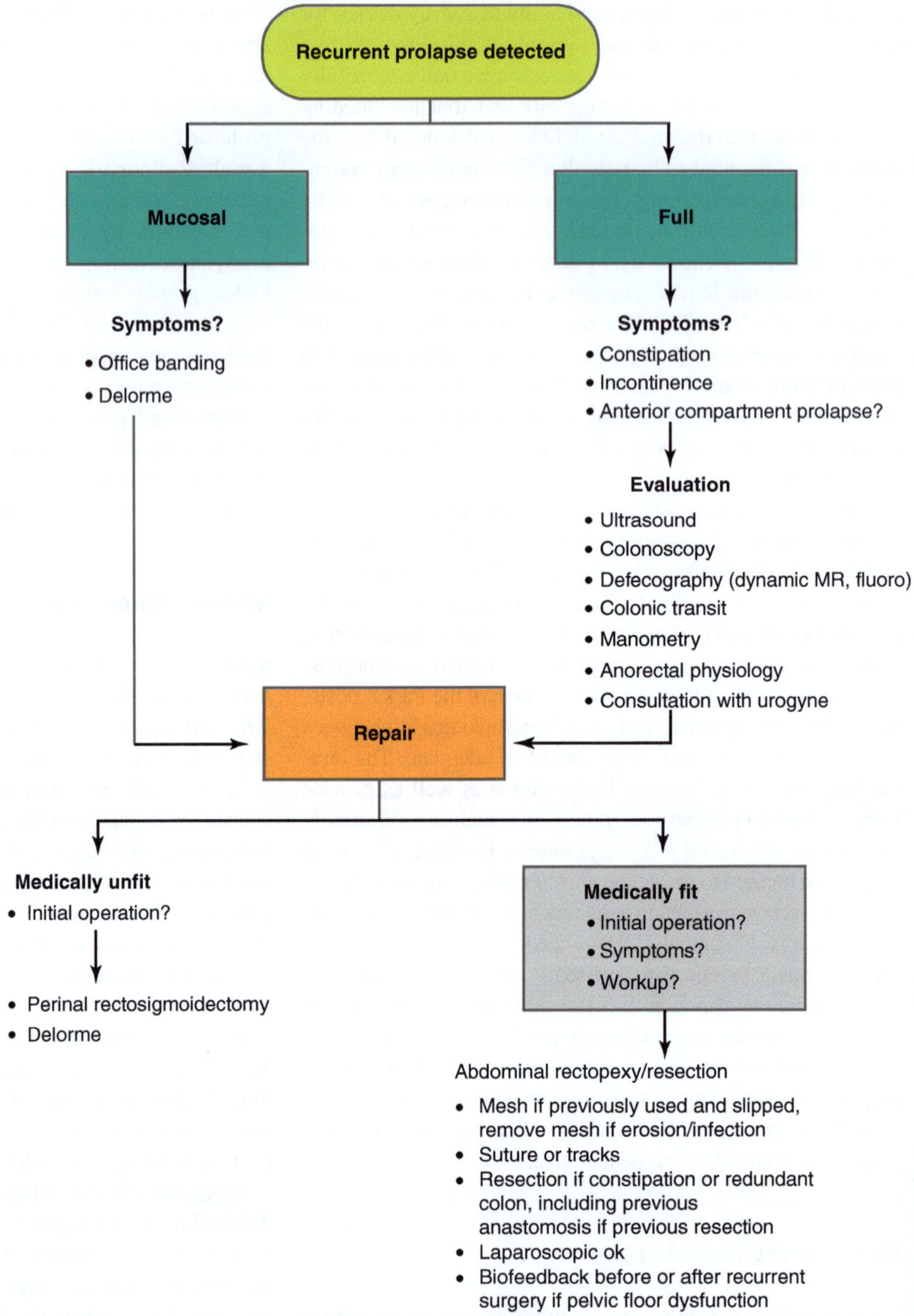

Fig. 11.8 Treatment algorithm for recurrent rectal prolapse

cannot be transanally resected or if the blood supply appears questionable, we would perform a Delorme procedure.

If the patient had a previous laparoscopic rectopexy with or without resection, we would consider a laparoscopic approach to repair the recurrence. We always perform laparoscopy using the open Hasson technique; however, in the case of a previous operation, an open technique is mandatory. If the patient had multiple abdominal operations or evidence of significant scar tissue at previous incisions on abdominal exam, we would likely perform an open procedure. Due to the reoperative nature of the surgery for recurrence, we would likely use ureteral stents for a transabdominal approach.

Summary Pearls

Patients' expectations should be managed from the initial encounter. An honest discussion regarding the risk of recurrence after the initial and second repair (not higher than after the initial operation according to the literature) is essential, using information provided in the individual patient's evaluation. Nonoperative management of recurrence is generally recommended only if the patient is unfit for even a perineal repair or if the symptoms are minimal and not too bothersome to the patient. Limited mucosal prolapse after initial prolapse repair is not considered true recurrence in the literature; in-office banding procedures can be performed, or if more significant, a Delorme procedure can be attempted if the patient is willing to undergo another operation.

They should also understand that the ultimate functional outcome of the procedure cannot be expected in less than 1–2 years after surgery. It is best to include not only the patient but, if the patient consents, also the family in these discussions. The postoperative function can sometimes be optimized by a combination of anti-motility agents, fiber, and pelvic floor retraining for the immediate postoperative period and potentially for the first 1–2 years. Regardless of the technique used, understanding the pearls and pitfalls for each procedure and sharing realistic expectations with the patient regarding both function and recurrence will prove extremely beneficial in managing rectal prolapsed (Fig. 11.8).

References

1. O'Brien D. Rectal prolapse. Clin Colon Rectal Surg. 2007;20(2):125–32.
2. Altomare D, Binda G, Ganio E, De Nardi P, Giamundo P, Pescatori M. Long-term outcome of Altemeier's procedure for rectal prolapse. Dis Colon Rectum. 2009;52(4):698–703.
3. Purkayastha S, Tekkis P, Athanasiou T, et al. A comparison of open vs. laparoscopic abdominal rectopexy for full-thickness rectal prolapse: a meta-analysis. Dis Colon Rectum. 2005;48(10):1930–40.
4. Varma M, Rafferty J, Buie WD. Practice parameters for the management of rectal prolapse. Dis Colon Rectum. 2011;54(11):1339–46.
5. Papaconstantinou HT. Recurrent rectal prolapse. In: Billingham RP, Kobashi KC, Peters WA, editors. Reoperative pelvic surgery. New York: Springer; 2009. p. 145–51.
6. Hool GR, Hull TL, Fazio VW. Surgical treatment of recurrent complete rectal prolapse: a thirty-year experience. Dis Colon Rectum. 1997;40(3):270–2.
7. Cirocco W. The Altemeier procedure for rectal prolapse: an operation for all ages. Dis Colon Rectum. 2010;53(12):1618–23.
8. Baig MK, Galliano D, Larach JA, Weiss EG, Wexner SD, Nogueras JJ. Pouch perineal rectosigmoidectomy: a case report. Surg Innov. 2005;12(4):373–5.
9. Raftopoulos Y, Senagore A, Di Giuro G, Bergamaschi R. Recurrence rates after abdominal surgery for complete rectal prolapse: a multicenter pooled analysis of 643 individual patient data. Dis Colon Rectum. 2005;48(6):1200–6.
10. Steele S, Goetz L, Minami S, Madoff R, Mellgren A, Parker S. Management of recurrent rectal prolapse: surgical approach influences outcome. Dis Colon Rectum. 2006;49(4):440–5.
11. Byrne C, Smith S, Solomon M, Young J, Eyers A, Young C. Long-term functional outcomes after laparoscopic and open rectopexy for the treatment of rectal prolapse. Dis Colon Rectum. 2008;51(11):1597–604.
12. Heemskerk J, de Hoog Dominique ENM, van Gemert W, Baeten CGMI, Greve JWM, Bouvy N. Robot-assisted vs. conventional laparoscopic rectopexy for rectal prolapse: a comparative study on costs and time. Dis Colon Rectum. 2007;50(11):1825–30.
13. Deen KI, Grant E, Billingham C, Keighley MR. Abdominal resection-rectopexy with pelvic floor repair versus perineal rectosigmoidectomy and pelvic floor repair for full-thickness rectal prolapse. Br J Surg. 1994;81(2):302–4.
14. Bachoo P, Brazzelli M, Grant A. Surgery for complete rectal prolapse in adults. Cochrane Database Syst Rev. 2000;(2):CD001758.
15. Glasgow S, Birnbaum E, Kodner I, Fleshman J, Dietz D. Recurrence and quality of life following perineal proctectomy for rectal prolapse. J Gastrointest Surg. 2008;12(8):1446–51.
16. Fengler SA, Pearl RK, Prasad ML, et al. Management of recurrent rectal prolapse. Dis Colon Rectum. 1997,40(7):832–4.
17. Pikarsky AJ, Joo JS, Wexner SD, et al. Recurrent rectal prolapse: what is the next good option? Dis Colon Rectum. 2000;43(9):1273–6.
18. Tsugawa K, Sue K, Koyanagi N, et al. Laparoscopic rectopexy for recurrent rectal prolapse: a safe and simple procedure without a mesh prosthesis. Hepatogastroenterology. 2002;49(48):1549–51.

Obstructive Defecation

12

Ann C. Lowry and Jennifer Lynn Irani

Key Points

- Obstructed defecation is defined by patient symptoms.
- Adjunctive tests such as transit studies, anorectal manometry, balloon expulsion, EMG, fluoroscopic (conventional) defecography, MR defecography, and perineal ultrasound may be useful in identifying a potential cause for a patient's symptoms but ought to be interpreted cautiously.
- Treatment depends on the etiology of obstructed defecation and is initially nonoperative. Fiber, improved toileting habits, and biofeedback are generally the primary approach.
- Obstructive defecation symptoms improve with rectocele repair, but optimal surgical approach remains uncertain.
- Preliminary results for ventral rectopexy and STARR for internal intussusception are emerging.

A.C. Lowry, MD (✉)
Division of Colorectal Surgery, Department of Surgery,
University of Minnesota, 1055 Westgate Drive, Suite 190,
St. Paul, Minneapolis, MN 55114, USA
e-mail: alowry@crsal.org

J.L. Irani, MD
Department of Surgery,
Harvard Medical School,
Brigham and Women's Hospital,
75 Francis Street, Boston, MA 02115, USA
e-mail: jirani@partners.org

Evaluation

History

Key Concept: Obstructive defecation is defined by patient symptoms.

The prevalence of constipation ranges from 0.7 to 79 %, with a median of 16 % worldwide, and patients with outlet dysfunction (i.e., obstructive defecation) make up a significant portion [1]. While differentiating among the various etiologies of constipation can be difficult, a careful history remains the key aspect. Patients with obstructive defecation complain of the need for prolonged straining and of a sense of incomplete rectal evacuation. Frequently they report spending up to 30 min in the bathroom attempting to defecate. They often use laxatives or enemas; they may use digital extraction and vaginal or perineal pressure to aid evacuation. Some patients may complain of both an infrequent urge to defecate and difficulty evacuating stool that reaches the rectum. While abdominal discomfort may accompany these symptoms, it is not the dominant complaint, as opposed to patients with slow-transit constipation or irritable bowel syndrome. Nausea and emesis are rare. Rectal pain is unusual unless the etiology is sphincter spasm related to an anal fissure.

Physical Examination

Key Concept: Obstructive defecation has a large differential diagnosis. It is critical to exclude mechanical causes of obstruction such as anal or rectal cancers.

The term obstructive defecation covers a set of symptoms that may be caused by rectal prolapse, internal rectal prolapse, rectocele, enterocele, pelvic organ prolapse, solitary rectal ulcer syndrome, descending perineum syndrome, and pelvic floor muscle dysfunction. The portion of the syndrome that relates to pelvic floor muscle dysfunction is also known as paradoxical puborectalis contraction, non-relaxing

S.R. Steele et al. (eds.), *Complexities in Colorectal Surgery*,
DOI 10.1007/978-1-4614-9022-7_12,

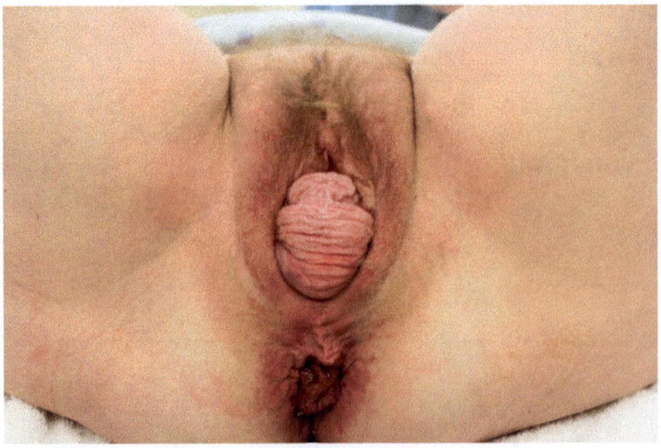

Fig. 12.1 Rectocele. Rectal prolapse can also seen at the verge that was easily visualized with straining (*Courtesy of M. Shane McNevin, MD*)

puborectalis syndrome, outlet obstruction, anismus, pelvic floor dyssynergia, spastic pelvic floor syndrome, and dyschezia. The first step in the evaluation is a careful physical examination. The purpose of the examination of these patients is to exclude other abnormalities and to identify the underlying cause. Inspection of the perianal area may reveal a patulous anus, skin irritation, or an anal fissure. The perianal and perineal regions should be examined at rest and with straining for perineal descent, rectal prolapse, and vaginal bulge (Fig. 12.1). The digital examination may reveal stenosis or a mass causing the symptoms. Attention should be paid to resting tone, squeeze, and sphincter response to Valsalva during the digital examination. The sphincter muscles and puborectalis muscle normally relax with straining. The examiner should also be aware to check for rectal wall descending during Valsalva (i.e., intussusception or prolapse) or a bulging from above in the rectovaginal septum (i.e., enterocele). Pressure on the anterior rectal wall during the examination may also identify a rectocele. Examination on the commode after bearing down may reveal a rectal prolapse or significant vaginal prolapse.

A careful urogynecologic examination is also important, particularly in any patient with a suggestion of rectal or other pelvic organ prolapse. If prolapse is visible at the vaginal introitus or a bulge is noted during the Valsalva maneuver, a systematic examination should be performed. With the patient in a supine position and the head of the examination table elevated to 45°, an appropriately sized vaginal speculum is placed in the vagina to view the cervix or vaginal cuff. While the patient is performing the Valsalva maneuver, the speculum is slowly removed. The extent to which the cervix or the vaginal vault follows the speculum through and out of the vagina is noted. The speculum is disassembled and the posterior or fixed blade is used for examination. To examine the anterior vaginal wall, the posterior vaginal wall is retracted with the fixed blade and the extent of any anterior vaginal prolapse during the Valsalva maneuver is noted. To examine the posterior vaginal wall, the fixed blade is inverted, the anterior vaginal wall is retracted, and the patient is instructed to repeat the Valsalva maneuver. Any resulting prolapse or bulge is noted. Bimanual and rectovaginal examinations help identify any coexisting pelvic abnormalities, including those of the perineal body. If pelvic organ prolapse is not evident, especially in a woman feeling a bulge, the patient should be examined in the standing position while she performs the Valsalva maneuver [2].

Endoscopy

The next step in evaluation of these patients is anoscopy and flexible sigmoidoscopy or colonoscopy. Anoscopy may identify circumferential folds in the rectal wall descending from above indicating a possible prolapse or intussusception. While the choice of endoscopic procedure is determined by the patient's age and interval since last screening examination, it is necessary to exclude polyps or neoplasm as the cause of the obstructive symptoms. The examination may also identify a solitary rectal ulcer, colitis cystica profunda, or any suspicious lesion that should be biopsied to exclude a neoplastic process and confirm the diagnosis. If the endoscopy is negative, the next step depends upon your clinical suspicion for another diagnosis and the patient's response to conservative therapy

Adjunctive Tests

Key Concept: *Additional testing is useful if the patient has mixed symptoms of infrequent urge and obstructed defecation. The testing is also performed to confirm findings on physical examination as the source of the symptoms or to identify the cause if there is uncertainty on the physical examination.*

There is no single test that is able to definitively diagnose obstructive defecation or the underlying etiology. Several adjunctive studies may be performed to help arrive at a diagnosis, including transit studies, anorectal manometry, balloon expulsion, EMG, fluoroscopic (conventional) defecography, MR defecography, and perineal ultrasound [3, 4]. If the patient complains of an infrequent urge to defecate, as well as difficult evacuation, colonic transit time and balloon expulsion tests may be useful to determine the primary problem.

Colonic Transit Study

Colonic transit can be evaluated with a colonic marker study (Fig. 12.2a, b) [3]. This test involves asking the patient to swallow a capsule containing radiopaque rings

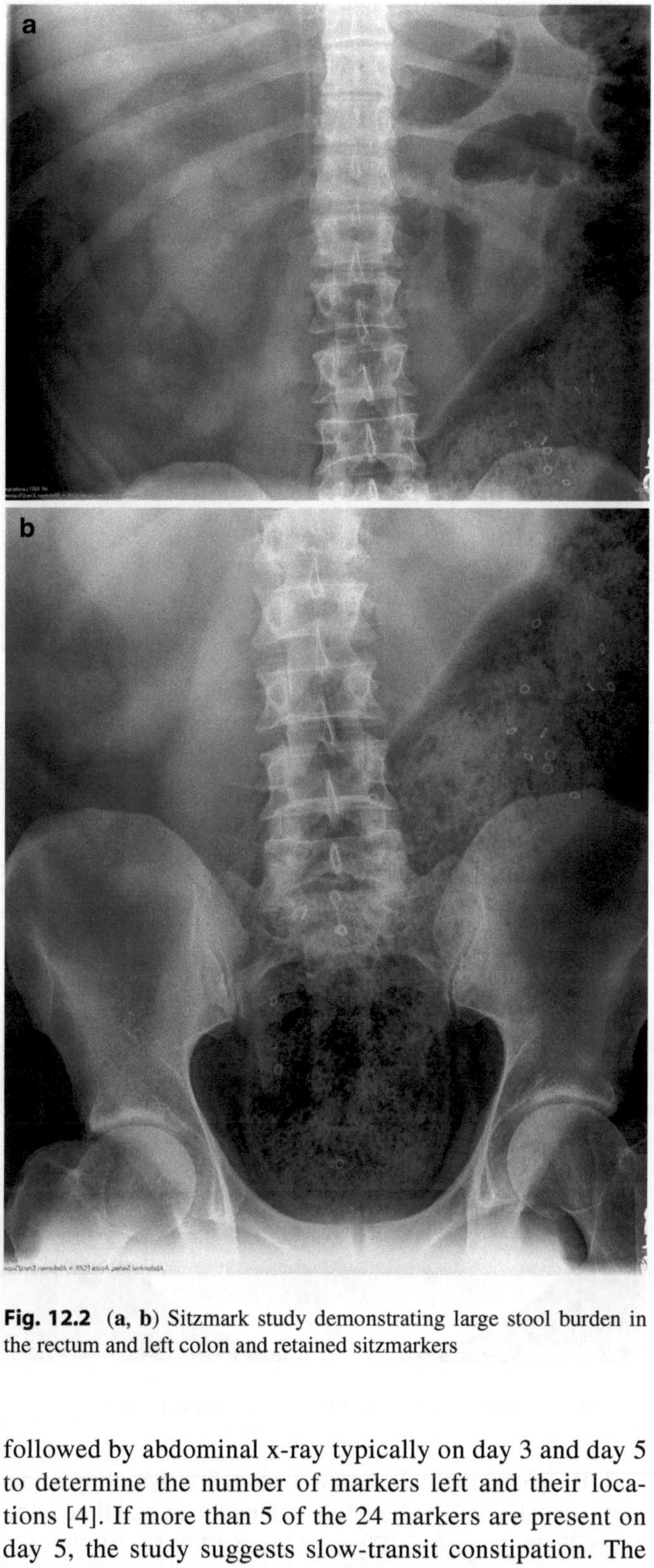

Fig. 12.2 (**a**, **b**) Sitzmark study demonstrating large stool burden in the rectum and left colon and retained sitzmarkers

followed by abdominal x-ray typically on day 3 and day 5 to determine the number of markers left and their locations [4]. If more than 5 of the 24 markers are present on day 5, the study suggests slow-transit constipation. The distribution of the markers may also suggest an etiology, with a diffuse pattern suggesting colonic inertia, and markers predominantly present in the distal colon and rectum suggesting that pelvic outlet obstruction is the primary problem, rather than abnormal transit through the colon [5].

Balloon Expulsion

A balloon expulsion test involves inflation of a rubber balloon inserted into the rectum; the patient is then asked to expel the balloon. Normal subjects can expel the balloon in 1 min. While a positive test (i.e., inability to expel) indicates obstructive defecation, some patients with obstructive defecation may still be able to expel the balloon. Although a simple test, the methods for performing the balloon expulsion test are not standardized in regard to the filling volume of the balloon, position of the patient, and expulsion time [6]. It also does not define the mechanism of obstructed defecation, but simply helps confirm it is the cause of the patient's symptoms. Therefore, it is best used as a screening test for a functional defecation disorder [7].

Key Concept: The primary purpose of some tests is to identify pelvic floor dyssynergia. One of the tests, manometry, also excludes Hirschsprung's disease.

If the patient complains only of obstructive defecation symptoms, the goal of additional testing is to identify the underlying etiology. More than one contributing factor may be seen on the testing. The following tests may be useful:

Anorectal Manometry

Anorectal manometry testing will tell you the resting anal pressure, squeeze pressure, rectoanal inhibitory reflex, rectal sensations (first and maximum tolerable), rectal compliance, and rectal and anal pressure during attempted defecation [6, 7]. Abnormalities in these parameters may direct the clinician towards potential pathophysiology causing obstructive defecation. The main abnormality in obstructive defecation is absent or inadequate relaxation of the anal sphincter, sometimes associated with contraction during straining [6]. An absent rectoanal inhibitory reflex (RAIR) is an indication of Hirschsprung's disease, which is usually diagnosed in childhood, rather than obstructive defecation. Elevated sensory thresholds, increased compliance, and rectal motor dysfunction may be seen with obstructive defecation and can be treated with biofeedback [6, 8]. You should be aware that manometry may overdiagnose dyssynergia. Paradoxical sphincter contraction has been shown in 22 % of asymptomatic controls, and the rate was not statistically different in constipated patients [7, 9]. The finding may be due to the horizontal patient position and simulated environment.

Electromyography (EMG)

EMG is a direct and specific test for the examination of somatic muscular activity of the external anal sphincter, puborectalis muscle, and pubococcygeus muscle during attempted defecation [10]. EMG may be performed with a needle study, but more frequently EMG recruitment testing is done with a sponge for the patient's comfort. With either method, the patient is asked to tighten the sphincter

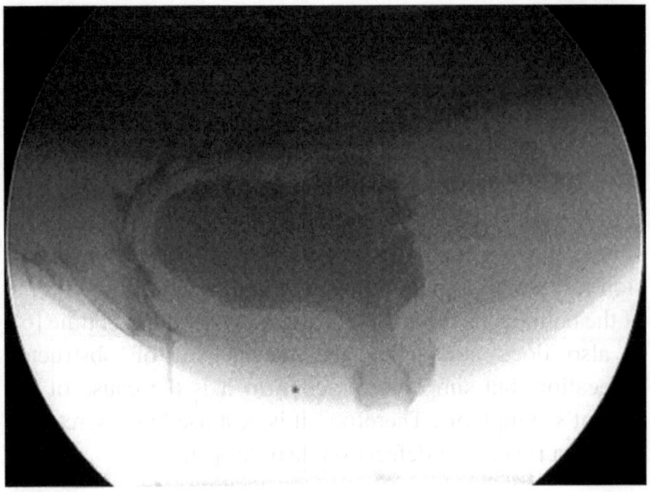

Fig. 12.3 Defecography of rectocele

muscle and then to bear down. Myoelectrical activity at rest, during squeeze, and push are recorded. Non-relaxation, or even increased activity, in these muscles during attempted defecation is considered abnormal and may indicate that the patient's symptoms are secondary to dysfunctional muscle. However, paradoxical activation of the puborectalis and external sphincter has been observed in disorders other than obstructive defecation and in normal subjects [11, 12]. Also, some patients with symptoms of obstructive defecation demonstrate normal inhibition of external sphincter and puborectalis activity [11, 13, 14], suggesting another etiology.

Imaging

Key Concept: Imaging is used when rectal prolapse, rectocele, solitary rectal ulcer syndrome, or findings suggestive of pelvic organ prolapse are seen on examination. Imaging may also confirm or refute the presence of non-relaxation of the puborectalis muscle.

Defecography

Defecography can identify structural abnormalities and also assess functional parameters [15]. Defecography may allow diagnosis of several problems that may be contributing to the patient's symptoms such as internal intussusception, external rectal prolapse, rectocele, sigmoidocele, enterocele, and paradoxical contraction of the puborectalis muscle (Figs. 12.3, 12.4 and 12.5) [6, 7]. However, other than rectal prolapse, many of these findings are present in asymptomatic controls, so the defecography findings ought not to be the sole indication for surgery [6, 16, 17]. Anorectal angle measurements among observers are greatly variable, as there is no consensus on whether the rectal axis should be drawn through the anterior, central, or posterior wall [7, 18].

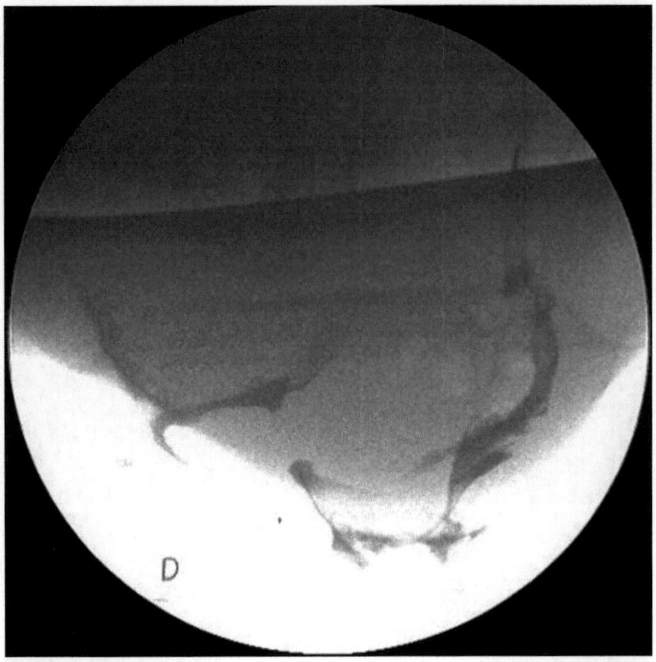

Fig. 12.4 Defecography of rectal prolapse with enterocele

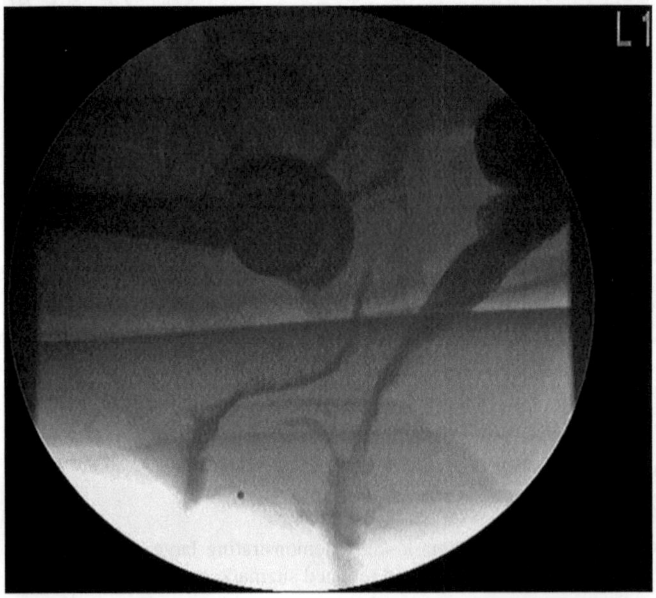

Fig. 12.5 Defecography of deep internal intussusception

MR defecography is a newer modality that allows anatomic and dynamic pelvic floor evaluation in real time without radiation exposure (Figs. 12.6 and 12.7) [7, 19]. Several studies have compared conventional defecography to MR defecography with differing results. MR defecography, unless open, requires a horizontal positioning of the patient, which is not a physiologic defecatory position but, however, has shown more reproducible results, compared to conventional fluoroscopic defecography [6, 20]. In a small study, seated open MR defecography compared to closed supine

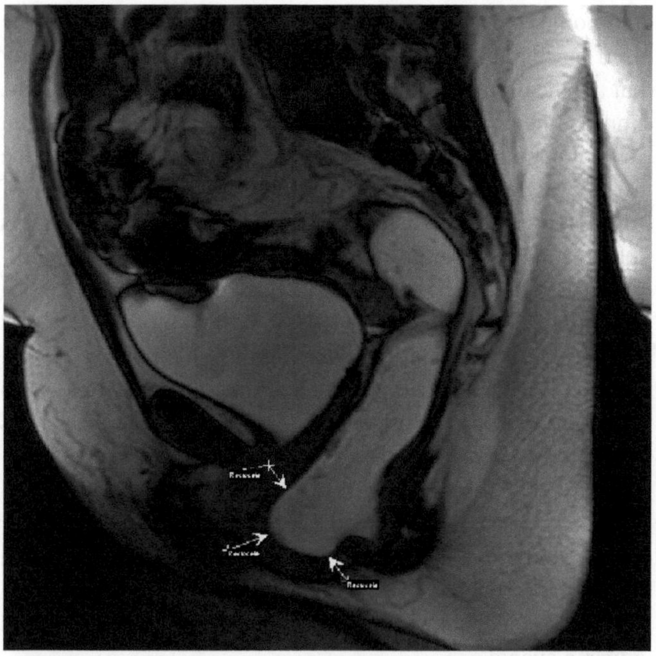

Fig. 12.6 MRI defecography of rectocele

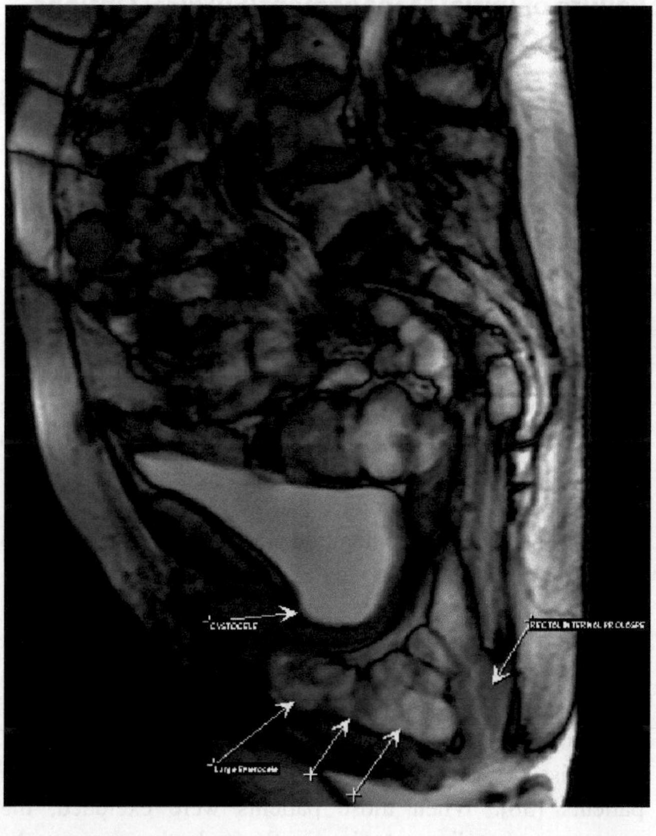

Fig. 12.7 MRI defecography of enterocele, cystocele, and rectal invagination

MR defecography shows similar detection of most clinically relevant findings. Rectal intussusception was seen only on seated MR [21]. Studies comparing conventional defecography and supine MR with evacuation phase showed no significant differences in sphincter hypotonia, dyssynergia, rectocele, or rectal prolapse [22, 23]. In contrast, a small study comparing dynamic pelvic MRI and videoproctography showed videoproctography to be more sensitive in detecting anterior and posterior rectoceles, rectoanal intussusceptions, sigmoidoceles, and perineal descent [24]. A different small study showed dynamic cystocolpoproctography and dynamic pelvic MR to be concordant for rectocele, enterocele, cystocele, and perineal descent; dynamic MR was the only modality that identified levator ani hernias; dynamic cystocolpoproctography identified sigmoidoceles and internal rectal prolapse more often than dynamic MR [25]. Likely, your local expertise will dictate the appropriate imaging modality at your institution.

Perineal Ultrasound

Dynamic perineal ultrasound is performed by placing a probe on the perineum, between the anus and the introitus. Compared to healthy controls, patients with symptoms of obstructive defecation demonstrate significantly greater absence of relaxation of the puborectalis muscle on straining and significantly higher incidence of rectal internal mucosal prolapse on dynamic perineal ultrasound [26]. There is good concordance between dynamic transperineal ultrasound and defecography for identifying rectocele, rectoanal intussusception, anorectal angle, and dyssynergic contraction of the puborectalis [27, 28]. Like many studies of this nature, the performance and interpretation are reliant on the experience and expertise of the user.

Our Recommendations

Key Concept: The choice of adjunctive tests depends upon the patient's symptoms and the findings on physical examination.

In our practice, after thorough history, physical examination, and endoscopy, we start with conservative management, including stool bulking and osmotic laxatives. If the patient has combined symptoms, we perform transit studies to help qualify the type of constipation the patient may be experiencing: slow transit vs. pelvic outlet obstruction vs. combination. Currently defecography is done for patients with demonstrated or suspected rectal prolapse or solitary rectal ulcer syndrome, as well as patients with symptomatic rectocele or enterocele. The goals are better understanding of the anatomy and exclusion of concomitant abnormalities. Admittedly, defecography is readily available at our site; however, when it is not, dynamic MRI is an option, but it is important to have a radiologist with the interest and training for appropriate interpretation. It is possible that in the future perineal ultrasound will replace both tests for radiation exposure and cost reasons, but at the present, there is only limited experience. EMG recruitment is done on patients with obstructive defecation unless full-thickness rectal prolapse is present. In all other patients, non-relaxation would be addressed first even if an indication for surgery was present. In addition, EMG recruitment helps to confirm or refute the diagnosis of anismus. We perform manometry on these patients but largely for research purposes rather than as aid for clinical decision-making. Balloon expulsion testing is rarely done. It is helpful however when the diagnosis is uncertain or if the patient is diverted.

Etiology and Treatment Options

Key Concept: Treatment decisions depend upon the etiology of obstructive defecation.

If a full-thickness rectal prolapse is diagnosed, surgical correction is performed; any persistent evacuation difficulties are addressed postoperatively. Please see Chap. 11 where Drs. Wexner and Hayden address the options for repair. If non-relaxation of the puborectalis muscle is identified on testing, particularly if seen on two tests, that issue is addressed first even if a rectocele, internal intussusception, or enterocele is also identified. If a rectocele is the only abnormality identified, it is addressed; the same is true for enterocele and sigmoidocele in some circumstances.

Non-relaxing Puborectalis

Key Concept: Non-relaxation of the puborectalis muscle may be an isolated finding or seen in combination with other abnormalities. Initial treatment is medical management including dietary recommendations and possible recommendation of fiber supplements or osmotic laxatives combined with biofeedback therapy.

Non-relaxation of the puborectalis may be diagnosed on EMG recruitment, defecography, balloon expulsion tests, and ultrasound. There is controversy about the diagnostic criteria and even the existence of this finding [9, 12]. The false-positive rate is poorly documented but false positives do occur, likely secondary to a poor understanding of instructions or embarrassment [9]. In our institution, 15 % of patients were able to demonstrate appropriate puborectalis function during their first biofeedback appointment, suggesting a false-positive diagnosis (unpublished data).

Our preferred initial treatment of non-relaxation of the puborectalis is biofeedback therapy. Regardless of the technique utilized, the goals of biofeedback therapy are to correct the lack of appropriate coordination of the abdominal muscles and sphincter mechanism and to enhance rectal sensory perception. Published methods include manometry-based biofeedback, EMG biofeedback, balloon defecation, and home device training. Surface EMG electrodes may be used on the abdominal and gluteal muscles. Protocols vary but typically include four to six training sessions. Improvement of symptoms varies between 44 and 100 % in several uncontrolled trials [29]. The wide range is likely due to the vague definition of endpoints, variable duration of follow-up, and inconsistent patient selection. What is clear is that results are better in patients who complete the full-prescribed course of treatment [30]. There have been several randomized controlled trials [31–36] where biofeedback was compared to medical management, polyethylene glycol, diazepam/placebo, balloon defecation treatment, and sham feedback therapy. In all of these studies, biofeedback was found to be superior to the other treatment options. An additional 1-year long-term follow-up study reported that biofeedback was superior to medical management [34]. Another recent study showed benefit in patients with anismus with and without IBS [37]. Overall, in addition to the positive outcomes, biofeedback is inexpensive and safe without reported adverse events.

Failure of Initial Management/Surgical Options

Key Concept: If symptoms do not resolve with biofeedback therapy, reported alternative treatments include botulinum neurotoxin injection and surgical division of the puborectalis muscle. Botulinum neurotoxin appears to be safe, while surgical division of the puborectalis muscle is no longer recommended because of reported complications.

If obstructive defecation symptoms persist in patients whose only abnormality is non-relaxation of the puborectalis muscle, then botulinum neurotoxin injection may be considered. In reported studies two bilateral injections of botulinum neurotoxin into the puborectalis and external sphincter muscles are performed with total amounts varying from 60 to 100 units [38–44]. The injections are done under either digital or ultrasound guidance and with either local or general anesthesia. Improvement in symptoms varies from 33 to 79 % [38, 40–45]. In the studies with postoperative evaluation, the sphincter pressures and anorectal angle decreased. The improvement typically lasts only 3 months, so repeat injections are often required. Careful selection of patients is important. In one study, examination under anesthesia of nonresponders revealed significant abnormalities (rectal prolapse, fissure, internal anal sphincter myopathy) in 97 % of patients [38]. When those patients were excluded, the response to botulinum toxin was 96 %. In that same study, gender and presenting symptoms were the only factors predictive of success, with men and patients presenting with obstructive defecation symptoms alone more likely to respond. A randomized study compared biofeedback to botulinum neurotoxin injection in treatment of anismus [39].

Initial improvement was significantly better in the injection group, but there was no difference in long-term success or patient satisfaction. None of the studies reported serious complications, though temporary incontinence of flatus is reported in several studies. Our feelings are that while the primary disadvantage of botulinum neurotoxin injection is the potential need for repeat treatment, it appears to be safe and a reasonable option in the treatment of these patients.

On the other hand, surgical division of the puborectalis muscle, a previously reported option has been largely abandoned because of the high rate of incontinence [46–48]. However, one recent study compared biofeedback, botulinum neurotoxin injection, and surgical division of the puborectalis muscle [49]. Patients undergoing surgical treatment had the best long-term improvement, with 70 % improvement at 1 year vs. biofeedback (30 %) or botulinum toxin injection (35 %). Incontinence was reported in 13 %. Outpatient anal dilatation is described as another option. Thirteen patients performed daily insertion of anal dilatators for 30 min for 3 months [50]. At 6 months from the end of treatment, all patients reported improvement. For patients who prefer or do not respond to other treatments, the remaining surgical option is diversion.

Our Recommendations

In our practice, patients with non-relaxation of the puborectalis muscle, either as an isolated or combined abnormality, are referred for biofeedback. For those patients with isolated non-relaxation that persists after biofeedback, botulinum neurotoxin injection is offered. We do not recommend division of the puborectalis muscle because of the risk of irreversible incontinence. Diversion is rarely indicated but may be offered when the impact on the symptoms severely impair patient's quality of life.

Rectoceles

Key Concept: *Rectoceles are common findings in parous women; caution must be exercised in attributing symptoms to them.*

The prevalence of rectoceles is poorly documented, as many women are asymptomatic, with reported rates varying from 18 to 40 % in limited studies (Fig. 12.8) [17, 51]. Confounding this, rectoceles are seen on defecography in 81 % of asymptomatic women [17]. Because rectoceles are quite common, you should be cautious about attributing symptoms to that finding alone. In addition, a recent review demonstrated variable association of the degree of posterior compartment prolapse and symptoms of obstructive defecation [52].

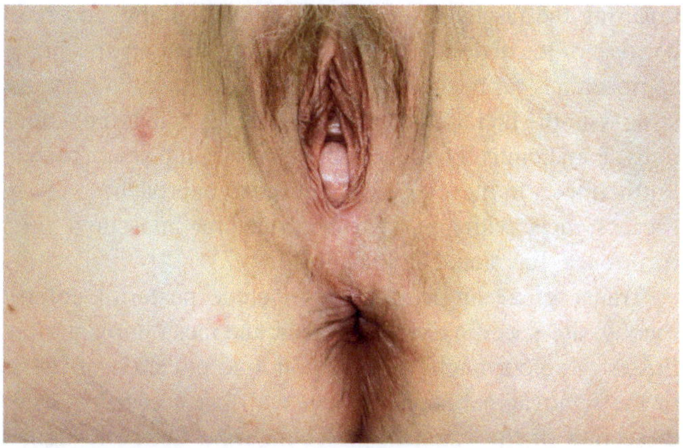

Fig. 12.8 Rectocele (*Courtesy of M. Shane McNevin, MD*)

Surgical Indications

Key Concept: *Surgery is indicated for persistent obstructive defecation symptoms and/or a symptomatic vaginal bulge.*

Women with obstructive defecation secondary to a rectocele typically complain of a sense of incomplete evacuation with a sensation of stool trapped in a visible vaginal bulge or rectal pocket. Perineal or posterior vaginal wall pressure facilitates evacuation and may serve as an indication that rectocele repair will alleviate the symptoms. While some surgeons use rectocele size over 3 cm as a criterion for surgery [53], others have found that this does not correlate well with the extent of symptoms [54]. Some authors believe that retention of dye in the rectocele is an indication of the clinical significance of the rectocele, while others maintain that this finding does not relate to the relief of symptoms postoperatively [55–57].

Key Concept: *A number of surgical options are available for rectocele repair; there is no clear evidence of superiority of one approach.*

Rectoceles occur because of disruption or diffuse thinning of the fascial tissue between the rectum and the vagina. They are essentially a hernia. In other areas of the body, mesh is frequently utilized now to reduce recurrence rates. Similarly, because of recurrence rates with traditional native tissue repairs of rectoceles, repairs utilizing mesh were developed. Some of those repairs, with the use of synthetic mesh, for example, have been complicated by persistent pain, mesh erosion, and infection. Another approach, stapled transanal resection of the rectum (STARR procedure) involves resection of redundant tissue in the rectum without repair of the fascia using linear staplers. While certain patients benefit, the procedure does not resolve symptoms in all women with rectoceles, and there is a generalized paucity of data describing the results in patients with rectoceles alone.

Ventral rectopexy with mesh anchored to the perineal body is also currently being evaluated with the goal of repairing the fascial defect with reduced complication rates because of the abdominal approach. Unfortunately, no single approach has yet been shown to be superior to the others. An issue with the literature regarding rectocele is that the definition of anatomically successful repair is not standardized. Furthermore, in most cases, the different approaches vary in success rates with regard to the outcome measured (i.e., recurrence, function, complications).

Transvaginal surgical choices include posterior colporrhaphy, site-specific rectocele repair, and mesh implantation. Posterior colporrhaphy involves midline plication of tissue in the rectovaginal septum often with perineoplasty. After dissection of the vaginal epithelium from the rectovaginal septum, the fascia, and in some hands the levator ani muscles, is plicated in the midline. The fibromuscular tissue adjacent to the perineal skin is also plicated to complete the perineoplasty. Generally, the anatomic abnormality is successfully repaired, but dyspareunia is common and the functional results variable [58–64]. Recurrence of symptoms appears to increase with the length of follow-up [65].

Site-specific repairs consist of identification and repair of the fascial defect in the rectovaginal septum [66–71]. A further modification added a perineal repair [72]. These repairs also result in acceptable anatomic correction with less sexual consequences, but the recurrence rates appear to be higher. A randomized trial of posterior colporrhaphy compared to site-specific repair with and without graft augmentation demonstrated slightly better anatomic success in the posterior colporrhaphy patients with no difference in functional outcome or dyspareunia [58]. Another comparative study confirmed those findings [73]. Overall, relief of defecation symptoms varies from 46 to 72 % [72–74].

Disappointing recurrence rates motivated the search for alternative repairs [65, 75, 76]. The third vaginal approach option is mesh implantation, which can occur either through use of a mesh-kit technique or as a supplement to any of the other procedures. Synthetic permanent, synthetic absorbable, and biologic meshes have been used. A number of comparative studies of synthetic mesh demonstrated comparative anatomic results to native tissue repair [77–81]. Four randomized controlled trials comparing transvaginal permanent synthetic mesh to traditional native tissue repair have been published; two of the studies involved the use of mesh kits [82–85]. One reported fewer recurrences with the use of mesh, while the other three reported no differences. The rate of mesh extrusion ranged from 5.6 to 16.9 %. Interestingly, the study with the positive results also revealed a much higher rate of new prolapse in an untreated compartment than with traditional repair [86]. Complications related to the mesh including mesh extraction, mesh retraction, pelvic pain, and sexual dysfunction were reported. Recent concerns about vaginal erosions of the mesh and mesh contractions resulting in chronic pain and vaginal shortening resulted in an update warning from the FDA in 2011 counseling surgeons about the risks and need for informed consent [87]. Your patients should be informed that surgical intervention may be necessary to correct the mesh extrusion and pain secondary to the mesh, should it occur. At the present there appears to be additional risk and insufficient benefit for recommending the use of synthetic mesh [88].

Those findings and recommendations led to use of other materials. One randomized controlled trial comparing synthetic absorbable mesh to native tissue found no difference in recurrence rates [89]. Unfortunately, the authors did not report bowel or sexual functional outcomes. There is some evidence that the complication rate is lower with biologic mesh than with other mesh. However, two studies comparing its use to native tissue found either no benefit [85] or a higher recurrence rate [58].

Transperineal repairs of rectoceles involve a perineal incision with subsequent dissection of the rectovaginal septum separating the posterior vaginal wall from the external sphincter distally and rectal wall proximally. The dissection proceeds cephalad to the posterior fornix. Imbrication of the fascial tissue, along with a site-specific repair or insertion of mesh, completes the repair [90–93]. A levatorplasty may also be added. A randomized controlled trial compared transanal repair, transperineal repair alone, and transperineal repair with levatorplasty [94]. Defecography revealed a reduction in the size of the rectocele in all groups, but functional scores improved only in the two transperineal groups. The combination of a transperineal approach with levatorplasty yielded the most improvement in functional outcome.

Transanal repair of rectocele involves the elevation of rectal mucosal flaps for the length of the rectocele [53, 95, 96]. The tissue in the rectovaginal septum is then imbricated; anterior levatorplasty and internal sphincter muscle plication may be added. The mucosal flaps are then re-approximated. Several investigators report high rates of symptomatic improvement after transanal repair [53, 95–101]. Typically, low rates of dyspareunia are demonstrated. However, a randomized controlled trial comparing vaginal to rectal repairs found a higher recurrence rate (7 % vs. 40 %) and more frequent incontinence of flatus after the transanal repair [102]. As noted above, the trial comparing transanal and perineal approaches demonstrated better functional results with the transperineal approach [94]. Yet, a recent Cochrane review found lower recurrence rates with a vaginal approach compared to transanal repairs, highlighting the differences among the various approaches for each of the outcomes assessed [103].

Regardless of the type of repair, most studies demonstrate improvement in obstructive defecation symptoms including splinting [85, 94, 104]. On the downside, those same studies also reveal a persistence of some symptoms in about 50 % of patients. This data, in addition to the frequency of the anatomic finding in asymptomatic women, emphasizes the importance of careful selection and informed consent for these patients. This is especially pertinent when considering that conservative management, including dietary, medication, and lifestyle changes and possibly a pessary, results in improvement in ~50 % of patients [105].

Our Recommendations

Recognizing there is not an optimal repair, our preferred approach is a site-specific repair if the defect can be identified and the surrounding tissue seems adequate. If the defect cannot be identified clearly, then a native tissue imbrication with the possible addition of biologic mesh (per surgeon preference) is utilized. Restoration of the perineal body is included. At the present time, we are avoiding the use of synthetic mesh.

Internal Intussusception

Key Concept: If internal intussusception is the only abnormality identified, medical management is the first-line treatment.

Internal intussusception (i.e., rectoanal intussusception, internal rectal prolapse, occult rectal prolapse) is full-thickness, circumferential prolapse of the rectum during evacuation that does not protrude through the anus [106, 107]. Defecography is the best way to diagnose internal intussusception. Importantly, it is unclear whether internal intussusception is pathologic or is a normal variation, as rectal intussusception is seen in 50 % of asymptomatic patients on defecography during defecation [17]. Interestingly, there is no difference in the speed or effectiveness of evacuation between asymptomatic volunteers with and without rectal intussusception. Likewise, symptomatic patients with intussusception did not have significantly different evacuation parameters compared to either asymptomatic group [108]. Furthermore, some authors believe it is a consequence of obstructed defecation rather than a cause of it [109]. The frequency with which obstructed defecation is associated with internal intussusception is unknown [110].

Rectal intussusception may cause symptoms of obstruction by blocking the rectal ampulla during defecation; this may cause a persistent urge to defecate as well as pain in the anal canal [111].

The treatment of internal intussusception is controversial. Initial management is always conservative. Therefore, we and most authors recommend conservative treatment consisting of fiber supplementation, refraining from straining, and biofeedback [3, 109, 112–114]. Over 50 % of patients with rectal intussusception experience complete or partial resolution of constipation symptoms with biofeedback [110].

Surgical Treatment

Key Concept: Caution must be exercised before the recommendation of surgical intervention as the outcomes after traditional surgical correction were disappointing. While more recent results from two new procedures are more encouraging, the role of surgery for this diagnosis is unclear.

Surgery for internal intussusception should be approached with caution. Adequate repair, as evidenced by elimination of the intussusception on defecography, may not equal symptom relief for the patient, and likewise, despite persistence of an anatomic problem (i.e., surgical failure), patients may feel symptomatic relief [109, 111]. Furthermore, the risk of internal prolapse progressing to total rectal prolapse is low [113, 115].

Various surgical techniques have been employed to treat internal intussusception associated with obstructed defecation including traditional rectopexy, ventral rectopexy, and stapled transanal resection of the rectum (STARR). In a survey of constipated patients who underwent laparoscopic resection rectopexy after biofeedback failed, 53 % reported improvement in bowel frequency [116]. In another small study, the majority of patients who underwent resection rectopexy reported an improvement in constipation symptoms [117]. However, others have found rectopexy to be an ineffective treatment for obstructed defecation that may even worsen constipation or tenesmus [118, 119]. Because the functional outcomes of traditional rectopexy (± resection) are unacceptably poor and patients with internal intussusception are unlikely to see improvements in their obstructive defecation with this procedure, a very frank discussion with the patient must precede surgical intervention [120].

Until recently, we, along with most surgeons, avoided surgery for internal intussusception because of the high likelihood of persistent symptoms. A small percentage of patients underwent stoma formation because their symptoms were so troublesome and prior repairs had been ineffective. Recently, however, outcomes from two procedures have been more encouraging. Laparoscopic ventral rectopexy, performed by dissecting exclusively anterior to the rectum, preserving the lateral stalks, and using polypropylene mesh for rectal fixation, has been used for internal intussusception with good results. At 3 months postoperative, 86 % of patients reported improvement in their obstructed defecation, and there were no mesh-related complications [120]. Others have found similar results [119]. Yet, many surgeons fear placing a permanent mesh directly on the bowel due to the potential for erosion or infection. At 6-month follow-up from laparoscopic ventral rectopexy using biologic mesh (Permacol) in patients with internal rectal prolapse and constipation, 82 % reported cured or improved constipation. There were no mesh-related complications [121]. While still in its infancy, ventral rectopexy has promising initial results.

As previously described, stapled transanal resection of the rectum (STARR) has emerged as another possible technique to treat obstructed defecation secondary to multiple causes, including internal intussusception. Notably, the presence of a coexisting enterocele, however, is a relative contraindication to the STARR procedure [122]. One hundred nineteen women suffering from obstructed defecation with associated rectocele and rectal intussusception were randomized to biofeedback or STARR; there was a significant improvement in symptoms in the STARR group compared to the biofeedback group after 1-year follow-up (81 % vs. 33 %, respectively). Fifteen percent of STARR patients experienced an adverse event (local infection, anorectal pain, incontinence, bleeding, urinary infection, or depression) [123]. Similarly, 85 % of 14 patients with intussusception (± rectocele) reviewed retrospectively who underwent the STARR procedure had significant improvement in stool evacuation at 68-month follow-up; however, three required reoperation [124]. Although 81 % of 326 patients who underwent STARR were highly satisfied and would recommend it or have it again, 72 % reported fecal urgency at 8 weeks (which declined over time) and 10 % reported recurrent symptoms postoperatively [125]. In another small study, 24 patients underwent pre- and postoperative MR defecography; an intussusception was observed in 20 patients, 18 of whom also had an anterior rectocele. Following the STARR procedure, 79 % of patients reported that the main symptoms disappeared (excessive straining, need for digital assistance during defecation, or incomplete evacuation), and MR revealed a correction of intussusception in 75 %. Furthermore, these patients had a significantly improved Cleveland Constipation Score compared to those without radiographic evidence of correction of intussusception [108]. In a retrospective review of 123 patients with obstructive defecation and rectocele and/or intussusception, 65 % had subjective improvement after STARR; however, 28 % had recurrent intussusception, 24 % required reoperation, and the postoperative complication rate was high, including one death following reoperation for necrotic rectum and uterus [126].

Although good results can often be enjoyed following the STARR procedure, several possible complications have been reported including urinary retention, severe pain, infection, fecal incontinence, stenosis, rectovaginal fistula, peritonitis, fecal urgency, bleeding, hematoma, and necrotizing fasciitis [122, 124, 126–128].

Our Recommendations

We currently treat internal intussusception primarily with conservative management. For patients with significant persistent symptoms, we are now trying ventral rectopexy after careful informed consent about the relative lack of published data. We have avoided the STARR procedure after balancing the risk of complications with the likelihood of improvement.

Enterocele

Key Concept: Enterocele is usually present with other pelvic floor findings, making the exact symptoms attributable to enterocele indecipherable.

Enterocele is a peritoneum-lined sac usually containing small bowel that herniates into the rectogenital septum [114, 129]. Characteristic symptoms of enterocele may be as follows: difficulty emptying, post-evacuation discomfort, and pelvic pain or heaviness [130]. Symptoms may be exacerbated by standing, may worsen as the day goes by, and are relieved by laying down [130]. Nevertheless, it is controversial whether or not enterocele causes difficulty evacuating and obstructed defecation [130, 131]. When comparing 77 women with enteroceles to 233 women without enteroceles, there were no significant differences in symptoms related to bowel function, such as infrequent bowel movements, straining, manual evacuation, and fecal incontinence [132].

With opacification of the bowel (using oral and rectal contrast), enterocele can be seen on defecography, when present [114, 130]. Enterocele is often not the sole finding on pelvic floor studies. In 104 patients with an enterocele, 76 % had concomitant findings such as perineal descent, rectocele, and rectal intussusception [130]. Since it is unclear what specific symptoms are caused by enterocele, initial management should be nonsurgical. We advise these patients to increase fiber and water intake, avoid straining, and initiate biofeedback [133]. Surgical repair may be more effective at relieving pelvic pain rather than obstructed defecation [130]. In 20 patients who underwent obliteration of the pelvic inlet with nonabsorbable mesh, symptoms of obstructed defecation persisted in all 15 patients with evacuation difficulties preoperatively [131].

Surgical Treatment

Enterocele repair can be undertaken from a transvaginal or transabdominal approach. Both yield excellent anatomic results; however, evaluating functional outcomes is more difficult, given that the majority of enteroceles are seen in women with other pelvic floor pathology [133]. Transvaginal repair is traditionally performed in patients with uterovaginal prolapse (Fig. 12.9a, b). Looking at abdominal approaches, there are definitively pros and cons when evaluating the outcomes. Abdominal

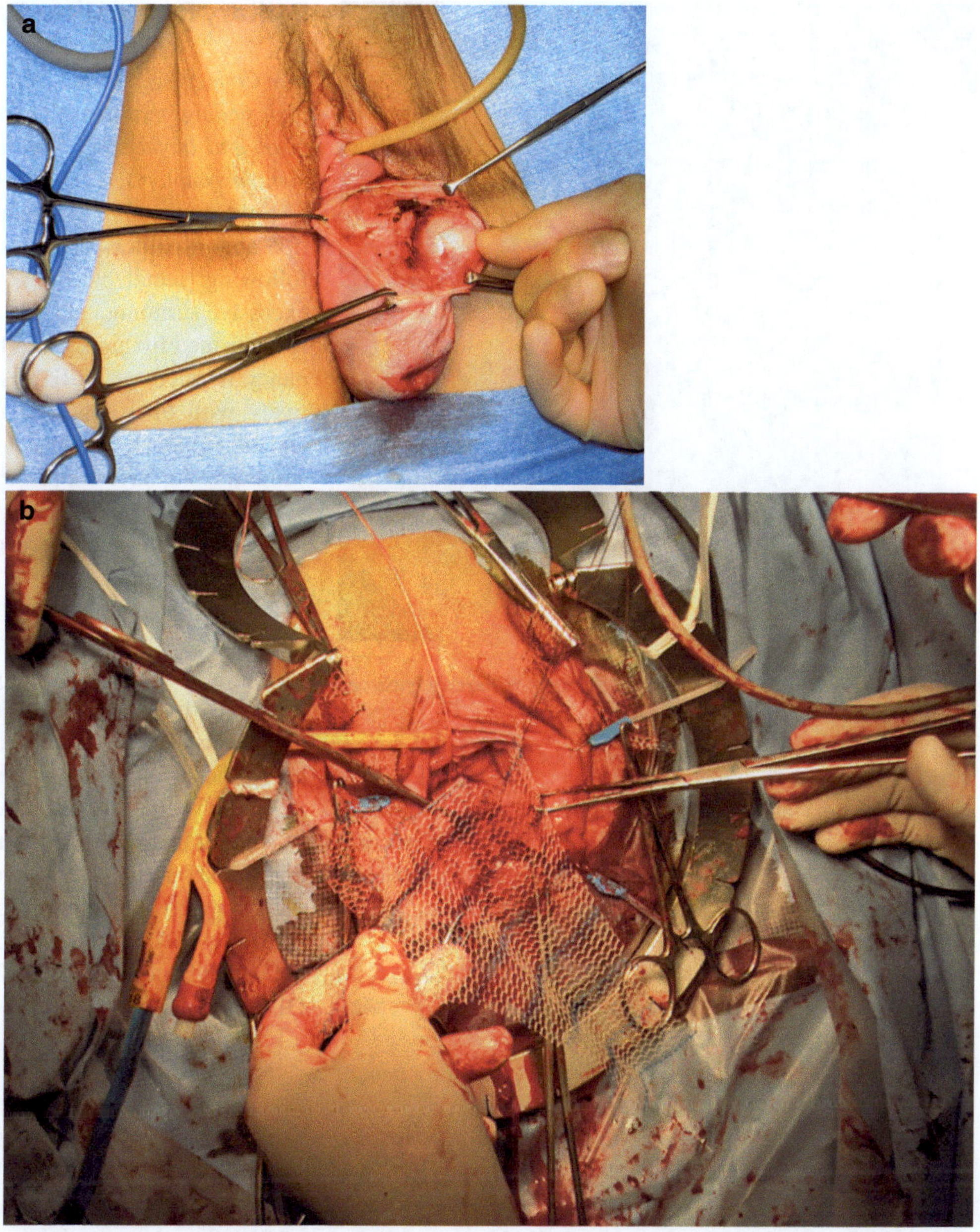

Fig. 12.9 (**a**, **b**) Vaginal vault prolapse with enterocele and mesh repair

colporectosacropexy with nonabsorbable mesh anatomically corrected the enterocele in 58 of 59 study patients; however, the number of patients with obstructed defecation was not different before and 27 months after surgery [134]. Obliteration of the pelvic inlet with U-shaped nonabsorbable mesh adequately corrected the enterocele in 91 % of patients; however, obstructed defecation persisted in 75 % of patients who presented with this problem before the procedure [135]. Some authors feel enterocele is a contraindication to the STARR procedure [122, 128, 136], while others have shown no difference in functional outcome and postoperative complications in patients with and without enterocele undergoing STARR for obstructed defecation syndrome [137]. Although studies are few, a combined laparoscopic and STARR procedure may ultimately prove beneficial to patients with enterocele [138, 139].

Our Recommendations

Based on the available data, it is unlikely that repairing an enterocele alone will benefit a patient complaining of obstructed defecation. Most repairs are performed in patients with additional indications for surgery such as rectal prolapse and rectal intussusception [134, 140]. For patients with

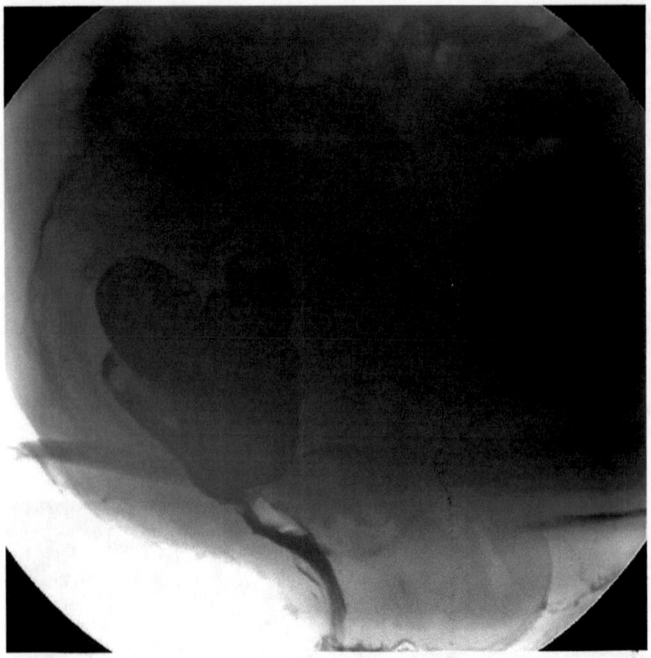

Fig. 12.10 Sigmoidocele seen on defecography (*Courtesy of Steven D. Wexner, MD*)

mild symptoms and relatively limited enterocele, medical management with an adequate bowel regimen is recommended. If concomitant anismus is identified, then a trial of biofeedback may be warranted.

Sigmoidocele

Key Concept: Patients with large sigmoidoceles may benefit from surgical correction, although data is sparse.

Sigmoidocele is similar to enterocele; however, the peritoneal sac contains sigmoid colon that herniates into the rectogenital septum [141]. There is a paucity of studies on this entity. In 1994, Jorge et al. [142] noted 24 sigmoidoceles out of 463 (5 %) cinedefecographies performed for constipation, incontinence, and chronic idiopathic rectal pain. Sigmoidocele was classified based on the degree of descent of the lowest portion of the sigmoid: 1st degree = above the pubococcygeal line, 2nd degree = below the pubococcygeal line but above the ischiococcygeal line, and 3rd degree = below the ischiococcygeal line (Fig. 12.10). Six patients with either 2nd- or 3rd-degree sigmoidocele underwent colectomy with or without rectopexy, and all reported improvement in constipation. The authors conclude that there is correlation among the mean level of sigmoidocele, percentage of redundancy, and clinical symptoms [142]. Nevertheless, there have been no further published data evaluating sigmoidocele in relation to obstructed defecation; thus, we cannot provide evidence-based recommendations on its treatment.

Solitary Rectal Ulcer Syndrome (SRUS)

Key Concept: SRUS is a rare entity with characteristic histologic findings that should be treated with behavior modification, fiber, and biofeedback. Ventral rectopexy may offer improvement in symptoms, although experience is limited thus far.

Solitary rectal ulcer syndrome is associated with evacuation abnormalities. Vague associated symptoms include the following: rectal bleeding, passage of mucus, rectal pain, excessive straining, and tenesmus [114]. Once the diagnosis is confirmed by biopsy and histological analysis and malignancy is ruled out, SRUS is traditionally treated conservatively with fiber supplementation, avoidance of straining, and biofeedback. Topical applications, such as steroids or sulfasalazine, have not proven effective [114].

Ulceration, if present, is typically anterior and low in the rectum making resection a difficult proposition, especially since the syndrome is strongly associated with chronic straining. Targeting therapy towards this abnormality (i.e., avoidance straining) is generally effective and avoids a large operation [114, 143]. We generally counsel the patients regarding dietary management, regular attempts to defecate, avoidance of prolonged time on the toilet, and appropriate toiling posturing. If non-relaxation is present on testing, biofeedback is also recommended.

Ventral rectopexy is emerging as a possible surgical option should conservative measures fail. Forty-eight patients who underwent laparoscopic ventral mesh rectopexy for SRUS after initial biofeedback were evaluated: 100 % had epithelial ulcer healing, and 68 % had improved ODS symptoms [144].

Our Recommendations

Once malignancy is ruled out, we target the potential causes of SRUS such as straining and prolapse (internal) through the use of a bowel regimen and potentially biofeedback. Although uncommon, if external rectal prolapse is present, it is repaired. Ventral rectopexy may become a reasonable surgical intervention for patients with persistent symptomatic ulceration although insufficient data exists at present to recommend it. Surgical resection has been utilized, but the operations are often technically challenging and frequently symptoms persistent. Occasional patients require diversion. The optimal timing for surgery and most effective surgical procedure are not known at this time.

Persistent Symptoms

It should be clear from the discussion that some patients will have persistent symptoms. They should be evaluated for missed diagnoses, failed surgical correction of the identified problem,

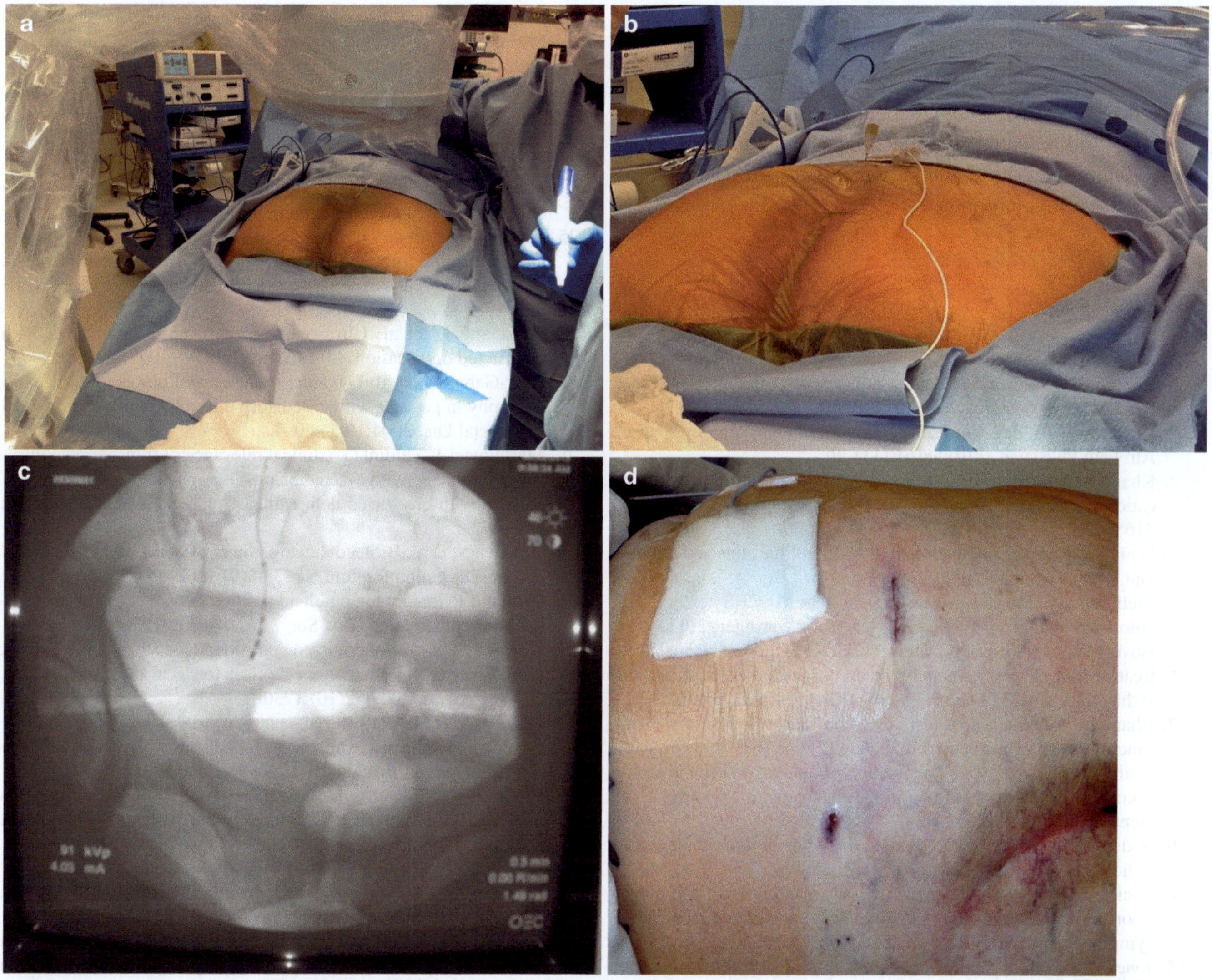

Fig. 12.11 Sacral nerve stimulation. (**a**) Accessing the correct sacral level. (**b**) Lead in place. (**c**) Fluoroscopy to confirm lead placement. (**d**) Completed in place with final wound closure

and new abnormalities that arose after surgical intervention. Attention is then directed to a recognized etiology for the symptoms. If that evaluation is not rewarding, then conservative management including dietary, lifestyle, and medication management should be recommended. Biofeedback may be helpful. A new option, sacral nerve stimulation is being investigated.

Sacral Nerve Stimulation

Key Concept: Sacral nerve stimulation (SNS) is not currently US FDA approved for constipation but may be an option in the future.

Most studies evaluating SNS for constipation are uncontrolled, retrospective case series that combine patients with slow-transit constipation and evacuatory dysfunction and have short durations of follow-up. Nevertheless, success rates (mostly defined as increase in defecatory frequency) in patients who went on to permanent implant range from 42 to 100 % [145]. Although it is difficult to interpret the current results, SNS offers a test period prior to permanent implantation, thus reducing the expense for patients who fail to respond. Risks from the procedure are often minimal and include infection and pain. Therefore, given the paucity of effective surgical treatments for obstructive defecation syndrome, SNS may emerge as a promising intervention to offer patients who fail conservative therapy and do not have other specific anatomic causes (Fig. 12.11a–d).

Summary Pearls

Symptoms of obstructive defecation are relatively common and may be the result of a number of different etiologies. Your history and physical examination will not only help determine the cause but also guide your subsequent evaluation. Remember first and foremost that conservative management benefits a significant percentage of patients, and this should be balanced against any attempt at surgical intervention. Operative therapy can be effective in select individuals, but persistent symptoms are a frequent occurrence. Therefore, frank discussion with your patient regarding the expected outcomes and potential complications is imperative. A careful evaluation is critical for the ones with persistent symptoms in order to appropriately determine their treatment.

References

1. Mugie SM, Benninga MA, Di Lorenzo C. Epidemiology of constipation in children and adults: a systematic review. Best Pract Res Clin Gastroenterol. 2011;25(1):3–18.
2. Kuncharapu I, Majeroni B, Johnson DW. Pelvic organ prolapse. Am Fam Physician. 2010;58(6):1111–7.
3. Khaikin M, Wexner SD. Treatment strategies in obstructed defecation and fecal incontinence. World J Gastroenterol. 2006;12(20):3168–73.
4. Whitehead WE, et al. Functional disorders of the anus and rectum. Gut. 1999;45 Suppl 2:II55–9.
5. Mellgren AF. Physiologic testing. In: The ASCRS textbook of colon and rectal surgery. 2nd ed. New York: Springer; 2011.
6. Bove A, et al. Consensus statement AIGO/SICCR: diagnosis and treatment of chronic constipation and obstructed defecation (part I: diagnosis). World J Gastroenterol. 2012;18(14):1555–64.
7. Bharucha AE. Update of tests of colon and rectal structure and function. J Clin Gastroenterol. 2006;40(2):96–103.
8. Andromanakos N, et al. Constipation of anorectal outlet obstruction: pathophysiology, evaluation and management. J Gastroenterol Hepatol. 2006;21(4):638–46.
9. Voderholzer WA, et al. Paradoxical sphincter contraction is rarely indicative of anismus. Gut. 1997;41(2):258–62.
10. Fucini C, Ronchi O, Elbetti C. Electromyography of the pelvic floor musculature in the assessment of obstructed defecation symptoms. Dis Colon Rectum. 2001;44(8):1168–75.
11. Jones PN, et al. Is paradoxical contraction of puborectalis muscle of functional importance? Dis Colon Rectum. 1987;30(9):667–70.
12. Schouten WR, et al. Anismus: fact or fiction? Dis Colon Rectum. 1997;40(9):1033–41.
13. Duthie GS, Bartolo DC. Anismus: the cause of constipation? Results of investigation and treatment. World J Surg. 1992;16(5):831–5.
14. Miller R, et al. Anismus in patients with normal and slow transit constipation. Br J Surg. 1991;78(6):690–2.
15. Bharucha AE, et al. Functional anorectal disorders. Gastroenterology. 2006;130(5):1510–8.
16. Hiltunen KM, Kolehmainen H, Matikainen M. Does defecography help in diagnosis and clinical decision-making in defecation disorders? Abdom Imaging. 1994;19(4):355–8.
17. Shorvon PJ, et al. Defecography in normal volunteers: results and implications. Gut. 1989;30(12):1737–49.
18. Ferrante SL, et al. The reproducibility of measuring the anorectal angle in defecography. Dis Colon Rectum. 1991;34(1):51–5.
19. Fletcher JG, et al. Magnetic resonance imaging of anatomic and dynamic defects of the pelvic floor in defecatory disorders. Am J Gastroenterol. 2003;98(2):399–411.
20. Kruyt RH, et al. Normal anorectum: dynamic MR imaging anatomy. Radiology. 1991;179(1):159–63.
21. Bertschinger KM, et al. Dynamic MR imaging of the pelvic floor performed with patient sitting in an open-magnet unit versus with patient supine in a closed-magnet unit. Radiology. 2002;223(2):501–8.
22. Foti PV, et al. Pelvic floor imaging: comparison between magnetic resonance imaging and conventional defecography in studying outlet obstruction syndrome. Radiol Med. 2013;118:23–39.
23. Vitton V, et al. Dynamic anal endosonography and MRI defecography in diagnosis of pelvic floor disorders: comparison with conventional defecography. Dis Colon Rectum. 2011;54(11):1398–404.
24. Matsuoka H, et al. A comparison between dynamic pelvic magnetic resonance imaging and videoproctography in patients with constipation. Dis Colon Rectum. 2001;44(4):571–6.
25. Kaufman HS, et al. Dynamic pelvic magnetic resonance imaging and cystocolpoproctography alter surgical management of pelvic floor disorders. Dis Colon Rectum. 2001;44(11):1575–83; discussion 1583–4.
26. Brusciano L, et al. Ultrasonographic patterns in patients with obstructed defaecation. Int J Colorectal Dis. 2007;22(8):969–77.
27. Beer-Gabel M, et al. Dynamic transperineal ultrasound vs. defecography in patients with evacuatory difficulty: a pilot study. Int J Colorectal Dis. 2004;19(1):60–7.
28. Martellucci J, Naldini G. Clinical relevance of transperineal ultrasound compared with evacuation proctography for the evaluation of patients with obstructed defaecation. Colorectal Dis. 2011;13(10):1167–72.
29. Heymen S, et al. Biofeedback treatment of constipation: a critical review. Dis Colon Rectum. 2003;46(9):1208–17.
30. Gilliland R, et al. Outcome and predictors of success of biofeedback for constipation. Br J Surg. 1997;84(8):1123–6.
31. Heymen S, et al. Randomized controlled trial shows biofeedback to be superior to pelvic floor exercises for fecal incontinence. Dis Colon Rectum. 2009;52(10):1730–7.
32. Heymen S, et al. Randomized, controlled trial shows biofeedback to be superior to alternative treatments for patients with pelvic floor dyssynergia-type constipation. Dis Colon Rectum. 2007;50(4):428–41.
33. Chiarioni G, Salandini L, Whitehead WE. Biofeedback benefits only patients with outlet dysfunction, not patients with isolated slow transit constipation. Gastroenterology. 2005;129(1):86–97.
34. Rao SS, et al. Long-term efficacy of biofeedback therapy for dyssynergic defecation: randomized controlled trial. Am J Gastroenterol. 2010;105(4):890–6.
35. Rao SS, et al. Randomized controlled trial of biofeedback, sham feedback, and standard therapy for dyssynergic defecation. Clin Gastroenterol Hepatol. 2007;5(3):331–8.
36. Hart SL, et al. A randomized controlled trial of anorectal biofeedback for constipation. Int J Colorectal Dis. 2012;27(4):459–66.
37. Patcharatrakul T, Gonlachanvit S. Outcome of biofeedback therapy in dyssynergic defecation patients with and without irritable bowel syndrome. J Clin Gastroenterol. 2011;45(7):593–8.
38. Hompes R, et al. Excellent response rate of anismus to botulinum toxin if rectal prolapse misdiagnosed as anismus ('pseudoanismus') is excluded. Colorectal Dis. 2012;14(2):224–30.
39. Farid M, et al. Comparative study between biofeedback retraining and botulinum neurotoxin in the treatment of anismus patients. Int J Colorectal Dis. 2009;24(1):115–20.
40. Ron Y, et al. Botulinum toxin type-A in therapy of patients with anismus. Dis Colon Rectum. 2001;44(12):1821–6.
41. Joo JS, et al. Initial North American experience with botulinum toxin type A for treatment of anismus. Dis Colon Rectum. 1996;39(10):1107–11.
42. Hallan RI, et al. Treatment of anismus in intractable constipation with botulinum A toxin. Lancet. 1988;2(8613):714–7.
43. Maria G, et al. Experience with type A botulinum toxin for treatment of outlet-type constipation. Am J Gastroenterol. 2006;101(11):2570–5.
44. Maria G, et al. Botulinum toxin in the treatment of outlet obstruction constipation caused by puborectalis syndrome. Dis Colon Rectum. 2000;43(3):376–80.

45. Friedenberg F, Gollamudi S, Parkman HP. The use of botulinum toxin for the treatment of gastrointestinal motility disorders. Dig Dis Sci. 2004;49(2):165–75.
46. Nyam DC, et al. Long-term results of surgery for chronic constipation. Dis Colon Rectum. 1997;40(3):273–9.
47. Kamm MA, Hawley PR, Lennard-Jones JE. Lateral division of the puborectalis muscle in the management of severe constipation. Br J Surg. 1988;75(7):661–3.
48. Barnes PR, et al. Experience of posterior division of the puborectalis muscle in the management of chronic constipation. Br J Surg. 1985;72(6):475–7.
49. Faried M, et al. Comparative study between surgical and non-surgical treatment of anismus in patients with symptoms of obstructed defecation: a prospective randomized study. J Gastrointest Surg. 2010;14(8):1235–43.
50. Maria G, et al. Treatment of puborectalis syndrome with progressive anal dilation. Dis Colon Rectum. 1997;40(1):89–92.
51. Hendrix SL, et al. Pelvic organ prolapse in the Women's Health Initiative: gravity and gravidity. Am J Obstet Gynecol. 2002; 186(6):1160–6.
52. Grimes CL, Lukacz ES. Posterior vaginal compartment prolapse and defecatory dysfunction: are they related? Int Urogynecol J. 2012;23(5):537–51.
53. Hammond KL, Ellis CN. Outcomes after transanal repair of rectoceles. Dis Colon Rectum. 2010;53(1):83–7.
54. Altman D, et al. Assessment of posterior vaginal wall prolapse: comparison of physical findings to cystodefecoperitoneography. Int Urogynecol J Pelvic Floor Dysfunct. 2005;16(2):96–103; discussion 103.
55. Sarles JC, et al. Endo-rectal repair of rectocele. Int J Colorectal Dis. 1989;4(3):167–71.
56. Murthy VK, et al. Excellent outcome using selective criteria for rectocele repair. Dis Colon Rectum. 1996;39(4):374–8.
57. Infantino A, et al. Does surgery resolve outlet obstruction from rectocele? Int J Colorectal Dis. 1995;10(2):97–100.
58. Paraiso MF, et al. Rectocele repair: a randomized trial of three surgical techniques including graft augmentation. Am J Obstet Gynecol. 2006;195(6):1762–71.
59. Kahn MA, Stanton SL. Posterior colporrhaphy: its effects on bowel and sexual function. Br J Obstet Gynaecol. 1997;104(1):82–6.
60. Lopez A, et al. Durability of success after rectocele repair. Int Urogynecol J Pelvic Floor Dysfunct. 2001;12(2):97–103.
61. Yamana T, Takahashi T, Iwadare J. Clinical and physiologic outcomes after transvaginal rectocele repair. Dis Colon Rectum. 2006;49(5):661–7.
62. Mellgren A, et al. Results of rectocele repair. A prospective study. Dis Colon Rectum. 1995;38(1):7–13.
63. Cundiff GW, Fenner D. Evaluation and treatment of women with rectocele: focus on associated defecatory and sexual dysfunction. Obstet Gynecol. 2004;104(6):1403–21.
64. Arnold MW, Stewart WR, Aguilar PS. Rectocele repair. Four years' experience. Dis Colon Rectum. 1990;33(8):684–7.
65. Chung CS, et al. Comparison of long-term clinical outcomes according to the change in the rectocele depth between transanal and transvaginal repairs for a symptomatic rectocele. J Korean Soc Coloproctol. 2012;28(3):140–4.
66. Richardson AC. The rectovaginal septum revisited: its relationship to rectocele and its importance in rectocele repair. Clin Obstet Gynecol. 1993;36(4):976–83.
67. Cundiff GW, et al. An anatomic and functional assessment of the discrete defect rectocele repair. Am J Obstet Gynecol. 1998;179 (6 Pt 1):1451–6; discussion 1456–7.
68. Singh K, Cortes E, Reid WM. Evaluation of the fascial technique for surgical repair of isolated posterior vaginal wall prolapse. Obstet Gynecol. 2003;101(2):320–4.
69. Kenton K, Shott S, Brubaker L. Outcome after rectovaginal fascia reattachment for rectocele repair. Am J Obstet Gynecol. 1999;181(6):1360–3; discussion 1363–4.
70. Porter WE, et al. The anatomic and functional outcomes of defect-specific rectocele repairs. Am J Obstet Gynecol. 1999;181(6):1353–8; discussion 1358–9.
71. Milani AL, et al. Midline fascial plication under continuous digital transrectal control: which factors determine anatomic outcome? Int Urogynecol J. 2010;21(6):623–30.
72. Schmidlin-Enderli K, Schuessler B. A new rectovaginal fascial plication technique for treatment of rectocele with obstructed defecation: a proof of concept study. Int Urogynecol J. 2013;24: 613–9.
73. Abramov Y, et al. Site-specific rectocele repair compared with standard posterior colporrhaphy. Obstet Gynecol. 2005;105(2): 314–8.
74. Sardeli C, et al. Outcome of site-specific fascia repair for rectocele. Acta Obstet Gynecol Scand. 2007;86(8):973–7.
75. Fialkow MF, Newton KM, Weiss NS. Incidence of recurrent pelvic organ prolapse 10 years following primary surgical management: a retrospective cohort study. Int Urogynecol J Pelvic Floor Dysfunct. 2008;19(11):1483–7.
76. Olsen AL, et al. Epidemiology of surgically managed pelvic organ prolapse and urinary incontinence. Obstet Gynecol. 1997;89(4): 501–6.
77. Lim YN, Rane A, Muller R. An ambispective observational study in the safety and efficacy of posterior colporrhaphy with composite Vicryl-Prolene mesh. Int Urogynecol J Pelvic Floor Dysfunct. 2005;16(2):126–31; discussion 131.
78. de Tayrac R, et al. Prolapse repair by vaginal route using a new protected low-weight polypropylene mesh: 1-year functional and anatomical outcome in a prospective multicentre study. Int Urogynecol J Pelvic Floor Dysfunct. 2007;18(3):251–6.
79. de Tayrac R, et al. A 2-year anatomical and functional assessment of transvaginal rectocele repair using a polypropylene mesh. Int Urogynecol J Pelvic Floor Dysfunct. 2006;17(2):100–5.
80. Milani R, et al. Functional and anatomical outcome of anterior and posterior vaginal prolapse repair with prolene mesh. BJOG. 2005;112(1):107–11.
81. Simon M, Debodinance P. Vaginal prolapse repair using the Prolift kit: a registry of 100 successive cases. Eur J Obstet Gynecol Reprod Biol. 2011;158(1):104–9.
82. Carey M, et al. Vaginal repair with mesh versus colporrhaphy for prolapse: a randomised controlled trial. BJOG. 2009;116(10): 1380–6.
83. Sokol AI, et al. One-year objective and functional outcomes of a randomized clinical trial of vaginal mesh for prolapse. Am J Obstet Gynecol. 2012;206(1):86.e1–9.
84. Withagen MI, et al. Trocar-guided mesh compared with conventional vaginal repair in recurrent prolapse: a randomized controlled trial. Obstet Gynecol. 2011;117(2 Pt 1):242–50.
85. Sung VW, et al. Porcine subintestinal submucosal graft augmentation for rectocele repair: a randomized controlled trial. Obstet Gynecol. 2012;119(1):125–33.
86. Withagen MI, et al. Development of de novo prolapse in untreated vaginal compartments after prolapse repair with and without mesh: a secondary analysis of a randomised controlled trial. BJOG. 2012;119(3):354–60.
87. FDA Safety Communication. UPDATE on serious complications associated with transvaginal placement of surgical mesh for pelvic organ prolapse, FDA, editor 2011: http://www.fda.gov/MedicalDevices/Safety/AlertsandNotices/ucm262435.htm.
88. Marks BK, Goldman HB. What is the gold standard for posterior vaginal wall prolapse repair: mesh or native tissue? Curr Urol Rep. 2012;13(3):216–21.

89. Sand PK, et al. Prospective randomized trial of polyglactin 910 mesh to prevent recurrence of cystoceles and rectoceles. Am J Obstet Gynecol. 2001;184(7):1357–62; discussion 1362–4.
90. Lehur PA, Kahn X, Hamy A. Surgical treatment of anterior rectoceles in women. The perioneal-vaginal approach. Ann Chir. 2000; 125(8):782–6.
91. Leventoglu S, et al. Transperineal rectocele repair with polyglycolic acid mesh: a case series. Dis Colon Rectum. 2007;50(12): 2085–92; discussion 2092–5.
92. Watson SJ, et al. Transperineal repair of symptomatic rectocele with Marlex mesh: a clinical, physiological and radiologic assessment of treatment. J Am Coll Surg. 1996;183(3):257–61.
93. Smart NJ, Mercer-Jones MA. Functional outcome after transperineal rectocele repair with porcine dermal collagen implant. Dis Colon Rectum. 2007;50(9):1422–7.
94. Farid M, et al. Randomized controlled trial between perineal and anal repairs of rectocele in obstructed defecation. World J Surg. 2010;34(4):822–9.
95. Khubchandani IT, et al. Endorectal repair of rectocele revisited. Br J Surg. 1997;84(1):89–91.
96. Khubchandani IT, et al. Endorectal repair of rectocele. Dis Colon Rectum. 1983;26(12):792–6.
97. Heriot AG, Skull A, Kumar D. Functional and physiological outcome following transanal repair of rectocele. Br J Surg. 2004; 91(10):1340–4.
98. Sehapayak S. Transrectal repair of rectocele: an extended armamentarium of colorectal surgeons. A report of 355 cases. Dis Colon Rectum. 1985;28(6):422–33.
99. Block IR. Transrectal repair of rectocele using obliterative suture. Dis Colon Rectum. 1986;29(11):707–11.
100. Roman H, Michot F. Long-term outcomes of transanal rectocele repair. Dis Colon Rectum. 2005;48(3):510–7.
101. Tjandra JJ, et al. Transanal repair of rectocele corrects obstructed defecation if it is not associated with anismus. Dis Colon Rectum. 1999;42(12):1544–50.
102. Nieminen K, et al. Transanal or vaginal approach to rectocele repair: a prospective, randomized pilot study. Dis Colon Rectum. 2004;47(10):1636–42.
103. Maher C, et al. Surgical management of pelvic organ prolapse in women. Cochrane Database Syst Rev. 2010;(4):CD004014.
104. Gustilo-Ashby AM, et al. Bowel symptoms 1 year after surgery for prolapse: further analysis of a randomized trial of rectocele repair. Am J Obstet Gynecol. 2007;197(1):76.e1–e5.
105. Murad-Regadas SM, et al. Management of patients with rectocele, multiple pelvic floor dysfunctions and obstructed defecation syndrome. Arq Gastroenterol. 2012;49(2):135–42.
106. Jones OM, Cunningham C, Lindsey I. The assessment and management of rectal prolapse, rectal intussusception, rectocoele, and enterocoele in adults. BMJ. 2011;342:c7099.
107. Tsiaoussis J, et al. Rectoanal intussusception: presentation of the disorder and late results of resection rectopexy. Dis Colon Rectum. 2005;48(4):838–44.
108. Dindo D, et al. Clinical and morphologic correlation after stapled transanal rectal resection for obstructed defecation syndrome. Dis Colon Rectum. 2008;51(12):1768–74.
109. Christiansen J, et al. Internal rectal intussusception: results of surgical repair. Dis Colon Rectum. 1992;35(11):1026–8; discussion 1028–9.
110. Hwang YH, et al. Biofeedback therapy for rectal intussusception. Tech Coloproctol. 2006;10(1):11–5; discussion 15–6.
111. Dvorkin LS, et al. Rectal intussusception: characterization of symptomatology. Dis Colon Rectum. 2005;48(4):824–31.
112. Steele SR, Mellgren A. Constipation and obstructed defecation. Clin Colon Rectal Surg. 2007;20(2):110–7.
113. Choi JS, et al. Outcome and management of patients with large rectoanal intussusception. Am J Gastroenterol. 2001;96(3):740–4.
114. Felt-Bersma RJ, Tiersma ES, Cuesta MA. Rectal prolapse, rectal intussusception, rectocele, solitary rectal ulcer syndrome, and enterocele. Gastroenterol Clin North Am. 2008;37(3):645–68, ix.
115. Mellgren A, et al. Internal rectal intussusception seldom develops into total rectal prolapse. Dis Colon Rectum. 1997;40(7):817–20.
116. von Papen M, et al. Functional results of laparoscopic resection rectopexy for symptomatic rectal intussusception. Dis Colon Rectum. 2007;50(1):50–5.
117. Johnson E, et al. Resection rectopexy for internal rectal intussusception reduces constipation and incomplete evacuation of stool. Eur J Surg Suppl. 2003;588:51–6.
118. Orrom WJ, et al. Rectopexy is an ineffective treatment for obstructed defecation. Dis Colon Rectum. 1991;34(1):41–6.
119. Slawik S, et al. Laparoscopic ventral rectopexy, posterior colporrhaphy and vaginal sacrocolpopexy for the treatment of recto-genital prolapse and mechanical outlet obstruction. Colorectal Dis. 2008;10(2):138–43.
120. Collinson R, et al. Laparoscopic ventral rectopexy for internal rectal prolapse: short-term functional results. Colorectal Dis. 2010; 12(2):97–104.
121. Sileri P, et al. Laparoscopic ventral rectopexy for internal rectal prolapse using biological mesh: postoperative and short-term functional results. J Gastrointest Surg. 2012;16(3):622–8.
122. Farouk R, Bhardwaj R, Phillips RK. Stapled transanal resection of the rectum (STARR) for the obstructed defaecation syndrome. Ann R Coll Surg Engl. 2009;91(4):287–91.
123. Lehur PA, et al. Outcomes of stapled transanal rectal resection vs. biofeedback for the treatment of outlet obstruction associated with rectal intussusception and rectocele: a multicenter, randomized, controlled trial. Dis Colon Rectum. 2008;51(11):1611–8.
124. Ommer A, Rolfs TM, Walz MK. Long-term results of stapled transanal rectal resection (STARR) for obstructive defecation syndrome. Int J Colorectal Dis. 2010;25(11):1287–92.
125. Goede AC, et al. Medium-term results of stapled transanal rectal resection (STARR) for obstructed defecation and symptomatic rectal-anal intussusception. Colorectal Dis. 2011;13(9):1052–7.
126. Gagliardi G, et al. Results, outcome predictors, and complications after stapled transanal rectal resection for obstructed defecation. Dis Colon Rectum. 2008;51(2):186–95; discussion 195.
127. Pescatori M, Gagliardi G. Postoperative complications after procedure for prolapsed hemorrhoids (PPH) and stapled transanal rectal resection (STARR) procedures. Tech Coloproctol. 2008; 12(1):7–19.
128. Corman ML, et al. Consensus conference on the stapled transanal rectal resection (STARR) for disordered defaecation. Colorectal Dis. 2006;8(2):98–101.
129. Aigner F, et al. The rectogenital septum: morphology, function, and clinical relevance. Dis Colon Rectum. 2004;47(2):131–40.
130. Takahashi T, et al. Enterocele: what is the clinical implication? Dis Colon Rectum. 2006;49(10 Suppl):S75–81.
131. Gosselink MJ, et al. Treatment of enterocele by obliteration of the pelvic inlet. Dis Colon Rectum. 1999;42(7):940–4.
132. Chou Q, Weber AM, Piedmonte MR. Clinical presentation of enterocele. Obstet Gynecol. 2000;96(4):599–603.
133. Ellis CN. Treatment of obstructed defecation. Clin Colon Rectal Surg. 2005;18(2):85–95.
134. Jean F, et al. Treatment of enterocele by abdominal colporectosacropexy – efficacy on pelvic pressure. Colorectal Dis. 2002;4(5): 321–5.
135. Oom DM, et al. Enterocele repair by abdominal obliteration of the pelvic inlet: long-term outcome on obstructed defaecation and symptoms of pelvic discomfort. Colorectal Dis. 2007;9(9):845–50.

136. Boccasanta P, et al. Stapled transanal rectal resection for outlet obstruction: a prospective, multicenter trial. Dis Colon Rectum. 2004;47(8):1285–96; discussion 1296–7.
137. Reibetanz J, et al. Enterocele is not a contraindication to stapled transanal surgery for outlet obstruction: an analysis of 170 patients. Colorectal Dis. 2011;13(6):e131–6.
138. Carriero A, et al. Laparoscopic correction of enterocele associated to stapled transanal rectal resection for obstructed defecation syndrome. Int J Colorectal Dis. 2010;25(3):381–7.
139. Petersen S, et al. Stapled transanal rectal resection under laparoscopic surveillance for rectocele and concomitant enterocele. Dis Colon Rectum. 2006;49(5):685–9.
140. Mellgren A, et al. Enterocele is correctable using the Ripstein rectopexy. Dis Colon Rectum. 1994;37(8):800–4.
141. Fenner DE. Diagnosis and assessment of sigmoidoceles. Am J Obstet Gynecol. 1996;175(6):1438–41; discussion 1441–2.
142. Jorge JM, Yang YK, Wexner SD. Incidence and clinical significance of sigmoidoceles as determined by a new classification system. Dis Colon Rectum. 1994;37(11):1112–7.
143. Malouf AJ, Vaizey CJ, Kamm MA. Results of behavioral treatment (biofeedback) for solitary rectal ulcer syndrome. Dis Colon Rectum. 2001;44(1):72–6.
144. Badrek-Amoudi A, et al. Laparoscopic ventral mesh rectopexy (LVMR) in the management of solitary rectal ulcer syndrome (SRUS): a cause for optimism? Colorectal Dis. 2013;15: 575–81.
145. Thomas GP, et al. Sacral nerve stimulation for constipation. Br J Surg. 2013;100(2):174–81.

Fecal Incontinence

13

Tracy L. Hull

Key Points

- The history is the most important aspect in planning treatment for fecal incontinence, which includes the patient's perception of the problem.
- Health-care providers and patients many times have divergent views as to the definition and severity of fecal incontinence.
- Quantitative tools of evaluation such as incontinence scores and quality of life scales are helpful when looking for improvement or change after a treatment intervention, but do not replace a thorough history and physical examination.
- The goal is to improve quality of life—a cure with "perfect" bowel control is usually not realistic. You should emphasize improvement and improvement in quality of life as the goals.
- There is no one treatment for fecal incontinence. Rather, therapy must be individualized, perhaps combining several methods for optimal improvement.
- Successful outcomes revolve around you having a clear understanding of the pathophysiology and any associated underlying conditions.
- While several operative and nonoperative options exist, ultimately a stoma may be the best option for certain patients who fail or are not candidates for these treatment strategies.

Evaluation

Fecal continence is a complex disorder. Controlled elimination of fecal matter and gas relies on a coordination of many facets of physiology to work in concert, automatically, and dependently until it reaches the distal rectum. At that time, human volition intervenes until the circumstances are socially acceptable to expel gas, liquid, or solid waste. Problems at any level of this process can lead to fecal incontinence. This can range from soiling of the anal skin to inability to control flatus to loss of an entire bowel motion—all either with or without knowledge that this horrifying event is occurring. Health-care providers and patients many times have divergent views as to the definition and severity of fecal incontinence. This is highlighted when considering the fecal incontinence severity index, as there are two formulas for determining scores based on whether the surgeon or the patient is completing the form [1]. When the tool was being developed, it was discovered that patients and colorectal surgeons rate and view the severity of accidental loss of solid stool differently. Therefore, all treatment of fecal incontinence begins with a comprehensive history, which must include the patient's perception of the problem.

History

Key Concept: A critical aspect to accurately determining the origin of fecal incontinence involves a thorough review of the patient's entire history. This includes evaluating for concomitant pelvic floor disorders that may change your treatment.

A comprehensive history starts with discovering exactly what the patient defines as loss of stool, the frequency, the urgency associated with defecation, and how it affects them. Precise questioning clarifies someone who plans their daily life around their bowels (i.e., does not eat for a day before they go to the grocery store or will not travel due to concerns of stool control) such that they have few incontinent episodes but at the cost of an extremely poor quality of life. It is

Electronic supplementary material The online version of this chapter (doi: 10.1007/978-1-4614-9022-7_13) contains supplementary material, which is available to authorized users. Videos can also be accessed at http://www.springerimages.com/videos/978-1-4614-9021-0.

T.L. Hull, MD
Department of Colon and Rectal Surgery,
Digestive Disease Institute, The Cleveland Clinic Foundation,
9500 Euclid Ave, Cleveland, OH 44195, USA
e-mail: hullt@ccf.org

S.R. Steele et al. (eds.), *Complexities in Colorectal Surgery*,
DOI 10.1007/978-1-4614-9022-7_13, © Springer Science+Business Media New York 2014

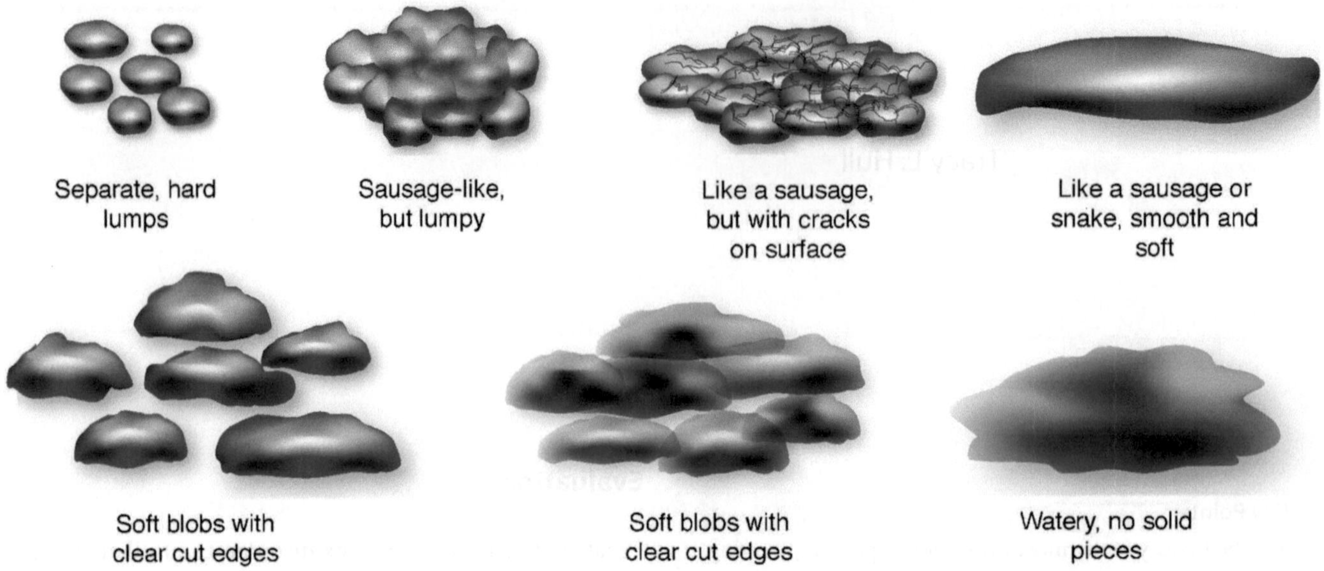

Fig. 13.1 Bristol stool scale (From Lewis and Heaton [52]. Reproduced with permission of Informa Healthcare © 1997)

also helpful to clarify the stool character. Using an aid such as the Bristol stool scale provides an easy visual method (Fig. 13.1; see also Table 20.2) [2]. Questions regarding changes in bowel habits over time (i.e., bowel habits when a teen and then changes during each decade of their life) provide clues to "normal" changes in women's bowels with aging [3]. Men can also have changes with their bowels as they age, but it many times is not as pronounced as in women. Many women may also experience typical changes during their hormonal menstrual cycle that stress a fragile balance in defecation and lead to gas/stool control issues.

Defining exactly when the problem with fecal control occurs is another important clue. For instance, do they feel like they fully empty their rectum (as may be seen when stool is trapped in a rectocele and may leak out after they leave the bathroom)? Do they have soilage or leakage in the first several hours after defecation (again stool trapped in a rectocele or stool retained in the rectum after evacuation)? Do they have loss of stool while sleeping (very unusual)?

Obstetrical history is also crucial, including number/weight of children, unusual presentation at delivery, prolonged labor, episiotomy, or tears of the perineum. Basic language helps to delineate some of these issues, such as asking if the doctor needed to use sutures in the vaginal area. Also most women remember if they had changes in bowel or bladder control after a delivery and if this had fully resolved.

Dietary choices can greatly affect stool quality, and a review of what, how much, when, and changes may elucidate a culprit that can be modified.

Many systemic diseases affect defecation and stool evacuation, especially diabetes, scleroderma, and multiple sclerosis. Also other central nervous system problems, which include back surgery or back injury, may lead to alterations in nerve signals to the intestine and the pelvis and should be investigated. Medications, including some herbal/health food store brands, change stool character, and ascertaining exactly when they were started and the relationship to any perceived changes in stool consistency should be sought. Many patients do not link the two, so careful questioning can assist in this endeavor.

Anal, pelvic, or abdominal surgery may also influence defecation, along with any anal trauma or injury. This would include anal intercourse or sexual abuse—both areas that surgeons typically are uncomfortable to investigate, though are crucial to ask about. Additionally, prior radiation treatment to the pelvis or a congenital malformation in the pelvis should be noted.

A large percentage of women may be experiencing other pelvic floor problems such as urinary incontinence, dysfunctional uterine bleeding, or vaginal prolapse. While these may not directly affect fecal control, your treatment options may be influenced by other pelvic disorders.

As a general rule, questions about alcohol, tobacco, illegal drug use, family history of bowel problems, and general health care (including colonoscopy) are important as they may provide clues that tailor which treatment options would be optimal for an individual patient.

Although not often as publicized, men experience problems with fecal control as well. Life-changing events such as loss of a spouse or divorce (i.e., diet may then have changed after spouse no longer cooks for them) or change in job (additional stress leads to a change in stool character) are particularly important to note along with all other points outlined above that would pertain to men. One study that

Table 13.1 Key concepts to be covered when obtaining the history

Clarify what the patient perceives as lack of fecal control
Clarify what and when the fecal incontinence occurs
How often does this occur
Associated fecal urgency
Affect on daily activities
Character of stool
Changes in pattern of defecation over decades of life
Changes in defecation with menstruation
Obstetrical history
Dietary history and relation to bowel issues
Other systemic diseases (i.e., diabetes, scleroderma, multiple sclerosis)
History of back injury or back surgery
Medications including herbal and over the counter and the temporal relationship to medication changes and the start of fecal incontinence
Anal surgery or trauma including anal intercourse
History of sexual abuse
Abdominal or pelvic surgery
History of radiation treatment to the pelvis
Congenital malformations (especially in the pelvis)
Other pelvic floor problems (i.e., urinary incontinence, dysfunctional uterine bleeding, vaginal prolapse)
Life-changing events (i.e., death of spouse or life partner, change in job)

specifically examined 43 males with fecal incontinence found that 77 % were classified as having fecal leakage and 23 % fecal incontinence [4]. Forty percent of those with leakage had a sphincter defect compared with 70 % in the fecal incontinent group. All patients with leakage improved with lifestyle changes and biofeedback, while 6/10 in the fecal incontinent groups required surgical intervention such as sacral nerve stimulation or other involved treatments. The authors concluded that males with fecal incontinence (versus leakage) had some type of sphincter weakening that typically requires surgical treatment. Table 13.1 summarizes the key elements that need to be discussed during the history.

Physical Examination

Key Concept: A thorough examination involves evaluation of everything from the undergarments and perineal skin to the perineum, including both rectal and vaginal examinations, and abdomen. Validated scoring systems will assist in quantifying and tracking progress.

The physical examination focuses generally on the abdomen and perineum. The abdominal exam generally keys on scars, masses, distension, and tenderness. When looking at the perineum, I first note the underclothes and perianal skin for any signs of soilage, along with any skin irritation (Fig. 13.2) or anal scars over the perineal body or over the anal skin. I typically examine patients in the left lateral

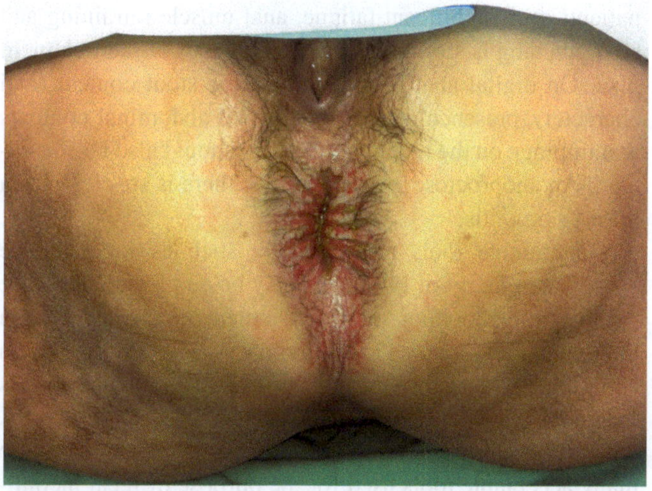

Fig. 13.2 This patient has severe anal excoriation from leakage of mucus and liquid stool at her anal verge. The other marks across her skin and buttocks are classic from continuous sitting on a heating pad in an unsuccessful attempt to alleviate the discomfort (Reproduced with permission from Tracy Hull, MD The Cleveland Clinic Foundation Cleveland, Ohio)

position. In women I look in the vagina and note, with strain, any descent of the vaginal wall. I may also digitize the vagina again to clarify vaginal descent or simultaneously digitate the anus and vagina to again clarify descent. I ask them to strain and also note anal descent. When I see that the anal area move 4–5 cm and take on the shape of a bowel, this may be associated with damaged support structures, straining, and defecation problems. While there are patients that have descent and no defecation issues, it is something to keep in mind in combination with the history as clues to the etiology of the fecal incontinence. These patients may not be totally emptying their rectum or have an element of internal prolapse that may be adding to their symptoms. The anal and perianal skin requires close inspection first looking at the length of the perineal body. I ask them to squeeze and look for anal muscle movement. Many times there is excessive buttock movement as patients have gotten into the habit of squeezing all muscles in that region in an effort to avoid the horrifying aftermath of fecal leakage. To determine if they can contract their anal muscle, touching the skin over the anal muscle and asking them to pull only that muscle toward their umbilical area will clarify for them the muscle to contract and allow you to detect anal sphincter movement. On digital anal exam, differentiating between movement of the levator muscle and anal sphincter when squeezing should be noted, as you may be falsely believe the patient has sphincter tone when in fact is coming from higher in the canal. Again asking them to pull the muscle to their umbilical area may assist in detecting anal sphincter movement. Also important is anal muscle fatigue, which may be detected after several prolonged (about 15 s) anal sphincter contractions. For patients with significant fatigue, anal muscle retraining and strengthening is strongly considered as part of the treatment plan. On digital anal exam, a mass, the stool content (and character), presence of a rectocele, and abdominal contents that impinge on the rectum with strain should also be considered. An anoproctoscopy is helpful if there is suspicion of a mass or proctitis.

Quantitative tools of evaluation such as incontinence scores and quality of life scales may be employed. They are helpful when looking for improvement or change after a treatment intervention. However, they should never replace a comprehensive history. Some form of incontinence tool is mandatory to determine using sacral nerve stimulation, which will be discussed in more detail below. As there are many acceptable tools used for the purpose of fecal incontinence, choosing one that works for you and your office staff and administering the questionnaires before seeing the patient and after treatment interventions will allow familiarity with its nuances and use. One study looked at the current popular tools to score fecal incontinence (Rothenberger, Wexner, Vaizey, and Fecal Incontinence Severity Index) and found the Wexner scale correlated most closely with subjective perception of severity of symptoms by patients [5]. Another study looked at "responsiveness and interpretability" of the Vaizey score, Wexner score, and Fecal Incontinence Quality of Life scale [6]. These researchers felt none of these popular tools attain the high levels of psychometric soundness needed to be recommended as the best tool to use. They also echo the notion previously stated, that what a patient views as important may be different from the physician. While the Wexner score was felt to be the most suitable for severity assessment, they recommended that several tools should be used for evaluation in an attempt to circumvent these issues. An overview of each tool and its pros and cons are beyond the scope of this paper, but an excellent overview was written by Wang and Varma [7], which outlines some of the commonly used tools.

Testing

Key Concept: Testing is meant to augment or clarify findings on history and physical examination. Ultrasonography is my preferential test to help guide therapy.

Testing is individualized based on the history and physical exam. In appropriate patients, a colonoscopy would be ordered. In some patients where I question their ability to control stool, a fiber enema is administered (Fig. 13.3). This consists of fiber (i.e., a packet or large tablespoon of Metamucil^R, Citrucel) that is poured into an empty container and mixed with about 50 cc of water and quickly instilled in the rectum before it has time to gel. Then the patient walks around, bends over, and generally has sustained non-strenuous activity for 5 min to determine if they have leakage of this mixture from their anus.

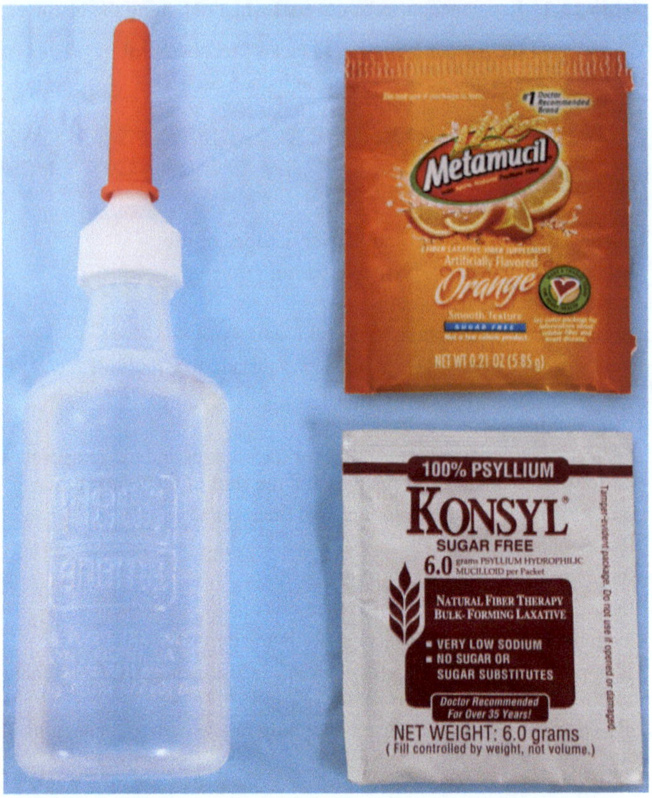

Fig. 13.3 Fiber enema: a packet of fiber or a large tablespoon is placed in an empty enema dispensing container. An empty Fleet Enema^R container works well. Then about 50 cc of tap water is added, and the mixture is quickly shook and then inserted into the rectum. The goal is to insert the mixture before the fiber has a chance to gel making insertion impossible (Reproduced with permission from Tracy Hull, MD The Cleveland Clinic Foundation Cleveland, Ohio)

The utility of anorectal physiology testing was questioned by our center and found not to correlate with incontinence scores [8]. Also ultrasound findings did not correlate with manometry results. We felt that preoperative anal manometry and endoanal ultrasound should be used to guide treatment, but improvement after an overlapping sphincter repair should not be assessed by changes in manometry pressures. This somewhat contradicts data from another unit; however, their aim was somewhat different. They looked at whether anal manometry could separate those patients with fecal incontinence from healthy individuals [9]. They found that patients with fecal incontinence had lower rest and squeeze pressures and lower urge sensation along with a higher volume of first sensation pressures. Overall they found that single studies were not helpful, but the entire panel of anal physiology studies had excellent sensitivity, moderate specificity, and convincing accuracy.

My feeling is that overall anal physiology testing may guide therapy, but I am not sure it is always needed. We rarely order needle EMG looking for neurological damage as it has not proved useful in guiding treatment. Perhaps looking for a sacral reflex before considering sacral nerve stimulation may be a consideration. I am also not sure that pudendal nerve terminal motor latency offers much assistance. Previously we used nerve prolongation, particularly bilaterally, to counsel patients that results after sphincter repair most likely would be poor. However, I have seen patients without prolongation of their pudendal nerves when tested, where absolutely no anal muscle moves when I ask them to squeeze on physical exam. Anal endosonography on the other hand provides a useful road map when considering treatment, and I usually rely on this test (making sure I perform it myself or know that the endosonographer is experienced in accurately depicting sphincter defects). Our unit still typically orders anorectal physiology on most patients because we maintain extensive databases that we may use in future studies; however, we only use the data to selectively counsel patients. For instance, a patient with a low maximal tolerated volume and low anal pressures may not achieve the expected short-term benefit from an overlapping sphincter repair. We would use this information to preoperatively discuss expected outcomes with the patient and aid in navigating the treatment plan. While pelvic magnetic resonance imaging is a consideration instead of or with anal endosonography, I am not convinced it adds enough information to justify the expense. I do not routinely order a defecating proctogram unless there is an accompanying problem with stool expulsion during defecation. Dudding and Vaizey wrote an excellent overview of testing for fecal incontinence and other pelvic floor disorders, and the reader is directed to this review for more in-depth descriptions of the various tests [10].

Treatment Options

Key Concept: From the very beginning, set realistic expectations with your patient and ensure they understand this may involve several different treatment modalities.

The next step in management involves an individual treatment plan for the patient. This does not encompass *only one* intervention, but could involve several combined modalities customized for the patient and revolves around a clear understanding of the pathophysiology and underlying conditions. Fecal incontinence should be viewed as a chronic disease like diabetes or hypertension. Similarly, in these chronic diseases, several treatment modalities may be needed for optimal control of the disease process and optimization of the patient's quality of life. Similarly management of fecal incontinence is a long-term notion, and adjustment in the treatment plan will be necessary as needed. This also involves setting realistic expectations for the patient and the surgeon (i.e., some health-care provider must be prepared to assist and manage this patient long term). Society typically views defecation issues as voluntary (i.e., mind over matter) which adds to unrealistic goals determined by the patient. Therefore, attaining "perfect" bowel function may not be a realistic goal, and the health-care provider should emphasize improvement and improvement in quality of life as the goals.

Conservative Management

Key Concept: Almost every patient will require medical management, which typically involves dietary supplements and one (or more) of several classes of medications.

Most treatment plans include some element of conservative management. Any issues with loose or soft stool can contribute to problems with control. Evaluation and treatment alone of diarrhea (or just loose stool) can sometimes greatly improve the patient's situation. These include fiber supplementation (taken with the least amount of water) pectin, and medication. Loperamide is a typical medication used, and instructions for use must be carefully discussed as the instructions on the package may not be appropriate for each patient's problem. Depending on the pattern of defecation, perhaps starting with one pill/capsule (2 mg) each morning could be the initial recommendation for this medication. The goal is titration to avoid fecal incontinence but not too much that produces constipation; however, this may not be possible. If one pill is too much, the liquid form administered to children can be used so the dose can be decreased. Also if constipation is an issue, using the medication every other day or every 3 days per week may allow therapeutic benefit for the incontinence without precipitating constipation.

Skin irritation frequently accompanies fecal incontinence or may even be the true reason a patient seeks medical assistance. Counseling regarding skin care therefore is also part of conservative treatment. Barrier creams that typically employ zinc (such as Calmoseptine^R, Calmoseptine, Inc., Huntington Beach, California) and lanolin (make sure they are not allergic to wool) may be lathered onto the anal skin like frosting (i.e., a thick layer). Patients should place these creams up to the dentate line for complete protection. They may stain underclothes, so patients should be warned of this possibility. Antibiotic ointments are rarely required, and occasionally an antifungal powder may need to be dusted on the skin if Candida is detected. This can be applied using a cotton ball (dusted over the barrier cream) and then leaving the cotton ball by the anus to wick away moisture (similar to cotton socks used in athletic activity). Since anal irritation may lead some patients to feel that their anal area is unclean, they may wipe that region excessively (similar to polishing furniture but instead polishing their anus). Advising them to wipe with unscented baby wipes or wet paper towel and avoid using soap and a washcloth in the shower along with minimal wiping after defecation can aid in improving anal irritation from excessive wiping.

Dietary manipulation may be advised if certain foods lead to loose, urgent, or uncontrolled stools. A food diary that corresponds to incontinent episodes may clarify offending foods. Fresh fruit and vegetables can make stools loose and add to urgency. Many patients have concerns with excessive or uncontrollable flatus. A low carbohydrate diet may reduce flatus. While many anti-gas (over-the-counter) medications can be recommended, many patients find these unhelpful with flatal incontinence. For severe problems with excessive flatus, an intermittent short course of antibiotics (rifaximin [Xifaxan^{R}] is a popular choice) can be prescribed, but many effective agents are very expensive. Metronidazole is another choice that is less expensive, but side effects such as an Antabuse effect, tin taste in the mouth, or peripheral neuropathy must be considered before prescribing. These agents will change the flora and decrease intestinal gas temporarily. Therefore, the medication must be repeated with the goal of the least days per month possible to attain relief. One way I advise taking antibiotics for this purpose is 1 week out of every month, which in my experience seems to adequately reduce issues with excessive flatus. Probiotics also are helpful for some patients with excessive gas issues.

Since a lot of information may be recommended regarding conservative therapy, it is extremely helpful to give precise *written* instructions for skin care and bowel-altering medication so the patient has exact instructions to follow and does not need to rely on memory to implement suggested changes or treatment. Since it is important to individualize the treatment, we do not use standardized forms and actually type out the instructions that are also filed in their chart.

For some patients with leakage, especially when it seems to occur directly after they leave the bathroom, a tap water or rinsing enema after defecation will eliminate any retained material and alleviate the problem. While many patients do not prefer this approach, if explained in a positive light and the patient successfully uses this treatment, they may change their mind. I typically recommend that an empty phosphate soda enema container be used (they can use the actual phosphate enema for irrigation rather than discarding it, then the container can be filled with water and used five to eight times again before the material cracks). Alternatively, a large catheter can be used to instill 50–200 cc of tepid tap water. I emphasize it is like "rinsing" out the rectum.

For some, a large volume water enema may be needed if they are using this treatment for more than minor leakage. For those patients, my nurse will discuss using a large volume enema consisting of 500–1,000 cc or water. This is delivered via a 28-Fr Foley catheter (as this has a 30-cc balloon that can be inflated if necessary) (Fig. 13.4). The fluid is placed in a tube feeding administration bag as this has a valve to regulate the inflow of fluid rather than straight tubing which otherwise allows the liquid to run in quickly. The catheter must be well lubricated and this is emphasized. We ask them to start with 500 cc and increase the amount weekly over 4–6 weeks. They are also counseled to allow 45–60 min to perform the irrigation and evacuation daily. It also tends to be more successful if performed at the same time daily (typically in the early morning). Encouragement and patience is provided by my nurse, and this seems to enhance success with this treatment. An extension of this thought process is the antegrade continence enema. A surgical procedure is performed where the appendix or a tapered segment of terminal

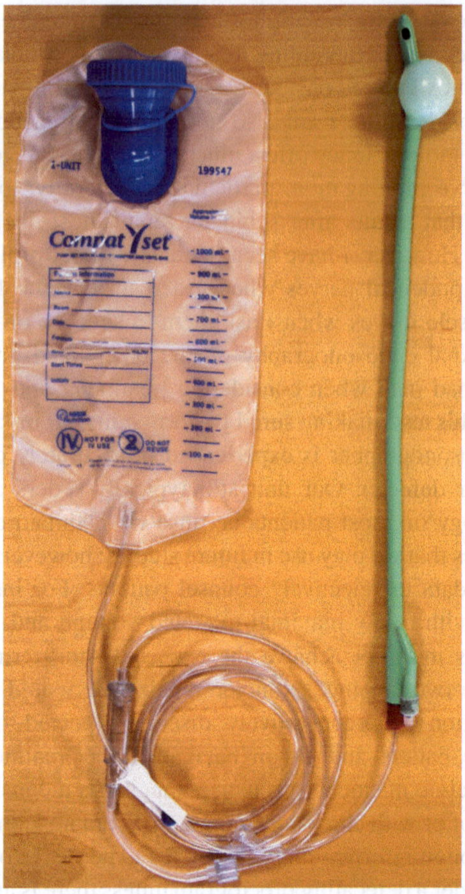

Fig. 13.4 For a large volume enema, a 28-Fr Foley is lubricated and inserted into the anus. For patients who cannot retain fluid, the balloon can be inflated with up to 30 cc and pulled back to rest against the pelvic floor. Then 500–1,000 cc of water is placed in the bag. Tubing connects the bag to the Foley. There is a control valve on the tubing. Fluid can be instilled under direct control of the patient via the control valve into the rectum and left colon (Reproduced with permission from Tracy Hull, MD The Cleveland Clinic Foundation Cleveland, Ohio)

ileum is brought to the surface to form a flush stoma about the size of a 10-French catheter. Water is instilled via the small stoma, which then flushes out the entire colon via the antegrade approach. While this therapy tends to be more popular in the pediatric population, selected adults are quite satisfied doing irrigation by this method.

Other Therapies

Key Concept: Progressively invasive treatment options are available. Each has its own strength and weaknesses, depending on the severity of incontinence and underlying pathology.

Physical Retraining (Biofeedback)

Physical retraining of the pelvic floor is also a treatment that may improve the patient's situation (and does not worsen) and should be considered. It is important to be alert to the fact that some insurance companies will not reimburse for this treatment. Also a therapist (whether a physical therapist, nurse, or other interested health-care provider) may not have specialized specific training for pelvic floor issues and may not provide the most optimal teaching. The Cochrane review done by Norton and Cody identified 21 studies with a total of 1,525 patients [11]. They found severe methodological weaknesses in nearly all studies reviewed but concluded that perhaps some portions of biofeedback and sphincter exercises may have therapeutic effect. The authors emphasized that this was not definitely shown in their review and larger well-designed trials were needed.

Anal Plug

For minor leakage, the anal plug may be considered. The recent Cochrane review looked at four studies of 136 patients [12]. They noted that the rate of intolerance or ineffectiveness from reviewed studies was 35 %. In the short-term (not considering any long-term results), anal plugs, when tolerated, could provide continence. They also noted that overall satisfaction was better when polyurethane plugs were used versus polyvinyl-alcohol plugs. Experience worldwide with plugs is limited. This device should be considered in patients with minor leakage, but dislodgement or intolerance is an issue. They can be obtained in various types, designs, and sizes. Insurance coverage may be limited. They also may be considered as part of a larger treatment plan for a patient.

Radiofrequency Energy (RFE)

Radiofrequency treatment of the anal sphincter has been available for over a decade and is administered per the SECCA^{R} machine and protocol (Figs. 13.5 and 13.6). Two

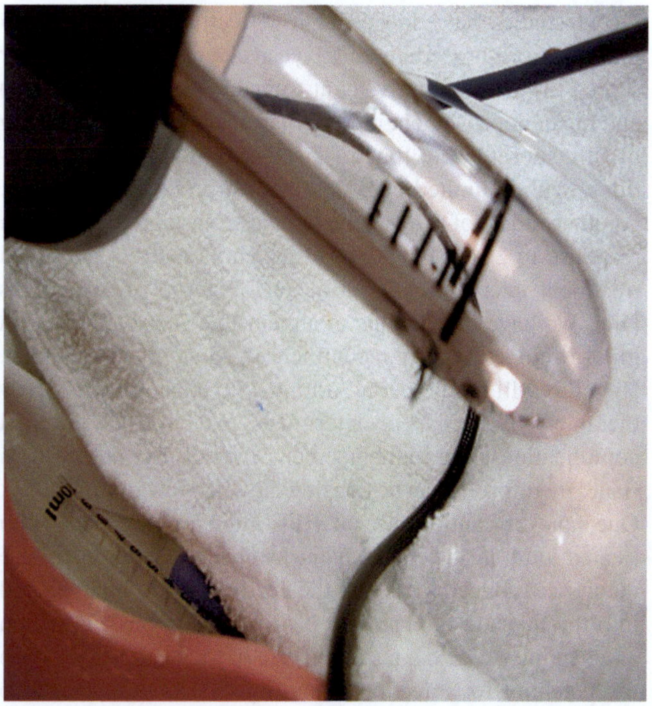

Fig. 13.5 The handpiece for the SECCA® procedure shown with the needles deployed. The handpiece is inserted in the anal canal starting at the dentate line and the four needles deployed into the tissue. Radiofrequency is then delivered for 90 s. The needles are retracted and the probe is rotated 90° and the process repeated until all four quadrants are treated. Then the probe is moved 5 mm proximal, and those four quadrants are treated. The process starts at the dentate line, and typically, there are 4 rows of treatment (Reproduced with permission from Tracy Hull, MD The Cleveland Clinic Foundation Cleveland, Ohio)

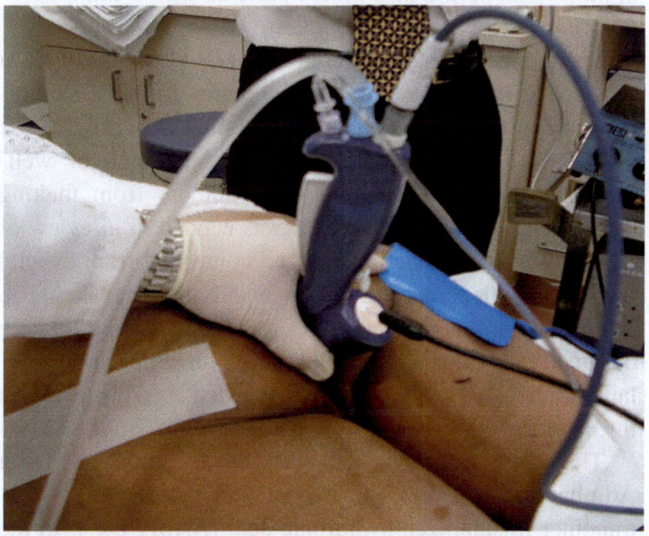

Fig. 13.6 Shown is the handpiece inserted in the anal canal with the attachments (Reproduced with permission from Tracy Hull, MD The Cleveland Clinic Foundation Cleveland, Ohio)

recent studies have looked at its effectiveness. One study looked at pre-procedure and 1-year changes in the Wexner score [13]. Mean improvement from 15.6 to 12.9 ($p=0.035$) and mean improvement in 3 of 4 Fecal Incontinence Quality of Life subsets were found. There were minimal complications, with 3 limited episodes of post-procedure bleeding. Another study of 27 patients found a sustained long-term response in 22 %, but 52 % of patients required additional treatment interventions at a mean follow-up of 40 months [14]. We have offered this treatment to select patients with mild-to-moderate fecal incontinence and an intact sphincter. How this will fit into our algorithm with the approval of new therapies will need to be determined. We have had minimal complications, and reimbursement, overall, has not been an issue; therefore, it can be considered when few options exist. One note of caution, use of RFE after a patient has been treated with an injectable agent has been discouraged. The theoretical concerns are that the needles would be deployed into the injected implant and have no effect on stimulation and heating of the connective tissue in the anal region. Also the potential for infection of the injected implant has also been raised as a possible complication. I am not aware of any studies definitively reporting this as happening, but this possibility has been raised and should be acknowledged. Therefore, if the use of RFE is being contemplated, its use should be considered *before* treating with an injectable agent.

Injectables

Key Concept: While preliminary results have shown success in small studies, several questions remain regarding the ideal substance, technique, and population. I prefer to use it in mild-to-moderate incontinent patients with a thinning or fibrotic internal sphincter complex.

There are over ten different materials that have been reported as injectables into the anal region for fecal incontinence. The Cochrane review of this subject highlights the diversity of this material, along with the lack of well-designed studies, prohibiting these authors from making definitive conclusions [15]. This was echoed in a review of 13 case series and one randomized controlled trial, in total involving 420 patients, by Luo and Samaranayake [16]. These authors also concluded that future appropriately designed randomized controlled trials with large study populations and longer follow-up are needed to truly evaluate injectables.

The only injectable that has been Food and Drug Administration (FDA) approved in the United States is dextranomer in stabilized hyaluronic acid (NASA Dx^{R}). In the randomized monitored study for FDA approval, 52 % of patients being injected had >50 % reduction in fecal incontinence episodes compared to 31 % of those receiving a sham injection who reported the same degree of improvement [17]. The high degree of improvement in the sham group is curious, but placebo treatments for fecal incontinence for unclear reasons seem to have up to a 30 % improvement rate. These results were sustained at 36 months, and all of the quality of life scores showed significant improvement at 36 months [18]. This is a safe procedure with minor bleeding being the most common complication although 2/278 patients in the FDA-monitored study developed an abscess (one rectal, one prostatic) [17].

Besides the lack of sufficient data to guide treatment, other controversies surrounding injectable agents involve technique. Currently, there are seven different techniques found in the literature to administer the agent. The procedure typically involves one cc of this material injected into the submucosal space in four areas at the top of the anal canal. While many inject in the submucosal space, the intersphincteric space may be better. Yet, there are several additional questions that remain unanswered. Would the use of ultrasound to guide injection be superior to blinded injection? This procedure is typically done in the outpatient setting, but would the results improve if done in the OR? Additionally should the needle go through the anal mucosa or be inserted from the perianal skin to the target location? The size of the needle is typically 21 gauge, which seems necessary as the material is quite viscous and difficult to push through the needle. However, is this size of needle correct, as some of the material can be seen oozing out of the injection site at times after the treatment? The exact optimal patient who will benefit from this treatment is also unclear. Some of the patients in the FDA-monitored trial had severe fecal incontinence [17], but would patients with mild-to-moderate incontinence or leakage be better candidates? Also can injectable material be used to augment a defect in the internal sphincter (such as after a lateral sphincterotomy that has leakage) or a divot in the smooth contour of the anal canal, which is leading to leakage? All these questions surround using this material.

Our practice continues to be performing this procedure in the outpatient setting. We target patients with mild-to-moderate fecal incontinence. Also we would offer this to a patient with internal sphincter thinning or fibrosis as seen on anal endosonography. The patient receives a phosphate enema before and then is typically positioned in the left lateral position. Using a long beveled anoscope, Betadine is swabbed in the anal canal (a plain wet swab is used if the patient reports an iodine sensitivity that is concerning). The nurse steadies the anoscope after it is placed in position. The physician steadies the needle with one hand and injects with the other. The material is injected about 1 cm cephalad to the dentate line. We use digital guidance to inject in the submucosal space in four quadrants and turn the needle a quarter turn before withdrawal in attempt to prevent material leakage. Postoperatively, we do not issue any restrictions in activity and give advice on keeping stools soft. We ask patients to call immediately if they have pain, bleeding, or fever.

Sphincter Repair

Key Concept: Sphincter repair still plays a role in the management of incontinence, though long-term results remain disappointing. Preoperative biofeedback may be considered to improve results.

For patients with an anterior sphincter defect, typically from childbirth trauma, an overlapping sphincter repair has been advocated. The initial enthusiasm for this operation has been tempered with the realization that long-term results tend to be abysmal [19]. A systematic review of 16 studies with nearly 900 patients concluded worsening results over time with no predictive factors identified [20]. Technical factors have been blamed for these poor results, but even with verification of an intact overlap, the long-term results remain poor. Even when pudendal nerve terminal motor latency is not affected, the results tend to be disappointing. The exact reason remains elusive. Since some women have no issues with fecal control until years after the delivery trauma, there may be intrinsic damage to the sphincter besides the structural damage. Hence, when a sphincter is damaged during childbirth, the scar and fibrosis may eventually interfere with optimal function even if the sphincter has been repaired and the repair remains intact.

In many countries sphincter defects are not repaired in favor of sacral nerve stimulation. However, there may still be a place for this procedure. It is a relatively easy procedure, requiring no extra equipment, lower cost than many other procedures for fecal incontinence, and can be performed globally in any OR. In a young woman who has a significant symptomatic childbirth injury, our unit prefers a sphincter repair as the initial recommended treatment. Additionally, many women may be averse to having a permanent device implanted (sacral nerve stimulation or artificial bowel sphincter) at a young age. Full disclosure regarding the possibility of poor long-term results is also part of the preoperative discussion. Another consideration is that many women who have had fecal control issues for any length of time have forgotten how to contract their anal sphincter muscles. They may pull their buttocks together to avoid stool loss. Therefore, planning some lessons regarding anal sphincter movement (physical therapy retraining) before the repair and then after the surgery has healed may be beneficial.

In an attempt to improve long-term results, our center proposed using a biological graft to reinforce the two overlapped ends [21]. In a pilot study of ten women, there were no complications. These patients were compared to ten matched patients who had undergone a traditional overlapping repair. At 1 year, significant improvement in continence and quality of life was seen over baseline and compared to results from traditional repair. The question is whether these improvements will be sustained as these patients age and that will require long-term studies.

For young women who have an obstetrical injury, timing is frequently questioned. If we see them within weeks of the injury, it is important for the tissue to fully heal before any repair is attempted. This typically takes 3–6 months for the scar to become soft and pliable. For women who desire more children, the questions comes up regarding repair now versus waiting until after they have finished having all their children. This is discussed extensively with the patient along with the infringement that the fecal incontinence has on their quality of life. It is unclear if waiting versus immediate repair makes a difference, so it is a decision that the patient will make. However, if they have more children, they should still have a C-section to avoid further injury to their anal muscles. I have seen women with a sphincter injury who defer repair and then have another vaginal delivery. On many occasions they return with worse problems such as no muscle movement in their entire perineal area or further injury of the muscle complex.

I prefer a full bowel preparation before this procedure and the prone position. However, successful results have been accomplished without a bowel prep or in the lithotomy position. A Foley catheter is inserted. For the procedure, typically a transverse incision is made across the perineal body. The ends of the muscle must be dissected out to allow overlap. There is some literature that end-to-end repair may be superior [22, 23], but I still prefer a careful overlap using 2-0 polydioxanone. While the internal and external muscle can be separated and repaired individually, I prefer to overlap them together in bulk. Another unanswered question is if a levatorplasty will improve the longevity of a repair. A word of caution regarding the levatorplasty is that it may lead to a bridge of tissue across the vagina and dyspareunia. Therefore, I will add a levatorplasty if it does not narrow the vagina, lead to a bridge of tissue that feels like a tight band across the posterior vagina, and not require extensive further dissection of tissue. I take special precaution when raising the flap of anorectal skin and mucosa to avoid making the flap too thin (or it will become ischemic) and also avoid using excessive trauma with pickups, which would pinch this fragile area. Irrigation with antibiotic solution is used throughout. The horizontal incision is closed transversely over the anal sphincter and vagina. I typically will leave the central portion open for drainage. Invariably the wound rarely heals in a straightforward manner when the skin is closed. The most important thing is to make sure there is an outlet for drainage of any fluid that may be trapped or is a transudate into the deep wound area. The goal is to avoid drainage into the anal area that could lead to a fistula or destroy the muscle repair. I try to make the environment such that the fluid drains out the perineal area or closer to the vagina. Drains are used selectively (by me, although one of my partners always uses a drain) particularly if there is a lot of dead space. In the postoperative period up to about 3 weeks, if fluid becomes trapped beneath the repair, it is crucial that it is evacuated to avoid an abscess. To this end the wound is examined if possible on a weekly or 2-week basis in the outpatient clinic to ensure fluid does not become trapped. After the surgery, if possible I admit the patient for 1–2 days. Many insurance companies will only approve 23-h stay, so adjustment to this time frame is needed.

There is no clear evidence as to postoperative care, so experience- versus evidence-based approach is taken. I administer IV antibiotics while the patient is hospitalized and then oral antibiotics for 5 more days. Women prone to vaginal yeast infections also are given an oral antifungal agent during this time. Postoperative bowel management is crucial and often neglected. Besides exogenous fiber and a regular diet, I ask patients to ingest 30 cc of mineral oil daily, warning them that they will have an orange discharge on their underclothes. If they do not have a stool by 3 days after starting an oral diet, then they are advised to take milk of magnesia, one ounce twice daily until they stool. I prefer very soft stools versus a hard stool bolus that is difficult to pass. They can take a shower, but no baths or sitz baths to avoid excessive skin maceration for 2–3 weeks. Leaving the anal skin incision open over part of the perineal body infers that it will heal by secondary intention from the bottom up. Warning patients that the wound may be open for 4 weeks and they may note blood with wiping or on their underclothes avoids alarming calls by patients. I allow them to walk and sit on the first postoperative day and also ask them to avoid lifting over 20–25 lb for 4–6 weeks as lifting or excessive exercise inadvertently will bear down on the pelvic floor and may put pressure on the repair. I also ask them not to sit on a doughnut to avoid pulling the buttock cheeks apart and hence pull on the repair.

Artificial Bowel Sphincter

Key Concept: While still plagued by increased complication rates, ABS may be an option for select, motivated patients. Several technical tips are useful to minimize the morbidity associated with ABS implantation.

There is still a place in the surgical armamentarium for the artificial bowel sphincter. This treatment may be offered to patients born without a functioning anal muscle, those that have traumatic loss of the anal muscle, or those that fail or are not candidates for other treatments. Even after the learning curve, this procedure has a significant infection rate, reported to be around 40 % in two single-institution studies [24, 25]. One unit that divided their cases by experience reported a 50 % failure rate for the first 12 cases but 80 % success in the last 25 [26]. Most recently this center reported implantation via the vaginal approach and a 22 % rate of adverse septic events in 32 patients. Of note, these were in women with severe damage and scarring of the perineum, and a vaginal approach was chosen due to concern regarding the feasibility of implantation via the perineal route [27]. Whether routine transvaginal implantation in women will improve results will need further study. Even with the high complication rate, up to 50–70 % can achieve success—defined as an activated working device and improved continence [25, 28] in centers with experience in implantation. Additionally, all studies report significantly reduced fecal incontinent episodes and improved quality of life in those with an activated device [25–28]. One further issue noted in patients with an activated device may be empting difficulties reported in 28–57 % [26, 29]. This may be due to a new "dam" on the rectum where it was freely open to evacuate before or overall congenital problems affecting rectal function.

I continue to offer this treatment to appropriate patients. I discuss in depth the issues of infection, complications, and explantation. While these are serious issues, they are almost never life-threatening. I also discuss the problems with evacuation that require considerable counseling and typically laxatives or enemas to ensure adequate evacuation. The device initially is not activated after implantation to allow all wounds to heal. During this time, I still recommend 30 cc of oral mineral oil to prevent impaction as the device itself coupled with postoperative swelling and use of narcotic pain medication may lead to new evacuation problems. If a patient has uncontrollable diarrhea, the mineral oil is discontinued, but otherwise I recommend that it be continued for two more weeks beyond the 6-week mark when I activate the device. I find in patients with severe fecal incontinence, especially when a stoma is their only alternative, the high failure rate does not deter them regarding this device.

Some technical tips that I have found helpful include, during the procedure, employing two teams for implantation, one for the perineal portion to implant the cuff and the other team for the abdominal portion to implant the pump and balloon. There has been speculation that this will reduce rates of infection, and while I do not know if this is true, it does reduce the operative time. I make sure the cuff around the anus when in the open position is just barely snug when buttoned, but not too tight to help lessen evacuation problems. I also insist on an experienced company representative being present with entirely new inventory in every size of each part of the device for several reasons. Since limited numbers are done in a year, I do not like to use inventory that has been on our hospital shelf for an extended period of time. At one point in my past experience, I had difficulty activating the pump on three consecutive cases, and it was theorized that shelf stock, which was up-to-date but not new, may have been the culprit. I additionally want an experienced company representative present to answer the multiple questions that nurses usually have about preparation of the device. This is a complex procedure with many steps, and even the experienced nurses will not be involved in many cases per year. I use a full bowel prep before the surgery, as one study showed that an independent risk factor for infection was short time from implant to first bowel motion [24]. Patients receive IV antibiotics before the implant that cover gram-negative, gram-positive, and anaerobic bacteria. They continue these antibiotics until discharge, which can be up to 5 days in the hospital. They then go home on oral antibiotic to total 10 days IV plus oral. The night before the procedure, they also wash with antiseptic soap. Women are cautioned not to shave their pubic hair for 5 days prior, and in the OR, hair is clipped and not shaved over the suprapubic region. Ice packs are used on the perineal wound for 24 h postoperatively, and bacitracin topical ointment is applied to the perineal wound directly after surgery and for the first week.

If an inadvertent opening is made in the rectum while developing the plane anterior to the rectum for cuff placement, then the insertion is abandoned. To attempt to avoid this situation, the rectovaginal septum in women or anterior anal area in men must be developed deeply enough (I prefer ~6 cm) to allow subcutaneous tissue to easily cover the device and be closed in layers prior to skin closure. If a vaginotomy occurs, in selected situations if I can place the device well cephalad to the vaginal opening, and the vaginotomy is repaired and then the anal cuff inserted. All skin incisions are closed in layers with polyglactin suture. I also irrigate the perineal wound with antibiotic irrigation during the procedure. Placement of the cuff from the abdominal incision into the labia or scrotum can be difficult. It is crucial to develop the tract via the abdominal incision with a large Kelley clamp and make it large enough to allow the device to easily slide to the desired level of the scrotum or labia. The activation button should be turned to face laterally, and the tissue just cephalad to the pump is snugged down with a suture to ensure the pump does not migrate toward the abdominal incision or change orientation. Care is taken when placing this suture to avoid needle penetration of the tubing. Which side to place the pump is chosen in the office preoperatively with the patient's input to ensure ease of manipulation of the pump with their preferred hand. Morbidly obese patients that cannot reach their labia or scrotum or patients with debility in hand coordination should be cautioned against an ABS.

Long-term activity restrictions are controversial. I ask them to avoid riding a bike but otherwise have not been restrictive. Avoidance of anal intercourse is also discussed.

Sacral Nerve Stimulation (SNS)

Key Concept: SNS has an evolving role in these patients. The ability to observe improvement during a test phase makes this is an attractive alternative.

While considerable experience has been reported since 1995 with sacral nerve stimulation (SNS) for fecal incontinence, it is one of the newer modalities available in the United States being FDA approved in 2011. The exact therapy has been used for urinary incontinence for the past two decades, and there is extensive data published in that arena. A unique aspect to SNS is that the device can be tested as stage 1 of a two-stage procedure to assess improvement before a permanent device is implanted (Video 13.1). Stage 1 can be done in two ways. Currently in the United States, a tined lead is inserted (typically in the S3 sacral foramina under fluoroscopic assistance) and connected to a temporary neurostimulator device. If there is a reduction in 50 % of incontinent episodes, then this lead is disconnected from the external neurostimulator device and a new connection is performed to a permanent neurostimulator device that is implanted in the subcutaneous fat of the upper buttock region. If there is no improvement, the lead can be removed. In many centers outside the United States, and gaining in popularity with urologists worldwide, is the alternative stage 1 method called percutaneous nerve evaluation (PNE). For PNE a temporary thin wire is threaded into the S3 foramen and secured at the exit site with tape onto the skin. It is connected to the same temporary neurostimulator device, and the patient is monitored for improvement in fecal incontinent episodes. If therapeutic success is reached, the temporary wire is removed and the permanent lead and permanent neurostimulator is implanted as the second stage of the procedure. This can occur at a later date after the PNE wire is removed.

At this point, I do not find the latter method as attractive because the PNE wire can easily become dislodged and the therapy deemed unsuccessful. Also the implanted tined lead may not be exactly in the same position as a successful PNE wire and that also can lead to failure when the permanent device is inserted. The popularity of PNE is related to the fact that it costs less to insert and can be removed easily. If successful, the plans for placement of the permanent device can be readily scheduled or delayed to the far future. With the permanent implantation of the tined lead during stage 1, the lead should be internalized or removed within 2–3 weeks to avoid infection. Compared to the ABS, the infection rate overall is less and reported to be 11 % in the monitored study for FDA approval in the United States [30].

Recently, success for therapies involving fecal incontinence has been defined as 50 % reduction in fecal incontinent episodes, which concurs with FDA requirements for approval in the United States. It is debated whether this truly improves a patient's suffering with fecal incontinence, but most results are reported in this fashion. In the multicentered prospective study conducted under a strict protocol for FDA approval mentioned above, 285 patients were screened and 133 met criteria for stage 1. Of those, 120 were successfully implanted during stage 2. At 1 year, 83 % had >50 % reduction in incontinent episodes [31], at 3 years 86 % [32], and at 5 years 89 % ($p<0.0001$) [33]. Overall, approximately 40 % were totally continent at these time points. Looking at the data another way, the number of incontinent episodes per week at baseline before this treatment was 9.1. At 1 year it dropped to 1.9 [31] and 1.7 at 5 years ($p<0.0001$) [33]. At 5 years, 44 patients had left the study, but only 15 exited due to lack of efficacy or patient-related issues with the device [33]. Quality of life was also found to significantly improve and remained sustained over the study period [34]. Overall, these results mirror other reports from centers outside the United States regarding the improvement in continence and quality of life [35–38].

Improvement is also seen when studies are done that include patients with an anterior sphincter defect [39]. Based on relevant studies, a consensus panel felt SNS could be offered to patients with 120° external sphincter defect [40]. Additionally this panel felt SNS was a good option to treat patients with combined fecal and urinary incontinence.

Unsolved issues in implantation include use of antibiotics. There are many protocols used by various centers. After an informal poll of urologists at our institution and various centers implanting SNS, we have elected to use cefazolin (Ancef^{R}) for stage 1 and vancomycin and gentamicin for stage 2. Another unsolved issue is whether or not to impose activity restrictions in the immediate postoperative period and long term. While we do not advise any long-term restrictions, after stage 1 we ask them not to shower, reduce physical activity to avoid pulling on the wire or dislodging it, and keep the device beneath clothing.

Controversies in Fecal Incontinence Management

Does Age Influence Choice of Treatment?

All treatment for fecal incontinence should be individualized and tailored to the patient. Generally, as stated above, we have advised young women with an obstetrical injury to have their sphincter repaired as the initial procedure. However, this may not be the recommendation at other centers—particularly outside the United States. When compared to younger patients with a median age of 38 years, older patients (median age 56) reported subjectively worse outcomes and tended to have worse incontinence scores and quality of life measures [41]. This study was based on a postal survey, which had a 55 % useable response rate and no preoperative scoring tool as a comparison. The introduction of injectables and SNS may change the algorithm, but anecdotally I have performed a sphincter repair on a woman in her late 80s with a satisfactory result. I prefer to look at their physiologic status and their stool and bowel consistency. In a woman with no muscle movement and typically loose stool that cannot be improved, I feel will fare poorly with a sphincter repair—particularly if older. Alternatively, whether SNS will be offered to older patients (older perhaps meaning in their 80s) remains to be defined. For an active patient, I believe age will not be the limiting issue.

Repeat Overlapping Sphincter Repair

Repeat overlapping sphincter repair is a feasible option when a defect is identified on anal endosonography. With US approval of SNS and injectable agents—combined with the realization that a sphincter defect does not preclude "success"—a repeat repair does not look as attractive. If they are eligible for SNS, I would favor that treatment.

Managing Expectations of Outcome

Perhaps one of the most important aspects of working with patients who experience fecal incontinence is setting realistic expectations. The notion of perfect continence like they probably experienced in their youth is rarely obtained. The goal should be improvement, particularly in their quality of life. Attempting to fully explain in layman terms the advantages and disadvantages of each procedure is challenging; therefore, most patients will rely on our assessment of their individual problem and our recommendation for improvement. Again, the concept that a combination of procedures may be necessary for improvement, and viewing incontinence as a chronic disease requiring lifelong adjustments, should be introduced.

What Findings on Testing Influence Certain Choices?

The history and physical exam is usually the most important determinant in providing a tailored treatment option. The most important test is usually anal endosonography because a defect in the muscle may influence what is recommended.

I may be hesitant to recommend SNS for a patient who has had a traumatic pelvic injury and hence no spinal reflex, but that again is not definite, as the first stage can be done to look for a response when the sacral foramina are stimulated.

For patients that seem to have a component of irritable bowel syndrome and fecal incontinence, SNS may be the preferred recommendation. We do not know how SNS truly works, but an intriguing study showed that chronic stimulation seems to affect the learning and reward center of the brain [42]. This potentially could have a positive effect on the mechanism of irritable bowel syndrome, but definitely more studies are required to confirm these thoughts.

Is a Stoma Ever the Best Option?

Absolutely! For some patients a permanent stoma is their best option—they may simply not want to hear or believe that. This includes patients who fail all therapy or are not candidates for lesser therapies for various reasons. While a stoma is usually my treatment of last resort, this allows patients to function outside their home. Additionally patients who want the most reliable "fix" may opt for a stoma since it involves one procedure with the most predictable outcome. Consultation with an enterostomal therapist is also helpful to answer questions and to mark the patient before surgery. After surgery, as equipment requires adjustment, these nurses can continue to answer questions and provide specialized advice. I try to steer wheelchair-dependent patients toward this option, and marking in the wheelchair is crucial for the correct position.

When patients choose this option, it is paramount that the best stoma be constructed. If this requires an open procedure, the approach (laparoscopic versus open) should not compromise the end result. I typically attempt to perform an end colostomy in the left colon making sure the bowel used is soft and pliable, or distal transverse colon if necessary, to attain the best stoma.

Defects in the Internal Sphincter Only or Other Types of Lateral Sphincter Defects

Select patients have defects in the internal sphincter only that lead typically to debilitating fecal leakage. Most commonly I see these patients after an internal sphincterotomy that changes the contour of their oval anus, leading to a deep crevice that allows escape of typically liquid stool or mucus. While I have no data to support this approach, I favor trying to re-approximate the internal sphincter in order to change the topography of that area.

The exact approach to address the lateral internal sphincter defect is a separate dilemma, as I have found that there is usually a thick scar over the area. I have tried a semicircular incision at the anal verge and creating a flap to the sphincter and repairing via this approach, but I have almost abandoned this, as the scar over the area of repair typically will become ischemic and necrotic. Therefore, when faced with these patients, I presently will incise longitudinally over the scar and dissect until each limb of the internal sphincter is identified. I try to limit the amount of dissection because the goal is to change the contour and eliminate the divot while trying to limit the amount of dead space created.

A similar type of topography issue can be seen in select cases after a fistulotomy or traumatic (slice/stab type) injury of the anus. This type of injury is not located anteriorly, and repair is not as straightforward as the typical anterior overlapping sphincter repair done for an obstetrical injury. Again this is typically a contour problem, and the goal is usually to create a smooth contour that will not allow liquid stool or mucus to seep through. Anal endosonography is crucial in providing a road map prior to surgery. A linear incision is made over the scar and the muscle ends are identified. In specific cases, especially if the defect in the sphincter is close to 180°, the scar (rather than the retracted muscle) can be used as one end of the circular repair, which is sewn to other end of muscle to improve function. I attempt to bring muscle across the anterior or posterior aspect of the anal circle where the sphincter would be and thus try to orient the scarred portion on the lateral sides. This seems to provide a more oval contour.

If optimal improvement is not seen, injectable therapy may be a consideration, although I have not used it in this type of patient as of yet. Also SNS or ABS may be a consideration if all other forms of therapy are unsuccessful.

How to Manage Concomitant Pelvic Floor Disorders (i.e., Rectal Prolapse, Rectocele) if Repairing the Sphincter

Typically I favor repair of associated pelvic floor disorders when a sphincter repair is planned in most instances. Over 10 years ago when our results were examined, there was no difference in outcome improvement if a sphincter repair was done at the same operation combined with an anterior pelvic procedure (with the urologist or urogynecologist) versus a sphincteroplasty alone [43, 44]. Combined surgery with the anterior pelvic surgeons requires a team approach and may involve a position change if you prefer to repair the anal sphincter in the prone position. Therefore, the anesthesiologist must also be agreeable to the position change.

I have performed several sphincter repairs when an abdominal procedure was done at the same setting for rectal prolapse repair. These were typically more difficult and very bloody repairs, such that I currently hesitate to perform simultaneous repairs in this setting as rule. Most women have improvement in their anal sphincter when their rectal prolapse no longer chronically stretches the muscle, so I wait and reassess at about 6 months.

Future Treatments

Key Concept: Several treatments have been reported that are currently not available in the United States.

Magnetic Ring

One described treatment involves a titanium wire containing magnetic beads threaded around the anus. When the pressure in the rectum during straining reaches a certain threshold, the magnetic beads spring open allowing defecation. Currently one company (Torax Shoreview, Minn) makes the device, which they have called Fenix™. They have conducted a feasibility study with this device [45] demonstrating ease of implantation and no requirement for adjustments by the physician or patient. Of 14 implanted devices, 3 were removed. Short-term results showed a decrease of the mean number of weekly incontinent episodes from 7.2 to 0.7. One group outside the United States that participated in this study compared their results in 10 patients implanted with the magnetic ring matched to 10 with an ABS [46] and 12 with the magnetic ring matched to 16 with SNS [47]. They found that the magnetic ring was as effective as SNS in improving continence scores and quality of life with similar morbidity. Regarding ABS, the magnetic ring patients had similar quality of life and less constipation versus ABS. It did show that the ABS patients tended to have better incontinence scores ($p=0.0625$). This device certainly looks promising with a relatively simple method of implantation and acceptable and comparable results compared to other treatments [48]. Further studies are needed to define its role and gain FDA approval in the United States.

Anal Sling

For urinary incontinence, slings have been used extensively to improve control. Similarly a U-shaped sling has been devised that goes behind the lowest part of the anorectum with the ends being brought out through small incisions lateral to the vagina at the medial notch of the obturator foramen. The tension is adjusted on the posterior anorectum and the excess "arms" clipped at the skin and the skin closed over them, to create a sling like support of the anus (Patents/US20110046436). A multicenter study has been completed and is awaiting adequate follow-up prior to publication of results.

Posterior Tibial Stimulation

Posterior tibial stimulation of the posterior tibial nerve at the medial ankle either by needle or surface electrode has been proposed to treat fecal incontinence. It is currently being studied for urinary incontinence in the United States and not approved or trialed as of this writing for fecal issues in the United States. There are eight studies from outside the United States, and all vary regarding treatment protocol (i.e., frequency of stimulation (20–30 Hz), timing (daily, alternate days, weekly, every other week), and duration (20–30 min)), but all use external portable pulse generators [49, 50]. Five studies had 60 % of patients reach the primary endpoint they set before starting and defined these patients as having a successful outcome. Again, all of these published studies all had varied protocols for treatment. A recent randomized, blinded, sham-controlled study of 144 patients from nine centers failed to show any benefit versus sham particularly in median number of fecal incontinent episodes per week [50]. This well-conducted study does cast some doubt toward its usefulness in individuals with fecal incontinence.

Summary Pearls

Fecal incontinence is a complex chronic disease. Many treatments are available, and individualization typically based on history and sphincter integrity currently aids in making treatment choices. Treatment choices revolve around conservative, nonsurgical, and surgical treatments (see Table 13.2). The surgical procedures aim to correct a defect, augment the sphincter, or change the "wiring" of the pelvic area. There is no panacea for treatment—which is a key concept. The Cochrane review for fecal incontinence in adults seemed to compare all treatments together, which proved to be unhelpful for providing guidance due to many reasons including the poor design of most trials [51]. But more importantly, the authors did not recognize that a crucial part of the question is which patient characteristics should steer health-care providers toward which treatments. More importantly, it failed to identify the reality that a combination of treatments may provide the best outcome. With all these unknown variables, future study should include discovering which patient characteristics are important to give optimal results for each individual therapy. A more difficult aspect for future study is

Table 13.2 Treatment options for fecal incontinence

Conservative (important to provide precise written instructions regarding the conservative treatment advised for the patient)
– Control diarrhea
– Address anal skin problems
– Counsel on avoiding excessive wiping
– Dietary manipulation
– Enema therapy
Nonsurgical
– Physical retraining (biofeedback)
– Anal plug
– Radiofrequency energy (SECCA[R])
– Injectables (NASHA Dx [R] in the United States)
Surgical
– Sphincter repair
– Artificial bowel sphincter
– Sacral nerve stimulation
– Diverting stoma
Future treatments
– Magnetic anal ring
– Anal sling
– Posterior tibial stimulation

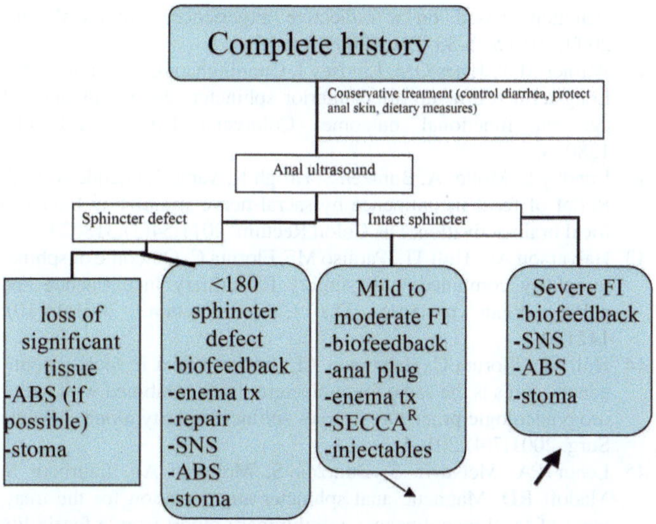

Fig. 13.7 My current algorithm when considering treating patients with fecal incontinence. *ABS* artificial bowel sphincter, *SNS* sacral nerve stimulation, *Tx* treatment, *FI* fecal incontinence

what combination of treatments will provide the best outcome for individual patients. In the meantime, providers treating these patients must be familiar with all treatments and prepared to offer various treatments, perhaps in combination, to optimize quality of life with the caveat that this is a lifelong problem and adjustments in treatment approaches will be necessary (Fig. 13.7).

References

1. Rockwood TH, Church JM, Fleshman JW, Kane RL, Mavrantonis C, Thorson AG, et al. Patient and surgeon ranking of the severity of symptoms associated with fecal incontinence: the fecal incontinence severity index. Dis Colon Rectum. 1999;42(12):1525–32.
2. O'Donnell LJD, Heaton KW. Pseudo-diarrhea in the irritable bowel syndrome: patients' records of stool form reflect transit time while stool frequency does not. Gut. 1988;29:A1455.
3. Bohle B, Belvis F, Vial M, Maestre Y, Pera M, Castillo M, Grande L, Parés D. Menopause and obstetric history as risk factors for fecal incontinence in women. Dis Colon Rectum. 2011;54(8):975–81.
4. Qureshi MS, Rao MM, Sasapu KK, Casey J, Qureshi MU, Sadat U, et al. Male faecal incontinence presents as two separate entities with implications for management. Int J Colorectal Dis. 2011;26(12):1589–94.
5. Seong MK, Jung SI, Kim TW, Joh HK. Comparative analysis of summary scoring systems in measuring fecal incontinence. J Korean Surg Soc. 2011;81(5):326–31.
6. Bols EM, Hendriks HJ, Berghmans LC, Baeten CG, de Bie RA. Responsiveness and interpretability of incontinence severity scores and FIQL in patients with fecal incontinence: a secondary analysis from a randomized controlled trial. Int Urogynecol J. 2013;24(3):469–78.
7. Wang JY, Varma MG. Measures for fecal incontinence, constipation, and associated quality of life. Semin Colon Rectal Surg. 2010;21:22–6.
8. Zutshi M, Salcedo L, Hammel J, Hull T. Anal physiology testing in fecal incontinence: is it of any value? Int J Colorectal Dis. 2010;25(2):277–82.
9. Pehl C, Seidl H, Scalercio N, Gundling F, Schmidt T, Schepp W, Labermeyer S. Accuracy of anorectal manometry in patients with fecal incontinence. Digestion. 2012;86(2):78–85.
10. Dudding TC, Vaizey CJ. Current concepts in evaluation and testing of posterior pelvic floor disorders. Semin Colon Rectal Surg. 2010;21:6–21.
11. Norton C, Cody JD. Biofeedback and/or sphincter exercises for the treatment of faecal incontinence in adults. Cochrane Database Syst Rev. 2012;(7):CD002111.
12. Deutekom M, Dobben AC. Plugs for containing faecal incontinence. Cochrane Database Syst Rev. 2012;(4):CD005086.
13. Ruiz D, Pinto RA, Hull TL, Efron JE, Wexner SD. Does the radiofrequency procedure for fecal incontinence improve quality of life and incontinence at 1-year follow-up? Dis Colon Rectum. 2010;53(7):1041–6.
14. Abbas MA, Tam MS, Chun LJ. Radiofrequency treatment for fecal incontinence: is it effective long-term? Dis Colon Rectum. 2012;55(5):605–10.
15. Maeda Y, Laurberg S, Norton C. Perianal injectable bulking agents as treatment for faecal incontinence in adults. Cochrane Database Syst Rev. 2010;(5):CD007959.
16. Luo C, Samaranayake CB, Plank LD, Bissett IP. Systematic review on the efficacy and safety of injectable bulking agents for passive faecal incontinence. Colorectal Dis. 2010;12(4):296–303.
17. Graf W, Mellgren A, Matzel KE, Hull T, Johansson C, Bernstein M, NASHA Dx Study Group. Efficacy of dextranomer in stabilised hyaluronic acid for treatment of faecal incontinence: a randomised, sham-controlled trial. Lancet. 2011;377(9770):997–1003.
18. Melgren A, Matzel KE, Pollack J, Hull T, Bernstein M, Graf W, forthe Solesta Study Groups. Long term efficacy of NASATM Dx injection therapy (Solesta R) for treatment of fecal incontinence. Podium presentation American Society of Colon and Rectal Surgeons, San Antonio, Texas. June 5, 2012.
19. Zutshi M, Hull TL, Bast J, Halverson A, Na J. Ten-year outcome after anal sphincter repair for fecal incontinence. Dis Colon Rectum. 2009;52(6):1089–94.
20. Glasgow SC, Lowry AC. Long-term outcomes of anal sphincter repair for fecal incontinence: a systematic review. Dis Colon Rectum. 2012;55(4):482–90.
21. Zutshi M, Ferreira P, Hull T, Gurland B. Biological implants in sphincter augmentation offer a good short-term outcome after a sphincter repair. Colorectal Dis. 2012;14(7):866–71.
22. Tjandra JJ, Han WR, Goh J, Carey M, Dwyer P. Direct repair vs. overlapping sphincter repair: a randomized, controlled trial. Dis Colon Rectum. 2003;46(7):937–42.
23. Farrell SA, Flowerdew G, Gilmour D, Turnbull GK, Schmidt MH, Baskett TF, et al. Overlapping compared with end-to-end repair of complete third-degree or fourth-degree obstetric tears: three-year follow-up of a randomized controlled trial. Obstet Gynecol. 2012;120(4):803–8.
24. Wexner SD, Jin HY, Weiss EG, Nogueras JJ, Li VK. Factors associated with failure of the artificial bowel sphincter: a study of over 50 cases from Cleveland Clinic Florida. Dis Colon Rectum. 2009;52(9):1550–7.
25. Wong MT, Meurette G, Wyart V, Glemain P, Lehur PA. The artificial bowel sphincter: a single institution experience over a decade. Ann Surg. 2011;254(6):951–6.
26. Michot F, Costaglioli B, Leroi AM, Denis P. Artificial anal sphincter in severe fecal incontinence: outcome of prospective experience with 37 patients in one institution. Ann Surg. 2003;237(1):52–6.
27. Michot F, Lefebure B, Bridoux V, Gourcerol G, Kianifard B, Leroi AM, Tuech JJ. Artificial anal sphincter for severe fecal incontinence implanted by a transvaginal approach: experience with 32 patients treated at one institution. Dis Colon Rectum. 2010;53(8):1155–60.
28. Ruiz Carmona MD, Alós Company R, Roig Vila JV, Solana Bueno A, Pla MV. Long-term results of artificial bowel sphincter for the

treatment of severe faecal incontinence. Are they what we hoped for? Colorectal Dis. 2009;11(8):831–7.
29. Gallas S, Leroi AM, Bridoux V, Lefebure B, Tuech JJ, Michot F. Constipation in 44 patients implanted with an artificial bowel sphincter. Int J Colorectal Dis. 2009;24(8):969–74.
30. Wexner SD, Hull T, Edden Y, Coller JA, Devroede G, McCallum R, et al. Infection rates in a large investigational trial of sacral nerve stimulation for fecal incontinence. J Gastrointest Surg. 2010;14(7): 1081–9.
31. Wexner SD, Coller JA, Devroede G, Hull T, McCallum R, Chan M, et al. Sacral nerve stimulation for fecal incontinence: results of a 120-patient prospective multicenter study. Ann Surg. 2010;251(3): 441–9.
32. Mellgren A, Wexner SD, Coller JA, Devroede G, Lerew DR, Madoff RD, Hull T, SNS Study Group, Collaborators. Long-term efficacy and safety of sacral nerve stimulation for fecal incontinence. Dis Colon Rectum. 2011;54(9):1065–75.
33. Hull T, Giese C, Wexner SD, Mellgren A, Devroede G, Madoff R, et al. Long-term durability of SNS therapy for chronic fecal incontinence. Dis Colon Rectum. 2013;56(2):234–45. doi:10.1097/DCR.0b013e318276b24c.PMID: 23303153.
34. Devroede G, Giese C, Wexner SD, Mellgren A, Coller JA, Madoff RD, et al. Quality of life is markedly improved in patients with fecal incontinence after sacral nerve stimulation. Female Pelvic Med Reconstr Surg. 2012;18(2):103–12.
35. Matzel KE, Lux P, Heuer S, Besendörfer M, Zhang W. Sacral nerve stimulation for faecal incontinence: long-term outcome. Colorectal Dis. 2009;11(6):636–41.
36. Altomare DF, Ratto C, Ganio E, Lolli P, Masin A, Villani RD. Long-term outcome of sacral nerve stimulation for fecal incontinence. Dis Colon Rectum. 2009;52(1):11–7.
37. George AT, Kalmar K, Panarese A, Dudding TC, Nicholls RJ, Vaizey CJ. Long-term outcomes of sacral nerve stimulation for fecal incontinence. Dis Colon Rectum. 2012;55(3):302–6.
38. Damon H, Barth X, Roman S, Mion F. Sacral nerve stimulation for fecal incontinence improves symptoms, quality of life and patients' satisfaction: results of a monocentric series of 119 patients. Int J Colorectal Dis. 2013;28(2):227–33.
39. Chan MK, Tjandra JJ. Sacral nerve stimulation for fecal incontinence: external anal sphincter defect vs. intact anal sphincter. Dis Colon Rectum. 2008;51(7):1015–24; discussion 1024–5.
40. Leroi AM, Damon H, Faucheron JL, Lehur PA, Siproudhis L, Slim K, et al. Sacral nerve stimulation in faecal incontinence: position statement based on a collective experience. Colorectal Dis. 2009;11(6):572–83. Epub 2009 Apr 15.
41. Warner MW, Jones OM, Lindsey I, Cunningham C, Mortensen NJ. Long-term follow-up after anterior sphincter repair: influence of age on functional outcome. Colorectal Dis. 2012;14(11): 1380–8.
42. Lundby L, Møller A, Buntzen S, Krogh K, Vang K, Gjedde A, et al. Relief of fecal incontinence by sacral nerve stimulation linked to focal brain activation. Dis Colon Rectum. 2011;54(3):318–23.
43. Halverson AL, Hull TL, Paraiso MF, Floruta C. Outcome of sphincteroplasty combined with surgery for urinary incontinence and pelvic organ prolapse. Dis Colon Rectum. 2001;44(10): 1421–6.
44. Hull TL, Floruta C, Halverson AL. Improvement in fecal incontinence scores is the same for sphincteroplasty combined with major urogynecologic procedures versus sphincteroplasty alone. J Pelvic Surg. 2001;7(4):201–4.
45. Lehur PA, McNevin S, Buntzen S, Mellgren AF, Laurberg S, Madoff RD. Magnetic anal sphincter augmentation for the treatment of fecal incontinence: a preliminary report from a feasibility study. Dis Colon Rectum. 2010;53(12):1604–10.
46. Wong MT, Meurette G, Stangherlin P, Lehur PA. The magnetic anal sphincter versus the artificial bowel sphincter: a comparison of 2 treatments for fecal incontinence. Dis Colon Rectum. 2011;54(7): 773–9.
47. Wong MT, Meurette G, Wyart V, Lehur PA. Does the magnetic anal sphincter device compare favourably with sacral nerve stimulation in the management of faecal incontinence? Colorectal Dis. 2012;14(6):e323–9.
48. Mantoo S, Meurette G, Podevin J, Lehur PA. The magnetic anal sphincter: a new device in the management of severe fecal incontinence. Expert Rev Med Devices. 2012;9(5):483–90.
49. Findlay JM, Maxwell-Armstrong C. Posterior tibial nerve stimulation and faecal incontinence: a review. Int J Colorectal Dis. 2011;26(3):265–73.
50. Leroi AM, Siproudhis L, Etienney I, Damon H, Zerbib F, Amarenco G, et al. Transcutaneous electrical tibial nerve stimulation in the treatment of fecal incontinence: a randomized trial (Consort 1a). Am J Gastroenterol. 2012;107(12):1888–96.
51. Brown SR, Wadhawan H, Nelson RL. Surgery for faecal incontinence in adults. Cochrane Database Syst Rev. 2010;(9):CD001757.
52. Lewis SJ, Heaton KW. Stool form scale as a useful guide to intestinal transit time. Scand J Gastroenterol. 1997;32(9):920–4.

Local Treatment of Rectal Cancer (TEM Versus TAMIS Versus Transanal Excision)

14

John H. Marks and Harry Reynolds

Key Points

- Local treatment options for rectal cancers vary markedly depending on the following: level of cancer in rectum, extent of lymph node involvement, and the T stage of the cancer.
- Initial thorough evaluation of the rectal lesion is critical and must assess position, level in rectum, size, ulceration, and clinical stage of the cancer and must include a digital rectal exam.
- Endoluminal surgery combined with neoadjuvant therapy offers an exciting option in select rectal cancers.

Introduction

Key Concept: The emergence of local therapies for rectal cancer is a paradigm similar to breast cancer treatment.

The search for the ideal treatment of rectal cancer continues to evolve. With advances in our understanding of the disease, the treatment algorithms available have become ever more complex. A multidisciplinary team approach is now the standard of care, but surgeons treating rectal cancer are responsible for understanding and directing all aspects of these ever-evolving multidisciplinary care paths. Staging modalities, though not yet perfected, continue to advance, allowing us to more carefully tailor care to our patients. Neoadjuvant chemoradiation is selectively used and with much success. Surgical options continue to expand as well, ranging from local resection techniques to total mesorectal excision, utilizing open, laparoscopic, and, now, robotic approaches. Local resection options include standard transanal excision (TAE), transanal minimally invasive techniques (TAMIS), and transanal endoscopic microsurgery (TEM).

An ideal treatment strategy would be curative while preserving sphincter function with minimal perioperative morbidity and mortality. Local excision techniques seem ideal in that they are sphincter preserving and can be accomplished with minimal morbidity and mortality when skillfully performed. Local excision of rectal cancer offers the promise of truly the ultimate application of minimally invasive surgery. Addressing a cancer transanally is really the longest standing application of true natural orifice surgery, or "NOTES," which has recently been spoken of so greatly. The question that arises when you talk about a local excision for rectal cancer is: is this a good idea or really just a leap of faith by the clinicians hoping to avoid the trauma and the difficulty of a radical resection for a difficult rectal cancer? The trends in oncologic surgery have been evermore focused upon not only curing the cancer but also doing so with the highest quality of life. Using breast cancer as a comparator, we have really seen a very similar evolution in rectal cancer. Breast cancer has seen the transition of the standard treatment from the radical

Electronic supplementary material The online version of this chapter (doi: 10.1007/978-1-4614-9022-7_14) contains supplementary material, which is available to authorized users. Videos can also be accessed at http://www.springerimages.com/videos/978-1-4614-9021-0.

J.H. Marks, MD, FACS, FASCRS (✉)
Division of Colorectal Surgery, Department of Surgery, Main Line Health Systems, Lankenau Medical Center, Wynnewood, PA, USA

Division of Colorectal Surgery, Lankenau Medical Center, 100 E Lancaster Ave, MOBW Suite 330, Wynnewood, PA 19096, USA
e-mail: marksj@mlhs.org

H. Reynolds, MD, FACS, FASCRS
Colon and Rectal Cancer Surgery, Case Western Reserve University, University Hospitals Case Medical Center, Cleveland, OH, USA
e-mail: harry.reynolds@uhhospitals.org

S.R. Steele et al. (eds.), *Complexities in Colorectal Surgery*,
DOI 10.1007/978-1-4614-9022-7_14,

mastectomy in 1960s and 1970s, to modified radical mastectomy, to lumpectomy and axillary dissection with external beam radiation, and now to lumpectomy and sentinel node resection with external radiation. Similarly, rectal cancer's evolution has progressed markedly over the past 100 years. Miles first described the abdominoperineal resection in 1907 [1]. This has remained the bulwark of treatment for rectal cancer, even up to the present day. However, in the mid- to late 1970s, sphincter preservation was first being described for lower rectal cancers, even after radiation therapy [2]. Having moved from postoperative radiation therapy to preoperative radiation therapy in the treatment of rectal cancer, there has been noted a regression of tumor size. In turn, this has led to a question of local excision after neoadjuvant therapy. Additionally, for early rectal cancer, there is a question if a local excision alone is a sufficient treatment of the cancer.

The issue with rectal cancer is, of course, that not all rectal cancers are the same. There is no cookie cutter approach to the treatment of this disease, which not only threatens the patient's life but also impacts so dramatically their quality of life. The significant risks of bladder and sexual dysfunction, need for a permanent colostomy, issues regarding body image, and complications of major surgery and stomas require us to reassess our approach to rectal cancer.

In looking at rectal cancer, it is obvious that not all of them are created equal. Treatment options will vary markedly depending on the level of the cancer in the rectum, whether lymph nodes are involved and clearly what the T stage of the cancer is. In fact, we always joke that Sigmund Freud would state that surgeons dealing with low rectal cancers are highly conflicted, even schizophrenic, in their approach to the T1 rectal cancer. What that means, and how we approach that, represents really the basis of this chapter. Our goal is to review the indications for, and contraindications to, local excision; discuss technical pearls for success; and review outcomes reported with traditional TAE, TAMIS, and TEM.

Patient Selection

Key Concept: Proper patient evaluation, staging, and selection of patients for a transanal approach are the first, and likely the most crucial, aspects to optimize outcomes. Beware—not all T1 lesions are the same!

We are going to initially focus on the following areas of conflict for T1 cancers:

1. Radical total mesorectal excision (TME) surgery: when is it needed? When is an APR needed?
2. When is a local excision adequate? When is it not? What constitutes an adequate local excision, and who is going to benefit from TEM/TEO or TAMIS surgery?
3. The role of radiation or chemoradiation in the T1 rectal cancer: when is that applied? What is the rationale for it?

While the approach of transanal excision has traditionally been limited to cancers in the distal rectum, with the advent of TEM [3] and TAMIS [4], the ability to operate endoluminally has applied these approaches to the entirety of the rectum. The initial evaluation of the rectal lesion is critical, as there are marked differences between various T1 cancers. Oftentimes, we refer to this in our unit as the difference between a polyp with a small focus of cancer and a polypoid cancer, based on the amount of involvement of the cancer in the submucosa. The central aspect of the preoperative evaluation is that it is thorough. As with any colorectal cancer patient, a CT of the chest, abdomen, and pelvis is performed for staging, and a baseline carcinoembryonic antigen is obtained. A thorough assessment of the patient's comorbidities and fitness for surgery is undertaken because a key factor in surgical decision-making is whether the patient will tolerate a formal proctectomy.

An essential tool for evaluation is a careful digital rectal examination. Status of the sphincter tone (both at rest and with squeeze), position of the mass, and level in the rectum—both distal and cephalad—are of central importance. The size of the tumor, whether or not it is ulcerated, and the clinical stage of the disease are all important variables that must be noted and recorded. In addition, fixation, adjacent organ involvement, and relationship to the peritoneal reflection are considered and documented. Tumors which are fixed and deeply ulcerated or involve adjacent organs are not suited for local excision. Likewise, tumors greater than 3–4 cm in diameter can be difficult to locally excise, as the defects created are typically greater than half circumferential and can be challenging to close. Anterior, posterior, or lateral location of the tumor is particularly important to ascertain as patient positioning at surgery is determined by tumor location. Anteriorly based tumors are approached in a prone jackknife position, and posterior tumors are typically approached from lithotomy. Anteriorly based tumors above the middle rectal valve must be approached with caution as they may lie above the peritoneal reflection. It is also important to recognize that many female patients may have deep cul-de-sacs that may cause the intraperitoneal location to be more caudal than expected. This can result in a challenging closure if the peritoneal cavity is breeched but oftentimes is better dealt with if you are not surprised by this occurrence. Ideal tumors for local excision are exophytic or pedunculated, small, mobile, in the distal rectum, and posteriorly located. Relative contraindications to local excision include poorly differentiated histology or the presence of lymphovascular invasion [5].

Staging the Lesion

Key Concept: Know the limitations of your institution, as both MRI and ERUS have a component of "user" variability to accurate staging. Your digital examination can often give you the most reliable and helpful information.

A radiographic evaluation of the level of penetration is best carried out using endorectal ultrasound and/or MRI evaluation. Endorectal ultrasound (ERUS) is helpful in delineating the depth of invasion in early-stage rectal cancers with approximately 90 % accuracy and in identifying mesorectal adenopathy with 70 % accuracy. ERUS is useful in establishing if a tumor breeches the muscularis propria (T3). It can also be helpful in sorting whether a tumor extends into the submucosa (T1) or involves the muscularis propria (T2). Nodes visualized on ERUS are likely metastatic and in fit patients should preclude consideration of local excision of the primary tumor without using neoadjuvant chemoradiation in favor for more "radical" abdominal surgery.

Pelvic MRI is becoming more commonly used for staging rectal lesions. It is very useful in the case of locally advanced cancers in determining relationships with the mesorectal margin and assessing for adjacent organ involvement (circumferential resection margin). Unfortunately, both of these will be altered in their accuracy, dependent upon previous biopsies and/or if the patient has had a snare polypectomy or partial snare polypectomy prior to being referred to your office. The thermal injury that results from these energy sources can potentially obscure the differentiation between the mucosa and submucosa, submucosa and muscularis propria, and even muscularis propria and perirectal fat. Additionally, the resolution of MRI does not typically allow delineation of the layers of the rectal wall, thus making it difficult to distinguish T1 from T2 cancers. This limited resolution, along with the unreliability of MRI to differentiate benign from malignant nodes, often makes it of limited value in determining suitability for local excision. Endorectal ultrasound and/or MRI should be added to the clinical evaluation with a flexible or rigid sigmoidoscope. We often find it very helpful to use both in those tumors that are above the reach of the finger. We find the flexible scope very helpful in gaining a better view of the lesion itself. However, position of the mass that cannot be palpated can only reliably be determined with a rigid sigmoidoscope as orienting a lesion anterior, posterior, left, and right with a flexible scope is often difficult. While it is usually not emphasized, a careful digital examination probably represents the single most important component of the evaluation.

The second issue that should be addressed if one is looking at a lesion, and there is some question as to whether or not there is an invasive component to it, is what will be the preferred approach for this patient should there be an underlying cancer. In this fashion, sometimes we advocate a submucosal excision using a transanal or TEM/TAMIS/TEO approach in order to have an effective excisional biopsy on a lesion if it is felt from clinical and radiographic evaluation to be benign and if the determination is that more dramatic surgery would be entertained if there was an invasive component to the lesion. Further pathologic subclassification of T1 tumors has been performed looking at the depth of invasion into the submucosa. The depth of invasion can be designated as SM1, SM2, or SM3, in accordance with what "third" of the submucosa the lesion extends. This pathologic subclassification can provide further information regarding the risk of lymph node metastases and, thus, local recurrence. Kikuchi et al. reported that in a study of 182 patients, no patients with SM1 lesions had lymph node metastasis, but 10 % of SM2 patients and 25 % of SM3 patients did have metastases to the lymph nodes. They found that SM3 was an independent, statistically significant risk factor for lymph node metastases (Table 14.1) [6].

Table 14.1 Risk of lymph node metastases in T1 rectal lesions by submucosal invasion

	% of patients with lymph node metastases
SM1	0 %
SM2	10 %
SM3	25 %

Why Do Lesions Recur After Local Excision?

Key Concept: Under-staging, tumor biology, and technical factors all play a role in the development of recurrence following local excision for rectal cancer.

Reasons for "local recurrence" for local therapy of rectal cancer are fourfold. Oftentimes, these include:

1. Untreated involved lymph nodes
2. Tumor implantation at the time of surgery
3. Tubular lymphatic spread or persistence at the time of surgery
4. A positive margin leaving a residual cancer (i.e., an R1 resection)

Local recurrence in these settings has more to do with local persistence of the cancer as the lymph nodes have not been treated either surgically or sterilized with radiation. The reasons for these issues being central to local recurrence of rectal cancer have to do with the challenge of local therapy. First, working transanally, it is difficult to gain adequate resection of the cancer. This must entail clearance distally, cephalad, and in the deep fashion. It is often difficult for the surgeon operating transanally to gain a good cephalad margin, and this is the main reason why the higher incidence of failure exists for transanal incision as opposed to other techniques. Additionally, in operating endoluminally with an intact cancer, there is a much higher risk of tumor implantation. The basic tenets of colon and rectal surgery are to exclude the cancer with a clamp or stapler and then irrigate and have your margin of resection at that point, distal to the clamp. Unfortunately, when operating within the lumen of the rectum with a live cancer in place, this is always a challenge and speaks of the need for irrigation of the operative field once the tumor is out with a tumoricidal agent. Third, lymph node resection in an endoluminal fashion can be carried out only for the few perirectal nodes that may be found immediately deep to the cancer itself. However, a real thorough mesorectal excision is never carried out using a traditional local excision or TEM/TAMIS/TEO approach. The last challenge, of course, is that of lymph node staging. The ability to identify which patients being operated on have lymph node metastases impacts markedly the way the patient is addressed. Any evidence of lymph node metastases should make you highly question the indication of a transanal approach—especially in the absence of combined modality therapy.

Location

Key Concept: Distal lesions recur at higher rates and have overall worse survival.

In looking at matters of failure of treatment of rectal cancer more closely, the level of the cancer becomes of primary importance. Following radical surgery, Wibe in 2004 found the failure rate of low rectal cancers to be statistically significantly worse. In a study of over 2,000 patients, they demonstrated a statistically significant increase in local failure of cancers in the distal third of the rectum (0–5 cm level), with a 15 % local recurrence rate compared to a 9 % failure rate for tumors in the upper third of the rectum in the same study. This correlated with a significantly worse survival for cancers in the distal third of the rectum (59 % in the distal rectum vs. 69 % in the upper rectum and 62 % in the mid-rectum) [7]. The reason for this is not surprising and has to do with the issues brought up earlier. As one gets down further into the pelvis, it is more difficult to operate cleanly without compromising the lateral margins. Additionally, even when operating in the proper TME plane, the mesorectum is much thinner as the rectum prepares to traverse the sphincter mechanism, so the lateral aspect of the tumor, and the deep margin, would put a cancer cell directly against the levators, increasing the likelihood of failure. These same factors are in play when addressing a low rectal cancer transanally.

Impact of Lymph Nodes

Key Concept: Accurate staging dramatically predicts lymph node positivity and guides proper selection of patients. Unfortunately, limitations with both MRI and ERUS make this more inherently difficult.

The next challenge for local therapy of rectal cancer has to do with lymph nodes. The best predictor for lymph node involvement, even in the year 2013, unfortunately, is still the tumor T stage. Controversy exists as to which T stages are appropriate for local excision techniques. Studies of patients undergoing proctectomy show disturbingly high rates of mesorectal node positivity: for a T1 cancer, nodal involvement ranges between 5 and 12 %; for T2 cancers, in the range of 17–25 %; and for T3 cancers, between 40 and 60 % (Table 14.2) [7–11].

Table 14.2 Rate of mesorectal node positivity by pathologic T stage

Pathologic T stage	Pathologic N stage (%)
pT1	6–12
pT2	17–22
pT3	>60

This being the case, the clinician has predictably fallen back on staging mechanisms focused on evaluating T stage. Unfortunately, ERUS is our best preoperative imaging modality for determining node positivity, and it is only approximately 70 % sensitive. To date, endorectal ultrasound remains the gold standard, although as previously mentioned, more and more interest has been raised by excellent results by Gina Brown and her group looking at MRI studies of rectal cancer [12]. T stage accuracy has been reported between 80 and 90 % with N stage accuracy between 70 and 80 %. However, even noted by such distinguished experts as the late Doug Wong, "unfortunately, fine distinction between deep tumors of one T stage and early tumors of the next T stage … are often difficult to make. Additionally regional lymphatic involvement is often difficult to determine because endorectal ultrasound cannot detect nodes further away in the mesorectum or find micrometastatic disease in a perirectal lymph node" [13]. When one looks at a gross specimen on a radical resection after neoadjuvant therapy and TME resection, one can see why it is difficult to find small microscopic deposits that would reside in the perirectal fat or the muscularis propria (Fig. 14.1). It was Fidler who described "the metastatic decathlon" through which a primary cancer anywhere in the body, not just the rectum, liberated tumor cells created via a vascularity entrance into the bloodstream, interacting with the intravascular immunocompetent cells, gaining endothelial contact, and either taking a hold in the lymph nodes or proliferating and having metastases develop [14]. To detect scant cells in a lymph node that have completed this course remains a challenge for all staging strategies to date.

So Whom Should You Select for a Transanal Approach (for Cure)?

Key Concept: In general, T1 lesions with no evidence of lymph node metastases and good histopathological factors are the best patients. However, there will still be a small percentage of patients that will recur.

As we look at some of the larger trials of rectal cancer treated locally, we see alarmingly high rates of failure.

Bleday and Steele in the late 1990s reported on 48 patients treated with full-thickness local excision and noted a 10 % failure rate in the T1 cancers and a 40 % failure rate in the T3 cancers. Fifteen percent of these patients developed some form of fecal fistula [15]. The CALBG group in 1999 reported on 110 patients treated locally with local excision for rectal cancer. The T1 cancers in that group had a 6 % failure rate and the T2 cancers a 14 % failure rate. Additionally, 15 % of the patients in this group had positive margins at the time of surgery [16]. Rothenberger in 2000 reported on 108 patients with rectal cancer treated locally from the University of Minnesota and showed an 18 % failure rate for T1 cancer and a 47 % failure rate for T2 cancer [17]. The University of Minnesota data was updated in 2005, showing 101 T1 cancers operated on with a 19 % local recurrence rate and 50 T2 cancers operated on with a 45 % local recurrence rate [18]. Additionally, the Cleveland Clinic reported on their failure rate in T1 cancers, and this showed a striking 29.4 % local recurrence rate in 52 patients with T1 cancers treated locally [19]. These experiences led the University of Minnesota to conclude in their paper that oncologic outcomes in T1 cancers may be compromised by local excision alone and that local excision alone is inappropriate for T2 patients for surgery (Table 14.3).

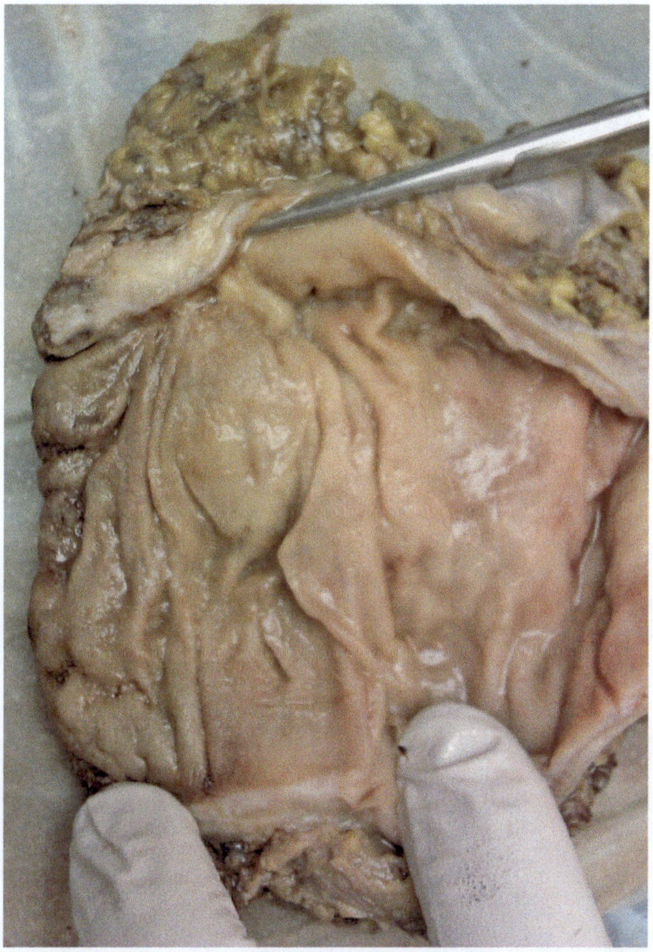

Fig. 14.1 Gross specimen on radical resection after neoadjuvant therapy and TME resection

The Norwegian rectal cancer group reported their T1 cancers operated upon either radically or with local excision [20]. It is noteworthy that in 256 patients who had radical resection, as would be expected in these early cancers, there was 100 % R0 resection. An 11 % rate of node positivity was also found. The local failure rate in that group was 6 % compared to the 38 patients in the local excision group of which there was a 17 % R2 resection and a 12 % local recurrence rate. In looking at this data more closely, it is actually somewhat surprising that there was not a higher failure rate due to a high rate of positive margins. What is noteworthy is that the failure rate for local excision is nearly exactly the same as the node positivity rate for T1 cancers undergoing radical resection. Looking at the data regarding local recurrence rate and lymph nodes together, we see lymph node involvement in between 6 and 12 % in the radically resected groups, and the failure rate with local recurrence after transanal excision in these experiences remains between 6 and 29 %. The conclusion we have reached in evaluating this data is that there are two possibilities for this. One is the persistence of untreated cancer in the lymph nodes, and two is the disturbance of the specimen cancer with incomplete resection and handling of the tissue transanally resulting in implantation of tumor at the time of surgery.

So whom should you select for a transanal approach? This obviously is a complex question with no quick and easy answer. In general, the decision to pursue local treatment of rectal cancer has to do both with the patient's comorbid conditions and the stage of the cancer. For a polyp with a small focus of cancer, this is an ideal approach for a full-thickness local excision. Patients with higher comorbidities such as obesity and preoperative pelvis are going to have a higher-risk profile for a major operative procedure. A greater

Table 14.3 Local recurrence rates by T stage

	Bleday et al. (1997) [15] (*n*=48)	Steele et al. CALBG (1999) [16] (*n*=110)	Mellgren et al. (2000) [17] (*n*=108)	Mellgren et al. (2005) [18] (*n*=151)	Madbouly et al. (2005) [19] (*n*=52)
T1	10 %	6 %	18 %	19 %	29.4 %
T2	0 %	14 %	47 %	45 %	
T3	40 %				

consideration of local excision would be entertained. Ultimately, our approach in general for local excision alone is only early T1 cancers with low risk for lymph node spread. That would be an SM1 with no lymphovascular invasion or poor differentiation.

Operative Approaches

"Traditional" Local Excision

Key Concept: More distal lesions that can be more easily directly visualized to ensure negative resection margins provide the best patients for this approach.

In patients deemed appropriate for local excision, a variety of approaches are available. Preoperative evaluation is undertaken as outlined above. Patient positioning is determined by tumor location as emphasized previously. Anteriorly based tumors necessitate prone positioning, while posteriorly based tumors are approached via lithotomy. Standard transanal techniques are best suited for middle and lower third lesions. A safe, reproducible operative technique is discussed below. A set of multiple operating proctoscopes of varying lengths and diameters is essential (Fig. 14.2). Anal effacement sutures are placed to facilitate exposure and placement of operating proctoscopes (Fig. 14.3). A headlight is essential if lighted proctoscopes are not available. An appropriately sized proctoscope is chosen which centers the lesion in the operative field (Figs. 14.4 and 14.5). Dissection can be performed with the use of standard long instruments. However, laparoscopic instruments can be very helpful. Stay sutures are placed at the lateral borders of the lesion. A dissection margin of one cm is marked with the cautery, and the excision is begun, proceeding with a full-thickness excision (Figs. 14.6 and 14.7). The deep margin extends to the mesorectal fat (Fig. 14.8). Care is taken to ensure the specimen is not fragmented. The lesion is retrieved and pinned on a foam board and the margins oriented (Fig. 14.9). The surgeon carefully reviews the margins with the pathologist and takes additional tissue if necessary. The defect is closed transversely. The previously placed stay sutures facilitate the closure (Fig. 14.10). The closure is examined with the proctoscope to ensure adequacy of the closure and patency of the rectal lumen. Proximal, anteriorly based lesions are particularly challenging. If above the peritoneal reflection, one must be sure of adequate closure. A preoperative discussion should be done with the patient regarding the possible need for laparoscopy or laparotomy and the potential need for proximal diverting loop ileostomy. If the integrity of the anastomosis is unclear, laparoscopy with proctoscopy and leak testing can be performed. Revision of the closure or formal proctectomy with or without diversion may be necessary if an intraperitoneal leak is found.

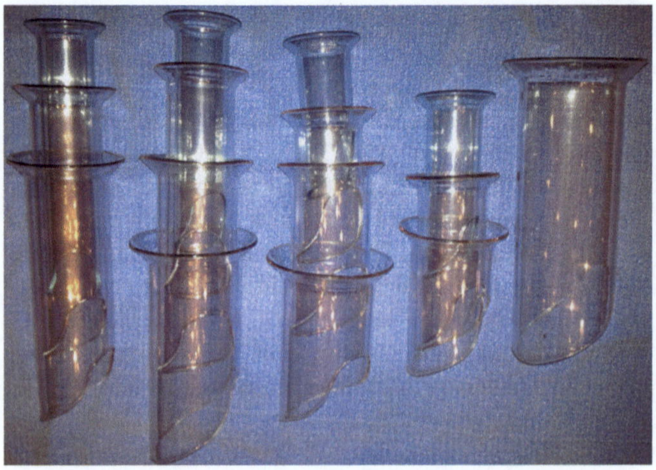

Fig. 14.2 Operating proctoscopes

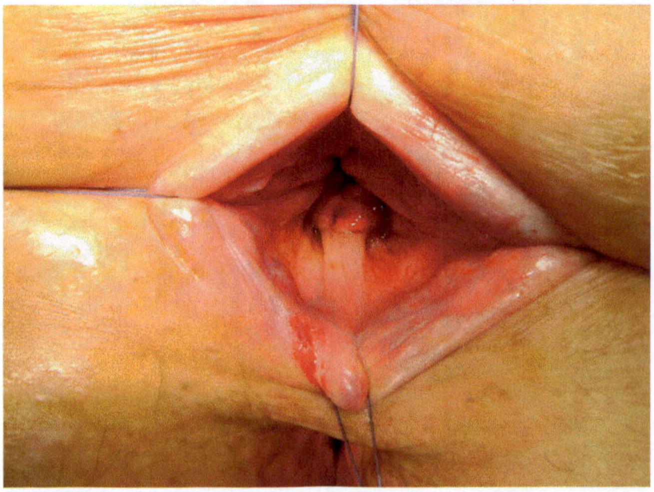

Fig. 14.3 Prone for anterior tumor, anal effacement sutures

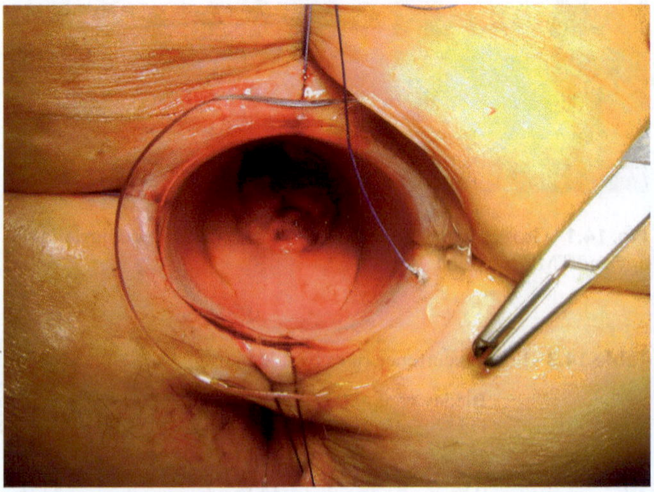

Fig. 14.4 Operating proctoscope placed and secured

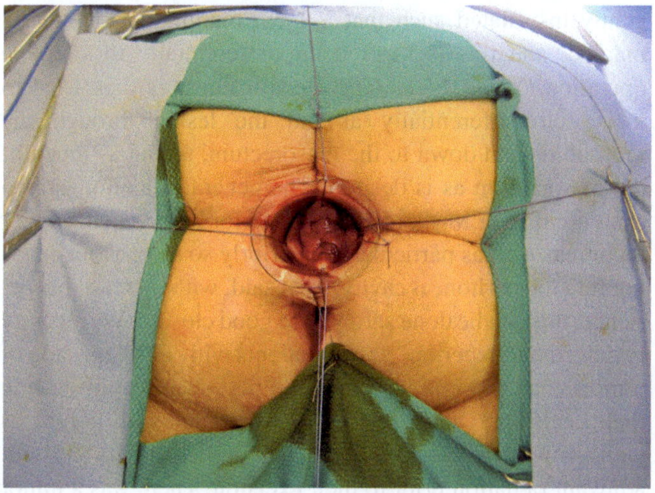

Fig. 14.5 Tumor viewed

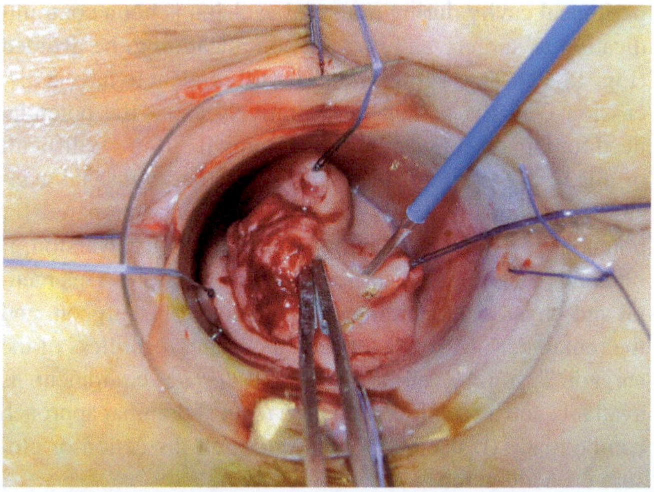

Fig. 14.6 Setup for excision

Minimally Invasive Options

Key Concept: Both TEM and TAMIS provide transanal approaches to higher lesions that were previously not possible with traditional transanal excision. For anterior and more proximal lesions, you should counsel the patient as to the possible need for a laparotomy/laparoscopy or possible diversion if the intraperitoneal cavity is breached.

Particularly with middle and upper third lesions, the question that comes to mind is whether the operative approach can be improved, and if so, how? This begs the question about the role of endoluminal surgery, be it TAMIS or TEM.

Transanal Endoscopic Microsurgery (TEM)

The technique of TEM uses an operating proctoscope 4 cm in diameter, which is attached to the table with a Martin's Arm. Using a video attachment or an operating microscope,

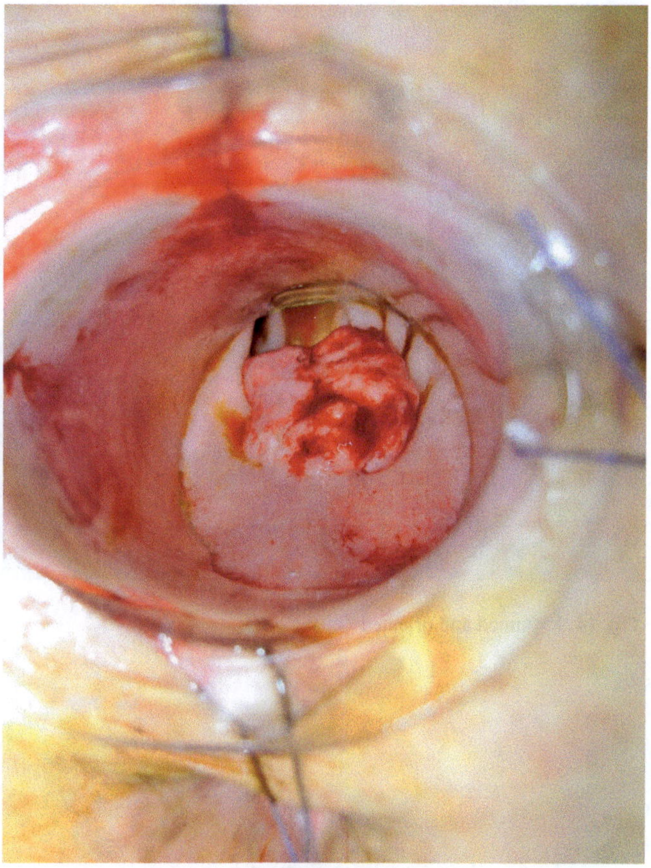

Fig. 14.7 Stay sutures and margin marking

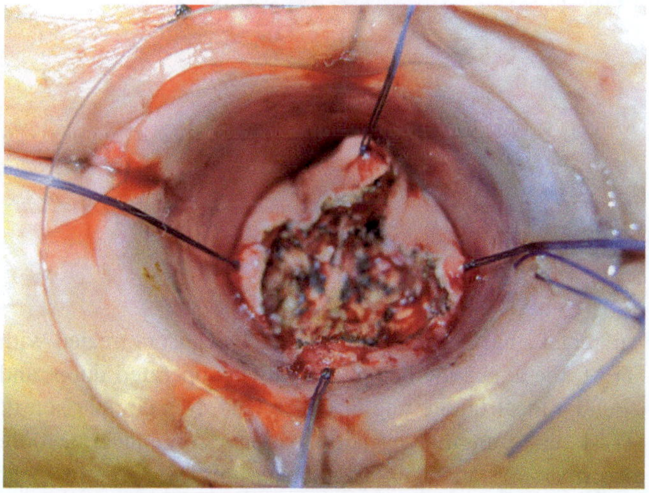

Fig. 14.8 Full-thickness excision

an airtight insufflation is gently placed, and this gives access to the rectum from the anal canal up to the rectosigmoid or at times even higher (Fig. 14.11). The equipment comes with three types of shafts: a beveled 20 cm shaft for higher lesions, a 15 cm shaft for smaller lesions, and a 10 cm flat TEM equipment for lesions with an inferior margin at the

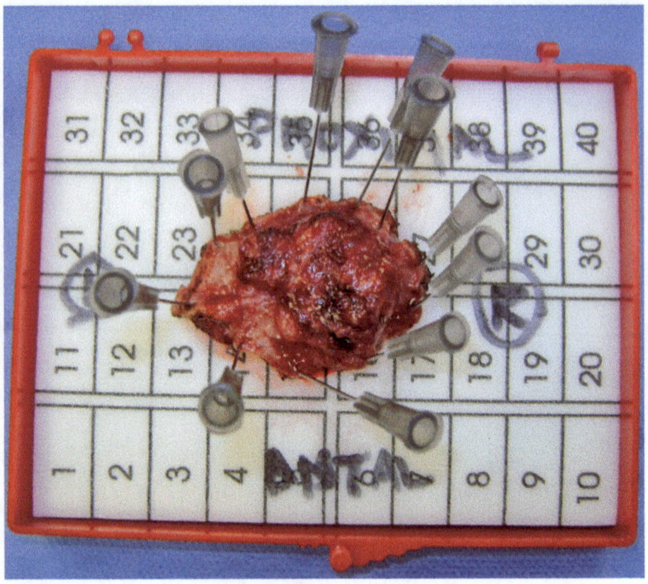

Fig. 14.9 Pinned and oriented

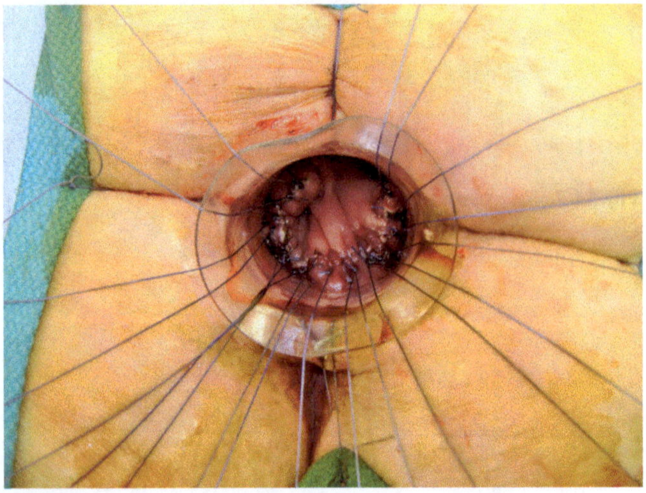

Fig. 14.10 Transverse closure

anorectal ring. Saclarides looked at T1 cancers treated with TEM, the aggregate being 221 patients operated upon, and found a local failure rate of 6.3 % [21]. In a comparison of TEM and transanal excision patients for cancer, Moore described a statistically significant improvement in clear margins with TEM as well as the ability to avoid fragmentation of the specimen using a TEM compared to a transanal operation [22]. While this has not been, and likely will not be, done with a TAMIS approach, it is predictable that a similar outcome would be achieved as this technique also permits pneumo-distention of the rectum with excellent optics and reach of the instruments.

From a technical standpoint, the operating microscope allows clear visualization of the lesion, and the rectum is gently insufflated such that a 1 cm margin can be clearly marked, and this is marked circumferentially to start the operation (Video 14.1). The electrocautery is then used to incise circumferentially around the lesion through the muscularis and down to the mesorectum, taking as much of the mesorectum as is desired. The general rules for indications are that TEM should be avoided for lesions in the upper rectum as well as particularly anteriorly so as to avoid entering into the peritoneal cavity. That said, with increased experience, this can be done safely with good closure. We recently reviewed our experience of 26 patients with TEM excision of tumors that had entrance into the peritoneal cavity during their excision. The group included patients with polyps as well as invasive cancer. Fifty percent of the patients had neoadjuvant radiation prior to their excision. There was a minor morbidity rate of 7 and 3 % wound disruptions, all of whom had radiation prior to surgery and all of whom were treated conservatively. In our hands, the threat of entrance into the peritoneal cavity during transanal excision is not a contraindication to surgery and is not a complication to be avoided (Fig. 14.12). That being said, it is still prudent to have a discussion with the patient preoperatively about the potential need for laparoscopy and/or laparotomy if closure is difficult or a leak is suspected. Just as with standard transanal excision techniques, it is always important to be prepared for potential revision or resection, with or without diversion, if one finds a particularly difficult tumor or closure. This mental and physical preparation of the patient, the surgeon, and the remainder of the OR team is important, regardless of the surgeon's skill level, so that appropriate equipment is available and a seamless transition to an abdominal approach can be made (if needed) when a difficult dissection or closure is encountered.

Transanal Minimally Invasive Surgery (TAMIS)

First described in 2009, transanal minimally invasive surgery (TAMIS) coupled the experiences built on the emerging single-port technology with traditional laparoscopic equipment [23]. As most operating rooms possess standard laparoscopic equipment and insufflation, and surgeons are becoming increasingly familiar with the technical skills required to resect the specimen and close the resultant defect, TAMIS allows for another minimally invasive means to reach of tumors as high as 15 cm from the anal verge without the expensive equipment required for TEM (Videos 14.2 and 14.3). More recently, TAMIS platforms, such as the SILS™ port (Covidien, Mansfield, MA) and Gelpoint Path (Applied Medical, Rancho Santa Margarita), provide standardized endoluminal rectal access to aid in ease of the procedure.

TAMIS outcomes thus far have been similar to both transanal and TEM approaches, though lack the long-term follow-up. Albert and colleagues reported on their first 50 patients (56 % malignant) undergoing a TAMIS procedure

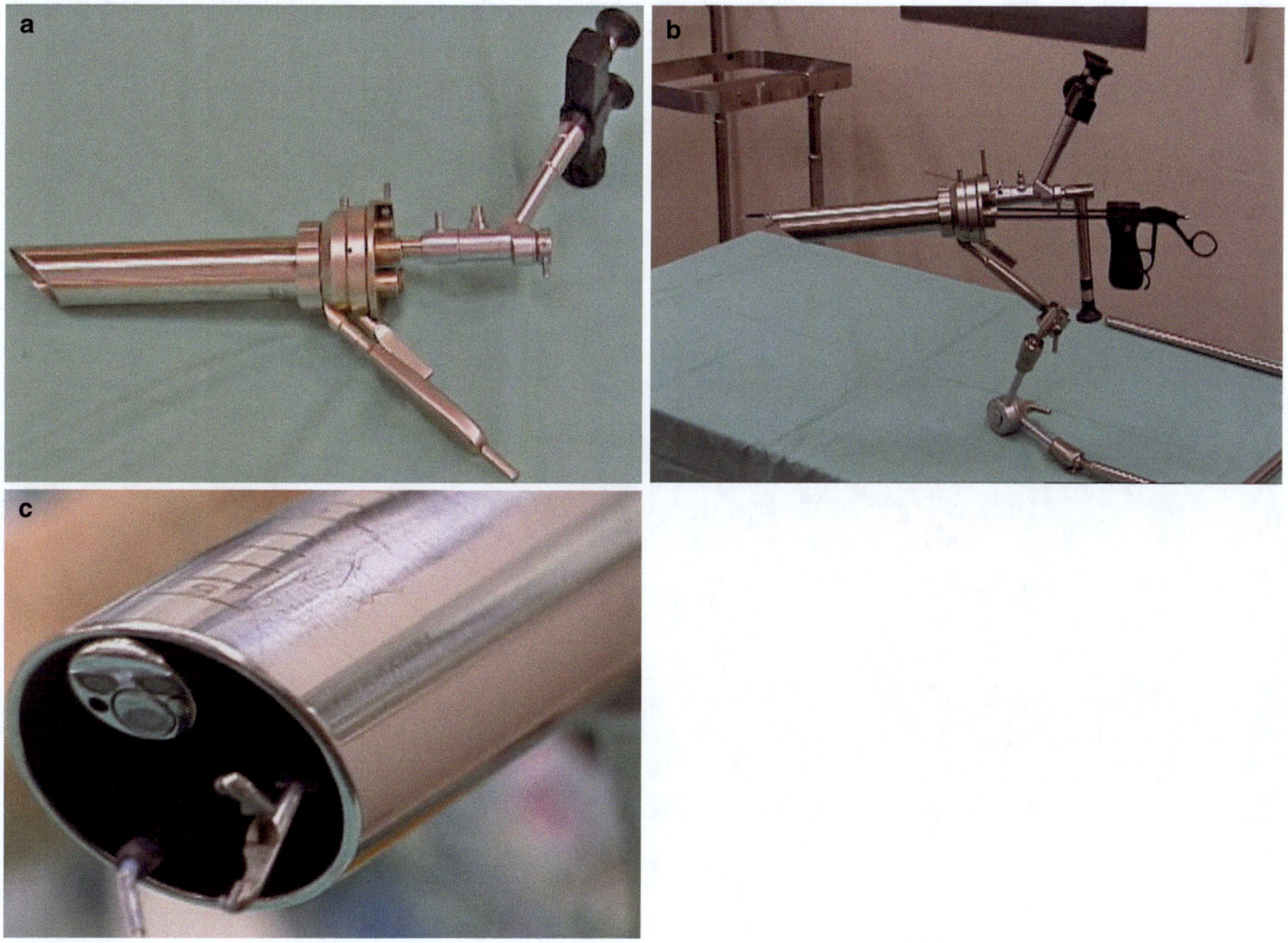

Fig. 14.11 TEM apparatus. (**a**) Operating proctoscope. (**b**) Proctoscope with Martin's Arm. (**c**) Proximal end of proctoscope, showing TEM instruments and camera

in one of the largest series to date. Overall, a recurrence occurred in 4 %, with positive margins occurring in 6 %, and development of early (6 %) and long-term (0 %) complications at a median follow-up of 20 months [24]. The authors concluded that operative times are faster than TEM, with overall outcomes being equivalent to TEM, and improved when compared to local excision series. Other TAMIS series have reported conversion to laparotomy for resection or diverting stoma (0–10 %), bleeding [5–10], perforation, infection (<5 %), and temporary incontinence (10–30 %) [25]. Late complications including stricture, fistula, and recurrence have been reported, though are generally rare. Technical tips for intraperitoneal entry involve a two-layer closure, placement of the patient in steep Trendelenburg position to facilitate retraction of the abdominal viscera from the pelvis, and a water-soluble enema in the early post-operative period to confirm absence of a leak. Another option is to perform laparoscopy at the time of the peritoneal entry to help with repair and placement of a drain and to perform a leak test [25].

The Role of Radiation Therapy

Key Concept: Radiation therapy decreases local recurrence for stages 1–3 lesions, and we feel it should be given for all patients preoperatively. Postoperative radiation therapy should be reserved only for select cases.

Regardless of local excision technique chosen, what is the role of radiation for stage I rectal cancer? Should preoperative radiation be utilized in early-stage cancers in the rectum if local excision is being considered? In looking at the MRC CR07 trial, comparing preoperative radiotherapy versus selective postoperative radiotherapy, interesting results were found. This was a multicenter randomized trial involving 1,350 patients who were operated on radically. It is noteworthy that there was a 31.5 % abdominoperineal resection rate in these patients. It is also of note that the local failure rate at 3 years for T1 cancers treated with preoperative radiation was 1.9 %, compared to 2.8 % treated postoperatively. For T2 lesions, local failure with preoperative radiotherapy was 1.9 % compared with a 6.4 % local failure rate with

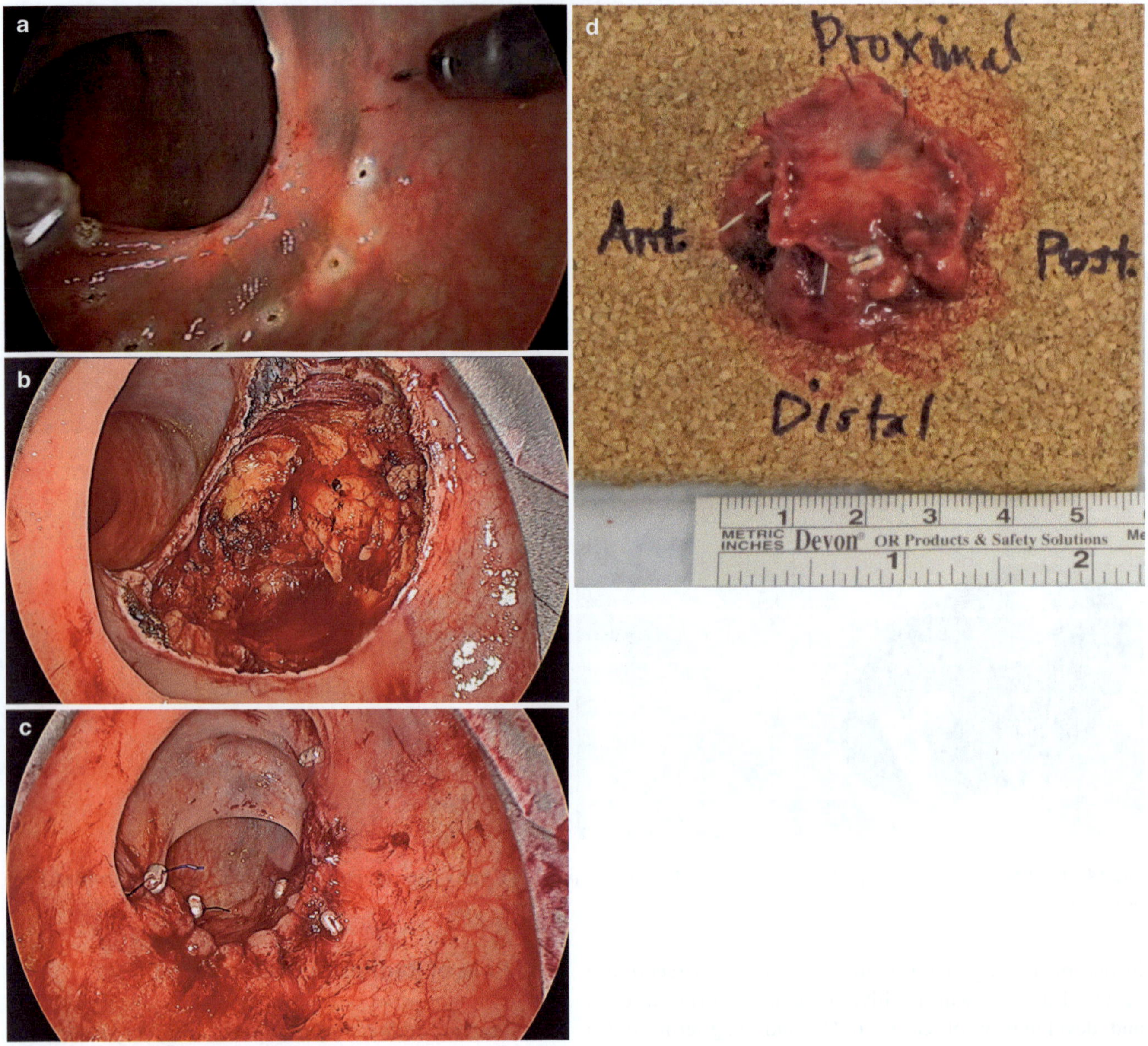

Fig. 14.12 (**a**) Margin marked by electrocautery. (**b**) Full-thickness, hemi-circumferential local excision. (**c**) TEM anastomosis. (**d**) Specimen, oriented and pinned out on cork board

postoperative treatment for selective postoperative treatment. Additionally, the failure rate for T3 cancers was down to 7.4 % when compared to 15.4 % in the postoperative radiotherapy group. All of these were statistically significant. This led the authors to conclude that for stage I as well as stage II and III disease, their data showed statistical improvement in terms of local control for cancers treated preoperatively with radiation therapy and advocated preoperative radiation treatment [26].

Our experience with radiation therapy followed by local excision dates back to 1984. This was the first experience in the world of local excision after preoperative radiation therapy. This was performed at Jefferson with the Marks and Mohiuddin method [27, 28]. In 2004, we reported on 44 patients treated with T2, N0 cancer in the distal 7 cm and found an overall local recurrence rate of 6.9 %. Twenty-three percent of these patients had complete responses, and there were no failures in that group. There was a 91 % 5-year survival rate [29]. Only a quarter of those patients were operated on using TEM. The others were done in transanal approaches. As we compared our experience with T2 rectal cancers following neoadjuvant treatment with TEM versus total mesorectal excision (TME), we found in 73 patients the local recurrence rate was not statistically different. It was 3.3 % for the TEM group compared with 2.3 % for the TME group. Additionally, survival was no different: 95 % in the TEM group compared with 97 % in the TME group [30]. Lezoche published similar results for full-thickness local excision

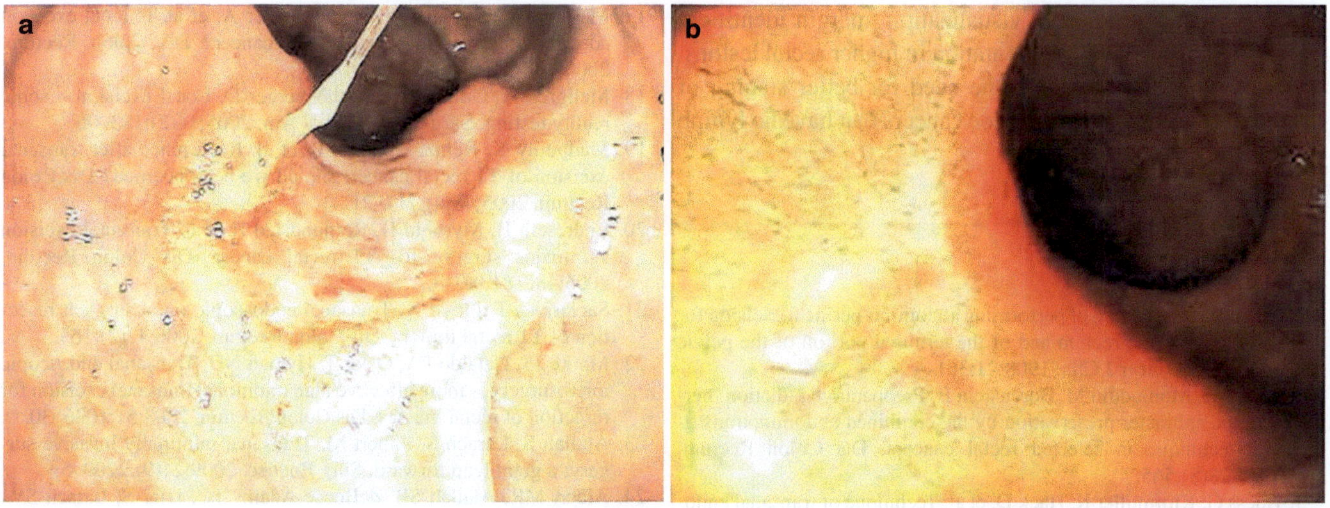

Fig. 14.13 Endoscopic images of rectal lesion before and after neoadjuvant chemoradiation. (**a**) Before, (**b**) after

after chemoradiation: 5 % local recurrence rate and an 89 % survival rate [31] (Fig. 14.13).

In general, postoperative radiation is never, in our minds, the ideal treatment plan. The only time this is employed has to do when there is a more advanced local stage of disease than originally anticipated by preoperative staging. For patient staged as an early T1 cancer or polyp that ends up having a T2 cancer but clean deep margins, I would consider postoperative radiation therapy as an option as opposed to proceeding always to radical surgery. Again, a discussion regarding the risk profile of the patient and the risk of leaving not fully treated lymph nodes in place has to be undertaken with the patient.

Summary Pearls

In conclusion, local excision for early-stage cancer is generally not sufficient. In a select case of medically compromised patients, of course, this is an ideal approach. For early T1 cancers or polyps with a small focus of cancer, local excision is clearly sufficient. However, for significant T1 cancers, a more aggressive approach is necessary. Undoubtedly, surgical technique matters, whether standard transanal excision techniques or TEM/TAMIS is utilized. One of the authors prefers a selective approach to the use of TEM/TAMIS versus standard TAE, reserving TEM/TAMIS for middle third and higher lesions. The other prefers the routine use of TEM for all levels. The choice of approach should be based not only on the location and characteristics of the tumor but also on the skill set of the operating surgeon and the equipment that is available. Selected reports of TEM results suggest improved local recurrence rates with TEM versus TAE; however, others suggest similarly high rates with TEM (10–20 % local recurrence rates with T1 lesions) [32, 33]. Chemoradiation holds promise to diminish the high failure rate for T1 and T2 cancers. Our general treatment algorithm is to treat high-risk unfavorable patients with rectal cancer with chemoradiation preoperatively. High-risk patients are defined as any T3 or node-positive patients and all cancers in the distal third of the rectum. The tumor's response to radiation therapy dictates whether a local approach to their cancer is warranted. In general, the tumor must have regressed to a size less than 4 cm without deep ulceration and felt to be confined to the bowel wall. The local excision is carried out. If there is full-thickness penetration or node positivity, radical surgery is then recommended. If there is a ypT1 or T2 cancer present, this serves as definitive therapy.

By combining local excision techniques and chemoradiation, the problem of persistent disease from untreated lymphatics is addressed. In higher lesions, TEM/TAMIS helps address the problem of specimen fragmentation and the challenge of achieving clear margins by operating with an endoluminal approach. With the combination of these approaches, the patient has an increased chance for success with an expanded role of local therapy for stage I rectal cancer. The challenge that persists, unfortunately, remains to better stage rectal cancers, so we can clearly identify those that have no lymphatic involvement. With more reliable information on staging in hand, we would have the technical ability with TEM and TAMIS to treat cancers in the upper rectum itself. Unquestionably, the future will see wider application of these techniques as additional work with these multidisciplinary, minimally invasive approaches to rectal cancer progresses.

Take-Home Points

1. Local excision is sufficient for early T1 cancers/polyps with a small focus of cancer.
2. Combining local excision and chemoradiation may address the problem of persistent disease from untreated lymphatics.

3. TEM/TAMIS addresses visualization, margin identification, and specimen fragmentation in higher rectal lesions.
4. A continued challenge is the need for better staging of rectal cancers to identify those cancers that have no lymph node involvement.

References

1. Miles WE. A method of performing abdomino-perineal excision for carcinoma of the rectum and of the terminal portion of the pelvic colon. CA Cancer J Clin. 1908;21:361–4.
2. Marks G, Mohiuddin M, Borenstein B. Preoperative radiation therapy and sphincter preservation by the combined abdominotranssacral technique in selected rectal cancers. Dis Colon Rectum. 1985;28(8):565.
3. Buess G, Kipfmuller K, Hack D, et al. Technique of transanal endoscopic microsurgery. Surg Endosc. 1988;2(2):71–5.
4. Atallah S, Albert M, Larach S. Transanal minimally invasive surgery: a giant leap forward. Surg Endosc. 2010;24(9):2200–5.
5. Saclarides T. Transanal endoscopic microsurgery: a single surgeon's experience. Arch Surg. 1998;133(6):595–9.
6. Kikuchi R, Takano M, Takagi K, et al. Management of early invasive colorectal cancer. Dis Colon Rectum. 1995;38(12):1286–95.
7. Wibe A, Syse A, Andersen E, et al. Oncological outcomes after total mesorectal excision for cure for cancer of the lower rectum: anterior vs. abdominoperineal resection. Dis Colon Rectum. 2004;47(1):48–58.
8. Sitzler PJ, Seow-Choen F, Ho YH, et al. Lymph node involvement and tumor depth in rectal cancers: an analysis of 805 patients. Dis Colon Rectum. 1997;40:1472–6.
9. Brodsky JT, Richard GK, Cohen AM, et al. Variables correlated with the risk of lymph node metastasis in early rectal cancer. Cancer. 1992;69:322–6.
10. Killingback M. Local excision of carcinoma of the rectum: indications. World J Surg. 1992;16:437–46.
11. Blumberg D, Paty P, Guillem J, et al. All patients with small intramural rectal cancers are at risk for lymph node metastasis. Dis Colon Rectum. 1999;42:881–5.
12. Brown G, Radcliffe A, Newcombe R, et al. Preoperative assessment of prognostic factors in rectal cancer using high-resolution magnetic resonance imaging. Br J Surg. 2003;90:355–64.
13. Kim HJ, Wong WD. Role of endorectal ultrasound in the conservative management of rectal cancers. Semin Surg Oncol. 2000;19:358–66.
14. Fidler IJ. Critical factors in the biology of human cancer metastasis: twenty-eighth G.H.A. Clowes memorial award lecture. Cancer Res. 1990;50:6130–8.
15. Bleday R, Breen E, Jessup JM, et al. Prospective evaluation of local excision for small rectal cancers. Dis Colon Rectum. 1997;40: 388–92.
16. Steele GD, Herndon JE, Bleday R, et al. Sphincter-sparing treatment for distal rectal adenocarcinoma. Ann Surg Oncol. 1999;6: 433–41.
17. Mellgren A, Sirivongs P, Rothenberger A, et al. Is local excision adequate therapy for early rectal cancer? Dis Colon Rectum. 2000;43(8):1064–71.
18. Mellgren A, Goldberg J, Rothenberger D. Local excision – some reality testing. Surg Oncol Clin N Am. 2005;14(2):183–96.
19. Madbouly K, Remzi F, Erkek B, et al. Recurrence after transanal excision of T1 rectal cancer: should we be concerned? Dis Colon Rectum. 2005;48(4):711–21.
20. Endreseth B, Myrvold H, Romundstad P, et al. Transanal excision vs. major surgery for T1 rectal cancer. Dis Colon Rectum. 2005;48(7):1380–8.
21. Saclarides T, Floyd N. Transanal endoscopic microsurgical resection of T1 rectal tumors. Dis Colon Rectum. 2006;42(2):165.
22. Moore JS, Cataldo PA, Osler T, Hyman NH. Transanal endoscopic microsurgery is more effective than traditional transanal excision for resection of rectal masses. Dis Colon Rectum. 2008;51:1026–30.
23. Atallah S, Larach S, Albert M. Transanal minimally invasive surgery: a giant leap forward. Surg Endosc. 2009;24(9):2200–5.
24. Albert MR, Atallah SB, deBeche-Adams TC, Izfar S, Larach SW. Transanal minimally invasive surgery (TAMIS) for local excision of benign neoplasms and early-stage rectal cancer: efficacy and outcomes in the first 50 patients. Dis Colon Rectum. 2013;56(3):301–7.
25. Albert M, Atallah S, Larach S, deBeche-Adams T. Minimally invasive anorectal surgery: from Parks local excision to transanal endoscopic microsurgery to transanal minimally invasive surgery. Semin Colorectal Surg. 2013;24(1):42–9.
26. Sebag-Montefiore D, Stephens R, Steele R, et al. Preoperative radiotherapy versus selective postoperative chemoradiotherapy in patients with rectal cancer (MRC CR07 and NCIC-CTG C016): a multicenter, randomised trial. Lancet. 2009;373(9666):811–20.
27. Marks G, Mohiuddin M, Masoni L, et al. High-dose preoperative radiation and full-thickness local excision. Dis Colon Rectum. 1990;33(9):735–9.
28. Mohiuddin M, Marks G, Bannon J. High-dose preoperative radiation and full thickness local excision: a new option for selected T3 distal rectal cancers. Int J Radiat Oncol. 1994;30(4):845–9.
29. Annamaneni R, Marks J, Hamdan W, Curran T, Mohiuddin M, Marks G. Full thickness local excision of prospectively staged T2 rectal cancers after neoadjuvant radiation/chemoradiation. Poster presented at: Society of Surgical Oncology annual cancer symposium; Atlanta, GA: 2005.
30. Mizrahi B, Marks J, Marks G, et al. T2 rectal cancer: a comparison of radical surgery and local excision by transanal endoscopic microsurgery following neoadjuvant therapy. Poster presented at: American Society of Colon & Rectal Surgeons annual scientific meeting; Hollywood, FL: 2009.
31. Lezoche E, Guerrieri M, Paganini A, et al. Long-term results in patients with T2-3 N0 distal rectal cancer undergoing radiotherapy before transanal endoscopic microsurgery. Br J Surg. 2005;92(12):1546–52.
32. Doornebosch P, Ferenschild F, de Wilt J, et al. Treatment of recurrence after transanal endoscopic microsurgery (TEM) for T1 rectal cancer. Dis Colon Rectum. 2010;53(9):1234–9.
33. Tsai B, Finne C, Nordenstam J, et al. Transanal endoscopic microsurgery resection of rectal tumors: outcomes and recommendation. Dis Colon Rectum. 2010;53(1):16–23.

Recurrent Rectal Cancer

15

Todd D. Francone and Martin R. Weiser

Key Points

- Preoperative considerations in the setting of locally recurrent rectal cancer are extensive. Meticulous evaluation before surgery is necessary to determine if the patient is medically fit and the tumor is resectable. In some cases, determination of resectability can only be made intraoperatively.
- Proper radiographic imaging can demonstrate the local extent of tumor recurrence, facilitating a detailed operative plan for en bloc resection.
- The single most important factor in optimizing outcomes is complete excision of the tumor with negative macroscopic and microscopic margins.
- Management of recurrent rectal cancer is often complex, requiring the involvement of a multidisciplinary team. Designing a care plan should be based not only on clinical, diagnostic, and physical findings but also on the individual patient's goals and expectations.

Introduction

Key Concept: Pelvic recurrence of rectal cancer is one of the most challenging clinical situations you may encounter. While multiple factors contribute to recurrence, technical factors, including the ability to achieve negative margins, are imperative to limit recurrent disease and improve long-term outcomes following operative therapy for recurrent rectal cancer.

Rectal cancer reportedly recurs within the pelvis at a rate of 4–33 % following curative-intent resection of the primary lesion. Recurrence typically presents within 5 years of the index operation; however, later recurrences are possible. Pelvic recurrence is associated with a poor prognosis and distressing symptoms that are difficult to palliate.

Multiple factors, including surgeon experience, have been shown to influence oncologic outcomes [1]; surgeons who perform more than 12 cases per year appear to have lower local recurrence rates than those who operate less [2]. Pathologic factors such as lymphovascular invasion and poor differentiation also increase the risk of local recurrence [3, 4]. Although the reasons for recurrence are numerous, extent of resection is the most critical factor; positive distal and/or positive circumferential margins are associated with local recurrence rates as high as 55 % [2, 3, 5]. Conversely, negative microscopic resection margins (R0) are associated with the lowest recurrence rates and the most favorable prognosis [6].

For patients with recurrence limited to the pelvis, multivisceral/extended rectal resection is the definitive surgical therapy. However, in recurrent disease, the surgical planes are disrupted by initial resection of the primary tumor, making re-resection significantly more challenging. These procedures are associated with considerable morbidity and require extensive surgical planning. A multidisciplinary team including surgeons, medical and radiation oncologists, radiologists, intensivists, specialized nurses, and occupational and physical therapists should be assembled to address the multifaceted issues that are likely to arise. The surgical team alone may include specialists in colorectal, urologic, gynecologic, orthopedic, neurologic, and plastic/reconstructive surgery. Multimodal therapy has played an essential role in the trend towards improved oncologic outcomes, including re-irradiation with external beam and intraoperative radiotherapy (IORT).

In this chapter, we will discuss the diagnosis, evaluation, and multimodal management of locally recurrent rectal cancer, as well as the associated perioperative and oncologic outcomes.

T.D. Francone, MD, MPH
Division of Surgery, Department of Colon and Rectal Surgery, Lahey Clinic, 41 Mall Road, Burlington, MA 01805, USA
e-mail: todd.d.francone@lahey.org

M.R. Weiser, MD (✉)
Department of Surgery, Memorial Sloan-Kettering Cancer Center, 1275 York Avenue, New York, NY 10021, USA
e-mail: weiser1@mskcc.org

S.R. Steele et al. (eds.), *Complexities in Colorectal Surgery*,
DOI 10.1007/978-1-4614-9022-7_15, © Springer Science+Business Media New York 2014

Presentation

Key Concept: Identifying local recurrence is challenging, as patients can present with or without symptoms.

Locally recurrent rectal cancer usually manifests months to years after the initial operation, with a mean time to recurrence of 25–36 months [6–11]. In a population-based study by Palmer et al. of 141 patients with locally recurrent rectal cancer, 70 % presented within the first 2 years and 85 % within 3 years after initial surgery [9]. The majority presents with symptoms, precipitating work-up and diagnosis. The most common symptoms are pain, rectal bleeding, or changes in bowel habits. Thirty-five percent or fewer are asymptomatic, and the recurrence is discovered on routine surveillance follow-up [8, 9]. Pelvic pain indicates possible involvement of other organs, bones, or nerves. Therefore, pain as a presenting symptom is of concern and portends a poor prognosis. If the initial operation was abdominoperineal resection (APR), a palpable mass in the perineum or nonhealing wound may indicate perineal recurrence. Small bowel obstruction suggests involvement of the small intestine.

Preoperative Evaluation and Staging

Preoperative Planning

Key Concept: Prior to embarking on surgery for recurrence, you must determine the feasibility of resecting all disease with negative margins. Patients must be evaluated for comorbid conditions, and their ability to tolerate and recover from reoperative surgery.

Proper preoperative evaluation is imperative when contemplating radical surgery for recurrent rectal cancer. A thorough examination of the patient's medical records, including operative reports and history of previous chemoradiation treatments, provides valuable information regarding anatomy and prognosis and helps determine a plan of care. Patients of advanced age, with significant comorbidities or poor performance status (ASA IV–V), are rarely candidates for the extensive surgery that is necessary. Appropriate risk assessment requires consideration of patient cognitive function as well. Distant metastatic disease must also be ruled out. In the presence of distant metastasis, such potentially morbid surgery offers little possibility of cure.

Physical Examination

Key Concept: Physical examination is an important part of the work-up of recurrent disease.

A proper physical evaluation (including digital rectal and vaginal examination) is crucial. Whenever possible, rectal examination with proctoscopy should be done. This may reveal the level, position and extent of tumor, as well as its fixation to adjacent organs and/or the bony pelvis. In addition, you will be able to get a sense for the response to any prior chemotherapy or additional radiation therapy. Vaginal exam in female patients is essential in order to clarify posterior vaginal wall involvement that may require en bloc resection. Additionally, it will highlight the need to involve your plastic surgery colleagues for a potential flap to close the resultant defect. In patients whose initial operation was an APR, careful examination of the perineum and surgical scar may reveal the presence of a palpable mass. A thorough pelvic exam is often the simplest, most direct method of determining whether sphincter-sparing surgery is feasible, or multivisceral resection or exenteration necessary. A complete colonoscopy should also be done whenever possible, to rule out synchronous primary tumors. Tissue diagnosis is typically necessary to differentiate scar from recurrent disease, especially if the tumor extends intraluminally.

Carcinoembryonic Antigen

Key Concept: Although CEA monitoring is controversial, persistently elevated levels of CEA warrant work-up for recurrent and metastatic disease.

The American Society of Clinical Oncology currently recommends that postoperative serum carcinoembryonic antigen (CEA) testing be performed every 2–3 months, for ≥3 years after diagnosis, in patients with stage II or III disease [12]. An elevated CEA level warrants further evaluation for metastatic as well as locally recurrent disease. The relevance of CEA in evaluating recurrence remains controversial. A few studies demonstrate significant association between high levels of CEA and poor prognosis, including decreased overall survival [7, 13–15].

Radiologic Imaging

Key Concept: Radiologic imaging is the most commonly used tool in staging locally recurrent rectal cancer. Accurate imaging can clarify the size, location, level, and extent of recurrence (both local and extrapelvic); delineate potential invasion into adjacent structures; and help determine appropriate patient selection for resection.

Local Disease

Verification of recurrent disease, often done by computed tomography (CT)-guided biopsy, is recommended before undertaking surgery. However, the challenge of imaging recurrent disease is complicated by the fact that previous surgery for the primary tumor makes it difficult to differentiate recurrent tumor from fibrosis. Magnetic resonance imaging (MRI), if available, is often the tool of choice.

Computed Tomography (CT)

Key Concept: While not as accurate as MRI, CT is a great initial examination to assess the gross extent of local disease and rule out distant recurrence.

Contrast-enhanced CT scanning and MRI are the imaging tools most often used to diagnose recurrent rectal cancer. The accuracy of CT in showing tumor invasion (in both primary and recurrent rectal cancer) has consistently proven inferior to the accuracy of MRI. For example, in a study by Beets-Tan et al., the sensitivity of CT in predicting tumor invasion was 70 %, with an associated specificity of 85 % [16]. This is because CT does not accurately differentiate between fibrosis, normal tissue, and recurrent tumor. Nevertheless, in our experience, CT has been very useful in the initial work-up of a locally recurrent tumor mass, or when distant disease in the abdomen is suspected.

Magnetic Resonance Imaging (MRI)

Key Concept: MRI has better accuracy than CT in detecting recurrent disease and delineating pelvic anatomy.

At the present time, MRI provides the best imaging of pelvic and extra-rectal involvement available. The inherently high soft tissue contrast resolution of MRI enables it to differentiate between normal tissue, scar tissue, and tumor. This is because tumor has a relatively high water content, and therefore a high T2w image; scar tissue has a comparatively low water content, and low signal intensity, on both T_1-weighted and T_2-weighted images.

Although MRI is consistently more accurate than CT in identifying local recurrence, it has limitations. In the setting of primary rectal cancer, MRI has demonstrated a sensitivity of 95 % and a specificity of 85–100 % in identifying local invasion [16, 17]. However, recent literature suggests that MRI may not be as reliable in evaluating locally recurrent rectal cancers, showing a sensitivity of 77–100 % and a specificity of 29–92 % [18–22]. A few studies have concluded that the accuracy of MRI varies according to anatomical location, with lower accuracy as regards the pelvic sidewall and pelvic floor. Messiou et al. reported their experience using MRI phased-array coil to identify recurrent tumor invasion at specific sites in the pelvis, prior to salvage surgery, in 49 patients over a 6-year period. In 30 of these patients, pelvic sidewall invasion was identified with MRI before surgery, but only 21 were confirmed on histologic examination. The authors concluded that tumor detection with MRI showed a sensitivity of 70 % and a specificity of 94 % [20].

As is the case with other imaging modalities, inaccuracy in MRI may be due to disruption of the anatomic planes from previous surgery (which increases the likelihood of fibrosis, granulation, and hematoma formation) or to radiation-induced inflammatory changes [22, 23]. Tumor tissue and fibrosis commonly coexist, resulting in relatively low signal intensity on T_2-weighted imaging. This is true not only in recurrent disease but in tumor radiated before the index surgery; in either case, it may result in a false negative. These limitations support the practice of biopsying any fibrotic tissues suspicious for malignancy. Dynamic MR has been utilized to distinguish fibrosis from tumor, based on the principle that recurrent tumor tissue shows earlier and greater degrees of enhancement than fibrosed tissue. The results for dynamic MR vary in the literature, with reported sensitivity ranging from 83 to 97 % and specificity from 81 to 100 % [19, 21, 24].

FDG-PET

Key Concept: FDG-PET can help distinguish benign fibrosis from recurrent disease.

Fluorine-18 fluorodeoxyglucose positron emission tomography (FDG-PET) may also be of value in the preoperative staging of locally advanced and recurrent rectal cancer. FDG-PET identifies changes in tumor glucose metabolism [25] and can be useful in the setting of recurrent disease [26–30]. Furthermore, FDG-PET may supplement other imaging modalities in distinguishing viable tumor from scar. In a meta-analysis by Huebner et al. including 366 patients with local pelvic recurrence, FDG-PET showed an overall sensitivity of 94.5 % (95 % CI, 90.8–98.2 %) and a specificity of 97.7 % (95 % CI, 95.7–99.7 %). The authors found that—when added to standard imaging techniques in diagnostic work-up—FDG-PET findings led to a change in clinical management in about 30 % of patients with recurrent disease [31].

Integrated FDG-PET/CT combines the benefits of functional and anatomical/morphological imaging, and appears to hold additional promise in distinguishing benign from viable malignant tumor. In a study by Votruba et al. of 84 patients with suspected colorectal cancer recurrence, FDG-PET demonstrated overall sensitivity and specificity of 80 and 69 %, respectively. When integrated FDG-PET/CT was used, sensitivity and specificity increased to 89 and 92 %, respectively [32]. Similarly, in a study of 62 patients with local recurrence after APR or low anterior resection, Evan-Sapir et al. reported that integrated FDG-PET/CT demonstrated better accuracy than FDG-PET in differentiating between malignant and benign lesions, with an overall accuracy of 74 and 92 %, respectively [27].

Distant Disease

The usefulness of CT scans of the chest and abdomen in identifying hepatic metastases is well accepted. However, CT reportedly misses or underestimates extent of disease in a significant proportion of patients [33]. Several recent studies have suggested that FDG-PET/CT is superior to CT, EUS, and MRI in this regard [34–36]. A meta-analysis by Kinkel et al. concluded that FDG-PET/CT is more sensitive than ultrasound, CT, or MRI in detecting gastroesophageal and colorectal hepatic metastases [34], and studies by Bipat et al. [36] and Mainenti et al. [35] concluded that PET/CT showed superior sensitivity in detecting colorectal hepatic metastases. In a study comparing FDG-PET and CT findings in 103 patients with suspected colorectal cancer recurrence, Flamen et al. concluded that FDG-PET had higher sensitivity than CT in identifying metastatic lymph nodes, as well as lung and peritoneal disease [37]. Because of its ability to detect early metastatic disease, FDG-PET/CT has influenced clinical management in up to 40 % of patients with recurrent colorectal cancer [38–40].

Imaging Summary Recommendations

In our experience, most patients will present after undergoing imaging with an abdominopelvic CT. We use this as a general guide to look for gross disease, pelvic sidewall involvement, or other indications of potentially non-resectable disease (i.e., bilateral hydroureter, extensive iliac involvement). We routinely use MRI to give us a preoperative roadmap for helping with fascial planes or in cases where there is still a question regarding differentiation between recurrent disease and post-therapeutic changes. In our hands, FDG-PET is most useful both in differentiating benign from malignant disease locally in the pelvis and determining the activity of small distant lesions (i.e., liver, lung) that may represent metastatic disease.

Histology

Key Concept: Tissue confirmation should be attempted whenever possible, before subjecting a patient to radical surgery for a suspected local recurrence.

In the event of an intraluminal recurrence, endoscopic retrieval of a tissue specimen is the obvious choice. When a suspected pelvic recurrence is not amenable to endoscopic biopsy, radiographic-guided biopsy is recommended. CT and MRI have both been used in tissue sampling. In some circumstances, however, tissue diagnosis is not feasible, or biopsy results are inconclusive. Nevertheless, if there is convincing radiologic evidence for recurrence, it is reasonable to proceed with surgical exploration. The patient should be properly educated and counseled preoperatively. He or she must be willing to accept the risks of the procedure despite the possibility that tumor will not be found within the surgical specimen.

Classification and Patterns of Recurrence

Key Concept: The pattern of recurrence is a factor when determining resectability.

Patterns of recurrence significantly influence the possibility of achieving an R0 resection. A useful and simple classification system by Moore et al. [6] utilized anatomical location to categorize tumors: (1) axial, not involving anterior, posterior, or lateral pelvic walls (this includes anastomotic recurrence after low anterior resection, local recurrence after transanal or transsphincteric excision, and perineal recurrence after APR); (2) anterior, involving the urinary bladder, vagina, uterus, seminal vesicles, or prostate; (3) posterior, involving the sacrum and coccyx; and (4) lateral, involving the bony pelvic sidewall or sidewall structures, including the iliac vessels, pelvic ureters, lateral lymph nodes, pelvic autonomic nerves, and sidewall musculature. This system contributes to a standardized approach in the pre- and postoperative management of local recurrence.

Defining Resectability

Key Concept: Resectability pertains not only to the pattern of recurrent disease but also to the individual patient's ability to tolerate the morbidity of the operation and the potential functional challenges that may occur postoperatively.

Resectable recurrent rectal cancer is defined as tumor that may be completely removed with curative intent (i.e., with histologically negative margins (R0)). The literature is consistent in this regard [6]. Because of the rigors involved, however, resectability should also be defined in terms of acceptable morbidity for the individual patient. Careful patient selection and proper risk assessment are critical. Patients with significant comorbidities or poor performance status (ASA IV–V) are rarely candidates for the extensive surgery that is required. Several other patient-related factors associated with decreased probability of an R0 resection include male gender [41], advanced age at initial diagnosis [42], advanced stage of the primary tumor [42], and previous APR [41, 42].

In a series of 116 patients treated at Memorial Sloan-Kettering Cancer Center, Moore et al. [6] found that tumors confined to the axial location, or to the axial and anterior locations, were more likely to be completely resectable than tumors involving the pelvic sidewall or lateral structures. The authors reported that negative margins were achieved in 90 % of patients with axial recurrences only (anastomotic recurrence), and in 71 % of patients with axial and anterior recurrences only. Negative margins were also achieved in 64 % of patients with lateral involvement by tumor, and in 55 % of patients without iliac vessel involvement. However, negative margins were obtained in only 43 % of patients with tumor located *anywhere but* axially and anteriorly. Where there was lateral involvement by tumor, negative margins were achieved in only 35 % (and reportedly in as few as 0 %, in other studies) [43]. Involvement of the ureter with hydronephrosis or iliac vessel involvement was associated with an R0 resection in only 17 and 29 % of patients, respectively. Other studies have supported these findings, suggesting that bilateral hydronephrosis and tumor encasement of the iliac vessels are contraindications to re-resection.

Posterior recurrence is associated with an even lower probability of R0 resection [43–45]. Complete removal of these tumors requires technically challenging procedures involving en bloc resection of the tumor and part of the sacrum. The major sequelae associated with such operations include neurologic defects involving the bladder, anorectal and sexual function, and potential musculoskeletal defects related to wound dehiscence. High sacrectomy (S1/S2) is associated with greater morbidity than mid-level or low sacrectomy. Nerve root involvement is a contraindication to resection because of the potential for resulting neurologic defects. Although bony and neurologic constraints may preclude resection, when curative-intent surgery is feasible and an R0 resection accomplished, there are lower recurrence rates and improved survival [44]. As the sacrectomy level decreases, the possibility of a complete resection increases. In a recent study by Sagar and colleagues [46], R0 resection was achieved in 13 of 40 patients undergoing abdominosacrectomy for recurrent rectal cancer. Complete resection was associated with a significantly improved median survival (56 months for R0 vs. 32 months for R1; $p = 0.048$). Moriya et al. described abdominosacral resection in 69 patients with recurrent rectal cancer, reporting an R0 rate of 83 % and 3-year disease-specific survival of 62 % in patients with negative margins [47].

The degree of tumor fixation within the pelvis significantly influences the feasibility of curative surgery and overall survival. In 2003, Hahnloser and associates demonstrated that patients with two or more sites of fixation had a significantly worse outcome compared to patients with mobile tumors or only one site of fixation. Degree of fixation was determined on preoperative imaging or at the time of surgery. Local recurrences were classified as not fixed (F0), fixed at one site (F1), fixed at 2 sites (F2), or fixed at three or more sites (F3). A greater number of fixation sites indicated more extensive, locally advanced tumors requiring technically more challenging radical surgery, and outcomes were worse with respect to local failure and long-term survival [8].

Other factors associated with poor long-term outcomes include APR as the original procedure, elevated preoperative CEA, preoperative pain, vascular invasion, and aggressive tumor biology [6, 10, 48].

For patients deemed to be resectable, counseling regarding the impact of surgery on quality of life is critical. While a low anterior resection restores intestinal continuity, it may also result in significant urgency or incontinence. Patients undergoing an APR with end colostomy should receive proper preoperative teaching and counseling regarding the potential physical, social, and psychological difficulties associated with having a stoma. However, surgery should generally be avoided in patients with disease characterized by circumferential pelvic sidewall involvement, bilateral ureteral obstruction, S1 or S2 bony or neural involvement, sciatic pain and pelvic imaging evidence of sciatic nerve involvement, or unresectable extrapelvic metastases. Patients who are not resectable should be counseled regarding the eventual worsening of their symptoms, including pain, bleeding, and obstruction. Palliative care professionals can help provide some relief of symptoms, as well as psychosocial and supportive care for patients and their families. Management of patient expectations in these circumstances requires understanding and compassion on the part of the surgeon and multidisciplinary team.

Multimodal Therapy

Role of Neoadjuvant Therapy

Key Concept: Neoadjuvant chemoradiation therapy plays a significant role in the setting of recurrent disease, as it does in primary rectal cancer. Prior treatment and total dosage will help determine appropriate selection of agents and treatment strategies.

In both primary and recurrent rectal cancer, multimodality therapy including chemotherapy and radiation is the standard of care. In primary disease, preoperative chemoradiation has been shown to reduce local recurrence more effectively than postoperative chemoradiation [49]. Preoperative chemoradiotherapy may effect tumor downsizing [49, 50], potentially facilitating complete resection of locally advanced disease. Therefore, neoadjuvant chemoradiation has become a standard practice in the treatment of locally advanced rectal cancers.

Most patients presenting with locally recurrent cancer have already been irradiated. Patients with pelvic recurrence who have not previously received radiation for their primary tumor should be considered for preoperative chemoradiotherapy. Treatment usually consists of external beam radiation up to a dose of 50.4 Gy, with concurrent 5-flourouracil (5-FU)-based chemotherapy [49, 50]. Because of the risk of late toxicity, fistula formation, and bowel obstruction, radiation is generally contraindicated in patients who have already received radiotherapy to a total dose up to or greater than 50.4 Gy. However, recent studies demonstrate that re-irradiation is reasonably well tolerated if the previous dose was less than 50.4 Gy, and a significant percentage of re-irradiated patients go on to radical surgical salvage. The American College of Radiology recommends that additional doses of radiation be based on the initial dose given, amount of small bowel in the treatment field, length of time to recurrence, size of the previously treated cancer, and size of the recurrent tumor. The dose typically ranges from 20 to 40 Gy, with acceptable late toxicity rates of 12 and 21 %, respectively [51]. A study by Valentini et al. evaluated the response rate, resectability rate, local control, and treatment-related toxicity of preoperative hyperfractionated chemoradiotherapy in patients with locally recurrent rectal cancer who had previously received radiation. They found that 86.4 % of patients completed treatment without interruption, with a 5.1 % rate of acute lower GI toxicity and no grade 4 toxicity. More than 44 % had either a complete or partial response after re-irradiation [52].

In a study by Pacelli and colleagues involving 58 patients with recurrent rectal cancer, the authors found that patients who had undergone previous radiotherapy tolerated either 23.4 Gy in 1.8 Gy fractions, or 1.2 Gy BID to 40.8 Gy preoperatively. Radiation treatment was completed in all patients, with no major complications reported. In 2002, Mohiuddin and colleagues [53] reported on the long-term results of re-irradiation in patients with recurrent rectal carcinoma. A total of 103 patients with recurrent rectal carcinoma received re-irradiation with concurrent 5-FU-based chemotherapy. After a median dose of 3,480 cGy, 34 patients underwent surgical resection for residual disease. The median and 5-year survival of patients undergoing surgical resection after re-irradiation was 44 months and 22 %, compared with 14 months and 15 % for patients treated with re-irradiation only ($p = 0.001$).

Patients who cannot undergo any additional radiation may be candidates for aggressive chemotherapy. First-line multi-agent chemotherapy typically includes a combination of oxaliplatin or irinotecan along with the 5-FU/leucovorin regimen. Second-line regimens may include a combination of other targeted agents, including bevacizumab and cetuximab.

Imaging should be done at 4–6 weeks from the completion of treatment to rule out interval progression of local disease or development of distant metastasis. If the patient remains a candidate for potential curative resection, surgery is typically performed 6–8 weeks after therapy. Intraoperative radiation therapy (IORT), if used, may provide additive tumoricidal effect.

Intraoperative Radiation Therapy (IORT)

Key Concept: Although controversial, IORT is an evolving intraoperative treatment modality for patients with recurrent rectal cancers, including those who have received prior external beam pelvic radiation.

A major goal of radiation oncologists is to increase the dose delivered to tumor, relative to the dose delivered to normal adjacent tissues. As Willett and colleagues noted, this has led to the use of field-shaping techniques with multi-leaf collimation, multiple field techniques, and intensity-modulated radiotherapy, as well as intracavitary and interstitial brachytherapy [54]. IORT delivers radiation to the tumor bed while normal tissue is shielded. Two alternative but complementary IORT techniques have evolved: intraoperative electron radiation (IOERT), which uses a linear accelerator to deliver electron particles, and high-dose-rate brachytherapy (HDR-IORT), which delivers an iridium seed (192-Ir) along after-loading catheters. In either technique, normal tissues are simultaneously moved aside or physically shielded. Because the tumor can be visualized intraoperatively, it is possible to more accurately define areas at risk for tumor involvement [54].

The decision to perform IORT is based on anticipated risk of residual microscopic disease. Intraoperative frozen section analysis can help identify at-risk margins (<5 mm) that may benefit from IORT [55]. The dose of IORT (10–20 Gy) depends on the amount of residual disease and, in some cases, the dose of external beam radiation delivered preoperatively (Table 15.1) [54, 59–61].

Table 15.1 Outcomes following intraoperative radiation therapy (IORT) for rectal cancer

Study	Patients (*n*)			IORT dose (Gy)			5-y local recurrence (%)			5-y overall survival (%)		
	R0	R1	R2	R0	R1	R2	R0	R1	R2	R0	R1	R2
Haddock et al. (2009) [56]	227 (37)	224 (37)	156 (26)	12.5	15	20	28	32	32	46	27	16
Pacelli et al. (2009) [15]	–	–	–	10–15	10–15	10–15	–	–	–	–	–	–
Dreseen et al. (2008) [57][a]	84 (57.2)	34 (23/1)	29 (19.7)	10	12.5	15–17.5	25	29.2	28.5	58.7	26.5	24.1
Heriot et al. (2007) [58][a]	98 (61.3)	40 (25)	14 (8.8)	10	10	10	–	–	–	–	–	–
Hahnloser et al. (2002) [8]	138 (45)	27 (3.3)	139 (45.7)	–	–	–	–	–	–	27	–	–
Wiig et al. (2002) [59]	18	29	12	15	15	17.5–20	30	50	–	60	20	0
Shoup et al. (2002) [48]	64 (64)	30 (30)	6 (6)	12.5–15	15–17.5	15–17.5	–	–	–	31.2[b]	9[b]	14[b]

Abbreviations: dash(–) not reported, *y* year
[a]3-year OS, LR
[b]Disease-free survival

Haddock et al. [56] recently reported on a retrospective analysis of 607 patients with recurrent colorectal cancer who received IORT. IORT was preceded or followed by external radiation in 583 patients (96 %), 70 % of whom had tumors located within the pelvis. The median IORT dose was 15 Gy (range, 7.5–30 Gy). Survival estimates at 5 years were 46, 27, and 16 % for R0, R1, and R2 resections, respectively. On multivariate analysis, R0 resection was the only independent factor associated with improved survival. Although no randomized trials evaluating IORT have been performed to date, data from large single institution studies suggest that IORT may influence local control and survival. As one would expect, multiple studies suggest that the extent of surgical resection, and therefore the volume of residual disease, is an important factor in improving local control with IORT. The experience with intraoperative brachytherapy at the Memorial Sloan-Kettering Cancer Center was reported by Alektiar et al. [62] in a study of 74 patients treated from 1992 to 1998. Median follow-up was 22 months. Fifty of these patients had negative margin (R0) resection. Five-year local control was 39 %; 5-year disease-free and overall survival was 23 %. Negative margins predicted local control: a 5-year rate of 43 % in patients with R0 resection vs. 26 % in those with R1 resection. Patients with negative margins had 5-year survival of 36 %, compared to only 11 % in patients with positive margins. More recently, Dresen et al. [57] reported on 57 patients receiving re-irradiation of 30.6 Gy with IORT, in addition to preoperative re-irradiation with external beam radiotherapy. The IORT dose was dependent upon completeness of resection. Five-year overall survival was 48 % in patients with an R0 resection. On univariate analysis, R0 resection was more likely in patients receiving re-irradiation, compared to patients who had previously received radiotherapy and were treated with surgery alone. In addition, patients who were re-irradiated with IORT had improved overall survival and decreased local and distant recurrence. Radical resection and stage of the primary tumor were the only factors predicting overall survival on multivariate analysis [56].

The morbidities associated with IORT are generally acceptable, but may be difficult to distinguish from disease-related toxicity. Common side effects include wound infection, ureteral obstruction, gastrointestinal complications such as obstruction or fistula, and peripheral neuropathy. In the series reported by Alektiar et al., morbidities included wound complications (24 %), bladder complications (20 %), ureteral stricturing (23 %), and peripheral neuropathy (16 %) [62]. In the study of over 600 patients by Haddock et al. [56], 32 % of patients developed neuropathy, the most common radiation-induced toxicity. Seven patients developed ureteral narrowing or obstruction.

We currently use IORT in cases in which there are anticipated close margins. Care must be taken to shield radiation-sensitive structures; input from the surgeon is critical.

Surgical Technique

Key Concept: Distinguishing tumor invasion from adherence is difficult, and wide resection provides the best chance for a margin negative resection. While it is important to preserve as much healthy anatomy as possible, these procedures typically require extensive resection and subsequent surgical reconstruction.

In order to achieve complete resection of tumor with negative margins, all organs involved by tumor must also be resected. Therefore, these extensive procedures often require the coordinated involvement of surgical specialists in urology, gynecology, orthopedics, neurology, radiation oncology, vascular surgery, and plastic surgery. In the absence of the rectum after APR, recurrent cancers are more likely to invade adjacent organs such as the sacrum and sacral nerves posteriorly, the vagina and uterus, or seminal vesicles and prostate, and the bladder anteriorly, and the ureters, autonomic nerve plexus, internal ileac lymph nodes, and vessels laterally.

Tumor that adheres to regional anatomic structures is generally assumed to invade them; all or part of these organs must be removed en bloc with the tumor. Focal invasion of adjacent organs, or metastatic lymph nodes in the pelvic sidewall, requires extended resection. The type of procedure—total pelvic exenteration, posterior exenteration, anterior exenteration, APR with sacrectomy, and sacropelvic exenteration—depends on the extent of tumor spread as well as distance of tumor from the anal sphincter musculature.

Preoperative Regimen

Key Concept: Developing a routine is important to achieving intraoperative success and minimizing morbidity.

Preoperative evaluation, including physical examination and imaging, will determine the need for additional studies such as pelvic ultrasound, cystoscopy, or dedicated sacral bone evaluation. Cystoscopy may be performed before resection or intraoperatively. Placement of ureteral stents can be done preoperatively to help identify and protect the ureters. Patients undergo bowel prep the day before surgery. Antibiotics are delivered in the operating room along with anesthesia. The patient is placed in the lithotomy position, giving the surgeon anterior access to the pelvis and perineum. Surgery will be performed in one or two stages, depending on the type of resection.

Rectal Washout

Key Concept: Rectal washout has theoretical advantages to reduce tumor shedding, with minimal downside.

The practice of rectal washout remains controversial. Some have theorized that viable exfoliated tumor cells implant at distant sites of bowel mucosa, potentially resulting in some anastomotic and/or various locoregional recurrences. A few studies suggest that free malignant cells collect on circular stapling devices during anterior resection [63, 64], implanting during construction of the anastomosis.

A number of small studies suggest that rectal irrigation may eliminate the free cells collected on circular staplers, reducing implantation and potential spillage into the pelvis [65, 66]. The type of rectal irrigation—saline vs. cytocidal—also remains a point of contention. Although cytocidal rectal washouts comprising solutions such as cetrimide or povidone-iodine are used more commonly, there is no data confirming that these are more effective than simple saline wash. A study by Church et al. concluded that rectal irrigation probably eliminates exfoliated malignant cells by mechanical cleansing, rather than through any cytocidal effect [67]. Similarly, Jenner and colleagues showed that saline wash effectively removes exfoliated malignant cells from the distal rectum mechanically [68]. Even so, no study to date has demonstrated the clinical relevance of rectal washout in reducing the incidence of local recurrence. In 2005, the American Society of Colon and Rectal Surgeons published practice parameters for the management of rectal cancer, stating that there was insufficient evidence to recommend intraoperative rectal washout [69]. However, given the minimal time involved and lack of detriment to the impending procedure, it is our practice to irrigate the rectum with 500 cc of 5 % povidone-iodine solution prior to incision.

Resection

Key Concept: You must maintain flexibility during the operation. This includes making an early decision as to whether you have the ability to perform an adequate resection that will benefit the patient.

Intraoperatively, you should first examine the abdomen for disseminated peritoneal disease, which would prevent a curative resection. This can be done via diagnostic laparoscopy, when possible, thus avoiding the morbidity associated with a major midline laparotomy. A laparotomy is often necessary, however, especially in the setting of adhesions.

The retroperitoneal lymph nodes should be examined for metastasis, which—especially if the nodes cannot be completely removed—may indicate incurable disease. The ureters are identified and preserved, and will not be transected until resectability is confirmed. Following abdominal inspection, the recurrent tumor is assessed. Dissection ideally begins in an extraperitoneal plane free of adhesions and scar tissue (Fig. 15.1). The inferior mesenteric artery is ligated and transected, followed by transection of the descending colon. The surgeon dissects posteriorly down to the levator ani, taking care to avoid the pelvic nerves whenever possible. The bladder is now mobilized from the retropubic space (Fig. 15.2). The bladder pillars attached to the lateral pubic rami are transected. In a female patient, the cardinal supporting ligaments are ligated and transected at the pelvic sidewall. In a male patient, dissection continues anteriorly and includes the prostate.

A decision must now be made. Will you proceed with a low anterior resection, or an APR? In recurrent rectal cancer,

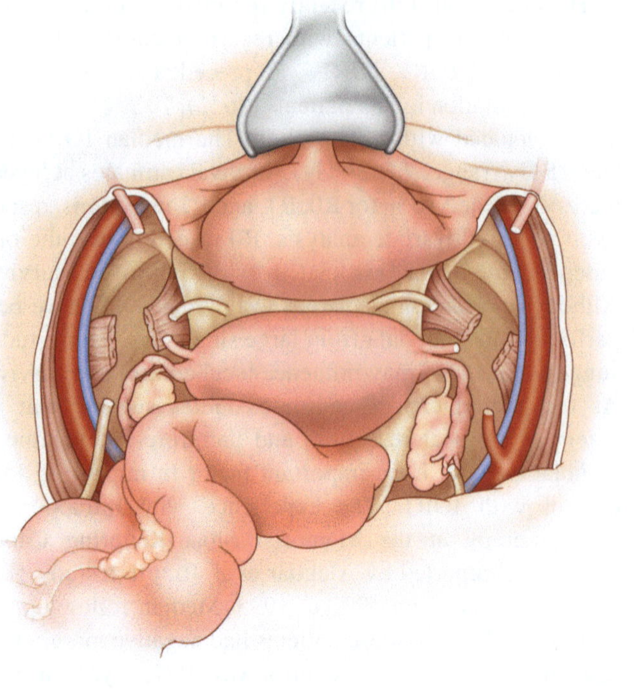

Fig. 15.1 In TPE, lateral dissection begins on the common and external iliac vessels, which are lateral to the parietal layer of the endopelvic fascia. The internal iliac artery and vein are clamped, cut, and tied distal at their origin. The ureter is cut in the pelvis, with care taken to preserve ureteral length for reconstruction

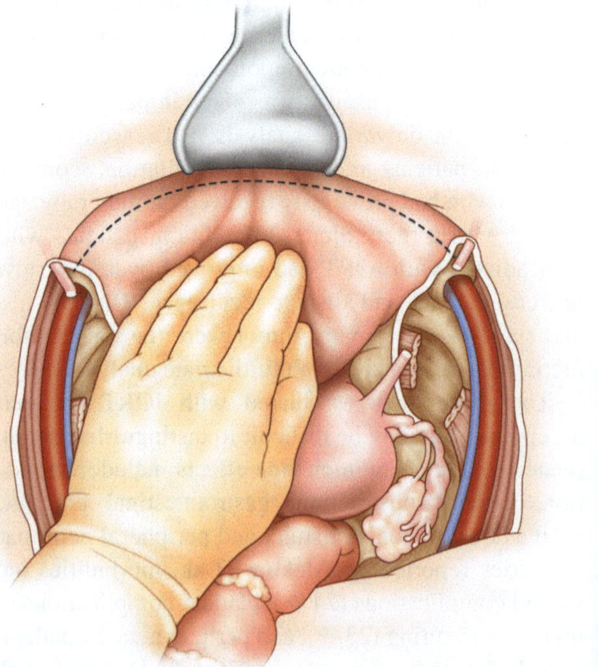

Fig. 15.2 The surgeon may perform dissection of the bladder before or after posterior dissection of the pelvic organs. The bladder is dissected from the symphysis and pubic rami, with dissection in the space of Retzius. The bladder is freed by dividing the lateral peritoneal attachments

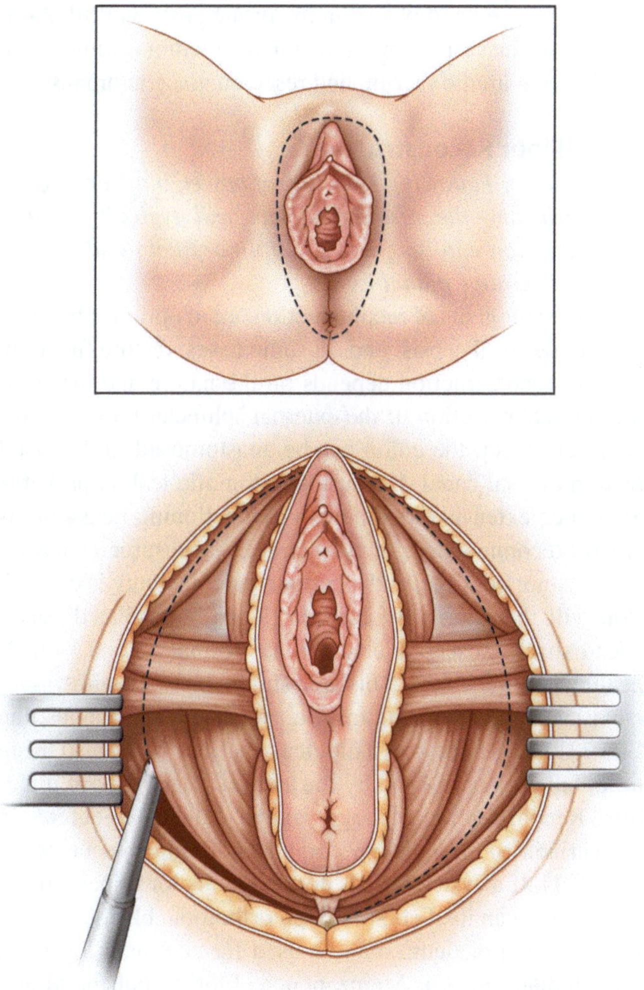

Fig. 15.3 Perineal dissection is necessary in TPE that includes the intra-levator organs (anal canal, labia majora, urethra). An elliptical incision is made from the tip of the coccyx to the pubic symphysis. The incision ends at the bulb of the penis (in a male patient), with the urethra previously divided in the pelvis. The pelvic floor attachments are divided widely, freeing the vagina (in a female patient), the urethra, and the rectum

an APR is usually necessary. If it is determined that an APR is required, dissection continues to the levator ani muscles, and then perineal dissection begins. The anal canal and lower rectum are dissected and removed through the ischiorectal fossa and urogenital diaphragm (Fig. 15.3). Wide lateral dissection of the pelvic floor (cylindrical dissection) is necessary to clear tumor. If tumor is extensively invasive in a female patient, the vagina, vulva, and urethra may have to be removed. The entire specimen can then be extracted through an abdominal or perineal incision.

Types of Procedures

Key Concept: The tumor location and extent of invasion will determine the type of procedure you perform.

Total exenteration is usually done in the setting of large, bulky lesions that invade the bladder or prostate. This procedure involves removal of the rectum, bladder, prostate, and seminal vesicles in male patients, and removal of the rectum, bladder, vagina, uterus, cervix, and parametrium in female patients.

Anterior exenteration is done when cancer invades the posterior bladder wall, anterior uterine wall, and organs in the anterior plane of the pelvis.

Posterior exenteration is done in a female patient if tumor invades the uterus. This procedure can be accomplished only if the bladder is not involved by tumor. Uterus, cervix, adnexa, and vagina (if required) are removed with the rectum. The operation is similar to total exenteration; however, instead of dissecting anterior to the bladder in the retropubic space, the peritoneum is incised over the bladder, and the bladder is dissected sharply off the anterior surface of the cervix and vagina and (depending on the level of tumor) down to or beyond the levator ani muscles. The ureters are dissected free from the anterior parametria distally, over the ureteral tunnel running along the uterine artery.

APR or LAR with partial cystectomy or vaginectomy may be considered if tumor does not extend into the bladder [involving the trigone] or the vagina far enough to require total removal of these organs. A partial cystectomy and reimplantation of the ureters can be done with a psoas hitch reconstruction. If only part of the vagina is involved by tumor, local resection of the invaded portion may suffice. If the resulting vaginal defect is too large for primary closure, reconstruction can be achieved using a myocutaneous rectus abdominis flap.

Sacral Resections

Key Concept: Sacral resections are generally done if tumor broadly adheres to or invades the sacrum or coccyx.

APR with sacrectomy begins in the same manner as a total pelvic exenteration: dissection in the ventral plane anteriorly, preserving the bladder, female reproductive organs, or prostate, if possible. Dissection takes place in a dorsal and dorsolateral fashion, following the presacral plane down to the level of the sacral transection. If transection of the sacrum at the S2/S3 level (or lower) clears disease, the cancer is resectable. Resection above S2 involves significant morbidity; the need for tumor clearance at that level often indicates unresectable disease. The level of sacral transection is marked on the anterior cortex of the sacrum using osteotome or K-wire. Gauze may be packed into the presacral space to reduce bleeding. The patient is turned and placed in the prone position. A dorsal longitudinal incision is made, starting at the level of L5 down to and around the anal canal. The gluteus maximus and gluteus minimus muscles are dissected off the sacrum, and the flaps are raised bilaterally. Transection of the sacrotuberous and sacrospinous ligaments is done at the

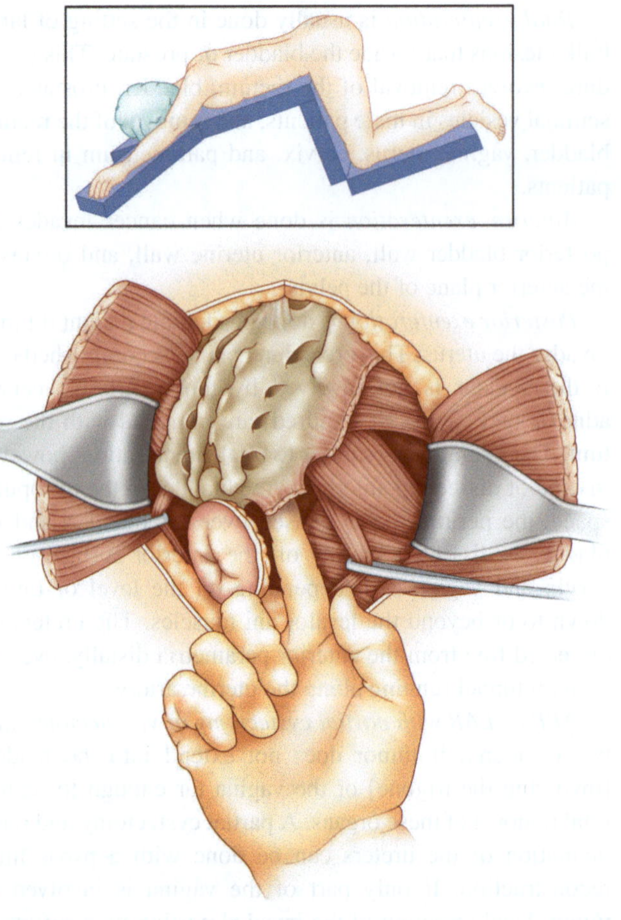

Fig. 15.4 After anterior dissection, the patient is placed in the prone position for sacral resection. A posterior sacral incision is made with excision of the anus. Flaps are raised to the lateral extent of the sacrum. The gluteus maximus and gluteus medius muscles are dissected from their sacral origins. The sciatic nerve is located by retracting the gluteus maximus and underlying piriformis muscle superiorly, at the lateral aspect of the mid-sacrum. The nerve is superficial to the obturator internus muscle, coursing inferolaterally between the ischial tuberosity and greater trochanter. The sacrotuberous and sacrospinous ligaments are incised at their attachments to the ischial tuberosity and ischial spine. The surgeon inserts a finger anteriorly from the medial aspect of the sciatic nerve, facilitating dissection beneath the piriformis muscle and through the underlying endopelvic fascia. This exposure directs the sacral ostectomy, ensuring sufficient tumor clearance

sacrum, facilitating access to the pelvic floor muscles and infra-piriformis opening. Medial to the infra-piriformis, you should insert a finger into the presacral space to identify the level of resection (Fig. 15.4). The sacrum is now resected, with care taken to protect the nerve roots within the proximal (preserved) sacrum. The distal sacrum, lateral pelvic walls, and rectum are removed en bloc.

Sacropelvic exenteration is undertaken only in the setting of very bulky tumors involving the lower sacrum and invading the reproductive organs in a female patient, the prostate in a male patient, and the bladder. This is a two-stage procedure: posterior dissection for distal sacrectomy and anterior dissection for pelvic exenteration. In the second stage, the patient is turned and placed in the prone position [70]. After division of the sacrum in stage two, the rectum is removed in continuity with the sacrum and resected visceral organs.

Pelvic Floor Reconstruction

Key Concept: Following resection of bowel, bladder, vagina, and perineum, the resultant defect will typically require reconstruction entailing multidisciplinary help and meticulous preoperative planning.

The major goals of reconstruction are to optimize healing, prevent perineal sepsis, and, in some cases, restore function. Type of reconstruction depends on the nature and extent of the surgical resection. If the external sphincter muscles have been left intact, the colon can be anastomosed to the distal rectum or anal canal. Because anastomotic leak is probable after such extensive treatment, a defunctioning ileostomy is always recommended. In most circumstances, rectal anastomosis is not possible, and a permanent colostomy is created. You will then normally confront a large, irradiated pelvic "dead space" susceptible to abscess formation and wound-healing complications. This area should be filled with vascular tissue such as omentum or a rotated myocutaneous flap [71–73]. Prosthetic or biological meshes have also been used, but are not favored by the authors due to risk of infection. Reconstruction of large vaginal defects, or defects in the perineal skin, is best accomplished with myocutaneous flaps [71]. If a cystectomy is done, options for urinary diversion include an ileal conduit or an orthotopic bladder substitution. Colon or ileum may be used for continent diversion (i.e., Indiana pouch, Mainz pouch, Florida pouch, Miami pouch). An ileal conduit, colonic conduit, or ureterocolostomy can also be constructed for urinary diversion [70].

Postoperative Complications

Key Concept: Due to the nature of the operation required for optimal outcomes, morbidity rates are significant, and you should have a plan for early identification and management of morbidity.

Most of the recent literature reporting on radical resection for locally recurrent rectal cancer describes acceptable perioperative mortality but significant morbidity (Table 15.2). Potential morbidities include surgical site infection, sepsis (usually related to the non-collapsible empty pelvis), complications related to urinary diversion, and complications related to IORT, including peripheral neuropathy and ureteral stenosis (Table 15.3). Dresen et al. [57] reported an overall complication rate of 59 % in their series of 144 patients undergoing radical resection for local recurrence. Nineteen percent suffered urinary retention and required prolonged catheterization. Fifteen percent developed pelvic abscess, requiring intervention. In another series of 160 patients undergoing radical or extended radical resection for recurrence, Heriot et al. [58] reported a relatively low morbidity of 27 % and minimal mortality of 0.6 %. Although it was not statistically significant, complications were more common in patients undergoing extended resections (requiring removal of at least one of the adjacent organs); the majority of these were perineal wound complications or pelvic abscess. A study from the Mayo Clinic reported 0.3 % in-hospital mortality and a 32 % rate of major complications in 304 patients undergoing resection for recurrent rectal cancer [8].

Complications and perioperative mortality increase with more radical procedures, such as sacropelvic resection. In 1994, Wanebo et al. reported 8.5 % perioperative mortality in 47 patients undergoing exenteration for recurrent rectal cancer [75]. The majority of complications were related to perineal and abdominal wound sepsis. It should be noted that a significant proportion of these procedures involved relatively high sacrectomies (S1 and S2). A 2006 study from the Memorial Sloan-Kettering Cancer Center reported on complications following sacropelvic resection in 29 patients with recurrent rectal cancer. Sacral resection was performed at the S2/S3 level in 55 % and at the S4/S5 level in 45 % of the study cohort. Previous surgery predicted the type of salvage operation required: total exenteration with sacrectomy was performed in 69 % of patients who had previously undergone APR; a less radical procedure was done for those who had undergone sphincter-saving surgery. In 59 % of patients, pedicle flaps were used to reconstruct the pelvis. The total complication rate was 59 %; 45 % were major complications, and most involved perineal wound breakdown and pelvic sepsis. There was one perioperative death [76].

Table 15.2 Postoperative complications (%)

Wound infection [56, 58, 59]	3.1–13
Obstruction [7, 8, 56]	5.3–13
Pelvic abscess [7, 8, 57–59]	4–26
Urinary complications [7, 56–59]	4.4–23
Enterocutaneous fistula [8, 58]	1.2–4.3
Perineal wound complications [8, 58]	4.6–9.4
Neuropathy [56]	15

Stoma

Key Concept: Permanent or temporary diversion is routine in these cases and is associated with its own set of

Table 15.3 Summary of long-term outcomes for multimodality therapy of recurrent rectal cancer

Study	Pts	Resected	Cases (%R0)	IORT +/– (*n*)	EBRT +/– (*n*)	Median survival (mos)	Morb. (%)	Mort. 30 d (%)	LR (%)	LR (R0)	DR (%)	OS (%)	5-y OS R0
Haddock et al. (2009) [56]	607[a]	427 (rectum)	37	+ (586)	+ (228)	36	50	1	28	28	53	30	46
Pacelli et al. (2009) [15]	58	44	62.5	+ (20)	+	–	20.9	7	25.7	11.5	-	54.2	72.4
Hansen et al. (2009) [74]	577	185	52.4	–	+	48 (R0)	–	1.6		17.5	25.1	14.9	62
Dresen et al. (2008) [57]	184	147	57.2	+ (136)	+ (39)	28	58.5	4.8 %	45.9	31	20.4[b]	28	48.4
Heriot et al. (2007) [58]	160	153	61.2	+ (12)	–	43	27	0.6	–	–	–	36.6	50
Asoglu et al. (2007) [7]	72	50	48	–	–	19	24	0.0	12.5	33	33.3	33	36
Boyle et al. (2005) [45]	64	57	36.8	–	–	33.6	43.9	1.6	–	49	–	40[b]	–
Valentini et al. (2004) [52]	59	30	35.6	–	+ (59)	42	15.4	2.6	31	17.8	30.5	39.3	66.8
Hahnloser et al. (2002) [8]	429	304	45	+ (131)	+ (244)	31	32	0.3	–	–	–	25	37
Wiig et al. (2002) [59]	107	107	36	+ (59)	+	40	44	1.6	50	30	–	30	60
Shoup et al. (2002) [48]	634[c]	111	64	+ (111)	–	31.2	–	0	33	–	45	22[d]	31.2[d]

Abbreviations: dash(-) not reported, *y* year, *OS* overall survival, *LR* local recurrence, *DR* distant recurrence, *IORT* intraoperative radiotherapy, *EBRT* irradiation in those patients who had already received radiation therapy with their primary tumor, *morb* morbidity, *mort* mortality

[a]Contains both colon and rectum; 427 (70 %) rectum

[b]3 years

[c]Study only includes those who underwent intraoperative radiation (111 of 634)

[d]Disease-free survival

complications, which you should be prepared to manage. Proper marking, preoperative involvement of an enterostomal therapist, and adequate technical construction can minimize stoma-related morbidity.

The reported incidence of ostomy complications has varied over the past three decades, ranging from 14 to 70 % [77–81]. Retrospective studies have identified several risk factors associated with increased overall stomal complications: poor perioperative siting, lack of stoma education by an enterostomal therapist [82, 83], height of the stoma (<10 mm) [84], creation of a stoma after emergency surgery [78], and patient comorbidities such as obesity [83, 85], Crohn's disease [83], and advanced age. Diabetes and smoking are associated with poor wound healing and, on several univariate analyses, have been found to play a potential role in ostomy separation, retraction, and parastomal hernia [78, 86].

Stoma-related complications can be categorized as early or late. The most common complications occur in the immediate postoperative period (less than 30 days) and include peristomal skin breakdown, stomal retraction, stomal necrosis, mucocutaneous separation, poor location, surgical wound infection, and sepsis. Late complications (typically 6–12 weeks after surgery) include parastomal hernia, prolapse, retraction, stenosis, obstruction, and stomal bleeding.

Preoperative counseling has been shown to help patients adapt psychologically to the significant lifestyle changes associated with having a stoma. Patients experience physical, psychosocial, and emotional stress, often because of changes in sexual function, self-esteem, social acceptance, and economic burden [87]. An enterostomal therapist should educate patients about their upcoming surgery and prepare them for what to expect afterwards. Counseling is not limited to preoperative education but also includes stoma site selection, pre- and postoperative technical advice, emotional support for the patient and family, discharge planning, outpatient follow-up, and ongoing rehabilitation [88]. Appropriate preoperative counseling has been associated with decreased stoma-related complications [78, 82], better postoperative stoma proficiency, earlier discharge from hospital [89], and overall improvement in quality of life.

Oncologic Outcomes of Multimodal Therapy

Key Concept: With proper patient selection and (most importantly) the ability to achieve negative surgical margins, substantial improvements in survival and local control can be achieved.

Results from multimodality treatment of locally recurrent rectal cancer are encouraging, demonstrating improved survival and local control in select patients (Table 15.2). The recent literature reports a broad range of 5-year overall survival ranging from 15 to 50 %, with local recurrence rates between 12 and 50 % (Table 15.2). This wide variation may be related to different regimens of multimodal therapy used at different institutions. That being said, it is vital to reiterate that the most important factor influencing prognosis in recurrent rectal cancer is complete surgical resection [13, 15]. Multiple studies have linked R0 resection with 5-year local recurrence rates as low as 12 % and 5-year overall survival as high as 70 % [15].

Salo et al. [90] completed a 10-year retrospective analysis of 131 patients with locally recurrent rectal cancer undergoing curative-intent surgery at the Memorial Sloan-Kettering Cancer Center from 1986 to 1995. The goals of this study were to determine predictors of resectability and assess post-salvage survival. Resection was accomplished in 79 % of patients. Median hospital stay was 14 days. Overall 5-year survival was 31 %. Concomitant salvage procedures included sacrectomy (16 patients), partial vaginectomy [15], hysterectomy [9], and pelvic sidewall dissection [21]. APR was performed in 46 patients, low anterior resection in 20, total pelvic exenteration in 18, Hartmann's resection in 11, perineal sacrectomy in 3, perineal excision in 3, and abdominal resection in 2. Fifty-two patients received IORT. Of the 71 patients who had R0 resection, median survival was 42 months; 3-year survival was 57 %; 5-year survival was 35 %. In patients with R1 resection, median survival was 32 months; 3-year survival was 38 %; 5-year survival was 23 %. In patients with an incomplete R2 resection (with gross residual disease), median survival was 27 months; 3-year survival was 36 %; 5-year survival was 9 %. In the 28 patients who were not resected, median survival was 16 months; 3-year survival was 4 %; 5-year survival was 0 % [90]. In a study of 29 patients undergoing sacropelvic resection, Melton et al. reported a median disease-specific survival of 49 months for patients with R0 resection and 23 months for those with R1/R2 resection [76].

Palliative Management

Key Concept: You and your patients should have realistic expectations when dealing with recurrent rectal cancer. Patients who are not viable candidates for surgery, or for whom the desired surgical results cannot be achieved, should undergo individualized palliative therapy based on their symptoms.

Despite progress in multimodality therapy, R0 resection is achieved in 60–65 % of patients at best, and many patients with recurrent disease are not eligible for surgery. Palliative treatment strategies should be considered for those who are not candidates for a potentially curative resection. The goal of palliative therapy is to relieve symptoms—including bleeding, urinary or fecal obstruction, and pain secondary to nerve root or bony involvement by tumor—and improve quality of life. A palliative care plan should be tailored to the individual patient, taking symptoms, age, comorbidities, and extent of disease into account. For patients who are unresectable due to diffuse metastatic disease or failure to meet resection criteria, chemotherapy remains the first-line treatment. Management of symptomatic patients is challenging and may require multimodal interventions, including radiation, endoscopic stenting, fecal diversion, and laser or argon photocoagulation.

Radiation

Key Concept: In the setting of unresectable disease, re-irradiation (delivered with palliative intent) may provide symptomatic relief.

As part of palliative management, radiation has been shown to improve pain and bleeding in patients with or without a prior history of radiotherapy. Re-irradiation is generally well tolerated. A retrospective study by Mohiuddin et al. of 103 patients receiving re-irradiation for recurrent rectal cancer demonstrated that bleeding was palliated in 100 % of patients, and that this was durable in 80 %, until death. Pain was also well controlled, although only 39 % were completely relieved of their discomfort [51, 53, 91]. In a study by Valentini et al., 83 % of patients who had previously been irradiated obtained pain relief from combined chemotherapy and re-irradiation [52].

Self-expanding Metallic Stents (SEMS)

Key Concept: Stents may be used for palliation of obstructing rectal cancer in select patients.

In patients under close surveillance after their index operation, rectal obstruction is rare. This is because, before developing obstruction, the majority present with symptoms such as changes in bowel habits or rectal pressure. In the event of an obstructing recurrent tumor, there are several treatment options, including self-expanding metallic stents (SEMS), operative fecal diversion, or palliative resection (Fig. 15.5a, b). Stents may provide a less invasive alternative to palliative surgery, resulting in shorter hospital stays and less morbidity and mortality. Data on stents in the setting of

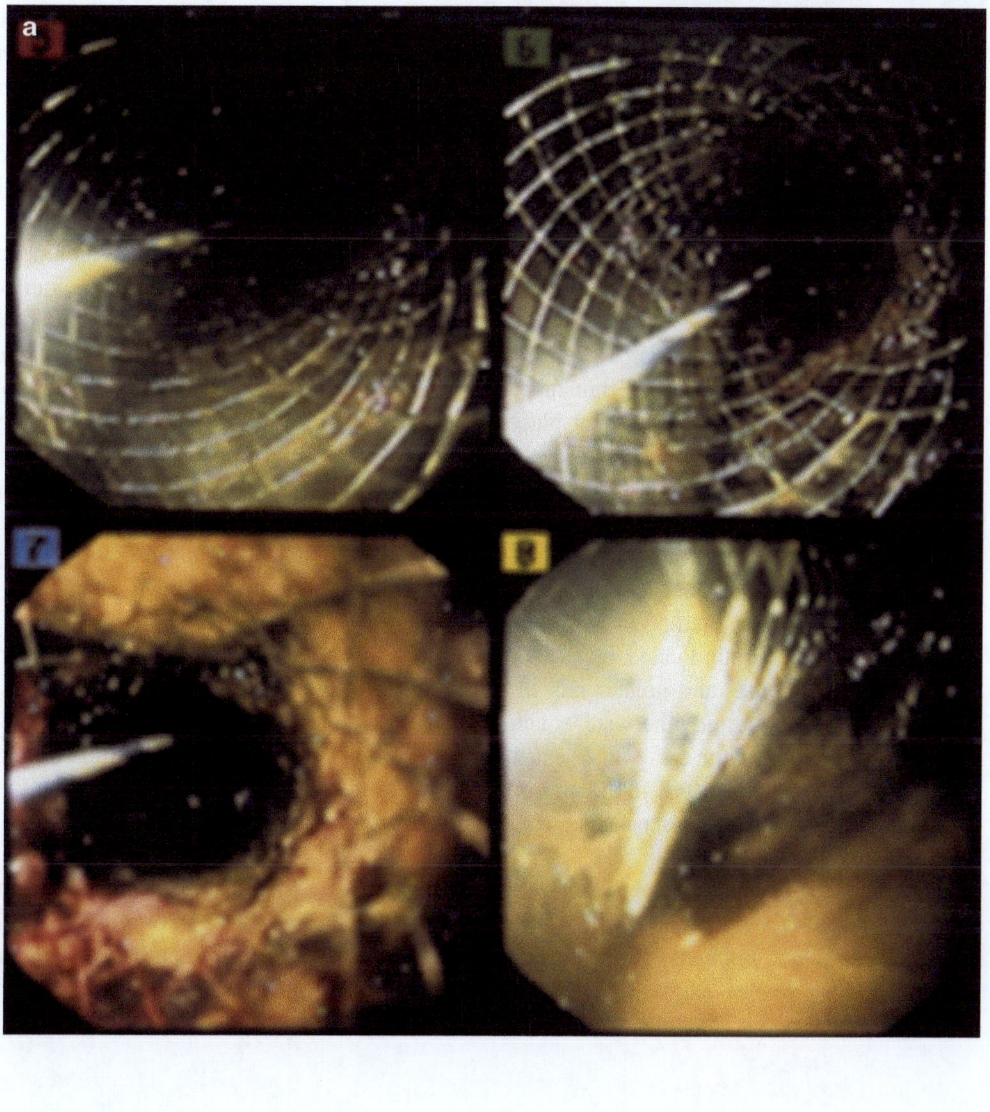

Fig. 15.5 (a) Endoscopic view of a stent or near-obstructing rectal cancer (Courtesy of W. Brian Sweeney, MD). (b) Plain radiograph demonstrating the stent in place (Courtesy of W. Brian Sweeney, MD)

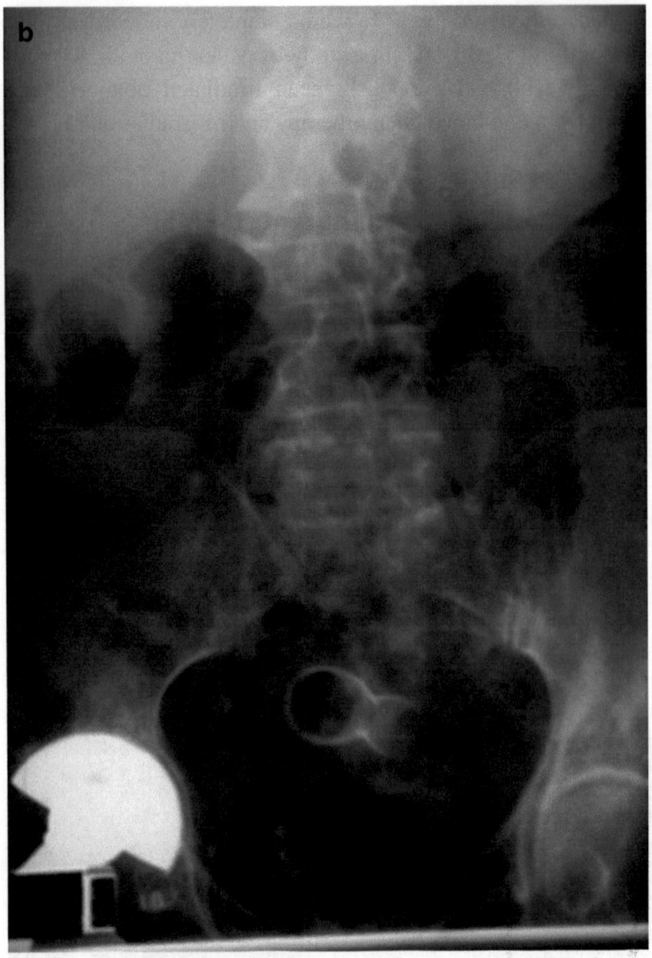

Fig. 15.5 (continued)

recurrent rectal cancer is limited, but in primary stage IV rectal cancer, the success rate of stent placement is reportedly as high as 95 %, and SEMS have been found to provide long-term relief in a majority of patients [92, 93]. Stent failure may occur, however. Early complications include malposition or perforation, and long-term complications include stent migration or occlusion. Stent placement in obstructing low rectal cancers (less than 5 cm from the anal verge) has traditionally been contraindicated because of increased pain, tenesmus, incontinence, and greater risk of migration. One small 2008 study suggested otherwise, concluding that stents placed within 5 cm of the anal verge can be tolerated and provide acceptable relief [94]. In either case, a stent failure rate of approximately 20 % can be expected, and this requires surgical intervention [92, 93].

Surgery: Fecal Diversion vs. Palliative Resection

A diverting stoma is preferred to palliative resection, and is a helpful alternative to endoscopic stenting if obstruction has occurred.

Fecal diversion can be accomplished effectively with an ileostomy or colostomy, though a sigmoid colostomy is preferable and more commonly used. The stoma can be created via a laparoscopic or open approach. The laparoscopic approach is more difficult in the setting of severely dilated intestine; however, given the numerous benefits such as reduction of pain and shorter hospital stay, a minimally invasive approach is preferred whenever feasible.

Palliative resection to relieve symptoms should generally be avoided in patients with incurable disease. Such procedures are associated with increased morbidity, but provide little improvement in quality of life.

Multidisciplinary Approach

Key Concept: Optimal decision-making requires interdisciplinary communication and coordination among multidisciplinary teams (MDTs).

Ideally, all treatment should be individually tailored, based on clinical, diagnostic, and physical findings, as well as on the patient's values and overall quality of life. A multidisciplinary approach is the most effective way to meet these goals. The importance of formal multidisciplinary meetings has been acknowledged in many European countries since the late 1990s and is gaining favor in the United States. The National Institute for Clinical Excellence in London has published updated guidelines for organizing MDTs (Improving Outcomes in Colorectal Cancers) [95]. Recommendations include a designated team coordinator and weekly meetings, attended by core members, providing peer review of tumor pathology and radiology.

Although there is limited data on MDTs in colorectal surgery, the evidence from esophageal, gastric, hepatobiliary, breast, and ovarian cancer surgery suggests that this approach improves patient selection and overall survival [96–99]. Multidisciplinary teams also provide a framework for assessing quality assurance. Outcomes such as TME grading, positive circumferential margins, and sphincter-sparing techniques have been used as surrogates to determine if MDTs are beneficial. In 2007, an audit by the National Health Service Team in Yorkshire, UK, demonstrated that the presence of MDTs is associated with increased use of preoperative radiation and higher rates of anterior resection in patients with primary rectal cancer, and a [nonsignificant] trend towards increased survival rates [100]. A recent retrospective case–control study by MacDermid and colleagues [101] examined the impact of MDTs on outcomes in 310 patients undergoing colectomy for colorectal cancer. Patients in the MDT cohort were more likely to receive adjuvant chemotherapy, and this may have contributed to a significant survival advantage: a 3-year survival of 58 % for Dukes C patients in the control group, and a 3-year survival of 66 % in the MDT group ($p=0.023$). On hazard regression analysis, MDT status was also shown to be an independent predictor of survival ($p=0.044$).

Centers of Excellence

Key Concept: While somewhat controversial, improved outcomes have been associated with high-volume, subspecialty-trained surgeons and designated centers.

The implementation of multidisciplinary teams may pose challenges with respect to hospital resource allocation, organization and coordination of specialists' schedules, attendance and participation in MDT meetings, and broad acceptance of the team approach. The MDT is more likely to exist in large academic institutions where there are more subspecialist physicians. Consequently, the data suggests that high-volume colorectal cancer centers with experienced subspecialty teams have better mortality and higher sphincter-sparing rates. Archampong et al. [102] performed a recent meta-analysis of 11 studies including over 18,000 patients, examining the relationship between surgeon caseload and patient outcomes. They demonstrated that high surgeon volume was associated with lower rates of permanent stomas and APRs, as well as improved 5-year survival. At Memorial Sloan-Kettering Cancer Center and other cancer specialty centers, multidisciplinary evaluation and discussion are considered part of the standard of care for all patients with rectal cancer.

Summary Pearls

The surgical management of recurrent rectal cancer is complex, requiring detailed preoperative work-up and careful selection of patients for resection. Proper radiologic imaging may provide critical information on the extent of local recurrence and tumor invasion, so that a detailed operative plan can be formulated. Resection of recurrent rectal cancer is characteristically extensive and associated with high morbidity. You should undertake it only when cure is considered possible. Even with combined modality treatments, including neoadjuvant therapy and complementary use of IORT, the ability to achieve adequate, microscopically negative margins is the single most important factor in achieving better outcomes, including cure.

The role of multidisciplinary teams in optimizing patient outcomes is evolving. Implementation of MDTs can provide the framework and the means for developing patient-tailored treatment strategies and a more seamless coordination of care. These teams include colorectal surgeons as well as urologists, gynecologists, orthopedic, neurologic, plastic and reconstructive surgeons, radiation and medical oncologists, and others. Input from stoma therapy nurses, dieticians, and preoperative counselors is also essential in preparing patients for the rigors of treatment. Patients must be psychologically prepared for extensive resection, prolonged hospital stay, a high incidence of morbidity, and the possibility that their disease will be found unresectable intraoperatively.

Multimodality treatment, including radical R0 surgery, offers the greatest potential for cure in patients with locally recurrent rectal cancer. Following combined modality treatment in carefully selected patients, a 5-year survival of up to 60 %, with acceptable morbidity, can be achieved.

References

1. Kim YW, Kim NK, Min BS, Huh H, Kim JS, Kim JY, et al. Factors associated with anastomotic recurrence after total mesorectal excision in rectal cancer patients. J Surg Oncol. 2009;99(1):58–64. doi:10.1002/jso.21166. PubMed PMID: 18937260. Epub 2008/10/22.
2. Birbeck KF, Macklin CP, Tiffin NJ, Parsons W, Dixon MF, Mapstone NP, et al. Rates of circumferential resection margin involvement vary between surgeons and predict outcomes in rectal cancer surgery. Ann Surg. 2002;235(4):449–57. PubMed PMID: 11923599; PubMed Central PMCID: PMC1422458. Epub 2002/03/30.
3. Stocchi L, Nelson H, Sargent DJ, O'Connell MJ, Tepper JE, Krook JE, et al. Impact of surgical and pathologic variables in rectal cancer: a United States community and cooperative group report. J Clin Oncol. 2001;19(18):3895–902. PubMed PMID: 11559727. Epub 2001/09/18.
4. Ogiwara H, Nakamura T, Baba S. Variables related to risk of recurrence in rectal cancer without lymph node metastasis. Ann Surg Oncol. 1994;1(2):99–104. PubMed PMID: 7834447. Epub 1994/03/01.
5. Moore HG, Riedel E, Minsky BD, Saltz L, Paty P, Wong D, et al. Adequacy of 1-cm distal margin after restorative rectal cancer resection with sharp mesorectal excision and preoperative combined-modality therapy. Ann Surg Oncol. 2003;10(1):80–5. PubMed PMID: 12513965. Epub 2003/01/07.
6. Moore HG, Shoup M, Riedel E, Minsky BD, Alektiar KM, Ercolani M, et al. Colorectal cancer pelvic recurrences: determinants of resectability. Dis Colon Rectum. 2004;47(10):1599–606. PubMed PMID: 15540287. Epub 2004/11/13.
7. Asoglu O, Karanlik H, Muslumanoglu M, Igci A, Emek E, Ozmen V, et al. Prognostic and predictive factors after surgical treatment for locally recurrent rectal cancer: a single institute experience. Eur J Surg Oncol. 2007;33(10):1199–206. doi:10.1016/j.ejso.2007.02.026. S0748-7983(07)00103-5 [pii]. Epub 2007/04/03. PubMed PMID: 17400423.
8. Hahnloser D, Nelson H, Gunderson LL, Hassan I, Haddock MG, O'Connell MJ, et al. Curative potential of multimodality therapy for locally recurrent rectal cancer. Ann Surg. 2003;237(4):502–8. doi:10.1097/01.SLA.0000059972.90598.5F. PubMed PMID: 12677146; PubMed Central PMCID: PMC1514480. Epub 2003/04/05.
9. Palmer G, Martling A, Cedermark B, Holm T. A population-based study on the management and outcome in patients with locally recurrent rectal cancer. Ann Surg Oncol. 2007;14(2):447–54. doi:10.1245/s10434-006-9256-9. PubMed PMID: 17139457. Epub 2006/12/02.

10. Park JK, Kim YW, Hur H, Kim NK, Min BS, Sohn SK, et al. Prognostic factors affecting oncologic outcomes in patients with locally recurrent rectal cancer: impact of patterns of pelvic recurrence on curative resection. Langenbecks Arch Surg. 2009;394(1):71–7. doi:10.1007/s00423-008-0391-6. PubMed PMID: 18663464. Epub 2008/07/30.
11. Pilipshen SJ, Heilweil M, Quan SH, Sternberg SS, Enker WE. Patterns of pelvic recurrence following definitive resections of rectal cancer. Cancer. 1984;53(6):1354–62. PubMed PMID: 6692324. Epub 1984/03/15.
12. Desch CE, Benson 3rd AB, Somerfield MR, Flynn PJ, Krause C, Loprinzi CL, et al. Colorectal cancer surveillance: 2005 update of an American Society of Clinical Oncology practice guideline. J Clin Oncol. 2005;23(33):8512–9. doi:10.1200/JCO.2005.04.0063. JCO.2005.04.0063 [pii]. PubMed PMID: 16260687. Epub 2005/11/02.
13. Caricato M, Borzomati D, Ausania F, Valeri S, Rosignoli A, Coppola R. Prognostic factors after surgery for locally recurrent rectal cancer: an overview. Eur J Surg Oncol. 2006;32(2):126–32. doi:10.1016/j.ejso.2005.11.001. S0748-7983(05)00318-5 [pii]. PubMed PMID: 16377120. Epub 2005/12/27.
14. Onodera H, Maetani S, Kawamoto K, Kan S, Kondo S, Imamura M. Pathologic significance of tumor progression in locally recurrent rectal cancer: different nature from primary cancer. Dis Colon Rectum. 2000;43(6):775–81. PubMed PMID: 10859076. Epub 2000/06/20.
15. Pacelli F, Tortorelli AP, Rosa F, Bossola M, Sanchez AM, Papa V, et al. Locally recurrent rectal cancer: prognostic factors and long-term outcomes of multimodal therapy. Ann Surg Oncol. 2010;17(1):152–62. doi:10.1245/s10434-009-0737-5. PubMed PMID: 19834766. Epub 2009/10/17.
16. Beets-Tan RG, Beets GL, Borstlap AC, Oei TK, Teune TM, von Meyenfeldt MF, et al. Preoperative assessment of local tumor extent in advanced rectal cancer: CT or high-resolution MRI? Abdom Imaging. 2000;25(5):533–41. doi:10.1107/s002610000086 [pii]. PubMed PMID: 10931993. Epub 2000/08/10.
17. Markus J, Morrissey B, deGara C, Tarulli G. MRI of recurrent rectosigmoid carcinoma. Abdom Imaging. 1997;22(3):338–42. PubMed PMID: 9107664. Epub 1997/05/01.
18. Titu LV, Nicholson AA, Hartley JE, Breen DJ, Monson JR. Routine follow-up by magnetic resonance imaging does not improve detection of resectable local recurrences from colorectal cancer. Ann Surg. 2006;243(3):348–52. doi:10.1097/01.sla.0000201454.20253.07. 00000658-200603000-00010 [pii]. PubMed PMID: 16495699; PubMed Central PMCID: PMC1448927. Epub 2006/02/24.
19. Torricelli P, Pecchi A, Luppi G, Romagnoli R. Gadolinium-enhanced MRI with dynamic evaluation in diagnosing the local recurrence of rectal cancer. Abdom Imaging. 2003;28(1):19–27. doi:10.1007/s00261-001-0127-3. PubMed PMID: 12483379. Epub 2002/12/17.
20. Messiou C, Chalmers AG, Boyle K, Wilson D, Sagar P. Preoperative MR assessment of recurrent rectal cancer. Br J Radiol. 2008;81(966):468–73. doi:10.1259/bjr/53300246. 53300246 [pii]. PubMed PMID: 18347028. Epub 2008/03/19.
21. Muller-Schimpfle M, Brix G, Layer G, Schlag P, Engenhart R, Frohmuller S, et al. Recurrent rectal cancer: diagnosis with dynamic MR imaging. Radiology. 1993;189(3):881–9. PubMed PMID: 8234720. Epub 1993/12/01.
22. Popovich MJ, Hricak H, Sugimura K, Stern JL. The role of MR imaging in determining surgical eligibility for pelvic exenteration. AJR Am J Roentgenol. 1993;160(3):525–31. PubMed PMID: 8430546. Epub 1993/03/01.
23. Robinson P, Carrington BM, Swindell R, Shanks JH, O'Dwyer ST. Recurrent or residual pelvic bowel cancer: accuracy of MRI local extent before salvage surgery. Clin Radiol. 2002;57(6): 514–22. doi:10.1053/crad.2002.0933. S0009926002909335 [pii]. PubMed PMID: 12069470. Epub 2002/06/19.
24. Kinkel K, Tardivon AA, Soyer P, Spatz A, Lasser P, Rougier P, et al. Dynamic contrast-enhanced subtraction versus T2-weighted spin-echo MR imaging in the follow-up of colorectal neoplasm: a prospective study of 41 patients. Radiology. 1996;200(2):453–8. PubMed PMID: 8685341. Epub 1996/08/01.
25. Cascini GL, Avallone A, Delrio P, Guida C, Tatangelo F, Marone P, et al. 18F-FDG PET is an early predictor of pathologic tumor response to preoperative radiochemotherapy in locally advanced rectal cancer. J Nucl Med. 2006;47(8):1241–8. doi: 47/8/1241 [pii]. PubMed PMID: 16883000. Epub 2006/08/03.
26. Bellomi M, Rizzo S, Travaini LL, Bazzi L, Trifiro G, Zampino MG, et al. Role of multidetector CT and FDG-PET/CT in the diagnosis of local and distant recurrence of resected rectal cancer. Radiol Med. 2007;112(5):681–90. doi:10.1007/s11547-007-0172-2. PubMed PMID: 17657420. Epub 2007/07/28.
27. Even-Sapir E, Parag Y, Lerman H, Gutman M, Levine C, Rabau M, et al. Detection of recurrence in patients with rectal cancer: PET/CT after abdominoperineal or anterior resection. Radiology. 2004;232(3):815–22. doi:10.1148/radiol.2323031065. 2323031065 [pii]. PubMed PMID: 15273334. Epub 2004/07/27.
28. Keogan MT, Lowe VJ, Baker ME, McDermott VG, Lyerly HK, Coleman RE. Local recurrence of rectal cancer: evaluation with F-18 fluorodeoxyglucose PET imaging. Abdom Imaging. 1997;22(3):332–7. PubMed PMID: 9107663. Epub 1997/05/01.
29. Nakamoto Y, Sakamoto S, Okada T, Senda M, Higashi T, Saga T, et al. Clinical value of manual fusion of PET and CT images in patients with suspected recurrent colorectal cancer. AJR Am J Roentgenol. 2007;188(1):257–67. doi:10.2214/AJR.05.0708. 188/1/257 [pii]. PubMed PMID: 17179375. Epub 2006/12/21.
30. Schmidt GP, Baur-Melnyk A, Haug A, Utzschneider S, Becker CR, Tiling R, et al. Whole-body MRI at 1.5 T and 3 T compared with FDG-PET-CT for the detection of tumour recurrence in patients with colorectal cancer. Eur Radiol. 2009;19(6):1366–78.
31. Huebner RH, Park KC, Shepherd JE, Schwimmer J, Czernin J, Phelps ME, et al. A meta-analysis of the literature for whole-body FDG PET detection of recurrent colorectal cancer. J Nucl Med. 2000;41(7):1177–89. PubMed PMID: 10914907. Epub 2000/07/29.
32. Votrubova J, Belohlavek O, Jaruskova M, Oliverius M, Lohynska R, Trskova K, et al. The role of FDG-PET/CT in the detection of recurrent colorectal cancer. Eur J Nucl Med Mol Imaging. 2006;33(7):779–84. doi:10.1007/s00259-006-0072-z. PubMed PMID: 16565845. Epub 2006/03/28.
33. Stevenson G. Radiology in the detection and prevention of colorectal cancer. Eur J Cancer. 1995;31A(7–8):1121–6. PubMed PMID: 7577005. Epub 1995/07/01.
34. Kinkel K, Lu Y, Both M, Warren RS, Thoeni RF. Detection of hepatic metastases from cancers of the gastrointestinal tract by using noninvasive imaging methods (US, CT, MR imaging, PET): a meta-analysis. Radiology. 2002;224(3):748–56. PubMed PMID: 12202709. Epub 2002/08/31.
35. Mainenti PP, Mancini M, Mainolfi C, Camera L, Maurea S, Manchia A, et al. Detection of colo-rectal liver metastases: prospective comparison of contrast enhanced US, multidetector CT, PET/CT, and 1.5 Tesla MR with extracellular and reticulo-endothelial cell specific contrast agents. Abdom Imaging. 2010;35(5):511–21. PubMed PMID: 19562412. Epub 2009/06/30.
36. Bipat S, van Leeuwen MS, Comans EF, Pijl ME, Bossuyt PM, Zwinderman AH, et al. Colorectal liver metastases: CT, MR imaging, and PET for diagnosis – meta-analysis. Radiology. 2005;237(1):123–31. doi:10.1148/radiol.2371042060. Epub 2005/08/16. doi: 2371042060 [pii]. PubMed PMID: 16100087.
37. Flamen P, Hoekstra OS, Homans F, Van Cutsem E, Maes A, Stroobants S, et al. Unexplained rising carcinoembryonic antigen

(CEA) in the postoperative surveillance of colorectal cancer: the utility of positron emission tomography (PET). Eur J Cancer. 2001;37(7):862–9. doi: S0959804901000491 [pii]. PubMed PMID: 11313174. Epub 2001/04/21.
38. Fong Y, Saldinger PF, Akhurst T, Macapinlac H, Yeung H, Finn RD, et al. Utility of 18F-FDG positron emission tomography scanning on selection of patients for resection of hepatic colorectal metastases. Am J Surg. 1999;178(4):282–7. doi: S0002-9610(99)00187-7 [pii]. PubMed PMID: 10587184. Epub 1999/12/10.
39. Ruers TJ, Langenhoff BS, Neeleman N, Jager GJ, Strijk S, Wobbes T, et al. Value of positron emission tomography with [F-18]fluorodeoxyglucose in patients with colorectal liver metastases: a prospective study. J Clin Oncol. 2002;20(2):388–95. PubMed PMID: 11786565. Epub 2002/01/12.
40. Faneyte IF, Dresen RC, Edelbroek MA, Nieuwenhuijzen GA, Rutten HJ. Pre-operative staging with positron emission tomography in patients with pelvic recurrence of rectal cancer. Dig Surg. 2008;25(3):202–7. doi:10.1159/000140690. 000140690 [pii]. PubMed PMID: 18577865. Epub 2008/06/26.
41. Lopez-Kostner F, Fazio VW, Vignali A, Rybicki LA, Lavery IC. Locally recurrent rectal cancer: predictors and success of salvage surgery. Dis Colon Rectum. 2001;44(2):173–8. PubMed PMID: 11227932. Epub 2001/03/03.
42. Garcia-Aguilar J, Cromwell JW, Marra C, Lee SH, Madoff RD, Rothenberger DA. Treatment of locally recurrent rectal cancer. Dis Colon Rectum. 2001;44(12):1743–8. PubMed PMID: 11742153. Epub 2001/12/14.
43. Yamada K, Ishizawa T, Niwa K, Chuman Y, Akiba S, Aikou T. Patterns of pelvic invasion are prognostic in the treatment of locally recurrent rectal cancer. Br J Surg. 2001;88(7):988–93. doi:10.1046/j.0007-1323.2001.01811.x. bjs1811 [pii]. PubMed PMID: 11442533. Epub 2001/07/10.
44. Bhangu A, Brown G, Akmal M, Tekkis P. Outcome of abdominosacral resection for locally advanced primary and recurrent rectal cancer. Br J Surg. 2012;99(10):1453–61. doi:10.1002/bjs.8881. PubMed PMID: 22961529. Epub 2012/09/11.
45. Boyle KM, Sagar PM, Chalmers AG, Sebag-Montefiore D, Cairns A, Eardley I. Surgery for locally recurrent rectal cancer. Dis Colon Rectum. 2005;48(5):929–37. doi:10.1007/s10350-004-0909-0. PubMed PMID: 15785880. Epub 2005/03/24.
46. Sagar PM, Gonsalves S, Heath RM, Phillips N, Chalmers AG. Composite abdominosacral resection for recurrent rectal cancer. Br J Surg. 2009;96(2):191–6. doi:10.1002/bjs.6464. PubMed PMID: 19160364. Epub 2009/01/23.
47. Moriya Y, Akasu T, Fujita S, Yamamoto S. Total pelvic exenteration with distal sacrectomy for fixed recurrent rectal cancer. Surg Oncol Clin N Am. 2005;14(2):225–38. doi:10.1016/j.soc.2004.11.014. S1055-3207(04)00128-0 [pii]. PubMed PMID: 15817236. Epub 2005/04/09.
48. Shoup M, Guillem JG, Alektiar KM, Liau K, Paty PB, Cohen AM, et al. Predictors of survival in recurrent rectal cancer after resection and intraoperative radiotherapy. Dis Colon Rectum. 2002;45(5):585–92. PubMed PMID: 12004205. Epub 2002/05/11.
49. Sauer R, Becker H, Hohenberger W, Rodel C, Wittekind C, Fietkau R, et al. Preoperative versus postoperative chemoradiotherapy for rectal cancer. New Engl J Med. 2004;351(17):1731–40. doi:10.1056/NEJMoa040694. PubMed PMID: 15496622. Epub 2004/10/22.
50. Quah HM, Chou JF, Gonen M, Shia J, Schrag D, Saltz LB, et al. Pathologic stage is most prognostic of disease-free survival in locally advanced rectal cancer patients after preoperative chemoradiation. Cancer. 2008;113(1):57–64. doi:10.1002/cncr.23516. PubMed PMID: 18442099. Epub 2008/04/30.
51. Konski AA, Suh WW, Herman JM, Blackstock Jr AW, Hong TS, Poggi MM, et al. ACR Appropriateness Criteria(R)-Recurrent Rectal Cancer. Gastrointest Cancer Res. 2012;5(1):3–12. PubMed PMID: 22574231; PubMed Central PMCID: PMC3348710. Epub 2012/05/11.
52. Valentini V, Morganti AG, Gambacorta MA, Mohiuddin M, Doglietto GB, Coco C, et al. Preoperative hyperfractionated chemoradiation for locally recurrent rectal cancer in patients previously irradiated to the pelvis: a multicentric phase II study. Int J Radiat Oncol Biol Phys. 2006;64(4):1129–39. doi:10.1016/j.ijrobp.2005.09.017. S0360-3016(05)02705-7 [pii]. PubMed PMID: 16414206. Epub 2006/01/18.
53. Mohiuddin M, Marks G, Marks J. Long-term results of reirradiation for patients with recurrent rectal carcinoma. Cancer. 2002;95(5):1144–50. doi:10.1002/cncr.10799. PubMed PMID: 12209702. Epub 2002/09/05.
54. Willett CG, Czito BG, Tyler DS. Intraoperative radiation therapy. J Clin Oncol. 2007;25(8):971–7. doi:10.1200/JCO.2006.10.0255. 25/8/971 [pii]. PubMed PMID: 17350946. Epub 2007/03/14.
55. Nuyttens JJ, Kolkman-Deurloo IK, Vermaas M, Ferenschild FT, Graveland WJ, De Wilt JH, et al. High-dose-rate intraoperative radiotherapy for close or positive margins in patients with locally advanced or recurrent rectal cancer. Int J Radiat Oncol Biol Phys. 2004;58(1):106–12. doi: S0360301603014949 [pii]. PubMed PMID: 14697427. Epub 2003/12/31.
56. Haddock MG, Miller RC, Nelson H, Pemberton JH, Dozois EJ, Alberts SR, et al. Combined modality therapy including intraoperative electron irradiation for locally recurrent colorectal cancer. Int J Radiat Oncol Biol Phys. 2011;79(1):143–50. doi:10.1016/j.ijrobp.2009.10.046. doi: S0360-3016(09)03516-0 [pii]. PubMed PMID: 20395067. Epub 2010/04/17.
57. Dresen RC, Gosens MJ, Martijn H, Nieuwenhuijzen GA, Creemers GJ, Daniels-Gooszen AW, et al. Radical resection after IORT-containing multimodality treatment is the most important determinant for outcome in patients treated for locally recurrent rectal cancer. Ann Surg Oncol. 2008;15(7):1937–47. doi:10.1245/s10434-008-9896-z. PubMed PMID: 18389321; PubMed Central PMCID: PMC2467498. Epub 2008/04/05.
58. Heriot AG, Byrne CM, Lee P, Dobbs B, Tilney H, Solomon MJ, et al. Extended radical resection: the choice for locally recurrent rectal cancer. Dis Colon Rectum. 2008;51(3):284–91. doi:10.1007/s10350-007-9152-9. PubMed PMID: 18204879. Epub 2008/01/22.
59. Wiig JN, Tveit KM, Poulsen JP, Olsen DR, Giercksky KE. Preoperative irradiation and surgery for recurrent rectal cancer. Will intraoperative radiotherapy (IORT) be of additional benefit? A prospective study. Radiother Oncol. 2002;62(2):207–13. doi: S0167814001004868 [pii]. PubMed PMID: 11937248. Epub 2002/04/09.
60. Lindel K, Willett CG, Shellito PC, Ott MJ, Clark J, Grossbard M, et al. Intraoperative radiation therapy for locally advanced recurrent rectal or rectosigmoid cancer. Radiother Oncol. 2001;58(1):83–7. doi: S0167814000003091 [pii]. PubMed PMID: 11165686. Epub 2001/02/13.
61. Bouchard P, Efron J. Management of recurrent rectal cancer. Ann Surg Oncol. 2010;17(5):1343–56. doi:10.1245/s10434-009-0861-2. PubMed PMID: 20041351. Epub 2009/12/31.
62. Alektiar KM, Zelefsky MJ, Paty PB, Guillem J, Saltz LB, Cohen AM, et al. High-dose-rate intraoperative brachytherapy for recurrent colorectal cancer. Int J Radiat Oncol Biol Phys. 2000;48(1):219–26. doi: S0360-3016(00)00634-9 [pii]. PubMed PMID: 10924992. Epub 2000/08/05.
63. Gertsch P, Baer HU, Kraft R, Maddern GJ, Altermatt HJ. Malignant cells are collected on circular staplers. Dis Colon Rectum. 1992;35(3):238–41. PubMed PMID: 1740068. Epub 1992/03/01.
64. Umpleby HC, Fermor B, Symes MO, Williamson RC. Viability of exfoliated colorectal carcinoma cells. Br J Surg. 1984;71(9):659–63. PubMed PMID: 6478151. Epub 1984/09/01.

65. Agaba EA. Does rectal washout during anterior resection prevent local tumor recurrence? Dis Colon Rectum. 2004;47(3):291–6. doi:10.1007/s10350-003-0046-1. PubMed PMID: 14991490. Epub 2004/03/03.
66. Terzi C, Unek T, Sagol O, Yilmaz T, Fuzun M, Sokmen S, et al. Is rectal washout necessary in anterior resection for rectal cancer? A prospective clinical study. World J Surg. 2006;30(2):233–41. doi:10.1007/s00268-005-0300-x. PubMed PMID: 16425079. Epub 2006/01/21.
67. Church JM, Gibbs P, Chao MW, Tjandra JJ. Optimizing the outcome for patients with rectal cancer. Dis Colon Rectum. 2003;46(3):389–402. doi:10.1097/01.DCR.0000054884.45152.15. PubMed PMID: 12626917. Epub 2003/03/11.
68. Jenner DC, de Boer WB, Clarke G, Levitt MD. Rectal washout eliminates exfoliated malignant cells. Dis Colon Rectum. 1998;41(11):1432–4. PubMed PMID: 9823812. Epub 1998/11/21.
69. Tjandra JJ, Kilkenny JW, Buie WD, Hyman N, Simmang C, Anthony T, et al. Practice parameters for the management of rectal cancer (revised). Dis Colon Rectum. 2005;48(3):411–23. PubMed PMID: 15875292. Epub 2005/05/06.
70. Smith JD, Paty PB. Extended surgery and pelvic exenteration for locally advanced rectal cancer. What are the limits? Acta Chir Iugosl. 2010;57(3):23–7. PubMed PMID: 21066979. Epub 2010/11/12.
71. Bell SW, Dehni N, Chaouat M, Lifante JC, Parc R, Tiret E. Primary rectus abdominis myocutaneous flap for repair of perineal and vaginal defects after extended abdominoperineal resection. Br J Surg. 2005;92(4):482–6. doi:10.1002/bjs.4857. PubMed PMID: 15736219. Epub 2005/03/01.
72. Klaassen RA, Nieuwenhuijzen GA, Martijn H, Rutten HJ, Hospers GA, Wiggers T. Treatment of locally advanced rectal cancer. Surg Oncol. 2004;13(2–3):137–47. doi:10.1016/j.suronc.2004.08.004. S0960-7404(04)00033-7 [pii]. PubMed PMID: 15572096. Epub 2004/12/02.
73. Madoff RD. Extended resections for advanced rectal cancer. Br J Surg. 2006;93(11):1311–2. doi:10.1002/bjs.5637. PubMed PMID: 17058323. Epub 2006/10/24.
74. Hansen MH, Balteskard L, Dorum LM, Eriksen MT, Vonen B. Norwegian colorectal Cancer Group. Locally recurrent rectal cancer in Norway. Br J Surg. 2009;96(10):1176-82. doi:10.1002/bjs.6699. PMID:19787766 [PubMed-indexed for MEDLINE]
75. Wanebo HJ, Koness RJ, Vezeridis MP, Cohen SI, Wrobleski DE. Pelvic resection of recurrent rectal cancer. Ann Surg. 1994;220(4):586–95; discussion 95–7. PubMed PMID: 7524455; PubMed Central PMCID: PMC1234440. Epub 1994/10/01.
76. Melton GB, Paty PB, Boland PJ, Healey JH, Savatta SG, Casas-Ganem JE, et al. Sacral resection for recurrent rectal cancer: analysis of morbidity and treatment results. Dis Colon Rectum. 2006;49(8):1099–107. doi:10.1007/s10350-006-0563-9. PubMed PMID: 16779712. Epub 2006/06/17.
77. Park JJ, Del Pino A, Orsay CP, Nelson RL, Pearl RK, Cintron JR, et al. Stoma complications: the Cook County Hospital experience. Dis Colon Rectum. 1999;42(12):1575–80. PubMed PMID: 10613476. Epub 1999/12/29.
78. Arumugam PJ, Bevan L, Macdonald L, Watkins AJ, Morgan AR, Beynon J, et al. A prospective audit of stomas – analysis of risk factors and complications and their management. Colorectal Dis. 2003;5(1):49–52. doi: 403 [pii]. PubMed PMID: 12780927. Epub 2003/06/05.
79. Leong AP, Londono-Schimmer EE, Phillips RK. Life-table analysis of stomal complications following ileostomy. Br J Surg. 1994;81(5):727–9. PubMed PMID: 8044564. Epub 1994/05/01.
80. Londono-Schimmer EE, Leong AP, Phillips RK. Life table analysis of stomal complications following colostomy. Dis Colon Rectum. 1994;37(9):916–20. PubMed PMID: 8076492. Epub 1994/09/01.
81. Porter JA, Salvati EP, Rubin RJ, Eisenstat TE. Complications of colostomies. Dis Colon Rectum. 1989;32(4):299–303. PubMed PMID: 2924670. Epub 1989/04/01.
82. Bass EM, Del Pino A, Tan A, Pearl RK, Orsay CP, Abcarian H. Does preoperative stoma marking and education by the enterostomal therapist affect outcome? Dis Colon Rectum. 1997;40(4):440–2. PubMed PMID: 9106693. Epub 1997/04/01.
83. Duchesne JC, Wang YZ, Weintraub SL, Boyle M, Hunt JP. Stoma complications: a multivariate analysis. Am Surg. 2002;68(11):961–6; discussion 6. PubMed PMID: 12455788. Epub 2002/11/29.
84. Cottam J, Richards K, Hasted A, Blackman A. Results of a nationwide prospective audit of stoma complications within 3 weeks of surgery. Colorectal Dis. 2007;9(9):834–8. doi:10.1111/j.1463-1318.2007.01213.x. doi: CDI1213 [pii]. PubMed PMID: 17672873. Epub 2007/08/04.
85. Leenen LP, Kuypers JH. Some factors influencing the outcome of stoma surgery. Dis Colon Rectum. 1989;32(6):500–4. PubMed PMID: 2791788. Epub 1989/06/01.
86. Nastro P, Knowles CH, McGrath A, Heyman B, Porrett TR, Lunniss PJ. Complications of intestinal stomas. Br J Surg. 2010;97(12):1885–9. doi:10.1002/bjs.7259. PubMed PMID: 20872841. Epub 2010/09/28.
87. Holzer B, Matzel K, Schiedeck T, Christiansen J, Christensen P, Rius J, et al. Do geographic and educational factors influence the quality of life in rectal cancer patients with a permanent colostomy? Dis Colon Rectum. 2005;48(12):2209–16. doi:10.1007/s10350-005-0194-6. PubMed PMID: 16228820. Epub 2005/10/18.
88. National guidelines for enterostomal patient education. Prepared by the Standards Development Committee of the United Ostomy Association with the Assistance of Prospect Associates. Dis Colon Rectum. 1994;37(6):559–63. PubMed PMID: 8200234. Epub 1994/06/01
89. Chaudhri S, Brown L, Hassan I, Horgan AF. Preoperative intensive, community-based vs. traditional stoma education: a randomized, controlled trial. Dis Colon Rectum. 2005;48(3):504–9.
90. Salo JC, Paty PB, Guillem J, Minsky BD, Harrison LB, Cohen AM. Surgical salvage of recurrent rectal carcinoma after curative resection: a 10-year experience. Ann Surg Oncol. 1999;6(2):171–7. PubMed PMID: 10082043. Epub 1999/03/19.
91. Hu JB, Sun XN, Yang QC, Xu J, Wang Q, He C. Three-dimensional conformal radiotherapy combined with FOLFOX4 chemotherapy for unresectable recurrent rectal cancer. World J Gastroenterol. 2006;12(16):2610–4. PubMed PMID: 16688811. Epub 2006/05/12.
92. Ptok H, Meyer F, Marusch F, Steinert R, Gastinger I, Lippert H, et al. Palliative stent implantation in the treatment of malignant colorectal obstruction. Surg Endosc. 2006;20(6):909–14. doi:10.1007/s00464-005-0594-7. PubMed PMID: 16738981. Epub 2006/06/02.
93. Hunerbein M, Krause M, Moesta KT, Rau B, Schlag PM. Palliation of malignant rectal obstruction with self-expanding metal stents. Surgery. 2005;137(1):42–7. doi:10.1016/j.surg.2004.05.043. doi: S0039606004003113 [pii]. PubMed PMID: 15614280. Epub 2004/12/23.
94. Song HY, Kim JH, Kim KR, Shin JH, Kim HC, Yu CS, et al. Malignant rectal obstruction within 5 cm of the anal verge: is there a role for expandable metallic stent placement? Gastrointest Endosc. 2008;68(4):713–20. doi:10.1016/j.gie.2007.12.051. S0016-5107(07)03360-3 [pii]. PubMed PMID: 18561924. Epub 2008/06/20.
95. Excellence NIfC. Improving outcomes in colorectal cancers: manual update [Published guidelines]. http://www.nice.org.uk/nicemedia/pdf/CSGCCfullguidance.pdf.
96. Davies AR, Deans DA, Penman I, Plevris JN, Fletcher J, Wall L, et al. The multidisciplinary team meeting improves staging accuracy and treatment selection for gastro-esophageal cancer. Dis Esophagus. 2006;19(6):496–503. doi:10.1111/j.1442-2050.2006.00629.x. DES629 [pii]. PubMed PMID: 17069595. Epub 2006/10/31.

97. Junor EJ, Hole DJ, Gillis CR. Management of ovarian cancer: referral to a multidisciplinary team matters. Br J Cancer. 1994;70(2):363–70. PubMed PMID: 8054286; PubMed Central PMCID: PMC2033481. Epub 1994/08/01.
98. Stephens MR, Lewis WG, Brewster AE, Lord I, Blackshaw GR, Hodzovic I, et al. Multidisciplinary team management is associated with improved outcomes after surgery for esophageal cancer. Dis Esophagus. 2006;19(3):164–71. doi:10.1111/j.1442-2050.2006.00559.x. DES [pii]. PubMed PMID: 16722993. Epub 2006/05/26.
99. Morris E, Haward RA, Gilthorpe MS, Craigs C, Forman D. The impact of the Calman-Hine report on the processes and outcomes of care for Yorkshire's breast cancer patients. Ann Oncol. 2008;19(2):284–91. doi:10.1093/annonc/mdm432. mdm432 [pii]. PubMed PMID: 17785759. Epub 2007/09/06.
100. Morris E, Haward RA, Gilthorpe MS, Craigs C, Forman D. The impact of the Calman-Hine report on the processes and outcomes of care for Yorkshire's colorectal cancer patients. Br J Cancer. 2006;95(8):979–85. doi:10.1038/sj.bjc.6603372. 6603372 [pii]. PubMed PMID: 17047646; PubMed Central PMCID: PMC2360721. Epub 2006/10/19.
101. MacDermid E, Hooton G, MacDonald M, McKay G, Grose D, Mohammed N, et al. Improving patient survival with the colorectal cancer multi-disciplinary team. Colorectal Dis. 2009;11(3):291–5. doi:10.1111/j.1463-1318.2008.01580.x. CDI1580 [pii]. PubMed PMID: 18477019. Epub 2008/05/15.
102. Archampong D, Borowski D, Wille-Jorgensen P, Iversen LH. Workload and surgeon's specialty for outcome after colorectal cancer surgery. Cochrane Database Syst Rev. 2012;(3):CD005391. doi:10.1002/14651858.CD005391.pub3. PubMed PMID: 22419309. Epub 2012/03/16

The Approach to the Rectal Cancer Patient with a Suspected Complete Clinical Response: Selection of Patients to the Watch and Wait Strategy

16

Rodrigo O. Perez and Angelita Habr-Gama

Key Points

- Tumor response following neoadjuvant chemoradiation will help determine the subsequent management for locally advanced rectal cancer.
- Classical indications for neoadjuvant chemoradiation need to evolve to include earlier stage tumors to achieve maximal effectiveness and avoid radical surgery.
- Stringent criteria and appropriate evaluation are critical to determining who can effectively and successfully partake in the watch and wait strategy.
- Your history and physical examination should be the major determinant of clinical response, followed by adjuvant laboratory and radiological testing to confirm or refute your clinical findings.

Introduction

Rectal cancer management has become increasingly complex over the last few decades [1]. The widespread use of neoadjuvant therapies has introduced a new variable, tumor response, which may dramatically change ultimate surgical decision from radical surgery to local excision, transanal endoscopic microsurgery, or even no surgery at all for the management of these patients. In this setting, surgeons have to consider many aspects of the disease prior to deciding on a definitive treatment approach.

R.O. Perez, MD, PhD (✉)
Division of Colorectal Surgery, Department of Gastroenterology, University of São Paulo School of Medicine, São Paulo, Brazil

Angelita and Joaquim Gama Institute, São Paulo, Brazil
e-mail: rodrigo.operez@gmail.com

A. Habr-Gama, MD
Department of Colorectal Surgery, Angelita and Joaquim Gama Institute, Rua Manoel da Nóbrega 1564, São Paulo, Brazil

Department of Gastroenterology, University of São Paulo School of Medicine, São Paulo, Brazil

Indications for Neoadjuvant Therapy

Key Concept: Earlier stage tumors (cT2N0) may be more likely to develop complete clinical response and benefit the most from neoadjuvant CRT.

Classical indications for neoadjuvant therapy in rectal cancer are mostly derived from randomized controlled studies that showed a local control benefit among patients with cT3-4 or cN+ treated with radiation or chemoradiation followed by radical surgery [2, 3]. However, recent updates with longer follow-up of these same cohorts suggest that the benefits in local disease control following neoadjuvant CRT and radical surgery are marginal or even outweighed by treatment-related toxicities [4–6]. Therefore, except for circumferential margin positivity, local control is not expected to be significantly increased with the use of neoadjuvant CRT provided appropriate total mesorectal excision is performed, even for cT3 or cN+ disease.

On the other hand, neoadjuvant radiation alone, chemoradiation, or even chemotherapy alone may lead to significant tumor regression resulting in significant changes in tumor size, depth of penetration, nodal sterilization, and even complete tumor disappearance, also known as complete pathological response (pCR) [7, 8]. Not only does this latter group of patients with pCR have improved oncological outcomes but also the opportunity of being spared from radical surgery and its associated immediate morbidity, mortality, functional disorders, and need for stomas [9–11].

The problem is that if you give neoadjuvant therapy only for advanced stage disease patients, very few will develop complete tumor response (up to 30 %). However, neoadjuvant therapy may be extremely useful for the selection of those patients

S.R. Steele et al. (eds.), *Complexities in Colorectal Surgery*,
DOI 10.1007/978-1-4614-9022-7_16, © Springer Science+Business Media New York 2014

that may safely avoid a radical operation, and thus may be used more effectively if more widely adopted to include patients with earlier disease stages. If earlier disease stages are offered this treatment strategy (including cT2N0), complete response may develop more frequently, reaching up to 42 % of patients, and would allow more patients to benefit from avoiding radical surgery and associated morbidities [12–16].

Types of Neoadjuvant Therapy

Key Concept: Considering downstaging is required for a complete response, long-course CRT seems to be a better option for this purpose.

Considering neoadjuvant therapy will be used for the purpose of tailoring surgical therapy for patients based on tumor response, strategies associated with significant tumor regression are preferred [1]. Therefore, combined association of chemotherapy and radiation (i.e., long course with hyperfractionated RT doses) has been shown to result in greater tumor regression rates and increased chance of a complete response [7, 13]. In contrast, short-course RT alone may only lead to significant tumor regression if longer intervals between RT completion and assessment of response are allowed [17]. The standard 1-week interval will lead to virtually no chance of developing a pCR [18].

Finally, even though most studies have dealt with radiation or chemoradiation therapies in the neoadjuvant setting, there is a suggestion that chemotherapy alone could provide similar outcomes in terms of rates of pathological response, therefore sparing patients from potentially unnecessary radiation-related toxicities [8]. In fact, a regimen with radiation and increased number of cycles of chemotherapy has resulted in surprisingly high rates of complete tumor regression (57 % complete clinical response). It has been our practice to offer patients this extended CRT regimen, especially considering that chances of having a complete response are higher [19, 20].

Assessing Tumor Response: Why?

Key Concept: Final treatment should be based on its status post-CRT. Therefore, assessment of response is crucial.

The rationale for assessing tumor response after neoadjuvant therapy is to define final treatment strategy based upon the current status of the tumor—that is, after therapy. Assessment of tumor response is important even if you are not ultimately changing the type of resection. After neoadjuvant therapy, tumors present significant changes in size, depth, and proximity to the mesorectal fascia. Even if total mesorectal excision will be the definitive treatment strategy, it may be considerably useful to know ahead of time what challenges are expected during surgical resection.

In up to 42 % of patients undergoing neoadjuvant CRT, however, complete tumor regression may develop. The problem is that most of the time, radical surgery is required to appropriately confirm the presence of complete pathological response. In an effort to spare patients from potentially unnecessary surgery, colorectal surgeons have attempted to assess tumor response in order to estimate pathological response by clinical, endoscopic, and radiological means. In this setting, the term complete clinical response has been used for patients with no clinical evidence of residual cancer after neoadjuvant therapy. However, the features of a complete clinical response may be quite subjective and depends on surgeon's experience, different diagnostic tools, and treatment-related factors. Attempts to standardize the definition of a complete clinical response are already available, particularly with the use of endoscopic and radiological imaging [21]. Still, clinical assessment remains highly subjective and surgeon dependent.

It has been suggested that patients with complete clinical response (*using very stringent criteria*) could be offered no immediate radical surgery. Instead, a strict surveillance program, also known as the "watch and wait" strategy, with frequent visits to the colorectal surgeon and the use of multiple staging modalities could provide safe follow-up. Initial studies trying to estimate the accuracy of clinical assessment in predicting pathological response were disappointing [22]. However, more recent studies have shown that clinical assessment can accurately detect pathological response when stringent criteria are used [23].

Assessing Tumor Response: When and How?

Key Concept: You should assess tumor response at 8–12 weeks following the completion of neoadjuvant therapy. The presence of an incomplete clinical response leads the patient away from any possibility of watch and wait alone.

Intervals between CRT completion and assessment of response may also be relevant. Studies suggest that longer intervals are associated with higher pCR rates [24–26]. Initially, 2 weeks was used and then 6 weeks, and now intervals as long as 12 weeks are being considered [27]. There are ongoing randomized studies to address these issues that will provide us further information on the ideal interval between CRT and assessment of response, in an effort to maximize the chances of a patient developing complete response. There is a chance, however, that intervals will need to be tailored or individualized for each patient, as tumors may respond differently as a function of time to treatment [28]. It has been our practice to assess tumor response at least 8 weeks from CRT completion. More recently however, longer intervals (up to 12 weeks) have been used for the majority of patients unless there is worsening of symptoms or radiological

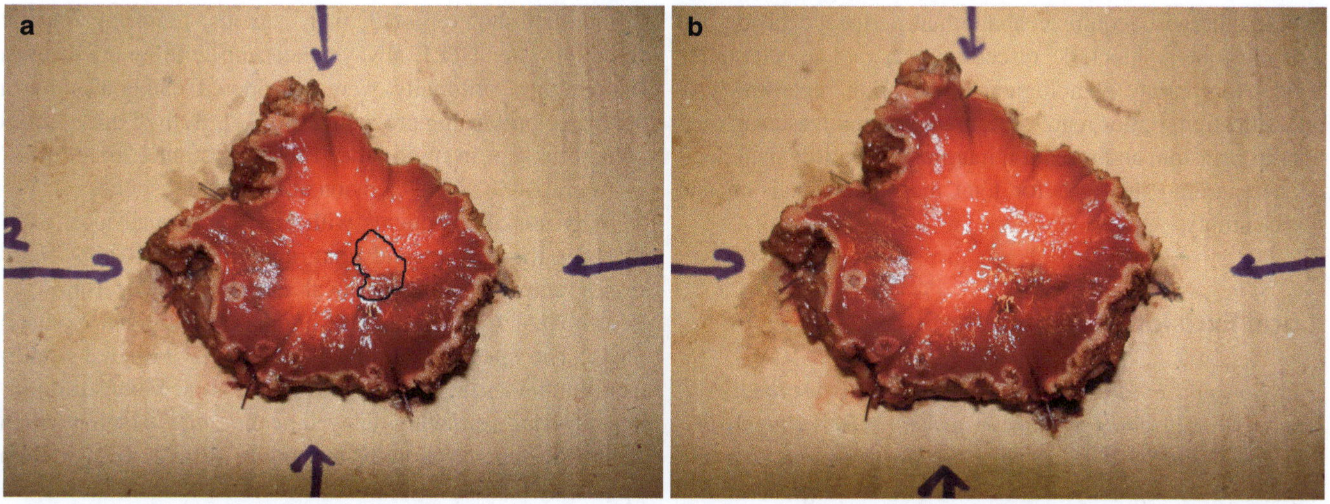

Fig. 16.1 (**a**) Area of irregularity detected at digital rectal examination that prompted full-thickness excisional biopsy with TEM. (**b**) Final pathology revealed the presence of residual cancer cells (ypT2)

evidence of disease progression even though this is rarely seen, it is not impossible.

Key Concept: Endoscopic biopsies may be misleading, particularly when negative. Do not rely solely on them. Clinical assessment should be enough to rule out a complete clinical response.

Response assessment always begins with characterization of symptoms. Symptomatic patients rarely have complete tumor regression, even though this feature has very low specificity. Digital rectal examination is perhaps one of the most relevant tools in tumor response assessment. There is currently no single diagnostic tool that can possibly replace the information given by DRE. Very frequently, irregularities of the rectal wall are better felt than seen and should be considered as highly suspicious for residual cancer (Fig. 16.1a, b). *No patient is considered for nonoperative approach in the presence of rectal wall irregularities, mass ulceration, or stenosis*. A complete clinical response is the absence of any irregularity of the rectal wall. The area can be thickened and firm, but to be considered a complete clinical response, the surface has to be regular and smooth [21].

Endoscopic assessment is also very important. Whitening of the mucosa and telangiectasia are usually seen in patients with a complete clinical response (Fig. 16.2). The presence of any ulceration or mucosal irregularity missed on DRE should prompt additional investigations and usually rule out a complete clinical response. Frequently, DRE may have to be reassessed after endoscopic guidance of any findings suggestive of residual cancer. During flexible or rigid proctoscopy, biopsies are frequently considered for assessment of response. If there is clinical evidence (DRE and endoscopic) of a cCR, forceps biopsies should be interpreted with caution since a negative biopsy cannot rule out microscopic residual

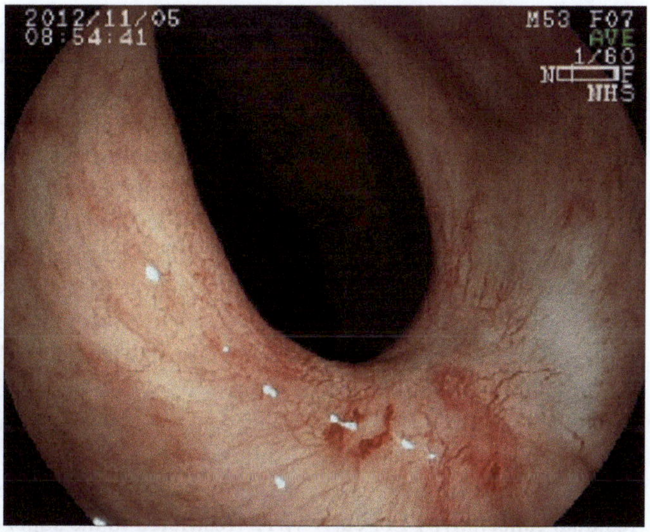

Fig. 16.2 Endoscopic view of a complete clinical response with obvious whitening of the mucosa and the presence of significant telangiectasia

cancer [29]. On the other hand, in the presence of clinical evidence of residual cancer (incomplete response), endoscopic biopsies are also rarely useful, except for convincing patients that there is residual disease there! Even in the presence of negative endoscopic biopsies, patients with incomplete clinical response should not be offered a nonoperative approach [29]. If they are resistant to radical resection or medically unfit, the least we would offer is a full-thickness excisional biopsy, preferably with the use of transanal endoscopic microsurgery. This "excisional biopsy," primarily considered as a diagnostic procedure, may be appropriate for patients with small (≤3 cm) lesions. However, we would restrict this to patients with low residual lesions that would otherwise require an abdominal-perineal excision or a coloanal intersphincteric resection as a radical alternative [30]. Appropriate pathological information regarding ypT classification, tumor regression grade, lymphovascular/perineural invasion, and resection margins may allow final decision regarding the need for total mesorectal excision and proctectomy.

Local Excision of the Tumor Site

Key Concept: Final pathological assessment after local excision will help guide your management. Use "diagnostic" TEM judiciously. Postoperative healing problems and significant scarring may lead to untoward surgical consequences if further resection is needed.

It has been our policy to offer strict follow-up to patients with final pathological specimen showing ypT0 after this "diagnostic" transanal local excision. This is due to the fact that the risk of lymph node metastases among these patients has been shown to be very low in the setting of neoadjuvant CRT and long (≥8 weeks) intervals. This is already true for unselected patients with ypT0, where the risk of nodal metastases is well under 10 % and in most cases less than 5 % [31–33]. However, with the significant improvements in radiological imaging, particularly with high-resolution magnetic resonance (MR) with the use of diffusion-weighted series and other lymphotropic agents, selection of patients with ycT0N0 is expected to further improve [34]. On the other end of the spectrum, patients with unsuspected residual ypT3, lymphovascular invasion, positive resection margins, and more than 10 % of viable residual cancer cells have been recommended immediate radical surgery.

Equally challenging cases are those with intermediate residual cancers: ypT1 or early ypT2 (restricted to the superficial muscular layer) cancers without lymphovascular invasion or other unfavorable pathological features. In the presence of negative margins (≥5 mm), it has been our policy to follow up these patients without immediate radical surgery, only if they would otherwise require an abdominal-perineal excisions or coloanal anastomosis. In this strategy of offering patients with small superficial residual cancers, radiologically staged as ycN0, a local procedure is quite appealing. However, there are at least two main drawbacks to this treatment strategy. First, healing of the rectal defects determined by local excision after neoadjuvant CRT is quite challenging and painful, particularly those closer to anal verge [35, 36]. Healing problems are much more frequent and may take as long as 8 weeks to completely heal. Even though severe complications are not frequent, pain is significant. The second drawback is that sphincter preservation may be compromised after performance of full-thickness local excision in this setting. A few studies have addressed this issue and reported that patients requiring radical resection after FTLE always ended up with an APR, even though they originally were considered candidates for a sphincter-preserving procedure [30, 37]. Both of these issues should be kept in mind when offering patients "diagnostic" or "therapeutic" local excision after partial response.

Why not offer patients with a cCR transanal local excision for the histological confirmation of ypT0? As mentioned above, healing of local excision defects following neoadjuvant CRT is not as simple as after local excision alone. The rates of wound dehiscence may be quite significant. In this setting, not only is pain an issue, but also significant scarring following delayed healing may develop which will make patient follow-up even more difficult. Even though ypT0 may be associated with lower risk of local failures, the risk is not zero and the patient still requires appropriate follow-up. Distinction between local recurrence in a rectal wall following wound dehiscence after a local excision with or without rectal stenosis may be quite challenging. Therefore, we believe that follow-up is considerably facilitated by preservation of rectal wall integrity with the watch and wait approach allowing for earlier detection of eventual recurrences in addition to superior functional outcomes.

Radiological Imaging

Key Concept: Radiological imaging should be used to confirm clinical findings. In the absence of complete clinical response, do not look for radiological evidence to support nonoperative management. It is better to fail identification of complete response in favor of radical surgery and end up with a pCR than to miss residual cancer and end up with an early local recurrence or tumor regrowth.

Radiological assessment of response is of paramount importance to appropriately select patients for an alternative treatment strategy such as the "watch and wait" approach following a complete clinical response. As a matter of fact, the developments in radiological imaging, including both PET/CT and MR, have been quite significant. Proper magnetic resonance imaging with the use of diffusion-weighted techniques is now used routinely for the assessment of response in these patients. Currently, we would only consider a true complete responder (1) in a patient showing low signal intensity area replacing the area of the previous tumor or (2) in a patient with no detectable abnormalities in standard MR associated with no evidence of disease on clinical and endoscopic examination (Fig. 16.3). A recent publication has reported three different patterns of low signal intensity that are compatible with a complete clinical response: minimal fibrosis, transmural fibrosis, and irregular fibrosis [38]. Others have attempted to estimate tumor regression grades (as described for pathological assessment) [39] by

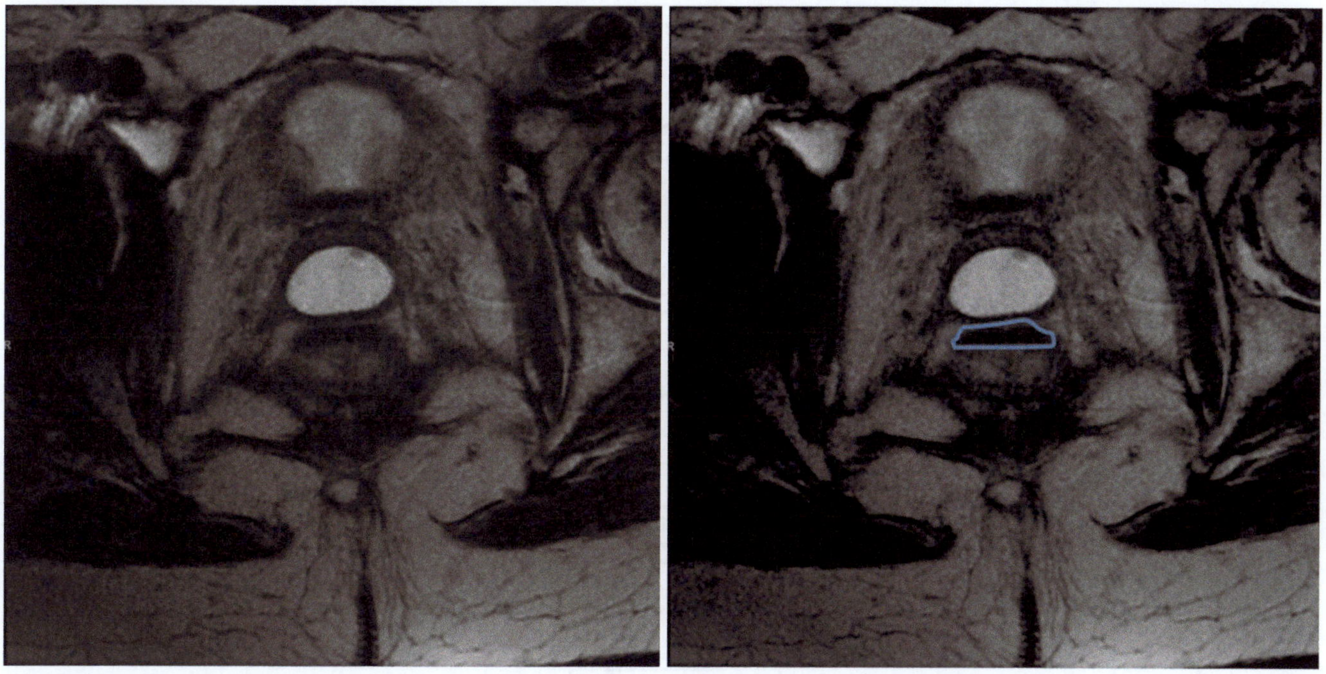

Fig. 16.3 Magnetic resonance of a patient with a complete clinical response and low signal intensity area within the rectal wall (transmural fibrotic pattern). Such radiological finding is consistent with a complete clinical response

standard MR imaging. [40] In addition, diffusion-weighted MR series should provide evidence of absence of restriction to diffusion to fulfill the criteria for a radiological complete response [41]. In our previously reported experiences with this "watch and wait" treatment strategy, MR imaging was not available to a significant proportion of patients [42]. Therefore, there is a hope that incorporation of these findings for the selection of patients with complete clinical response will significantly impact the outcomes of the watch and wait strategy. The presence of mixed signal intensity (Fig. 16.4) within the area of the previous cancer should raise a suspicion of an incomplete clinical response (Fig. 16.5). In addition to the assessment of the rectal wall, the mesorectum is also at risk for the presence of residual cancer despite complete primary regression (ypT0N1). Therefore, MR imaging should also provide the colorectal surgeon with information regarding possible mesorectal (or even lateral node) involvement regardless of primary tumor response (Fig. 16.6).

Molecular imaging may also play a role in the assessment of tumor response. PET/CT imaging offers information on tumor metabolism in addition to standard radiological anatomical features. In this setting, PET/CT has been used for the assessment of tumor response to neoadjuvant chemoradiation therapy [12, 43]. In addition to the visual identification of FDG uptake within the area of the rectal wall harboring the tumor or within the mesorectum, PET/CT allows the estimation of the metabolism profile. Standard uptake values are direct estimations of tissue metabolism and may be used for the distinction of residual inflammatory changes and residual cancer. Measurement of SUV in two different intervals from FDG injection is routinely performed (at 1 and 3 h) and allows two distinct patterns (dual time) of metabolism. Increases in SUVs

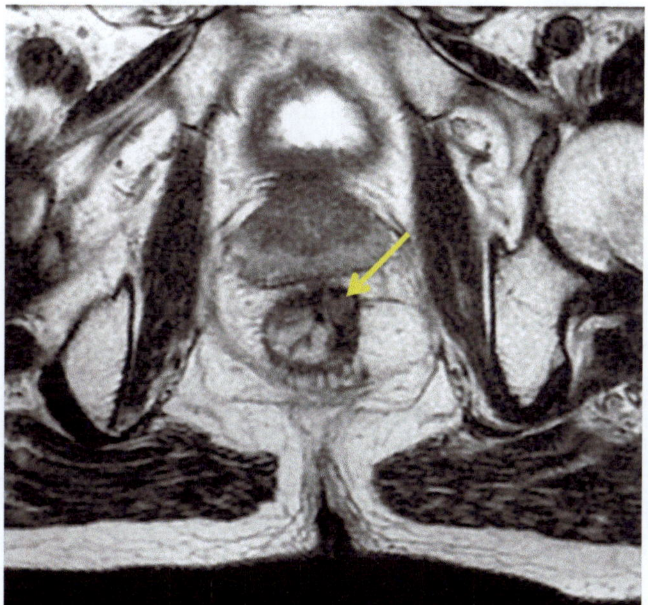

Fig. 16.4 Magnetic resonance of a patient with a complete clinical response but mixed signal intensity (*arrow*) within the rectal wall. PET/CT showed FDG uptake and radical surgery confirmed the presence of residual cancer ypT2N0

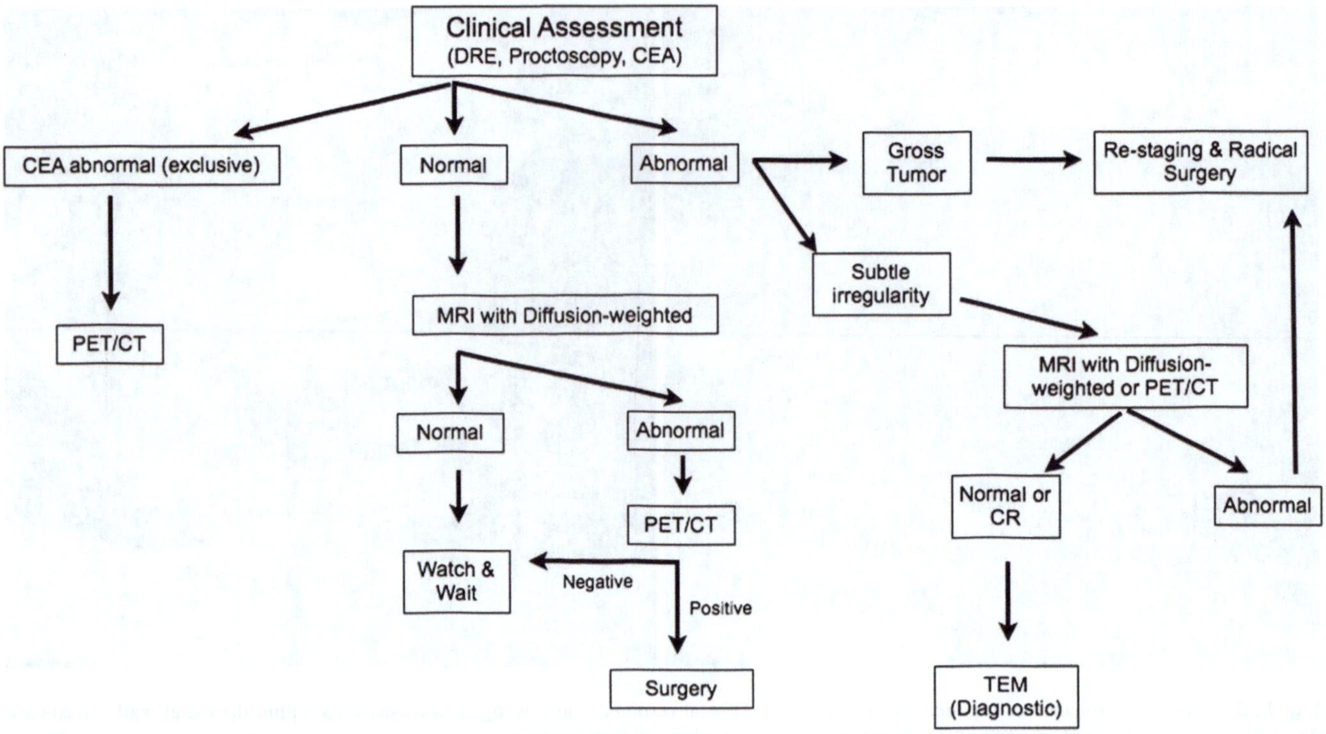

Fig. 16.5 Flowchart of the watch and wait strategy

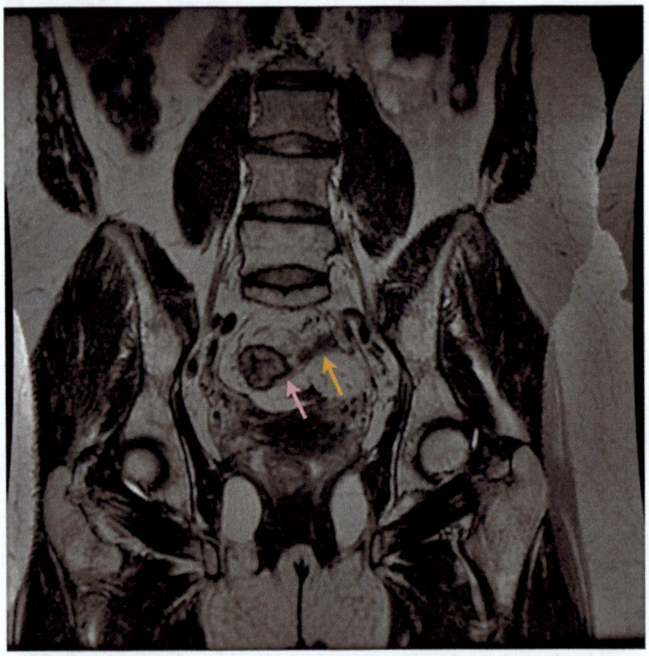

Fig. 16.6 Magnetic resonance showing the presence of mesorectal involvement (*orange arrow*) despite complete clinical response (*pink arrow*) of the primary tumor (ycT0N1). Radical surgery confirmed the presence of ypT0N1 disease

(between 1 and 3 h) suggest the presence of residual cancer whereas decreases suggest inflammatory or fibrotic changes [28]. Even though we have used PET/CT to distinguish between complete and incomplete responses in the setting of a prospective study with acceptable overall accuracy (85 %), PET/CT may not be appropriate for routine use for this purpose, mainly due to increased cost and need for multiple studies with significant radiation exposure [12]. Instead, the use of this molecular imaging modality should perhaps be considered for patients with significant discordant results between studies, particularly between clinical and radiological findings.

Carcinoembryonic Antigen (CEA)

Key Concept: Pre- and posttreatment CEA can help determine clinical response and may guide additional evaluation.

Pretreatment CEA levels have been shown to be predictors of response to neoadjuvant CRT and ultimately survival [39, 44]. Posttreatment CEA levels are also relevant and normal levels after CRT have been associated with increased complete clinical response rates [45]. Abnormal CEA levels before or after CRT should raise the suspicion of incomplete response to CRT and/or metastatic dissemination. In this setting, abnormal CEA levels should lead to a more liberal use of PET/CT imaging for the assessment of tumor response since it may also allow detection of unsuspected metastatic disease in addition to the diagnosis of incomplete response (Fig. 16.5).

Summary Pearls: Final Decision Management

Key Concept: Putting it altogether to determine the optimal management requires consideration of the clinical, endoscopic, radiological, and laboratory findings, in addition to the patient's overall health and desires.

Patients are usually assessed for tumor response to neoadjuvant chemoradiation at least 8–10 weeks from treatment completion regardless of the exact treatment regimen used. Clinical and endoscopic features are assessed in the clinic using digital rectal examination and rigid proctoscopy. Flexible proctoscopy is used solely for video documentation or for situations where endoscopic biopsies are required. Again, endoscopic biopsies are rarely useful due to the considerably low negative predictive values. Still, they may be useful to convince the patient that there is residual cancer. Colorectal surgeons should not be obsessed for the obtainment of positive biopsies prior to indication for radical surgery. Clinical assessment showing incomplete response should suffice. CEA levels should be normal both before and after treatment; otherwise, additional studies are strongly recommended.

If a patient has clinical evidence of a complete response, radiological assessment should be performed for two purposes. First, confirmation of findings consistent with a complete response within the rectal wall should be present; second, confirmation of the absence of dissemination to the mesorectal/lateral nodes is also required. Usually, MR with diffusion-weighted series is sufficient for most cases. In patients with an incomplete clinical response due to subtle mucosal irregularities, radiological staging that indicates complete response, and a normal CEA (prior to and after CRT), transanal local excision (preferably using TEM) may be used primarily as a diagnostic procedure. In patients with a complete clinical response but with radiological evidence of residual disease on MRI or abnormal CEA levels (pre- or posttreatment), PET/CT may be a useful assessment tool. A normal PET/CT may still allow consideration of a nonoperative approach in select cases after discussion with the patient. Abnormal PET/CT in this setting should be viewed as highly suspicious for residual cancer. Incomplete clinical response (gross residual cancer or ulceration) should prompt restaging to allow proper determination of final surgical approach, but never to suggest a nonoperative approach.

Patients suspected for a complete clinical response are closely followed and reassessed for tumor response every 1–2 months for the first year, every 3 months for the 2nd year, and every 6 months thereafter. If initial radiological assessment of response is normal (MR) or consistent with a complete response, radiological reassessment may be performed at 6 months from initial assessment.

Additional Therapy

Key Concept: Future treatment regimens may include adjuvant systemic chemotherapy following cCR.

Until now, patients with a complete clinical response have not been offered adjuvant systemic therapy of any kind following nonoperative management. However, the risk of systemic recurrence among these patients is still significant and may ultimately justify its use in selected patients according to baseline radiological features such as nodal positivity. Therefore, even though high-risk patients (cT3N+ at baseline staging) may still be considered for a nonoperative approach after a cCR following CRT, adjuvant systemic chemotherapy may prove to be beneficial. Even though this may sound appropriate, it warrants further investigation in properly designed prospective studies.

References

1. Kosinski L, Habr-Gama A, Ludwig K, Perez R. Shifting concepts in rectal cancer management: a review of contemporary primary rectal cancer treatment strategies. CA Cancer J Clin. 2012;62(3): 173–202.
2. Sauer R, Becker H, Hohenberger W, et al. Preoperative versus postoperative chemoradiotherapy for rectal cancer. N Engl J Med. 2004;351(17):1731–40.
3. Kapiteijn E, Marijnen CA, Nagtegaal ID, et al. Preoperative radiotherapy combined with total mesorectal excision for resectable rectal cancer. N Engl J Med. 2001;345(9):638–46.
4. Sauer R, Liersch T, Merkel S, et al. Preoperative versus postoperative chemoradiotherapy for locally advanced rectal cancer: results of the German CAO/ARO/AIO-94 randomized phase III trial after a median follow-up of 11 years. J Clin Oncol. 2012;30(16): 1926–33.
5. Peeters KC, van de Velde CJ, Leer JW, et al. Late side effects of short-course preoperative radiotherapy combined with total mesorectal excision for rectal cancer: increased bowel dysfunction in irradiated patients – a Dutch colorectal cancer group study. J Clin Oncol. 2005;23(25):6199–206.
6. van Gijn W, Marijnen CA, Nagtegaal ID, et al. Preoperative radiotherapy combined with total mesorectal excision for resectable rectal cancer: 12-year follow-up of the multicentre, randomised controlled TME trial. Lancet Oncol. 2011;12(6):575–82.
7. Bosset JF, Calais G, Mineur L, et al. Enhanced tumoricidal effect of chemotherapy with preoperative radiotherapy for rectal cancer: preliminary results–EORTC 22921. J Clin Oncol. 2005;23(24): 5620–7.
8. Schrag D, Weiser MR, Goodman KA, et al. Neoadjuvant FOLFOX-bev, without radiation, for locally advanced rectal cancer. J Clin Oncol. 2010;28(15s):(suppl; abstr 3511).
9. Maas M, Nelemans PJ, Valentini V, et al. Long-term outcome in patients with a pathological complete response after chemoradiation for rectal cancer: a pooled analysis of individual patient data. Lancet Oncol. 2010;11(9):835–44.
10. Smith FM, Waldron D, Winter DC. Rectum-conserving surgery in the era of chemoradiotherapy. Br J Surg. 2010;97(12):1752–64.
11. Habr-Gama A, Perez RO. Non-operative management of rectal cancer after neoadjuvant chemoradiation. Br J Surg. 2009;96(2):125–7.
12. Perez RO, Habr-Gama A, Gama-Rodrigues J, et al. Accuracy of positron emission tomography/computed tomography and clinical

assessment in the detection of complete rectal tumor regression after neoadjuvant chemoradiation: long-term results of a prospective trial (National Clinical Trial 00254683). Cancer. 2012; 118(14):3501–11.
13. Sanghera P, Wong DW, McConkey CC, et al. Chemoradiotherapy for rectal cancer: an updated analysis of factors affecting pathological response. Clin Oncol (R Coll Radiol). 2008;20(2):176–83.
14. Garcia-Aguilar J, Shi Q, Thomas Jr CR, et al. A phase II trial of neoadjuvant chemoradiation and local excision for T2N0 rectal cancer: preliminary results of the ACOSOG Z6041 trial. Ann Surg Oncol. 2012;19(2):384–91.
15. Lezoche E, Baldarelli M, Lezoche G, et al. Randomized clinical trial of endoluminal locoregional resection versus laparoscopic total mesorectal excision for T2 rectal cancer after neoadjuvant therapy. Br J Surg. 2012;99(9):1211–8.
16. Habr-Gama A, Perez RO, Nadalin W, et al. Operative versus non-operative treatment for stage 0 distal rectal cancer following chemoradiation therapy: long-term results. Ann Surg. 2004;240(4): 711–7; discussion 717–8.
17. Radu C, Berglund A, Pahlman L, Glimelius B. Short-course preoperative radiotherapy with delayed surgery in rectal cancer – a retrospective study. Radiother Oncol. 2008;87(3):343–9.
18. Bujko K, Nowacki MP, Nasierowska-Guttmejer A, et al. Long-term results of a randomized trial comparing preoperative short-course radiotherapy with preoperative conventionally fractionated chemoradiation for rectal cancer. Br J Surg. 2006;93(10):1215–23.
19. Habr-Gama A, Sabbaga J, Gama-Rodrigues J, et al. Watch and Wait Approach Following Extended Neoadjuvant Chemoradiation for Distal Rectal Cancer: Are We Getting Closer to Anal Cancer Management? Dis of Colon Rectum. 2013;56(10):1109–17.
20. Habr-Gama A, Perez RO, Sabbaga J, et al. Increasing the rates of complete response to neoadjuvant chemoradiotherapy for distal rectal cancer: results of a prospective study using additional chemotherapy during the resting period. Dis Colon Rectum. 2009;52(12):1927–34.
21. Habr-Gama A, Perez RO, Wynn G, et al. Complete clinical response after neoadjuvant chemoradiation therapy for distal rectal cancer: characterization of clinical and endoscopic findings for standardization. Dis Colon Rectum. 2010;53(12):1692–8.
22. Hiotis SP, Weber SM, Cohen AM, et al. Assessing the predictive value of clinical complete response to neoadjuvant therapy for rectal cancer: an analysis of 488 patients. J Am Coll Surg. 2002;194(2):131–5; discussion 135–6.
23. Smith FM, Chang KH, Sheahan K, et al. The surgical significance of residual mucosal abnormalities in rectal cancer following neoadjuvant chemoradiotherapy. Br J Surg. 2012;99(7):993–1001.
24. Kalady MF, de Campos-Lobato LF, Stocchi L, et al. Predictive factors of pathologic complete response after neoadjuvant chemoradiation for rectal cancer. Ann Surg. 2009;250(4):582–9.
25. Tulchinsky H, Shmueli E, Figer A, et al. An interval >7 weeks between neoadjuvant therapy and surgery improves pathologic complete response and disease-free survival in patients with locally advanced rectal cancer. Ann Surg Oncol. 2008;15(10):2661–7.
26. Francois Y, Nemoz CJ, Baulieux J, et al. Influence of the interval between preoperative radiation therapy and surgery on downstaging and on the rate of sphincter-sparing surgery for rectal cancer: the Lyon R90-01 randomized trial. J Clin Oncol. 1999;17(8):2396.
27. Evans J, Tait D, Swift I, et al. Timing of surgery following preoperative therapy in rectal cancer: the need for a prospective randomized trial? Dis Colon Rectum. 2011;54(10):1251–9.
28. Perez RO, Habr-Gama A, Sao Juliao GP, et al. Optimal timing for assessment of tumor response to neoadjuvant chemoradiation in patients with rectal cancer: do all patients benefit from waiting longer than 6 weeks? Int J Radiat Oncol Biol Phys. 2012;84(5):1159–65.
29. Perez RO, Habr-Gama A, Pereira GV, et al. Role of biopsies in patients with residual rectal cancer following neoadjuvant chemoradiation after downsizing: can they rule out persisting cancer? Colorectal Dis. 2012;14(6):714–20.
30. Perez RO, Habr-Gama A, Lynn PB, et al. Transanal endoscopic microsurgery for residual rectal cancer (ypT0-2) following neoadjuvant chemoradiation therapy: another word of caution. Dis Colon Rectum. 2013;56(1):6–13.
31. Mignanelli ED, de Campos-Lobato LF, Stocchi L, et al. Downstaging after chemoradiotherapy for locally advanced rectal cancer: is there more (tumor) than meets the eye? Dis Colon Rectum. 2010;53(3):251–6.
32. Bujko K, Nowacki MP, Nasierowska-Guttmejer A, et al. Prediction of mesorectal nodal metastases after chemoradiation for rectal cancer: results of a randomised trial: implication for subsequent local excision. Radiother Oncol. 2005;76(3):234–40.
33. Kim DW, Kim DY, Kim TH, et al. Is T classification still correlated with lymph node status after preoperative chemoradiotherapy for rectal cancer? Cancer. 2006;106(8):1694–700.
34. Lambregts DM, Beets GL, Maas M, et al. Accuracy of gadofosveset-enhanced MRI for nodal staging and restaging in rectal cancer. Ann Surg. 2011;253(3):539–45.
35. Marks JH, Valsdottir EB, DeNittis A, et al. Transanal endoscopic microsurgery for the treatment of rectal cancer: comparison of wound complication rates with and without neoadjuvant radiation therapy. Surg Endosc. 2009;23(5):1081–7.
36. Perez RO, Habr-Gama A, Sao Juliao GP, et al. Transanal endoscopic microsurgery for residual rectal cancer after neoadjuvant chemoradiation therapy is associated with significant immediate pain and hospital readmission rates. Dis Colon Rectum. 2011;54(5):545–51.
37. Bujko K, Richter P, Kolodziejczyk M, et al. Preoperative radiotherapy and local excision of rectal cancer with immediate radical re-operation for poor responders. Radiother Oncol. 2009;92(2):195–201.
38. Lambregts DM, Maas M, Bakers FC, et al. Long-term follow-up features on rectal MRI during a wait-and-see approach after a clinical complete response in patients with rectal cancer treated with chemoradiotherapy. Dis Colon Rectum. 2011;54(12):1521–8.
39. Restivo A, Zorcolo L, Cocco IM, et al. Elevated CEA levels and low distance of the tumor from the anal verge are predictors of incomplete response to chemoradiation in patients with rectal cancer. Ann Surg Oncol. 2013;20(3):864–71.
40. Patel UB, Taylor F, Blomqvist L, et al. Magnetic resonance imaging-detected tumor response for locally advanced rectal cancer predicts survival outcomes: MERCURY experience. J Clin Oncol. 2011;29(28):3753–60.
41. Lambregts DM, Vandecaveye V, Barbaro B, et al. Diffusion-weighted MRI for selection of complete responders after chemoradiation for locally advanced rectal cancer: a multicenter study. Ann Surg Oncol. 2011;18(8):2224–31.
42. Habr-Gama A, Perez RO, Nadalin W, et al. Long-term results of preoperative chemoradiation for distal rectal cancer correlation between final stage and survival. J Gastrointest Surg. 2005;9(1):90–9; discussion 99–101.
43. Kristiansen C, Loft A, Berthelsen AK, et al. PET/CT and histopathologic response to preoperative chemoradiation therapy in locally advanced rectal cancer. Dis Colon Rectum. 2008;51(1):21–5.
44. Das P, Skibber JM, Rodriguez-Bigas MA, et al. Predictors of tumor response and downstaging in patients who receive preoperative chemoradiation for rectal cancer. Cancer. 2007;109(9):1750–5.
45. Perez RO, Sao Juliao GP, Habr-Gama A, et al. The role of carcinoembriogenic antigen in predicting response and survival to neoadjuvant chemoradiotherapy for distal rectal cancer. Dis Colon Rectum. 2009;52(6):1137–43.

Ileal Pouch Complications

17

Ravi Pokala Kiran and Victor W. Fazio

Key Points

- Taking the time at the initial IPAA operation to attend to all the small details goes a long way in the prevention of IPAA complications and avoids having to deal with the difficulties of managing these.
- Difficulties with creation of the pouch are mitigated by ensuring proper length, investigating the staple line, and use of diversion to allow for initial healing.
- Prompt and successful management of early complications will often minimize the development of long-term pouch complications and maintain long-term pouch function.
- Late complications of IPAA include pouch-vaginal fistula, pouch sinus, and change in diagnosis to Crohn's disease. A thorough evaluation and stepwise approach to treatment will help minimize pouch loss.
- Pouch salvage is a viable option for a majority of patients, though this needs to be individualized, as certain patients may benefit from conversion to a permanent stoma.

R.P. Kiran, MBBS, MS (Gen Surgery), FRCS (Eng), FRCS (Glas), FACS, MSc (EBM) (✉)
Division of Colorectal Surgery, Department of Surgery, New York-Presbyterian/Columbia University Medical Center, 177 Fort Washington Avenue, 7 South Knuckle, NewYork, NY 10032, USA
e-mail: rpk2118@columbia.edu

V.W. Fazio, AO, MB, MS, FRACS, FACS, FRCS (Ed Hon), MD (Pol Hon), FRCSI (Hon)
Division of Colorectal Surgery, Department of Surgery, Cleveland Clinic Lerner College of Medicine of Case Western University, Cleveland Clinic Foundation, Cleveland, OH 44195, USA
e-mail: faziov@ccf.org

Introduction

For patients undergoing proctocolectomy, the ileal pouch-anal procedure (IPAA) is currently the favored operation since this allows the maintenance of intestinal continuity with defecation by the normal route. The procedure is durable and associated with excellent satisfaction, given the acceptable functional outcomes in terms of fecal continence, and the ability to maintain a good quality of life (QOL) with minimal restrictions. While the majority of patients do well with the procedure, a proportion of patients develop early or long-term problems related to the pouch. Since some of these problems are avoidable, the clinician should adopt a decision-making strategy that incorporates the pre- and intraoperative consideration of factors associated with the risk for early and late complications when preoperatively evaluating patients for an IPAA. Since some factors are modifiable, measures aimed at addressing these prior to IPAA may prevent some of these complications. Prompt and successful management of some of the complications that occur early after surgery may prevent the adverse consequences of these with regard to long-term pouch preservation and maintenance of function. Thus, an awareness of the impact of such conditions on long-term function and the institution of measures aimed at the prompt management of perioperative complications when they do occur may promote pouch salvage and outcomes. On the other hand, when pouch failure does occur, management needs to be individualized based on a consideration of the potential effect of poor function or pouch disorders on a particular patient's health, desires, and quality of life.

Factors associated with pouch failure, preoperative predictors that may foretell worse outcomes over the long-term, and the influence of certain perioperative complications on long-term pouch retention and function are examined below.

S.R. Steele et al. (eds.), *Complexities in Colorectal Surgery*,
DOI 10.1007/978-1-4614-9022-7_17, © Springer Science+Business Media New York 2014

Factors Associated with Pouch Failure

Key Concept: Patients can be risk stratified into good or poor candidates for IPAA based on readily available preoperative and postoperative factors and counseled appropriately regarding expected outcomes, surgical options, and risk of early and late pouch failure.

Several factors likely influence pouch failure and may vary for the individual patient. A previous study from the Cleveland Clinic [1] evaluated risk factors associated with ileal pouch failure and accurately predicted the risk of failure in individual patients based on a combination of preoperative and postoperative factors. Patient diagnosis, prior anal pathology, abnormal anal manometry, patient comorbidity, pouch-perineal or pouch-vaginal fistulae, pelvic sepsis, and anastomotic stricture and separation were all factors that were included into a model that accurately predicted the risk of ileal pouch failure to various degrees. The Cleveland Clinic Foundation ileal pouch failure score was developed to accurately predict pouch failure at 1, 2, 5, 10, and 15 years. A subsequent study [2] included only preoperative factors that may be associated with this risk and identified the type of resection (total proctocolectomy vs. completion proctectomy), type of anastomosis (stapled vs. hand sewn), patient diagnosis (mucosal ulcerative colitis and others vs. Crohn's disease), and comorbidity as having the strongest effect on pouch survival. Currently, our preference is to perform a primary ileoanal pouch by a stapled technique, with a hand-sewn anastomosis being reserved for redo pouches, a strategy that is supported by the findings of this study. Since urgent colectomy was associated with pouch failure, appropriate medical treatment of disease to prevent acute colitis and/or adopting surgery before patients need an urgent subtotal colectomy or develop complications of medical therapy or poor general state from poorly controlled disease may be associated with improved outcomes. Crohn's disease was also associated with worse pouch survival; thus, steps to identify this condition prior to IPAA are important.

Pelvis Sepsis

Key Concept: Pelvic sepsis is associated with worse functional outcomes and a higher rate of pouch loss.

Pelvic sepsis that develops after IPAA is a significant complication that may be associated with adverse outcomes. Although previous studies [3–6] relating to the association between pelvic sepsis and pouch outcomes have reported disparate results, our experience [7] suggests adverse outcomes for patients who develop sepsis: defined as the development of an abdominal, pelvic, or perianal infectious process detected by clinical, radiologic, or operative means occurring within 3 months of loop ileostomy closure or within 3 months of restorative proctocolectomy when stoma diversion has not been performed. Patients who developed pelvic sepsis experienced worse functional outcomes and quality of life even when it did not lead to pouch failure. Close attention to preoperative and intraoperative planning during restorative proctocolectomy and the adoption of strategies to reduce this complication after IPAA are hence important. Pelvic sepsis has previously been shown to be independently associated with the presence of higher body mass index, final pathologic diagnosis of ulcerative/indeterminate colitis or Crohn's disease, and intraoperative and postoperative transfusions on multivariate analysis in our patients [8]. Furthermore, there was also an independent association among individual surgeons, suggesting room for improvement in planning for surgery to reduce the occurrence of this complication.

Evaluation of Pouch Dysfunction

Key Concept: While pouch function varies among individuals, dysfunction should be assessed with a thorough and systematic history and physical examination, along with a directed endoscopic and radiologic evaluation.

The function of the normal pouch is variable and differs among patients. In general, patients experience six to eight bowel movements over a 24-h period with acceptable control. The majority of patients do not need to wear pads, can defer defecation, and do not have episodes of urgency or incontinence. Quality of life is high and most patients deny physical, social, work-related, or sexual restrictions.

When patients develop pouch dysfunction, evaluation should include a thorough history that details the function of the pouch and assesses symptoms that might provide a clue to the capacity, compliance, and emptying of the pouch. You also need to assess as to whether this represents a recent change or rather if patients experienced these symptoms from the time of IPAA creation. A careful physical examination of the anoperineum, including an assessment of the integrity of the sphincter mechanism, needs to be performed. Pouchoscopy helps determine the size, configuration, and compliance of the pouch, as well as the degree of inflammation, if any, of the anal canal, pouch, and afferent limb. Biopsies at pouchoscopy may confirm or rule out pouchitis or cuffitis and Crohn's disease and demonstrate indirect evidence of infectious complications. Stool and blood tests can further determine an infectious etiology as the cause of the changes in pouch function. The typical pouch is about 15-cm long, with good capacity and compliance, with an "owl's-eye appearance" at the upper portion bearing the tip of the J of the pouch and the afferent limb on either side of the septum (beak). The normal cuff varies in length but usually measures from 3 to 5 cm and has minimal inflammation. Several additional tests are available that are useful in determining the underlying etiology for pouch dysfunction.

Gastrografin Enema

This procedure helps identify fistulae between the pouch and vagina (Fig. 17.1) or perineum, the conformation of the pouch, and the presence of any narrowing of the afferent limb, inlet, or outlet (at the IPAA) of the pouch.

MRI Pelvis

This is a good test for the evaluation of abnormalities relating to the structure of the pouch and pelvis and the identification of any persistent presacral collections, abscesses, or fistulae that could be contributing to the patient's symptoms. Pelvic sepsis due to chronic leaks related to the pouch or suture and staple lines may be responsible for indolent infection in the presacral space, which may manifest as low- or high-grade sepsis and poor pouch function.

CT Enterography

This is a good test for the evaluation of the condition of the small intestine proximal to the pouch and especially helps to clarify the presence or absence of inflammatory bowel disease, particularly in the setting of underlying Crohn's disease that can lead to strictures or fistulae. Pelvic abnormalities related to the pouch and the state of the perineum and associated abnormalities can also be assessed.

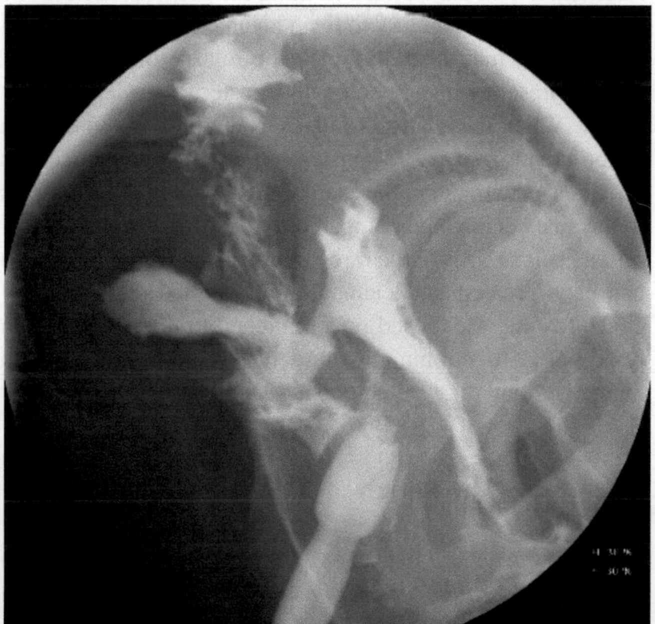

Fig. 17.1 Gastrografin enema demonstrating a pouch-vaginal fistula

Tests of Anorectal Physiology

Anorectal manometry evaluates resting and squeeze tone of the sphincter mechanism. The presence of paradoxical pressures, when correlated with difficulties with evacuation, may confirm outlet obstruction that is either organic or functional.

Endorectal ultrasound helps assess the integrity of the sphincters in patients with incontinence.

EMG/pudendal nerve terminal motor latency (PNTML) testing may help identify a neuropathy or sphincter dysfunction, though are often not as useful in this setting.

A *defecating pouchogram* identifies any problems with evacuation.

Surgical Decision-Making

Key Concept: The majority of patients undergo a multistage procedure to mitigate the risk of pouch problems from an unprotected pouch anastomotic leak.

As previously discussed, certain perioperative complications likely influence long-term pouch outcomes and function. Thus, avoiding such complications may preserve function over the long term. The ability to stage the proctocolectomy and IPAA allows for the gradation of the severity of surgical insult, and thus, the choice of the extent of the procedure can be individualized for each patient, depending upon anticipated outcomes. While suitable patients who are well nourished, of average build with mild colitis, and not on immunosuppression may be candidates for a one-stage pouch procedure, this is rarely employed in our practice. Although a one-stage operation may minimize the cumulative influence of multiple operations, in terms of complications and risks, a leak from an unprotected anastomosis may have devastating complications, including loss of the pouch. We hence very selectively perform a single-stage restorative proctocolectomy, and the majority of even such good-risk patients undergo a two-stage restorative proctocolectomy where the IPAA is defunctioned by a proximal loop ileostomy (Fig. 17.2). For patients who are sicker, more malnourished, with severe colitis, or under treatment with large doses of steroids and immunosuppression, a three-stage procedure is chosen since this likely minimizes complications. The rationale for such an approach is that an initial colectomy with an end ileostomy eliminates the inflamed colon without adding the risk of an intestinal anastomosis when tissues are still inflamed and nutrition is inadequate. This strategy also allows pelvic dissection to be deferred until the rectum is less inflamed, since this minimizes the potential risk of injury to the pelvic nerves. An initial subtotal colectomy is also a good option in patients with a suboptimal body mass index (BMI), since this allows for the institution of nutritional intervention and exercise to optimize weight prior to IPAA creation.

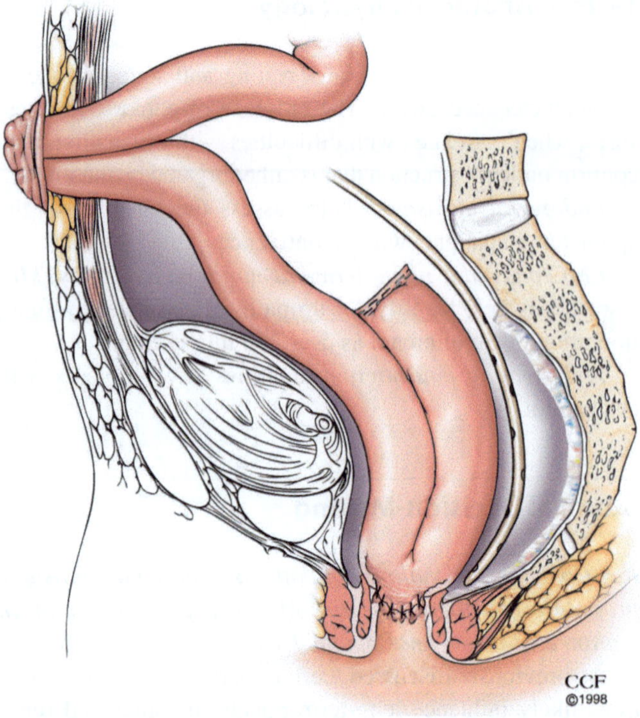

Fig. 17.2 Ileal J-pouch-anal anastomosis with defunctioning loop ileostomy (Reprinted with permission, Cleveland Clinic Center for Medical Art & Photography © 2012. All Rights Reserved)

Intraoperative Challenges During Ileoanal Pouch Creation and Anastomosis

Key Concept: Several potential technical challenges, ranging from achieving a tension-free anastomosis to inducing an iatrogenic fistula, are present during pouch construction that you need to be aware of and have a plan to overcome or avoid altogether.

Commonly employed options with regard to pouch configuration and anastomosis include a J or S pouch and a stapled or hand-sewn anastomosis (Fig. 17.3). Our current preference for a primary ileoanal pouch is a J pouch 20 cm long with a stapled IPAA. The option of mucosectomy with a hand-sewn anastomosis is in general reserved for specific circumstances such as for a redo IPAA, colitis with high-grade dysplasia or cancer involving the distal rectum, or when patients with FAP have extensive carpeting of the distal rectum with polyps. During IPAA creation, close attention needs to be directed towards the avoidance of anastomotic tension, maintenance of appropriate orientation and blood supply of the pouch and the residual anorectum, and the avoidance of the incorporation of the vagina/prostate and seminal vesicles in the staple line.

Problems with Reach of the Pouch

Key Concept: Prior to transecting the rectum, evaluate for potential problems with length, and when there is an issue, proceed through a series of maneuvers to ensure a tension-free anastomosis.

The length and orientation of the small bowel and the anatomy of the pelvis and mesentery are variable in different patients. Thus, difficulty with reach of the pouch to the anal canal for an anastomosis is expected in some circumstances. Tall patients and those with a high BMI are particularly at risk. Thus, weight loss before surgery may be helpful. In the operating room, various maneuvers may be employed to facilitate reach. High ligation of the ileocolic vessels, release of the small bowel mesentery from the retroperitoneum, mobilization of the duodenum, excision of the redundant mesenteric tissue lateral to the superior mesenteric vessels ("jib-sail"), and performing releasing incisions along the mesenteric edge of the small intestine also facilitate reach of the pouch to the anal canal. Although ligation of some of the branches of the SMA (or the main trunk of the SMA) has also been described, we rarely employ this maneuver due to the risk for compromise of blood supply to the entire small intestine.

Difficulty with reach of the pouch to the anal canal can be anticipated before rectal transection during proctectomy and the operation accordingly modified to promote the chance for a successful IPAA. Prior to transaction of the rectum, an IPAA can be simulated with the most dependent portion of the pouch held in a Babcock forceps that is delivered into the pelvis. A bimanual palpation with the gloved finger passed into anal canal prior to IPAA helps confirm reach of the Babcock to the intended level of division of the rectum (Fig. 17.4). In certain circumstances, such as patients with a high BMI, difficulties with reach of the pouch to the anal canal may persist. In this, and other similar instances, the rectal stump may be intentionally left slightly long to minimize tension on the IPAA. Orienting the pouch in such a way as to direct the mesentery to lie in an anterior location during anastomosis may also allow for the release of tension that may be present with a pouch with a posteriorly oriented mesentery. When these efforts fail, consideration may be given to the creation of an "S" instead of a "J" pouch since this provides an extra 2 cm of reach of the pouch for anastomosis to the anal canal when compared to the other pouch configurations (Fig. 17.5). In the rare circumstance where the pouch has been created and cannot be anastomosed to the anal canal, leaving the closed pouch hitched to the pelvis with a proximal defunctioning ostomy has been described as a maneuver that allows the pouch to lengthen with time.

Ischemia of the Pouch

Key Concept: Avoid overaggressive dissection of the pouch blood supply or inadvertent pouch rotation that may result in devascularization or kinking of the arterial inflow to the pouch and resultant ischemia.

This is a rare occurrence and is usually related to an overzealous skeletonization of the blood vessels that supply the

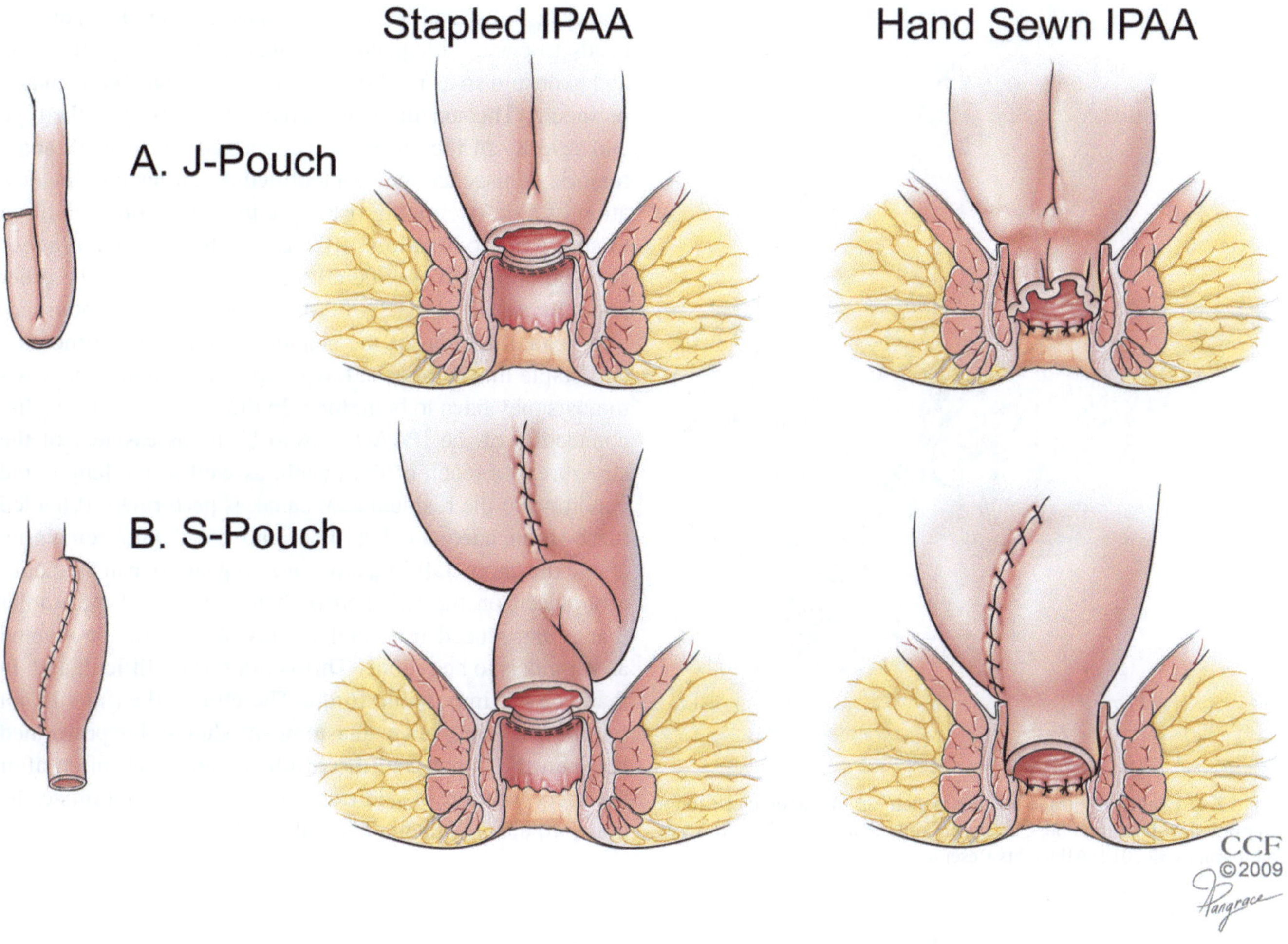

Fig. 17.3 (**a**, **b**) Commonly used pouch configurations and anastomoses (Reprinted with permission, Cleveland Clinic Center for Medical Art & Photography © 2012. All Rights Reserved)

pouch or damage to the blood supply of the pouch by direct injury or traction due to tension. Additionally, inadvertent twisting of the pouch as it is brought down into the pelvis can block arterial blood flow to the pouch. When ischemia occurs, pouch excision with the creation of a new pouch with an additional length of small intestine proximal to the pouch can be undertaken. This, however, may sometimes be associated with difficulty of reach of the pouch to the anal canal.

Problems with Stoma Creation

Key Concept: Certain patients may be expected to have difficulties with diversion and you should have a plan ahead of time to deal with this situation.

The defunctioning ileostomy can be difficult to create in patients who have had difficulty with reach of the pouch or those with a high BMI. Creation of the ostomy in a more proximal portion of the small intestine in these circumstances minimizes tension on the IPAA. This can, however, be associated with a high ostomy output and thus requires the careful monitoring of volume of output and fluid and electrolyte balance with the concomitant use of bowel stoppers until ostomy closure. While in many cases this may be unavoidable, anticipating diversion difficulties and discussing potential strategies to alleviate them with the patient will allow for realistic expectations. This may include mandating weight loss prior to surgery, trading off the ideal location of the stoma for one that is functionally better, using an end-loop versus a loop stoma, or instituting a medical regimen early to slow effluent and improve absorption.

Problems with the Anastomosis and Stapler Misfire

Key Concept: Mechanical difficulties with a stapler may be managed with a redo stapled or conversion to a hand-sewn anastomosis. You must ensure adequate length is available to avoid tension at the anastomosis.

Problems associated with the anastomosis and stapler misfire that occur in the operating room can be disheartening;

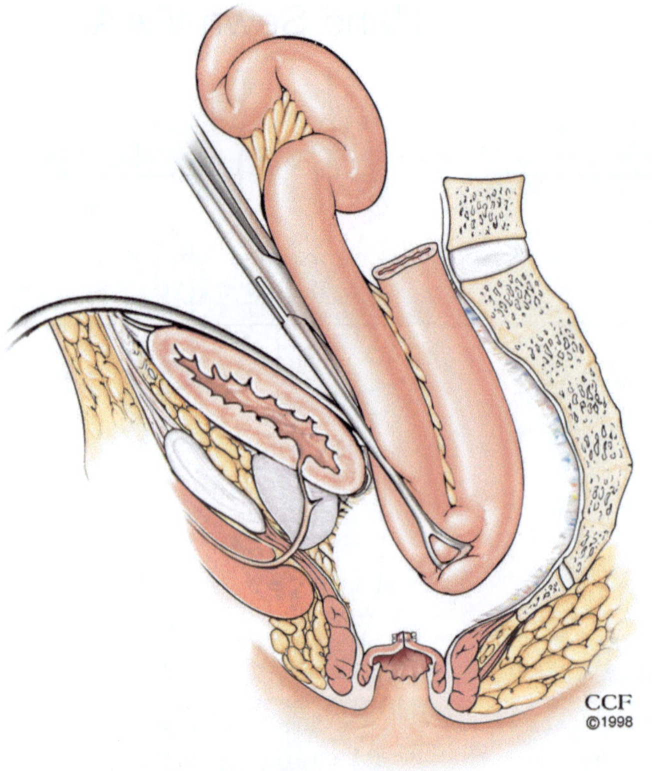

Fig. 17.4 Evaluating reach of the pouch to the anorectal stump (Reprinted with permission, Cleveland Clinic Center for Medical Art & Photography © 2012. All Rights Reserved)

however, the situation is usually salvageable. The surgeon needs to ensure adequate assistance to facilitate retraction and exposure so as to allow access to both the abdomen and perineum. The specific management depends upon the type and severity of the problem encountered. For a small anastomotic dehiscence that is identified on air testing, the creation of a defunctioning ostomy either alone or in addition to suture approximation of the defect by the abdominal or perineal approach may be all that is required. On the other hand, for a major breach of the anastomosis, when nonfunction or malfunction of the stapler occurs or when the anal cuff staple line is breached by the inserted stapler, the anastomosis may have to be redone. In these circumstances, disconnection of the IPAA followed by an assessment of the structure and reach of the pouch, as well as the length and condition of the residual anal canal, is performed. Provided there is an adequate length of the rectal cuff remaining above the anorectal ring, a purse-string suture can be manually placed on the cuff and is then tied around the stapler that is introduced transanally. This allows for the stapled anastomosis to be redone. This is often very difficult and, in many cases, impossible to do. Therefore, when this is not feasible, a hand-sewn anastomosis should be performed between the pouch and the residual anal canal, often after the incorporation of additional maneuvers to mobilize the pouch to ensure adequate length.

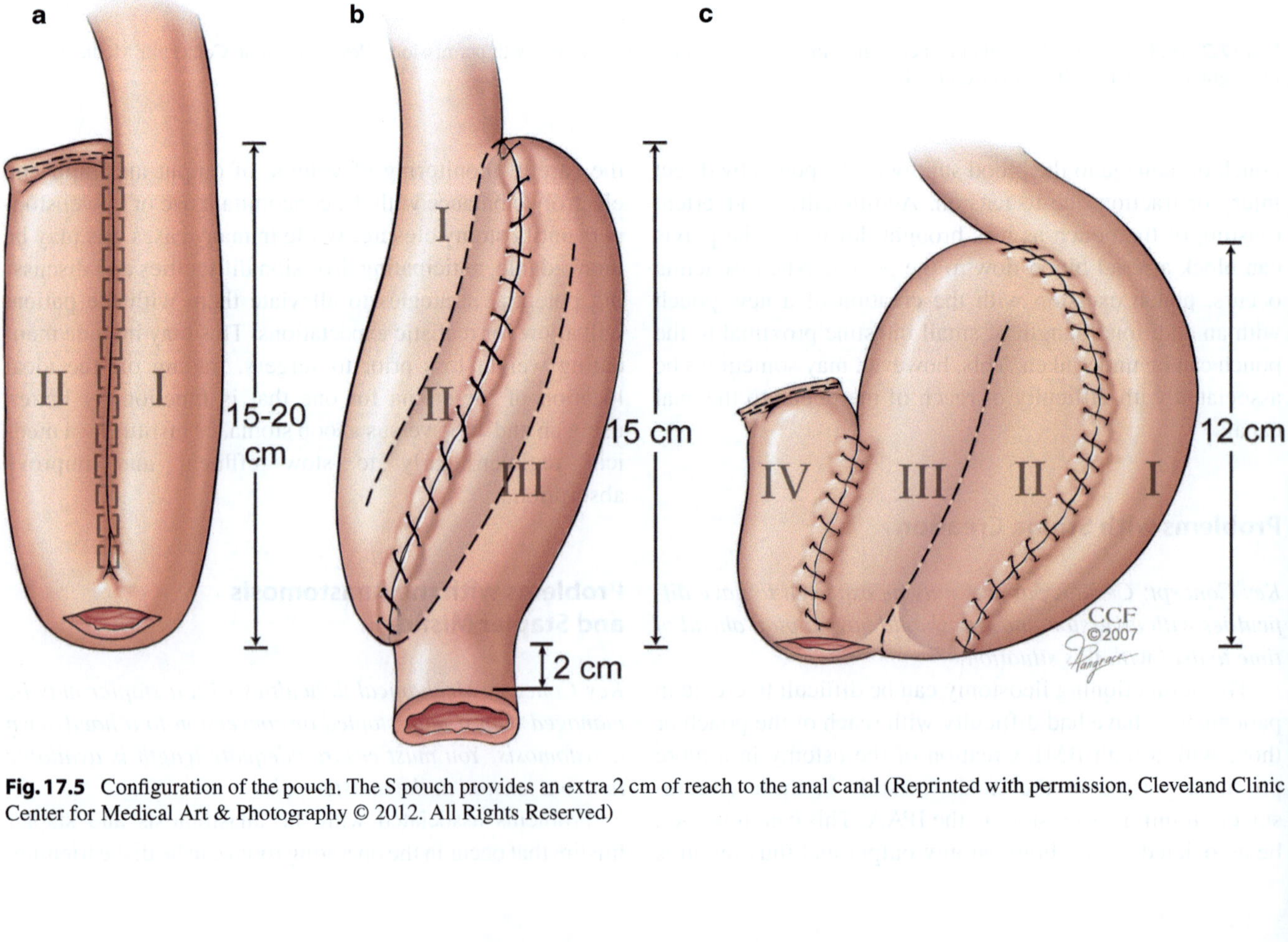

Fig. 17.5 Configuration of the pouch. The S pouch provides an extra 2 cm of reach to the anal canal (Reprinted with permission, Cleveland Clinic Center for Medical Art & Photography © 2012. All Rights Reserved)

Management of Surgical Complications Related to the Pouch

Early Complications

As previously discussed, some of the complications, especially those related to the anastomosis and pelvic sepsis, may affect the long-term function of the pouch. Thus, the prompt identification of these complications and their management is required so as to preserve a functional pouch.

Anastomotic Disruption and Pelvic Abscess

Key Concept: Whether through a transanal, transabdominal, or trans-anastomotic route, prompt drainage of pelvic abscesses (often along with appropriate diversion) is crucial to preserving pouch function.

These conditions are often interrelated. An anastomotic disruption may be isolated or associated with sepsis and may be silent or present with pelvis sepsis and abscess. Patients with a pelvic abscess usually present with fever, leukocytosis, and other signs of infection or sepsis. However, the findings may sometimes be indolent and manifest as a persistent ileus or prolonged recovery in the postoperative period. A CT scan of the abdomen and pelvis with oral, intravenous, and rectal contrast helps delineate the presence and location of any abscess and any associated anastomotic leak. Hemodynamic instability and peritonitis mandate an exploratory laparotomy with peritoneal washout and the creation of an ostomy when the pouch was not defunctioned at IPAA. Conversion of a loop ileostomy above a pouch to an end ostomy allows for complete diversion of enteric contents from the pouch and may occasionally be required. In stable patients, the prompt institution of percutaneous drainage of any identified abscesses and treatment with intravenous antibiotics allows for the control of sepsis and may minimize long-term ill-effects on the pouch due to persistent sepsis.

When a pelvic abscess or presacral collection is detected after IPAA, prompt surgical drainage of the abscess with eradication of sepsis may help conserve the pouch. When such abscesses are associated with an anastomotic leak detected on CT scan, whether drainage should be by the transanal route or by percutaneous CT-guided drainage is often a dilemma. A transanal/trans-anastomotic drainage of the abscess through the breached suture or staple line may be more comfortable for the patient and takes advantage of the conditions already present. However, whether a trans-anastomotic drain interferes with anastomotic healing and, consequently, pouch retention is a potential concern. In contrast, CT-guided drainage may be more uncomfortable and be associated with concerns for the development of an extrasphincteric fistula. The results of a review of our experience [9] with 71 patients suggest that pouch failure is high for patients with pelvic abscess associated with an anastomotic leak, but the success rates for the transanal and percutaneous drainage procedures in terms of long-term pouch retention (75.5 and 83 % respectively) and pouch function are similar. Thus, management of the patients needs to be individualized based on a determination of the relative ease and efficacy of the two procedures and the comfort of the patient based on the location and size of the abscess and the anastomotic defect.

Postoperative Bleeding from the Pouch

Key Concept: Identify staple line bleeding during pouch construction. For those manifesting in the postoperative setting, endoscopic control is diagnostic and therapeutic.

This complication can be minimized by inspecting the back row of staples aligned along the mesentery of the small bowel after the pouch has been created. Our practice is to oversew any bleeding areas that are identified in the staple line with interrupted sutures placed in a figure-of-eight fashion. When bleeding occurs postoperatively, this may manifest as bleeding through the anal canal or into the ileostomy. Pouch endoscopy with cauterization of any identified bleeding points or the application of hemostatic clips or injection of epinephrine usually controls bleeding. When there is diffuse oozing, the instillation of ice-cold saline with epinephrine into the pouch facilitates control of bleeding [10].

Late Complications

Many of these late complications manifest following takedown of the ileostomy and restoration of stool through the pouch.

Pouch-Vaginal Fistula (PVF)

Key Concept: While investigative studies are available to help guide treatment, EUA is the gold standard for evaluating PVF. Management options range from local options with or without diversion to redo IPAA.

This complication is potentially disabling and can cause significant impingement on quality of life. However, its presentation and the extent of its effect vary among patients. Common symptoms include discomfort, irritation, incontinence, as well as recurrent vaginal and urinary infections.

Investigations

These are chosen so as to assess the size, nature, and location of the fistula; state of the anoperineum and sphincter mechanism; configuration, size, and state of the pouch; and the presence or absence of any associated disease of the small intestine. The potential diagnosis of Crohn's disease needs to be considered in any patient who develops fistulous and septic complications after IPAA, since this determines the management and also the eventual outcomes. Differentiating septic complications related to IPAA creation from Crohn's disease is important; however, this is

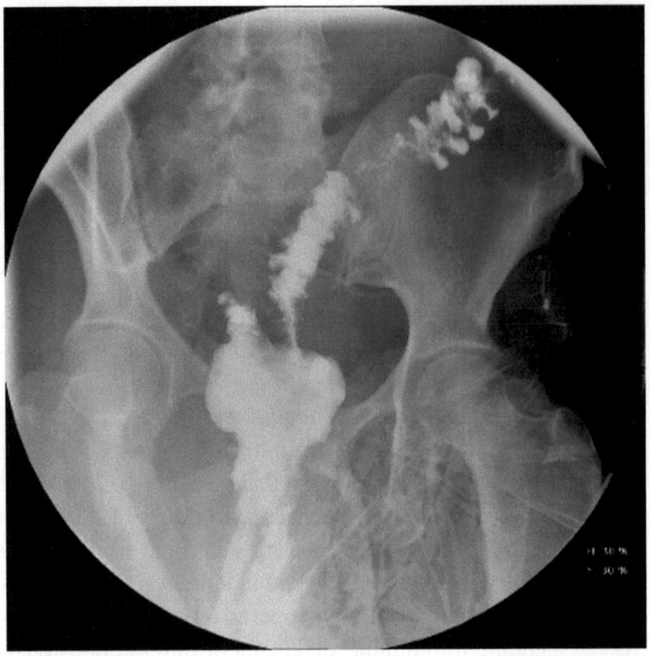

Fig. 17.6 Gastrografin study demonstrating a pouch-vaginal fistula with contrast filling both structures

often easier said than done. It is especially difficult when distinct clinical and histopathological features of Crohn's disease are absent. In general, septic complications that occur within 1 year of IPAA creation or closure of a defunctioning ostomy are likely to be due to perioperative IPAA complications. On the other hand, their occurrence after 1 year of IPAA construction suggests the possibility of a diagnosis change to Crohn's disease when the initial diagnosis was ulcerative or indeterminate colitis.

A thorough review of the history and medical records relating to the IPAA surgery and the postoperative course is required since this may provide insight into the potential differential diagnoses that may have caused the fistula. A review of pathology relating to the biopsies, even prior to surgery and of the colectomy or proctocolectomy specimen, additionally helps assess the possibility of Crohn's disease as the correct diagnosis. General, abdominal, and perineal examination for clinical harbingers of Crohn's disease and evaluation of the tone of the sphincter at rest and with squeeze provide useful information. Vaginoscopy and pouchoscopy may allow for the identification of the fistula and an assessment of the location, number, nature, and size of any fistula as well as the physical state of the pouch, anal canal, and vagina. Examination under anesthesia provides excellent information and is currently the gold standard test in the evaluation of a pouch-vaginal fistula. As stated previously, other tests that should be considered include gastrografin enema, vaginogram, and MRI of the pelvis since these help to further characterize the anatomy of the fistula. CT or MR enterography also helps delineate the anatomy of the pouch and the state of the small bowel above the pouch (Fig. 17.6).

The final decision relating to the management of the pouch-vaginal fistula depends upon the severity of the symptoms and their effect on the patient's quality of life (QOL). Examination under anesthesia allows for a better assessment of the fistula tract and the state of the associated tissues. If there is evidence of active inflammation, sepsis, and induration in the tract or adjoining abscess cavity and surrounding tissues, the placement of a seton allows for the reduction in the ongoing sequestration of infection and further damage of tissues. The seton also allows for the normalization of the tissues so that a better assessment of the area may subsequently be feasible. Adequate drainage also allows for the tissues surrounding the fistula to become healthy, with an improvement in the elasticity and tensile strength of anorectal and pouch-related tissues that may be utilized in the definitive repair of the pouch-vaginal fistula. The additional use of medical treatment with antibiotics, anti-inflammatory agents, and anti-Crohn's disease medication may be required to reduce inflammation before the consideration of repair, especially for those involving local procedures.

Some patients with pouch-vaginal fistulae are candidates for perineal procedures. A redo IPAA is an option when repair by the perineal approach is unlikely to be successful or when local procedures have failed. Although there is a relatively high risk for pouch failure for patients with a pouch-vaginal fistula, up to 85 % of pouch-vaginal fistulae can be healed using these approaches [11–14].

Treatment Options for PVF

Local Procedures

These include pouch or vaginal advancement flap repairs, perineal pouch advancement, fistula plugs, and gracilis flap repair. Local repair may be considered for low, simple fistulae that are not associated with florid inflammation.

Advancement Flap Repair

Technique: We prefer the prone jackknife position in the operating room, with the patient under general anesthesia and skeletal muscle relaxation to provide the best exposure to the area. The procedure is covered with intravenous antibiotics, and a Foley catheter is placed into the bladder. Although the Lone Star Retractor System™ (CooperSurgical Inc, Trumbull, CT) is an option for anoperineal exposure, our preference is the placement of effacement sutures in the four quadrants of the perineum, which provide equivalent exposure to the anal verge and canal. A Hill-Ferguson retractor introduced into both the vagina and anal canal facilitates exposure of the fistula tract. A malleable probe such as a lacrimal probe or instead a Lockhart-Mummery probe facilitates identification of the tract. If there is no evidence of festering sepsis and the surrounding tissues are supple and noninflamed, consideration may be given to the creation of a flap for repair. The os of the fistula on the side of the pouch is circumscribed, and a U-shaped curvilinear broad-based flap incorporating the mucosa and submucosa of the pouch wall is raised with the os at its apex. The fistula tract is dissected into the pouch-vaginal septum and excised. The tissue surrounding the excised fistula tract is approximated using #2-0 Vicryl sutures with sutures that incorporate the sphincter mechanism. The flap is developed upwards and sutured to the pouch-anal mucosa, the sutures placed in such a way as to incorporate the adjoining sphincter mechanism on their deep aspect, ensuring a tension-free repair. Our preference is to keep patients on strict bed rest in the hospital for the first 24 h after the procedure. The Foley catheter is discontinued on the second postoperative day and limited mobility of the patient to the bathroom allowed until the return of bowel function. The use of preoperative bowel preparation delays the return of bowel function. Patients are usually discharged on oral antibiotics.

Fibrin Glue, Fistula Plug, Biologic Mesh Repair, and Gracilis Muscle Interposition

These perineal procedures [15–17] have been described for the management of pouch-vaginal fistulae. Considering the variable success reported with these procedures, we do not routinely use these techniques.

Failure of Flap Repair

Redo flap procedures may be considered in some patients who have had failure with a flap repair provided the basic principles of avoidance of sepsis, maintenance of tensile strength, and control of ongoing inflammation can be ensured. Repeat flap procedures facilitate healing of some fistulae which initially failed repair and thus improve the cumulative success of the flap procedure [12, 13].

Perineal Pouch Advancement

This can be accomplished by the perineal route, whereby the anterior half of the pouch is disconnected from the anal canal and the pouch mobilized transanally and approximated to the anal canal.

Redo IPAA

This is the most definitive option in patients with a pouch-vaginal fistula who have previously had failure of local procedures. The procedure can be considered in patients who otherwise have a healthy pouch, anoperineum, and sphincter mechanism. Details of the redo pouch procedure per se are discussed elsewhere in the text. The technique, as it pertains to a pouch-vaginal fistula, is slightly modified depending upon the location of the fistula. When the fistula involves the IPAA or is proximal to the IPAA, abdominoperineal disconnection of the pouch, followed by revision of the pouch after excision and debridement of the portion involved in the fistula tract, is completed. The defect in the rectovaginal septum is repaired, followed by the performance of mucosectomy with a hand-sewn anastomosis at the anal verge. The previous pouch may be utilized if it's noted to be healthy and of adequate capacity, or augmented or refashioned prior to anastomosis, if required. A neoileal pouch creation after excision of the previous pouch may be required if the pouch is damaged or inflamed. Additionally, the use of an omental pedicle flap, when feasible, to separate the pouch from the vagina allows for extra protection between the pouch and the vagina. When the pouch-vaginal fistula is located below the IPAA, either at the dentate line or in the anal canal, mucosectomy with pouch-anal anastomosis of the previously revised, or a new, pouch to the perianal skin allows the use of the full thickness of the pouch wall as a natural flap over the vaginal opening.

Loop Ileostomy

A defunctioning ileostomy can be considered as a temporizing maneuver to divert the fecal stream either prior to or concomitantly with the local repair of a pouch-vaginal fistula. This may also be a suitable option as a first step to improve quality of life that is affected by the irritating and infectious effects of the chronic fecal drainage into the vagina and perineum. Finally, pouch excision with end ileostomy and conversion of the J pouch to a K pouch are other options that can be considered in the individual patient.

Pouch-Perineal Fistula (PPF)

The evaluation, management, and surgical options for pouch-perineal fistulae are similar to those for pouch-vaginal fistulae. Figure 17.7 demonstrates the steps of an advancement flap repair as it pertains to a pouch-perineal fistula.

Pouch Sinus

Key Concept: *Pouch sinus presentation varies widely, helps dictate therapy, and is the best predictor of outcome.*

An anastomotic sinus of the pouch is a condition about which there is minimal information in the literature. It is known to occur in 2.8–8 % of patients after an IPAA procedure and is related to the development of an anastomotic leak that is confined to a blind-ending track. The problem can be puzzling since presentation and outcomes may vary. The sinus tract may be asymptomatic and incidentally detected on imaging studies or cause symptoms, which may extend from minor to more major including sepsis, pelvic pain, pouch dysfunction, and pouch failure. Its occurrence is also associated with widely differing outcomes-from a condition without any consequence in some patients to pouch failure in others. Several therapies including debridement, unroofing, occlusive treatment with fibrin glue, pouch revision, and redo pouch [18–20] have been described. A recent review of the presentation,

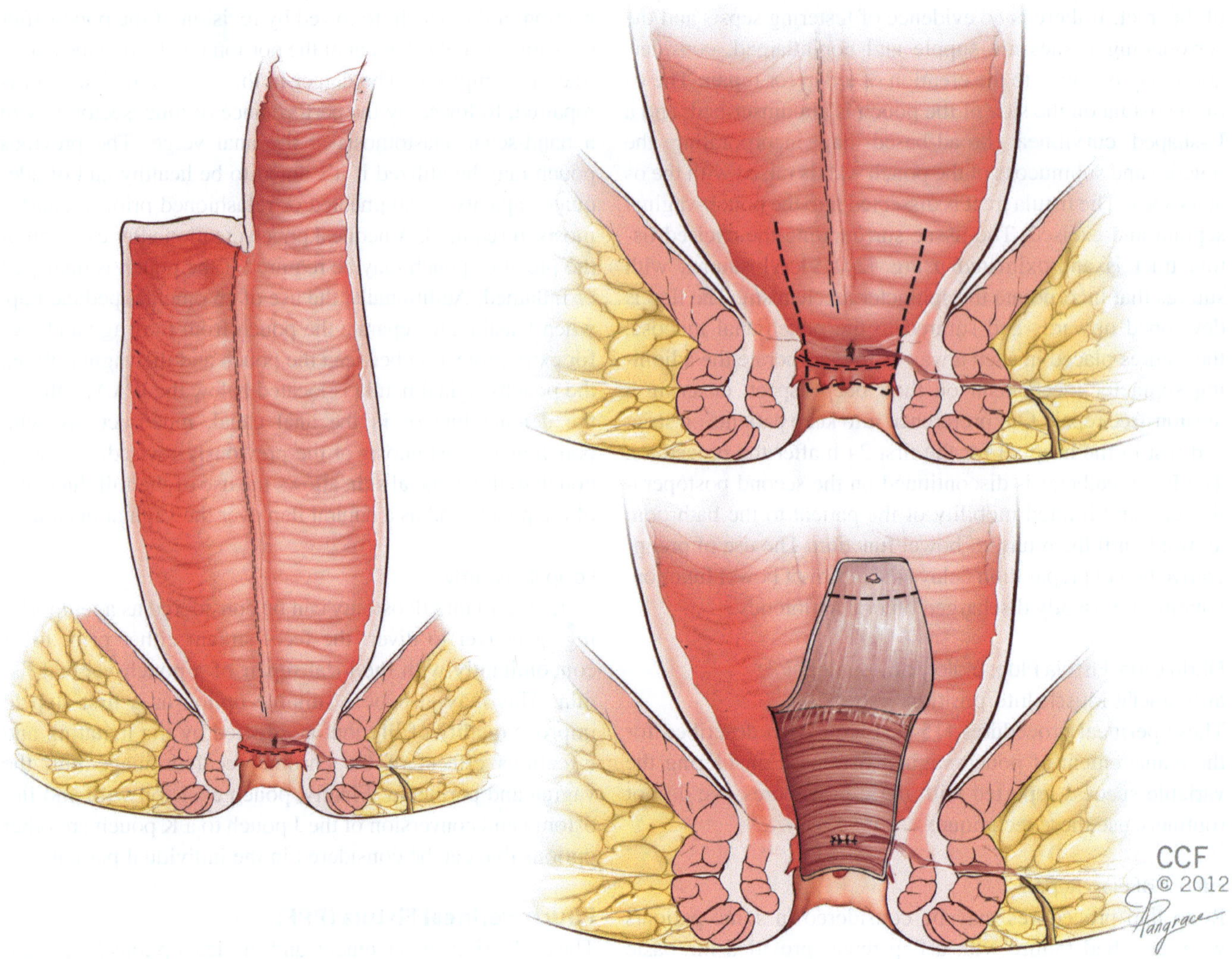

Fig. 17.7 Advancement flap repair of pouch-perineal fistula (Reprinted with permission, Cleveland Clinic Center for Medical Art & Photography © 2012. All Rights Reserved)

management, and outcomes for 45 (2 %) patients who developed a pouch sinus after IPAA [21] suggests that diagnosis is usually established at pouchoscopy, gastrografin enema, CT scan, or MRI of the pelvis. Symptomatic presentation is a significant predictor for low healing rates and is associated with a high risk of pouch failure. Management depends upon the presentation, size, location, and presence of other associated factors such as whether or not the patient is defunctioned. Observation and watchful monitoring is the initial treatment of choice when permitted by the patient's condition. The overall healing rate for the 45 patients in this study was about 60 %, with a healing rate of 84 % for asymptomatic patients. Unroofing of the sinus was helpful in asymptomatic sinuses (81 % healed) but less so in symptomatic patients (18 % healed). Fibrin glue, used in three patients, resulted in complete healing in two (66 %) patients. With transanal drainage of the sinuses, 66 % patients eventually healed. Again, healing rate in asymptomatic patients was much higher (100 %) compared to symptomatic patients (20 %). When other measures fail, a redo pouch is an option for these patients. Of three patients who underwent a redo pouch, two (66 %) achieved successful healing with a functional pouch.

Based on these results, an algorithm was proposed for the management of pouch sinuses, which is discussed below.

Incidentally detected sinus: Sinuses detected in patients without an ostomy who are asymptomatic are best left alone without intervention.

Sinus detected on routine Gastrografin enema prior to stoma closure after IPAA: In such patients, delaying ileostomy closure for a few months until healing of the sinus is demonstrated is the best strategy.

Symptomatic and persistent sinus: Symptomatic sinuses and those that are defunctioned, but nonhealing on watchful waiting alone, may be managed by transanal drain placement, unroofing of the sinus, or injection of fibrin glue to facilitate healing. Simple closure of the ileostomy may be considered in selected asymptomatic patients with a small persistent sinus. When eventual healing of the sinus is expected, a loop ileostomy with further local procedures to facilitate closure is an option in patients who are not defunctioned. When there is failure of healing, especially in symptomatic patients, a redo IPAA or the alternatives of a conventional or continent ileostomy may be considered.

Crohn's Disease of the Pouch

Key Concept: The ultimate diagnosis of Crohn's disease in pouch patients can present in a variety of locations and manifestations. In addition to endoscopic and surgical therapy, aggressive medical therapy should be instituted.

Crohn's disease may affect the body, afferent limb, or IPAA of the pouch, perineum, or small intestine proximal to the pouch. Management depends upon the phenotype, whether inflammatory, fibrostenotic, or fistulous, and the resultant symptoms. Medical management includes medical treatment with steroids, immunosuppressive medication, and/or biologics. Endoscopic intervention including dilatation may be used for isolated short-segment strictures of the IPAA, pouch body, or afferent limb. Surgical treatment is required for strictures not amenable to endoscopic therapy and when there is failure of endoscopic therapy. When surgery is performed, preservation of intestinal continuity is feasible in the majority of patients with localized fibrostenosing disease. Strictures of the afferent limb may require small bowel resection or stricturoplasty or rarely a side-to-side anastomosis between the strictured segment and the top of the pouch. Strictures of the pouch body can similarly be managed with stricturoplasty. Such treatment is usually combined with a defunctioning ostomy above the pouch and medical treatment of the Crohn's disease. More extensive disease involvement of the pouch may necessitate pouch excision or permanent defunction. Strictures of the IPAA may similarly be managed with dilatation, stricturoplasty, or diversion. Perianal disease may be managed with drains or setons for loculated abscesses or fistulae and coupled with medical treatment. Advancement flap repair may be a suitable option for Crohn's-related pouch-perineal or pouch-vaginal fistulae after control of sepsis and medical treatment of inflammation. Extensive perineal disease and recurrent abscesses or fistulae resistant to local measures may necessitate a temporary or permanent ostomy. Such patients may rarely be candidates for a continent ileostomy when the pouch and the proximal small intestine are free of Crohn's disease (though caution should be exercised). Despite the potential problems related to the nipple valve with a continent ileostomy and the risk of reoperations relating to this complication, the procedure may be suitable for Crohn's patients with an adequate length of small intestine at surgery, especially when this can be maintained, even if eventual resection of the continent reservoir were to occur. In such patients, conversion of the ileoanal pouch to a continent ileostomy, in fact, conserves small intestinal length and absorptive capacity in contrast to pouch excision. When an ileoanal pouch is salvaged or continent ileostomy is created in patients with Crohn's disease, the use of suppressive medication to reduce the risk of recrudescence of the Crohn's disease needs to be carefully considered.

Incontinence

Key Concept: In pouch patients with incontinence, the cause of the incontinence determines management and outcomes.

Incontinence may be due to abnormalities of the pouch including pouchitis, cuffitis, presacral sinus, or chronic presacral cavity related to an anastomotic leak. Alternatively, this can be due to weakness of the sphincter mechanism from either patient-specific factors or postsurgical changes. Evaluation of the pouch and the anal canal and sphincter mechanism reveals potential causes. Minor degrees of incontinence and those relating to inflammation of the pouch or cuff may improve with medical therapy. When incontinence occurs as a complication of these complications, the surgical treatment of the complications corrects the incontinence. Isolated sphincter defects can be managed with sphincter repair. However, when sphincter compromise is severe, options include pouch excision with permanent ileostomy or a continent ileostomy.

Outlet Dysfunction

Key Concept: Difficulty in evacuation may be due to structural or functional disorders and can often be managed successfully by nonoperative means.

Problems with pouch evacuation may be due to a wide range of causes such as IPAA stricture or pouch prolapse. Strictures from scar tissue or Crohn's disease can be managed by dilatation or stricturoplasty. For outlet dysfunction that occurs in the absence of an anatomic cause, biofeedback is an option. Enemas and intermittent self-intubation of the pouch with irrigation may be useful in both organic and functional obstructive disorders. Finally, sacral nerve stimulation may play a role in the future but has little data supporting its efficacy.

Pouchitis and Cuffitis

Key Concept: Bleeding, pain, and increased stool frequency from residual inflammation at the IPAA or in the pouch itself should initially be approached with medical management. Surgical options to include ablation, diversion, or excision should be considered second-line or last-resort options for recalcitrant disease.

These conditions relate to inflammation of the pouch or the lining of the residual anal canal and are diagnosed at pouchoscopy and biopsy (Fig. 17.8). Treatment is primarily

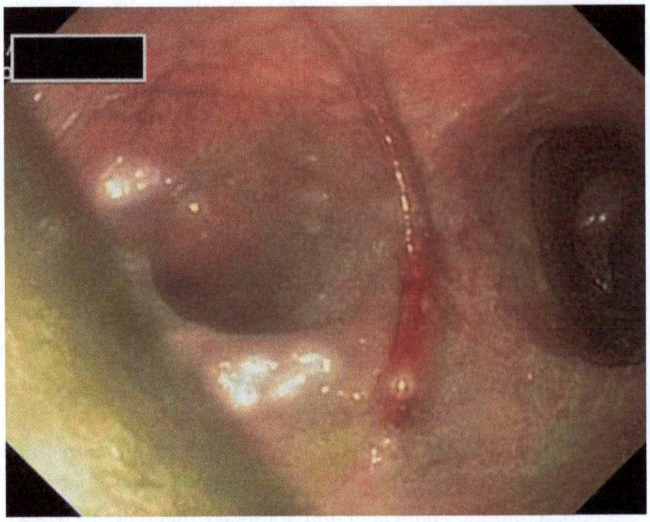

Fig. 17.8 Pouchitis on flexible sigmoidoscopy. Notice the erythematous mucosa and the watery stools present in the pouch

medical. Small areas of cuff inflammation may be approached through ablative or excisional means, though often require multiple attempts. A defunctioning ostomy or pouch excision with an end ileostomy may however be required for recalcitrant pouchitis or cuffitis unresponsive to medical treatment. Corrective surgery or redo IPAA may also be required for the management of pouchitis secondary to pouch-related conditions such as chronic presacral abscess, pouch sinus, small pouch size, or obstruction due to stricture or pouch prolapse. Redo IPAA is also an option for persistent cuffitis secondary to a long segment of anal canal and rectal remnant retained at the time of IPAA.

Pouch Prolapse

Key Concept: This rare condition should be treated primarily with dietary management and avoidance of straining. Pexy of the pouch is reserved for severe cases.

This is a rare complication of the ileoanal pouch, with few reports examining the presentation, investigation, and management of the condition. Ehsan et al. [22] conducted a survey on pouch prolapse and indicated an incidence of 0.3 % for the condition, which was similar to our experience (11 patients, 0.3 %). Seven of the patients in our experience had full-thickness pouch prolapse while four had mucosal prolapse. Diagnosis in ten patients was based on symptoms and examination, while in one patient was diagnosis was made at pouchography performed to investigate pouch dysfunction. Our experience suggests that the first line of treatment for patients with mucosal prolapse is stool bulking agents and biofeedback so as to avoid excessive straining. In two patients, this was successful in relieving symptoms while the other two patients underwent a local perineal procedure with pouch advancement after the excision of redundant mucosal tissue. None of these patients subsequently developed full-thickness prolapse. Patients with full-thickness pouch prolapse were treated with definitive transabdominal surgery. Pouchpexy using a transabdominal approach, with fixation of pouch to the sacrum using nonabsorbable sutures, was used in the first six patients, while one patient needed mesh fixation of the pouch for recurrent pouch prolapse.

Leak from the Tip of the "J"

Key Concept: Leaks in this location most often follow an indolent course but may require operative therapy and can even lead to loss of the pouch.

This is a rare and indolent complication related to the pouch. Leaks from suture lines in the pouch itself and from the tip of the J pouch (Fig. 17.9a) are less likely than anastomotic leaks but are also associated with pouch failure. A review of our experience related to the diagnosis and management of leaks from the tip of the J in 27 patients [23] suggested that the frequency of this condition for patients who underwent primary IPAA is very low (0.5 %). Patients present with variable symptoms such as abdominal pain, fever, or diarrhea—making the diagnosis difficult to establish. Further, in some patients, leaks may present with a fistula rather than a pelvic abscess, a presentation usually suggestive of an anastomotic leak or Crohn's disease. A leak could be detected on gastrografin enema ($n=4$) or pouchoscopy ($n=4$) in only 8 of the 27 patients. In one patient, an abscess was detected during emergent laparotomy for acute peritonitis due to leak from the tip of the J pouch. The majority of patients had a long median time between primary IPAA and salvage surgery suggesting that a leak from the tip of the J pouch leads to an indolent course. This is further corroborated by the fact that in six patients (22 %), the ultimate diagnosis could only be made at the time of salvage surgery. These six patients underwent salvage surgery due to their symptoms and the suspicion of a septic complication after primary IPAA. A high degree of suspicion is hence required for its diagnosis, since pouch leaks are associated with pouch failure after IPAA. When a leak from the tip of the J pouch is detected, management depends upon the nature and degree of the defect and associated findings in the pouch and pelvis. Salvage surgery may require pouch repair with suture (Fig. 17.9b) or stapled (Fig. 17.9c) repair of the leak site with or without a redo IPAA or pouch resection with redo IPAA.

J-Pouch to K-Pouch (Continent Ileostomy) Conversion

Key Concept: Select, highly motivated patients may undergo conversion of their IPAA to a continent ileostomy, though commonly associated with a higher rate of complications.

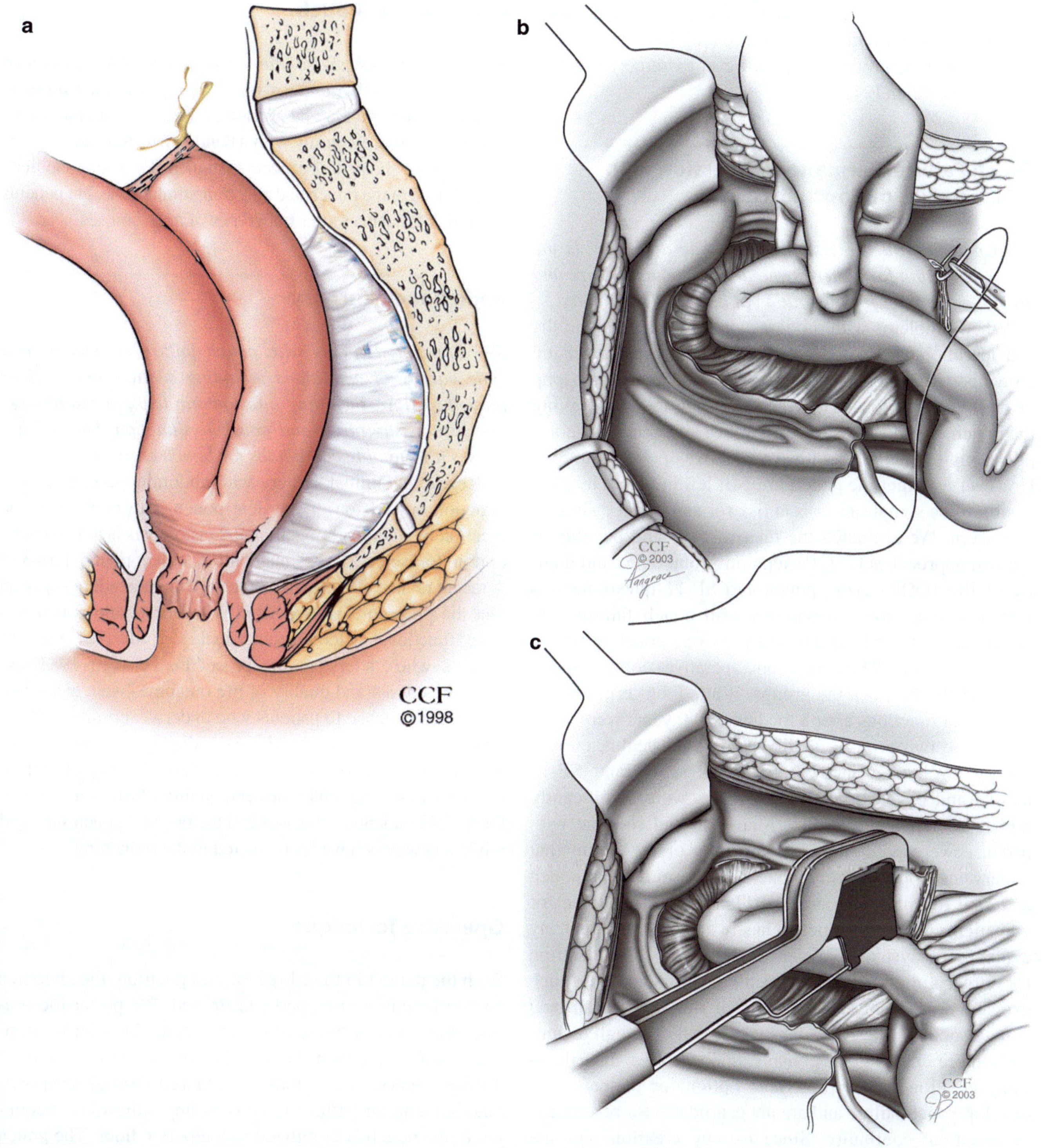

Fig. 17.9 (**a**) Leak from the tip of the J pouch (Reprinted with permission, Cleveland Clinic Center for Medical Art & Photography © 2012. All Rights Reserved). (**b**) Suture repair of a leak from the tip of the J pouch (Reprinted with permission, Cleveland Clinic Center for Medical Art & Photography © 2012. All Rights Reserved). (**c**) Stapled repair of the tip of the J pouch (Reprinted with permission, Cleveland Clinic Center for Medical Art & Photography © 2012. All Rights Reserved)

For patients with pouch failure secondary to problems with the anal canal and perineum and patients with pouch failure who may be suitable candidates for a redo IPAA but elect not to continue to maintain defecation by the normal route, conversion of the J pouch to a K pouch is an option. The procedure is complex and associated with a high frequency of complications since it incorporates the additional technical challenges of the continent ileostomy reservoir creation to the operative difficulties of reoperative abdominal and pelvic surgery required for pouch mobilization. Patients who undergo the procedure are however extremely satisfied with the operation [24].

Pouch Failure: Permanent Diversion with Pouch In Situ or Pouch Excision?

Key Concept: Pouch excision, rather than diversion, is the preferred option for patients who develop pouch failure and are not candidates for restoration of intestinal continuity.

When problems with the ileoanal pouch necessitate the consideration of an ostomy, options include pouch excision with a permanent end ileostomy or instead an ostomy (loop or end) above a pouch, leaving the pouch in situ. Leaving the pouch in situ avoids the difficulties and hence the complications associated with reoperative pelvic surgery. However, whether the pouch itself (if left in place) leads to troublesome symptoms or is at risk for malignant change is a concern. We evaluated the relative risks and benefits of the two approaches [25]. Perioperative outcomes and quality of life (QOL) using pouch and SF-12 questionnaires were evaluated for 136 patients with pouch failure who underwent either a loop ileostomy above a pouch in situ or pouch excision. Thirty-day postoperative complications were similar between the groups. While long-term urinary and sexual functions after a median of 9.9 years were similar for the two groups, quality of life and health, current energy level, Cleveland Global QOL score, and SF-12 mental and physical component scales were significantly higher after pouch excision. Anal pain and seepage with pad use were predominant complaints of the group that underwent loop ileostomy alone. Long-term data on pouch and anal transitional zone surveillance were available for 18 patients who had the pouch in situ and did not reveal any evidence of dysplasia or cancer. However, the indication for surgery in eight of the patients who underwent pouch excision was dysplasia or cancer of the anal transitional zone or pouch. These results suggest that although technically more challenging, pouch excision, rather than ileostomy creation, is the preferable option for patients who develop pouch failure and are not candidates for restoration of intestinal continuity. Since ostomy creation was not associated with neoplasia in the pouch left in situ, this option may be a reasonable intermediate- or long-term alternative when pouch excision is not feasible or advisable and when concerns about reoperation in the pelvis are significant. An ostomy creation in other circumstances also offers some patients the anticipation of eventual correction of the pouch-related complication and reestablishment of intestinal continuity. Pouch surveillance, however, bears consideration when the pouch is left in situ.

Cancer of the Pouch

Key Concept: This rare condition may occur with both stapled and hand-sewn IPAA and warrants appropriate surveillance.

This is rare and may be located in the pouch or anal transitional zone. Mucosectomy with a hand-sewn anastomosis does not eliminate the risk of cancer. A stapled IPAA may facilitate surveillance of the pouch and anal transitional zone, but patients are at risk for cancer after both types of anastomoses.

Redo Pouch Surgery

Key Concept: Patients with pouch failure secondary to a wide variety of conditions including septic complications related to IPAA including anastomotic leak, pelvic abscess and fistula, strictures, and pouch dysfunction due to other causes are suitable candidates for pouch excision.

Repeat abdominal surgery with abdominoperineal reconstruction or revision of the ileal pouch with or without the creation of a neoileal pouch-anal anastomosis is a reasonable option for selected patients with a failed pouch [26–32]. A recent review of our experience with the procedure suggests that the procedure is associated with acceptable pouch salvage, functional outcomes, and quality of life [33]. For 241 patients who underwent the procedure between 1983 and 2007, functional and quality of life outcomes were encouraging. When matched to patients who underwent primary IPAA, redo pouch patients reported greater daytime and night seepage and daytime pad usage after a median follow-up of 5 years, but other functional outcomes and quality of life were similar. Of the 241 patients, 170 cases had the original pouch salvaged while a new pouch was constructed in the remaining.

Operative Technique

With the patient in the Lloyd-Davies position, the abdomen and perineum are prepped and draped. We prefer the routine placement of bilateral ureteral stents in order to minimize injury and identify any damage to these structures during surgery. The abdomen is entered through the previous incision, and after the lysis of any adhesions encountered, the pouch is mobilized to the pelvic floor. The pouch is disconnected from the anastomosis, delivered into the abdomen, and evaluated. The state and residual capacity of the pouch, the length of remaining small intestine, and anticipated challenges with reach of the pouch to the anal canal determine whether the old pouch is revised or instead excised with a new pouch created prior to reanastomosis. If the redo IPAA is performed for pouch failure secondary to a chronic presacral abscess cavity (Fig. 17.10a), the detritus within the cavity is excised or drained (Fig. 17.10b).

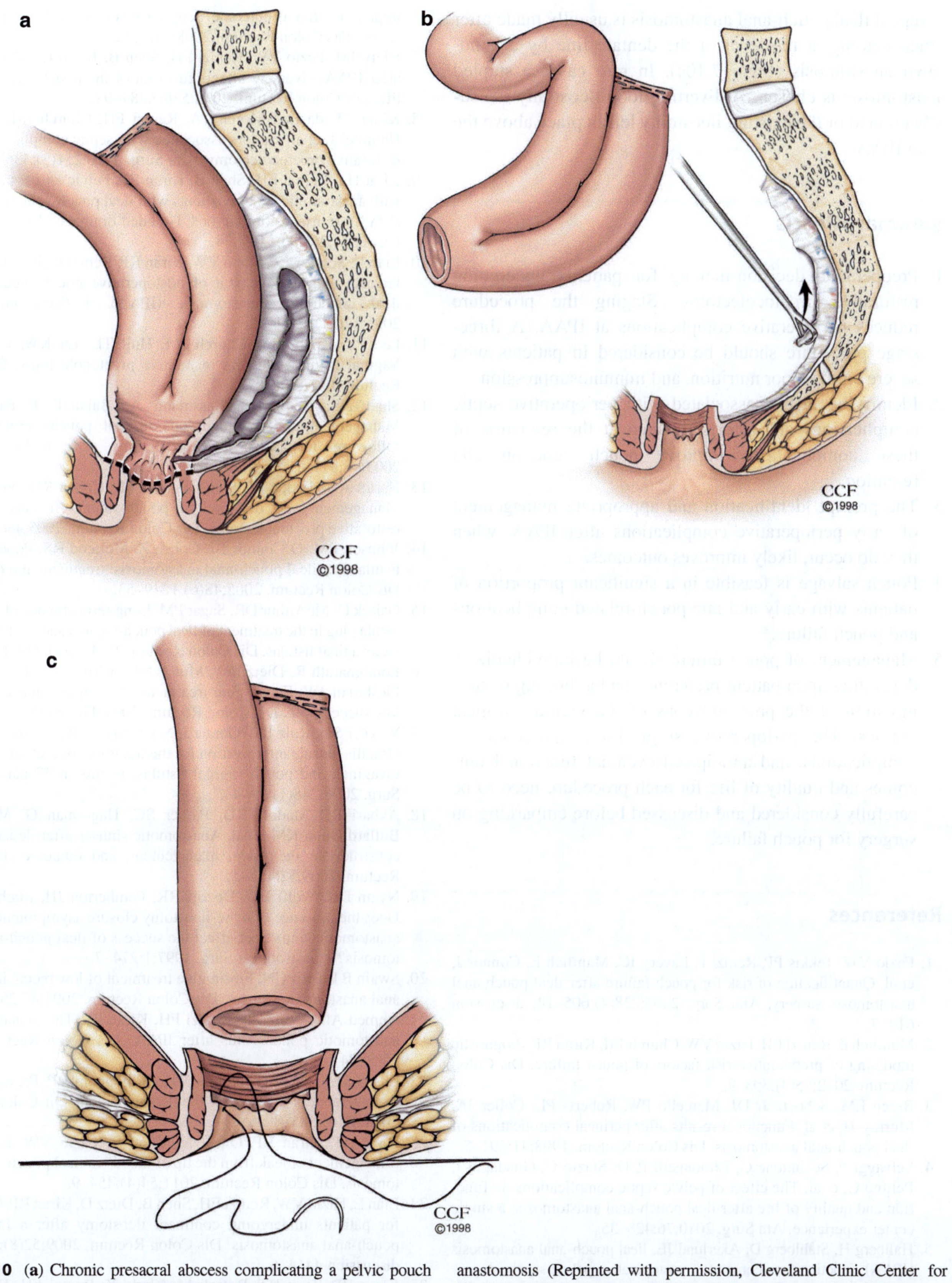

Fig. 17.10 (**a**) Chronic presacral abscess complicating a pelvic pouch (Reprinted with permission, Cleveland Clinic Center for Medical Art & Photography © 2012. All Rights Reserved). (**b**) Debridement of the presacral abscess cavity after disconnection of the pouch from the anastomosis (Reprinted with permission, Cleveland Clinic Center for Medical Art & Photography © 2012. All Rights Reserved). (**c**) Hand-sewn redo pouch-anal anastomosis (Reprinted with permission, Cleveland Clinic Center for Medical Art & Photography © 2012. All Rights Reserved)

A repeat ileal pouch-anal anastomosis is usually made after mucosectomy at the level of the dentate line by a hand-sewn anastomosis (Fig. 17.10c). In rare cases a stapled anastomosis is chosen. A diverting loop ileostomy is usually created or the existing ileostomy left in place above the redo IPAA.

Summary Pearls

1. Preoperative decision-making for patients undergoing restorative proctocolectomy: Staging the procedure reduces perioperative complications at IPAA. A three-stage procedure should be considered in patients with severe colitis, poor nutrition, and immunosuppression.
2. Identifying factors associated with perioperative septic complications and efforts directed at the reduction of these complications improve pouch function and retention.
3. The prompt identification and appropriate management of early perioperative complications after IPAA, when they do occur, likely improves outcomes.
4. Pouch salvage is feasible in a significant proportion of patients with early and late pouch-related complications and pouch failure.
5. Management of pouch failure should be individualized, depending upon patient preference and a thorough determination of the pros and cons of the various surgical options. The perioperative surgical risk, potential for complications, and anticipated eventual functional outcomes and quality of life for each procedure need to be carefully considered and discussed before embarking on surgery for pouch failure.

References

1. Fazio VW, Tekkis PP, Remzi F, Lavery IC, Manilich E, Connor J, et al. Quantification of risk for pouch failure after ileal pouch anal anastomosis surgery. Ann Surg. 2003;238(4):605–14; discussion 614–7.
2. Manilich E, Remzi FH, Fazio VW, Church JM, Kiran RP. Prognostic modeling of preoperative risk factors of pouch failure. Dis Colon Rectum. 2012;55(4):393–9.
3. Breen EM, Schoetz Jr DJ, Marcello PW, Roberts PL, Coller JA, Murray JJ, et al. Functional results after perineal complications of ileal pouch-anal anastomosis. Dis Colon Rectum. 1998;41:691–5.
4. Selvaggi F, Sciaudone G, Limongelli P, Di Stazio C, Guadagni I, Pellino G, et al. The effect of pelvic septic complications on function and quality of life after ileal pouch-anal anastomosis: a single center experience. Am Surg. 2010;76:428–35.
5. Hallberg H, Ståhlberg D, Akerlund JE. Ileal pouch-anal anastomosis (IPAA): functional outcome after postoperative pelvic sepsis. A prospective study of 100 patients. Int J Colorectal Dis. 2005;20:529–33.
6. Chessin DB, Gorfine SR, Bub DS, Royston A, Wong D, Bauer JJ. Septic complications after restorative proctocolectomy do not impair functional outcome: long-term follow-up from a specialty center. Dis Colon Rectum. 2008;51:1312–7.
7. Kiely JM, Fazio VW, Remzi FH, Shen B, Kiran RP. Pelvic sepsis after IPAA adversely affects function of the pouch and quality of life. Dis Colon Rectum. 2012;55(4):387–92.
8. Kiran RP, da Luz Moreira A, Remzi FH, Church JM, Lavery I, Hammel J, et al. Factors associated with septic complications after restorative proctocolectomy. Ann Surg. 2010;251(3):436–40.
9. Kirat HT, Remzi FH, Shen B, Kiran RP. Pelvic abscess associated with anastomotic leak in patients with ileal pouch-anal anastomosis (IPAA): transanastomotic or CT-guided drainage? Int J Colorectal Dis. 2011;26(11):1469–74.
10. Lian L, Serclova Z, Fazio VW, Kiran RP, Remzi F, Shen B. Clinical features and management of postoperative pouch bleeding after ileal pouch-anal anastomosis (IPAA). J Gastrointest Surg. 2008;12(11):1991–4.
11. Lee PY, Fazio VW, Church JM, Hull TL, Eu KW, Lavery IC. Vaginal fistula following restorative proctocolectomy. Dis Colon Rectum. 1997;40(7):752–9.
12. Shah NS, Remzi F, Massmann A, Baixauli J, Fazio VW. Management and treatment outcome of pouch-vaginal fistulas following restorative proctocolectomy. Dis Colon Rectum. 2003;46:911–7.
13. Heriot AG, Tekkis PP, Smith JJ, Bona R, Cohen RG, Nicholls RJ. Management and outcome of pouch-vaginal fistulas following restorative proctocolectomy. Dis Colon Rectum. 2005;48(3):451–8.
14. Johnson PM, O'Connor BI, Cohen Z, McLeod RS. Pouch-vaginal fistula after ileal pouch-anal anastomosis: treatment and outcomes. Dis Colon Rectum. 2005;48(6):1249–53.
15. Gajsek U, McArthur DR, Sagar PM. Long-term efficacy of the button fistula plug in the treatment of Ileal pouch-vaginal and Crohn's-related rectovaginal fistulas. Dis Colon Rectum. 2011;54(8):999–1002.
16. Loungnarath R, Dietz DW, Mutch MG, Birnbaum EH, Kodner IJ, Fleshman JW. Fibrin glue treatment of complex anal fistulas has low success rate. Dis Colon Rectum. 2004;47(4):432–6.
17. Wexner SD, Ruiz DE, Genua J, Nogueras JJ, Weiss EG, Zmora O. Gracilis muscle interposition for the treatment of rectourethral, rectovaginal, and pouch-vaginal fistulas: results in 53 patients. Ann Surg. 2008;248(1):39–43.
18. Akbari RP, Madoff RD, Parker SC, Hagerman G, Minami S, Bullard Dunn KM, et al. Anastomotic sinuses after ileoanal pouch construction: incidence, management, and outcome. Dis Colon Rectum. 2009;52:452–5.
19. Nyam DC, Wolff BG, Dozois RR, Pemberton JH, Mathison SM. Does the presence of a pre-ileostomy closure asymptomatic pouch-anastomotic sinus tract affect the success of ileal pouch-anal anastomosis? J Gastrointest Surg. 1997;1:274–7.
20. Swain BT, Ellis CN. Fibrin glue treatment of low rectal and pouch-anal anastomotic sinuses. Dis Colon Rectum. 2004;47:253–5.
21. Ahmed Ali U, Shen B, Remzi FH, Kiran RP. The management of anastomotic pouch sinus after IPAA. Dis Colon Rectum. 2012; 55(5):541–8.
22. Ehsan M, Isler JT, Kimmins MH, Billingham RP. Prevalence and management of prolapse of the ileoanal pouch. Dis Colon Rectum. 2004;47(6):885–8.
23. Kirat HT, Kiran RP, Oncel M, Shen B, Fazio VW, Remzi FH. Management of leak from the tip of the "J" in ileal pouch-anal anastomosis. Dis Colon Rectum. 2011;54(4):454–9.
24. Lian L, Fazio VW, Remzi FH, Shen B, Dietz D, Kiran RP. Outcomes for patients undergoing continent ileostomy after a failed ileal pouch-anal anastomosis. Dis Colon Rectum. 2009;52(8):1409–14; discussion 4414–6.
25. Kiran RP, Kirat HT, Rottoli M, Xhaja X, Remzi FH, Fazio VW. Permanent ostomy after ileoanal pouch failure: pouch in situ or pouch excision? Dis Colon Rectum. 2012;55(1):4–9.

26. Ogunbiyi OA, Korsgen S, Keighley MR. Pouch salvage. Long-term outcome. Dis Colon Rectum. 1997;40:548–52.
27. Dehni N, Remacle G, Dozois RR, Banchini F, Tiret E, Parc R. Salvage reoperation for complications after ileal pouch-anal anastomosis. Br J Surg. 2005;92:748–53.
28. MacLean AR, O'Connor B, Parkes R, Cohen Z, McLeod RS. Reconstructive surgery for failed ileal pouch-anal anastomosis: a viable surgical option with acceptable results. Dis Colon Rectum. 2002;45:880–6.
29. Baixauli J, Delaney CP, Wu JS, Remzi FH, Lavery IC, Fazio VW. Functional outcome and quality of life after repeat ileal pouch-anal anastomosis for complications of ileoanal surgery. Dis Colon Rectum. 2004;47:2–11.
30. Sagar PM, Dozois RR, Wolff BG, Kelly KA. Disconnection, pouch revision and reconnection of the ileal pouch-anal anastomosis. Br J Surg. 1996;83:1401–5.
31. Tekkis PP, Heriot AG, Smith JJ, Das P, Canero A, Nicholls RJ. Long-term results of abdominal salvage surgery following restorative proctocolectomy. Br J Surg. 2006;93:231–7.
32. Fazio VW, Wu JS, Lavery IC. Repeat ileal pouch-anal anastomosis to salvage septic complications of pelvic pouches: clinical outcome and quality of life assessment. Ann Surg. 1998;228:588–97.
33. Remzi FH, Fazio VW, Kirat HT, Wu JS, Lavery IC, Kiran RP. Repeat pouch surgery by the abdominal approach safely salvages failed ileal pelvic pouch. Dis Colon Rectum. 2009;52(2):198–204.

The Failed Anastomosis

18

Nathan Smallwood, Matthew G. Mutch, and James W. Fleshman

Key Points

- Be aware of the propensity for poor perfusion at the splenic flexure, especially during high ligation, and the posterior rectal stump following TME.
- Preventive measures for anastomotic leaks are more likely to be identified preoperative for a right colectomy and intraoperative for left.
- Simplify your decision on whether to perform proximal diversion by answering three questions. What is the risk based upon location? Can the patient tolerate a leak? What are the patient wishes?
- With a leaking anastomosis, proximal diversion many times is just as effective as resection and end ostomy, but with less associated morbidity and risk of permanent stoma.
- Even in the diverted patient, inadequate treatment of a leak can lead to chronic pelvic sepsis causing increased morbidity and poor long-term anorectal function.
- Most leaks can be managed with a minimally invasive approach and an ostomy avoided.

The Healing Anastomosis

As we explore the causes of anastomotic failure and ways to prevent and manage the failure, it is important to have a thorough understanding of the normal healing process. With this fundamental knowledge, we can better understand how our operations positively and negatively alter the natural process of anastomotic healing.

The Anatomical Perspective

Key Concept: One of the fundamental principles of a healthy anastomosis is understanding bowel wall anatomy, and while the submucosa provides "strength," each layer impacts outcomes for both stapled and hand-sewn anastomoses.

There are specific characteristics of each layer of the intestinal wall that have a profound influence on an anastomosis. In 1887, Halsted revealed that the submucosa provided the strength for a sutured anastomosis. This concept, though simple today, was revolutionary and had a dramatic impact on the success of intestinal anastomoses. In fact, anastomotic failures were so common in 1887 that the advisability of performing a bowel anastomosis was in question [1].

Mucosa

The innermost layer of the colon, the mucosa, consists of an epithelial layer composed of columnar absorptive epithelium and mucin cells intermixed with openings from mucosal crypts. At the base of these crypts are pluripotent stem cells that give rise to epithelial cells, which migrate towards the lumen. The lamina propria is situated between the inner mucosa and outer muscularis propria and contains much of the immune cells of the colon along with loose connective tissue and capillaries. The connective tissue of the lamina propria does not provide any strength to the intestinal anastomosis [2]. Lymphatic vessels are located just inside a thin

N. Smallwood, MD
Department of Surgery, Baylor University Medical Center, 3500 Gaston Ave., Dallas, TX 75246, USA
e-mail: cottonsmallwood@yahoo.com

M.G. Mutch, MD
Department of Surgery, Section of Colon and Rectal Surgery, Washington University School of Medicine, 660 South Euclid Ave Campus, 8109, St. Louis, MO, USA
e-mail: mutchm@wustl.edu

J.W. Fleshman, MD (✉)
Department of Surgery, Baylor University Medical Center, 3500 Gaston Ave., Dallas, TX 75246, USA
e-mail: james.fleshman@baylorhealth.edu

S.R. Steele et al. (eds.), *Complexities in Colorectal Surgery*,
DOI 10.1007/978-1-4614-9022-7_18, © Springer Science+Business Media New York 2014

layer of smooth muscle called the muscularis mucosa. This smooth muscle layer can undergo isolated thickening in cases of diverticular disease [3]. Apposition of the mucosa is an important part of anastomotic healing and allows for the normal reparative process to occur much more quickly. An intact mucosa is important in providing a barrier to bacteria and other intestinal contents [2].

Submucosa

This is the most important layer of the intestinal wall for the surgeon. This layer contains the bulk of all collagen found in the intestinal wall and consists of predominantly type I collagen, with lesser amounts of type III and V [3]. This layer provides most of the tensile strength and is the anchor for holding sutures [4]. The strength is dependent on both the amount of collagen and the degree of cross-linking [3]. Cross-linking of collagen is dependent on adequate oxygen tension. Tissues with a PO_2 less than 40 mmHg are unable to form mature collagen [5, 6]. The blood supply of the bowel terminates in the submucosa and spreads out in a fine mesh of capillaries critical in the delivery of oxygen and nutrients to the overlying mucosa.

Muscularis Propria

The muscle of the muscularis propria is separated into an inner circular muscle and an outer longitudinal muscle. The muscles function primarily for peristalsis. Even though this layer has some collagen content, it does not provide much additional strength to the anastomosis. In the chronic obstructive state, the collagen content can significantly increase along with the thickness of the hypertrophied muscular layers and the overall wall thickness [7]. In diverticulosis both layers of muscle are abnormal. The outer longitudinal layer becomes thickened due to an increase in elastic fibers, resulting in relative bowel shortening [8]. The inner circular layer thickness increases due to its chronic contractile state and not necessarily from hypertrophy [3]. Edema tends to separate the muscle bundles and weaken this layer. The pathophysiologic changes in diverticular disease and in chronic obstruction can set the stage for anastomotic failure if the anastomosis contains any part of this diseased portion, a largely preventable situation with adequate resection.

Serosa

This outermost very thin layer composed of mesothelial cells, blood vessels, and lymphatics is most useful in sealing the anastomosis. This is underscored by the fact that deserosalized areas of the intestine are at higher risk of a leak [2]. Direct apposition of this layer is therefore very important in order to promote sealing of the anastomosis [9]. Small subclinical leaks may occur even in the "perfect" stapled anastomosis; yet, adhesions on the serosal surface at the stapled anastomosis may function to seal the anastomosis by providing serosal gap coverage.

The layers of the intestine are made up of both solid and liquid elements and can be referred to as biphasic. This principle is important in a stapled anastomosis because pressure applied to the intestinal wall displaces the liquid component, resulting in compression and elongation of the solid component, which is known as tissue creep. Compression applied too rapidly results in shear stress. Optimal stapling consists of allowing adequate time for tissue compression and creep while not producing excessive tensile stress [10]. It is therefore important to know the appropriate staple height and compression time for a specific wall thickness during stapled anastomosis. Sutured anastomoses also require consideration of this principle since suture depth (ideally in the submucosa) varies with intestinal wall thickness and water content. Compression with knot tying can produce tissue tears or fracture.

The Physiologic Perspective

Key Concept: Wound healing at the anastomosis follows a set pattern similar to other parts of the body.

The GI tract undergoes the process of healing through an orderly and regulated series of steps designed first to establish an immune barrier and second to repair the injured area [5]. These series of steps have been traditionally broken down into three periods. The phases of inflammation, proliferation, and remodeling are as applicable to the GI tract as they are to healing in the skin and other tissues.

Inflammatory Phase

The inflammatory phase, referred to as the lag phase, begins with an initial hemostatic response and vasoconstriction. Following this, vasodilation allows for the influx and diapedesis of neutrophils. Neutrophils are the predominant cell within the first 24 h [2]. The primary role of the neutrophil is to decrease the bacterial burden of the wound. After the first 48 h, macrophages begin to populate the wound and release specific growth factors, such as platelet-derived growth factor, which allow further progression of the repair [5]. It is also during this period that a fibrin seal is formed at the serosal layer allowing for a watertight seal. The clinical significance of this is emphasized by the fact that parts of the GI tract without the intact serosal layer have a higher incidence of anastomotic leaks [2].

Proliferative Phase

Influx of fibroblasts and the appearance of granulation tissue mark the beginning of the proliferative phase. The function of fibroblasts during this phase is highly dependent on certain factors such as fibroblast growth factor and transforming growth factor beta. Both collagen synthesis and degradation take place during this period. Collagen breakdown is greater than synthesis in the first few days (Fig. 18.1). The risk of an anastomotic leak is highest during the first 3 days. Studies have shown that bursting strength (the amount of intraluminal pressure measured in mmHg needed for anastomotic disruption) is lovest in this time frame [2, 5]. It is at this time the strength of the anastomosis is entirely dependent on the mechanical strength of the suture or staple relationship with the adjacent uninjured intestinal wall. This initial loss in wound strength is much less pronounced in the small intestine. Collagen synthesis begins earlier and to a greater degree in the small intestine as compared to the colon [2]. This difference could explain the higher leak rate in colonic anastomosis (0.9 % vs. 2.4 %) compared to enteric [11].

Remodeling

The provisional matrix previously formed is remodeled into a stronger thinner area with fibroblast proliferation and transition in collagen formation from type III to type I [2]. This is the time period in which fibroblast-mediated wound contraction occurs. It has been suggested that fibrosis occurs because of reorganization of granulation tissue into scar that is likely more pronounced in more ischemic tissue. An increase in ischemic tissue is one possible explanation for the higher incidence of stenosis seen with stapled anastomosis compared to hand sutured [2, 12].

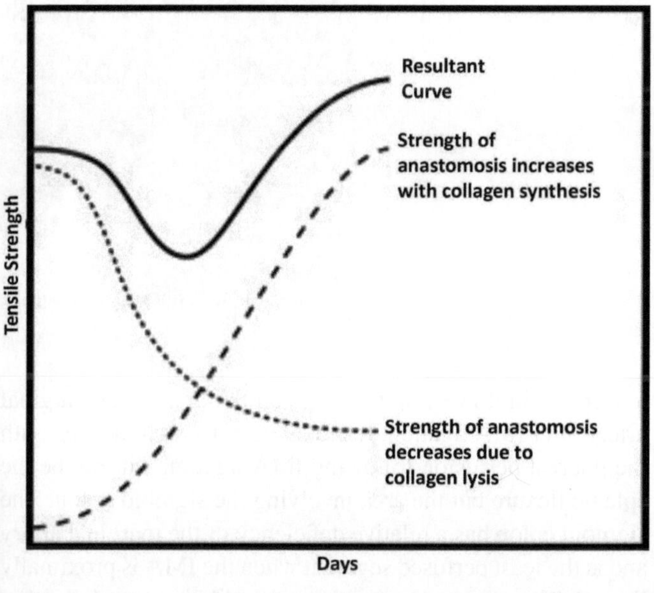

Fig. 18.1 The contribution of anastomotic collagen synthesis and lysis to overall anastomotic strength (With permission from Munireddy et al. [2])

Failed Anastomotic Healing

The healing of the gastrointestinal anastomosis is a timely and orderly process which occurs successfully the majority of the time. Failure of this process is caused by local or systemic factors that interrupt the "timely recovery of the injured tissue's mechanical integrity [13]." Tissue perfusion is a major factor that affects healing locally.

Tissue Perfusion

Key Concept: Macro- and microvascular blood flow provide the necessary factors to enable anastomotic healing. Avoid using the sigmoid colon, when possible, and fully mobilize the splenic flexure to provide a tension-free low colorectal anastomosis.

For the normal healing process of an anastomosis to take place, it must have ample tissue perfusion to deliver the influx of inflammatory cells, growth factors, and oxygen. Ample tissue perfusion of a healing anastomosis is determined by the macrovascular and microvascular anatomy as well as the arterial tissue oxygen saturation [5].

Macrovascular Anatomy

The mucosa, which receives two-thirds of the blood supply of the colon [14], is extremely sensitive to reducing blood flow. This leads to ischemia that can rapidly become transmural and irreversible. In addition, reperfusion of ischemic bowel can cause further tissue damage that extends beyond the boundaries of the previous injury. The vasculature of the colon and rectum, along with the multiple variations that exist, is well known to the surgeon. This knowledge is a necessity in order to perform a safe and successful oncologic resection, but for the purpose of the intestinal anastomosis and why it fails, it is far more instructive to focus on the specific areas of relative vascular insufficiency. These areas of vascular insufficiency can be congenital or specifically result from surgical resection. Below are the notable areas of concern.

Griffiths' Point

J. D. Griffiths described a "critical point" that exists at the splenic flexure where the marginal artery is often diminished. The marginal artery in this area is dependent on the left branch of the middle colic and branches of the ascending left colic artery to provide blood flow [15]. Indeed Griffiths' point

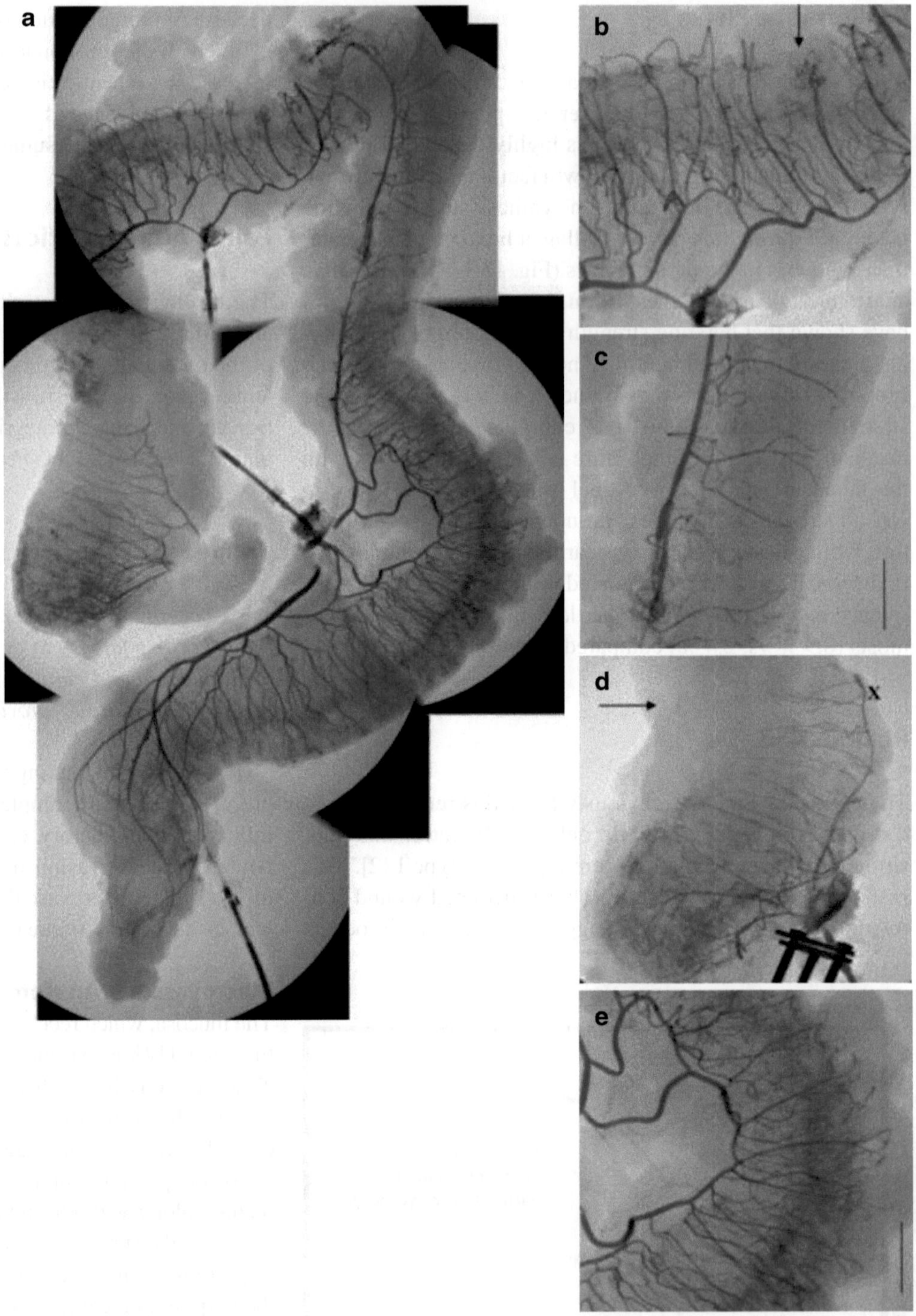

Fig. 18.2 Images (**a–e**) are angiographs taken of the entire colon and rectum. (**a**) Combined angiographic images of the colon and rectum. (**b**) Transverse colon. (**c**) Descending colon. In this portion of the descending colon, there is wide interspacing between vasa recta with relative absence of collaterals at the antimesenteric border. This is in comparison to the transverse and right colon (With permission from Allison et al. [15]). *Arrow* indicates point of ischemia in (**b, d**)

is one of the "water shed" areas that develops poor perfusion during systemic hypotension. This area of the splenic flexure, as well as the proximal and mid-descending colon, has also been shown to contain more widely spaced and infrequent vasa recta compared to more frequent and one centimeter apart spacing seen in other areas of the colon [15] (Fig. 18.2). Griffiths, along with other surgeons, has recommended that the branches of the left colic artery be preserved when ligating the inferior mesenteric artery (IMA) during a sigmoid or rectal resection [16]. The actual significance of left colic preservation remains to be proven at this time. It is clear that a decrease in flow of up to 50 % can be seen in the marginal artery after IMA ligation. It should be noted that the area with the poorest perfusion following IMA ligation will not be the splenic flexure but the area involving the sigmoid colon. The sigmoid colon has a relative deficiency of the marginal artery and is the least perfused segment when the IMA is proximally ligated. Therefore, as long as the sigmoid is resected, ligation of the IMA proximal to the left colonic branch (high ligation) should not result in colonic ischemia [15, 17].

Additionally, the marginal artery of Drummond may not exist or be patent in a significant number of patients.

The lack of blood flow to the left colon, via the marginal artery from the left middle colic artery, results in ischemia of the entire left colon after high ligation of the IMA at the aorta. This will be immediately apparent and should result in a change in plan to use more proximal colon for a colorectal anastomosis. It is the author's opinion that during a low anterior resection, the descending colon should be used as the proximal end of the anastomosis to the rectum and the splenic flexure should be routinely mobilized. In general, high ligation seems safe and potentially provides an oncological benefit, though one exception should be noted. Elderly males were shown in one study to have a much more reduced blood flow within the descending colon following high ligation than females. This is thought to be due to atherosclerotic changes. Men are known to have earlier development and more severe atherosclerotic lesions than do women [17]. The average age of a man with newly diagnosed colon and rectal cancer is 69, and therefore, most men with colon and rectal cancer are at risk of atherosclerotic lesions. This could explain why the male gender has been previously shown to be a risk factor for anastomotic leaks in low colorectal anastomosis. Elderly males undergoing a low anterior resection who have evidence of significant atherosclerosis could potentially benefit from a more distal ligation of the IMA in order to preserve the LCA and adequate distal perfusion. Intraoperative evaluation of perfusion could be of use in this subset of patients.

Sudeck's Point

This area is described as the point between the last sigmoidal branch and the left branch of the superior rectal artery [17]. Its main relevance has been seen in episodes of intestinal ischemia, commonly after abdominal aortic aneurysm repair and IMA ligation. However, this area may also be of significance if the majority of the sigmoid remains and is used in the anastomosis following rectal resections. It is therefore important to avoid using the sigmoid for the anastomosis for multiple reasons.

Rectal Stump

The rectum has been traditionally viewed as having a robust blood supply with a rich network of collaterals. This is based on the clinical finding that the rectum, as opposed to the colon, is very rarely involved in clinical episodes of intestinal ischemia. In reality, the distal rectum does not seem to have this robust blood supply nor the same degree of resistance to ischemia, following a low anterior resection (LAR). This observation was first described by Goligher in 1949. More recently Allison et al. [15] performed angiography of resected specimens' specific reasons for this phenomenon (Fig. 18.3). They observed that the upper rectum had an adequate network of collateral vessels based upon the superior rectal artery. In contrast, the lower rectum had a much poorer collateral network that mainly consisted of intramural vessels. Prior to the LAR, the blood flow from the rectum would preferentially travel down the posterior left and right branches of the superior rectal artery to end in the mesentery or rectal wall. The anterior left and right branches were the only vessels seen to give direct collaterals to the middle and inferior rectal arteries. Following LAR, the rectal stump is dependent upon flow from the middle and inferior rectal arteries. Angiography performed on the rectal stump using the middle rectal artery (Fig. 18.3) retrograde showed blood flow only through the anterior branch of the superior rectal artery. The posterior rectum was shown to be dependent upon a variable amount of intramural collaterals between the anterior and posterior branches. This results in a poorly perfused posterior-inferior rectal stump, and is likely why it is not too uncommon for leaks to occur at the posterior aspect of the anastomosis [15]. Another report did not show decreased perfusion specifically in the posterior-inferior rectum, but the rectal stump had a greater reduction in blood flow as compared to the proximal end [18]. In addition they found significantly more leaks in those patients where there was a blood flow reduction of 16 % or greater [18].

Microvascular Anatomy

Small vessel collaterals can be of significance at specific locations of the colon and rectum. Just as a decrease in the number of these collaterals can affect local tissue perfusion, local vasomotor control over these collaterals can also have a profound effect. This is most profound when splanchnic vasoconstriction occurs in the setting of blood loss and hypotension, as well as increased sympathetic activity, and can dramatically impact the healing anastomosis.

Arterial Oxygen Tension

As humans we are obligate aerobes. In addition to aerobic metabolism, oxygen is needed in collagen synthesis; however, when the oxygen tension drops below 40 mmHg, collagen synthesis ceases [5]. The amount of oxygen that is delivered to the tissues is dependent upon a multitude of factors that includes cardiac output, local vascular resistance, and hemoglobin content. Both cardiac output and local vascular resistance have a more profound impact on tissue oxygenation than hemoglobin as only a mere half of all oxygen-carrying hemoglobin is needed at any point in time for aerobic metabolism [19]. As such, anemia in and of itself is less likely a major contributing risk factor of anastomotic leaks.

Summary Pearl

Currently the list of identified risk factors for anastomotic leaks is extensive, and their exact relationship to, and significance in, anastomotic leaks is hard to define. You are therefore faced with a complex array of risk factors, all

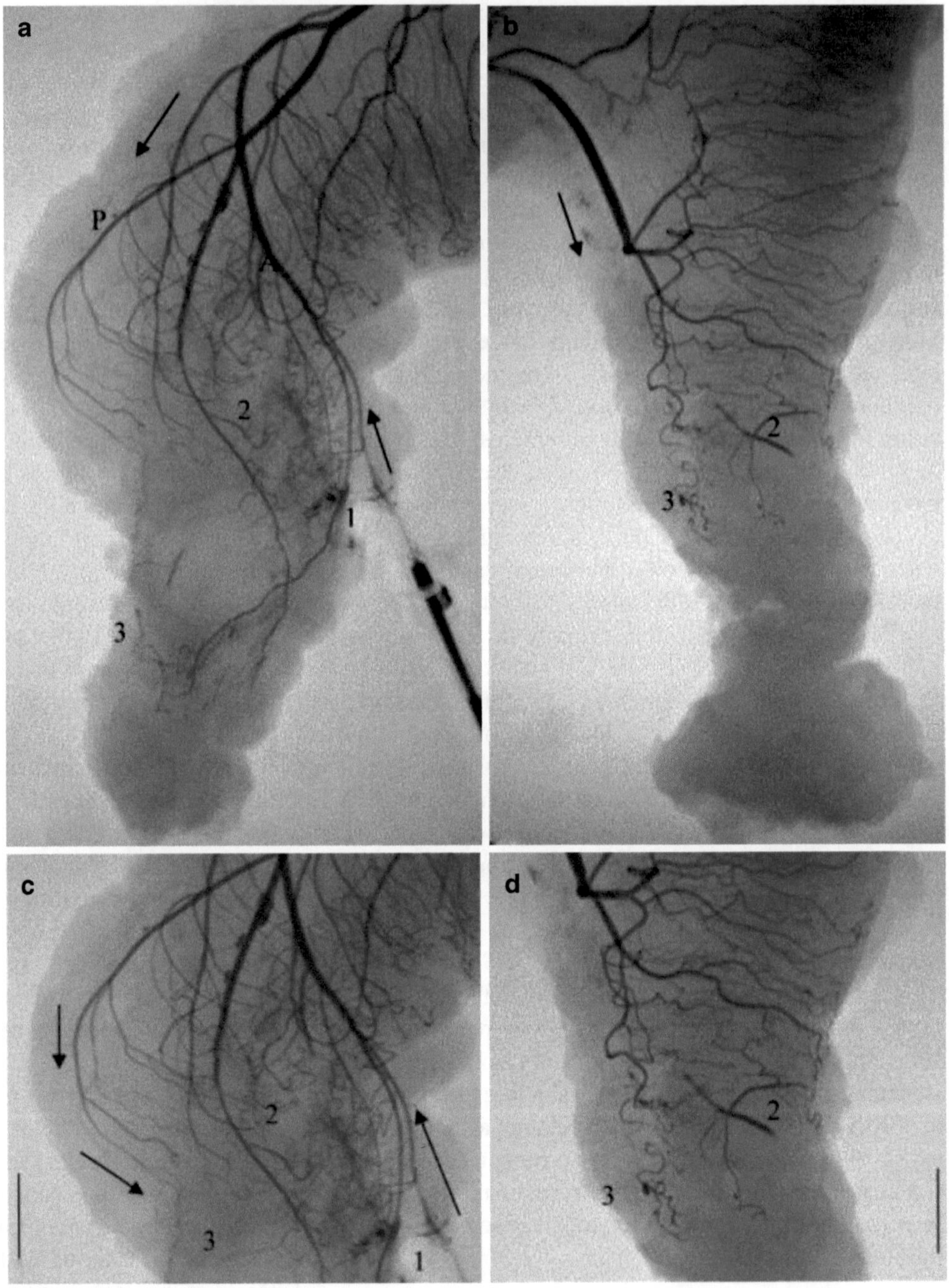

Fig. 18.3 The superior rectal artery (SRA) divides into a right and left branch in the upper mesorectum. Both the right and left branch give off smaller anterior and posterior arteries that supply the rectum. Only the anterior branches communicate directly with the middle rectal artery (With permission from Allison et al. [15]). (**a**) Injection through middle rectal artery. After rectal resection and sacrifice of the SRA, blood preferentially flows down the anterior branches (**a**) to the bifurcation point in the upper mesorectum. Blood then travels antegrade down the posterior branches (*P*) to the posterior portion of the rectum. (**b**–**d**) Rectal resections distal to the SRA bifurcation prevent direct flow from the anterior branches (1) to the posterior branches. Instead, the posterior rectum must rely on small vessel intramural collaterals (2) and inferior collaterals of the posterior branches (3) *Arrows* indicates blood flow

with varying degrees of importance, affecting to some degree one or more components of anastomotic healing, and you must decide which one is at play in a particular patient.

Risk Factors

Key Concept: *Risk factors for anastomotic leak fall into the three broad categories*: *patient-related, location-related, and intraoperative factors. Knowledge of such risk factors should ultimately provide the basis of future preventive techniques while currently highlighting those patients in whom proximal diversion may be warranted.*

Patient-Related

Key Concept: *Certain inherent risk factors are present with every operation, though identifying and targeting modifiable risk factors, when possible, may mitigate the development of leaks.*

Weakly associated patient-related risk factors include age, tobacco and alcohol use, and obesity [20]. Obesity is not felt to be a risk factor at all in right-sided resections; however, there tends to be a more significant association with rectal resections [21]. A combination of risk factors may yield even more significance. This is likely why a higher American Society of Anesthesia (ASA) classification (usually scores of 3 or more) is one of the more consistently found risk factors for leak [20]. Likewise, patients with Charleston Comorbidity Index scores of 3 or more have also been found to have significantly higher anastomotic leaks [17]. These and other types of scoring systems might be more useful indicators of a patient's risk of anastomotic leak.

Poor Nutritional Status

Key Concept: Nutrition is a potentially modifiable risk factor that can often be improved prior to surgery. Its impact on anastomotic leak is somewhat variable, but poor nutrition is commonly associated with higher rates of leak, specifically for right-sided resections.

Certain preventive measures can be taken even before the operation is begun to reduce the risk for leak, primarily in the elective setting. Wexner suggests that these preventive measures are more commonly encountered preoperatively in a right colectomy and intraoperatively in a left colectomy [22]. This statement has been further validated by other studies, including one multicenter prospective trial [23]. Identifying those patients who are of poor nutritional status and treating them preoperatively may reduce the risk for and the morbidity and mortality from anastomotic leaks [23]. Generally, poor nutritional status has been defined in the literature as weight loss ≥10 %, serum albumin <3.5, and serum proteins <5.5 g/dL [24–27]. It is important to define what level of severity of malnutrition requires preoperative nutritional support. Most studies have used a weight loss of ≥10 % to define malnutrition [28]. However, according to Jie et al., this only represents the cutoff value for which complications are seen to increase [28]. The nutritional risk score (NRS) may be a better indicator of severe malnutrition for which preoperative nutrition is indicated. Parameters which are used in the NRS include weight loss in the last 3 months, decrease in food intake, body mass index, severity of disease, and age. Thus, a 65-year-old patient with colon cancer who has greater than 15 % weight loss in the last 3 months and needs a right colectomy would have a score of 5. With this scoring system, Jie found that in those patients with a NRS ≥5 and a lower GI resection, preoperative nutrition decreased the complication rate from 45 % in the control group to 27 % in those patients with preoperative nutrition [28]. An in-depth discussion regarding the impact of nutritional support can be found in Chap. 3 by Dr. Maykel.

Immunosuppression

Key Concept: Patients with malignancy and inflammatory bowel disease often require surgical resection and are commonly immunosuppressed or taking immunosuppression agents preoperatively. You need to have a thorough understanding of how this can impact postoperative morbidity including anastomotic leaks.

Steroids

Corticosteroids decrease the activation and infiltration of inflammatory cells into wounds along with inhibiting certain growth factors that are necessary for collagen synthesis [29]. Intuitively it would seem that corticosteroids impair anastomotic healing; however, their exact effect on anastomotic leaks is less clear. Multiple studies have shown no increased risk with preoperative steroid use [30–34]. These studies are mainly retrospective and include patients with variable dose and duration of steroid usage and type of operation performed. A more recent prospective study found that both long-term and perioperative usage are associated with a higher risk of anastomotic leakage [35]. Steroids have also been shown to increase the rates of wound infections and septic complications [36, 37]. If possible steroids should be weaned preoperatively, and you should more readily consider proximal diversion (especially in the case of a rectal anastomosis).

Infliximab, AZA, 6-MP

There does not seem to be an association with anastomotic leaks or other postoperative complications with the use of infliximab, though this is controversial. This holds even when infliximab is used in combination with azathioprine or 6-mercaptopurine [32, 36]. There does not seem to be any benefit in stopping these medications preoperatively or delaying surgery in Crohn's patients. However, infliximab has been shown to negatively impact outcomes after operations for ulcerative colitis [38].

Crohn's Disease

Key Concept: In addition to the pathophysiology of the disease itself, the Crohn's patient is likely to present with other risk factors for anastomotic leaks including preoperative malnutrition and immunosuppressive medication use.

Multiple studies have shown a high risk of intra-abdominal septic complications in patients with Crohn's disease [39, 40]. Other risk factors which are much more specific to Crohn's disease include a hand-sewn anastomosis, end-to-end anastomoses, histologic positive margins, penetrating-type disease, and the need for sigmoid resection [20, 30, 34, 41]. We recommend stapled side-to-side anastomoses when performing an ileocolostomy and to highly consider performing proximal diversion in cases where both small bowel and sigmoid resections are needed. Grossly histologic negative margins are almost impossible to achieve in a patient with Crohn's disease without causing unnecessary bowel resection. A grossly negative margin, as indicated by the soft, thin mesentery at the point of resection, is adequate.

Radiation

Key Concept: Radiation alone may not increase the risk of leak, and does not mandate the need for diversion, typically, unless when combined with chemotherapy.

Neoadjuvant radiotherapy in the pelvis may result in increased risk of anastomotic leak; however, this belief has not been definitively established in the literature [42]. A study that looked at 1,338 patients with rectal cancer over a 30-year period was unable to find any significant association between neoadjuvant radiotherapy and anastomotic leaks. Other factors such as location and size of tumor were found to be of more significance. This has been confirmed in other reports, including a fairly large randomized trial [43]. There is no need for routine diversion in patients who have received neoadjuvant radiotherapy alone. If chemotherapy is added to the radiation, a higher risk is likely, and a diverting stoma is recommended. As will be further discussed later, proximal diversion does not prevent a leak but reduces its impact.

Diverticulitis and Emergency Surgery

Key Concept: Although emergent surgery is a well-known risk factor for complications, diverticulitis may be an independent risk factor for anastomotic leak.

Diverticulitis and emergency operations have previously been identified as risk factors for anastomotic leaks [44–47]. Emergency operations are at an increased risk of postoperative complications in general, which include wound infections, intra-abdominal abscesses, anastomotic leak, wound dehiscence, and mortality [44]. In addition, other risk factors such as the disease process itself, location of the anastomosis to be performed, and condition of the patient play a role in the development of a leak. Diverticulitis commonly involves some of these same factors but may be an independent risk factor for leak, even in nonemergent conditions. This increased risk may be due to persistent inflammation or unresolved abscesses at the time of the operation and decreased anastomotic strength due to an increase in wall thickness secondary to muscular hypertrophy and an inappropriate selection of staple height [23]. One preventable risk factor for leak is avoiding any retained sigmoid on the rectal stump. An anastomosis between the left colon and soft rectum is essential to cure diverticulitis and prevent an anastomotic leak.

Peritonitis

It is a commonly held belief that an anastomosis created in the setting of peritonitis will be at increased risk of anastomotic dehiscence [48, 49]. However, previous animal studies and other clinical studies have failed to show any increase in risk of leaks in the setting of peritonitis [49, 50]. There may be a difference between purulent versus fecal peritonitis (e.g., Hinchey III vs. IV) and the risk of leak, as previously reported by Biondo and colleagues [50]. In a follow-up study, they were able to perform a primary resection and anastomosis with a respectable 5.7 % leak rate without the use of proximal diversion in patients with purulent peritonitis. They excluded those with fecal peritonitis, as well as ASA IV, and unstable or immunocompromised patients. Of the remaining 208 patients, 50 % of the patients had peritonitis, of which half of these had diffuse peritonitis. Peritonitis was not found to be an independently associated risk factor for anastomotic leaks [47]. At present it does not appear that purulent peritonitis alone is a risk factor for anastomotic leak [47, 50–52].

"Loaded Colon"

One of the reasons why emergency surgery is felt to be associated with higher leaks is that these operations are performed on the unprepped colon. The "loaded colon" has been reported to have up to a threefold increase in anastomotic leaks [53]. This is contradictory to the most recent studies on mechanical bowel preparation that have concluded that it can be safely omitted. Methods such as intraoperative colonic lavage have been shown to have a positive effect on anastomotic integrity and collagen metabolism and can allow for a primary anastomosis to be performed without diversion in emergency operations for colonic obstruction [49, 54]. Until additional evidence to the contrary emerges, it is recommended that colonic lavage be performed when distal colon and rectal anastomoses are created in the "loaded colon." In contrast, elective operations to remove the left colon or rectum can be safely performed with only enemas (without a complete bowel preparation) to empty the stool.

Hemodynamic Instability

Since the healing anastomosis is extremely dependent upon adequate perfusion, episodes of hypotension, and especially those requiring vasopressors, should be an absolute indication for preventive measures. In fact, shock was one of the only two risk factors for which proximal diversion would be needed, according to an AAST multicenter trial, in the cases of traumatic injuries to the colon [55].

In the majority of emergency or diverticular operations—in the absence of either fecal peritonitis or shock—a primary resection and anastomosis can be performed safely. Lower rates of anastomotic leak, re-interventions, and other wound infections are seen with proximal diversion when other risk factors are present. As previously stated, intraoperative lavage is recommended for emergency resections involving the impacted left colon to allow primary anastomosis [20].

Location

The site of the anastomosis has been the most consistent and significant risk factor for anastomotic leak [56]. The further distal an anastomosis is created, the higher the risk of leak. An ileocolic anastomosis has a leak rate of 2–3 % compared to a 10–17 % leak rate in coloanal anastomosis. Even in rectal anastomoses, a significant difference can be seen the closer the staple line gets to the anal verge [56]. The highest risk of anastomotic leak can be seen for anastomoses at and below 5–8 cm from the anal verge [23].

There are several proposed reasons for the difference in leak rates between proximal and distal locations including:

1. *Increasing amount of intraluminal bacteria from proximal to distal colon* [23]
2. *Absence of peritoneal cover in distal rectum* [23]
3. *Compromised vascularity to distal rectal stump especially posterior* [23]
4. *Increased intraluminal pressure of rectum during a closed anal sphincter and defecation*

Obesity and Male Gender

Key Concept: These two risk factors for leak are primarily seen in association with a low rectal anastomosis.

Obesity is known to be a risk factor for postoperative wound infections, prolonged open operations for rectal resection, and conversion from laparoscopic to open [57]. While obesity is variably associated with anastomotic leakage, there is considerable evidence that obesity affects the leak rate for low rectal anastomoses. In several studies, obesity has been shown to be the strongest risk factor for the development of a leak [21, 58, 59]. Additionally, the male gender is mainly found as a risk factor for problems with low rectal anastomosis and usually is not found to be significant for more proximal anastomoses [23, 60–62]. Both obesity and male gender, and more specifically the deep narrow male pelvis, can make low rectal operations significantly more difficult. Men also may be at increased risk of poor anastomotic perfusion. It is known that men can have altered intestinal microcirculation in response to hormones and are at an increased risk of advanced atherosclerosis compared to women [63].

Operative Risk Factors

Key Concept: There is no method of intestinal anastomosis that is leak free. Although you have a somewhat limited ability to prevent anastomotic leaks, your performance at the time of the operation can have a major influence.

Blood Loss, Transfusions, and Operative Time

Key Concept: One way you can reduce the risk of anastomotic failure during the operation is by limiting intraoperative blood loss and the time it takes to perform the operation.

While both of these parameters have been confirmed to decrease leak rate on multivariate analysis [64, 65], the actual significance is not completely clear, as this has not been uniform across the literature [66, 67]. Furthermore, the actual amount of blood loss or duration of operation that matters is much less clear. Operative times found to be of significance ranged from 120 to 270 min [17, 24, 66, 67], while meaningful operative blood loss has been defined as that which requires blood transfusion—a highly variable definition [17]. What seems clearer is that increased operative time leads to more exposure of the patient to tissue trauma and bacteria [25] and correlates with hypothermia in most patients. Primary hypothermia correlates with increased infectious complications and hospital length of stay [68]. Even more, increased operative times and greater amounts of blood loss are surrogate markers for the degree of difficulty of the surgery. You must be mindful of these objective indicators of a more difficult operation in order to accurately decide whether or not to perform proximal diversion. While occasionally viewed as a "failure," it is never wrong to err on the side of diversion.

Intraoperative Complications

Key Concept: Adverse events during the operation, even if not directly involving the anastomosis, can increase the risk of anastomotic leak.

Trencheva et al. defined an intraoperative complication as injury to the bowel, other organs, or blood vessels. In addition, stapling device malfunction, hypotension, oxygen saturation less than 90 % for more than 5 min, pH less than 7.3, and even blood loss requiring intraoperative blood transfusion were also classified as an intraoperative complication. In their series, any patient with an intraoperative complication was four times as likely to have an anastomotic leak [17]. On one hand, this may again be a surrogate for a more difficult operation. More appropriately, this highlights the degree of interconnectivity among all aspects of an operation and the impact one problem can have on another.

Total Mesorectal Excision (TME)

Key Concept: Although oncologically sound, TME results in a lower anastomosis and the potential for loss of blood supply that may increase the leak rate.

During the widespread adoption of total mesorectal excision, there was a substantial rise in leak rates from the previously reported 9 to ~23 % [69]. Over the next 4 years following this initial study, the leak rate eventually did return to the level seen before TME [69]. A study looking at laparoscopic resections showed that the addition of TME more than doubled the leak rate for upper rectal cancer [67]. TME for high rectal cancer may result in insufficient blood supply to the posterior portion of the proximal rectum, which is further evidenced by the fact that tumor-specific mesorectal excisions have lower rates of anastomotic leaks [15, 70].

Tension and Splenic Flexure Mobilization

Key Concept: Avoiding tension has been classically viewed as one of the fundamental principles of a healing anastomosis and remains a significant preventative measure in reducing anastomotic leak.

The colon seems to be especially effected by applied tension, even more so than the small intestine. Blood flow did not return to preoperative levels until the seventh postoperative day following experimentally applied tension in animal studies [71]. Mobilization of the splenic flexure has commonly been used to decrease tension in the rectal anastomosis. Karanja et al. found a 9 % leak rate with splenic flexure mobilization compared to 22 % without mobilization [72]. Additional evidence supporting its actual significance is limited. The anastomosis is subjected to other sources of tension during peristalsis and defecation that result in radial tension for which splenic flexure mobilization would seem to provide less benefit. The major importance in splenic flexure mobilization may ultimately be improved blood supply of the descending colon (rather than the sigmoid) when used for the colorectal anastomosis.

Drains

Key Concept: Drains may be useful in low extraperitoneal anastomosis, but are not typically indicated when the anastomosis is intraperitoneal.

The use of drains has been extensively debated over the last decade, largely because they offer both real and theoretical benefits and risks, yet are only one of many factors that play a role in a proper anastomosis. Furthermore, they are widely variable in their use, type, and rationale for placement. There is extensive evidence that draining an intraperitoneal anastomosis is of no benefit [69]. In the case of gross contamination or abscess at the time of resection, the intraperitoneal anastomosis should be created in a less hostile location and after extensive contamination control. Draining the pelvic anastomosis may be of some benefit. The pelvis does seem to be unique as compared to the abdominal cavity in that fluid is much more likely to accumulate in the most dependent area of the pelvis around the anastomosis and the non-peritonealized pelvic floor fails to absorb fluid efficiently [47, 73]. However, it is unclear how effectively our drains remove this fluid or what impact this has on the healing anastomosis [17, 47, 74]. The other proposed benefit of draining the pelvic anastomosis is detection of an anastomotic leak. On one hand, studies have shown that drains have very poor detection rates and that other clinical signs are more likely to appear before any change in drain effluent [61]. Others have shown some benefit in leak detection where drains detected a leak in 80 % of patients and in 40 % of cases this preceded any other clinical signs [75]. In the most recent meta-analysis, there was not enough sufficient evidence to indicate that drains are able to prevent anastomotic leaks or other anastomotic complications; however, the authors acknowledged the need for more randomized control trials specifically looking at lower rectal anastomosis [66]. It is our practice to use drains selectively in cases where build up of fluid in the pelvis begins during the case despite good hemostasis or after a very bloody operation where every vessel could not have been controlled. In general, we remove the drains once the effluent is less than 15 cc/day or if clear.

Laparoscopy

Key Concept: Laparoscopic approaches with experienced surgeons may result in a decrease in leak rates.

A study using the Nationwide Inpatient Sample population database found a decrease in the rate of anastomotic leak along with a corresponding decrease in wound infection following laparoscopic surgery, despite an increased leak rate with conversion to open surgery [76]. The recently published Danish nationwide cohort study demonstrated an increase risk of leak with minimally invasive approaches; however, this study was performed during the period when the laparoscopic method was first being used [77]. While no definite conclusion can be drawn, this latter study does highlight the potential impact that inexperience can play in leak rates. Interestingly anastomotic leaks have been diagnosed earlier following laparoscopic surgery, and as a result of the primary operation being laparoscopic, laparoscopic management of the leak was possible [67]. A possible cause of low rectal anastomotic leaks in totally laparoscopic cases may be the use of multiple firings of the endoscopic stapler to transect the rectum. Crossing staple lines and poor perfusion always put an anastomosis at risk, regardless of the surgical approach.

Omental Wrapping

Key Concept: *Wrapping the anastomosis with a well-vascularized pedicle of omentum has been associated with decreased leaks in small studies.*

Animal studies have proven the unique ability of the omentum to adhere to and effectively bridge the anastomosis [78, 79] and allow for absorption of fluid [80]. Some have cautioned its use secondary to the likely negative impact in cases where the omental pedicle is devascularized [80]. The most recent meta-analysis found a significant reduction in clinical anastomotic leak only. Issues involving blinding and a small number of patients within each study limited the strength of the conclusion. Omentoplasty should be left up to the surgeon's personal experience.

Simultaneous Liver Resection

Key Concept: *Staged resections may decrease the overall morbidity and leak rate for extensive disease, while simultaneous resection is generally safe in carefully select patients.*

Synchronous liver metastases are present in 23–51 % of newly diagnosed patients [81], and liver resection remains the best option for those patients with resectable disease [82–84]. Staged procedures have been the traditional approach [83]. Most studies evaluating safety and efficacy are retrospective and therefore suffer from selection bias resulting in more extensive liver resections in the group of patients with a staged approach to extensive liver resections [83]. These studies do show that limited liver resections can be performed at the same time as the colon resections with equivalent morbidity and mortality [82–84]. With more extensive liver resections and in those 70 years or older, the morbidity and mortality significantly increase, favoring a staged approach [82]. Age and extensive liver resections seem to be the main factors to consider when deciding upon a staged versus simultaneous resection. Leak is just one of the many causes of postoperative morbidity and mortality. The only study focused on anastomotic leak after simultaneous liver resection showed an operative time greater than 8 h was the most significant risk factor for anastomotic leak regardless of the extent of the liver resection. The majority of leaks occurred with rectal resections (36 % leak rate). Patients with colonic resections were observed to have a 13 % leak rate, but this was still higher than those patients who only underwent a colonic resection [82].

Proximal Diversion

Key Concept: *Understand your goal with diversion, where it is a crucial part to minimizing morbidity and where it can be safely avoided. When you feel you need to proximally divert a patient, it is generally a good idea.*

The effectiveness of proximal diversion, whether a loop colostomy or loop ileostomy, is highly debated. Most studies have focused on whether proximal diversion can prevent anastomotic leak. Some have suggested that proximal diversion does not prevent, but only minimizes the clinical impact of leaks [85]. In a systematic review by Montedori, proximal diversion was found to be useful in preventing both anastomotic leak and the need for urgent reoperations [86]. Proximal diversion also minimizes the clinical impact of leaks by decreasing the leak rate and the need for laparotomy. Unfortunately, there is also added morbidity with proximal diversion. Problems ranging from dehydration and electrolyte abnormalities to mechanical problems can be as high as 30 % [86], resulting in an 18 % readmission rate [87]. In addition, there is a 15–20 % complication rate with ostomy closure [88, 89]. Because of its associated morbidity, proximal diversion should not be routinely performed. The decision for proximal diversion must be carefully weighed against the negative impact of leak and the morbidity of an ostomy. This decision-making process can be simplified by focusing on three key questions.

1. *What is the risk of leak based upon the location of the anastomosis?*

   Extraperitoneal anastomoses and those within 5–8 cm from the anal verge are at the highest risk of a leak and should generally be diverted [23]. Leaks at this level can negatively impact future bowel function and increase the risk of a permanent stoma [90]. The decision to divert more proximal anastomoses should be based upon the presence of other additional risk factors.

2. *Can the patient tolerate a leak?*

   Older patients and those with multiple medical comorbidities should be considered for proximal diversion. These patients typically have very little physiologic reserve to tolerate a leak.

3. *What are the patient wishes?*

   It is important to include the patient in your decision-making. Some patients are adverse to any stoma, temporary or not. Others may be more concerned with the complications from a leak than with having an ostomy. A fully informed patient will be able to better voice their own concerns and be much more satisfied with the eventual outcome. Knowing what the patient wants can simplify intraoperative decision-making.

Mechanical Bowel Preparation (MBP)

Key Concept: MBP does not significantly impact anastomotic leak rates in colon resection, but may decrease complications with rectal resections, and likely should be continued when possible for elective rectal cases.

Multiple studies have concluded that mechanical bowel preparation (MBP) in elective colon resections does not significantly impact anastomotic leaks [91]. The evidence is overwhelmingly in favor of abandoning the use of MBP in colon resections. There is less evidence for the effectiveness of MBP in rectal resections. Some studies have shown that MBP can be safely omitted in rectal resections [92, 93], but most studies have excluded patients with a rectal anastomosis [91]. A multicenter randomized controlled trial showed a higher risk of infectious complications without MBP [94]. They also showed a nonsignificant increase in clinical anastomotic leaks and pelvic sepsis [94]. For now, it would be wise to continue mechanical bowel preparation, when possible, for planned rectal resections.

The results of these studies also do not address some of the other potential benefits of mechanical bowel preparation. A well-prepped bowel allows for:

- Better visualization when intraoperative colonoscopy is needed
- Easier creation, visualization, and leak testing of an anastomosis when using an EEA stapler
- Easier bowel manipulation during laparoscopic surgery

Prevention

Dr. Abbas has questioned whether surgeons should continue to accept the risk of anastomotic leaks [95]. Surgeons have been faced with similar questions in the past. Early surgery for appendicitis was fraught with major difficulties due to poor diagnostic methods and no available methods of antisepsis. This was a time period when abdominal surgery was performed only as a last resort. In 1881, W.A. Byrd stated "I fail to find any recorded cases in which this procedure (laparotomy) has been attempted with success… medicine is useless in these cases except for the production of euthanasia, and surgery cannot even accomplish this." Six years after this statement, a successful appendectomy was performed by Thomas Morton [96]. It is important that we not become complacent but continually strive to break new barriers.

Intraoperative Anastomotic Assessment

Key Concept: Several methods are available for investigating the integrity of the anastomosis. Whatever method you choose, it should be, in general, a routine part of your practice for all left-sided anastomosis.

Laser Fluorescence Angiography

Following injection of fluorescent dye, a mounted camera with an infrared filter is used to view the resected ends or newly created anastomosis. Special software can be used to compare two different areas of perfusion. A study showed that using the IC-View system® (Pulsion Medical System, Munich, Germany) changed the site of resection in 16 % of patients [97]. Other available forms of fluorescence angiography include the Spy Elite® (Lifecell, Bridgewater, NJ) for open surgeries and the Firefly™ used in the DaVinci® Si™ Surgical System Robot (Intuitive Surgical, Sunnyvale, VA).

Intraoperative Air Leak Test

Studies assessing the effectiveness of air leak testing have shown mixed results [98–100], though typically demonstrate usefulness and no downside. In a large retrospective cohort [101], untested anastomoses had twice the rate of clinical leak than those that were tested. Patients who underwent suture repair after a positive air leak test had a clinical leak rate of 12.2 % compared to 3.8 % for patients with a negative air leak test. Patients who underwent anastomotic revision or proximal diversions after a positive air leak test had a 0 % clinical leak rate [101]. This study provides significant evidence for the use of intraoperative leak testing. A diverting ostomy should always be a consideration with positive air leaks.

Intraoperative Endoscopic Assessment

Li et al. [102] looked at the selective versus routine use of endoscopic examination in bowel resections. Endoscopic examination with air leak testing was performed on the pre-resected bowel, the rectal stump, and the post-anastomotic bowel. This study showed a nonsignificant increase in leaks (5.1 % vs. 0.9 %) with selective versus routine endoscopic examination. The endoscope compared to the proctoscope provides better visualization of the anastomosis and likely a better assessment of its integrity.

Intraoperative Dye Test

Using a 22 French Foley, a mixture of sterile water and blue dye is injected intraluminally, while the bowel proximal to the anastomosis is clamped. It takes a volume of 180–240 mL to adequately distend the anastomosis. A study using this method found that the dye test allowed for the easier detection and localization of leaks compared to air leak testing [103].

Intraluminal Devices

Key Concept: These devices are either early in their experience or have not demonstrated a marked benefit to reducing leaks.

Transanal Decompression Devices

These devices are believed to decrease intraluminal pressure by keeping the anal sphincter open. Rectal tubes, usually a Foley catheter, are placed 15 cm above the anastomosis. They provide for both decompression and antibiotic irrigation [104]. There are no comparative studies evaluating the use of rectal tubes. Transanal stents are 4 cm in length and left in place for 5–7 days following insertion [105]. A prospective randomized study in 2006 was prematurely stopped due to an increase in leaks in the stent group [106].

Intraluminal Barriers

Intraluminal barriers prevent the fecal stream from contacting the healing anastomosis. Animal studies have shown that fecal contact negatively impacts the healing [52]. In animal studies, the Coloshield and the Valtrec-Secured Intracolonic Bypass (VIB) have both been very effective in preventing leaks. Leaks were prevented even when an incomplete anastomosis was intentionally created [105]. Both devices are secured proximal to the anastomosis and are spontaneously expelled. Multiple small studies have shown a 0–8.7 % anastomotic leak rate with the use of the Coloshield. These authors claim the Coloshield is a viable alternative to fecal diversion [105, 107]. The VIB device was shown to have an equal rate of leaks in a head to head comparison with a loop ileostomy [108]. The C-seal® (Polyganics Groningen, the Netherlands) is the newest device and can be attached to the bowel proximal to the anastomosis with an EEA stapler. Clinical trials evaluating the C-seal are currently underway.

Compression Anastomosis

A sutureless anastomosis without the associated foreign body has its theorized advantage. It is not a new concept, as the idea dates as far back as 1826—long before Murphy's button [109]. In the largest study to date, there was a 3.2 % anastomotic leak rate among 1,180 elective open and laparoscopic colorectal anastomoses [109]. The authors concluded that the ColonRing device (novoGI Inc, Netanya, Israel) is feasible and safe and could be considered as an alternative to stapled end-end colorectal anastomosis. Further prospective studies directly comparing the two techniques are needed.

Extraluminal Devices

Methods used to bolster the staple line with bioabsorbable Seamguard® (W.L. Gore & Associates, Flagstaff, AZ) or meshed AlloDerm® (Lifecell, Bridgewater, NJ) have not improved the anastomotic strength [110, 111]. Clinical data evaluating the use of such tissue-bolstering devices for the colorectal anastomosis is limited. Staple line reinforcement has not had the same success in the colorectal anastomosis as is seen in the gastric bypass or sleeve, where there primary purpose is reduction in bleeding [112].

Managing the Failed Anastomosis

Key Concept: Any successful management strategy for anastomotic leak that results in reduced morbidity and mortality and improves the quality of life emphasizes early diagnosis and infectious source control through the use of methods that do not increase the risk of permanent stoma or negatively impact future bowel function.

Anastomotic Leaks

Anastomotic leaks account for a quarter of all deaths following colorectal surgery [45]. These mortality rates have changed very little over the last three decades despite the continuing improvements in critical care management. The mortality and morbidity from anastomotic leaks are greatly influenced by the duration of time before a diagnosis is made and the source of infection controlled [45]. Unfortunately many patients will be discharged home before a diagnosis is made, and others will be treated with more conservative therapies, both of which delay definitive therapy and extend the duration of infection and sepsis. Aside from morbidity and mortality, patients with anastomotic leaks can have a significant decrease in their quality of life, which is mainly due to the high rates of a permanent stoma (up to 72 % in some studies), especially when end ostomies are performed instead of proximal diversion [113].

Clinical Manifestations

Key Concept: Symptoms range widely from nonspecific cardiopulmonary and GI complaints to fever and septic shock. Watching for patients who begin to deviate from the standard postoperative course will aid in early diagnosis.

The timeframe in which patients present with anastomotic leaks follows a bimodal distribution, with symptomatic leaks occurring between 7 and 12 days and asymptomatic leaks diagnosed months later, usually during the evaluation for ostomy closure [45, 70]. The typical symptoms of an anastomotic leak include pulmonary, cardiac, and gastrointestinal symptoms that unfortunately are not too different from postoperative symptoms in patients without leaks. Indeed since these symptoms are not specific for an anastomotic leak, patients sometimes are treated by the surgeon for days to weeks before the anastomotic leak is finally diagnosed [114]. While cardiac, pulmonary, or gastrointestinal symptoms (individually) may be fairly nonspecific, there is evidence that the likelihood of an anastomotic leak significantly increases as a patient develops additional symptoms [115]. The return of bowel function has always been an important component in the postoperative management of the colorectal patient. Lack of bowel function beyond 6th postoperative day is highly predictive of an anastomotic leak, but the presence of bowel function alone is a poor negative predictor [115]. Fever and leukocytosis are fairly insensitive during the initial postoperative stay and are unlikely to reach predictive values while the patient is hospitalized [115]. Operatively placed drains can provide clues to the occurrence of a leak, but surgeons must not be completely dependent on them, as even patients with benign appearing drainage can have anastomotic leaks. Peritonitis is an obvious clinical sign but may not be present in diverted patients or those with an extraperitoneal anastomosis. Purulent anal discharge is fairly specific, but can easily go unnoticed by the surgeon or patient. Sometimes patients may not display any one sign or symptom, but simply fail to follow the standard postoperative course or meet discharge requirements. These patients which are "failing to progress" need to be promptly evaluated for an anastomotic leak.

Making a Timely Diagnosis

Key Concept: While several different tests and scoring systems are available to aid in the early diagnosis of leak, the most important factor is the surgeon's clinical awareness and acumen.

The importance of a timely diagnosis was shown in the study by Alves and colleagues [45] where the mortality rate increased from 0 to 18 % if the diagnosis was made after the fifth postoperative day. Leaks can be difficult to diagnose in the early postoperative period because signs and symptoms take time to progress. The use of water-soluble contrast enema or computed tomography is not sensitive enough to be used to screen for leaks. At the present time, there is ongoing research into other methods to accurately predict which patients have an anastomotic leak with the hope that this will prompt an earlier diagnosis. C-reactive protein (CRP) appears to be a very promising marker for anastomotic leaks. Almeida et al. [116] showed that serum CRP levels were elevated in all patients immediately postoperatively on and after the third day in all patients who had leaks. A total of four studies have all shown persistently elevated CRP levels after postoperative days 2–4 in colorectal patients diagnosed with anastomotic leaks [116, 117]. A CRP level of 190 mg/L or more on postoperative day 3 that fails to decrease in the following days is a very accurate predictor of anastomotic leak in colorectal patients [118]. High levels of sensitivity (>95 %) and diagnostic accuracy (88.5 %) were seen in esophageal leaks when using the scoring system, as seen below, based on the postoperative levels of CRP, WBC, and albumin [119].

$$\text{NUnScore} = 11.3894 + (0.005 \times \text{CRP}) + (\text{WCC} \times 0.186) - (0.174 \times \text{albumin})$$

Another scoring system that used 15 different clinical and laboratory parameters decreased the delay in diagnosing anastomotic leaks among colorectal patients [120]. While these studies are promising, the clinical use of these markers and scoring systems has not been widely established. Currently, the surgeon must rely on a heightened sense of awareness to signs and symptoms that, when present, should prompt further workup. Computed tomography with rectal contrast is proven to be better in identifying anastomotic leaks than water-soluble contrast enema and also allows for accurate identification of any abscess that may be amenable to percutaneous drainage [74]. Some surgeons advocate that contrast should be injected down the distal limb of the ostomy as opposed to through the rectum to prevent further disunion of the anastomosis [121]. Some patients will present with peritonitis and/or and septic shock and require an urgent laparotomy before any diagnostic studies can be performed. All efforts should be made to try and evaluate the anastomosis preoperatively, since intraoperative evaluation can be difficult especially when the leak creates an inflammatory mass that surrounds the anastomosis. In cases with no preoperative evaluation, the anastomosis must be grossly inspected during laparotomy and with the endoscope. If there is no evidence of any dehiscence during this inspection, the anastomosis should then be tested for a leak by insufflating air through an endoscope within the anal canal or by injecting Betadine into the rectum via the endoscope. Not all cases of postoperative sepsis are due to a leaky anastomosis, and it is important to correctly identify and control the source of infection to prevent recurrent sepsis. While it is also helpful to identify these cases preoperatively to avoid negative exploratory laparotomy, when there is a strong suspicion, the operating room is almost always the right call (even if no leak is found).

Determining the Appropriate Intervention

Key Concept: There are no guidelines, based upon high levels of scientific evidence, currently available for the surgeon to follow. However, adhering to important principles when faced with this situation will often minimize additional morbidity and mortality.

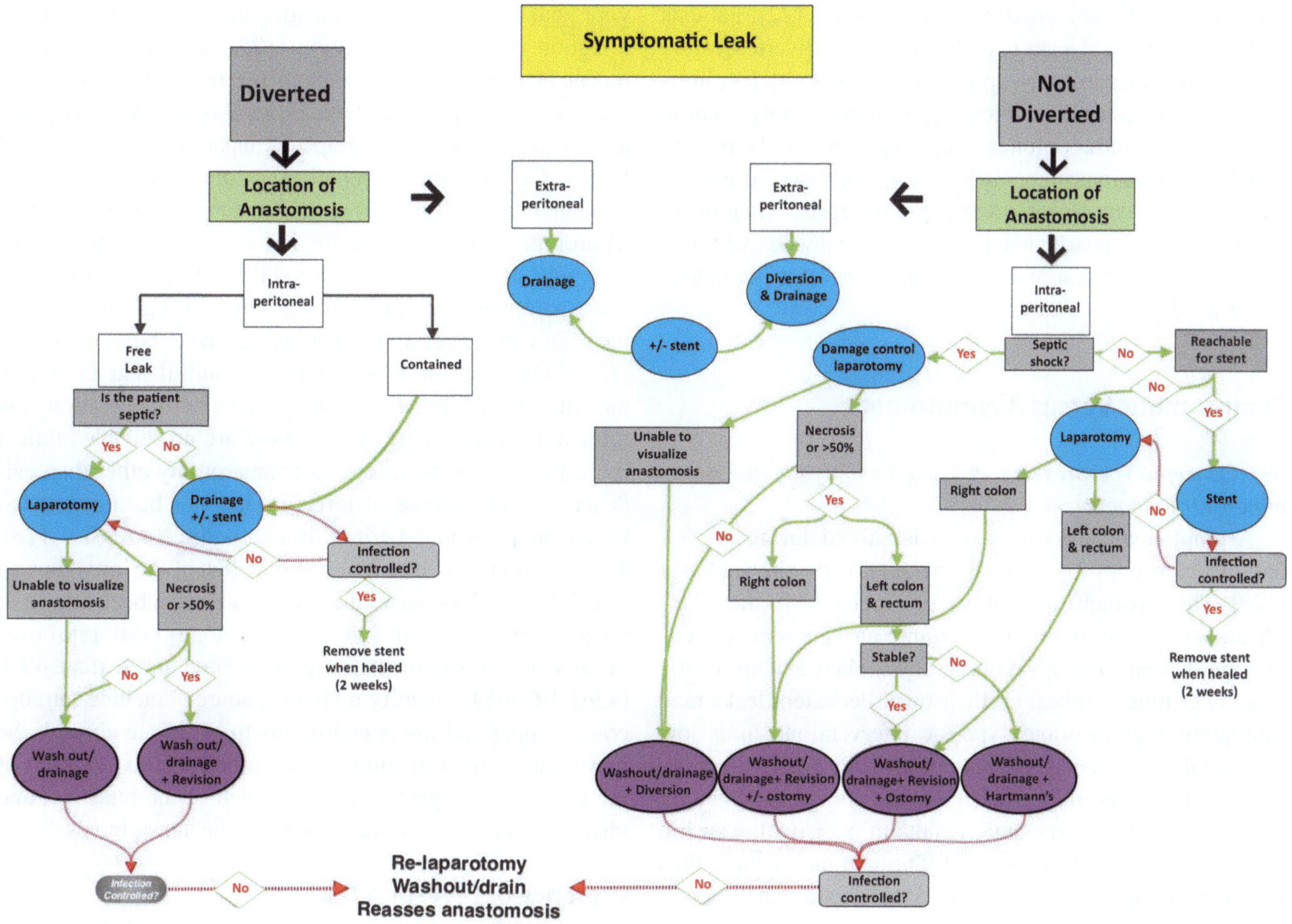

Fig. 18.4 Algorithm to treat a symptomatic leak

Anastomotic leaks vary in presentation, as do patients that suffer from them. Due to this variety seen in patients and the disease, multiple different types of interventions are possible. This poses a significant challenge to the surgeon when managing a problem unusual to the practice. The management of leaks has received very little attention in the literature with most studies being retrospective, underpowered, and suffering from bias. The following guidelines and algorithm, we have provided, are created from an extensive review of the literature combined with the authors' own clinical experience. Beyond the literature on colorectal leaks, we reviewed studies on the management of postoperative sepsis, damage control laparotomy, influence of different management techniques on definitive stoma rates, and other less invasive methods during the acute and chronic period. In reviewing these studies, in conjunction with our own clinical experience, we were able to delineate some key fundamental principles that are necessary in the effective management of anastomotic leaks which are further illustrated in our management algorithm (Fig. 18.4).

Identification and Location

Key Concept: With any peri-anastomotic abscess, you should rule out a concurrent anastomotic fistula. One of the most important first steps is to determine whether a leak is intraperitoneal or completely extraperitoneal.

The first step for any surgeon is to confirm that there is indeed a leak and determine its location. An abscess adjacent to anastomosis is not an anastomotic leak until it is proven to be so by CT, contrast enema, or in the operating room. Patients with abscesses, but without evidence of a leak, most likely can be treated with percutaneous drainage or antibiotics alone. Conversely, if these patients do not respond to drainage and antibiotics or recur after drain removal, they should be treated as if they have a leak since both CT and contrast enema can be falsely negative. Patients with anastomotic leaks located within the peritoneal cavity more often have diffuse contamination, peritonitis, and present with sepsis than those patients whose leaks are extraperitoneal. This is the likely explanation for an increase in mortality associated with right-sided colon resections [122]. Patients with extraperitoneal leaks usually are already diverted, rarely benefit from a laparotomy, and can be treated with less invasive therapies. If a patient does require a laparotomy because of significant intraperitoneal contamination, it is recommended that the anastomosis be revised or resected only in the case of severe necrosis and ongoing sepsis. Attempts to repair or revise a nearly intact anastomosis may be extremely difficult and may cause the patient to have a permanent ostomy [115].

Symptomatic Versus Asymptomatic

Key Concept: *The presence and degree of symptoms determine your management.*

Asymptomatic leaks are usually identified during an evaluation (endoscopy or contrast enema) for ostomy reversal [123]. These patients are not acutely at risk of further complications and therefore do not require any immediate intervention. The only therapy is observation. Many asymptomatic leaks over time will heal on their own. Persistent leaks may ultimately require some type of intervention. In a low colorectal anastomosis with ongoing local contamination, the resulting scar may impact pelvic floor and sphincter function, which unfortunately results in poor quality of life even though the leak heals [124]. Surgical judgment is thus important to avoid this scenario. Symptomatic patients will always require some form of intervention ranging from percutaneous drainage to exploratory laparotomy depending on other associated factors.

Postoperative Sepsis

Key Concept: *Evidence of sepsis or septic shock will require the use of more aggressive therapy, as the goal is early infection control and prevention of recurrent sepsis.*

Secondary peritonitis occurs in 12–16 % of patients undergoing elective abdominal operations and carries a high mortality rate (20–60 %) [125]. In a patient with postoperative sepsis, the three key components to infection control consist of draining the infected material, eradicating the source of infection, and preventing recurrent sepsis [126]. Early control of the infection improves mortality by minimizing the duration of sepsis and eliminating septic shock and multiple organ failure [127]. Diffuse peritonitis requires laparotomy and washout [115, 121, 126]. Laparoscopy, washout, and drain placement may be an option in selected patients treated initially with a laparoscopic resection. The most debatable issue involves whether a repeat laparotomy should be predetermined at the time of sepsis control or based upon signs of an ongoing infection (also referred to as laparotomy on demand) [128]. Currently, the best available evidence favors the use of the laparotomy on demand, where your goal as a surgeon is to identify and control the source of infection in a single operation [125]. The use of planned repeat laparotomies even though the infectious source has been controlled provides no additional benefit and is associated with increased nontherapeutic laparotomies (66 %) and longer ICU stays [125]. In patients with severe physiological derangements and hemodynamic instability, an abbreviated laparotomy is appropriate for initial control of peritonitis. This will allow for further correction of abnormal physiologic parameters in the intensive care setting while saving the definitive operation once these have been corrected [129]. The surgeon should also be mindful that in certain patients, even after a seemingly successful operation, the infectious source will persist. There are no reliable clinical indicators for the need for repeat laparotomy other than evidence that the source of infection has not been controlled based on persistent peritonitis or continued sepsis [128]. This decision should be made within 48 h of the initial operation for secondary peritonitis as patients have been shown to have a survival benefit (28 % vs. 77 % mortality rate) over those patients where the surgeon waited more than 48 h [126]. Efforts to identify a "hidden source" include intraoperative upper and lower endoscopy to insufflate air with the bowel submerged in saline (inner tube test), exploration of the lesser sac, inspection of every inch of the intestine, and visualization of the luminal aspect of the anastomosis.

Presence of Diverting Ostomy

Key Concept: *Patients with a previously created diverting ostomy are more likely to be asymptomatic, have an extraperitoneal anastomosis, and less likely to need a laparotomy. Do not be fooled by the "contained leak" in those patients without a diverting ostomy, as many of these will eventually need formal laparotomy/laparoscopy.*

Patients with symptomatic anastomotic leaks who have a diverting ostomy are less likely to present clinically with peritonitis and sepsis (10 % vs. 28 %) or require a laparotomy (8.6 % vs. 25.4 %) [90]. Those who do require a laparotomy, due to a diffuse leak or severe sepsis, will usually only need a thorough washout and placement of drains adjacent to the anastomosis [121, 130].

Symptomatic intraperitoneal leaks in patients that are not diverted nearly always require a laparotomy [121, 131]. In the subgroup of patients who are not diverted and have contained intraperitoneal leaks, it may be tempting to try percutaneous drainage and antibiotics alone, but evidence shows that this usually fails and will eventually require a laparotomy [131].

Extraperitoneal leaks are less likely to present with peritonitis or intra-abdominal sepsis than intraperitoneal anastomosis [121]. Instead extraperitoneal leaks may present as urinary symptoms, rectal drainage, and rectovaginal fistulas in addition to localized pain and tenderness [75, 121, 124].

Proximal diversion has improved mortality (15 % vs. 37 %) compared to anastomotic takedown and end colostomy (Hartmann's) [132]. Patients with proximal diversion are more likely to have their stomas reversed (100 % vs. 57 %) and with decreased morbidity (17.6 % vs. 71 %) compared to Hartmann's [132]. Proximal diversion can improve anastomotic healing and allow for the use of other interventions needed to repair the anastomosis [133, 134]. Local drainage alone without diversion risks prolonged pelvic sepsis causing fibrosis of the neorectum resulting in very poor function [135].

Diversion, Resection, and Revision

Key Concept: Unstable patients or those with low rectal anastomoses have better early and future outcomes if the anastomosis is left alone and only diversion and drainage is performed.

During the laparotomy, high-volume lavage with warm fluid and drainage of the infected material is the basis for successful infectious source control. In addition the surgeon can perform proximal diversion, anastomotic revision with or without proximal diversion, or resection of the anastomosis with Hartmann's stump and end ostomy. Several factors are against both you and the patient at this stage. Reoperations for anastomotic leaks take place in a hostile abdomen in the setting of a severe inflammatory response to the infection and usually encumbered by the dense adhesions of the postoperative period. Patients with septic shock are also not likely to tolerate the long operation needed for any formal revision. Additionally, the inflammatory mass around the anastomotic leak prevents any safe surgical dissection [91]. Many outside factors also influence your options (i.e., age, shock, immune status). Treatment of anastomotic leak accompanied by septic shock may benefit from a diverting colostomy or ileostomy, such as in the case of trauma or diverticulitis, as these adequately control the source of contamination and infection [115, 132, 136]. Diversion is particularly beneficial in patients with septic shock who might not tolerate a longer procedure or those cases where the peri-anastomotic inflammatory process does not permit a safe dissection of the anastomosis.

Resection of the low-lying rectal anastomosis and end colostomy can negatively impact a patient's ability to undergo future ostomy closure [132]. The literature confirms that an end colostomy with a Hartmann pouch causes increased morbidity and increases the permanent stoma rate without actually providing any significant benefit over a diverting ostomy [132]. Anastomotic revision under severe inflammatory conditions may adversely affect the blood supply at the anastomosis that could result in continued sepsis from the ensuing bowel necrosis. For this reason many advocate the use of diversion alone [113, 131].

In situations where there is necrosis or a greater than 50 % dehiscence of the anastomosis, a diverting ostomy may be inadequate in controlling the source of infection. Resection and reanastomosis with proximal diversion are recommended, if technically feasible, in a stable patient. However, if the blood supply still appears to be insufficient following resection or in any circumstance where a reanastomosis would be inappropriate, an end ostomy should be created. The exception to this is the circumstance where an extremely low rectal anastomosis has been constructed with proximal diversion. The addition of rectal lavage has been shown to be effective even in cases with >50 % dehiscence [74]. It is beneficial in the long term to preserve the anastomosis, but ongoing pelvic contamination or chronic infection can likewise have devastating consequences for future bowel function and quality of life [137]. In circumstances where that is likely, another approach may be considered. The Turnbull-Cutait pull-through of the left colon can eliminate the risk of poor blood supply or tension causing another anastomotic leak (Fig. 18.5a–d). This technique often requires extensive mobilization of the left and transverse colon to allow the bowel to be pulled though the short rectal stump. The mucosa is stripped to the dentate line, and the bowel is pulled through the anus to leave 7–10 cm hanging from the anus. A 34-French mushroom catheter is placed in the left colon to hang out of the anus and the bowel tied to the catheter to prevent slippage. The catheter is placed to closed drainage, and the externalized bowel is wrapped with Betadine soaked Kerlix and kept moist with fresh Betadine for 7 days. The patient returns to the OR on day 7 to amputate the external segment and suture the coloanal anastomosis.

Suture Repair

Key Concept: Do not give in to the allure of performing a simple suture repair.

Since many anastomotic dehiscences are small, it seems logical that they would be amenable to simple suture repair. Unfortunately sutures can decrease the blood supply to nearby tissues in an area of dehiscence that may already have a questionable blood supply, thus potentially making matters worse. Some surgeons are advocates of suture repair in minor defects (1 cm or less); however, there is limited evidence to support this recommendation. In fact, at least one study has questioned whether suture repair should be an option at all [112]. This study found that patients with a positive leak test during an elective colorectal resection had a much higher incidence of postoperative leaks with suture repair compared to revision [113]. If you do decide to perform a suture repair, you should consider performing a proximal diversion. In fact, with any positive leak test, the decision tree should almost always include a diverting stoma [138].

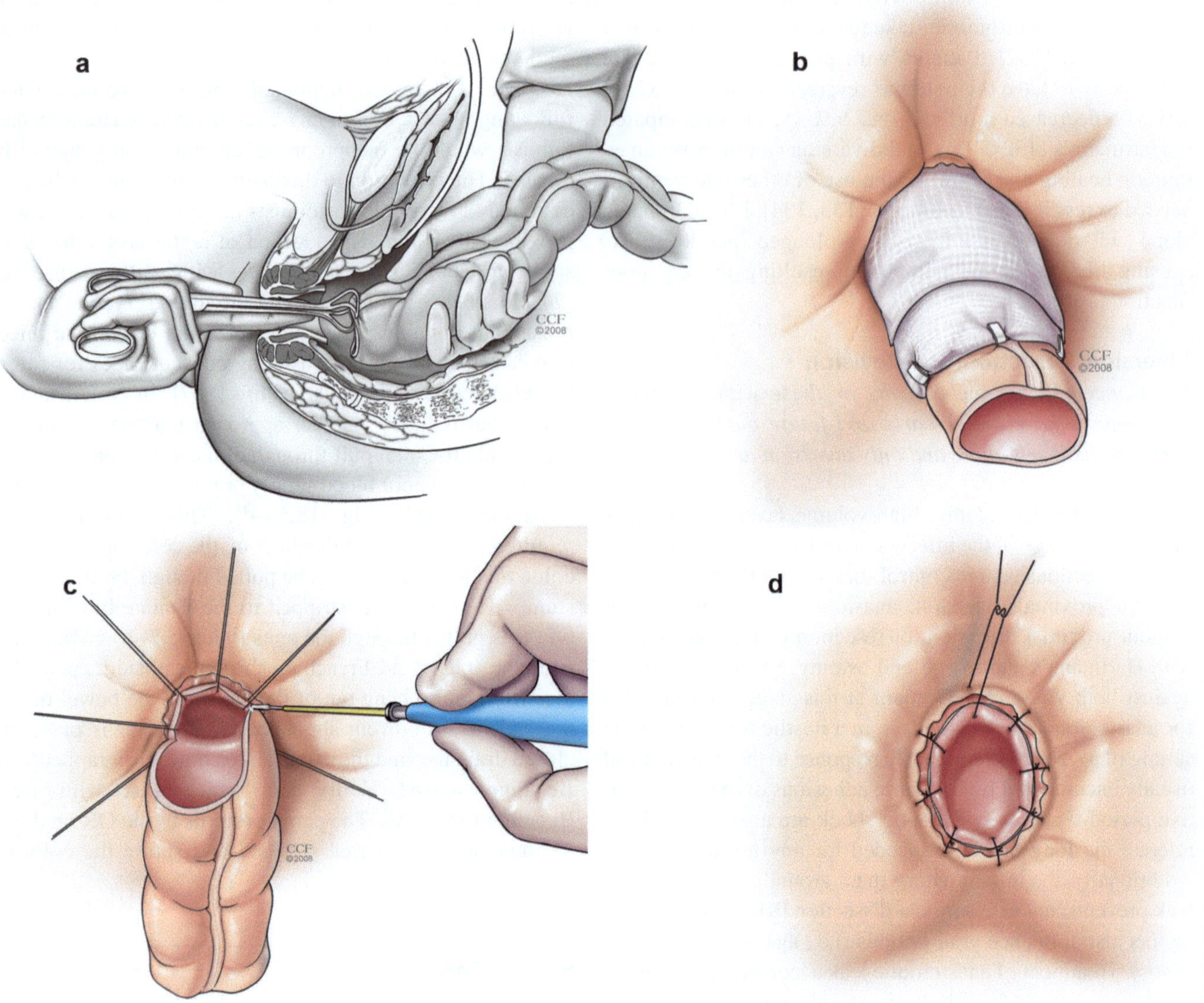

Fig. 18.5 Turnbull-Cutait pull-through. (**a**) The end of the colon is grasped from below and pulled through the anal verge. (**b**) Excess length is pulled through to the desired level and wrapped in dressing. (**c**) After time, the excess length is resected. (**d**) Final hand-sewn colo-anal anastomosis. (Reprinted with permission. © Cleveland Clinic Foundation, Cleveland, OH)

Management Unique to the Crohn's Patient

Key Concept: Crohn's patients with an ileocolic anastomotic leak behave differently and require different treatment than those with a colocolic anastomosis.

Anastomotic leaks can have a severe impact on the long-term outcome in patients with Crohn's disease. Only one study specifically focuses on the management of ileocolic and colocolic anastomotic leaks. The only apparent difference in Crohn's patients was seen in ileocolic leaks [139]. It was readily apparent in this study that resection with end ileostomy had far superior results in mortality (0 % vs. 21 %) and disease recurrence (0 % vs. 57 %) compared to methods which attempted to preserve or revise the anastomosis. Colo-colonic anastomotic-related complications were treated with methods of anastomotic preservation or takedown with end ostomies. Anastomotic-preserving methods included combined antibiotics, percutaneous drainage, and laparoscopic lavage or laparotomy with suturing of the leak site or resection and revision with or without proximal diversion. There was no difference in mortality, enterocutaneous fistula, or disease recurrence. Colo-colonic anastomotic leaks appeared to be a more localized process, with a much higher rate of spontaneous healing of enterocutaneous fistula. These results should be given consideration when faced with ileocolic anastomotic complications and warrant further studies. Most often, though, a conservative approach to managing the leak should be considered.

Establishment of drainage by percutaneous placement of pigtail catheters allows the sepsis to be treated and bowel rest to be applied in an attempt to close the leak without operating. This approach can successfully manage up to two-thirds of abscesses and fistulas [140].

Management After the Acute Setting

Key Concept: You are not finished treating a leak until after ostomy closure. Treating the area of dehiscence early on may allow for higher rates of ostomy closure and improved functional outcomes.

After the successful management of an anastomotic leak, the focus should shift to planning for the eventual restoration of intestinal continuity. This is an issue of equal importance, especially to the patient, and is best addressed early. Anastomotic defects, whether they are simple fistulas or large sinuses, can often spontaneously heal on their own if the patient is diverted [124, 130]. Unfortunately, not all defects will heal completely. Some will require additional months of diversion before they completely heal. The cavity around the leak must be completely healed before ostomy closure in order to prevent recurrent pelvic sepsis [134]. During this "healing period," chronic inflammation, and even low-grade infection, is allowed to persist while the defect undergoes secondary healing. The resulting fibrosis and scar formation can lead to persistent larger sinuses or ultimately to stenotic areas [141]. New methods of treating the local area of disrupted anastomosis may speed healing and reduce contamination to improve functional outcome.

Endoscopic Vacuum-Assisted Closure (Endoluminal VAC) or Endo-Sponge™

Key Concept: This negative pressure system may be useful for select low-lying anastomotic leaks; however, it should be applied within 6 weeks and will require several endoscopic changes.

Modification of the vacuum-assisted dressing to achieve endoluminal and endocavitary suction has been useful in closing low colorectal anastomotic leaks [141–144] (Fig. 18.6). The actual manufactured device currently available for use in treating gastrointestinal complications is the Endo-Sponge™ (B Braun Melsungen AG, Melsungen, Germany) [145], which has been available in Europe for more than a decade (Fig. 18.6). As of 2012 the FDA has approved it in the USA. Surgeons have adapted the current Wound V.A.C™ (Lifecell, Bridgewater, NJ) for use as an internal Wound V.A.C™ dressing. The amount of negative pressure to use when adapting the Wound V.A.C™ for anastomotic leaks is unknown. For the Endo-Sponge™ the negative pressure is set at a much lower negative pressure than the traditional Wound V.A.C™, but it appears that even −125 mmHg is well tolerated [141]. One purported advantage is the endoluminal VAC can drain intestinal contents before they are able to leak out into the adjoining abscess cavity. On the contrary, percutaneous drainage is unable to prevent this extravasation. Effective drainage and removal of necrotic material reduces the bacterial burden facilitating an increase in granulation tissue and a decrease in the size of the cavity [142]. The endoluminal VAC can at times even prevent the need for proximal diversion [142]. However, the endoluminal VAC is more effective at shrinking cavities if applied within 6 weeks after the anastomotic leak [143]. This is likely attributable to the increase in collagen deposition and scarring within the adjoining cavity which takes place over time. Once secondary healing occurs, the cavity is far less likely to undergo any significant cavity contraction [143]. Closure of presacral sinuses, abscess cavities, and fistulas occurs in 75–97 % of patients who began treatment within 6 weeks compared to 38 % in patients who began treatment after 6 weeks. Total number of VAC changes (endoscopic sessions) needed for successful closure was a median of 11–13 over a median time period of 34–40 days [142, 143]. At times patients may have very small fistula openings that feed larger sinuses. Endoluminal VAC placement into the abscess cavity is difficult or impossible through small fistula openings. For these small fistulae orifices that lead to larger sinuses, the endoluminal VAC can be applied over the fistula orifice within the rectum with or without percutaneous drainage of the sinus. The other option would be to expand the fistula orifice to allow sponge placement. Endoluminal VAC therapy is promising and seems to be very useful in the early setting—allowing for both healing and drainage, and even complete closure of anastomotic fistulas or sinuses. Even if the endoluminal VAC is unable to completely close a defect, it will still have resolved any infection and provided healthier tissue for use in other methods of repair.

Fibrin Glue

Key Concept: Fibrin glue is probably best used in the chronic setting to close small fistula openings before trying other more invasive options—so long as there is limited purulent material and a minimal amount of fecal or bacterial contamination.

Fibrin glue (combined thrombin and fibrinogen) or other types of nonbiologic glues have been used during anastomosis creation and for leaks and fistulas. Despite the early success showing an 85 % healing rate of anal fistulae, recent

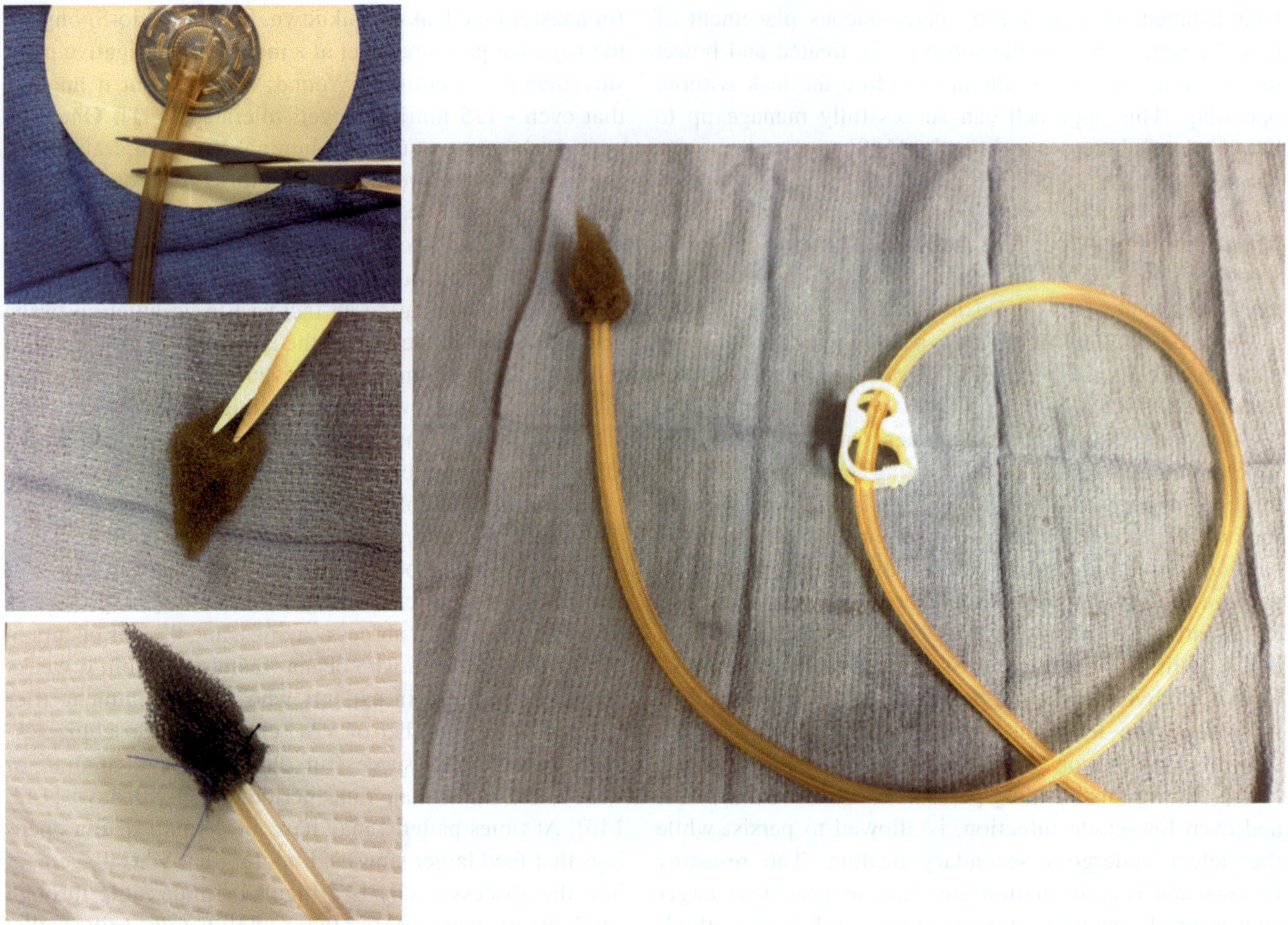

Fig. 18.6 Adaptation of KCI's proprietary V.A.C.® Therapy System for use as a type of endoluminal VAC. Images *A–D* are a pictorial guide in creating an endoluminal VAC. *Step A*: Cut the tubing close to the suction application pad to provide adequate length without requiring extra tubing. The KCI™ tubing can be directly applied to the sponge or if needed attached to a smaller diameter drain for smaller fistulas. Cut the sponge to the size of sinus or fistula tract keeping in mind the amount of magnification when viewed through the endoscope. Make sure the base is broader to allow a securer attachment of the tubing. *Step B*: Cut a circular area out of the base of the sponge extending about half the length of the sponge. *Steps C, D*: Secure the sponge with through and through bites of sponge and tubing. Three different horizontal mattress stitches using a Keith needle is a fairly easy and secure method. The remainder of the procedure is similar to placing the Endo-Sponge™

studies have failed to replicate these numbers. It also has been shown that fibrin glues are less effective in treating rectal complications compared to other areas like the esophagus. During the acute setting tissues have a significant amount of bacterial content and inflammation [146]. Currently, fibrin glue has a 25–33 % success rate as a single agent for treating rectal anastomotic complications [146, 147]. It is difficult to discern from the literature the exact role for fibrin glue. The two benefits in using fibrin glue are that it is fairly quick and easy to apply and it will not prevent the use of any other method if it fails. Fibrin glue is most useful in a chronic setting, especially with the low-volume small bowel fistula that is due to an anastomotic leak at an ileocolic staple line or strictureplasty. After removal of the percutaneous drain from the collapsed tract, the tract can be filled with fibrin glue to finish the healing.

Covered Stents

Key Concept: *While the emerging use of covered stents may dramatically change the way we treat certain leaks, for now they are relegated to treating those patients with a severe or complete disunion of their anastomosis, typically along with a proximal diverting ostomy, or in patients that have both a fistula and an adjacent stenotic area.*

Stents are beginning to be used in cases of malignant colorectal obstructions, with a very limited amount of use in colorectal anastomotic leaks. Much of what we know about the use of stents for anastomotic complications comes from treating esophageal anastomotic leaks. Covered stents, when used to treat esophageal anastomotic leaks, have been able to achieve complete resolution, in a minimally invasive fashion, within days to weeks. Studies show that esophageal stents allow much earlier resumption of oral intake, significant shorter hospital stays, and an 87–94 % success rate [148, 149]. The overall therapeutic principle behind stents is that they are able to effectively "bridge the breach" [150] and in doing so provide a scaffold which allows for reapproximation of the two ends, mucosal regeneration, and prevention of further drainage through the anastomotic defect and infectious complications.

Only a small number of studies, mainly composed of case series, include colorectal anastomotic leaks (Fig. 18.7). Studies show varying degrees of success in treating acute leaks, sometimes with almost complete anastomotic disunion as well as chronic fistulas [150, 151]. This is level IV evidence, at best, but we can draw some general conclusions.

1. Additional procedures, like percutaneous drainage, are very often still needed [150, 151].
2. The use of covered stents to cover the opening in the colorectal anastomosis may allow the fistula to heal without a diverting ostomy in up to 80 % of patients [151].
3. There is a high incidence of rectal pain if the distal aspect of the stent is within 5 cm of anal verge [152].
4. Migration is the #1 problem:
   - Full-thickness sutures or clips can help prevent migration.
   - Biodegradable and fully covered stents are more likely to migrate.
   - Patients who have stenosis in addition to a leak are less likely to have migration problems.
   - Due to these migration issues, using the stent to avoid proximal diversion could be technically challenging and may expose the patient to further infectious-related complications if migration does occur.
5. Partially covered stents migrate less, but allow for tissue in growth, and the eventual removal can at times be very difficult.

   Solution: *Stent Within a Stent Technique*

   Some gastroenterologists prefer to place a fully covered stent within the previously placed stent a few days before the stent will be removed. This will cause necrosis and sloughing of the mucosal in-growth and easier removal [153].
6. "Stent-guided regeneration and epithelialization" [150]—This is an interesting concept where stents, in cases of near-complete anastomotic disunion, act like scaffolds, allowing for approximation of the two bowel ends and reepithelialization.

Transanal Repair

Key Concept: *Different methods of transanal repair have been used in an attempt to close the unhealed fistula or sinus near the anal verge and allow for future ostomy closure. These include simple suturing, curettage, clips, marsupialization, plugs (for RVF,) and mucosal advancement—all with variable results and experience.*

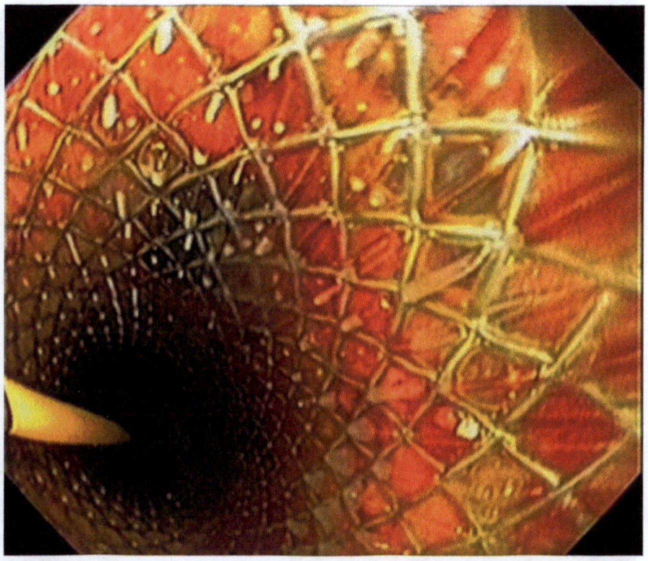

Fig. 18.7 Covered stent use for a colorectal anastomotic leak (Courtesy of Elisa Birnbaum, MD)

Transanal methods are technically more difficult to use for leaks higher up in the rectum and are prone to fail in patients who are not diverted. Simple suturing should only be attempted for small defects in tissues with minimal inflammation, and even then it is prone to fail. Some chronic small fistula tracts may be allowed to heal by performing local curettage to remove the epithelialized tract but more often is used as an adjunct to other procedures such as fistula plugs and endomucosal flaps [154]. Patients with chronic, large presacral sinuses, associated with small openings, may benefit from expanding the small opening in a procedure known as marsupialization where the rectal wall overlying the abscess cavity is incised and abscess cavity laid open. Marsupialization allows for better drainage and healing that can result in complete resolution of the sinus in a few months through reepithelialization. Marsupialization can be done endoscopically using an Olympus Triple Lumen Needle Knife [155], as well as with proctoscope or anoscope and the laparoscopic electrocautery scissors. Currently, this author, and others [156], uses a laparoscopic EndoGIA stapling device placed through the anus with the thin anvil in the fistula and the staple cartridge in the rectal lumen with good results, but it is conceivable that radiofrequency tissue sealing devices could work just as well. Flap advancement techniques more often have been used to treat rectovaginal fistulas, but can also be applied to any anastomotic fistula in close proximity to the anal verge [154, 157]. Flap advancement is akin to simple suturing but appears to have better results because it involves excising the fistula opening and

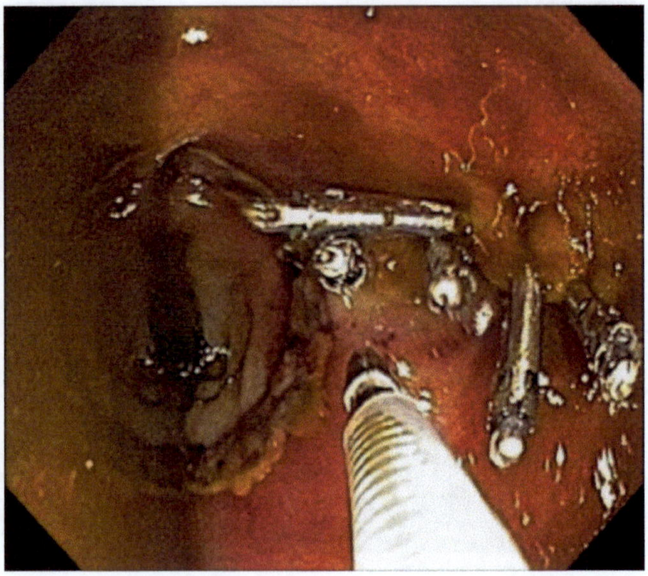

Fig. 18.8 Endoscopic clip placement for an anastomotic leak (Courtesy of Elisa Birnbaum, MD)

mobilizing the adjacent tissues, allowing for the approximation of healthy tissues without tension. Finally, there are limited reports of successful use of endoscopic clips to close the opening (Fig. 18.8).

Redo Surgery

Key Concept: Reoperative surgery should not be undertaken lightly, although it is sometimes the only way in which bowel continuity can be restored after other methods have failed.

Redo surgery is an *elective* surgery to restore intestinal continuity. It is associated with an approximately 20 % failure rate due to intraoperative failures or postoperative complications that ultimately result in a permanent stoma [158]. Anastomotic leaks occur with at least equal frequency as the initial operation; therefore, it is highly recommended to protect the new anastomosis with a diverting ostomy. This unfortunately will require an additional procedure, at a later date, for ostomy closure. Mortality is typically low with the appropriate patient selection, while morbidity is still typically high (32–55 %) [158, 159]. Some patients, even after a successful redo surgery, will have significant functional issues, such as increased frequency, incontinence, constipation, and difficult evacuation, following ostomy closure. Ureteral stent placement is recommended in the previously operated pelvis [159].

As a general rule of thumb, redo surgery is appropriate in patients:

- When other methods have failed
- Who have a minimal risk of perioperative mortality
- Who are not currently undergoing chemotherapy or radiation
- Nutritionally optimized
- Highly motivated for ostomy reversal
- Fully understand the risks involved and the possibility of failure

Anastomotic Stenosis

Key Concept: Anastomotic stenosis may be as significant as leaks because of the impact on a patient's quality of life, potential need for multiple revision attempts, and risk of permanent stoma.

Unfortunately for the colon and rectal surgeon, there are multiple ways an anastomosis can fail, with stenosis being a prominent one. It is a relatively common complication following colorectal surgery, reported in up to 20 % of patients [160]. Due to the wide variety of definitions used, the normally quoted incidence ranges from 3 to 30 % [161–163]. Using a single definition for "stenosis" as the inability to pass an 18- or 19 mm-diameter rigid rectoscope through an observed narrowing regardless of symptoms resulted in an incidence of 13–20 % [160, 161]. This number is likely to vary per surgeon and, in our own experience, does not seem to be as common. Many patients will have a fibrous stricture or web at the site of the anastomosis, sometimes appearing to be totally occluding the lumen. These are almost always easily broken up digitally or with the passage of the rigid proctoscope, and ultimately do not recur. Regardless of its true incidence, anastomotic stenosis is a challenge for the surgeon.

Pathophysiology

Key Concept: Several risk factors, including stapling devices, correlate with higher stenosis rates, while an intact mucosa may lead to lower rates of development.

Use of stapling devices, but not the size of stapler, is a risk factor for stenosis [161]. Necrotic tissue within the staple line and the small gap that is created between adjacent mucosa leads to an increased inflammatory response, collagen deposition, and secondary healing [101]. The significance of having an intact mucosa can further be derived from esophageal endomucosal resections where significant stenosis can occur in 75–80 % of patients who undergo more than 75 % circumferential resections of the mucosa [164]. An iatrogenically created mucosal defect in the esophagogastrostomy model in a dog resulted in higher degrees of stenosis and more scarring at the site of the anastomosis than those with an intact mucosa [164]. An intact mucosa and mucosa-to-mucosa apposition appear to be important in preventing stenosis. Other identified risk factors include anastomotic leaks, pelvic sepsis, long-term diversion, and radiotherapy [163, 165].

Symptoms and Clinical Course

Key Concept: Symptoms of anastomotic stenosis include bloating, constipation, and incomplete defecation. You should realize that the severity of symptoms will often not correlate with the degree of stenosis.

A clinical scoring system combines both the severity of symptoms with the necessary therapeutic intervention [160, 161]. Severe cases of stenosis in diverted patients will not be apparent until the patient undergoes hypaque enema evaluation for ostomy closure. Regardless of the absence of symptoms, the stenosis will need to be treated before ostomy closure. In general, though, patients should only be treated if they are symptomatic [160].

Treatment

Key Concept: Treatment for stenosis is accomplished using finger dilation, endoscopic balloon dilation, or stent placement.

Many stenoses will be amenable to finger fracture or endoscopic dilation alone; however, repeat procedures are commonly needed [161]. In some patients no method of treatment will work other than surgical revision. Most treatments are more effective if performed within the first few months postoperatively and seem to be much more refractory if performed later [161]. Some patients, despite problematic symptoms, will wait months to years before seeking help. Informing patients of the expected symptoms and changes in bowel function will speed diagnosis and treatment [161].

Balloon Dilation

Endoscopic balloon dilation, whether performed under fluoroscopy or through the scope, has up to a 90 % success rate with minimal associated morbidity. Patients should realize that multiple dilating procedures may be required before symptom resolution. This may be related to inadequate initial balloon dilatation [162]. Kim et al. [162] used a balloon dilation treatment algorithm that involved dilating a single 20 mm balloon followed by adding a second 10 mm balloon if no pain or blood was seen on the catheter. The 10 mm balloon was then changed out to a 15 mm and finally a 20 mm balloon as long as the patient did not experience pain or blood is not seen on the catheter. This method resulted in an 86 % success rate at long-term follow-up; however, there was no control group for comparison [162]. There is currently no consensus as to how many different dilation treatments are warranted before moving on to some other modality. A general rule is that after three endoscopic dilations, any symptomatic recurrent stenosis should be treated with a different method.

Stents

Stents were first used to treat cancer-related esophageal obstructions. Obstructive colorectal cancers are now being treated with soft expanding metal stents. The absolute effectiveness of this treatment modality is unknown at this time. It has been shown to be effective in the cases where both stenosis and a fistula or sinus exist as previously discussed. Successful stenting of anastomotic stricture has been reported [166]. Migration and in-growth of tissue are likely complications.

Complete Obstruction

There are other alternatives besides surgical revision that can potentially treat the totally occluded anastomosis. In addition to the circular stapled revision, which will be described later, one other alternative remains. This method explained by Curcio et al. [167] uses a suprapapillary puncture catheter to access the proximal lumen from the distal lumen under both endoscopic and fluoroscopic control. Placement of a 0.025 in. wire through the 18 gauge catheter allowed for progressive balloon dilation of the area up to a 20 mm balloon with good results. In circumstances where the ostomy proximal to the obliterated anastomosis is available to introduce an endoscope, the light of the proximally placed endoscope can guide recanalization using cautery or sharp dissection. Resection of the central scar and complete dilation are then possible.

Surgical Revision

Surgical revision should be considered should other less invasive modalities fail. The operation will be difficult with blood supply to the anastomosis tenuous, and similar to revision of anastomotic leaks, should not be taken lightly. There are two techniques that allow for surgical correction of the stenosis without formal resection and revision. These are stricturoplasty and circular stapled revision without resection. The stricturoplasty is similar to the Heineke-Mikulicz pyloroplasty on the anterior aspect of the anastomosis. The stapled revision requires a longitudinal incision on the anterior border of the proximal limb with insertion of the anvil, and under direct vision, the pin of the circular stapler is deployed through the stenotic or obstructed area and the anvil attached. McKee and colleagues described this method [168] by using a 29 mm circular stapler in a 51-year-old female. Success with these two methods needs to be further explored. However, they should remain in the surgeon's armamentarium, especially in cases where the complete dissection of the low rectal anastomoses is difficult. Anastomotic resection and reconstruction is preferred if soft tissue is not available or revision increases the likelihood of further complications due to poor blood supply. A low rectal anastomosis is an extremely difficult procedure in the reoperative pelvis and requires patience and experience to achieve success.

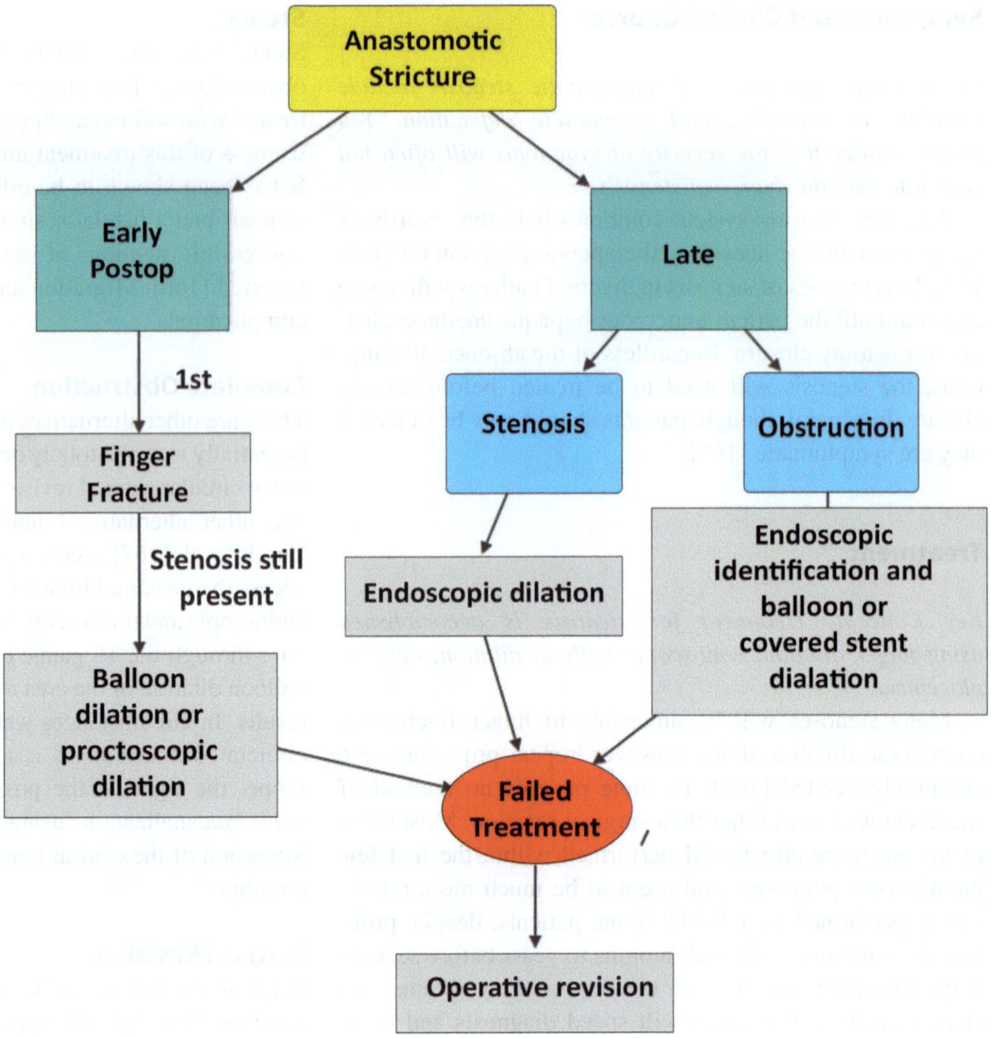

Fig. 18.9 Algorithm to treat an anastomotic stricture

Anastomotic Stenosis Summary

The severity of the problem with anastomotic stenosis in relation to its incidence is extremely variable. Since staplers appear to be the most important risk factor for anastomotic stenosis, future preventive measures will need to address the design of stapled anastomoses. There is no consensus that outlines management or treatment of stenosis. A treatment algorithm is presented in Fig. 18.9. Finally, anastomotic stenosis or recurrence of stenosis months to years after successful treatment may be due to cancer recurrence. It is therefore important to take biopsies upon the first identification of stenosis along with additional biopsies and/or imaging in cases of recurrent stenosis that follows a prolonged asymptomatic period.

References

1. Dietz UA, Debus ES. Intestinal anastomoses prior to 1882; a legacy of ingenuity, persistence, and research form a foundation for modern gastrointestinal surgery. World J Surg. 2005;29:396–401.
2. Munireddy S, Kavalukas SL, Barbul A. Intra-abdominal healing: gastrointestinal tract and adhesions. Surg Clin North Am. 2010;90(6):1227–36.
3. Brian WA. The pathology of diverticulosis: classical concepts and mucosal changes in diverticula. J Clin Gastroenterol. 2006;40 Suppl 3:S126–31.
4. Halsted WS. Circular suture of the intestine: an experimental study. Am J Med Sci. 1887;94:436–61.
5. Thompson SK, Chang EY, Jobe BA. Clinical review: healing in gastrointestinal anastomoses, part I. Microsurgery. 2006;26:131–6.
6. Kologlu M, Yorganci K, Renda N, et al. Effect of local and remote ischemia-reperfusion injury on healing of colonic anastomoses. Surgery. 2000;128(1):99–104.
7. Mast BA. Healing in other tissues. Surg Clin North Am. 1997;77:529–47.
8. Whiteway J, Morson BC. Elastosis in diverticular disease of the sigmoid colon. Gut. 1985;26:258–66.
9. Thornton FJ, Barbul A. Healing in the gastrointestinal tract. Surg Clin North Am. 1997;77:549–73.
10. Baker RS, Foote J, Kemmeter P, Brady R, Vroegop T, Serveld M. The science of stapling and leaks. Obes Surg. 2004;14:1290–8.
11. Hyman N. Anastomotic leaks after intestinal anastomosis: it's later than you think. Ann Surg. 2007;245:254–8.
12. Stewart D, Hunt S, Pierce R, et al. Validation of the NITI endoluminal compression anastomosis ring (EndoCAR) device and

comparison to the traditional circular stapled colorectal anastomosis in a porcine model. Surg Innov. 2007;14:252–60.
13. Dubay DA, Franz MG. Acute wound healing: the biology of acute wound failure. Surg Clin North Am. 2003;83:463–81.
14. Wiesner W, Khurana B, Ji H, Ros PR. CT of acute bowel ischemia. Radiology. 2003;226:635–50.
15. Allison AS, Bloor C, Faux W, et al. The angiographic anatomy of the small arteries and their collaterals in colorectal resections: some insights into anastomotic perfusion. Ann Surg. 2010;251(6): 1092–109.
16. Meyers MA. Griffiths' point: critical anastomosis at the splenic flexure. Significance in ischemia of the colon. AJR Am J Roentgenol. 1976;126:77–94.
17. Trencheva K, Morrissey KP, Wells M. Identifying important predictors for anastomotic leak after colon and rectal resection: prospective study on 616 patients. Ann Surg. 2013;257(1):108–13.
18. Vignali A, Gianotti L, Braga M, Radaelli G, Malvezzi L, Di Carlo V. Altered microperfusion at the rectal stump is predictive for rectal anastomotic leak. Dis Colon Rectum. 2000;43(1):76–82.
19. Marino PL. The ICU, book. Philadelphia: Lippincott Williams & Wilkins; 2006. p. 26–7.
20. Davis BD, Rivadeneira DE. Complications of colorectal anastomoses: leaks, strictures, and bleeding. Surg Clin North Am. 2013; 93(1):61–87.
21. Veyrie N, Ata T, Muscari F. Anastomotic leakage after elective right versus left colectomy for cancer: prevalence and independent risk factors. J Am Coll Surg. 2007;205:785–93.
22. Wexner S. Invited critique to article of Alves et al. Postoperative mortality and morbidity in French patients undergoing colorectal surgery. Arch Surg. 2005;140:284.
23. Benoist S, Panis Y, Alves A, Valleur P. Impact of obesity on surgical outcomes after colorectal resection. Am J Surg. 2000;179: 275–81.
24. Dana A, Edward H, Celia M. Risk factors for anastomotic leak following colorectal surgery. Arch Surg. 2010;145:371–6.
25. Mäkelä JT, Kiviniemi H. Risk factors for anastomotic leakage after left-sided colorectal resection with rectal anastomosis. Dis Colon Rectum. 2003;46(5):653–60.
26. Garcia-Botello SA, Garcia-Armengol J, Garcia-Granero E, et al. A prospective audit of the complications of loop ileostomy construction and takedown. Dig Surg. 2004;21(5–6):440–6.
27. Clinical Outcomes of Surgical Therapy Study Group. A comparison of laparoscopically assisted and open colectomy for colon cancer. N Engl J Med. 2004;350(20):2050–9.
28. Jie B, Jiang Z, Nolan M, Zhu S. Impact of preoperative nutritional support on clinical outcome in abdominal surgical patients at nutritional risk. Nutrition. 2012;28:1022–7.
29. Schacke H, Docke WD, Asadullah K. Mechanisms involved in the side effects of glucocorticoids. Pharmacol Ther. 2002;96(1): 23–43.
30. Shental O, Tulchinsky H, Greenberg R, Klausner JM, Avital S. Positive histological inflammatory margins are associated with increased risk for intra-abdominal septic complications in patients undergoing ileocolic resection for Crohn's disease. Dis Colon Rectum. 2012;55(11):1125–30.
31. Mascarenhas C, Nunoo R, Asgeirsson T, et al. Outcomes of ileocolic resection and right hemicolectomies for Crohn's patients in comparison with non-Crohn's patients and the impact of perioperative immunosuppressive therapy with biologics and steroids on inpatient complications. Am J Surg. 2012;203(3):375–8.
32. Bafford AC, Powers S, Ha C, et al. Immunosuppressive therapy does not increase operative morbidity in patients with Crohn's disease. J Clin Gastroenterol. 2012;47(6):491–5.
33. Colombel JF, Loftus Jr EV, Tremaine WJ, et al. Early postoperative complications are not increased in patients with Crohn's disease treated perioperatively with infliximab or immunosuppressive therapy. Am J Gastroenterol. 2004;99(5):878–83.
34. Fazio VW, Marchetti F, Church M, et al. Effect of resection margins on the recurrence of Crohn's disease in the small bowel. A randomized controlled trial. Ann Surg. 1996;224(4):563–71; discussion 571–3.
35. Slieker JC, Komen N, Mannaerts GH. Long-term and perioperative corticosteroids in anastomotic leakage: a prospective study of 259 left-sided colorectal anastomoses. Arch Surg. 2012;147(5):447–52.
36. Yamamoto T, Allan RN, Keighley MR. Risk factors for intra-abdominal sepsis after surgery in Crohn's disease. Dis Colon Rectum. 2000;43:1141–5.
37. Post S, Betzler M, von Ditfurth B, et al. Risks of intestinal anastomoses in Crohn's disease. Ann Surg. 1991;213:37–42.
38. Selvasekar CR, Cima RR, Larson DW, et al. Effect of infliximab on short-term complications in patients undergoing operation for chronic ulcerative colitis. J Am Coll Surg. 2007;204(5):956–62.
39. Subramanian V, Pollok RC, Kang JY, Kumar D. Systematic review of postoperative complications in patients with inflammatory bowel disease treated with immunomodulators. Br J Surg. 2006;93(7):793–9.
40. Alves A, Panis Y, Bouhnik Y, Pocard M, Vicaut E, Valleur P. Risk factors for intra-abdominal septic complications after a first ileocecal resection for Crohn's disease: a multivariate analysis in 161 consecutive patients. Dis Colon Rectum. 2007;50(3):331–6.
41. Heuman R, Boeryd B, Bolin T, Sjodahl R. The influence of disease at the margin of resection on the outcome of Crohn's disease. Br J Surg. 1983;70(9):519–21.
42. Nisar PJ, Lavery IC, Kiran RP. Influence of neoadjuvant radiotherapy on anastomotic leak after restorative resection for rectal cancer. J Gastrointest Surg. 2012;16(9):1750–7.
43. Sauer R, Becker H, Hohenberger W, et al. Preoperative versus postoperative chemoradiotherapy for rectal cancer. N Engl J Med. 2004;351(17):1731–40.
44. Kim J, Mittal R, Konyalian V, King J, Stamos MJ, Kumar RR. Outcome analysis of patients undergoing colorectal resection for emergent and elective indications. Am Surg. 2007;73(10):991–3.
45. Alves A, Panis Y, Trancart D, et al. Factors associated with clinically significant anastomotic leakage after large bowel resection: multivariate analysis of 707 patients. World J Surg. 2002; 26(4):499–502.
46. Choi HK, Law WL, Ho JW. Leakage after section and intraperitoneal anastomosis for colorectal malignancy: analysis of risk factors. Dis Colon Rectum. 2006;49(11):1719–25.
47. Biondo S, Pares D, Kreisler E, et al. Anastomotic dehiscence after resection and primary anastomosis in left-sided colonic emergencies. Dis Colon Rectum. 2005;48(12):2272–80.
48. Gooszen AW, Tollenaar RA, Geelkerken RH, et al. Prospective study of primary anastomosis following sigmoid resection for suspected acute complicated diverticular disease. Br J Surg. 2001; 88(5):693–7.
49. Forloni B, Reduzzi R, Paludetti A, Colpani L, Cavallari G, Frosali D. Intraoperative colonic lavage in emergency surgical treatment of left-sided colonic obstruction. Dis Colon Rectum. 1998;41(1):23–7.
50. Biondo S, Perea MT, Ragué JM, Parés D, Jaurrieta E. One-stage procedure in non-elective surgery for diverticular disease complications. Colorectal Dis. 2001;3:42–5.
51. Ravo B, Metwally N, Castera P, Polansky PJ, Ger R. The importance of intraluminal anastomotic fecal contact and peritonitis in colonic anastomotic leakages. An experimental study. Dis Colon Rectum. 1988;31(11):868–71.
52. Ravo B, Metwall N, Yeh J, Polansky P, Frattaroli FM. Effect of fecal loading with/without peritonitis on the healing of a colonic anastomosis: an experimental study. Eur Surg Res. 1991;23(2): 100–7.
53. Salem L, Flum DR. Primary anastomosis or Hartmann's procedure for patients with diverticular peritonitis? A systematic review. Dis Colon Rectum. 2004;47(11):1953–64.

54. Chiappa A, Zbar A, Biella F, Staudacher C. One-stage resection and primary anastomosis following acute obstruction of the left colon for cancer. Am Surg. 2000;66(7):619–22.
55. Demetriades D, Murray JA, Chan L, et al. Penetrating colon injuries requiring resection: diversion or primary anastomosis? An AAST prospective multicenter study. J Trauma. 2001;50(5):765–75.
56. Boccola MA, Buettnr PG, Rozen WM, et al. Risk factors and outcomes for anastomotic leakage in colorectal surgery: a single-institution analysis of 1576 patients. World J Surg. 2011; 35(1):186–95.
57. Gendall KA, Raniga S, Kennedy R, Frizelle FA. The impact of obesity on outcome after major colorectal surgery. Dis Colon Rectum. 2007;50(12):2223–37.
58. Jung SH, Yu CS, Choi PW, et al. Risk factors and oncologic impact of anastomotic leakage after rectal cancer surgery. Dis Colon Rectum. 2008;51(6):902–8.
59. Nesbakken A, Nygaard K, Westerheim O, et al. Audit of intraoperative and early postoperative complications after introduction of mesorectal excision for rectal cancer. Eur J Surg. 2002; 168(4):229–35.
60. Law WL, Chu KW, Ho J, Chan CW. Risk factors for anastomotic leakage after low anterior resection with total mesorectal excision. Am J Surg. 2000;179:92–6.
61. Yeh CY, Changchien CR, Wang JY, et al. Pelvic drainage and other risk factors for leakage after elective anterior resection in rectal cancer patients: a prospective study of 978 patients. Ann Surg. 2005;241(1):9–13.
62. Rullier E, Laurent C, Garrelon JL, Michel P, Saric J, Parneix M. Risk factors for anastomotic leakage after resection of rectal cancer. Br J Surg. 1998;85(3):355–8.
63. Ba ZF, Yokoyama Y, Toth B, Rue 3rd LW, Bland KI, Chaudry IH. Gender differences in small intestinal endothelial function: inhibitory role of androgens. Am J Physiol Gastrointest Liver Physiol. 2004;286(3):G452–7.
64. Telem DA, Chin EH, Nguyen SQ, et al. Risk factors for anastomotic leak following colorectal surgery: a case–control study. Arch Surg. 2010;145(4):371–6.
65. Lee MR, Hong CW, Yoon SN, et al. Risk factors for anastomotic leakage after resection for rectal cancer. Hepatogastroenterology. 2006;53(71):682–6.
66. Lipska MA, Bissett IP, Parry BR, Merrie AE. Anastomotic leakage after lower gastrointestinal anastomosis: men are at a higher risk. ANZ J Surg. 2006;76(7):579–85.
67. Choi DH, Hwang JK, Ko YT, et al. Risk factors for anastomotic leakage after laparoscopic rectal resection. J Korean Soc Coloproctol. 2010;26(4):265–73.
68. Kurz A, Sessler DI, Lenhardt R. Perioperative normothermia to reduce the incidence of surgical-wound infection and shorten hospitalization. Study of wound infection and temperature group. N Engl J Med. 1996;334(19):1209–15.
69. Karliczek A, Jesus EC, Matos D, Castro AA, Atallah AN, Wiggers T. Drainage or nondrainage in elective colorectal anastomosis: a systematic review and meta-analysis. Colorectal Dis. 2006;8(4):259–65.
70. Matthiessen P, Hallbook O, Andersson M, et al. Risk factors for anastomotic leakage after anterior resection of the rectum. Colorectal Dis. 2004;6:462–9.
71. Mansson P, Zhang XW, Jeppsson B, Thorlacius H. Anastomotic healing in the rat colon: comparison between a radiological method, breaking strength and bursting pressure. Int J Colorectal Dis. 2002;17(6):420–5.
72. Karanjia ND, Corder AP, Bearn P, Heald RJ. Leakage from stapled low anastomosis after total mesorectal excision for carcinoma of the rectum. Br J Surg. 1994;81(8):1224–6.
73. Tsujinaka S, Kawamura YJ, Konishi F, Maeda T, Mizokami K. Pelvic drainage for anterior resection revisited: use of drains in anastomotic leaks. ANZ J Surg. 2008;78(6):461–5.
74. Urbach DR, Kennedy ED, Cohen MM. Colon and rectal anastomoses do not require routine drainage: a systematic review and meta-analysis. Ann Surg. 1999;229(2):174–80.
75. Eckmann C, Kujath P, Schiedeck TH, Shekarriz H, Bruch HP. Anastomotic leakage following low anterior resection: results of a standardized diagnostic and therapeutic approach. Int J Colorectal Dis. 2004;19(2):128–33.
76. Kang CY, Chaudhry OO, Halabi WJ, et al. Outcomes of laparoscopic colorectal surgery: data from the nationwide inpatient sample 2009. Am J Surg. 2012;204(6):952–7.
77. Krarup PM, Jorgensen LN, Andreasen AH, Harling H, Danish Colorectal Cancer Group. A nationwide study on anastomotic leakage after colonic cancer surgery. Colorectal Dis. 2012;14(10):e661–7.
78. Moreaux J, Horiot A, Barrat F, Mabille J. Obliteration of the pelvic space with pedicled omentum after excision of the rectum for cancer. Am J Surg. 1984;148:640–4.
79. Merad F, Hay JM, Fingerhut A, Flamant Y, Molkhou JM, Laborde Y. Omentoplasty in the prevention of anastomotic leakage after colonic or rectal resection. A prospective randomized study in 712 patients. Ann Surg. 1998;227:179–86.
80. Tocchi A, Mazzoni G, Lepre L, et al. Prospective evaluation of omentoplasty in preventing leakage of colorectal anastomosis. Dis Colon Rectum. 2000;43(7):951–5.
81. Jemal A, Siegel R, Ward E, et al. Cancer statistics, 2008. CA Cancer J Clin. 2008;58(2):71–96.
82. Nakajima K, Takahashi S, Saito N, et al. Predictive factors for anastomotic leakage after simultaneous resection of synchronous colorectal liver metastasis. J Gastrointest Surg. 2012;16(4):821–7.
83. Martin 2nd RC, Augenstein V, Reuter NP, Scoggins CR, McMasters KM. Simultaneous versus staged resection for synchronous colorectal cancer liver metastases. J Am Coll Surg. 2009;208(5):842–50; discussion 850–2.
84. Roxburgh CS, Richards CH, Moug SJ, Foulis AK, McMillan DC, Horgan PG. Determinants of short- and long-term outcome in patients undergoing simultaneous resection of colorectal cancer and synchronous colorectal liver metastases. Int J Colorectal Dis. 2012;27(3):363–9.
85. Wong NY, Eu KW. A defunctioning ileostomy does not prevent clinical anastomotic leak after a low anterior resection: a prospective, comparative study. Dis Colon Rectum. 2005;48(11):2076–9.
86. Montedori A, Cirocchi R, Farinella E, Sciannameo F, Abraha I. Covering ileo- or colostomy in anterior resection for rectal carcinoma. Cochrane Database Syst Rev. 2010;5, CD006878.
87. Messaris E, Sehgal R, Deiling S, et al. Dehydration is the most common indication for readmission after diverting ileostomy creation. Dis Colon Rectum. 2012;55(2):175–80.
88. Bakx R, Busch OR, Bemelman WA, Veldink GJ, Slors JF, van Lanschot JJ. Morbidity of temporary loop ileostomies. Dig Surg. 2004;21:277–81.
89. Williams NS, Nasmyth DG, Jones D, Smith AH. Defunctioning stomas: a prospective controlled trial comparing loop ileostomy with loop transverse colostomy. Br J Surg. 1986;73:566–70.
90. Matthiessen P, Hallbook O, Rutegard J, Simert G, Sjodahl R. Defunctioning stoma reduces symptomatic anastomotic leakage after low anterior resection of the rectum for cancer: a randomized multicenter trial. Ann Surg. 2007;246(2):207–14.
91. Cao F, Li J, Li F. Mechanical bowel preparation for elective colorectal surgery: updated systematic review and meta-analysis. Int J Colorectal Dis. 2012;27(6):803–10.
92. Bretagnol F, Alves A, Ricci A, Valleur P, Panis Y. Rectal cancer surgery without mechanical bowel preparation. Br J Surg. 2007;94:1266–71.
93. Vlot EA, Zeebregts CJ, Gerritsen JJ, Mulder HJ, Mastboom WJ, Klaase JM. Anterior resection of rectal cancer without bowel preparation and diverting stoma. Surg Today. 2005;35:629–33.

94. Bretagnol F, Panis Y, Rullier E, et al. Rectal cancer surgery with or without bowel preparation: the French GRECCAR III multicenter single-blinded randomized trial. Ann Surg. 2010;252:863–8.
95. Abbas MA. Anastomotic leak: should we continue to accept the risks? Dis Colon Rectum. 2010;53(6):859–60.
96. Kelly H, Hurdon E. The vermiform appendix and its diseases. Philadelphia: WB Saunders and Company; 1905.
97. Kudszus S, Roesel C, Schachtrupp A, Hoer JJ. Intraoperative laser fluorescence angiography in colorectal surgery: a noninvasive analysis to reduce the rate of anastomotic leakage. Langenbecks Arch Surg. 2010;395(8):1025–30.
98. Yalin R, Aktan AO, Yegen C, et al. Importance of testing stapled rectal anastomoses with air. Eur J Surg. 1993;159(1):49–51.
99. Wheeler JM, Gilbert JM. Controlled intraoperative water testing of left-sided colorectal anastomoses: are ileostomies avoidable? Ann R Coll Surg Engl. 1999;81:105–8.
100. Schmidt O, Merkel S, Hohenberger W. Anastomotic leakage after low rectal stapler anastomosis: significance of intraoperative anastomotic testing. Eur J Surg Oncol. 2003;29(3):239–43.
101. Griffen FD, Knight CD, Whitaker JM, et al. The double stapling technique for low anterior resection. Ann Surg. 1990;211: 745–52.
102. Li VK, Wexner SD, Pulido N, et al. Use of routine intraoperative endoscopy in elective laparoscopic colorectal surgery: can it further avoid anastomotic failure? Surg Endosc. 2009;23(11): 2459–65.
103. Chen CW, Chen MJ, Yeh YS, Tsai HL, Chang YT, Wang JY. Intraoperative anastomotic dye test significantly decreases incidence of anastomotic leaks in patients undergoing resection for rectal cancer. Tech Coloproctol. 2013;17:579–83.
104. Gurjar SV, Forshaw MJ, Ahktar N, Stewart M, Parker MC. Indwelling trans-anastomotic rectal tubes in colorectal surgery: a survey of usage in UK and Ireland. Colorectal Dis. 2007;9: 47–51.
105. Morks AN, Havenga K, Ploeg RJ. Can intraluminal devices prevent or reduce colorectal anastomotic leakage: a review. World J Gastroenterol. 2011;17(40):4461–9.
106. Bulow S, Bulut O, Christensen IJ, Harling H, Rectal Stent Study Group. Transanal stent in anterior resection does not prevent anastomotic leakage. Colorectal Dis. 2006;8(6):494–6.
107. Ravo B. The intracolonic bypass procedure. Int J Colorectal Dis. 1987;2(1):38–42.
108. Ye F, Wang D, Xu X, Liu F, Lin J. Use of intracolonic bypass secured by a biodegradable anastomotic ring to protect the low rectal anastomosis. Dis Colon Rectum. 2008;51:109–15.
109. Masoomi H, Luo R, Mills S, Carmichael JC, Senagore AJ, Stamos MJ. Compression anastomosis ring device in colorectal anastomosis: a review of 1,180 patients. Am J Surg. 2013;205(4):447–51.
110. Fajardo AD, Chun J, Stewart D, Safar B, Fleshman JW. 1.5:1 meshed AlloDerm bolsters for stapled rectal anastomoses does not provide any advantage in anastomotic strength in a porcine model. Surg Innov. 2011;18(1):21–8.
111. Fajardo AD, Amador-Ortiz C, Chun J, Stewart D, Fleshman JW. Evaluation of bioabsorbable seamguard for staple line reinforcement in stapled rectal anastomoses. Surg Innov. 2012;19(3):288–94.
112. Stamou KM, Menenakos E, Dardamanis D, et al. Prospective comparative study of the efficacy of staple-line reinforcement in laparoscopic sleeve gastrectomy. Surg Endosc. 2011;25(11): 3526–30.
113. Thornton M, Joshi H, Vimalachandran C, et al. Management and outcome of colorectal anastomotic leaks. Int J Colorectal Dis. 2011;26(3):313–20.
114. Sutton CD, Marshall LJ, Williams N, Berry DP, Thomas WM, Kelly MJ. Colo-rectal anastomotic leakage often masquerades as a cardiac complication. Colorectal Dis. 2004;6(1):21–2.
115. Bellows CF, Webber LS, Albo D, Awad S, Berger DH. Early predictors of anastomotic leaks after colectomy. Tech Coloproctol. 2009;13(1):41–7.
116. Almeida AB, Faria G, Moreira H, Pinto-de-Sousa J, Correia-da-Silva P, Maia JC. Elevated serum C-reactive protein as a predictive factor for anastomotic leakage in colorectal surgery. Int J Surg. 2012;10(2):87–91.
117. Welsch T, Muller SA, Ulrich A, et al. C-reactive protein as early predictor for infectious postoperative complications in rectal surgery. Int J Colorectal Dis. 2007;22:1499–507.
118. Korner H, Nielsen HJ, Soreide JA, Nedrebo BS, Soreide K, Knapp JC. Diagnostic accuracy of C-reactive protein for intraabdominal infections after colorectal resections. J Gastrointest Surg. 2009;13(9):1599–606.
119. Noble F, Curtis N, Harris S, et al. Risk assessment using a novel score to predict anastomotic leak and major complications after oesophageal resection. J Gastrointest Surg. 2012;16(6):1083–95.
120. den Dulk M, Noter SL, Hendriks ER, et al. Improved diagnosis and treatment of anastomotic leakage after colorectal surgery. Eur J Surg Oncol. 2009;35(4):420–6.
121. Phitayakorn R, Delaney CP, Reynolds HL, et al. Standardized algorithms for management of anastomotic leaks and related abdominal and pelvic abscesses after colorectal surgery. World J Surg. 2008;32(6):1147–56.
122. Smith JJ, et al. The national bowel cancer audit project 2007. London: Association of Coloproctology of Great Britain and Ireland; 2007. p. 63–4.
123. Rahbari NN, Weitz J, Hohenberger W, et al. Definition and grading of anastomotic leakage following anterior resection of the rectum: a proposal by the international study group of rectal cancer. Surgery. 2010;147(3):339–51.
124. Lim M, Akhtar S, Sasapu K, et al. Clinical and subclinical leaks after low colorectal anastomosis: a clinical and radiologic study. Dis Colon Rectum. 2006;49(10):1611–9.
125. van Ruler O, Mahler CW, Boer KR, et al. Comparison of on-demand vs. planned relaparotomy strategy in patients with severe peritonitis: a randomized trial. JAMA. 2007;298(8):865–72.
126. Koperna T, Schulz F. Relaparotomy in peritonitis: prognosis and treatment of patients with persisting intraabdominal infection. World J Surg. 2000;24(1):32–7.
127. Ruttinger D, Kuppinger D, Holzwimmer M, et al. Acute prognosis of critically ill patients with secondary peritonitis: the impact of the number of surgical revisions, and of the duration of surgical therapy. Am J Surg. 2012;204(1):28–36.
128. Lamme B, Boermeester MA, Reitsma JB, Mahler CW, Obertop H, Gouma DJ. Meta-analysis of relaparotomy for secondary peritonitis. Br J Surg. 2002;89(12):1516–24.
129. Person B, Dorfman T, Bahouth H, Osman A, Assalia A, Kluger Y. Abbreviated emergency laparotomy in the non-trauma setting. World J Emerg Surg. 2009;4:41.
130. Hedrick TL, Sawyer RG, Foley EF, Friel CM. Anastomotic leak and the loop ileostomy: friend or foe? Dis Colon Rectum. 2006;49(8):1167–76.
131. Damrauer SM, Bordeianou L, Berger D. Contained anastomotic leaks after colorectal surgery: are we too slow to act? Arch Surg. 2009;144(4):333–8.
132. Fraccalvieri D, Biondo S, Saez J, et al. Management of colorectal anastomotic leakage: differences between salvage and anastomotic takedown. Am J Surg. 2012;204(5):671–6.
133. Verlaan T, Bartels SA, van Berge Henegouwen MI, Tanis PJ, Fockens P, Bemelman WA. Early, minimally invasive closure of anastomotic leaks: a new concept. Colorectal Dis. 2011;13 Suppl 7:18–22.
134. Whitlow CB, Opelka FG, Gathright Jr JB, Beck DE. Treatment of colorectal and ileoanal anastomotic sinuses. Dis Colon Rectum. 1997;40(7):760–3.

135. van Koperen PJ, van der Zaag ES, Omloo JM, Slors JF, Bemelman WA. The persisting presacral sinus after anastomotic leakage following anterior resection or restorative proctocolectomy. Colorectal Dis. 2011;13:26–9.
136. Cleary RK, Pomerantz RA, Lampman RM. Colon and rectal injuries. Dis Colon Rectum. 2006;49(8):1203–22.
137. Hallbook O, Sjodahl R. Anastomotic leakage and functional outcome after anterior resection of the rectum. Br J Surg. 1996; 83:60–2.
138. Ricciardi R, Roberts PL, Marcello PW, et al. Anastomotic leak testing after colorectal resection: what are the data? Arch Surg. 2009;144(5):407–11.
139. Iesalnieks I, Kilger A, Glass H, et al. Intraabdominal septic complications following bowel resection for Crohn's disease: detrimental influence on long-term outcome. Int J Colorectal Dis. 2008;23(12):1167–74.
140. Gutierrez A, Lee H, Sands BE. Outcome of surgical versus percutaneous drainage of abdominal and pelvic abscesses in Crohn's disease. Am J Gastroenterol. 2006;101(10):2283–9.
141. Nagell CF, Holte K. Treatment of anastomotic leakage after rectal resection with transrectal vacuum-assisted drainage (VAC). A method for rapid control of pelvic sepsis and healing. Int J Colorectal Dis. 2006;21(7):657–60.
142. Weidenhagen R, Gruetzner KU, Wiecken T, Spelsberg F, Jauch KW. Endoscopic vacuum-assisted closure of anastomotic leakage following anterior resection of the rectum: a new method. Surg Endosc. 2008;22(8):1818–25.
143. van Koperen PJ, van Berge Henegouwen MI, Rosman C, et al. The Dutch multicenter experience of the endo-sponge treatment for anastomotic leakage after colorectal surgery. Surg Endosc. 2009;23(6):1379–83.
144. Arezzo A, Miegge A, Garbarini A, Morino M. Endoluminal vacuum therapy for anastomotic leaks after rectal surgery. Tech Coloproctol. 2010;14(3):279–81.
145. Weidenhagen R, Wiecken F, Spelsberg K, Jauch W. User's report. Available at: www.aesculap.extranet.bbraun.com/public/frame_doc_index.html?med_id=1000007687. Accessed 9 Feb 2013.
146. Lippert E, Klebl FH, Schweller F, et al. Fibrin glue in the endoscopic treatment of fistulae and anastomotic leakages of the gastrointestinal tract. Int J Colorectal Dis. 2011;26(3): 303–11.
147. Gisbertz SS, Sosef MN, Festen S, Gerhards MF. Treatment of fistulas in ano with fibrin glue. Dig Surg. 2005;22(1–2):91–4.
148. Freeman RK, Ascioti AJ, Wozniak TC. Postoperative esophageal leak management with the polyflex esophageal stent. J Thorac Cardiovasc Surg. 2007;133:333–8.
149. Freeman RK, Van Woerkom JM, Ascioti AJ. Esophageal stent placement for the treatment of iatrogenic intrathoracic esophageal perforation. Ann Thorac Surg. 2007;83:2003–8.
150. Amrani L, Menard C, Berdah S, et al. From iatrogenic digestive perforation to complete anastomotic disunion: endoscopic stenting as a new concept of stent-guided regeneration and re-epithelialization. Gastrointest Endosc. 2009;69(7):1282–7.
151. DiMaio CJ, Dorfman MP, Gardner GJ, et al. Covered esophageal self-expandable metal stents in the nonoperative management of postoperative colorectal anastomotic leaks. Gastrointest Endosc. 2012;76(2):431–5.
152. Song H-Y, Kim JH, Kim KR, et al. Malignant rectal obstruction within 5 cm of the anal verge: is there a role for expandable metallic stent placement? Gastrointest Endosc. 2008;68:713–20.
153. Gornals JB, Golda T, Soriano A. Stent-in-stent technique for removal of a metal stent embedded in the colon wall by using a fully covered, self-expandable metal esophageal stent (with video). Gastrointest Endosc. 2012;76(3):695–6.
154. Blumetti J, Chaudry V, Prasad L, Abcarian H. Delayed transanal repair of persistent coloanal anastomotic leak in diverted patients after resection for rectal cancer. Colorectal Dis. 2012;14(10):1238–41.
155. Zhou JL, Shen B. Endoscopic needle knife therapy for anastomotic leakage following anterior resection for rectal cancer. Colorectal Dis. 2012;14(6):e365–6.
156. Stewart BT, Stitz RW. Marsupialization of presacral collections with the use of an endoscopic stapler. Dis Colon Rectum. 1999;42:264–5.
157. Fleshman JW, McLeod RS, Cohen Z, Stern H. Improved results following the use of an advancement technique in the treatment of ileoanal anastomotic complications. Int J Colorectal Dis. 1988; 3:161–5.
158. Pitel S, Lefevre JH, Tiret E, Chafai N, Parc Y. Redo coloanal anastomosis: a retrospective study of 66 patients. Ann Surg. 2012;256(5):806–10; discussion 810–1.
159. Lefevre JH, Bretagnol F, Maggiori L, Ferron M, Alves A, Panis Y. Redo surgery for failed colorectal or coloanal anastomosis: a valuable surgical challenge. Surgery. 2011;149(1):65–71.
160. Bannura GC, Cumsille MA, Barrera AE, Contreras JP, Melo CL, Soto DC. Predictive factors of stenosis after stapled colorectal anastomosis: prospective analysis of 179 consecutive patients. World J Surg. 2004;28(9):921–5.
161. Nguyen-Tang T, Huber O, Gervaz P, Dumonceau JM. Long-term quality of life after endoscopic dilation of strictured colorectal or colocolonic anastomoses. Surg Endosc. 2008;22(7):1660–6.
162. Kim PH, Song HY, Park JH, Kim JH, Na HK, Lee YJ. Safe and effective treatment of colorectal anastomotic stricture using a well-defined balloon dilation protocol. J Vasc Interv Radiol. 2012;23(5):675–80.
163. Polese L, Vecchiato M, Frigo AC, et al. Risk factors for colorectal anastomotic stenoses and their impact on quality of life: what are the lessons to learn? Colorectal Dis. 2012;14(3):e124–8.
164. Nieponice A, McGrath K, Qureshi I, et al. An extracellular matrix scaffold for esophageal stricture prevention after circumferential EMR. Gastrointest Endosc. 2009;69(2):289–96.
165. Schlegel RD, Dehni N, Parc R, et al. Results of reoperations in colorectal anastomotic strictures. Dis Colon Rectum. 2001;44: 1464–8.
166. Perez Roldan F, Gonzalez Carro P, Villafanez Garcia MC, et al. Usefulness of biodegradable polydioxanone stents in the treatment of postsurgical colorectal strictures and fistulas. Endoscopy. 2012;44(3):297–300.
167. Curcio G, Spada M, di Francesco F, et al. Completely obstructed colorectal anastomosis: a new non-electrosurgical endoscopic approach before balloon dilatation. World J Gastroenterol. 2010;16(37):4751–4.
168. McKee R, Pricolo VE. Stapled revision of complete colorectal anastomotic obstruction. Am J Surg. 2008;195(4):526–7.

Pelvic Bleeding

19

Amit Merchea and Bruce G. Wolff

Key Points

- Intraoperative presacral hemorrhage is a rare but potentially lethal complication.
- Most frequently, hemorrhage can be controlled by simple local means such as compression, electrocautery, or ligation.
- In laparoscopic cases, if control cannot be achieved, conversion to an open procedure should be expeditious and definitive.
- Surgeons should have an algorithm for treating bleeding that they and their operative team are comfortable enacting quickly and definitively.

Introduction

Key Concept: Hemorrhage is rare, but can be life-threatening. It is imperative to know the anatomy, remain calm, be meticulous, and know when to call for help.

Hemorrhage during pelvic surgery is a rare but potentially life-threatening phenomenon. The internal iliac (hypogastric) arteries supply the majority of blood flow to the pelvis. This vessel divides into anterior and posterior branches, with the anterior division providing the majority of the vascular supply to the pelvis and the posterior division largely providing collateral circulation. Areas of the pelvis that are potential sites of hemorrhage include the presacral space, iliac vasculature, retroprostatic or retrovaginal region, and gluteal vessels.

Presacral venous bleeding has a reported incidence in the literature of 3–9 % [1, 2]. The presacral venous plexus is covered by the presacral and pelvic fascia over the anterior sacrum. It is formed by two lateral sacral veins, the middle sacral vein, and many communicating veins. These ultimately communicate with the internal vertebral venous system via the basivertebral veins, which may be large-caliber and high-pressure vessels (Fig. 19.1) [3, 4]. It has been demonstrated that the adventitia of the presacral veins is adherent to the periosteum of the sacrum where the veins enter the sacral foramina – these areas are particularly vulnerable to tearing [5]. Mobilization of the rectum during proctectomy is usually performed with minimal bleeding; however, if the presacral fascia is breached, significant hemorrhage may ensue from the underlying presacral venous plexus or basivertebral veins [2, 4]. When the basivertebral veins are injured, these may retract into the sacral foramen making control difficult. Moreover, in the lithotomy position, the hydrostatic pressure in the sacral veins can be significantly higher than that of the inferior vena cava – thus increasing the potential rate of hemorrhage [4–6]. One must remember that it is very rarely necessary to violate the presacral fascia or to dissect upon the surface of the sacrum. Another caveat is careful placement of sutures in the presacral fascia during rectal rectopexy. During rectopexy, the presacral fascia is exposed and sutures are placed through this into the underlying periosteum. If bleeding is noticed with placement of these sutures, one can tie these down in an effort to ligate the injured vessel.

The overall incidence of vascular injury during pelvic operations is low (~1–2.3 per 100,000) [7, 8]. Dissection planes are often readily apparent in the normal patient; however, body habitus, previous surgery, large tumors, inflammation, radiation, and other factors may alter them and make these planes more difficult to discern. Adequate preoperative preparation, complete understanding of anatomic relations

A. Merchea, MD
Division of Colon and Rectal Surgery,
Department of Surgery, College of Medicine, Mayo Clinic,
4500 San Pablo Rd, Jacksonville, FL 32224, USA
e-mail: merchea.amit@mayo.edu

B.G. Wolff, MD (✉)
Division of Colon and Rectal Surgery,
Department of Surgery, College of Medicine,
Mayo Clinic, 200 First Street SW, Rochester, MN 55904, USA
e-mail: wolff.bruce@mayo.edu

S.R. Steele et al. (eds.), *Complexities in Colorectal Surgery*,
DOI 10.1007/978-1-4614-9022-7_19, © Springer Science+Business Media New York 2014

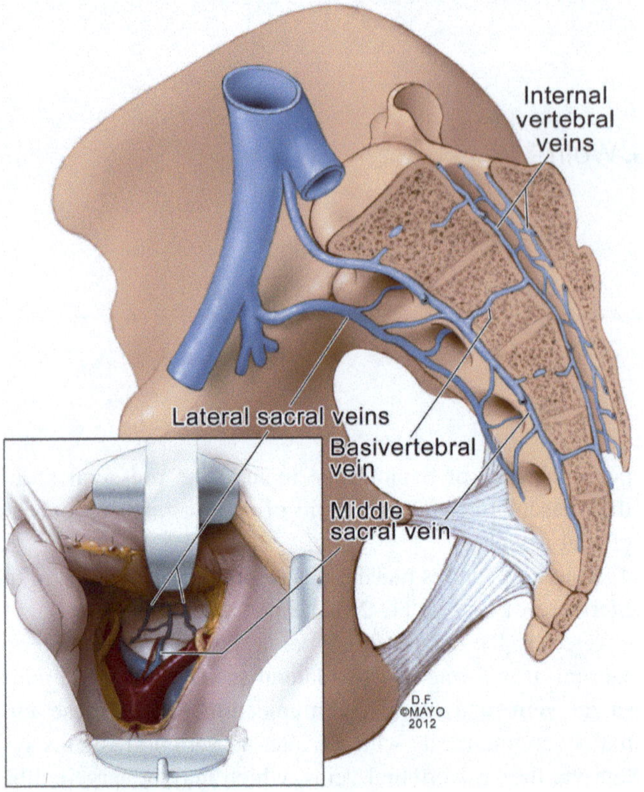

Fig. 19.1 The presacral venous plexus with communicating veins and basivertebral veins (With permission from Mayo Foundation for Medical Education and Research. All rights reserved)

within the pelvis, along with meticulous surgical technique and appropriate exposure, is essential to limit the risk of pelvic hemorrhage.

Risk Factors for Major Bleeding

Key Concept: Appropriately and completely evaluate the patient preoperatively and attempt to anticipate and plan for patients that may have an increased risk of bleeding.

The patient must be appropriately screened and examined preoperatively. Among the goals of this evaluation is to identify any comorbid condition that may influence the operative outcome. Within the context of bleeding, the patient must be screened in terms of their hematologic system – in particular, examining for any acquired or congenital coagulopathy (from inherited/acquired platelet disorders, factor deficiency, organ dysfunction, medications, etc.). In addition to a complete medication administration history, any prior kidney or liver dysfunction or malnutrition may impact the body's ability to form clot. Routine coagulation studies should be carried out prior to any procedure with the potential for blood loss. If a patient has an identified coagulation disorder, perioperative management of this may be best managed in concert with a hematologist.

Certain other patient factors may portend an increased risk of intraoperative hemorrhage. The re-operative pelvis requires a number of particular considerations. The surgeon must realize that anatomy may be altered or displaced secondary to adhesions and fixation of structures, including vasculature. Large, vascular tumors may pose a significant challenge for the surgeon [9]. Preoperative planning and potential coil embolization in these cases may temper the risk of intraoperative hemorrhage during resection. An intralesional resection may even be necessary *in large tumors that may distort the anatomy*, although in cases of malignancy this would be oncologically inappropriate [10].

Preoperative radiotherapy can increase the risk of bleeding compared to non-radiated cases [11]. Radiation therapy can lead to fibrosis and scarring, making identification of, and dissection in, appropriate tissue planes difficult. Tissues may become fixed and immobile, increasing the risk of inadvertent injury.

Limited literature exists concerning the characteristics and management of operative vascular injury. Oderich et al. have published a retrospective review spanning 18 years from the Mayo Clinic examining iatrogenic operative injuries of the abdominal and pelvic venous system. Of the 44 venous injuries identified, 30 involved the pelvic vasculature (most commonly, the external iliac vein). Perioperative mortality was 18 %, all attributed to the venous injury [7].

Prevention

Key Concept: Maintain adequate exposure (do not compromise safety for cosmesis) and have meticulous surgical technique.

Secondary to preoperative patient preparation, operative conduct is important in preventing hemorrhage. Adequate exposure and meticulous surgical dissection are essential. For open operations, a generous incision should be made to adequately visualize the anatomy. Laparoscopic or robotic approaches may improve visualization and dissection, particularly in a narrow pelvis, but control of hemorrhage once it occurs may be technically challenging.

Fundamental surgical principles of tension and countertension facilitate the identification and dissection in avascular planes. Eight avascular planes and spaces within the pelvis have been previously described (Table 19.1) [12]. Dissection

Table 19.1 Avascular planes and potential spaces of the pelvis

Retropubic space
Vesicovaginal space
Rectovaginal space
Retrorectal space
Pararectal spaces (two)
Paravesical spaces (two)

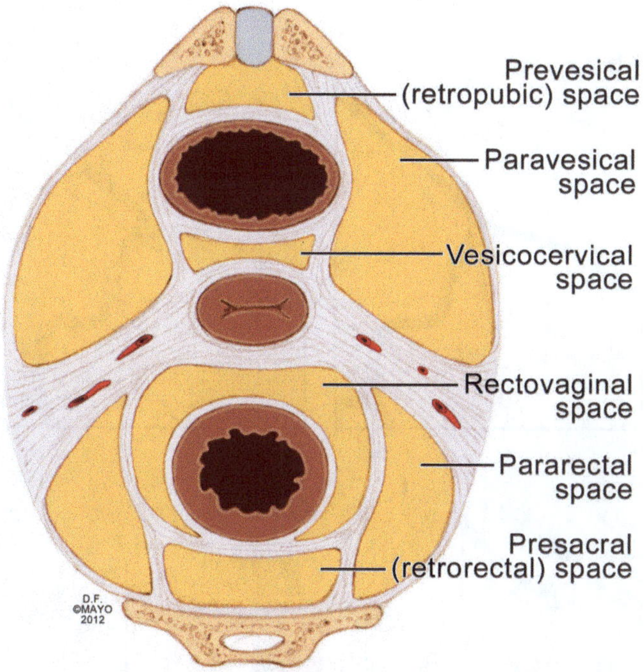

Fig. 19.2 The eight avascular planes of the pelvis (With permission from Mayo Foundation for Medical Education and Research. All rights reserved)

within these spaces can be expeditious and is generally safe (Fig. 19.2). When performing proctectomy, bluntly dissecting the posterior mesorectum from the sacrum with one's hand has been reported to be a common cause of presacral venous trauma and, in general, should be avoided [4].

Controlling Bleeding

Key Concept: Stay calm, have a stepwise algorithm for approaching various bleeding scenarios, and use the techniques you are comfortable with.

When a significant vascular injury occurs or brisk bleeding is evident, rapid and purposeful action must be taken to achieve control. Fundamental to achieving this is maintenance of composure and calm for the surgeon. Equally important is open communication with the anesthesiology team to alert them of significant hemorrhage so that more intensive monitoring can be initiated (hemodynamics, blood loss, urinary output, etc.) and blood products can be acquired from the blood bank. Methods of hemorrhage control include manual compression, electrocautery [13], vascular ligation, suture repair, use of topical coagulants [14, 15], damage-control techniques [5], and radiologic intervention. Whichever method is utilized, evacuation of blood from the operative field and securing adequate exposure of the bleeding site is imperative to accurately identify the source. Caution must be taken to protect vulnerable structures in the vicinity of the bleeding source as proximal and distal control is achieved, if possible.

The initial maneuver in controlling bleeding is often simple packing of the pelvis *with laparotomy sponges. Laparoscopically, a smaller sponge, such as a Ray-Tec, may be inserted through a 10/12 mm port and used to clear field or tamponade low-volume bleeding.* In many cases of low-pressure, low-volume bleeding, the hemorrhage will readily cease. Clips (or sutures) on visible presacral vessels may be feasible and must be placed on both sides of the vessel. *Sometimes further mobilization of the rectum or surrounding structures is necessary in order to adequately visualize the bleeding point.* Other unique and novel techniques have been described with varying success to halt presacral hemorrhage that could not be stopped with more conventional means (packing, electrocautery, suture ligature, clamping).

Many topical hemostatic agents have been described [14]. In our practice bone wax, gelatin foams (Gelfoam), oxidized cellulose (Surgicel), and thrombin with gelatin (FloSeal) are most commonly used. Bone wax exerts its effect through occlusion of bleeding orifices. This is not absorbed by the body and may become a nidus for infection [16]. Gelatin foams and oxidized cellulose act by providing a matrix for the initiation of coagulation [17, 18]. These are best used to control small vessel bleeding and are absorbed by the body within weeks. Thrombin with gelatin requires contact with blood to serve as the source for fibrinogen and can achieve reasonable control of moderate arterial bleeding [19].

Argon plasma coagulation is another thermal method of coagulation. In this modality, argon gas is ionized and used to deliver thermal energy to tissue adjacent to the probe with limited depth of penetration (2–3 mm). If readily available, this may be an effective tool.

The use of titanium thumbtacks inserted into the bleeding orifice of the sacrum has previously been reported (Fig. 19.3) [4, 20]. These thumbtacks, however, may not be readily available and a rare complication of erosion through the bowel wall has been reported [21]. Harrison et al. [22] reported on eight patients with massive bleeding treated with muscle fragment welding technique (Fig. 19.3), initially described by Xu in 1994 [23]. In this method a segment of rectus abdominis muscle is harvested from the patient's incision and placed over the bleeding region. Electrocautery on maximum is then applied to a forceps holding the muscle in place to "weld" the bleeding site. In all of these patients, hemostasis was successfully achieved after initial attempts at control via tamponade failed. Remzi et al. [24] describe securing a patch of harvested rectus abdominis to the bleeding point with absorbable sutures. While successful in their reported patients, suturing in a narrow, bleeding pelvis may be technically difficult and time consuming.

Other open surgical methods reported include the use of secured hemostatic sponges [1, 15], tissue expanders [25,

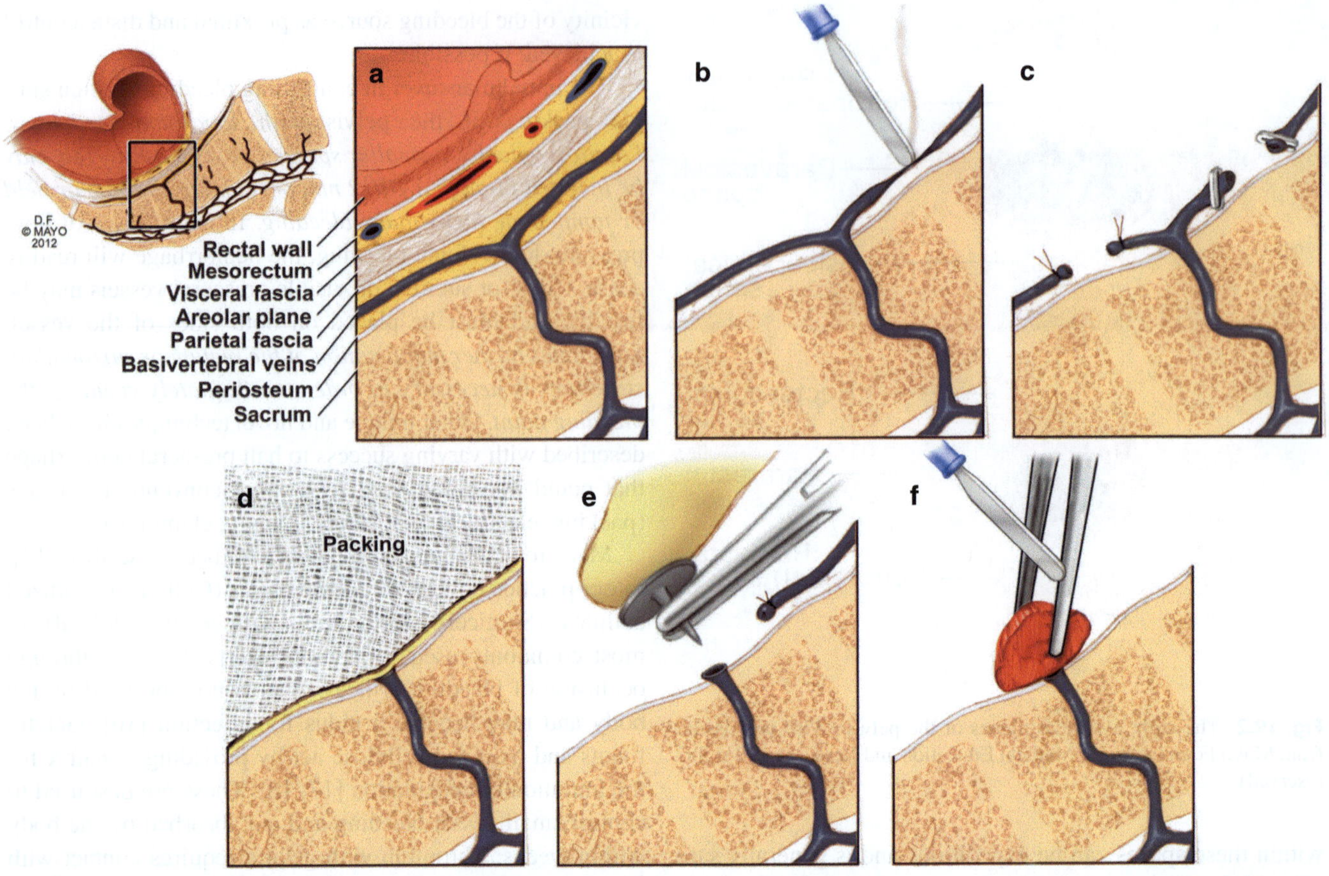

Fig. 19.3 Methods for control of hemorrhage. (**a**) Normal presacral venous plexus anatomy, (**b**) electrocautery, (**c**) suture ligature or clipping of transected vessels, (**d**) pelvic packing, (**e**) thumbtacks inserted into the sacrum, and (**f**) muscle welding (With permission from Mayo Foundation for Medical Education and Research. All rights reserved)

26], and saline bags [27]. Van der Vurst et al. [1] recently described the use of an endoscopic helical tacker to secure a sponge of Surgicel over the bleeding sacrum, thus eliminating the space beneath and providing tamponade. Tissue expanders and saline bags employ the same concept as packing in arresting hemorrhage. Proponents of these methods suggest that advantages include the ability to perfectly fit the concavity of the sacrum, the ability to increase the hemostatic pressure by increasing the fluid infused, and the potential ability to remove the devices at bedside, under local procedures [27]. While each of these alternative methods is reportedly effective, it is of our opinion that the simplest and most expeditious method that the operative team is comfortable with is initially chosen.

In the event of intractable pelvic hemorrhage, internal iliac artery ligation can increase the likelihood of control by decreasing the mean blood flow, mean arterial pressure, and overall pulse pressure within the pelvis [28, 29]. Care must be taken to identify the other branches of the iliac system to avoid inadvertent ligation of the common or external iliac arteries and to avoid injury to the hypogastric vein, which is deep and lateral, during ligation of the artery. *These vessels can be temporarily occluded with vessel loops or atraumatic vascular clamps to determine the level of effectiveness of this maneuver.* Ligation does not generally cause pelvic ischemia because of the extensive collaterals, unless the patient has significant peripheral arterial disease.

As laparoscopic and robotic methods are becoming more prevalent, surgeons must become facile with managing intraoperative complications, including bleeding. Management of this potentially lethal complication can be particularly challenging. Many of the same (or similar) techniques that are used in open approaches can be employed in laparoscopic operations [11]. However, if minimally invasive measures at controlling hemorrhage fail, the decision to convert to an open procedure must be made rapidly and without hesitation.

The initial maneuver laparoscopically often employs electrocautery to coagulate small bleeding vessels. Compression of the site with a gauze sponge inserted through one of the trocars can aide in compression, visualization, and exposure. Secondary to this, some authors have described harvesting an omental patch or epiploic fat and subsequently using bipolar cautery to "weld" this over the bleeding site, much like the rectus abdominis muscle patch. Bovine pericardial grafts have also been tacked to the bleeding site by endoscopic helical tackers to achieve tamponade [11]. Finally, argon beam coagulation is an alternative method that may be used [30]. It must be noted, however, that there should not be significant delay in enacting any of these methods. Not just the surgeon but the operating room staff must all be comfortable with the use of these tools. Given the potential lethality of presacral hemorrhage, surgeon judgment is the most important of the available tools – there should be no delay in converting to an open procedure if this is necessary to achieve hemostasis. The key is to minimize the blood loss – after control, set up remedial maneuvers methodically.

Massive, ongoing hemorrhage leads to acidosis, hypothermia, and coagulopathy – the so-called lethal triad [31]. In such circumstances the surgeon must consider "bailing out" and resuscitating the patient out of the operating room – particularly when the patient develops ongoing coagulopathy, despite blood product administration [5]. Originally described in the trauma literature [32, 33], the principles of "damage-control surgery" can be applied to other circumstances.

Pelvic packing with later reexploration is one form of damage control. Zama et al. [34] reported their experience in 93 patients with pelvic packing during abdominoperineal resection or low-anterior resection where packing was kept in place for up to 48 h. No patient in this series required any further intervention after removal of the packs, and there were no intra-abdominal or pelvic infectious complications or rebleeding. Our method of pelvic packing and temporary abdominal closure includes tightly packing multiple laparotomy pads within the pelvis; a sterile plastic drape is placed overlying the bowel to protect it, followed by suction drains and sterile towels. A sterile adhesive, occlusive drape is placed over this and suction applied to the drains. The patient is reexplored once physiologically stabilized in 24–48 h. Should bleeding persist or rebleeding occurs, transcatheter arterial embolization of the bleeding vessel can be attempted.

Summary Pearls

Pelvic and presacral bleeding is a rare and sometimes lethal event. The risk is limited by exquisite anatomic knowledge and careful dissection. However, they can occur and you need to be prepared that this may occur every time you perform a pelvic dissection. While you, as the surgeon, should have a stepwise algorithm to treat such episodes, you must have the instruments either readily available or nearby. Asking for tacks when no one is aware of where they are is futile. Finally, be comfortable with the techniques they employ, and do not hesitate in seeking assistance of more experienced colleagues, if necessary.

References

1. van der Vurst TJ, Bodegom ME, Rakic S. Tamponade of presacral hemorrhage with hemostatic sponges fixed to the sacrum with endoscopic helical tackers: report of two cases. Dis Colon Rectum. 2004;47(9):1550–3 [Case Reports].
2. Pollard CW, Nivatvongs S, Rojanasakul A, Ilstrup DM. Carcinoma of the rectum. Profiles of intraoperative and early postoperative complications. Dis Colon Rectum. 1994;37(9):866–74.
3. Baque P, Karimdjee B, Iannelli A, Benizri E, Rahili A, Benchimol D, et al. Anatomy of the presacral venous plexus: implications for rectal surgery. Surg Radiol Anat. 2004;26(5):355–8.
4. Wang QY, Shi WJ, Zhao YR, Zhou WQ, He ZR. New concepts in severe presacral hemorrhage during proctectomy. Arch Surg. 1985;120(9):1013–20.
5. McPartland KJ, Hyman NH. Damage control: what is its role in colorectal surgery? Dis Colon Rectum. 2003;46(7):981–6 [Review].
6. Hill AD, Menzies-Gow N, Darzi A. Methods of controlling presacral bleeding. J Am Coll Surg. 1994;178(2):183–4.
7. Oderich GS, Panneton JM, Hofer J, Bower TC, Cherry Jr KJ, Sullivan T, et al. Iatrogenic operative injuries of abdominal and pelvic veins: a potentially lethal complication. J Vasc Surg. 2004;39(5):931–6.
8. Nehler MR, Taylor Jr LM, Porter JM. Iatrogenic vascular trauma. Semin Vasc Surg. 1998;11(4):283–93 [Review].
9. Glasgow SC, Birnbaum EH, Lowney JK, Fleshman JW, Kodner IJ, Mutch DG, et al. Retrorectal tumors: a diagnostic and therapeutic challenge. Dis Colon Rectum. 2005;48(8):1581–7.
10. Dozois EJ, Malireddy KK, Bower TC, Stanson AW, Sim FH. Management of a retrorectal lipomatous hemangiopericytoma by preoperative vascular embolization and a multidisciplinary surgical team: report of a case. Dis Colon Rectum. 2009;52(5):1017–20 [Case Reports].
11. D'Ambra L, Berti S, Bonfante P, Bianchi C, Gianquinto D, Falco E. Hemostatic step-by-step procedure to control presacral bleeding during laparoscopic total mesorectal excision. World J Surg. 2009;33(4):812–5.
12. Gostout BS, Cliby WA, Podratz KC. Prevention and management of acute intraoperative bleeding. Clin Obstet Gynecol. 2002; 45(2):481–91 [Review].
13. Filippakis GM, Leandros M, Albanopoulos K, Genetzakis M, Lagoudianakis E, Pararas N, et al. The use of spray electrocautery to control presacral bleeding: a report of four cases. Am Surg. 2007;73(4):410–3.
14. Achneck HE, Sileshi B, Jamiolkowski RM, Albala DM, Shapiro ML, Lawson JH. A comprehensive review of topical hemostatic agents: efficacy and recommendations for use. Ann Surg. 2010;251(2):217–28 [Research Support, Non-U.S. Gov't Review].
15. Zhang CH, Song XM, He YL, Han F, Wang L, Xu JB, et al. Use of absorbable hemostatic gauze with medical adhesive is effective for achieving hemostasis in presacral hemorrhage. Am J Surg. 2012;203(4):e5–8.
16. Johnson P, Fromm D. Effects of bone wax on bacterial clearance. Surgery. 1981;89(2):206–9 [Research Support, U.S. Gov't, P.H.S.].
17. Wilkinson HA, Baker S, Rosenfeld S. Gelfoam paste in experimental laminectomy and cranial trephination: hemostasis and bone healing. J Neurosurg. 1981;54(5):664–7.
18. Frantz VK. Absorbable cotton, paper and gauze: (oxidized cellulose). Ann Surg. 1943;118(1):116–26.
19. Germanos S, Bolanis I, Saedon M, Baratsis S. Control of presacral venous bleeding during rectal surgery. Am J Surg. 2010;200(2): e33–5.
20. Nivatvongs S, Fang DT. The use of thumbtacks to stop massive presacral hemorrhage. Dis Colon Rectum. 1986;29(9):589–90.
21. Critchley AC, Holtham SJ. An unusual case of chronic anal pain–a pin in the bum? Ann R Coll Surg Engl. 2010;92(6):W27–8 [Case Reports].

22. Harrison JL, Hooks VH, Pearl RK, Cheape JD, Lawrence MA, Orsay CP, et al. Muscle fragment welding for control of massive presacral bleeding during rectal mobilization: a review of eight cases. Dis Colon Rectum. 2003;46(8):1115–7.
23. Xu J, Lin J. Control of presacral hemorrhage with electrocautery through a muscle fragment pressed on the bleeding vein. J Am Coll Surg. 1994;179(3):351–2.
24. Remzi FH, Oncel M, Fazio VW. Muscle tamponade to control presacral venous bleeding: report of two cases. Dis Colon Rectum. 2002;45(8):1109–11 [Case Reports].
25. Cosman BC, Lackides GA, Fisher DP, Eskenazi LB. Use of tissue expander for tamponade of presacral hemorrhage. Report of a case. Dis Colon Rectum. 1994;37(7):723–6 [Case Reports].
26. Braley SC, Schneider PD, Bold RJ, Goodnight Jr JE, Khatri VP. Controlled tamponade of severe presacral venous hemorrhage: use of a breast implant sizer. Dis Colon Rectum. 2002;45(1):140–2 [Case Reports].
27. Ng X, Chiou W, Chang S. Controlling a presacral hemorrhage by using a saline bag: report of a case. Dis Colon Rectum. 2008; 51(6):972–4 [Case Reports].
28. Burchell RC. Physiology of internal iliac artery ligation. J Obstet Gynaecol Br Commonw. 1968;75(6):642–51.
29. Tomacruz RS, Bristow RE, Montz FJ. Management of pelvic hemorrhage. Surg Clin North Am. 2001;81(4):925–48.
30. Kandeel A, Meguid A, Hawasli A. Controlling difficult pelvic bleeding with argon beam coagulator during laparoscopic ultra low anterior resection. Surg Laparosc Endosc Percutan Tech. 2011;21(1):e21–3.
31. Moore EE, Burch JM, Franciose RJ, Offner PJ, Biffl WL. Staged physiologic restoration and damage control surgery. World J Surg. 1998;22(12):1184–90; discussion 90–1.
32. Shapiro MB, Jenkins DH, Schwab CW, Rotondo MF. Damage control: collective review. J Trauma. 2000;49(5):969–78.
33. Stone HH, Strom PR, Mullins RJ. Management of the major coagulopathy with onset during laparotomy. Ann Surg. 1983;197(5): 532–5.
34. Zama N, Fazio VW, Jagelman DG, Lavery IC, Weakley FL, Church JM. Efficacy of pelvic packing in maintaining hemostasis after rectal excision for cancer. Dis Colon Rectum. 1988;31(12): 923–8.

Part IV

Anorectal Disease

Hemorrhoidal Disease: Postoperative Complications

20

Stefan D. Holubar and David E. Rivadeneira

Key Points

- In the United States, governmental and medical society recommendations suggest that Americans should ingest at least 25 g of dietary fiber (12 servings of fruits and/or vegetables per day). Many patients find this a difficult-to-obtain goal and is the basis for recommendations for supplemental soluble fiber to allow soft, bulky stool, which minimizes hemorrhoidal tissue trauma.
- When considering any operative approach to internal hemorrhoidal disease, proper patient selection is the crucial first step in avoiding complications. A complex interplay of factors such as age, gender, continence, comorbidities, and expected survival all play an important role in deciding on the optimal treatment.
- Despite the degree to which hemorrhoidal disease impacts patients' lives, surgeons and patients must be aware that postoperative complications may result in permanent quality of life consequences.

S.D. Holubar, MD, MS, FACS
Section of Colon and Rectal Surgery, Dartmouth-Hitchcock Medical Center, Geisel School of Medicine at Dartmouth, The Dartmouth Institute for Health Policy Research, One Medical Center Drive, Level 4C, Lebanon, NH 03756, USA
e-mail: stefan.holubar@dartmouth.edu, http://www.dhmc.org

D.E. Rivadeneira, MD, MBA, FACS, FASCRS (✉)
Division of Colorectal Surgery, Huntington and Southside Hospitals Northshore/LIJ Health System, Hofstra University School of Medicine, 755 New York Avenue, Suite 108, Huntington, NY 11743, USA
e-mail: drivadeneira@nshs.edu,
http://www.drdavidrivadeneira.com

The Hemorrhoidal Consult

Key Concept: When patients are referred to you with symptoms due to hemorrhoids, it is not hemorrhoidal pathology until you make the diagnosis.

"Hemorrhoids" are without a doubt the most common indication for referral to a colorectal surgeon. Due to several factors ranging from lack of experience to lack of a complete examination, you will often find that less than half of the patients referred for that indication actually have hemorrhoidal disease and only a minority (~10 %) of which will require intervention more than lifestyle modification [1, 2]. While this is more likely a reflection of improper training, it serves notice that you are the expert and need to be very familiar with anorectal anatomy and pathology. Given that half of the population of the United States over 50 are estimated to have hemorrhoidal bleeding at some point, likely due in part to lack of dietary fiber in the Western diet, the magnitude of the problem for both colorectal surgeons and as a public health concern should not be underestimated [3].

When approaching the hemorrhoidal consultation, one of the first things you as the consultant should consider is the patient's age. Aging results in physiologic changes that include pelvic floor laxity and constipation but also bring about a more sedentary lifestyle and the need for medications that can lead to excess straining. Similarly, patient gender has important implications. For females this includes a thorough gynecologic history focusing on prolonged labor, number of vaginal deliveries, episiotomies, and lacerations, as these can impact surgical decision-making and may contribute to otherwise avoidable complications. For example, a female patient with grade 3 hemorrhoids who had a previous third- or fourth-degree laceration may have an attenuated rectovaginal septum (Fig. 20.1). Depending on your findings, you may choose to perform a hemorrhoidectomy rather than a pexy, due to the risk of an iatrogenic rectovaginal

S.R. Steele et al. (eds.), *Complexities in Colorectal Surgery*,
DOI 10.1007/978-1-4614-9022-7_20, © Springer Science+Business Media New York 2014

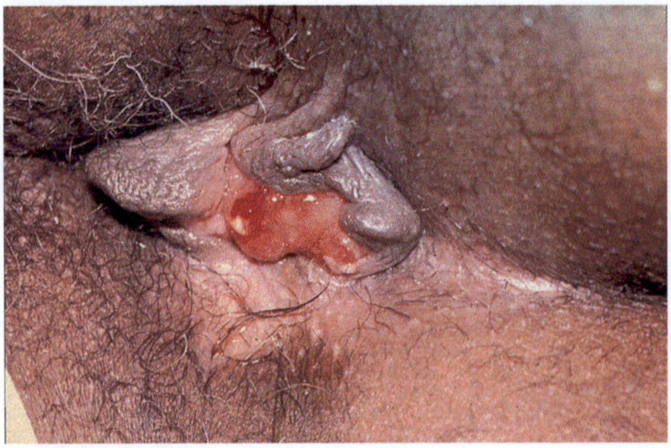

Fig. 20.1 Grade 3 hemorrhoids with attenuated RV septum (Courtesy of Richard Billingham, MD)

Table 20.1 Internal hemorrhoidal disease grading (classification)

Grade	Physical/anoscopic findings
I	No prolapse
II	Prolapse with spontaneous reduction
III	Prolapse requiring manual reduction
IV	Irreducible

fistula formation or sphincter disruption and the development of gross fecal incontinence. Most often a history of prolapse, along with the physical findings (Table 20.1) and the daily impact on the patient's quality of life, will guide the appropriate therapy.

Furthermore, you must always have a high index of suspicion for other competing etiologies of recurrent rectal bleeding such as other anorectal pathology, colorectal cancer, inflammatory bowel disease, COPD, or portal hypertension, mostly based on history, other symptoms, and family history (Fig. 20.2). Just because you see hemorrhoids on examination does not mean they are the underlying cause for your patient's symptoms.

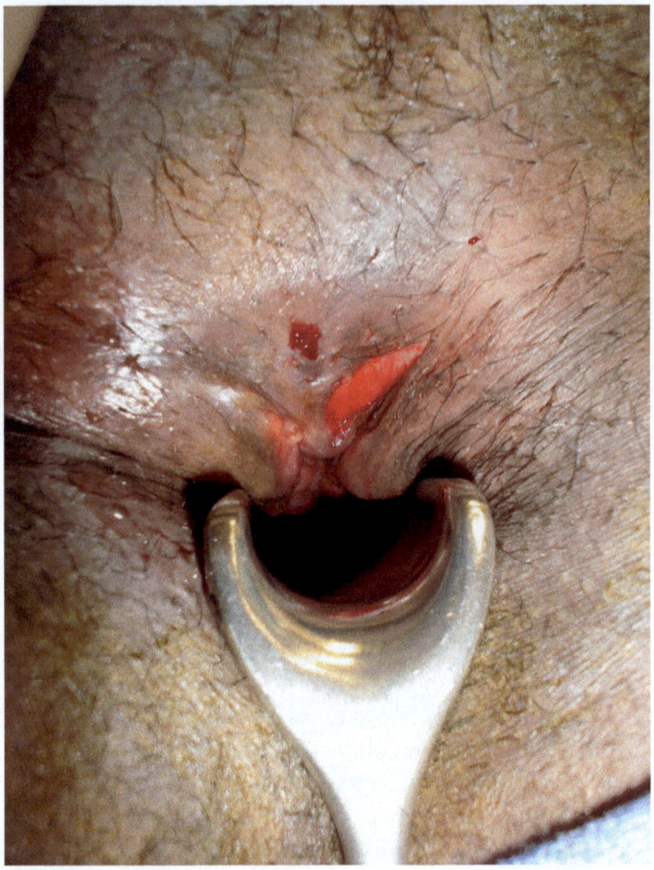

Fig. 20.2 Atypical anal fissure in a patient with concomitant hemorrhoids (Courtesy of Philip Y. Pearson, MD)

Table 20.2 Bristol stool form scale [4]

Type	Description
1	Nutlike nuggets, hard to pass
2	Tubular and lumpy, hard to pass
3	Tubular with cracks on surface
4	Tubular, soft, and smooth
5	Soft blobs with clear cut edges
6	Mushy, fluffy, ragged edge stool
7	Completely watery stool

Dietary and Bowel Habits

Key Concept: Every patient can benefit from supplemental fiber and education on proper bowel habits.

Focused history should quantify and qualify the patient's typical dietary and bowel habits. Almost all patients will initially state their diet is high in fiber. Yet, you should specifically determine whether or not a high-fiber diet (12 servings per day) or supplement is used and the frequency of stooling and the quality of stool using a standardize instrument (Bristol stool chart, Table 20.2; see also Fig. 13.1) [4]. This allows assessment of the size and shape (nuggets vs. large) as well as quality (soft vs. hard vs. watery diarrhea). It is also something you can characterize and follow over time to see their response to therapy. Hemorrhoid disease patients will often report habits, which include *straining* in order to affect a bowel movement, and often they will spend an inordinate amount of time on the commode. *Reading on the commode* while stooling is to be avoided. Likewise patients with *diarrheal stools* can have rectal bleeding that may be related to the frequency of wiping or competing etiology. It is important to exclude those causes. Another tool we find useful for assessing patients with constipation is the Rome-III criteria

Table 20.3 Rome-III criteria for functional constipation*

1	Must include *two or more* of the following: – Straining during at least 25 % of defecations – Lumpy or hard stools in at least 25 % of defecations – Sensation of incomplete evacuation for at least 25 % of defecations – Sensation of anorectal obstruction/blockage for at least 25 % of defecations – Manual maneuvers to facilitate at least 25 % of defecations (e.g., digital evacuation, support of the pelvic floor) – Fewer than three defecations per week
2	Loose stools are rarely present without the use of laxatives
3	Insufficient criteria for irritable bowel syndrome

*Criteria fulfilled for the last 3 months with symptom onset at least 6 months prior to diagnosis

Table 20.4 Side effects of common antiplatelet and anticoagulants

Medication	Selected side effects
Aspirin	Bronchospasm, allergy, PUD
Clopidogrel	Cytopenia (rare); TTP, PUD, angina, hypertension, headache
Prasugrel	Hypertension, TTP, cough, rash, nausea, headache
Dipyridamole	Cardiac ischemia/angina; nausea, vomiting, headache; least risk of bleeding
Glycoprotein IIb/IIIa antagonists	Thrombocytopenia; highest risk of bleeding
Coumadin	Several medication interactions

All can cause bleeding
PUD peptic ulcer disease, *TTP* thrombotic thrombocytopenic purpura

for functional constipation (Table 20.3) [5]. This is a helpful adjunct to classify the constipation, the usual root of the hemorrhoidal disease, as functional (slow transit or related to pelvic floor dysfunction) as opposed to irritable bowel syndrome type C.

Fecal continence (or lack thereof) also has a major impact on the development of and treatment recommendations for patients with symptoms attributable to hemorrhoidal disease. If intervention is required, an elderly female with frequent incontinence to gas, liquid, and occasionally solids may be better served by serial rubber band ligation, or hemorrhoidectomy, as opposed to hemorrhoidopexy, as cases of worsening continence after passage of the transanal stapling device has been observed.

Colonoscopy

Key Concept: Colonoscopy is not for diagnosing hemorrhoids but should be performed in at-risk patients, concerning findings, and those without resolution of their symptoms.

The role of colonoscopy has a definite place in the targeted evaluation and follow-up of rectal bleeding initially ascribed to hemorrhoids [6, 7]. Consider the case of an adopted 30-year-old man with a 2-year history of rectal bleeding. Most physicians would initially attempt a trial of fiber management and anoscopic rubber band ligation if you suspected internal hemorrhoids as the source. However, given the lack of family history, it is still crucially important that he have defined follow-up for the bleeding, as many colorectal surgeons have seen young patients with rectal bleeding, ascribed to as hemorrhoidal by the other providers, who then present much later with a locally advanced colorectal cancer after the bleeding never really resolves.

This is not to say that colonoscopy for rectal bleeding is the first diagnostic test, only that it must nonetheless be reserved for appropriate circumstances. Clearly all colorectal surgeons bear a shared responsibility for assessing adherence to national standard of care guidelines and at a minimum inquiring if their patients are up-to-date with screening colonoscopy [8].

Antiplatelet Agents and Anticoagulants

Key Concept: A number of both OTC and prescription medications can not only increase the risk of bleeding but also need to be addressed prior to intervention.

Hemorrhoidal disease is commonly seen in patients older than 50 years of age, the typical age of onset of symptomatic coronary artery disease and/or peripheral vascular disease. Given the side array of antiplatelet agents and anticoagulants (Table 20.4), colorectal surgeons must review their patient's medication lists and be familiar with these medications. As newer, more effective agents are added to the market, surgeons must also continuously be aware of the potential of bleeding events when operating on patients actively taking them, as well as the risk of thromboembolic events if they are held. A widely held tenet in medicine is that thromboembolic disease is more difficult to treat and more lethal than bleeding, which can generally be managed nonoperatively with transfusions in all but the most extreme circumstances.

One widely used medication is clopidogrel (Plavix TM), a potent antiplatelet agent that currently is without known antidote other than time and platelet transfusion. This medication, in conjunction with aspirin, is routinely given for 1 year after percutaneous vascular stenting in order to reduce thromboembolic events prior to endothelialization. It is recommended that the decision to hold this medication be made by the colorectal surgeon in conjunction with their cardiology colleagues, and studies suggest that for most patients after 5 days of cessation of therapy, surgery can be undertaken without increased risks [9].

"Every pain in the bottom is not a hemorrhoid" – How to deal with patients and referring providers when this is not hemorrhoids and they are convinced it is

Key Concept: You should take this opportunity to educate your referring physicians and patients, not chide them.

This is one of the most frustrating and most commonly encountered scenarios. As stated, as much as 50 % of symptoms such as rectal pain, bleeding, and prolapse are inappropriately attributed to hemorrhoids by the primary care physician, endoscopist, or the patient themselves. Therefore, part of the scope of practice is not to educate just the patients but the referring providers as well. It is also a bit of a balancing act between providing proper education and avoiding accusations or arguments. One thing we have found successful, even prior to an in-office enema administration or anorectal examination, is counseling patients that they should have an open mind as to what we will find. We often tell them about the 50 % statistic and ask them to keep in mind this may be the first time they are seeing a subspecialist. They should be aware that anorectal problems are commonly mistaken for each other, and they may be diagnosed with some competing etiology such as fissures, fistulas, infections, poor hygiene, or in a minority malignancy. Furthermore, we let them know that they may have hemorrhoids, but the symptoms are coming from something else. Most commonly, a simple question even without exam as to the quality of the pain (sharp as opposed to dull) gives a clue that one is dealing with a fissure as opposed to hemorrhoids (or infrequently both). Often patients have suffered for so long with "hemorrhoids" that they are quite relieved to not only finally have the proper diagnosis but also leave with what hopefully is an effective treatment plan. If they truly are convinced it to be a hemorrhoidal problem, you should consider a referral to another colorectal surgeon for a second opinion.

Similar to patient misperceptions, the flexible endoscopic appearance of anorectal pathology can be quite different than on anoscopic exam, and primary care providers (and even gastroenterology) who do not perform a high volume of anoscopy may be obviously trying to help but limited in their depth and breadth of anorectal experience. You must be careful not to offend the referring providers and ideally point out how common misperceptions of anorectal pathology occur in the copy of the note or letter that is sent back to the referring physician. Family Medicine and/or Gastroenterology Grand Rounds along with other educational venues are an ideal way to increase local provider awareness of common anorectal pathology. Certainly arming our colleagues with knowledge of optimal lifestyle modification is a crucial first step.

Table 20.5 Lifestyle modifications for patients with hemorrhoidal disease

	Lifestyle modification
Diet	High-fiber booklet
Soluble fiber supplement (bulking agent)	One heaping tablespoon in 8 oz of water once or twice daily with the goal of producing soft, bulky stool on a daily basis (ideally). Can reduce amount of water to 4 oz if loose stool
Fluids	2 l fluid intake by mouth per day
Straining	Avoid straining on the commode
Commode	Avoid reading on the commode or spending excessive time on the commode
Perianal hygiene	Avoid excessive cleansing; use a peri-bottle, sports bottle, sitz bath, detachable showerhead, or bidet. Apply zinc oxide or other diaper ointment before each bowel movement to protect perianal skin
Nothing per rectum	Avoid suppositories, digital dis-impaction, or any other transanal instrumentation or intervention
Kegel exercises	Age appropriate for borderline continence or incontinence
Pelvic floor retraining	If concomitant pelvic floor dysfunction

Lifestyle Modification

Key Concept: Fiber does really work, if your patients take adequate amounts on a regular basis.

In the United States, governmental and medical society recommendations suggest that Americans should ingest at least 25 g of dietary fiber (12 servings of fruits and/or vegetables per day). Many patients find the goal of 25 g of dietary fiber per day a difficult goal to obtain. Yet, it is also the basis for recommendations, based on level 1 data, for the use of supplemental soluble fiber to allow a soft, bulky stool, which minimizes hemorrhoidal tissue trauma. In a meta-analysis of seven randomized trials, Alonso-Coello et al. showed that fiber results in an approximate 50 % decrease in symptoms [10]. Most, if not all, patients should try lifestyle modification before any more invasive intervention. Table 20.5 lists examples of lifestyle modification.

Surgical Decision-Making: How to Decide on What Surgery to Do (Open, Closed, Energy, PPH, THD)

Key Concept: A number of surgical options exist for hemorrhoidectomy. Understand the risks and benefits with each one, and use them as appropriate in indicated patients.

In 1992, Bleday et al. reviewed the University of Minnesota experience with hemorrhoidal disease [11]. Of an initial 21,000 patients, 45 % were offered conservative therapy, 45 % rubber band ligation, and 9.3 % underwent operation.

Table 20.6 Surgeon- and patient-related factors that influence the choice of operative intervention for hemorrhoidal disease refractory to conservative treatment

Surgeon-related	Patient-related
Prior education and training	Age, gender, medications
Operative experience	Bowel and sphincter function
Local resources	Patient travel resources
Product availability	Patient work and family preferences
Confidence of diagnosis of isolated hemorrhoidal disease (i.e., concurrent pelvic floor dysfunction, fecal incontinence, IBD)	Red flag comorbidities: portal hypertension, Crohn, pregnancy, hx pelvic radiotherapy/radiation proctitis, immunosuppression/ immunocompromised, bleeding diatheses, poor functional status, limited life expectancy, others
Magnitude of hemorrhoidal disease burden (i.e., how big are they?)	Magnitude of the hemorrhoidal disease on the patient's daily quality of life (i.e., how bad is it?)

Certainly this experience suggests only 10 % of patients require more than lifestyle modification and/or rubber band ligation. If the surgeon and patient decide that more than conservative measures are warranted, many factors may influence the choice of intervention (Table 20.6). Clearly one size does not fit all, and treatment needs to be tailored and individualized for each patient based on the estimation of benefit and risk of the various surgical options and surgeon comfort and experience with chosen technique being crucial.

In general, grade II hemorrhoidal disease is treated with lifestyle modification and then banding, while the gold standard operation for grade III hemorrhoidal disease is the closed modification of the classic open Milligan-Morgan excisional hemorrhoidectomy (i.e., closed Ferguson excisional hemorrhoidectomy), due to its lowest recurrence rate. However, patients must be willing to sacrifice a significant amount of days off work (average of 2 weeks), and pain and discomfort may take 6 weeks or longer to subside with an excision. A common modification of this operation is the use of a Harmonic Scalpel® (Ethicon, Cincinnati, OH) or LigaSure™ device (Covidien, Mansfield, MA), even for grade IV disease [12, 13]. In general these adjuncts, despite their increased costs, decrease operative time and may result in less pain, fewer complications (less bleeding and urinary retention), and better patient satisfaction [12–16]. Initial concerns that the LigaSure may result in anal stenosis are likely due to lack of experience with the technique [17–19] and in experienced hands lead to equivalent outcomes as conventional hemorrhoidectomy. Although a meta-analysis of nine randomized trials from 2007 suggested that although use of the LigaSure hemorrhoidectomy reduced operative time and blood loss, it may not decrease pain or result in faster time to return to work [20]. Subsequently the Cochrane Collaboration meta-analysis from 2009 of 12 randomized studies on this topic suggested that given apparent equivalent outcomes with decreased pain and earlier return to work (4.8 days earlier), LigaSure hemorrhoidectomy appears superior to conventional excisional hemorrhoidectomy [21].

Compared with excisional hemorrhoidectomy, stapled hemorrhoidopexy is a relatively new, minimally invasive, technologically driven procedure. Despite it being a young procedure (approximately 10 years old), extensive level I data exists with which to guide optimal patient selection and educate expected outcomes [22, 23]. Due to its increased recurrence rate, the procedure for prolapse and hemorrhoids (PPH) should be used selectively as an alternative to conventional or bipolar excisional hemorrhoidectomy in patients with *circumferential* grade III hemorrhoidal disease without an especially large external component. Well-over a dozen randomized trials exist which usually show, similar to laparoscopic (minimally invasive surgery), that the PPH has a shorter operative time, less postoperative pain, and faster return to work compared to excisional hemorrhoidectomy [22]. In essence the device is a circular end-to-end anastomotic (EEA) stapler up-sized for the anorectal canal and specifically designed and intended for endoluminal supra-hemorrhoidal tissue mucosal resection (not full-thickness resection!). Thus, it results in pexying the prolapsing hemorrhoids higher in the anorectal canal ("face-lift for the anus" similar conceptually to serial rubber band ligation done all at once). The resultant mucosal resection should have very few if any muscle fibers in it and ideally should be symmetric and not be eccentric or "waisted." Median operative times should be around 30 min for those over the learning curve. Despite short operative times and less postoperative pain, widespread adoption has been limited over surgeon concern regarding (a) the different, potentially more serious complications and (b) lack of long-term data. The most recent meta-analysis on the topic showed that the PPH procedure has a higher recurrence rate, with need for more re-interventions, compared with excisional hemorrhoidectomy [24]. Thus, it would appear patients and surgeons must weigh the short-term gains vs. the long-term potential for recurrence.

A number of randomized trials have compared LigaSure hemorrhoidectomy to stapled hemorrhoidopexy [25, 26]. Arsiani recently randomized 98 patients and found that the stapled procedure had non-statistically significantly higher complication rate (24 % vs. 14 %) and recurrence rate (11 % vs. 2 %). These results are nearly identical to those of Sakr et al. who randomized 68 patients and found complications in 24 % vs. 6 % and residual prolapse in 12 % vs. 3 %.

Transanal Hemorrhoidal Dearterialization (THD)

Key Concept: THD appears to be effective for grade II and III hemorrhoids but has (at present) a niche role in the treatment of hemorrhoids.

The newest minimally invasive, alternative treatment option for hemorrhoidal disease for patients who defer or have contraindication to excisional hemorrhoidectomy is transanal hemorrhoidal dearterialization (THD) also known as Doppler-guided hemorrhoidal artery ligation (HAL*)*. Giordano et al. performed a systematic review of the procedure which reviewed 17 studies and almost 2,000 patients [27]. Although its place in the hemorrhoidal disease treatment algorithm remains uncertain, it appears to be an efficacious, minimally invasive option for grade II and grade III disease. As an outpatient procedure, operative times were typically less than 1 h, with most patients returning to work within a few days and only 18 % of patients experiencing pain. Acute hemorrhage was rare—seen in only three patients. Despite these excellent short-term outcomes, at 1-year symptom recurrence was relatively common—11 % for prolapse, 10 % for bleeding, and 9 % for painful defecation. Subsequently in a review of 170 patients, Ratto et al. reported bleeding in 1.2 %, confirmed residual prolapse in 10 %, and recurrent disease requiring operative intervention in 4 % [28]. In this at 1 year, bleeding and prolapse were controlled in 94 and 90 %, respectively. Clearly results are superior in grade II or II disease compared to grade IV disease, in which this therapy is likely a suboptimal choice [27, 28]. Given the paucity of high-quality data, this procedure will not be discussed in the remainder of this chapter.

Hemorrhoidal Crisis: What Do You Decide to Do at the Time?

Key Concept: When presented with this situation, it is not the time to be overly aggressive surgically. Stick to your basic principles of preserving anoderm, relieve the inflammation and clot, and do not damage the underlying sphincter.

Hemorrhoidal crisis, defined as acutely incarcerated or strangulated internal hemorrhoids with a component of secondary external thrombosis, requires expedient expert care (Figs. 20.3 and 20.4). These patients usually have a past history of constipation and prolapse and present with severe anorectal pain as well as urinary retention. In the past, patients were treated conservatively with analgesics, ice packs, and sitz baths given the major impendent to surgical intervention of distorted anatomy from both the underlying clot burden as well as the marked edema. However, true risk to patients, especially if diabetic, exists with nonoperative approach given necrotic tissue.

In order to expedite resolution of suffering, colorectal surgeons facile with excisional hemorrhoidectomy can and should intervene selectively in single or multiple quadrants as the distorted anatomy and comfort of the surgeon allows excising necrotic tissue, expressing thrombosis, and reducing prolapse. Optimal intervention includes either closed or, in the presence of significant necrotic tissue, open excisional hemorrhoidectomy (Fig. 20.5). In general, the authors would avoid stapled hemorrhoidopexy in these circumstances for

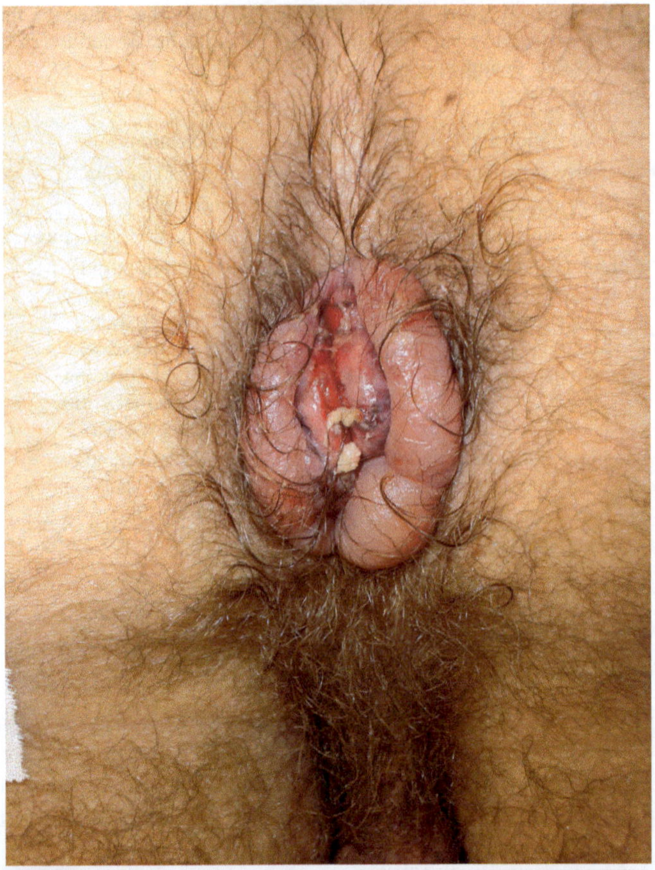

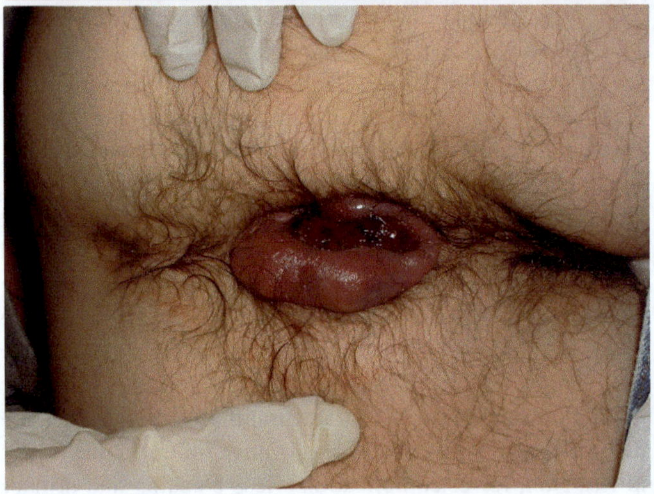

Figs. 20.3 and 20.4 Hemorrhoidal crisis (Courtesy of Richard Billingham, MD and Philip Y. Pearson, MD)

fear of the large 33-mm stapler or large dilator causing inadvertent sphincter damage. In addition, a large part of the symptoms from this situation is from the external component—something that the stapled pexy does not address.

In 1982, C. Wang from Taiwan reported on his experience with urgent closed hemorrhoidectomy in 56 patients [29]. The reported technique specifically used packing to push the mucosal flaps against the anorectal wall and to reduce hemorrhage, and he reported excellent outcomes. More recently

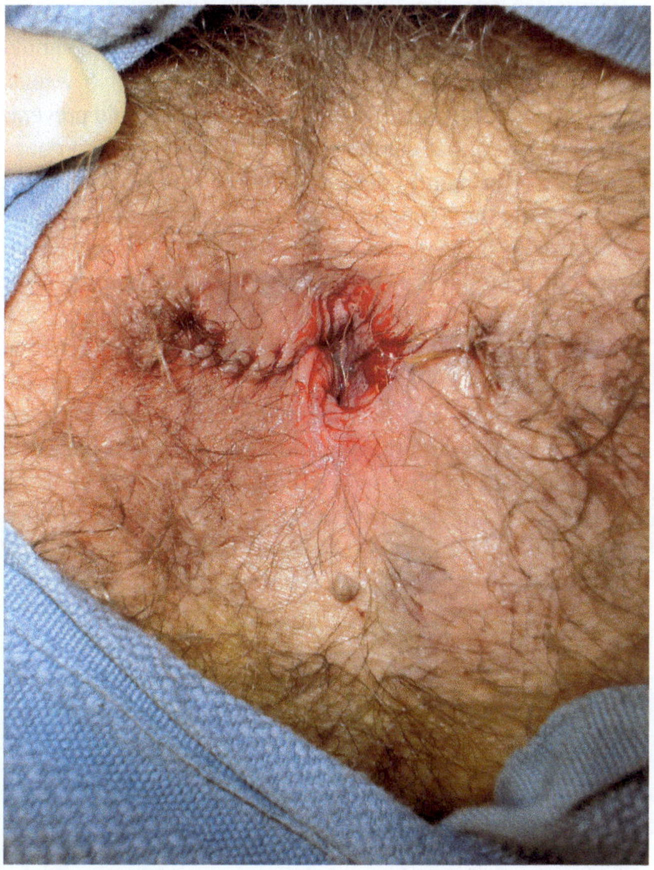

Fig. 20.5 Wounds following excision for hemorrhoidal crisis. This patient is the same as Fig. 20.2 for comparison (Courtesy of Philip Y. Pearson, MD)

a randomized trial of a potentially less morbid alternative of incising the mucosa overlying the clots (similar to as for external hemorrhoids) with rubber band ligation was shown to be safe and effective [30].

In our experience, the choice of what to offer the patient depends highly on the surgeon assessment of the degree of anatomic distortion and presence or absence of gangrenous changes—the latter a clear indication for excision. Also, if a less invasive approach is undertaken, without adequate assessment of gangrene or suboptimal results, a contingency plan for expeditious treatment must be in place if the patient decompensates (i.e., rural or unreliable patients may need to be admitted for observation).

Postoperative Regimen

Bowel Management and Avoiding Constipation

Key Concept: Ensure your patient is on a proper bowel regimen postoperatively or obstipation (or extreme pain with hard bowel movements days later) will ensue.

After elective hemorrhoidectomy, in addition to taking fiber and increased fluids, it is important for patients to preemptively treat and avoid narcotic-induced constipation. We recommend fiber twice daily, stool softener three times daily, and if no bowel movement within 48 h, then 60 cc of milk of magnesia every 12 h until a movement is achieved. An alternative regimen would be fiber in the morning and MiraLax (17 g in a tall glass of water) in the evening.

Pain Control with Narcotics, NSAIDS

Key Concept: Non-narcotics aid in reducing not only the pain but also decreasing the need and side effects from narcotics.

Optimal analgesia is achieved using a combination of nonnarcotics and narcotics including, for example, maximum dose Tylenol (recently reduced from 4 to 3 g per 24 h by the FDA due to concerns over hepatic toxicity) 750 mg by mouth every 6 h, alternating every 3 h with 600 mg of ibuprofen with food every 6 h. Opioid-naïve patients are then typically prescribed oxycodone 5–10 mg every hour as needed for breakthrough pain, with titration as needed. The amount of postoperative opioids may be reduced by the intraoperative use of ketorolac, as well as other newer adjuncts as described below [31].

Sitz Baths: Do They Work?

Key Concept: Despite lack of evidence, sitz baths are widely used and have little downside.

Used since ancient times, little level I data exist for the effect of warm sitz (from the German word "sit") baths on hemorrhoidal pain, but several studies have documented that warm water sitz baths do indeed result in a decrease in anorectal canal pressure for both fissure and hemorrhoid patients [32, 33].

Patients are counseled that soaking the buttocks and anus in warm water for 15 min four times a day is generally recommended and is thought to (1) aid in keeping the area clean, (2) increase perfusion to aid healing (3) reduce anorectal canal resting pressure, and (4) be soothing for most but not all patients. In our experience, sitz baths are effective for the stated reasons, and patients should be counseled that they are an important component of their optimal postoperative outcome and one which they need to take responsibility for.

Preoperative Counseling and Postoperative Instructions

Key Concept: Managing patients' expectations ahead of time and having preprinted instructions for the postoperative

Table 20.7 Post-hemorrhoidal banding patient instructions

	Self-care after banding
Discomfort in rectum	Sitz baths, Tylenol, ibuprofen
Constipation prevention	1st-line fiber, 2nd-line milk of magnesia
Bleeding	Minor bleeding expected
Infection	Rare; if delayed urinary retention or fever >101.3 °F (38.5 °C), then consider proceeding to the emergency department
Passing the band	Expect to not necessarily see the band(s) pass in the stool
Recurrent symptoms	Return to clinic no sooner than 6 weeks for consideration of additional banding

period that addresses many of the commonly encountered scenarios and questions go a long way in making this easier on your patient (and you).

Banding

As part of the informed consent process, patients should be counseled re: the likelihood of needing additional banding every 4–6 weeks until the problem is cured or the patient and the surgeon decide to try a different therapy. In addition, we cover the possibility of vasovagal reaction (relatively common) that they may experience some additional bleeding after the band falls off in 5–7 days, discomfort with the feeling that something is stuck in their rectum for approximately 24 h, feel the urge to defecate, and that rarely the rubber band application of the rubber band may result in perianal sepsis and risk of colostomy or death. Patients are counseled if they have fever or urinary retention to proceed to the emergency room for evaluation. Table 20.7 shows a sample of banding patient instructions.

Stapled Hemorrhoidopexy

Patients should be counseled that the first part of the operation is an exam under anesthesia, and sometimes those findings will steer us away from the stapled procedure; you and patient should, ahead of time, discuss the possibility that the EUA may change the operative plan, and the surgeon may recommend just banding at the time of EUA or excisional hemorrhoidectomy. Although stapled hemorrhoidopexy results in less discomfort relative to excisional procedure, patients may still experience significant discomfort that may last as long as 2 weeks (or permanently in the setting of complications) and should be given appropriate analgesics (i.e., narcotics) and bowel regimen. Also, most of the complications of stapled hemorrhoidopexy (see below) should be discussed with the patient, including chronic or permanent alterations in bowel habits and permanent pain and need for additional surgery. In general the recommendations from Table 20.7 apply, with the exception that patients may see staples as opposed to bands.

Excisional Hemorrhoidectomy

This procedure is notoriously painful, and patient should expect pain and discomfort for the better part of 6 weeks. Patients need to be committed to doing sitz baths and preventing constipation that can be anticipated due to the narcotics and also fear of painful defecation (fiber twice daily, Colace 100 mg orally three times daily at a minimum, increased fluid >2 l per day). If the patient does not have a bowel movement within 48 h of surgery despite the above regimen, then we recommend starting 60 cc of milk of magnesia every 12 h until a bowel movement is achieved. Use of ice packs (frozen peas which mold to the area as they soften) may also be used to treat discomfort and swelling. Patients also need to understand that after approximately 24–48 h, the wounds are likely to open up and significant swelling may occur. It is also a good idea to let your patient know they may have open wounds for weeks that will eventually heal in but may be left with small tags that can always be removed in the office.

Complications of Hemorrhoidectomy: What Are They, How Often Do They Occur, and How to Approach and Manage Them?

Key Concept: Hemorrhoidectomy typically goes very well, but it is not a benign operation. You need to be aware of not only how to avoid complications but also how to manage them.

Other than surgical texts which provide exhaustive reviews of complications [34, 35], some of the best available, real-world data on hemorrhoidectomy complications comes from the University of Minnesota experience in over 21,000 patients [11]. Overall a small percentage developed a complication of excisional hemorrhoidectomy. A similar, small but interesting study (largely due to the fact that they reported what the complications were attributable to) is a review of over 700 Russian patients that found complications occurred in 23.3 %—likely higher than many surgeons would estimate [36]. They found that one-quarter of these were attributable to occult concomitant anorectal pathology at the time of the hemorrhoidectomy, one-third attributable to the excision itself, and 36 % attributable to systemic disease. A summary of complications is shown in Table 20.8.

Urinary Retention

One of the more common occurrences after excisional hemorrhoidectomy, urinary retention can be a nuisance for patient but can also predispose to urinary tract infection secondary to repeated catheterization. The University of Minnesota study [11] reported that 20 % of patients developed either urinary retention or infection. Retention is

Table 20.8 Complications of excisional hemorrhoidectomy [36]

	Frequency	Possible preventive measures	Management
Pain	100 %	Preemptive analgesia, avoid excessive anoderm (skin) excision. Preoperative expectation management	Tylenol, NSAIDs, narcotics, bowel regimen
Skin tags	Common	Preoperative expectation management	Consider excision only if associated with exceptionally poor hygiene and/or quality of life and not stenotic
Urinary retention	2–36 %	Limit intraoperative fluids, mandatory voiding, and bladder scans prior to discharge	Intermittent clean catheterization, Foley catheterization, outpatient follow-up
Incontinence	2–12 %	Avoid incising sphincter muscle. Patient selection (avoid excision in patients with preexisting incontinence)	Seepage and soiling usually resolves by 8 weeks. Pads, bulking agents, antimotility agents. Kegel exercises, pelvic floor retraining
Recurrent hemorrhoids	<10 %	Optimal patient selection and technique, preoperative expectation management	Banding, redo excision
Hemorrhage	2–6 %	Completion anoscopy, packing, hold aspirin, NSAIDs, antiplatelet agents preoperatively	Exam under anesthesia, suture ligation
Stricture/severe anal stenosis	<6 %	Avoid excessive excision without adequate *mucosal* bridges between quadrants	Anal self-dilation, dermal advancement flaps/anoplasty
Infection/chronic open wounds	<6 %	Avoid excessive excision without adequate *skin* bridges between quadrants. Preoperative smoking cessation/nutritional optimization	Wound hygiene, bulking agents, nutritional optimization
Whitehead deformity	?	Do not excessively exteriorize the advanced mucosa beyond the dentate line	Dermal advancement flaps/anoplasty
Wet anus and pruritus ani	?	Do not excessively exteriorize the advanced mucosa beyond the dentate line. Avoid incising sphincter muscle. Patient selection (avoid excision in patients with preexisting incontinence)	Dietary changes, bulking agents, antimotility agents. If ectropion, then anoplasty with excess mucosal excision and anchoring of cut mucosal edge +/− dermal advancement flap
Chronic pain	?	Avoid excising posterior midline	Define and treat underlying source of pain

certainly multifactorial and related to excess IV fluids, rectal pain and spasm, and narcotics. (See preventative strategies at the end of this chapter and in Table 20.8.) Typically patients will require placement of a Foley catheter with a leg bag for 3–7 days, followed by successful resolution following a "fill and pull" in the clinic setting.

Hemorrhage

Early acute postoperative hemorrhage after excisional hemorrhoidectomy, defined as within the first 24 h, is a technical error from inadequate suture ligation of the apex of the hemorrhoidal pedicle. Delayed hemorrhage is typically reported at 2.4–6 % [11, 34] and may represent disruption of the pedicle suture by erosion or destruction by sepsis and is likely unavoidable in most cases. Although the vast majority of cases are self-limiting, moderate to severe stenosis will often require a repeat examination under anesthesia and suture ligation.

Whitehead Deformity

Mucosal ectropion (Fig. 20.6) is a complication most commonly seen after Whitehead operation, also known as circumferential hemorrhoidectomy. Currently, in the early twenty-first century, given the success and durability of 3-quadrant open or closed excisional hemorrhoidectomy, relatively few colorectal surgeons have been trained in the procedure or perform it commonly. Nonetheless, it can still result from excessive hemorrhoidectomy and/or improper technique of suturing the mucosa not approximately to, but distally to, the dentate line and or anal verge or suturing excessive/prolapsing mucosa. Such improper technique can also lead to anal stricture. When confronted with this situation, resection of the excess mucosa and bilateral flaps are often successful (Fig. 20.7).

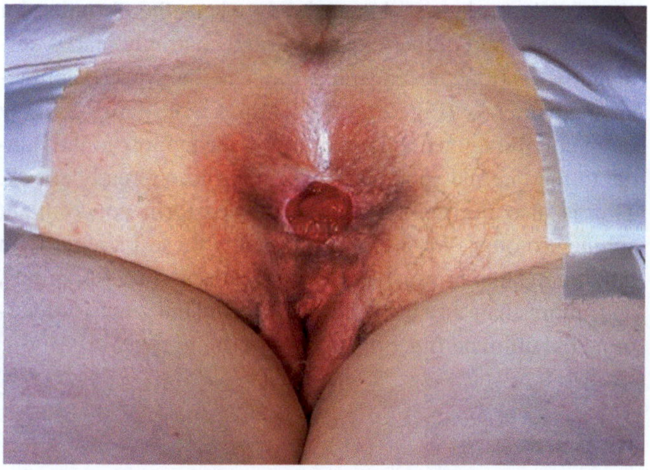

Fig. 20.6 Mucosal ectropion following circumferential hemorrhoidectomy (Courtesy of W. Brian Sweeney, MD)

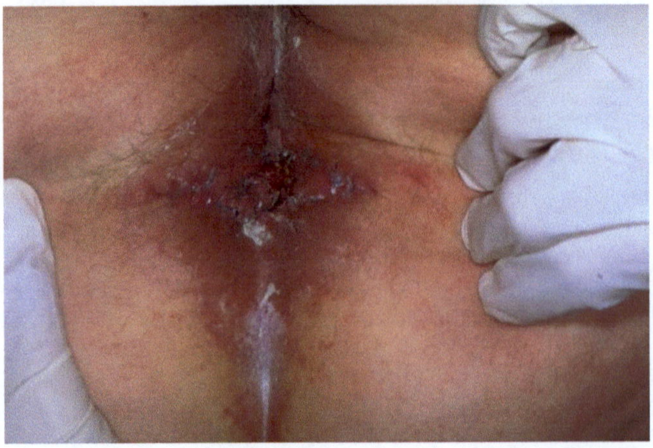

Fig. 20.7 Completed bilateral house flaps for mucosal ectropion (Courtesy of W. Brian Sweeney, MD)

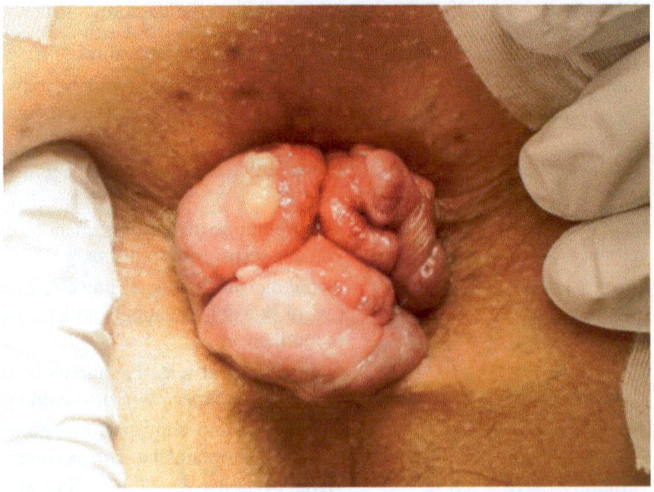

Fig. 20.8 Chronic grade three hemorrhoids. Note the chronic hypertrophic skin changes and mucosa with stigmata of recent bleeding

Fecal Incontinence

Frank fecal incontinence after hemorrhoidectomy is rare; however, continence alteration may be relatively common (2–12 %) and likely due to preexisting incontinence in older or female patients with altered pelvic floor. This may be partly attributable to anal retracting/exuberant exam under anesthesia or rarely can be seen in the case of massively chronically prolapsing hemorrhoids where the chronic clot has fibrosed and obliterated the normal anatomic planes sufficiently to allow the surgeon to damage the external sphincter inadvertently (Fig. 20.8). Incontinence to flatus is likely more common given the proximity of the hemorrhoidal bundle to the internal sphincter, especially those already at risk. This is also the main reason *not* to perform concomitant sphincterotomy. We prefer to approach these patients with bulking agents, bowel-slowing medications (i.e., Imodium), and, more than anything, allowing sufficient time to determine the ultimate function, as most will improve.

Anal Stricture

Anal stricture, estimated to occur in 0–6 % of patients after hemorrhoidectomy, represents the trading of one surgical disease for another (Fig. 20.9) [37]. Patients with very large essentially circumferential hemorrhoidectomy, in whom a three-quadrant or circumferential excision is undertaken and the wounds are closed under tension, are prone to develop this complication. It can certainly also develop in lesser cases in patient known to be predisposed to excess scar formation. The underlying pathophysiology is lack of elastic tissue encircling the sphincter complex, with removal of the anoderm, preventing iris-like dilation during defecation. Treatment is anoplasty with healthy elastic perianal skin is

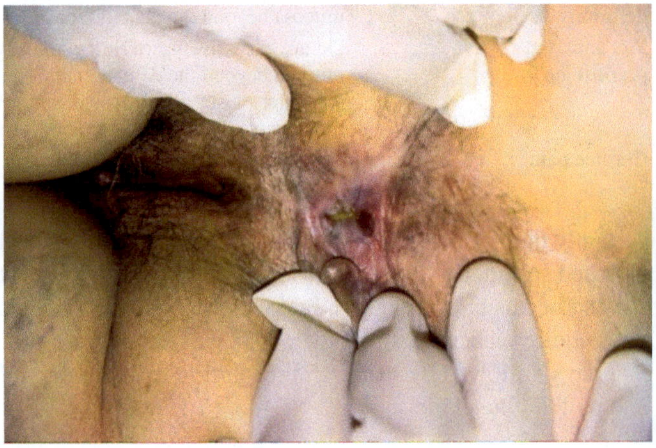

Fig. 20.9 Anal stenosis following hemorrhoidectomy. Note the small maximal diameter with eversion of the anal canal (Courtesy of W. Brian Sweeney, MD)

brought into the anal canal (Fig. 20.10). Severe, circumferential anal canal stenosis is rare and typically managed either by chronic self-dilation with Young's dilators [34] or dermal advancement flaps such as house, V-to-Y, or diamond flaps.

Chronic Open Wounds

In a review of 1,184 hemorrhoidectomies, Pattan-arun found that at 2 weeks, although wound dehiscence was found in 2 %, irrespective if the case was done urgently for hemorrhoidal crisis or electively, by the fourth postoperative week all had healed without stricture [38]. We have not always had this success rate at 4 weeks, and typically tell our patients their wounds may be open for 6–8 weeks prior to final closure. A small percentage of patients will continue to have

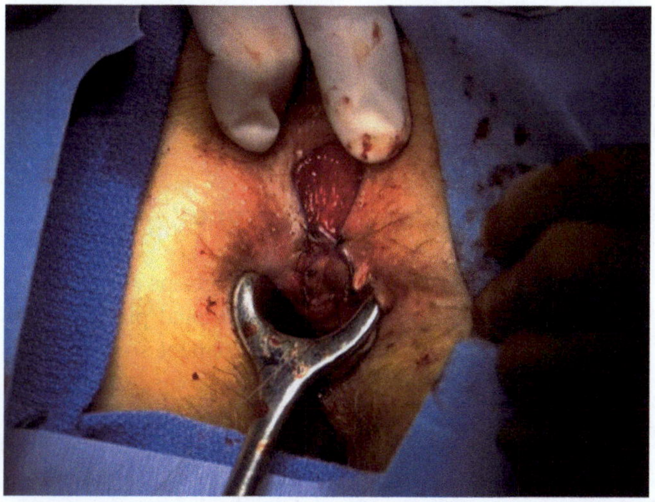

Fig. 20.10 House flap anoplasty for anal stenosis (Courtesy of W. Brian Sweeney, MD)

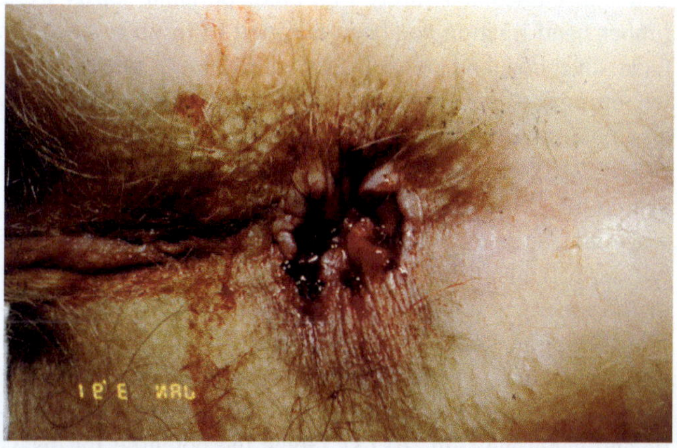

Fig. 20.11 Chronic open wounds following 3-quadrant hemorrhoidectomy (Courtesy of Richard Billingham, MD)

open wounds (Fig. 20.11). We have found anecdotally that 10 % metronidazole ointment applied bid has worked well in this situation. You should always consider the possibility of underlying Crohn's disease in these patients. Occasionally, in the absence of healing, you may need to perform a dermal flap.

Wet Anus and Pruritus Ani

This complication can result either from lack of approximation of the anal cushions resulting in mucus seepage, pH alterations, and chronic perianal itching or from mucosal ectropion. Depending on the source, this often resolves with complete healing of the wounds. Ectropion (as above) may require revisional surgery. While the causes of pruritus ani are extensive (and beyond the scope of this chapter), we have found good results with avoiding soaps and other methods in attempt to "clean" the area. Also, Calmoseptine® ointment (Calmoseptine Inc), using non-deodorant baby wipes, cotton balls at the anal verge for moisture wicking, and avoidance of scratching all are part of a regimen to relieve symptoms.

Chronic Pain

Chronic pain is rare. While it has been described more commonly following PPH, it may also be seen after hemorrhoidectomy. We refer you to the excellent chapter in this text by Drs. Bastawrous and Billingham on the approach to this condition.

Skin Tags (They Want It Flat!)

Excision of the external component of hemorrhoids is a standard part of excisional three-quadrant hemorrhoidectomy. However, patients must be counseled regarding the possibility of residual skin tags. While the patient or surgeon quest for "the perfect anus" is plausible, it may result in anal stenosis or anal fissuring—thus, trading one problem for another, potentially more troublesome, and more difficult to treat, problem. However, removal of small external tags following a hemorrhoidectomy is often easily accomplished in the clinic.

Recurrent Hemorrhoids

Management of recurrent disease may be strongly influenced by prior excisional hemorrhoidectomy. Reassessment of all the baseline characteristics is mandatory, including lifestyle modification and weight reduction and reevaluating the need for colonoscopy, as is obtaining the initial consultation and operative reports. Consideration of other previously recognized factors, which may be influencing the symptoms of bleeding, as simple as noncompliance, or as complex as unrecognized bleeding diatheses or original misdiagnosis is crucial prior to recommending optimal treatment.

Depending on the size of the problem, the recurrence may now be amenable to banding or in select cases a directed hemorrhoidectomy ensuring you leave enough anoderm to avoid stricture.

Banding Complications

Key Concept: While several of the complications seen with excisional hemorrhoidectomy can also occur with banding, unique complications do occur with this procedure that you need to be familiar with and counsel your patients accordingly.

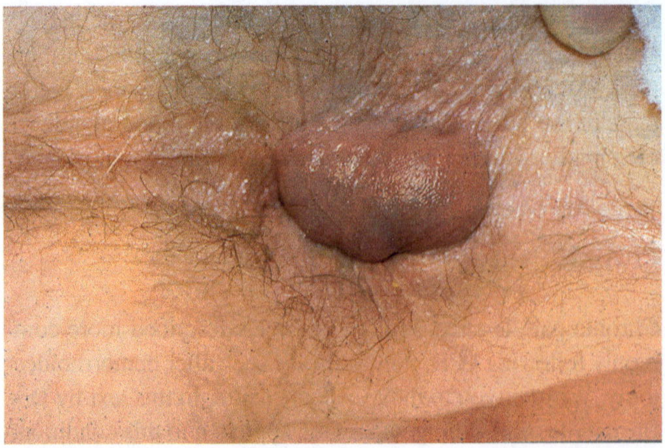

Fig. 20.12 Acute thrombosed hemorrhoid following banding (Courtesy of Richard Billingham, MD)

Pain

Discomfort and pain after rubber band ligation is common (5–60 %), but severe pain uncommon is estimated to occur in approximately 5 % and may be related to either anospasm or from placing the bands too close to the dentate line. In general, bands should be placed at least 1–2 cm proximal to the dentate line. If this is the case, the band should be immediately removed with a small blade. Occasionally, especially when patients re-present several hours later, there may be acute swelling that mandates examination under anesthesia to both remove the band and rule out signs of sepsis. Pain may also result from overzealous examination and resultant acute anal fissure. Typically this will get better on its own quickly, though may benefit from topical pain medications such as lidocaine.

In a prospective study of over 512 patients, 2.5 % were hospitalized—half due to delayed massive bleeding, the others for fever and urinary retention, and three with severe pain due to acute thrombosis of external hemorrhoids (Fig. 20.12) [39]. In this series, another 4.6 % developed minor complications, almost half of these for thrombosed external hemorrhoids, and even several for priapism.

Bleeding

After banding, bleeding may be immediate or delayed, minor or massive [40].

Some surgeons suggest that patients who are on anticoagulants or antiplatelet agents are best managed by excisional hemorrhoidectomy as compared with rubber band ligation as the excisional technique hemostasis would seem to be more reliable to avoid delayed bleeding. However, at least one large study suggests the risk of bleeding to be low (1–2 %) even if these medications are *not* held, with the exception of Plavix, which accounted for 50 % of the bleeding episodes [41]. In general, banding on anticoagulation medications and most antiplatelet agents is a relative contraindication [1].

Vasovagal Symptoms and Syncope

Placing patients in steep Trendelenburg's position for the several minutes required for exam and band placement, as well as the stress and severe embarrassment some patients experience, may result in vasovagal symptoms and even syncope. It is wise to have smelling salts within reach of the providers so as to recognize pre-syncope and hopefully avoid a traumatic fall off the table.

Sepsis

Often discussed but rarely observed, perianal sepsis from rubber band ligation has been reported to result in need for fecal diversion and potentially death, largely due to overwhelming sepsis from Fournier's gangrene. Of note, this has also been observed after excisional hemorrhoidectomy and PPH [42]. You must be familiar with presenting signs and symptoms, which include delayed urinary retention, fever, worsening/severe pain, excessive drainage, and shock. We tell our patients if they experience any one of these to report to the emergency department. Work-up may reveal leukemoid reaction and extraluminal (retroperitoneal) gas and fluid collections. Examination may range from relatively normal or a small amount of edema/inflammation to cellulitis and gangrene (Fig. 20.13). Given the potential for disastrous outcomes, broad-spectrum antibiotics and prompt examination under anesthesia with debridement of necrotic tissue are recommended (Fig. 20.14).

Recurrence

The durability of rubber band ligation is known to be inferior to excisional hemorrhoidectomy, especially for grade III disease. In many ways, recurrence can be more of an anticipated outcome than a complication, and patients should be counseled thusly [43]. Given a recurrence, we should note that prior banding is generally not a contraindication to additional banding. In fact, most banding patients are satisfied with this treatment option. The impact of disease on the patient's quality of life and ability to tolerate the increased time off work and pain associated with excisional hemorrhoidectomy need to be reassessed prior to choosing the next treatment option. Nonetheless, re-banding is generally safe and moderately efficaciousness as reported by

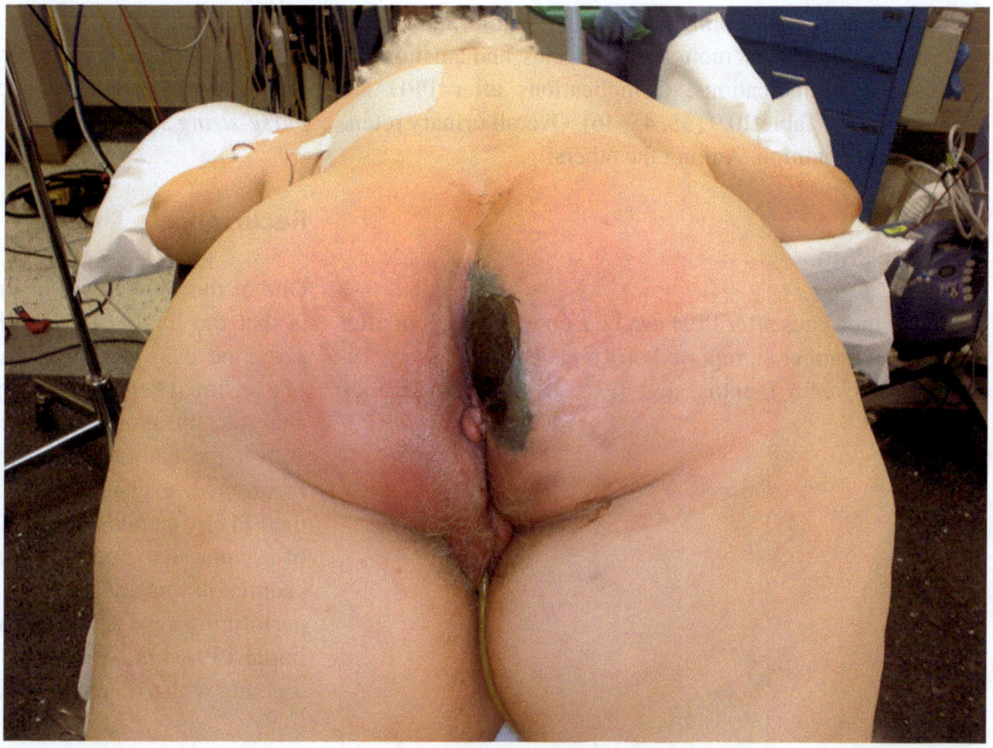

Fig. 20.13 Fournier's gangrene with cellulitis and ischemia (Courtesy of Philip Y. Pearson, MD)

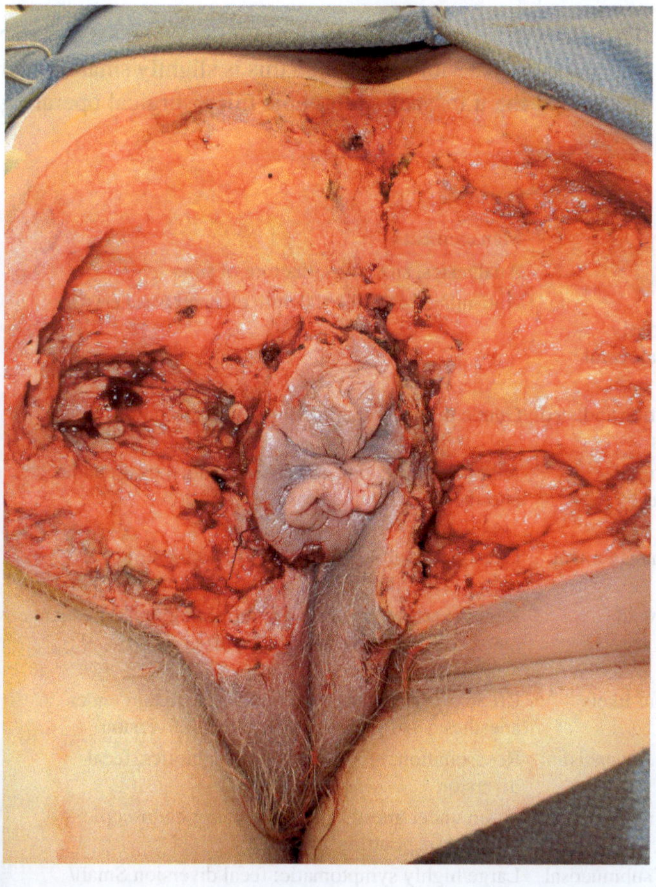

Fig. 20.14 Wide debridement of Fournier's gangrene (Courtesy of Philip Y. Pearson, MD)

Iyer et al. [44]. In their series of 805 patients and 2,114 bands, symptoms were successfully treated in 60–74 % of recurrences, with an overall cumulative success rate of 80 %.

Stapled Hemorrhoidopexy (PPH)

Indications: When Should We Be Using This Procedure?

Key Concept: There are a wide variety of opinions on the utility of stapled hemorrhoidopexy.

As mentioned in the surgical decision-making section earlier in the chapter, due to its increased recurrence rate, PPH should be used selectively as an alternative to conventional or bipolar excisional hemorrhoidectomy in patients with circumferential grade III hemorrhoidal disease without an especially large external component. PPH may also potentially be used in early grade IV hemorrhoidal disease, though we do not use it in these cases, or in the presence of gangrenous hemorrhoids (Fig. 20.15).

Pescatori et al. reviewed the literature on severe complications of PPH including chronic pain, rectal luminal obliteration, rectovaginal fistula, pelvic sepsis, and need for proximal fecal diversion [45]. Their review found that fourth-degree hemorrhoidal disease was a relative contraindication to PPH as the results are worse and complications rates higher than in third-degree disease. Another relative complication is poor sphincter function, while anticipated future anoreceptive intercourse, enteroceles, and anismus are absolute contraindications. Complications after PPH are summarized in Table 20.9 [35, 45, 46]. Overall urinary retention is most common. Among the others:

Chronic Pain

Pain and tenesmus after PPH can be a chronic problem after PPH. Cheetham et al. reported on 16 patients who were followed for over 6 months, and 1/3 had pain and urgency which lasted for as long as 15 months [47]. Most of these patients had muscle incorporated into the donut (Fig. 20.16), emphasizing the importance of *mucosal only bites on the purse-string suture*.

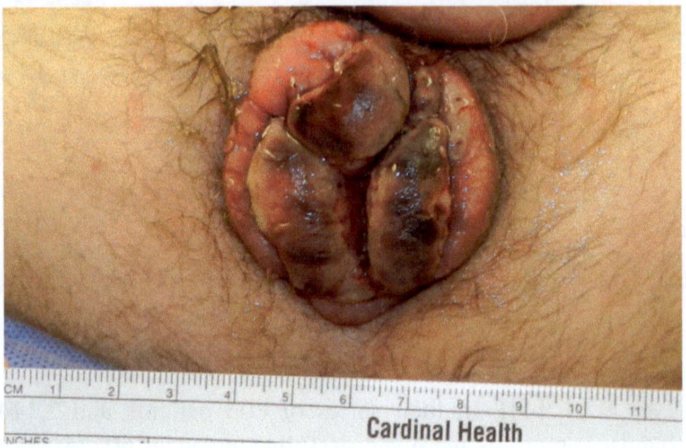

Fig. 20.15 Gangrenous hemorrhoids

Recurrence

One of the weaknesses of this minimally invasive approach is that the long-term durability is questionable, especially given the short- and medium-term results are inferior to that of excisional hemorrhoidectomy [23]. In the Cochrane meta-analysis, similar to the more recent meta-analysis described above, the authors found that for all outcomes related to recurrence, excisional hemorrhoidectomy was superior to the PPH by an odds ratio of 2.7–3.6, although the proportion of asymptomatic patients was no different between the procedures in this analysis. We also do not have experience in performing repeat stapled hemorrhoidopexy (following an initial PPH) but worry about leaving two staple lines close together with a potentially ischemic area of mucosa between.

Sphincter Damage

The width (size) of the PPH device is 33 mm and the circular anoscope up to 37 mm. Although this is slightly smaller than the size of the transanal endoscopic microsurgical operating

Table 20.9 Complications of stapled hemorrhoidopexy

Complication	Frequency	Possible preventive measures	Management
Acute pain	26–60 %	Avoid incorporating muscle	Analgesics, sitz baths, tincture of time
Chronic pain and/or urgency (post-PPH syndrome)	5–31 %	Avoid too low stapler placement, avoid incorporating muscle. Mucosal-submucosal purse-string/staple line should be in distal rectal mucosa *not* anal canal	Anti-inflammatories, calcium channel blockers
Rectal stenosis	<21 %	Fiber supplementation to avoid constipation-induced staple extrusion with subsequent fibrosis	Gentle digital rectal dilation without sedation
Delayed bleeding from staple line	1–13 %	Completion anoscopy with suture ligation of bleeders or hemostatic agents, i.e., FloSeal	Assess for unrecognized coagulopathy, exam under anesthesia, suture ligation
Recurrence	7.5 %	Optimal patient selection, expectation management, optimal technique	Lifestyle modification, rubber band ligation, THD, redo PPH, excisional hemorrhoidectomy?
Sphincter damage/ incontinence	1 %	Gentle serial dilation. Avoid in patients with borderline continence	Kegel exercises, pelvic floor retraining, bulking agents, antimotility agents, others as appropriate
Pelvic sepsis	Rare	Proper technique and patient selection but likely unpreventable	Broad-spectrum antibiotics, CT scan, exam under anesthesia +/– laparotomy and fecal diversion
Rectal perforation	Rare	All cases involved full-thickness wall rectal excision	Resuscitation, broad-spectrum antibiotics, fecal diversion
Rectal obstruction	Rare	Ensure proper purse-string suture placement so that both are cut by the stapler	Exam under anesthesia, transanal or endoscopic purse-strong cutting
Rectovaginal fistula	Rare	Ensure anterior purse-string in mucosal-submucosal and not full thickness. Double-check vagina before firing stapler	Large/highly symptomatic: fecal diversion Small/ mildly symptomatic: transvaginal/endorectal advancement flap(s)

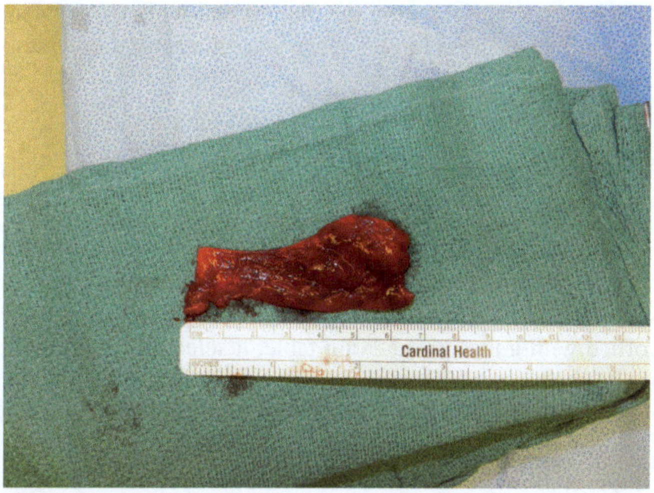

Fig. 20.16 Stapled hemorrhoidopexy specimen demonstrating varying degrees of thickness

proctoscope (40 mm), caution should still be used in those patients with preexisting sphincter injury or fecal incontinence. For those without these contraindications, slow, gentle, serial dilation from one-finger breathe to the size of the device is optimal. The other mechanism by which sphincter damage during PPH may occur is by placing the purse-string suture too deep. When fired, especially when the stapler is placed too low (i.e., in the anal canal), the staple line may incorporate muscle fibers. If this occurs, you have to fall back on medical management of bulking and bowel-slowing agents, and again, waiting to see their eventual function.

Too Low Stapler Placement: Post-PPH Syndrome

Proper technique suggests that the resulting staple line should be approximately 2 cm proximal to the apex of the hemorrhoidal bundles. Placing the purse-string and stapler too low will result in inadvertent excision of the hemorrhoidal tissues. Given their bulkiness, this is likely to result in an asymmetric resection of the mucosal ring that will increase recurrence rate (Fig. 20.16). However, low stapler placement may also cause internal sphincter spasm and inflammation, similar to low anterior syndrome following a proctectomy. This is typically treated with anti-inflammatory agents *per orum* or *per rectum* but in rare cases may require removal of the staples.

Bleeding

Bleeding from the staple line is relatively common after the PPH device is fired. This can be minimized by holding the stapler for a minimum of 20 s before firing. Post-firing careful, circumferential anoscopy to assess for bleeding from the staple line is a mandatory part of the procedure. We prefer a placement of hemostatic 3–0 vicryl sutures perpendicular to the staple line as needed to achieve optimal hemostasis. Mongardini et al. reported on 197 PPH procedures in which FloSeal™ was used as a hemostatic adjunct, instead of hemostatic sutures on the suture line, and no major postoperative bleeding was observed, compared to 1.3 % in other series [48].

Preventing Complications

Key Concept: Like most things, it is often easier to avoid complications than to manage them. Here are some helpful tips we have found regarding hemorrhoid management.

Technical Tips: Excisional Hemorrhoidectomy

Avoid inadvertent excessive excision (cushions vs. anoderm): In order to obtain the optimal exam under anesthesia, we recommend general anesthesia with neuromuscular blockade (paralysis). Similarly a four-quadrant intersphincteric block can aid in optimal exposure (we use a 50-50 mixture of Marcaine and lidocaine). Preemptive perianal skin block with this mixture may decrease postoperative discomfort. However, you must keep in mind that local may distort the normal anatomy, so consider using a marking pen to mark the anoderm to be excised prior to instillation of local anesthetic.

It should always be remembered and taught that the goal of excisional hemorrhoidectomy is to excise the optimal amount of hemorrhoidal cushions to prevent recurrence of the symptoms, while overzealous anodermal excision will invariably result in anal stenosis. When excising several columns, you should always leave a minimum of 1–2 cm of anoderm between columns.

Reduce the risk of intraoperative bleeding: In order to reduce the risk of bleeding *during* an excisional hemorrhoidectomy, some surgeons choose to place a ligating/pexying stitch at the apex of the hemorrhoidal bundle and nascent specimen prior to excision to decrease bleeding during excision.

Avoid sphincter injury: You can use large curved Mayo scissors to push the sphincters down against the anorectal wall during excision of the specimen to decrease likelihood of injury to the underlying sphincter.

Optimal analgesia: Several adjuncts exist that can help to reduce postoperative pain.

One includes performing a lateral internal sphincterotomy at the same time as the hemorrhoidectomy [49–55]. Data from randomized trials are few and have mixed results. In our opinion, especially given long-term outcomes after sphincterotomy for fissure with up to 10 % continence alternations, it cannot be recommended at present. Chemical sphincterotomy with Botox or calcium channel blockers may reduce pain in the first postoperative week and may be a seasonable albeit costly alternative [56].

Several randomized trials have examined the role of electrosurgical devices such as the LigaSure™ or Harmonic Scalpel™ to incrementally improve excisional hemorrhoidectomy. A meta-analysis from 2007 showed that although the LigaSure may decrease operative time and blood loss, it does so at increased cost without decrease in postoperative pain [20]. Another medical device reported to reduce post-hemorrhoidectomy are implantable local infiltration systems such as the On-Que™ and other pumps such as a subcutaneous morphine pump [57]. In general, lack of high-quality data, local availability, and cost all limit widespread adoption.

A recent, exciting development that holds promise in the reduction of post-hemorrhoidectomy pain is liposomal bupivacaine. The liposomes slowly dissolve, releasing the local anesthetic over 72 h. To date, several randomized trials of the effect of this medicine in this patient population have been published [58–60]. In a randomized trial of almost 186 patients, Gorfine et al. reported that this injection of 300 mg of liposomal bupivacaine, as compared to placebo, resulted in a statistically significant reduction in opioid use and improved patient satisfaction. In another randomized trial including 100 patients, Haas et al. demonstrated a similar effect on opioid use and also showed a dose-response curve up to 266 mg of the liposomal formula compared with 75 g of non-liposomal bupivacaine. This formulation, which appears effective as shown by these studies, holds promise. Due to its relative infancy, current widespread adoption is limited by the relative lack of literature, as well as its cost.

Prevention of early bleeding: At the conclusion of excisional hemorrhoidectomy, some surgeons use an anal pack or anal tampon to push the mucosa against the anorectal wall. This may be as simple as lubricated plain gauze with tie (tampon string) or as fanciful (and costly) as nonadherent dressing such as rolled-up "cigarette" of Telfa™ wrapped in Surgicel® (Ethicon Biosurgery, Cincinnati, OH). Although these measures provide some reassurance to the surgeon, they are likely excessive if increased attention is paid to hemostasis as viewed anoscopically at the end of the case.

Increase the detection of early bleeding: An alternative to anal packing is an anal dam, which keeps the anus open enough to allow blood to egress from the canal so as to allow timely recognition while the patient is still in the recovery room and hopefully before a patient develops hemorrhagic shock. The cut end of the surgeon's rubber glove, or a piece of Telfa, is placed with one end in the canal and the other outside of the body. This is felt to be critical important by some surgeons, following the dictum that with a competent (closed) anus, the colorectum can store the entire intravascular volume of blood.

Patient Selection

As mentioned throughout this chapter, patient selection is crucial for optimal outcomes. Optimal treatment recommendations start with a thorough examination, ideally in the office with a motorized exam table, a selection of different anoscopes, and high-quality lighting. Patient goals should also be carefully assessed prior to the examination and again prior to leaving. For example, a patient may successfully undergo lifestyle modifications and serial rubber band ligation for bleeding internal hemorrhoids. On follow-up, the bleeding is treated, but the patient still notices (yet does not complain of) prolapse. Despite the prolapse, from the patient's perspective, their goals may have been met without additional intervention. On the other hand, if a cirrhotic has chronic bleeding internal hemorrhoids, rubber banding may result in torrential, unstoppable bleeding, so the patient and other care provider expectation of no bleeding may not be reasonable, and simple suture ligation, transjugular intrahepatic portosystemic shunt (TIPS), or palliation of the anemia with transfusion of blood products may be the safest, most appropriate treatment (Fig. 20.17).

Fluid Restriction (Urinary Retention)

According to the American Society of Colorectal Surgeons recommendations, intraoperative fluid restriction will decrease the likelihood of urinary retention [1, 61]. Thus, it is important for you to communicate this to the anesthesia team who may not be aware of these recommendations. Protocols for early recognition prior to discharge need to be established at each surgeon's operative facility; we recommend mandatory void >100 cc plus a bladder scan to avoid unnecessary emergency room visits in those in whom it will develop.

Summary Pearls

Managing patients with hemorrhoidal disease will be a frequent occurrence for anyone treating patients with colorectal problems. Though difficult to summarize everything you will encounter, we leave you with a few final thoughts.

- Complications after treatment for hemorrhoidal disease, including recurrence, are relatively common and in many cases can be avoided by proper patient selection, preoperative optimization, and intervention tailored to the individual's goals and expectations.

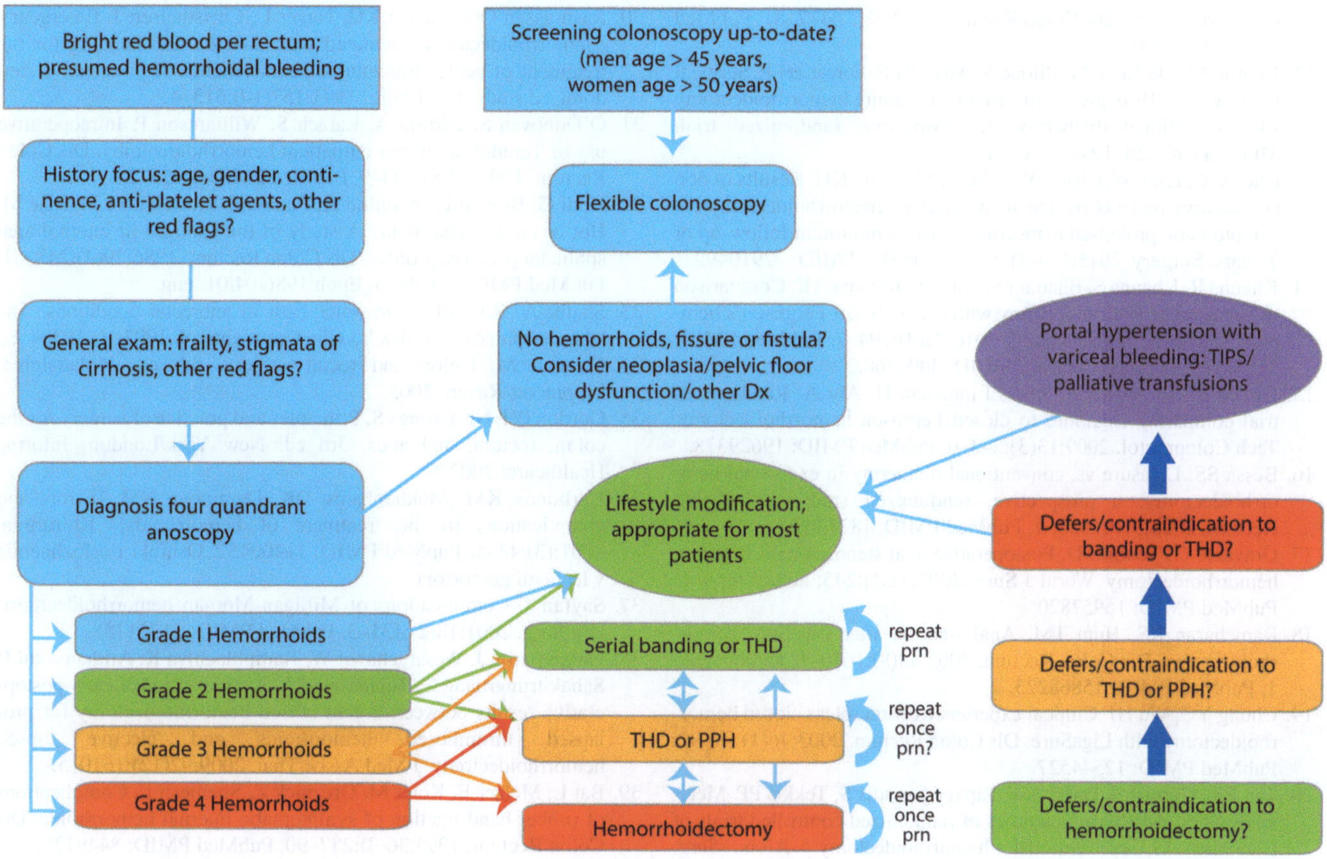

Fig. 20.17 Algorithmic approach to selection of hemorrhoidal operation

- Technical complications after operative intervention can result in permanent negative impact on patient quality of life. Therefore, it is imperative that you as the surgeon be competent, aware of the technical nuances of the procedures you offer, and familiar with the frequency and management of procedural-specific complication.

References

1. Rivadeneira DE, Steele SR, Ternent C, Chalasani S, Buie WD, Rafferty JL. Practice parameters for the management of hemorrhoids (revised 2010). Dis Colon Rectum. 2011;54(9):1059–64. PubMed PMID: 21825884. Epub 2011/08/10. eng.
2. Cataldo P, Ellis CN, Gregorcyk S, Hyman N, Buie WD, Church J, et al. Practice parameters for the management of hemorrhoids (revised). Dis Colon Rectum. 2005;48(2):189–94. PubMed PMID: 15711856. Epub 2005/02/16. eng.
3. Gencosmanoglu R, Sad O, Koc D, Inceoglu R. Hemorrhoidectomy: open or closed technique? A prospective, randomized clinical trial. Dis Colon Rectum. 2002;45(1):70–5. PubMed PMID: 11786767. Epub 2002/01/12. eng.
4. Lewis SJ, Heaton KW. Stool form scale as a useful guide to intestinal transit time. Scand J Gastroenterol. 1997;32(9):920–4. PubMed PMID: 9299672. Epub 1997/09/23. eng.
5. Longstreth GF, Thompson WG, Chey WD, Houghton LA, Mearin F, Spiller RC. Functional bowel disorders. Gastroenterology. 2006;130(5):1480–91. PubMed PMID: 16678561. Epub 2006/05/09. eng.
6. Cappell MS. Reducing the incidence and mortality of colon cancer: mass screening and colonoscopic polypectomy. Gastroenterol Clin North Am. 2008;37(1):129–60, vii-viii. PubMed PMID: 18313544. Epub 2008/03/04. eng.
7. Zauber AG, Winawer SJ, O'Brien MJ, Lansdorp-Vogelaar I, van Ballegooijen M, Hankey BF, et al. Colonoscopic polypectomy and long-term prevention of colorectal-cancer deaths. N Engl J Med. 2012;366(8):687–96. PubMed PMID: 22356322. Pubmed Central PMCID: 3322371. Epub 2012/02/24. eng.
8. Jover R, Herraiz M, Alarcon O, Brullet E, Bujanda L, Bustamante M, et al. Clinical practice guidelines: quality of colonoscopy in colorectal cancer screening. Endoscopy. 2012;44(4):444–51. PubMed PMID: 22438159. Epub 2012/03/23. eng.
9. Price MJ, Walder JS, Baker BA, Heiselman DE, Jakubowski JA, Logan DK, et al. Recovery of platelet function after discontinuation of prasugrel or clopidogrel maintenance dosing in aspirin-treated patients with stable coronary disease: the recovery trial. J Am Coll Cardiol. 2012;59(25):2338–43. PubMed PMID: 22698488. Epub 2012/06/16. eng.
10. Alonso-Coello P, Mills E, Heels-Ansdell D, Lopez-Yarto M, Zhou Q, Johanson JF, et al. Fiber for the treatment of hemorrhoids complications: a systematic review and meta-analysis. Am J Gastroenterol. 2006;101(1):181–8. PubMed PMID: 16405552.
11. Bleday R, Pena JP, Rothenberger DA, Goldberg SM, Buls JG. Symptomatic hemorrhoids: current incidence and complications of

operative therapy. Dis Colon Rectum. 1992;35(5):477–81. PubMed PMID: 1568400.
12. Gentile M, De Rosa M, Pilone V, Mosella F, Forestieri P. Surgical treatment for IV-degree hemorrhoids: LigaSure hemorrhoidectomy vs. conventional diathermy. A prospective, randomized trial. Minerva Chir. 2011;66(3):207–13.
13. Chen CW, Lai CW, Chang YJ, Chen CM, Hsiao KH. Results of 666 consecutive patients treated with LigaSure hemorrhoidectomy for symptomatic prolapsed hemorrhoids with a minimum follow-up of 2 years. Surgery. 2013;153(2):211–8. PubMed PMID: 22910492.
14. Khanna R, Khanna S, Bhadani S, Singh S, Khanna AK. Comparison of Ligasure hemorrhoidectomy with conventional Ferguson's hemorrhoidectomy. Indian J Surg. 2010;72(4):294–7. PubMed PMID: 21938191. Pubmed Central PMCID: 3002768.
15. Fareed M, El-Awady S, Abd-El monaem H, Aly A. Randomized trial comparing LigaSure to closed Ferguson hemorrhoidectomy. Tech Coloproctol. 2009;13(3):243–6. PubMed PMID: 19629378.
16. Bessa SS. Ligasure vs. conventional diathermy in excisional hemorrhoidectomy: a prospective, randomized study. Dis Colon Rectum. 2008;51(6):940–4. PubMed PMID: 18273670.
17. Gravante G, Venditti D. Postoperative anal stenoses with Ligasure hemorrhoidectomy. World J Surg. 2007;31(1):245; author reply 6. PubMed PMID: 16957820.
18. Ramcharan KS, Hunt TM. Anal stenosis after LigaSure hemorrhoidectomy. Dis Colon Rectum. 2005;48(8):1670–1; author reply 1. PubMed PMID: 15868225.
19. Chung YC, Wu HJ. Clinical experience of sutureless closed hemorrhoidectomy with LigaSure. Dis Colon Rectum. 2003;46(1):87–92. PubMed PMID: 12544527.
20. Tan EK, Cornish J, Darzi AW, Papagrigoriadis S, Tekkis PP. Meta-analysis of short-term outcomes of randomized controlled trials of LigaSure vs conventional hemorrhoidectomy. Arch Surg. 2007;142(12):1209–18; discussion 18. PubMed PMID: 18086990. Epub 2007/12/19. eng.
21. Nienhuijs S, de Hingh I. Conventional versus LigaSure hemorrhoidectomy for patients with symptomatic Hemorrhoids. Cochrane Database Syst Rev. 2009;(1):CD006761. PubMed PMID: 19160300.
22. Tjandra JJ, Chan MK. Systematic review on the procedure for prolapse and hemorrhoids (stapled hemorrhoidopexy). Dis Colon Rectum. 2007;50(6):878–92. PubMed PMID: 17380367.
23. Jayaraman S, Colquhoun PH, Malthaner RA. Stapled hemorrhoidopexy is associated with a higher long-term recurrence rate of internal hemorrhoids compared with conventional excisional hemorrhoid surgery. Dis Colon Rectum. 2007;50(9):1297–305. PubMed PMID: 17665254.
24. Giordano P, Gravante G, Sorge R, Ovens L, Nastro P. Long-term outcomes of stapled hemorrhoidopexy vs conventional hemorrhoidectomy: a meta-analysis of randomized controlled trials. Arch Surg. 2009;144(3):266–72. PubMed PMID: 19289667.
25. Arslani N, Patrlj L, Rajkovic Z, Papes D, Altarac S. A randomized clinical trial comparing Ligasure versus stapled hemorrhoidectomy. Surg Laparosc Endosc Percutan Tech. 2012;22(1):58–61. PubMed PMID: 22318061.
26. Sakr MF, Moussa MM, Elserafy M. Ligasure hemorrhoidectomy versus stapled hemorrhoidopexy: a prospective randomized clinical trial. Minerva Chir. 2010;65(3):251–8. PubMed PMID: 20668414.
27. Giordano P, Overton J, Madeddu F, Zaman S, Gravante G. Transanal hemorrhoidal dearterialization: a systematic review. Dis Colon Rectum. 2009;52(9):1665–71. PubMed PMID: 19690499.
28. Ratto C, Donisi L, Parello A, Litta F, Doglietto GB. Evaluation of transanal hemorrhoidal dearterialization as a minimally invasive therapeutic approach to hemorrhoids. Dis Colon Rectum. 2010;53(5):803–11. PubMed PMID: 20389215.
29. Wang CH. Urgent hemorrhoidectomy for hemorrhoidal crisis. Dis Colon Rectum. 1982;25(2):122–4. PubMed PMID: 7067546.
30. Rasmussen OO, Larsen KG, Naver L, Christiansen J. Emergency haemorrhoidectomy compared with incision and banding for the treatment of acute strangulated haemorrhoids. A prospective randomised study. Eur J Surg. 1991;157(10):613–4.
31. O'Donovan S, Ferrara A, Larach S, Williamson P. Intraoperative use of Toradol facilitates outpatient hemorrhoidectomy. Dis Colon Rectum. 1994;37(8):793–9. PubMed PMID: 8055724.
32. Dodi G, Bogoni F, Infantino A, Pianon P, Mortellaro LM, Lise M. Hot or cold in anal pain? A study of the changes in internal anal sphincter pressure profiles. Dis Colon Rectum. 1986;29(4):248–51. PubMed PMID: 3948615. Epub 1986/04/01. eng.
33. Shafik A. Role of warm-water bath in anorectal conditions. The "thermosphincteric reflex". J Clin Gastroenterol. 1993;16(4):304–8.
34. Corman M. Colon and rectal surgery. 5th ed. Philadelphia: Lippincott-Raven; 2005.
35. Gordon PH, Nivatvongs S. Principles and practice of surgery for the colon, rectum, and anus. 3rd ed. New York/London: Informa Healthcare; 2007.
36. Kurbonov KM, Mukhabbatov DK, Daminova NM. [Errors and complications in the treatment of hemorrhoids]. Khirurgiia. 2001;(3):43–5. PubMed PMID: 11400452. Oshibki i oslozhneniia v lechenii gemorroia.
37. Sayfan J. Complications of Milligan-Morgan hemorrhoidectomy. Dig Surg. 2001;18(2):131–3. PubMed PMID: 11351158.
38. Pattana-arun J, Wesarachawit W, Tantiphlachiva K, Atithansakul P, Sahakitrungruang C, Rojanasakul A. A comparison of early postoperative results between urgent closed hemorrhoidectomy for prolapsed thrombosed hemorrhoids and elective closed hemorrhoidectomy. J Med Assoc Thai. 2009;92(12):1610–5.
39. Bat L, Melzer E, Koler M, Dreznick Z, Shemesh E. Complications of rubber band ligation of symptomatic internal hemorrhoids. Dis Colon Rectum. 1993;36(3):287–90. PubMed PMID: 8449135.
40. MacRae HM, McLeod RS. Comparison of hemorrhoidal treatments: a meta-analysis. Can J Surg. 1997;40(1):14–7. PubMed PMID: 9030078. Epub 1997/02/01. eng.
41. Nelson RS, Ewing BM, Ternent C, Shashidharan M, Blatchford GJ, Thorson AG. Risk of late bleeding following hemorrhoidal banding in patients on antithrombotic prophylaxis. Am J Surg. 2008;196(6):994–9; discussion 9. PubMed PMID: 19095121. Epub 2008/12/20. eng.
42. McCloud JM, Jameson JS, Scott AN. Life-threatening sepsis following treatment for haemorrhoids: a systematic review. Colorectal Dis. 2006;8(9):748–55. PubMed PMID: 17032319. Epub 2006/10/13. eng.
43. Shanmugam V, Thaha MA, Rabindranath KS, Campbell KL, Steele RJ, Loudon MA. Rubber band ligation versus excisional haemorrhoidectomy for haemorrhoids. Cochrane Database Syst Rev. 2005;(3):CD005034. PubMed PMID: 16034963.
44. Iyer VS, Shrier I, Gordon PH. Long-term outcome of rubber band ligation for symptomatic primary and recurrent internal hemorrhoids. Dis Colon Rectum. 2004;47(8):1364–70. PubMed PMID: 15484351.
45. Pescatori M, Gagliardi G. Postoperative complications after procedure for prolapsed hemorrhoids (PPH) and stapled transanal rectal resection (STARR) procedures. Tech Coloproctol. 2008;12(1):7–19. PubMed PMID: 18512007. Pubmed Central PMCID: 2778725.
46. Correa-Rovelo JM, Tellez O, Obregon L, Miranda-Gomez A, Moran S. Stapled rectal mucosectomy vs. closed hemorrhoidectomy: a randomized, clinical trial. Dis Colon Rectum. 2002;45(10):1367–74; discussion 74–5. PubMed PMID: 12394436.
47. Cheetham MJ, Mortensen NJ, Nystrom PO, Kamm MA, Phillips RK. Persistent pain and faecal urgency after stapled haemorrhoidectomy. Lancet. 2000;356(9231):730–3. PubMed PMID: 11085693.
48. Mongardini M, Custureri F, Schillaci F, Cola A, Maturo A, Fanello G, et al. [Prevention of post-operative pain and haemorrhage in PPH (Procedure for Prolapse and Hemorrhoids) and STARR (Stapled Trans-Anal Rectal Resection). Preliminary results in 261 cases]. G Chir. 2005;26(4):157–61. PubMed PMID: 16035252. La prevenzione del dolore e dell'emorragia post-operatoria nella PPH

(Procedure for Prolapse and Hemorrhoids) e nella STARR (Stapled Trans-Anal Rectal Resection). Risultati su una serie di 261 pazienti.
49. Mathai V, Ong BC, Ho YH. Randomized controlled trial of lateral internal sphincterotomy with haemorrhoidectomy. Br J Surg. 1996;83(3):380–2. PubMed PMID: 8665199.
50. Galizia G, Lieto E, Castellano P, Pelosio L, Imperatore V, Pigantelli C. Lateral internal sphincterotomy together with haemorrhoidectomy for treatment of haemorrhoids: a randomised prospective study. Eur J Surg. 2000;166(3):223–8.
51. Khubchandani IT. Internal sphincterotomy with hemorrhoidectomy does not relieve pain: a prospective, randomized study. Dis Colon Rectum. 2002;45(11):1452–7. PubMed PMID: 12432291.
52. Kanellos I, Zacharakis E, Christoforidis E, Angelopoulos S, Kanellos D, Pramateftakis MG, et al. Usefulness of lateral internal sphincterotomy in reducing postoperative pain after open hemorrhoidectomy. World J Surg. 2005;29(4):464–8. PubMed PMID: 15770383.
53. Hosseini SV, Sharifi K, Ahmadfard A, Mosallaei M, Pourahmad S, Bolandparvaz S. Role of internal sphincterotomy in the treatment of hemorrhoids: a randomized clinical trial. Arch Iran Med. 2007;10(4):504–8. PubMed PMID: 17903056.
54. Chauhan A, Tiwari S, Mishra VK, Bhatia PK. Comparison of internal sphincterotomy with topical diltiazem for post-hemorrhoidectomy pain relief: a prospective randomized trial. J Postgrad Med. 2009;55(1):22–6. PubMed PMID: 19242074.
55. Diana G, Guercio G, Cudia B, Ricotta C. Internal sphincterotomy reduces postoperative pain after Milligan Morgan haemorrhoidectomy. BMC Surg. 2009;9:16. PubMed PMID: 19852840. Pubmed Central PMCID: 2774293.
56. Siddiqui MR, Abraham-Igwe C, Shangumanandan A, Grassi V, Swift I, Abulafi AM. A literature review on the role of chemical sphincterotomy after Milligan-Morgan hemorrhoidectomy. Int J Colorectal Dis. 2011;26(6):685–92. PubMed PMID: 21212965.
57. Goldstein ET, Williamson PR, Larach SW. Subcutaneous morphine pump for postoperative hemorrhoidectomy pain management. Dis Colon Rectum. 1993;36(5):439–46. PubMed PMID: 8482162.
58. Gorfine SR, Onel E, Patou G, Krivokapic ZV. Bupivacaine extended-release liposome injection for prolonged postsurgical analgesia in patients undergoing hemorrhoidectomy: a multicenter, randomized, double-blind, placebo-controlled trial. Dis Colon Rectum. 2011;54(12):1552–9. PubMed PMID: 22067185.
59. Haas E, Onel E, Miller H, Ragupathi M, White PF. A double-blind, randomized, active-controlled study for post-hemorrhoidectomy pain management with liposome bupivacaine, a novel local analgesic formulation. Am Surg. 2012;78(5):574–81. PubMed PMID: 22546131. Epub 2012/05/02. eng.
60. Bergese SD, Ramamoorthy S, Patou G, Bramlett K, Gorfine SR, Candiotti KA. Efficacy profile of liposome bupivacaine, a novel formulation of bupivacaine for postsurgical analgesia. J Pain Res. 2012;5:107–16. PubMed PMID: 22570563. Pubmed Central PMCID: 3346068. Epub 2012/05/10. eng.
61. Place R, Hyman N, Simmang C, Cataldo P, Church J, Cohen J, et al. Practice parameters for ambulatory anorectal surgery. Dis Colon Rectum. 2003;46(5):573–6. PubMed PMID: 12792430. Epub 2003/06/07. eng.

Fistula-in-Ano

21

David E. Beck

Key Points

- Although it seems very basic, correctly identifying the internal and external openings without missing secondary or high blind tracts or creating false passages is the key to minimizing failures and recurrences.
- Imaging studies are typically not required outside of complex and recurrent fistulae.
- While several methods are used in the surgical management of fistula-in-ano, they all work on the basic premise of destroying or sealing the internal opening.
- When in doubt, preserve the sphincter muscle complex.

Background

Fistula-in-ano is one of the most common anorectal disorders you will encounter. Many of them will be straightforward and heal without any recurrence or functional deficits. Others will be almost as trying on you as they are debilitating on your patient. It is important that you have a stepwise approach to anal fistulas and always consider the anatomy of the tract(s), sphincter complex involved, prior history of your patient (e.g., anorectal surgery continence status), and any underlying pathology (e.g., IBD). My goal in this chapter is to provide you with information regarding the diagnosis and treatment, and along the way give you some of my thoughts and biases about how I think about this problem.

D.E. Beck, MD, FACS, FASCRS
Department of Colon and Rectal Surgery,
Ochsner Clinic foundation, 1514 Jefferson Highway,
New Orleans, LA 70121, USA
e-mail: dbeckmd@aol.com

Pathophysiology

Key Concept: A cryptoglandular origin is the source of ~80 % of all anal fistulas.

A fistula-in-ano is an abnormal tract or cavity communicating with the rectum or anal canal by an identifiable internal and external opening. Most fistulas are thought to arise due to cryptoglandular infection and can be classified as described by Parks and colleagues (Fig. 21.1 and Table 21.1) [1]. Other causes include infections (e.g., HIV), inflammation (e.g., IBD), neoplasms, and trauma [2]. While these are fairly straightforward concepts, it is important to remember that approximately 30–50 % of anorectal abscesses will lead to an anal fistula. When draining an anorectal abscess, you should inform your patient of this fact, to both manage expectations and allow them to follow-up appropriately if this should occur.

Evaluation and Workup

History

Key Concept: Most routine fistulas you can elicit on history alone. Use the history to tease out those that are more concerning for sources other than cryptoglandular.

A patient with a fistula-in-ano will often recount a history of an abscess that has been drained either surgically or spontaneously. Patients may complain of drainage, pain with defecation, bleeding due to the presence of granulation tissue at either opening, swelling, and/or decrease in pain with drainage. Additional bowel or systemic symptoms (i.e., abdominal pain, bloody diarrhea, weight loss, immunosuppression) may be present when the fistula is not cryptoglandular.

S.R. Steele et al. (eds.), *Complexities in Colorectal Surgery*,
DOI 10.1007/978-1-4614-9022-7_21, © Springer Science+Business Media New York 2014

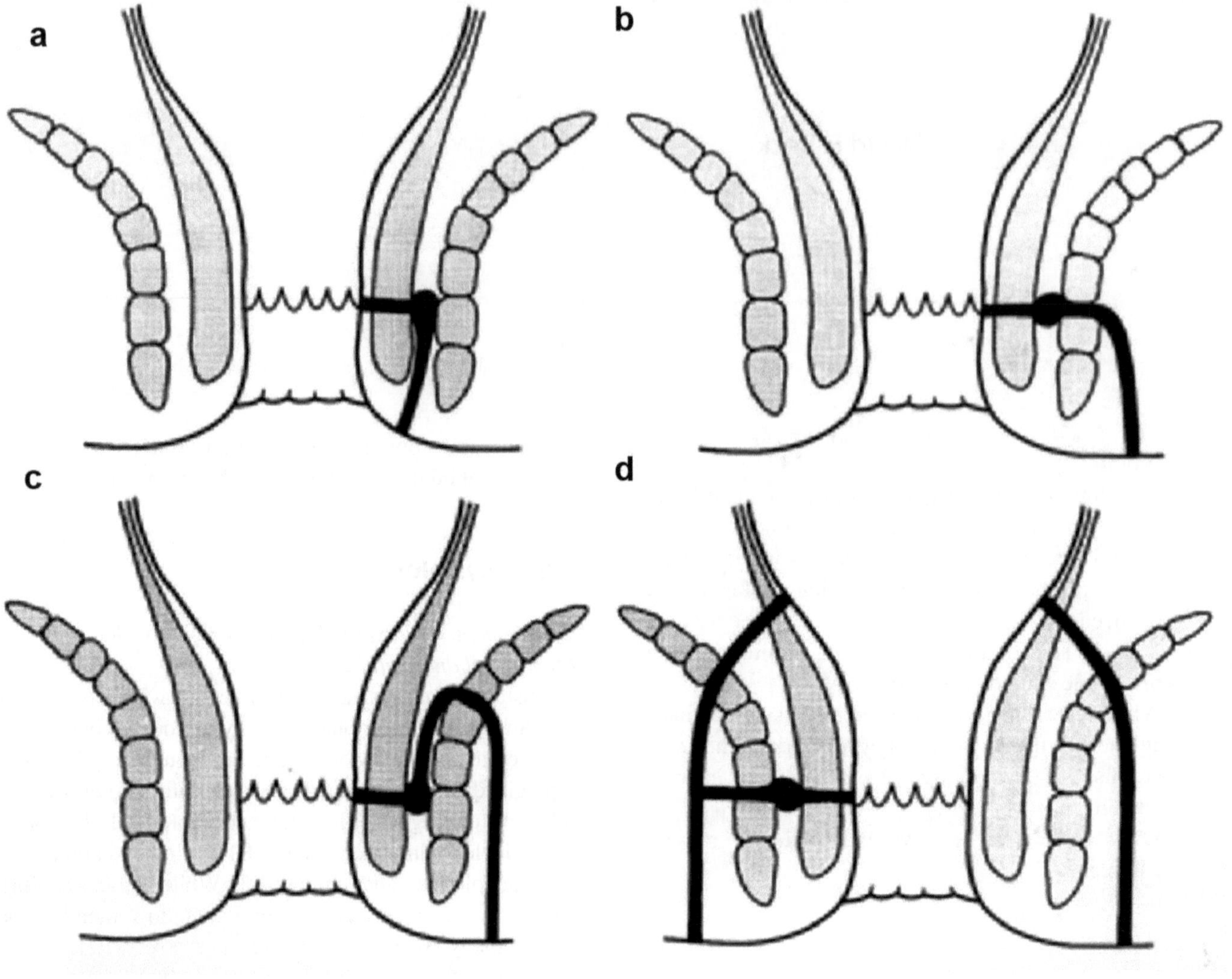

Fig. 21.1 Classification of fistula-in-ano. (**a**), Intersphincteric. (**b**), Transsphincteric. (**c**), Suprasphincteric. (**d**) Extrasphincteric (With permission from Vasilevsky [2])

Table 21.1 Classification of fistula-in-ano

Intersphincteric
Simple low tract
High blind tract
High tract with rectal opening
Rectal opening without perineal opening
Extrarectal extension
Secondary to pelvic disease
Transsphincteric
Uncomplicated
High blind tract
Suprasphincteric
Uncomplicated
High blind tract
Extrasphincteric
Secondary to anal fistula
Secondary to trauma
Secondary to anorectal disease
Secondary to pelvic inflammation

Physical Examination

Key Concept: Although you may not always readily find the internal opening on physical examination, you can often get a feel for the extent of the disease process and exclude other sources of pathology.

The external or secondary opening may be seen as an elevation of granulation tissue discharging pus. This may be elicited on digital rectal examination. In most cases, the internal or primary opening is not apparent. The number of external openings and their location may be helpful in identifying the primary opening. According to Goodsall's rule (Fig. 21.2), an opening seen posterior to a line drawn transversely across the perineum will originate from an internal opening in the posterior midline. An anterior external opening will originate in the nearest crypt. Generally, the greater the distance from the anal margin, the greater the probability of a complicated upward

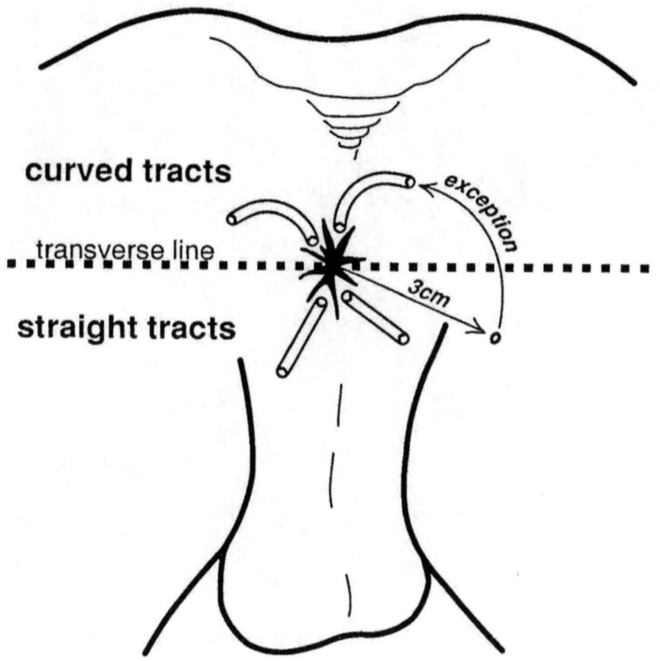

Fig. 21.2 Goodsall's rule (With permission from Vasilevsky [2])

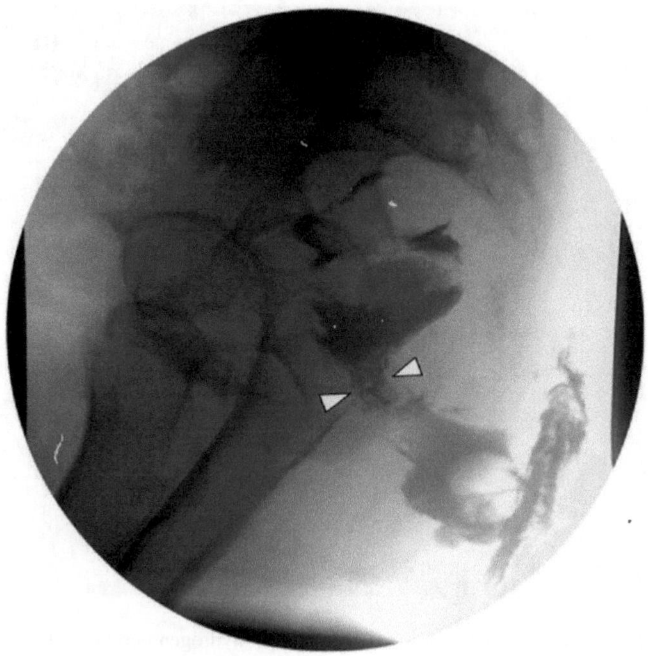

Fig. 21.3 Fistulogram (With permission from Vasilevsky [2]) (*White arrows* mark fistula tract)

extension [3]. Digital rectal examination may reveal an indurated cord-like structure beneath the skin in the direction of the internal opening with asymmetry between right and left sides. Internal openings may be felt as indurated nodules or pits leading to an indurated tract [3]. Look for posterior or lateral induration that may be palpable, as this may indicate fistulas deep in the postanal space or horseshoe fistulas [3, 4]. Bidigital rectal examination will define the relationship of the tract to the sphincter muscles and provides information as to preoperative sphincter tone, bulk, and voluntary squeeze pressure that need to be assessed.

Anoscopy is done prior to operation in an attempt to identify the primary opening, while sigmoidoscopy may locate a proximal internal opening and excludes underlying pathology such as proctitis or neoplasia. If you see either of these (or findings concerning for either), you need to redirect your workup and likely perform biopsies, cultures, etc., as appropriate. Colonoscopy or barium enema is indicated in patients with symptoms of inflammatory bowel disease, in patients with multiple or recurrent fistulas, and in patients who merit colorectal cancer screening. Anal manometry is normally not required, but may be useful in women with previous obstetric trauma, elderly patients, a patient with Crohn's disease or AIDS or in a patient with a recurrent fistula [5]. Preoperative imaging is used infrequently, with options including fistulography, CT scanning, endoanal ultrasound, and MRI.

Imaging Studies

Key Concept: I will use imaging studies in recurrent fistulas occasionally when I think it may be helpful to demonstrate clinically undetected sepsis, to serve as a guide at the time of the initial surgery, to determine the relationship of the fistula tract to the sphincter mechanism, and to reveal the site of sepsis in a recurrent fistula.

Fistulography

Key Concept: Although fistulography may help in select cases, it is plagued by difficulties, is invasive, and may result in the dissemination of sepsis.

Fistulography, which involves cannulation of the external opening with a small feeding tube or catheter and injection of water soluble contrast, may be useful in the evaluation of recurrent fistulas or in Crohn's disease where previous surgical forays or disease may have altered anorectal anatomy (Fig. 21.3) [6]. Contrast is introduced at low pressures to avoid tissue disruption and allow secondary tracts to fill. Localization of an associated abscess or the level of the internal opening may be difficult due to the absence of precise landmarks. Contrast may reflux into the rectum wrongly suggesting an extrasphincteric tract with a rectal opening. Accuracy rates in identifying the internal openings and extensions have ranged from 16 to 96 % with a false-positive rate of 12 % [6, 7].

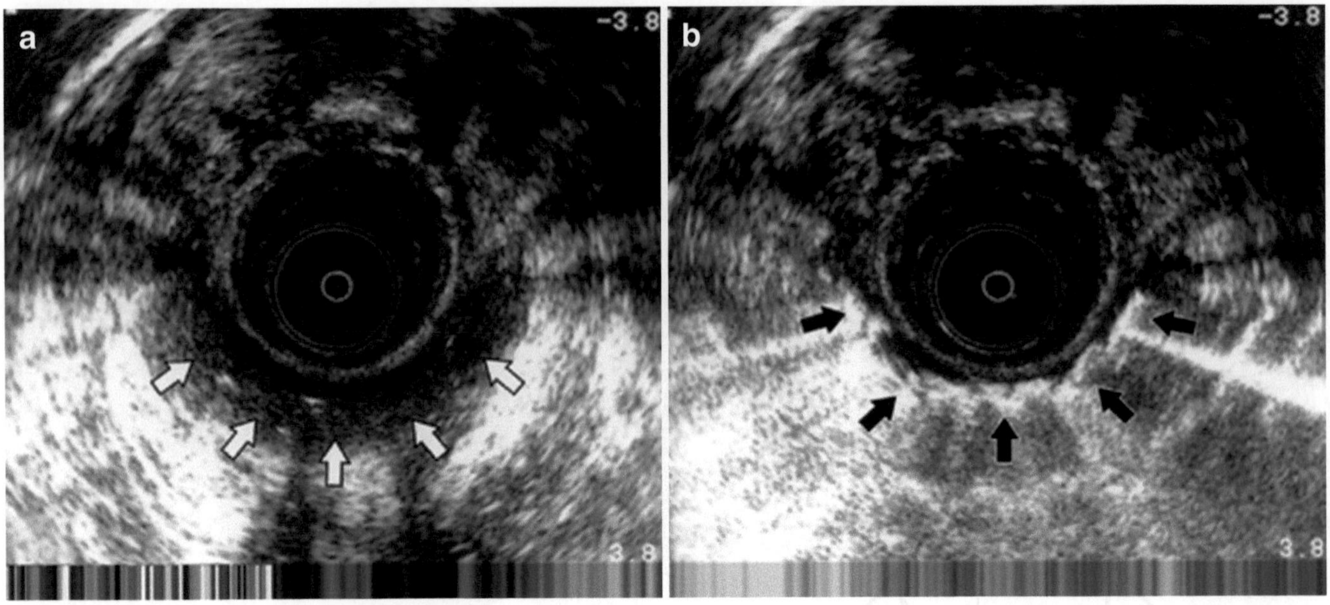

Fig. 21.4 (**a**) Anal endosonogram (**b**) with hydrogen peroxide. (Courtesy of Dr. Julio Faria) *White arrows* demonstrate unenhansed fistula tract. *Black arrows* highlight hydrogen peroxide enhansed fistula tract

CT Scan

Key Concept: CT is most helpful to look at surrounding structures rather than the fistula itself.

CT scanning performed with intravenous and rectal contrast is a less invasive method to assess the perirectal spaces and may differentiate an abscess from perirectal cellulitis [2]. It does not permit visualization of tracts in relation to the levators, but may be helpful in assessing the degree of rectal inflammation in patients with inflammatory bowel disease.

Endoanal Ultrasound

Key Concept: Ultrasound often can show you the presence and extent of the fistula, though should be interpreted by an experienced provider.

Endoanal ultrasound can establish the location of the primary opening and the relation of the primary tract to the anal sphincters, determine if the fistula is complex, and identify areas of suppuration [8]. A study conducted in 2002 using a 10 mHz probe along with injection of hydrogen peroxide was able to identify the internal opening in 93 % (Fig. 21.4) [8]. Ultrasound is rapid and well tolerated and can be transported to the operating room for challenging cases. Unfortunately, it is operator dependent, and scars or defects caused by previous sepsis, surgery, or trauma may confuse ultrasonographic interpretation [10].

MRI

Key Concept: MRI is becoming the preferred imaging technique in many centers for recurrent and complex fistulas.

MRI may be of value in the assessment of patients with complex fistulas and in those with anatomic distortion resulting from previous surgery (Fig. 21.5). MRI has been found to accurately delineate the site of the internal opening and the presence and course of primary and secondary fistulous tracts [11]. It may also significantly decrease recurrence rates in surgery for recurrent fistulas [12]. I find MRI to be useful in those cases that I feel require imaging and will often use it as a first modality.

Treatment

General Principles

Key Concept: The principles of fistula surgery are to eliminate the fistula, prevent recurrence, and preserve sphincter function. Success is usually determined by identification of the primary opening and dividing the least amount of muscle possible.

Several techniques can help you identify the primary opening in the operating room:

1. Passage of a probe or probes from the external to the internal opening or vice versa
2. Injection via a catheter inserted into the fistula tract of contrast such as hydrogen peroxide (Fig. 21.6) or dilute methylene blue and noting their appearance at the dentate line
3. Following the granulation tissue present in the fistula tract
4. Noting puckering of an anal crypt when traction is placed on the tract

Patients are educated on the challenges of fistula management and the different approaches available. Depending on the patient and their anatomy, success has varied from 60 to 90 %. In general, most surgeons prefer to accept a recurrence

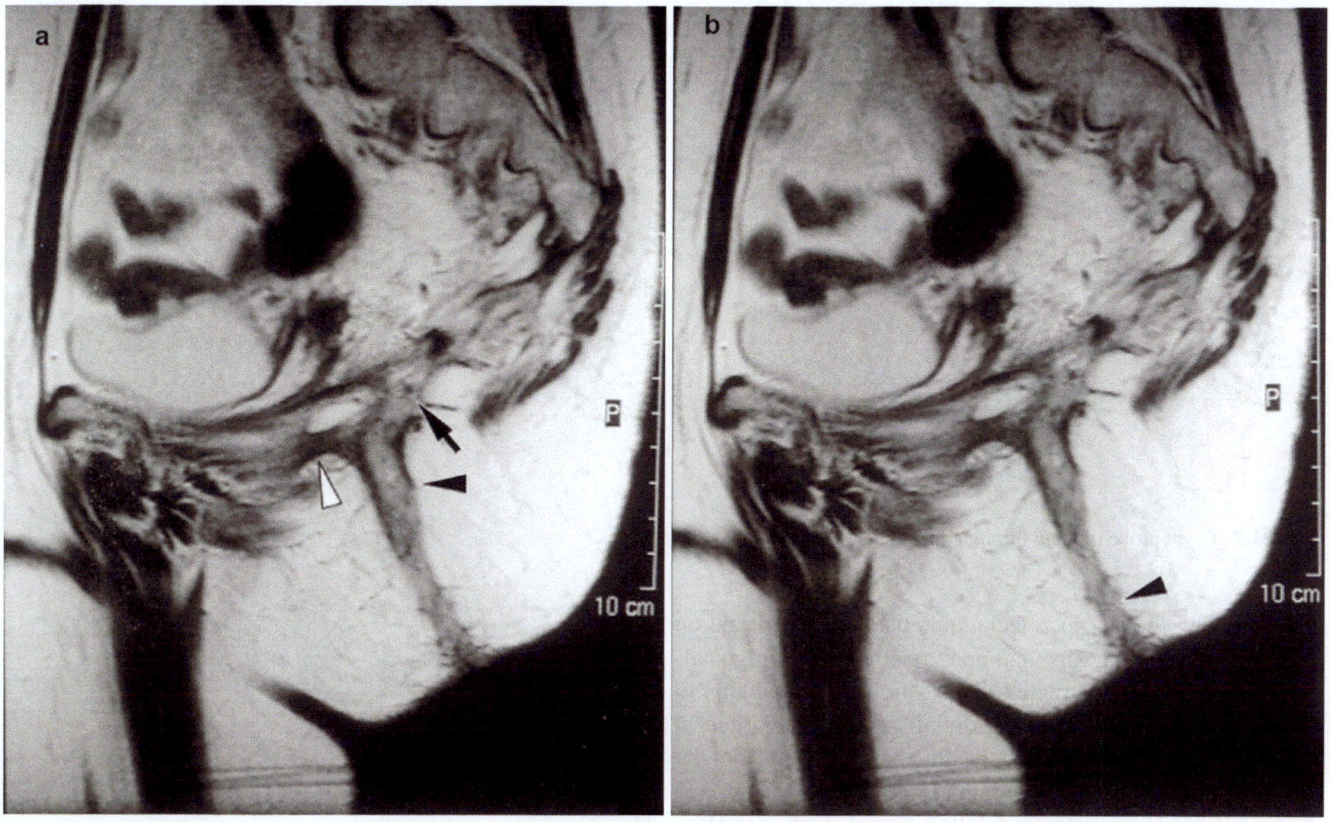

Fig. 21.5 Phase array MRI demonstrating the fistula opening (*black arrow*) and tract (*black arrow head*) (With permission from Vasilevsky [2]) *White arrow* demonstrates secondary entension

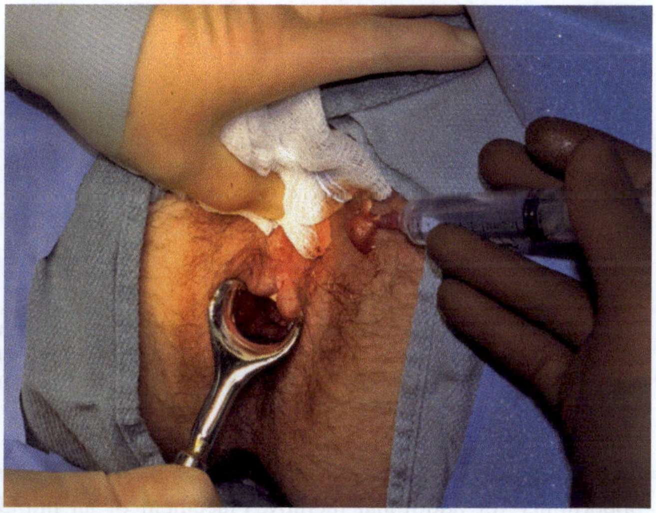

Fig. 21.6 Injection of dilute hydrogen peroxide to identify the internal opening (Courtesy of W. Brian Sweeney, MD)

over injury to the patient or their sphincters. For most surgical procedures the patient is placed in the prone jackknife or left lateral (Sims') position following induction of a general or regional anesthetic. Local anesthesia consisting of mixture of 0.5 % lidocaine or 0.25 % bupivacaine hydrochloride with 1:200,000 epinephrine is injected along the fistula tract for hemostasis following insertion of an anal speculum. The fistula is assessed to determine its location and relation to the sphincters using the techniques described above. Taking into account the characteristics of the fistula and the patient, several options are available.

Operative Management

Lay-Open Technique (Fistulotomy)

Key Concept: Fistulotomy provides the best success for low-lying fistulas, though you will have an open wound for a while that you need to follow-up on.

For simple intersphincteric and low transsphincteric fistulas, a probe is carefully inserted from the external opening through the tract to the internal opening at the dentate line (Fig. 21.7). The tissue overlying the probe is incised with electrocautery and any granulation tissue and the tract pseudoepithelium is curetted or fulgurated. Additional gentle probing is used to identify any high blind tracts or extensions, which are unroofed, if found. If you desire, the wound may be marsupialized on either edge by sewing the edges of the incision to the tract with a running absorbable suture. There is no need to insert packing if an adequate unroofing has been accomplished (Figs. 21.8 and 21.9).

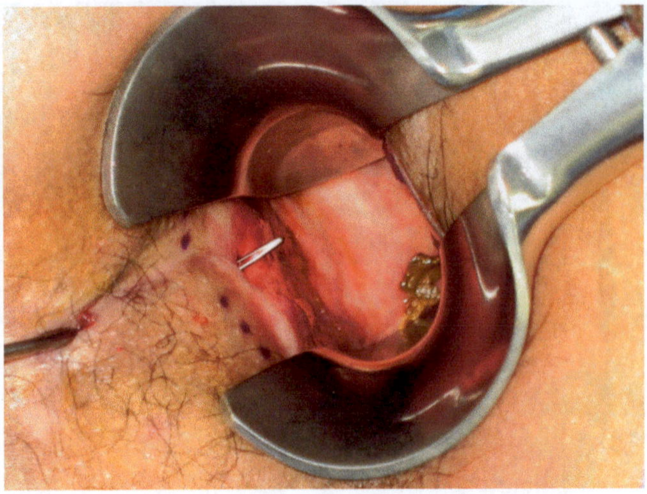

Fig. 21.7 Crypt probe running through the fistula tract

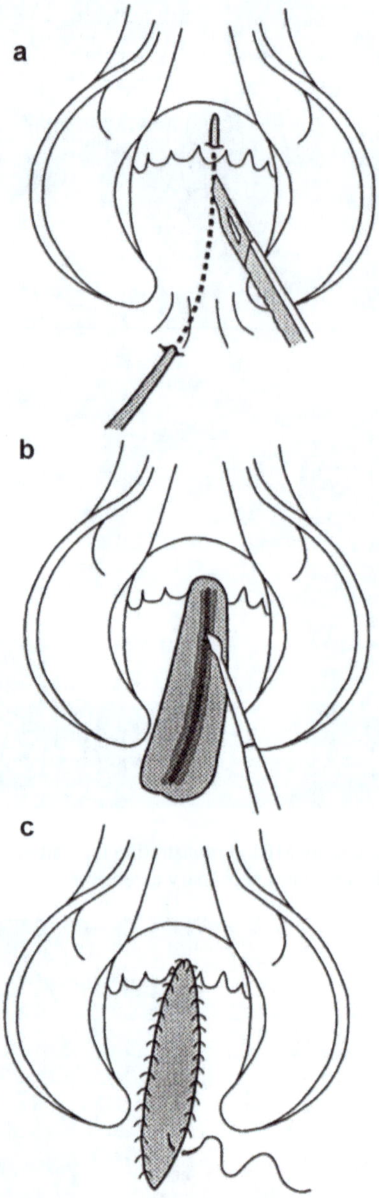

Fig. 21.8 Technique of laying open. (**a**) Insertion of probe and incision of tissue overlying probe. (**b**) Curettage of granulation tissue. (**c**) Marsupialization of wound edges (With permission from Vasilevsky [2])

Following the lay-open technique, patients are placed on regular diets, bulk agents, and non-codeine-containing analgesia. Patients are instructed to take frequent sitz baths to ensure perianal hygiene. I see them back in the office at 2-week intervals to ensure that healing has occurred from the depths of the tract. Granulation tissue can be cauterized using silver nitrate sticks, and cotton-tipped swabs are often used to probe the depths of the incision to ensure that adequate healing is occurring.

Fistulotomy has the highest success rate but leaves a wound that must heal by secondary intention. The amount of sphincter muscle that can be safely divided is a matter of surgical judgment that takes into account patient characteristics and the specifics of the fistula. In general, division of muscle distal to the dentate line will not have major alterations in continence. *Suprasphincteric* fistulas involve the entire external sphincter complex as well as the puborectalis muscle, and laying open the entire tract would render the patient incontinent. Thus other methods should be utilized.

Setons

Key Concept: Setons are great for allowing drainage, allowing the tract to fibrose, and preparing the fistula for a secondary procedure. Cutting setons aren't used much anymore.

If the fistula tract is seen to cross the sphincter muscle at a high level, the insertion of a seton is an option. A seton may be any foreign substance that can be inserted into the fistula tract to encircle the sphincter muscles. Materials commonly employed include silk or other nonabsorbable suture material, Penrose drains, rubber bands, or Silastic vessel loops. Setons may be used in two fashions.

A draining seton is placed through the tract and left loosely in place to act as a drain to facilitate drainage and delineate the tract (Fig. 21.10). In complex disease, prolonged drainage allows resolution of sepsis and provides an opportunity for additional therapy. Placement of an initial draining seton has improved the success of subsequent procedures (e.g., the LIFT or suprasphincteric fistulae), as described later in this chapter.

Prior to the development of additional surgical options, when a fistula involved a significant portion of the sphincter mechanism, a cutting seton was considered. With this technique, the lower portion of the internal sphincter is divided along with the skin to reach the external opening and a nonabsorbable or elastic suture is inserted into the fistulous tract. The ends of the suture are tied with multiple

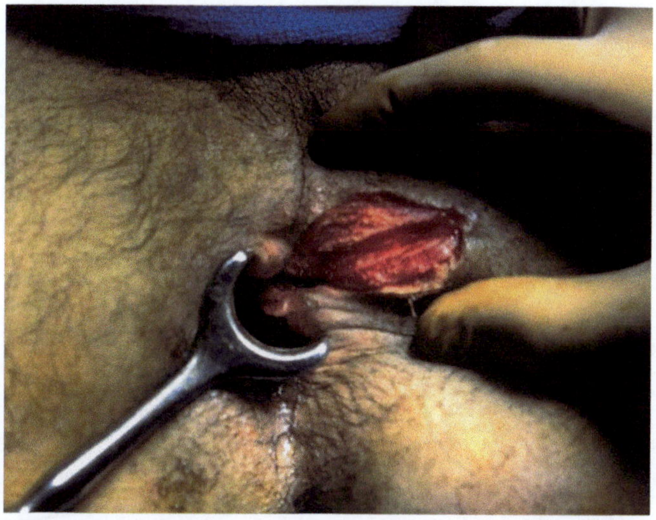

Fig. 21.9 Fistulotomy (Courtesy of W. Brian Sweeney, MD)

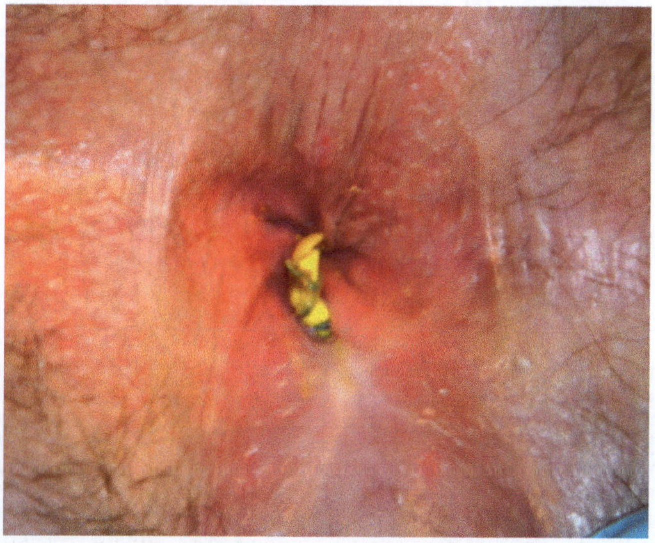

Fig. 21.10 Silastic vessel loop draining seton in place

knots to create a handle for manipulation (Figs. 21.11 and 21.12). The cutting seton was traditionally tightened at regular intervals to slowly cut through the sphincter. This allows the tract to become more superficial, converting a high fistula into a low one. The proximal fistulotomy subsequently heals by stimulating fibrosis behind it. This prevents separation or retraction of the sphincter muscle. The seton also allows delineation of the amount of remaining muscle that may be divided at a second operation several weeks later. The technique is very uncomfortable for the patient, and with the availability of other options, cutting setons are rarely used. A recent extensive literature search suggested abandoning the use of cutting setons because of sphincter damage and incontinence rates approaching 12 % [2].

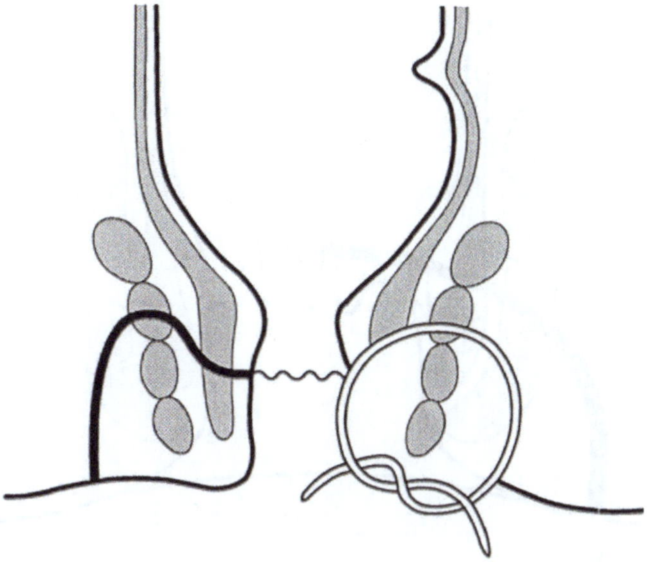

Fig. 21.11 Diagram of a cutting seton (With permission from Vasilevsky [2])

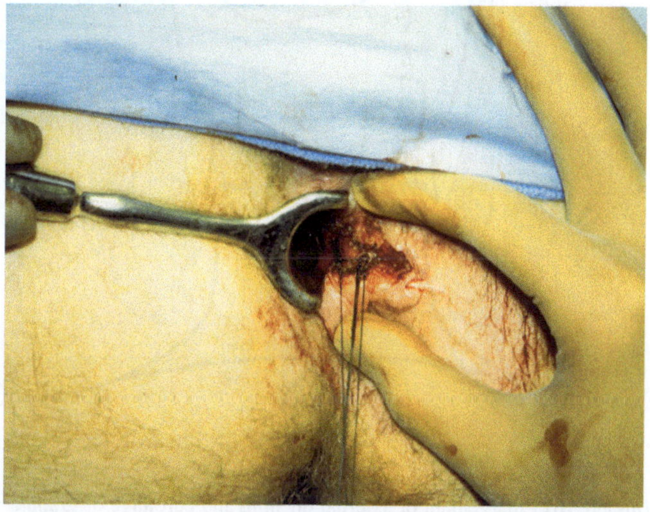

Fig. 21.12 Cutting seton in place (Courtesy of W. Brian Sweeney, MD)

Anorectal Advancement Flap

Key Concept: Anorectal advancement flaps provide a good option for difficult and recurrent fistulas. Ensure your flap is well vascularized by making it wide enough, including some of the underlying muscle and mobilize enough to make it tension-free.

The traditional laying-open technique is often inappropriate for anterior fistulas in women, in patients with inflammatory bowel disease, in patients with high transsphincteric and suprasphincteric fistulas, as well as in those with previous multiple sphincter operations and multiple and complex fistulas. For these patients, an anorectal advancement flap has been advocated (Figs. 21.13a–d and 21.14) [14]. Advantages

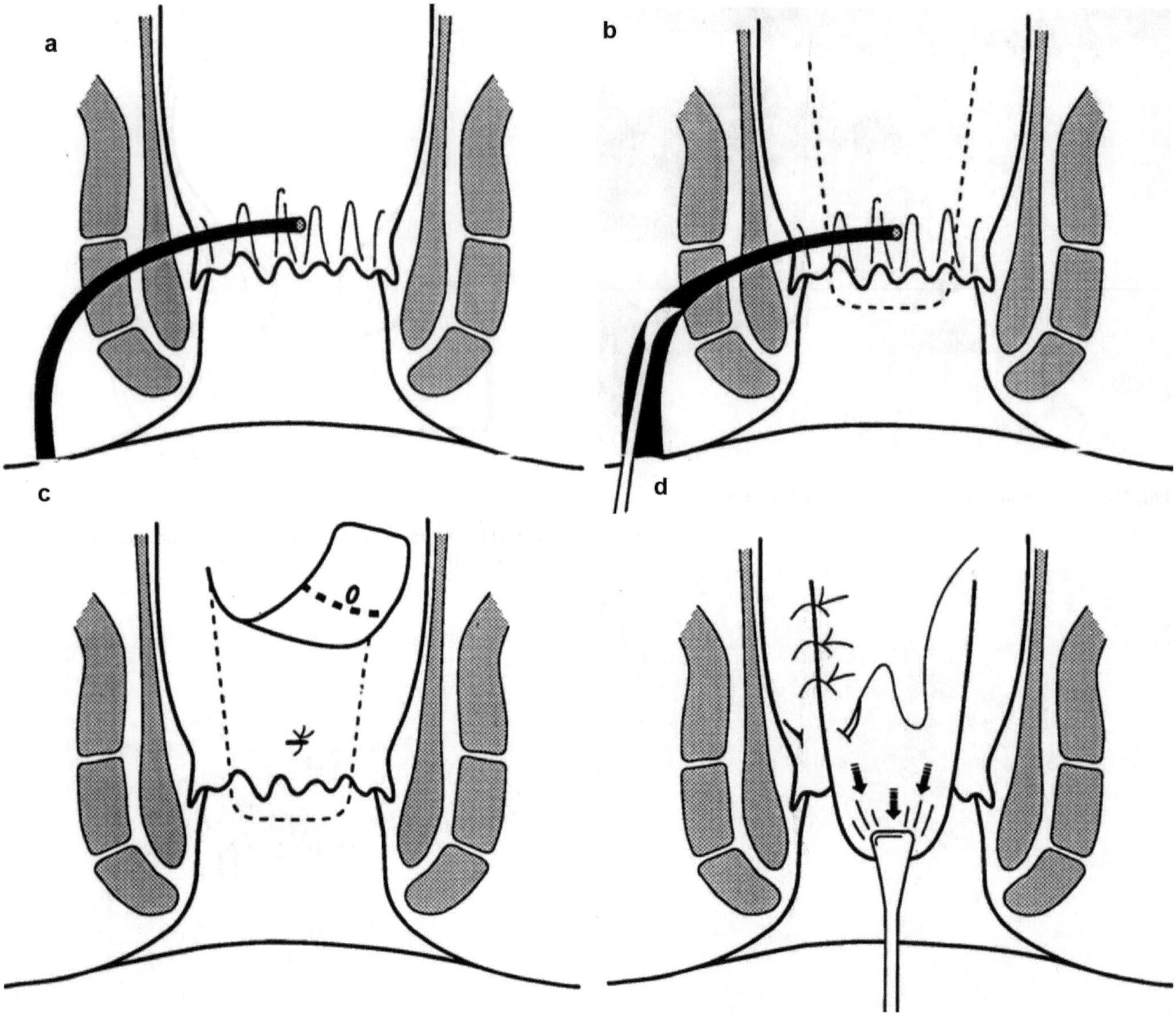

Fig. 21.13 Anorectal advancement flap. (**a**) Transsphincteric fistula-in-ano. (**b**) Enlargement of external opening and curettage of granulation tissue, (**c**) mobilization of flap and closure of internal opening, (**d**) suturing of flap in place covering internal opening (With permission from Vasilevsky [2])

of this technique include a reduction in the duration of healing, reduced associated discomfort, lack of deformity to the anal canal, as well as little potential additional damage to the sphincter muscles since no muscle is divided [2].

Following preparation and positioning, the fistula tract is identified with a probe and either cored out or curetted. The internal opening is identified and excised and the external opening is enlarged to allow for drainage. A full-thickness flap of rectal mucosa, submucosa, and part of the internal sphincter is raised. The residual internal opening is closed with absorbable suture. The flap is then advanced 1 cm below the internal opening. The tip of the flap containing the fistulous opening is excised, and the flap is sewn into place with absorbable sutures ensuring that the mucosal and muscular suture lines do not overlap. The base of the flap should be twice the width of the apex to maintain good blood supply. Successful results have reported in over 90 % of patients [15]. Factors associated with poor outcomes include Crohn's disease and steroids [16]. The flap is a great option for recurrent or difficult fistula-in-ano, but you need to ensure your technique allows for great mobilization and preservation of the blood supply to optimize your success.

Fibrin Glue

Key Concept: With time and experience, fibrin glue has had low rates of incontinence but high rates of failure and recurrence.

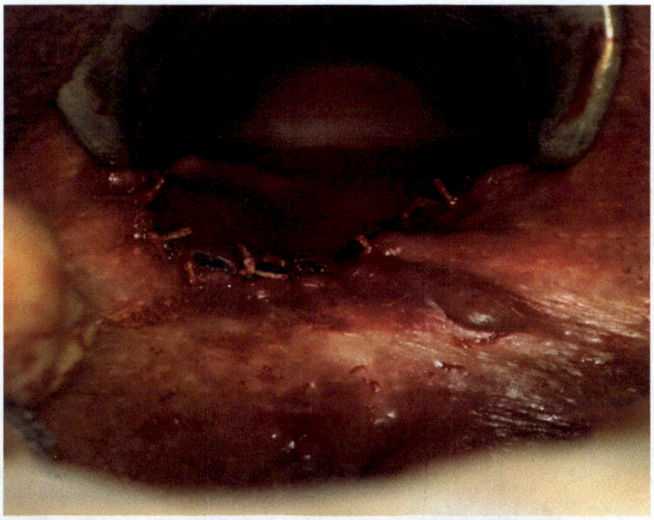

Fig. 21.14 Completed anorectal advancement flap (Courtesy of W. Brian Sweeney, MD)

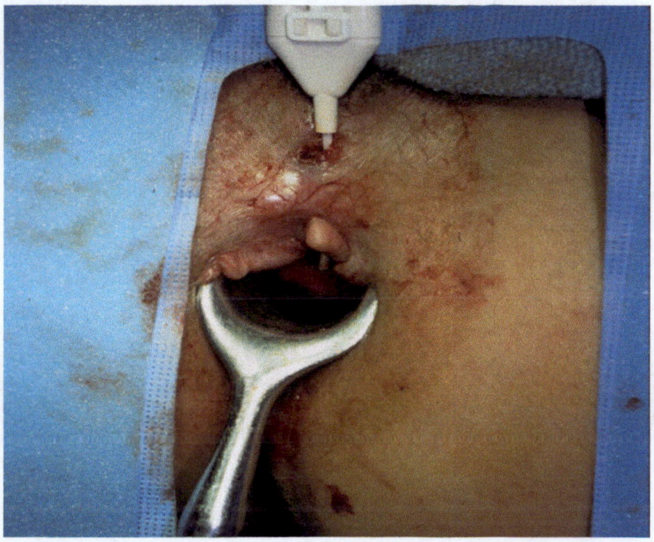

Fig. 21.15 Injection of fibrin glue down a fistula tract (Courtesy of W. Brian Sweeney, MD)

The use of fibrin glue as a primary treatment alone or in combination with an advancement flap was appealing since it is a simple, noninvasive approach that avoids the risk of incontinence associated with fistulotomy. In the case of failure, it may be repeated several times without jeopardizing continence. As with fistulotomy, the fistula tract along with its internal and external openings is identified and curetted (with curettes or flexible brushes). Fibrin glue is injected into the fistula tract through a Y connector so that the entire tract is filled and the glue can be seen emerging from the internal opening (Fig. 21.15). The injecting catheter is slowly withdrawn so that the entire tract is filled (Fig. 21.16).

Enthusiasm generated because of initial short-term success rates of 70–74 % has been tempered due to delayed fistula recurrence despite initial apparent healing [17–19]. Slightly better results were obtained with a 2-stage approach consisting of seton placement followed by glue injection at a second stage. Although the exact mechanisms responsible for failure have not been entirely appreciated, it has been suggested that curettage may not adequately remove all granulation or epithelialized tissue thus failing to provide the correct environment for the glue to work [20]. Other adverse factors shown to influence healing include the presence of a short tract which may make it easier for the fibrin glue plug to become dislodged as well as the presence of a cavity on endoanal ultrasound [21]. The latter was associated with a complication of perianal abscess since the tract may not have been entirely filled with glue [22]. Fibrin glue is associated with a low incontinence rate as well as a disappointing low cure rate and not used much anymore.

Anal Fistula Plug

Key Concept: Plugs provide an option for sphincter preservation, although recurrence and failure rates are 40–60 %.

Two bioprosthetic plugs are currently available to treat anal fistulas. The Biodesign® anal fistula plug (lyophilized porcine intestinal submucosal, Cook Biotech, West Lafayette, IN) and the Gore® Bio-A fistula plug (synthetic bioabsorbable, W L Gore, Flagstaff, AZ) provide a scaffold for colonized by host tissue cells, blood vessels, and connective tissue.

Following preparation and positioning, the internal and external openings are delineated. A probe is gently passed from the external to the internal opening to confirm the position of the tract and facilitate insertion of the plug. Debridement or curettage of the tract should not be performed. A seton should be used temporarily if there is acute inflammation or drainage. A 2-0 suture is placed through the tapered end of the plug and the ends of this suture are attached to the fistula probe at the primary opening. The suture is pulled from the primary opening, through the fistula tract to exit at the secondary opening. For patients with a "horseshoe" fistula, an incision may be made over the fistula tract distal to the anal verge to create a secondary opening that the ends of the suture are brought through. With gentle traction on the suture, the plug is pulled into the primary opening of the fistula until it is snug but not forced tightly. Excess plug is removed by transecting the plug at the level of the primary opening. The plug is secured in the primary opening using a 2-0 absorbable suture placed in a figure of 8 fashion with the suture crossing through the center of the plug and incorporating a generous portion of the sphincter mechanism on both sides. Any plug protruding through the secondary opening is also excised. The distal end of the plug is not sutured to the fistula tract and the distal opening is left open for drainage (Fig. 21.17). Patients are advised to avoid vigorous physical activity for 2 weeks after plug placement to minimize the chance of plug dislodgement. No dietary restrictions are necessary nor are topical antibiotics indicated.

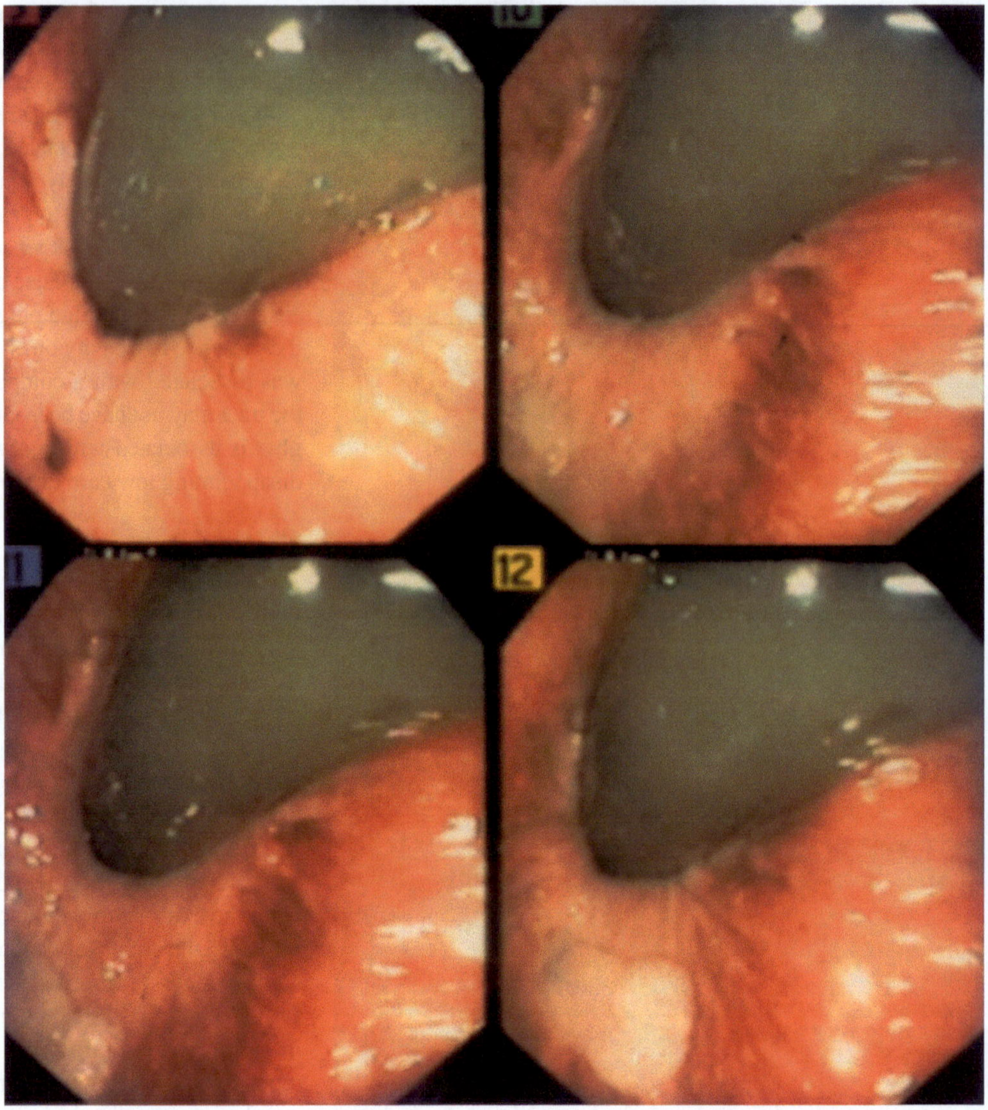

Fig. 21.16 Endoscopic view of fibrin glue filling the internal opening. The internal opening can be seen in the left upper picture as the dark area at ~7o'clock, with subsequent images showing the fibrin glue filling this opening (Courtesy of W. Brian Sweeney, MD)

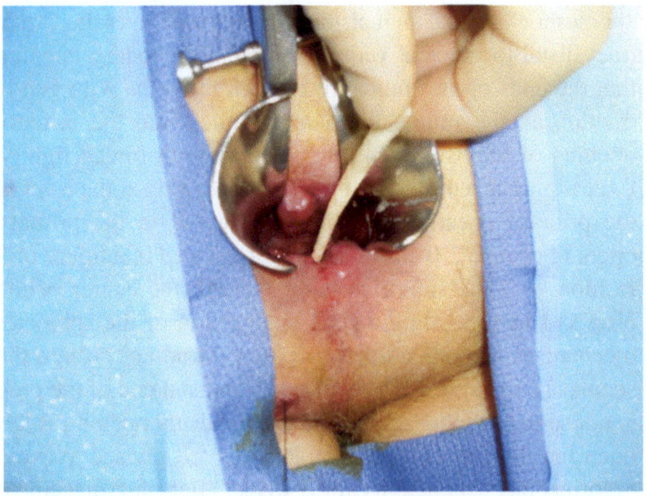

Fig. 21.17 Anal fistula plug (Courtesy of David Armstrong, MD, Atlanta, GA)

As with many of these alternative techniques, initial results were successful [23, 24]. Unfortunately, subsequent experience has been less successful with healing rates averaging 40–60 %. Contraindications for the use of the plug include fistulas with a persistent abscess cavity or infection, allergy to porcine products, and inability to identify both the external and internal openings. The latter constitutes an absolute contraindication for use of the plug. The plug is useful in certain situations of failure or recurrence or in people with borderline continence that you want to ensure no damage to the muscle occurs.

LIFT Procedure

Key Concept: The LIFT identifies and divides the fistula tract in the intersphincteric space. Readying the tract with use of a seton to allow for fibrosis will aid in success.

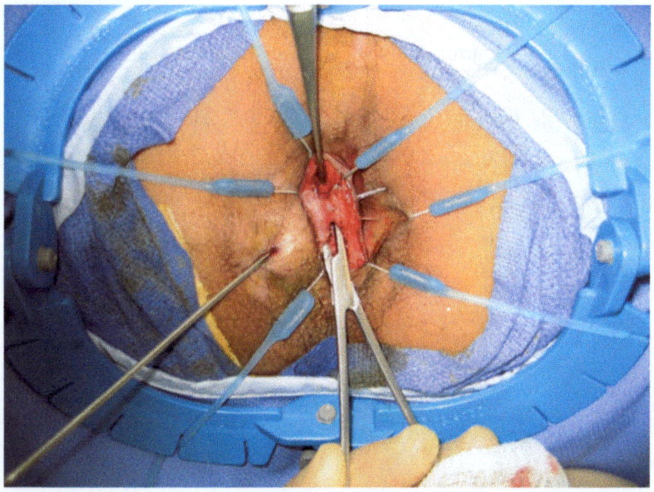

Fig. 21.18 LIFT procedure. Dissection of the fistula tract in the intersphincteric plane

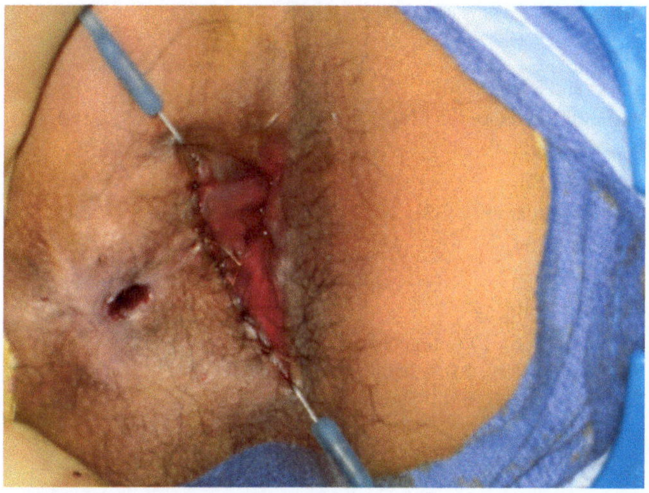

Fig. 21.19 Completed LIFT procedure

Recently a new sphincter-sparing technique has been introduced called the ligation of the intersphincteric fistula tract (LIFT) procedure [25]. This technique relies on the secure closure of the internal opening and removal of the infected cryptoglandular tissue in the intersphincteric space. Patients with early fistulous abscess in which the intersphincteric tract is not well formed and those with high internal openings are less suitable for this technique.

After preparation and positioning an anoscope is inserted into the anal canal and the internal opening is identified. A probe is gently passed through the fistula tract. A 1.5–2.0 cm curvilinear incision is made at the intersphincteric groove overlying the fistula tract and cautery is used to dissect into the intersphincteric plane. The intersphincteric tract that contains the probe is dissected (Fig. 21.18), divided, and ligated next to the internal opening with an absorbable suture. The residual tract distal to the suture is also ligated. Tract division may be confirmed by injection or probing of the external opening and granulation tissue may be curetted. The incision is closed with 3-0 absorbable suture (Fig. 21.19).

Initial reports in the literature include success rates of 58–94 % [25, 26]. The exact place where the LIFT fits into the algorithm for fistula management remains to be seen. Some surgeons are using the LIFT more and more as a primary option (following seton placement) for all high and complex fistulae that cannot be managed with a fistulotomy, while others reserve this procedure for failures or recurrences. While this is a promising technique, more experience and longer-term follow-up data is going to prove valuable.

Fistulectomy

Key Concept: Removal of the tract entirely should (in general) not be performed.

Excision of the fistula or fistulectomy is avoided as it produces larger wounds with prolonged healing time, a greater separation of muscle ends, a greater risk of injuring or excising underlying muscle, and a subsequent greater risk of incontinence [14, 27].

Dermal Flaps

Key Concept: Using the perineal skin for a flap, instead of anorectal mucosa, is useful for distal non-healing fistula.

Another option to treat transsphincteric fistulas without division of muscle involves the use of a dermal flap. This technique closes the internal opening using a variety of skin flaps, such as sliding (House) or island flaps. It is helpful in distal fistulas in which a mucosal advancement flap would produce an ectropia and in patients who have failed other techniques. Success has been reported as 77 % [28].

Results

My Approach

The author's preference is to select a fistulotomy for simple low fistulas. For more complicated fistulas, I would consider a draining seton if there is infection or inflammation present or either a plug or LIFT for the first attempt. Recurrences are offered a LIFT (if a plug was used previously or the tract is suitable for a LIFT) or an advancement flap. Next, for continued failures, a Martius flap with or without proximal diversion.

Complications

Key Concept: Similar to any procedure, both early and late complications can be expected in a small percentage of

Table 21.2 Results of fistula surgery

Author	Year	No. of patients	Recurrence %	Incontinence %
Marks and Ritchie [30]	1977	793	–	3, 17, 25[a]
Vasilevsky and Gordon [31]	1985	160	6.3	0.7, 2.0, 3.3[b]
Van Tets [29]	1994	19	–	33.0
Sangwan [32]	1994	461	6.5	2.8
Garcia-Aguilar et al. [33]	1996	293	7.0	42.0
Mylonakis [34]	2001	100	3.0	0, 6.0, 3.0[c]
Malouf [35]	2002	98	4.0	10
Westerterp [36]	2003	60	0	50

[a]3 % solid stool, 17 % liquid stool, 25 % flatus
[b]0.7 % solid stool, 2.0 % liquid stool, 3.3 % flatus
[d]0 solid stool, 6.0 % soiling, 3,0 % gas

patients. Using proper technique and placing the patient on a postoperative bowel and wound regimen will help to minimize these complications.

Early postoperative complications that have been reported following fistula surgery include urinary retention, hemorrhage, fecal impaction, and thrombosed external hemorrhoids, which were found to occur in less than 6 % of cases [2]. Later complications such as pain, bleeding, pruritus, and poor wound healing have been reported in ~9 % of patients [14]. Anal stenosis may occur and is usually the result of loose stools allowing healing of the anal canal by scar contracture. Mucosal prolapse due to extensive division of sphincter muscle may also occur and can be treated by band ligation, sclerosis, or excision [14]. With attention to both operative detail and postoperative follow-up, these complications can be reduced to a minimum.

Incontinence

Key concept: Incontinence after fistulotomy depends both on the amount of muscle divided at operation and on preexisting sphincter damage and scarring of the anal canal.

Minor disorders of continence following fistulotomy have been reported to range from 18 to 52 %, while soiling and insufficiency have been reported in as many as 35–45 % [29] (Table 21.2). The occurrence of continence disorders has been found to be related to the complexity of the fistula and to the level and location of the internal opening [29].

Patients with complicated fistulas, high openings, posterior openings, and fistula extensions have been found to be at higher risk [29]. In the treatment of complicated fistulas and those with high openings, more muscle is divided, thus decreasing anal pressures, while posterior fistula wounds have been associated with higher rates of incontinence because of their more circuitous routes [29]. Drainage of extensions may accidentally damage small nerves and create more scar tissue around the anorectum [29]. If the edges of the fistulotomy wound do not approximate precisely, the anus may be unable to properly close, resulting in intermittent leakage of gas and stool [37]. In addition to these factors, impaired continence was associated with increasing age [30] and female gender [29, 30]. The latter is probably the result of partial anal sphincter disruption and/or traction injury to the pudendal nerves sustained during vaginal delivery [30].

Although excellent results employing a seton have been reported [38], its use does not protect against the development of impaired continence [29]. Minor continence disorders were reported in 73 % [29] while Williams [39] reported minor disturbances in 54 %. Parks [40] found that minor incontinence occurred in 39 % with the two-stage approach versus 17 % when only the first stage was performed and the seton was removed rather than dividing the muscle. Major fecal incontinence was reported as 6.7 % in a review of several series [30]. The degree of incontinence is thought to be influenced by the patient's preoperative state of control as well as to how the anal wound heals [30]. Analysis of data compiled in a recent literature search found that a 12 % rate of incontinence with the rate increasing as the location of the internal opening moved more proximally [13].

Excellent results with respect to continence have been reported with the use of the advancement flap, although recent reports have observed disturbances in continence in 9–35 % attributed to overstretching of the sphincters by self-retaining retractors [16, 41, 42]. Disruption of the internal sphincter also occurs if some internal sphincter fibers are developed with the flap [43].

As would be expected, continence is unaffected with the use of fibrin glue and the fistula plug. In a study that looked at changes in anorectal morphologic and functional parameters after fistula surgery, it was found that fistulotomy and advancement flaps were most associated with changes in internal anal sphincter defects with decreased resting and squeeze pressure on manometry noted after fistulotomy while rectal advancement flaps were associated with decrease in resting pressure [44]. It therefore behooves you as the surgeon to recognize preexisting sphincter defects by endoanal ultrasound prior to embarking on fistula surgery.

Recurrence

Key Concept: Recurrence and failure of healing is inevitable in a small amount of patients. You can limit this by identifying the correct internal opening, determining the extent of the fistula, and proper wound care. Counsel your patients appropriately regarding the possibility of several operations and a need for long-term management for proper healing.

Recurrence rates following fistulotomy range from 0 to 18 % [32]. Results from selected references are cited in Table 21.2. Causes include failure to identify a primary opening or recognize lateral or upward extensions of a fistula [31, 32]. Inability to locate the primary opening may imply a circuitous tract, spontaneous closure of the primary opening, or a microscopic opening [32]. The presence of secondary tracts that can be easily missed accounted for early recurrence in 20 % [31, 32]. Premature closure of the fistulotomy wound can be obviated by producing an external wound twice the size of the anal wound resulting in proper healing of the internal wound prior to the external wound [32]. Diligent postoperative care can also reduce recurrence rates by avoiding bridging and pocketing of the wound [45]. Epithelialization of the fistula tract from internal or external openings rather than chronic infection of an anal gland has also been suggested as the cause of a persistent anal fistula [46].

Recurrence rates following staged repairs utilizing a seton range from 0 to 29 % [37]. Recurrence rates following anorectal advancement flaps were initially reported to be low; however, long-term follow-up recurrence rates of 40 % have been reported [42]. Recurrence can be minimized provided that care has been taken to avoid necrosis or retraction of the flap. The use of full-thickness rectal wall has been advocated to prevent ischemic necrosis of the flap [47].

Special Considerations

Key Concept: You should be aware of each of these situations that may require management in a different fashion, or bring up other considerations that may affect treatment, function, or recurrence rates.

The *horseshoe variety of the suprasphincteric fistula* presents the problem of complete sphincter involvement combined with the presence of multiple external openings a great distance from the cryptoglandular source. Treatment consists of identification of the internal opening and proper drainage of the postanal space. The horseshoe extensions are enlarged for counter-drainage and the granulation tissue is curetted (Fig. 21.20). Setons can be placed from the posterior drainage incision to the external openings (modified Hanley technique).

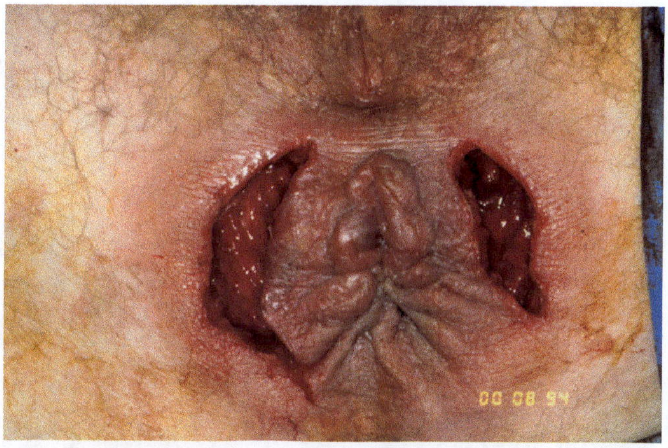

Fig. 21.20 Horseshoe fistula with counter-incisions (Courtesy of C. Os Finne, MD)

Extrasphincteric Fistula

Key Concept: The treatment of an extrasphincteric fistula depends on its etiology.

If the fistula arises secondary to an anal fistula, a secondary opening above the puborectalis is thought to be iatrogenic due to extensive probing of a transsphincteric fistula. The lower portion of the internal sphincter is divided and the rectal opening is closed with a nonabsorbable suture. A temporary colostomy may be necessary but a medical colostomy consisting of preoperative mechanical and antibiotic bowel preparation followed by enteral feeding may suffice. If the fistula is the result of entrance of a foreign body, it must be removed, drainage must be established, the internal opening closed, and a temporary colostomy constructed to decrease rectal pressure. This type of fistula may also be a manifestation of Crohn's disease. Treatment will depend on the nature of the anorectal mucosa, and drainage may be assisted by placement of a seton (Fig. 21.21). Finally the fistula may be the result of downward tracking of a pelvic abscess, which must be drained so that the fistula can heal.

Crohn's Disease

Key Concept: Combine medical therapy aimed at the Crohn's disease with surgical therapy that typically includes draining all abscesses and placement of setons in the acute setting.

Anal fistulas are the most difficult and challenging complication of Crohn's disease to manage. They constitute the most common perianal manifestations, occurring in 6–34 % of patients [48]. The location of Crohn's disease in the bowel has an impact on the frequency of fistulas. Patients with colonic Crohn's have a higher incidence with the rate approaching 100 % in those with rectal Crohn's [49].

As discussed previously, patients with Crohn's disease should undergo sigmoidoscopy, colonoscopy, and small bowel follow through to determine the extent of disease. Delineation

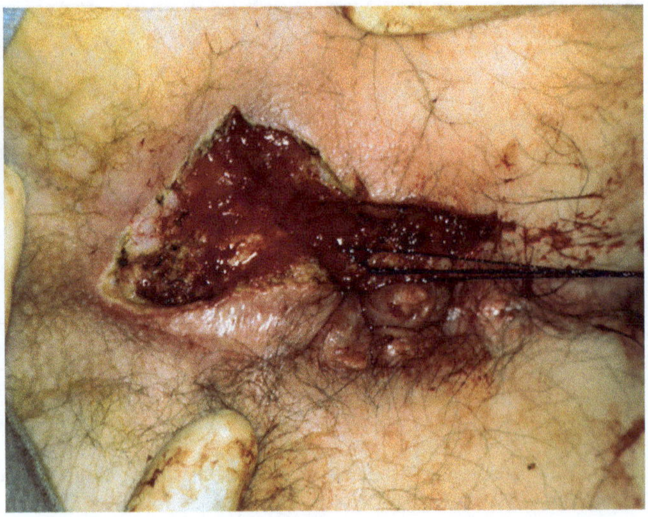

Fig. 21.21 Drainage of a suprasphincteric fistula with opening and division of the lower part of the tract and placement of a seton around the cephalad muscle (Courtesy of W. Brian Sweeney, MD)

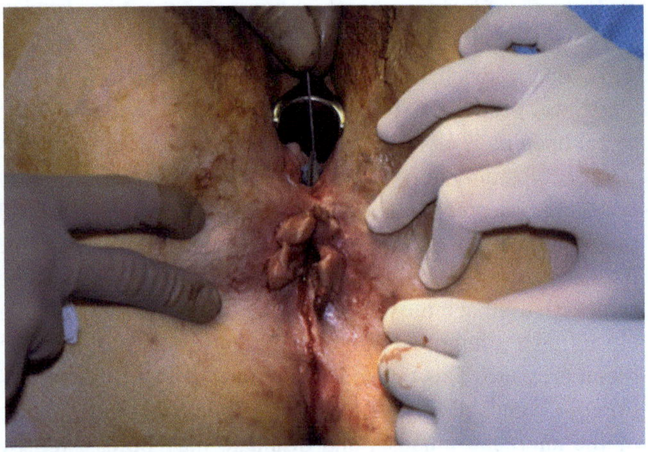

Fig. 21.22 Perianal Crohn's disease. Note the multiple tags and probe going through an anterior fistula (Courtesy of W. Brian Sweeney, MD)

of the fistulous tract is especially important in Crohn's disease since many fistulas may be complex in nature (Fig. 21.22). Endoanal ultrasound and MRI have been helpful in detecting abscesses that were clinically unsuspected on clinical examination and has been helpful in determining the relationship of the fistulous tract to the sphincter muscles [51]. Therapeutic goals in managing anorectal fistulas in Crohn's disease remain the alleviation of symptoms and preservation of continence. Fear of poor and delayed wound healing and the risk of sphincter injury have often suggested a conservative approach. Medications used in the treatment of fistulas include antibiotics such as metronidazole and ciprofloxacin and immunomodulators such as corticosteroids, 6 MP, azathioprine, and infliximab.

Prolonged healing and or incontinence have been associated with strictures, active rectal disease, and multiple operations [51]. Initial therapy should be directed at resolving inflammation in the rectum with the use of topical steroid or 5-acetylsalycylic enemas or suppositories. In addition oral medication may be necessary.

Regarding the actual fistula, remember to do what you can to promote drainage and avoid dividing muscle. Complex fistulas with high rectal openings might best be managed conservatively, because impaired continence may certainly result if the sphincter muscle is divided. Eradication of the fistula in this situation may not be possible because of the complexity of the tracts. Seton placement has been advocated to promote drainage, limit recurrent suppuration, and preserve sphincter function [52]. It is likely your best option in the acute setting. Rectal advancement flaps have been used in the absence of severe rectal disease [53], but you likely should not be performing a flap in patients with acute abscesses and fistulas. In general, these have been found to succeed in patients without concomitant small bowel Crohn's [54].

The presence of a protective stoma does not guarantee success, but may be beneficial in the patient who has undergone multiple unsuccessful repairs [46]. For severe intractable disease, an intersphincteric proctectomy may ultimately become necessary. The intersphincteric technique reduces the size of the resulting wound and reduces the incidence of unhealed sinuses. While your patient may not want to discuss a stoma or permanent loss of their rectum, for those with severe disease, it may be best to bring up the possibility of this early in course to allow time to sink in and discuss in the future.

Fistula-in-Ano in the HIV-Positive Patient

Key Concept: Severity of illness must be assessed prior to operative intervention since patients with more advanced disease are less likely to heal their wounds. Optimize their medical therapy, determine the complexity and how symptomatic the fistula is, and proceed accordingly.

Anal fistulas are prevalent in the anoreceptive HIV-positive individual [55]. Disturbed locoregional defenses may allow infection to occur. Although anal fistulas in HIV-positive patients arise from the dentate line similar to those in HIV negative patients, they are more likely to have incomplete anal fistulas leading to blind sinus tracts [56]. Concern for wound healing has tempered enthusiasm for operative intervention. However, selective operative management will result in a high rate of complete or partial wound healing with symptomatic relief without excessive morbidity or mortality [55]. Data are conflicting as to whether preoperative CD4+ lymphocyte counts can be related to poor wound healing; however, Consten found that low CD4+ lymphocyte counts in patients with perianal sepsis were a risk factor for disturbed wound healing [55, 56]. Use of highly active antiviral therapy (HAART) may reduce the incidence of opportunistic infections and anorectal disease and aid healing [57].

Asymptomatic fistulas require no treatment. Perioperative antibiotic therapy over a 5-day course has been recommended because of the high risk of infectious complications [55]. Care should be exercised to avoid creation of large wounds and to preserve as much sphincter muscle as possible since these patients may be prone to diarrhea, which may overwhelm a partially divided sphincter [55]. In patients who are good operative risks, fistulotomy is appropriate in patients with intersphincteric or low transsphincteric fistulas. For high or complex fistulas as well as for those patients who are poor operative risks, liberal use of draining setons is recommended [55]. It is important to realize that cellulitis may be seen with a fistula without concomitant underlying exudate [55].

Rectourethral Fistulas

Key Concept: These are difficult cases that may require both fecal and urinary diversion. It is helpful to enlist the help of a urologist. The anatomy of the fistula, its underlying cause, and degree of symptoms will determine the operative therapy.

Rectourethral fistulas are rare but devastating complications that may occur following radical open or laparoscopic prostatectomy, radiation treatment for prostate cancer, trauma, recurrent perineal abscess of cryptoglandular origin, Crohn's disease, or following treatment with radiofrequency hyperthermia for benign prostatic hypertrophy. The prostatic urethra is the most common site for fistulization to occur since this portion of the urethra is adjacent to the rectal wall.

The most common symptoms include leakage of urine through the rectum during voiding, pneumaturia, fecaluria, and recurrent urinary tract infections resistant to antibiotic treatment. PSA determination should be done to rule out recurrence of carcinoma. Digital rectal examination should always be performed to determine if there is any anorectal pathology that could be the cause. Sigmoidoscopy will show the fistula opening, which is located on the anterior rectal wall, and in addition rules out rectal pathology as a source. Cystoscopy and retrograde urethral cystography should be performed to determine the presence of a urethral stricture. Assessment of urinary continence should be also done prior to any attempt at surgical repair.

Operative repair of rectourethral fistulas is challenging due to technical difficulties and difficult exposure. Multiple repairs have been described, but there is no consensus as to which type of repair is best. You should also remember that small fistulas may be managed conservatively with an indwelling Foley catheter [58].

Treatment consisting of fecal diversion with either colostomy or ileostomy and urinary diversion with suprapubic catheterization under cover of antibiotics has been described in the management of rectourethral fistulas secondary to radiation when the urethral defect has been found to be too large to repair. Definitive repair options include the following: a transabdominal approach (abdomino-anal pull through in combination with omental interposition); perineal approaches using the gracilis muscle, dartos, or Martius flap; an anterior trans-anorectal approach; a posterior approach (Kraske laterosacral or York Mason (transsphincteric) approach); a transanal approach (endorectal advancement flap or transanal endoscopic microsurgery); and a cystectomy and ileal conduit [58–64]. Each option has proponents who maximizes the strength and minimizes disadvantages of each technique.

Summary Pearls

When dealing with anal fistula, and especially complex ones, it is always best to go back to the principles of fistula surgery: eliminate the fistula, prevent recurrence, and preserve sphincter function. An appropriate history and limited examination in the office is usually followed by an exam under anesthesia, where the internal and external openings and fistula tract are identified. Your operative therapy is selected based on patient characteristics, your experience, and, importantly, the operative findings regarding what type of fistula you are dealing with. Success is usually determined by proper identification of the primary opening – don't make one. There are occasions when the tract will go to what appears to be the appropriate crypt, and a few cell layers will be available at what appears to be the internal opening. Prior to just popping through, ensure you are not being fooled, and don't make a false passage. In the absence of anything else, first do what is right for the patient. Divide the least amount of muscle possible. Simple low fistulas are managed with a fistulotomy. The more complicated ones can be managed with a plug, LIFT, or advancement flap, depending on the prior history of the patient and pertinent anatomy. You are likely not going to have a successful endorectal advancement flap in someone with severe proctitis or prior radiation. So tailor your approach towards what you are given. Remember, recurrences can be managed with a similar or more extensive procedure, but often your first attempt is your best chance, so if it needs to be staged, do so.

References

1. Parks AG, Gordon PH, Hardcastle JD. A classification of fistula-in-ano. Br J Surg. 1976;63:1–12.
2. Vasilevsky CA. Anorectal abscess and fistula. In: Beck DE, Wexner SD, Roberts PL, Saclarides TJ, Senagore A, Stamos M, editors. ASCRS textbook of colorectal surgery. 2nd ed. New York: Springer; 2011.

3. Cirocco WC, Reilly JC. Challenging the predictive accuracy of Goodsall's rule for anal fistulas. Dis Colon Rectum. 1992; 35:537–42.
4. Wexner SD, Rosen L, Roberts PL, et al. Practice parameters for treatment of fistula-in-ano- supporting documentation. Dis Colon Rectum. 1996;39:1363–72.
5. Sainio P, Husa A. A prospective manometric study of the effect of anal fistula surgery on anorectal function. Acta Chir Scand. 1985;151:279–88.
6. Weisman RI, Orsay CP, Pearl RK, Abcarian H. The role of fistulography in fistula-in-ano. Report of five cases. Dis Colon Rectum. 1991;34:181–4.
7. Kuijpers HC, Schulpen T. Fistulography for fistula-in-ano: is it useful? Dis Colon Rectum. 1985;28:103–4.
8. Cataldo P, Senagore J, Luchtefeld MA, et al. Intrarectal ultrasound in the evaluation of perirectal abscesses. Dis Colon Rectum. 1993; 36:554–8.
9. Lengyel AJ, Hurst NG, William JG. Preoperative assessment of anal fistulas using endoanal ultrasound. Colorectal Dis. 2002;4:436–40.
10. Soew-Choen F, Burnett S, Bartram CI, Nicholls RJ. Comparison between anal endosonography and digital examination in the evaluation of anal fistulas. Br J Surg. 1991;78:445–7.
11. Barker PG, Lunniss PJ, Armstrong P, et al. Magnetic resonance imaging of fistula-in-ano: technique, interpretation and accuracy. Clin Radiol. 1994;49:7–13.
12. Buchanan G, Halligan A, Cohen CRG, et al. Effect of MRI on clinical outcome of recurrent fistula-in-ano. Lancet. 2002;360:1661–2.
13. Ritchie RD, Sackier JM, Hode JP. Incontinence rates after cutting seton treatment for anal fistula. Colorectal Dis. 2009;11:564–71.
14. Fazio VW. Complex anal fistulae. Gastroenterol Clin North Am. 1987;16:93–114.
15. Kodner IJ, Mazor A, Shemesh GI, et al. Endorectal advancement flap repair of rectovaginal and other complicated anorectal fistulas. Surgery. 1993;114:682–90.
16. Sonoda T, Hull T, Piedmonte MR, Fazio VW. Outcomes of primary repair of anorectal and rectovaginal fistulas using the endorectal advancement flap. Dis Colon Rectum. 2002;45:1622–8.
17. Cintron JR, Park JJ, Orsay CP, et al. Repair of fistula-in-ano using autologous fibrin tissue adhesive. Dis Colon Rectum. 1999;42:607–13.
18. Patrij L, Kooman B, Mortina CM, et al. Fibrin glue-antibiotic mixture in the treatment of anal fistulae:experience with 69 cases. Dig Surg. 2000;17:77–80.
19. Cintron JR, Park JJ, Orsay CP, et al. Repair of fistulas –in-ano using fibrin adhesive. Long term follow up. Dis Colon Rectum. 2000;43:944–50.
20. Buchanan GN, Bartram CI, Phillips RKS, et al. Efficacy of fibrin sealant in the management of complex anal fistulas. A prospective trial. Dis Colon Rectum. 2003;46:1167–74.
21. You SY, Mizrahi N, Zmora O, et al. The role of endoanal ultrasound as a predictive factor in endoanal advancement flap surgery (abstract). Colorectal Dis. 2001;3(Suppl):76.
22. Lindsey I, Smilgen-Humphreys MM, Cunningham C, et al. Randomized controlled trial of fibrin glue vs conventional treatment for anal fistula. Dis Colon Rectum. 2002;45:1608–15.
23. Johnson EK, Gaw JU, Armstrong DN. Efficacy of anal fistula plug vs fibrin glue in closure of anorectal fistulas. Dis Colon Rectum. 2006;49:371–6.
24. Garg P, Song J, Stat ABM. The efficacy of anal fistula plug in fistula-in-ano: a systematic review. Colorectal Dis. 2010;12(10): 965–70.
25. Rojanasakul A. LIFT procedure: a simplified technique for fistula-in-ano. Tech Coloproctol. 2009;131:237–40.
26. Moloo H, Goldberg SM. Novel correction of intersphincteric perianal fistulas preserves anal sphincter. Presented at the American College of Surgeons, San Francisco; Oct 2008.
27. Kronberg O. To lay open or excise a fistula-in-ano. Br J Surg. 1985;72:970.
28. Nelson RL, Cintron J, Abcarian H. Dermal- island flap anoplasty for transsphincteric fistula-in-ano: assessment of treatment failures. Dis Colon Rectum. 2000;43:681–4.
29. Van Tets WF, Kuijpers HC. Continence disorders after anal fistulotomy. Dis Colon Rectum. 1994;37:1194–7.
30. Marks CG, Ritchie JK. Anal fistulas at St. Mark's Hospital. Br J Surg. 1977;64:84–91.
31. Vasilevsky CA, Gordon PH. Results of treatment of fistula-in-ano. Dis Colon Rectum. 1985;28:225–31.
32. Sangwan YP, Rosen L, Riether RD, et al. Is simple fistula-in-ano simple? Dis Colon Rectum. 1994;37:885–9.
33. Garcia-Aguilar JC, Belmonte C, Wong WD, et al. Surgical treatment of fistula-in-ano. Factors associated with recurrence and incontinence. Dis Colon Rectum. 1996;39:723–9.
34. Mylonakis E, Katsios C, Godevenos D, et al. Quality of life of patients after surgical treatment of anal fistula; the role of anal manometry. Colorectal Dis. 2001;3:417–21.
35. Malouf AJ, Buchanan GN, Carapeti A, et al. A prospective audit of fistula-in-ano at St. Mark's Hospital. Colorectal Dis. 2002;4:13–9.
36. Westerterp M, Volkers NA, Poolman RW, van Tets WF. Anal fistulotomy between Skylla and Charybdis. Colorectal Dis. 2003;5:549–55.
37. Pearl RK, Andrews JR, Orsay CP, et al. Role of the seton in the management of anorectal fistulas. Dis Colon Rectum. 1993;36:573–9.
38. Ramanujam PS, Prasad ML, Abcarian H. The role of seton in fistulotomy of the anus. Surg Gynecol Obstet. 1983;157:419–22.
39. Williams JG, Macleod CAH, Goldberg SM. Seton treatment of high anal fistula. Br J Surg. 1991;78:1159–61.
40. Parks AG, Stitz RW. The treatment of high fistula-in-ano. Dis Colon Rectum. 1976;19:487–99.
41. Schouten WR, Zimmerman DD, Briel JW, Briel JW. Transanal advancement flap repair of transsphincteric fistulas. Dis Colon Rectum. 1999;42:1419–23.
42. Mizrahi N, Wexner SD, Zmora O, et al. Endorectal advancement flap: are there predictors of failure? Dis Colon Rectum. 2002;45:1616–21.
43. Wang JY, Garcia-Aguilar J, Sternberg JA. Treatment of transsphincteric anal fistulas. Are fistula plugs an acceptable alternative. Dis Colon Rectum. 2009;52:692–7.
44. Roig JV, Jordan J, Garcia-Armengol J. Changes in anorectal morphologic and functional parameters after fistula-in-ano surgery. Dis Colon Rectum. 2009;52:1462–9.
45. Soew-Choen F, Phillips RKS. Insights gained from the management of problematical anal fistulae at St. Mark's Hospital, 1984-88. Br J Surg. 1991;78:539–41.
46. Lunniss PJ, Sheffield JP, Talbot IC, et al. Persistence of idiopathic anal fistula may be related to epithelialization. Br J Surg. 1995;82:32–3.
47. Lewis P, Bartolo DCC. Treatment of trans-sphincteric fistulae by full thickness anorectal advancement flaps. Br J Surg. 1990;77:1187–9.
48. Williams JG, Rothenberger DA, Nemer FD, Goldberg SM. Fistula-in-ano in Crohn's disease. Results of aggressive surgical treatment. Dis Colon Rectum. 1991;34:378–84.
49. Schwartz DA, Pemberton JH, Sandborn WJ. Diagnosis and treatment of perianal fistulas in Crohn's disease. Ann Intern Med. 2001;135:906–18.
50. Jenss H, Starlinger M, Skaleij M. Magnetic resonance imaging in perianal Crohn's disease. Lancet. 1992;340:1286.

51. Levien DH, Surrell J, Mazier WP. Surgical treatment of anorectal fistula in patients with Crohn's disease. Surg Gynecol Obstet. 1989;169:133–6.
52. White RA, Eisenstat TE, Rubin RJ, Salvati EP. Seton management of complex anorectal fistulas in patients with Crohn's disease. Dis Colon Rectum. 1990;33:587–9.
53. Jones OJ, Fazio VW, Jagelman DG. The use of transanal rectal advancement flaps in the management of fistulas involving the anorectic. Dis Colon Rectum. 1987;30:919–23.
54. Joo JS, Weiss EG, Nogueras JJ, Wexner SD. Endorectal advancement flap in perianal Crohn's disease. Am Surg. 1998;64:147–50.
55. Savafi A, Gottesman L, Dailey TH. Anorectal surgery in the HIV+patient: update. Dis Colon Rectum. 1991;34:299–304.
56. Consten CJ, Siors FJM, Noten HJ, et al. Anorectal surgery in human immunodeficiency virus-infected patients. Dis Colon Rectum. 1995;38:1169–75.
57. Aleali M, Gottesman L. Anorectal disease in HIV-positive patients. Clin Colon Rectal Surg. 2001;14:265–73.
58. Blumberg JM, Lesser T, Tran VQ. Management of rectal injuries sustained during laparoscopic radical prostatectomy. Urology. 2009;73:163–6.
59. Thompson IM, Marx AC. Conservative therapy of rectourethral fistula: five-year follow up. Urology. 1990;6:533–6.
60. Zmora O, Potenti FM, Wexner SD, et al. Gracilis muscle transposition for iatrogenic rectourethral fistula. Ann Surg. 2003;237:483–7.
61. Parks AG, Motson RW. Peranal repair of rectoprostatic fistula. Br J Surg. 1983;70:725–6.
62. Garofalo TE, Delaney CP, Jones SM, et al. Rectal advancement flap repair of rectourethral fistula. A 20-year experience. Dis Colon Rectum. 2003;46:762–9.
63. Prasad ML, Nelson R, Hambrick E, Abcarian H. York Mason procedure for repair of postoperative rectoprostatic urethral fistula. Dis Colon Rectum. 1983;26:716–20.
64. Wilbert DM, Buess G, Bichler K-H. Combined endoscopic closure of rectourethral fistula. J Urol. 1996;155:256–8.

Anal Intraepithelial Neoplasia (AIN)/High-Grade Squamous Intraepithelial Lesion (HSIL)

22

Mark Lane Welton

Key Points

- Anal cancer can be prevented with treatment of HSIL.
- Anal cancer develops at higher rates in immunocompromised patients.
- Exact localization of lesions relative to accepted standardized landmarks is critical to improved understanding of squamous cell cancers of the anal and perianal regions.

Introduction and Controversy

Key Concept: While controversy regarding the definition, prognosis, method of diagnosis, surveillance, and treatment for AIN/HSIL exists, there is no doubt that the disparity that is present in its current management needs to be remedied.

Colorectal cancer incidence is decreasing while anal cancer is increasing in prevalence [1, 2]. Why? Is it improved healthy eating habits in Western cultures? This seems unlikely given the explosion of obesity and morbid obesity in Western Europe and the United States. Is it rather that colorectal surgeons, gastroenterologists, and most primary care physicians accept that early detection and endoscopic removal of polyps decreases the rate of colorectal cancer despite the lack of prospective randomized controlled trials to substantiate this theory? No one definitively asked the question "can we truly differentiate better which polyp will progress and which ones won't," although we know they don't all have the same biologic risk. We "know" they all need to be removed. Not removing polyps that technically could be removed would likely be considered below standard of care even though removal is associated with a finite bleeding and perforation rate and their associated morbidity and mortality. Despite these risks, no surgeon reading this chapter would suggest observation of a polyp in an otherwise healthy patient.

M.L. Welton, MD, MHCM, FACS, FASCRS
Department of Colon and Rectal Surgery,
Stanford University School of Medicine, Stanford Hospital and Clinics, 300 Pasteur Dr, Stanford, CA 94304, USA
e-mail: mwelton@stanford.edu

Defining AIN/HSIL

The conversation around the management of anal intraepithelial neoplasia (AIN heretofore referred to as HSIL) is raucous, and the data supporting clinical management is confusing, conflicting, and unclear [3]. And, as in the case of colonoscopy, the more you "know," the less certain you become in your knowledge. For instance, with regard to colonoscopy recommendations, should women at average risk be screened 10 years later than men for colorectal polyps? Should African-American men be screened earlier than average-risk patients? Data supports both these recommendations, and yet our practices are slow to shift, in part because of concerns about messaging and in part because individual and group practice behaviors are slow to change [4].

The challenge in changing practice behaviors regarding cancers of the anus and perianus and their precursor lesions may be attributed somewhat to the low prevalence of anal cancer, poor definitions of what constitutes an anal cancer, along with a reluctance of some to adopt newer treatment options such as high-resolution anoscopy (HRA). Regarding the former, I would agree that the low prevalence of anal cancers makes it difficult to develop a large enough experience to test hypotheses and make recommendations [1]. There is also no question that the definition of what really constitutes "anal" is confusing, even to experienced providers. For many it is "down there" or "near the rectum," and a skilled informative exam is often deferred. Treatment is based on being down there and the exact location of the lesion cannot be reconstructed from records blurring not

S.R. Steele et al. (eds.), *Complexities in Colorectal Surgery*,
DOI 10.1007/978-1-4614-9022-7_22, © Springer Science+Business Media New York 2014

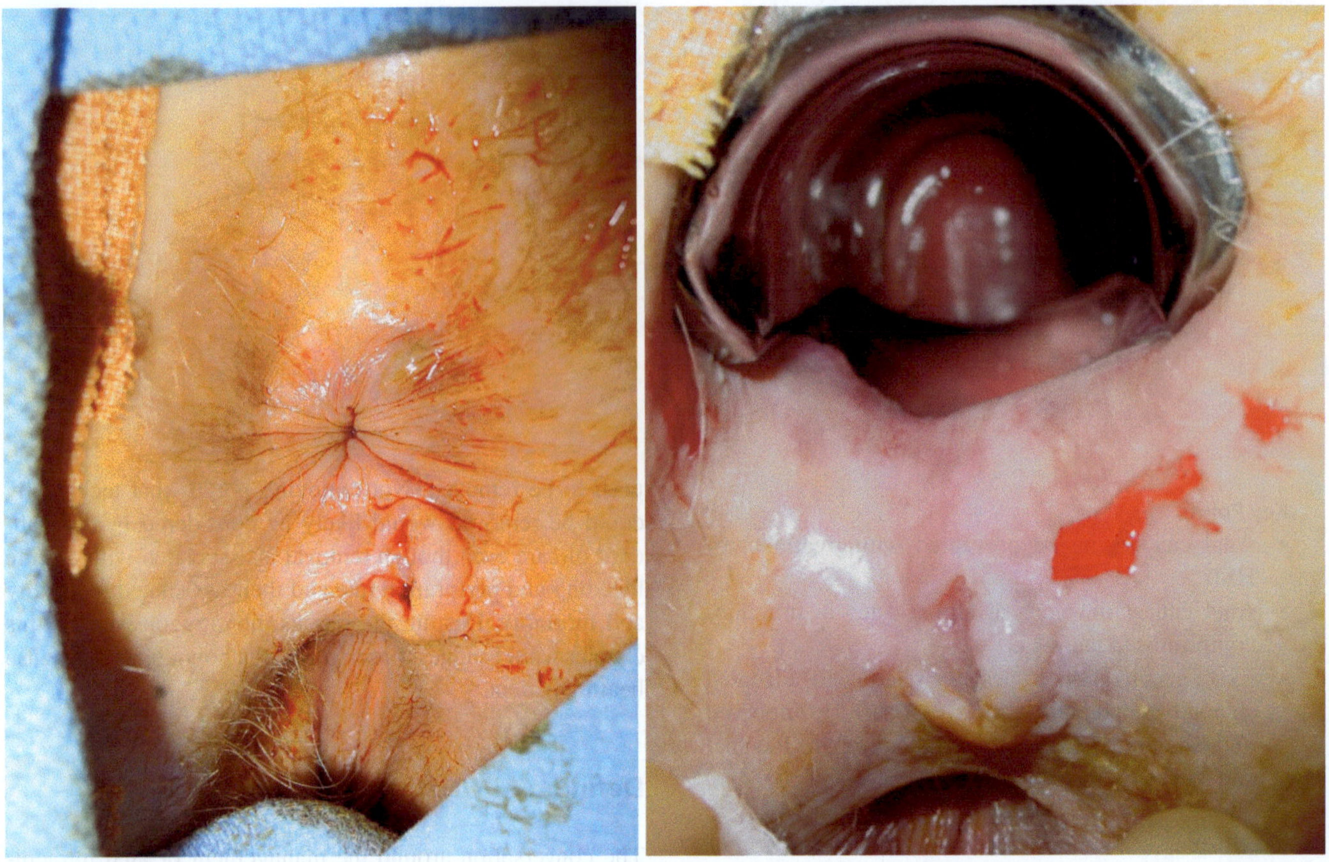

Fig. 22.1 Photograph of a lesion in a patient who sought a second opinion day before starting chemoradiation therapy for an anal cancer. I did not feel the lesion was an anal canal lesion. It was a perianal lesion and it was locally excised. Gynecological oncologists would consider this lesion vulvar. The patient is disease-free 12 years later

only the boundaries of anal and perianal (previously referred to as anal margin) lesions but also the data upon which recommendations and guidelines are based.

Further complicating the definition issue, the gynecological and colorectal terminologies overlap [5]. Gynecologists define the posterior limit of the vulva as the anus. This includes a broad swath of tissue that colorectal surgeons consider perineum and perianal. Lesions in this disputed region treated by a colorectal surgeon might simply be locally excised, whereas a gynecologist might treat the exact same lesion with a skinning vulvectomy and node dissection. Thus, experts in both fields familiar with "their" landmarks might be quite comfortable with the definition of the lesion and associated standard of care treatment plans, and yet they are radically different (Fig. 22.1).

Lack of Adoption

Finally, there has been a reluctance to learn HRA, a technique that allows for early detection and treatment of presumed premalignant lesions [6–8]. The premalignant lesions, HSIL, can be seen under direct visualization with either a colposcope or an operating microscope when the anal canal and distal rectal mucosa are treated with acetic acid. The technique is simple, can be done in the office or operating room, and uses equipment available in the operating room and in some offices. More importantly, this has been shown to decrease rates of progression to anal cancer in high-risk patients compared to historical controls of progression in average-risk patients and patients of undeclared risk [9–12]. And yet, the technique has not been widely adopted, with many citing a lack of evidence that HSIL progresses to cancer and concerns regarding the inability to accurately determine which patients need to be treated versus those that might otherwise be observed. Unfortunately for nonbelievers and more importantly HSIL patients, we now have data that untreated HSIL progresses to anal cancer [13].

The lack of adoption of HRA as a means for treating HSIL and preventing anal cancer raises the question as to why it hasn't been more broadly accepted? During the time that HRA has been advocated but not adopted by most, laparoscopic colectomy was adopted as the standard of care, despite confounding variables that make it difficult to attribute the benefits claimed for laparoscopy to laparoscopy [14–17].

Concomitant with the widespread take off of minimally invasive colectomy, we witnessed the institution of care pathways that feed patients earlier, remove urinary catheters earlier, manage pain differently, and set expectations of an earlier discharge. This has led to shorter lengths of stay and earlier return to work in both open and laparoscopic procedures [14–18]. Currently, robotic surgery and single-incision surgery are being advocated and advanced similarly despite absence of trials proving benefit [19].

The argument that we shouldn't treat anal HSIL because we don't know which lesion will progress to anal cancer, or because it is a "field defect" that is therefore untreatable and the cancer will develop somewhere else, is inconsistent with the rest of much of our colorectal and medical practice patterns, in general. We treat esophageal dysplasia without knowing which region will progress to cancer. Similarly we treat cervical dysplasia, bile duct dysplasia, and colonic dysplasia with procedures that are high risk and highly morbid. These are all diseases with a "field defect" like that seen in anal dysplasia. In all of these diseases, we currently lack the knowledge that would allow us to predict who will progress and yet we treat and in many cases, aggressively. For some reason, HSIL remains different.

Many arguments are advanced for this disparity. First, HRA is not well reimbursed and we presently only have a T, or trial code. Second, many surgeons report it is a painful procedure [20]. Although the latter may be valid, surgeons routinely perform hemorrhoidectomies, a procedure with a very similar, if not worse, postoperative pain profile. Third, many cite a lack of data to support that HRA can prevent cancer or that HSIL actually progresses to cancer. Papers from our institution and others refute this claim [9, 12, 13]. Additionally, the same surgeons who demand evidence prior to accepting HRA have adopted new technologies (i.e., PPH) with potentially more severe associated risks and significant complications without clinical trials supporting proven short- or long-term benefit. Finally and most troubling to me is the observation that adoption of laparoscopic surgery, single-incision surgery, robotic surgery, PPH, and other "new" interventions was driven in large part by industry and there is no industry driving HRA. Though this may be simple coincidence, the observation remains somewhat concerning.

HSIL and Anal Cancer: The Problem

Key Concept: Understanding the terminology along with proper documentation of the lesions and their locations is the first step in ensuring we have accurate data on the natural history of HSIL involving the various regions of the perianus.

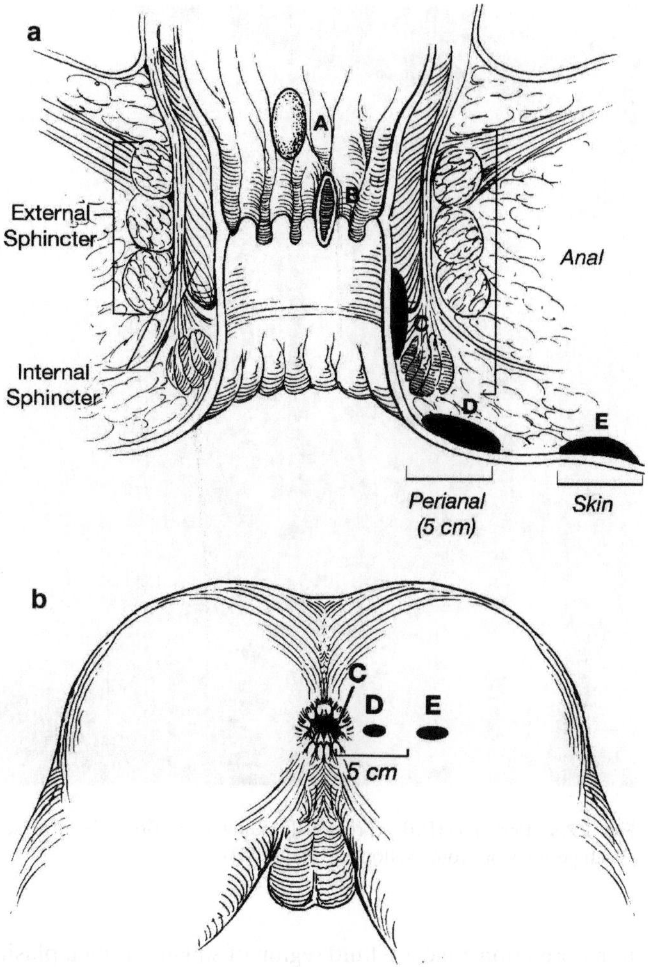

Fig. 22.2 (**a**, **b**) Classification scheme for defining lesions as anal or perianal that does not rely on relationship to dentate line. Tumors *A*, *B*, and *C* represent *anal* lesions that are not visible or are incompletely visible while gentle traction is placed on the buttocks. Tumor *D* is a perianal tumor because it is completely visible with gentle traction on the buttocks, and lesion *E* is a skin cancer (With permission from Welton and Raju [45])

There is no doubt that anal cancer is increasing in both genders and that it is increasing most rapidly in men [1, 21, 22]. Major challenges facing clinicians treating patients with anal and perianal HSIL and cancer are lack of clear terminology and natural history. The first challenge lies in defining anus and perianus. This issue has been addressed by adopting terminology that all clinicians can agree upon without reference to poorly understood specific landmarks. Thus, an *anal cancer* is defined as a squamous cell carcinoma that may *not* be seen at all or in its entirety while gentle traction is placed on the buttocks [23]. In contrast, a *perianal cancer* is a squamous cell carcinoma within 5 cm of the anus that *is completely visualized* while gentle traction is placed on the buttocks (Fig. 22.2). The *transformation zone* was introduced because many clinicians were confused by squamous cell carcinomas occurring in the distal rectal mucosa. The

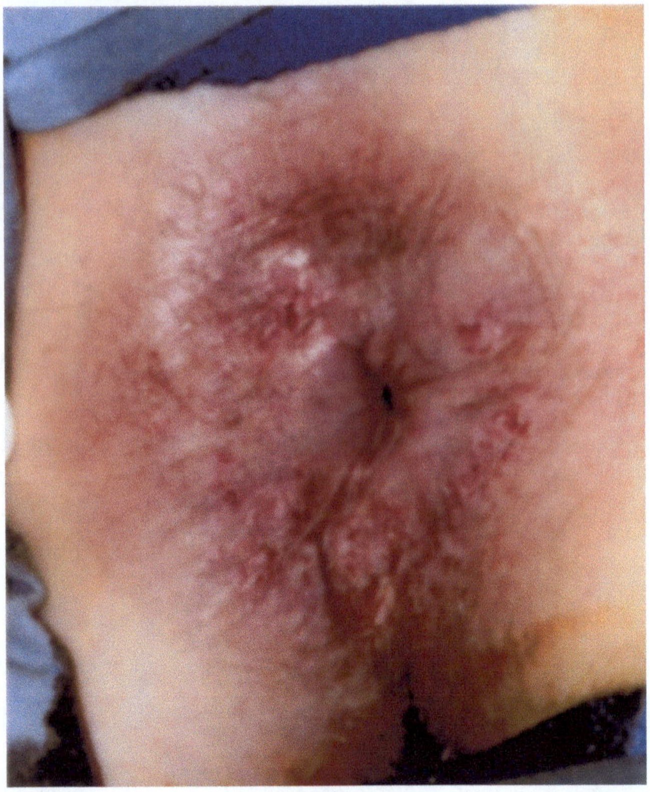

Fig. 22.3 Perianal HSIL (previously known as Bowen's disease) (With permission from Welton and Raju [45])

transformation zone is a fluid region of squamous metaplasia occurring 0–10 cm proximal to the dentate line where squamous metaplasia is commonly found. The metaplastic tissue is at particular risk for HPV infection.

A first step in understanding the natural history of anal and perianal cancers, and their precursor lesions, is an accurate reporting of exactly where the lesion was found. The current literature often confuses the two regions, leading to uncertainty as to how best to approach premalignant lesions in either zone. This confusion is evident while trying to reconcile the recommendations to treat Bowen's disease and observe HSIL [10, 24, 25]. Why would the recommendation be to treat patients with "Bowen's disease" with a highly morbid procedure – punch biopsies, frozen section-directed wide local excision, and flap reconstruction with proximal diversion if the recommendation was to observe HSIL of the distal rectal mucosa (Fig. 22.3)? We currently lack any data to support they are biologically different [26]. If the argument is that because of the field defect, we don't know which lesion will progress, then observation of a perianal skin lesion is much less risky and morbid as small perianal cancers can be easily identified and locally excised. In contrast, squamous cell carcinomas arising in the distal rectal mucosa are difficult to identify early, and all but the smallest and most superficial are treated with chemoradiation therapy. Similarly the argument to observe distal rectal and anal mucosal lesions because "the natural history of HSIL" is unclear fails to hold up to scrutiny. The natural history of perianal "Bowen's disease" is also unclear. Even with wide local excision, patients develop recurrent HSIL and cancer. This disparity in treatment recommendations for similar disease processes highlights our lack of understanding. Due to the confusion around histologic terminology for lower anogenital intraepithelial lesions involving the cervix, vagina, vulva, penis, scrotum, anus, and perianal skin, the Lower Anogenital Standard Terminology conference was held in March of 2012. This was a large multidisciplinary conference involving pathologists, gynecologists, infectious disease specialists, urologists, colorectal surgeons, and others in an effort to clarify and standardize terminology. The results of the consensus conference were published in June 2012 [3] and the recommendations for anal intraepithelial neoplasia were:

1. Standardize terminology using the above anatomic definitions.
2. Standardize pathology reporting into two categories low-grade squamous intraepithelial lesion (LSIL) and high-grade squamous intraepithelial lesion (HSIL) with modifiers of AIN II and III as needed.
3. Report lesions as microinvasive if ≤ 3 mm of invasion seen on histologic evaluation of completely excised lesions that are less than 7 mm in size.
4. Consider local excision adequate treatment of microinvasive lesions.
5. Consider p16 IHC evaluation to distinguish precancer from precancer mimics such as immature squamous metaplasia.

By using standardized terms that refer to standardized pathologic findings of tissues taken from known locations, we may develop a more robust understanding of which lesions of the anus and perianus will progress to cancer. Currently, the lack of a clear understanding of the natural history of HSIL is erroneously used as an argument for nontreatment [24, 25]. On the contrary, the natural history of untreated Bowen's disease is also unclear, and yet radical excision has been the standard treatment for a long time. Yet, despite this aggressive approach, some lesions still progress to cancer [10], just as some untreated HSIL will progress to cancer [9, 24, 25]. In a recent review, it was noted that progression rates appear to be lower in the anus than in the cervix [27]. Yet in the cervix, the natural history data looks at progression rates over 30 years, something we don't have for lesions of the perianus. Further, the natural history of untreated HSIL of the cervix and vulva suggests 30–50 % will progress to cancer over 30 years [28]. Looked at the other way, this means that 50–70 % *won't* progress to cancer over thirty years. As in the anus and perianus, it is undefined which gynecologic lesions will progress (and when), and yet there is uniform agreement to treat HSIL of the cervix, vagina, and vulva. I am not arguing that we shouldn't treat HSIL of the cervix. The huge drop in cervical cancers after the advent of cervical Pap smears and directed ablation is a modern medical success story. I am simply arguing for consistency in medical practice. Unfortunately, we now have clear documentation untreated anal HSIL progressing to cancer vacating the lack of data and progression argument [13].

Finally, if we can eventually distinguish anal and perianal cancers from premalignant lesions and each other, we may be able to address a suggestion from the gynecological literature regarding a possible difference between cervical and vulvar biology. In this paradigm, just as vulvar lesions are less aggressive than cervical, perianal squamous cell carcinomas may prove to have a less aggressive biology than those of the anal canal [21]. If this held true, perhaps this could lead to varying treatment recommendations based on the lesion location and inherent differences in rates of progression among them. Unfortunately, whether these differences exist, and if they do, whether they are due to differences in blood supply, lymphatic drainage, exposure to trauma, or immunologic differences in different types of squamous epithelia need to be more clearly elucidated. While we do know that risk factors for developing anal HSIL include HIV, HPV, anoreceptive intercourse, more than five anal sex partners, use of illicit drugs, older age at first anoreceptive act, infection with high number of HPV types, smoking, multiple partners, and a history of cervical dysplasia or cervical cancer, we lack accurate information on how these factors meld together to lead some lesions progressing while others do not [21, 29]. Furthermore, we don't know exactly why someone with no risk factors or high-risk behaviors may present with aggressive disease. Hopefully, going forward, more accurate and uniform documentation will result in answers to these questions.

Treatment

Key Concept: You cannot apply one set of rules uniformly across all risks categories. While you should follow general principles, treat each patient individually taking into account their risk profile, disease burden, treatment history, and your level of concern with the lesions present.

For those not familiar with managing this disease, it should be stated that treatment of anal and perianal HSIL is not technically challenging. In fact, often the only technically challenging aspect of the treatment is adequate visualization of the lesions. This skill set has been mastered by gynecologists, family practitioners, internist, oncologists, nurse practitioners, and some general and colorectal surgeons, and you can master it as well. Courses in how to perform HRA are taught at least twice each year by the American Society for Colposcopy and Cervical Pathology (ASCCP).

High-Resolution Anoscopy (HRA): Initial Examination and Technique

Briefly, HRA involves the magnified visualization of the distal rectal mucosa, anal mucosa, and perianal skin through an operative microscope or colposcope after pretreatment with 3 % acetic acid. HSIL will stand out against the background of acetowhitening as a distinct vascular pattern within the acetowhitened mucosa or skin. The vessel changes are characteristic of HSIL regardless of underlying tissue type – cervix, distal rectal mucosa, or anus (Fig. 22.4). These lesions are biopsied as needed and targeted for focal destruction while sparing the surrounding normal mucosa. In contrast to popular belief, when lesions in the insensate distal rectal mucosa are treated, the patient may experience essentially no postoperative pain. Treated lesions of the anus and perianus that involve the sensate anal mucosa and perianal skin result in postoperative pain similar to hemorrhoidectomies and other benign anorectal conditions that colorectal surgeons commonly treat.

I prefer the operating room for the initial examination and treatment as well as for re-treatment of extensive disease, disease overlying engorged hemorrhoidal cushions, and for disease complicating, or complicated by, other benign anorectal diseases [30]. The patient is treated in the prone jackknife position with the buttocks taped apart. Anesthesia is MAC local with 0.25 % Marcaine in the subcutaneous tissue and 0.5 % Marcaine in the sphincters for an anal block. This allows for excellent visualization of most lesions. A thorough digital rectal examination is carried out focusing on subtle changes in the skin, mucosa, and submucosa of the perianus and distal rectum. This initial exam often focuses my subsequent visual inspection. I examine the perianal skin looking for any hyperpigmentation, erythema, elevation, or scaling consistent with a lesion. I think conduct a routine anoscopy with a Hill Ferguson anoscope, visualizing the distal rectal mucosa and anal mucosa. Next, I place one acetic acid soaked raytec in the anal canal and distal rectum. I place another one over the anus and perianus. I position the operative microscope over the anus and begin with a thorough evaluation of the perianal skin, noting location of worrisome lesion for subsequent biopsy and destruction. I then thoroughly evaluate the anal mucosa and distal rectal mucosa in a circumferential fashion taking care to visualize any abnormalities palpated on digital rectal examination. All lesions concerning for HSIL are biopsied treated with needle tip electrocautery taking care to avoid burning deeply by moving the cautery tip quickly smoothly across the surface of the

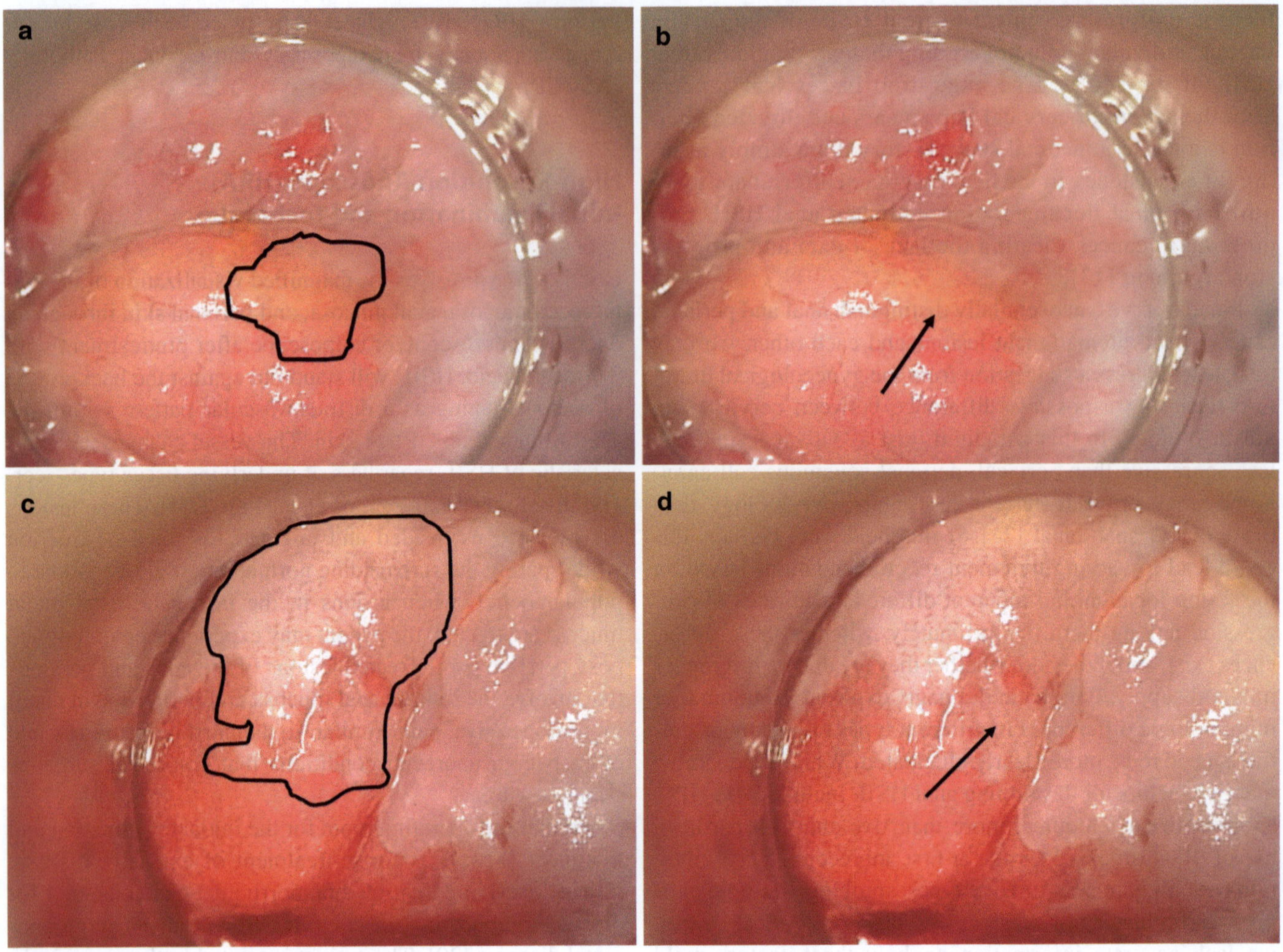

Fig. 22.4 High-resolution anoscopy images of LSIL and HSIL after the application of acetic acid. Biopsies of visualized lesions confirmed HRA appearances, and region biopsied is indicated with *arrows* in images (**b**) and (**d**). Panels (**a**) and (**b**) demonstrate anal LSIL in the distal rectal mucosa with subtle punctate vessel changes. The geography of the lesion is emphasized in the left frame with a *black border*. (**c, d**) Distal rectal mucosa where HSIL is visible. The *left* image has the lesion highlighted with a *black border* focusing the reader on the serpiginous, cerebriform vessels and the outline of the entire lesion. The *right* image demonstrates the mosaic pattern created by blood vessels in an acetowhite background (With permission from Welton and Raju [45])

lesion. If the underlying hemorrhoidal tissues are disrupted, this is generally controlled without difficulty using cautery alone. Very rarely I have had to control hemorrhoidal hemorrhage with a chromic catgut ligature placed at the apex of a hemorrhoidal cushion. Overall, I prefer the operating room, at least initially, to office-based therapies as I feel this allows for better visualization and determination of extent of disease. I have often found disease along the hemorrhoidal column that would not have been identified without the relaxation and visualization provided by MAC local. The relaxation of the sphincters allows for flattening of the distal rectal mucosa and improved lesion detection. Without this improved visualization, I believe lesions are missed and this results in the false impression that lesions have "returned" when in fact the lesion is persistent and was never adequately addressed in the first place.

Dealing with Recurrence

When lesions do recur, they may be treated in the office with trichloroacetic acid or infrared coagulation (IRC). As noted above, some recurrences are best treated in the operating room. More importantly, we, and others, have experienced excellent control of HSIL and minimal progression to cancer with this approach [6, 8, 9, 12].

Issues around HRA and cautery destruction that have discouraged more widespread adoption are the incorrect belief that all lesions recur (so why treat them in the first place and risk complications like nonhealing wounds or stenosis) and the patients experience significant pain (see above for this myth buster). Furthermore, reimbursement is poor, especially given the time and effort required to develop and hone the new skill set necessary to visualize and treat these lesions.

Our group and others have shown that despite initial recurrences, HSIL can be cleared in ~80 % of patients and progression to cancer can be significantly diminished (Pineda and Goldstone) [6, 8, 9, 12, 20]. This is done through targeted destruction in the operating room with follow-up destruction in clinic as needed. Admittedly, the patients do experience postoperative pain. Yet, this can be largely controlled with sitz baths (in a bathtub filled to the chest), LMX-5 % topical lidocaine cream, and a narcotic agent. I have found that the warm bath and LMX-5 % are the most effective methods of pain relief.

Coding

Reimbursement continues to be a challenge with no specific code available for the diagnosis and treatment of anal dysplasia. A trial code is available for HRA itself, but since I do this in the operating, I am not using that code alone. I use the codes for diagnostic anoscopy and destruction of condylomata – extensive. When I am destroying HSIL in the distal rectal mucosa, I am coding for transanal destruction of rectal neoplasia. I also note use of the operative microscope, but this is reportedly routinely included in diagnostic anoscopy.

Follow-Up

Follow-up anal cytology is a critical component of a successful program. The timing of the cytologic sampling is undefined and is even changing in the gynecology literature. My current practice is to see patients back 1 month after surgery to review pathology and see how they are progressing. If they were found to have HSIL and I felt I was able to completely clear the disease, I see them back in 6 months for a digital rectal exam and anoscopy in the office. If they are not involved in high-risk behaviors where I am concerned for persistence, inoculation or re-inoculation, I recommend a follow-up anal cytology at 1 year after treatment. If they are at high risk or continue to engage in high-risk behaviors, I recommend follow-up anal cytology and HRA at 1 year. If the patient is immunosuppressed from chronic disease or medication to control chronic illness, then more frequent follow-up (i.e., 3–6 months) is typically warranted with anal exams, anal cytology, and HRA as needed. These decisions are all informed by the patient's particular risk factors including the burden of disease, the severity and type of their immune-compromised state, the pace of their disease, the adequacy of my evaluation, and complicating associated anal pathology. Otherwise, if there was a normal examination, I recommend that surveillance be extended to every other year. Importantly, if I was unable to clear the disease at the first treatment, I will bring them back to the operating room in 3 months to complete treatment and then proceed with follow-up as detailed above.

Topical Agents

I have no personal experience with the dispensing of topical agents such as 5-FU and imiquimod. I have been referred to patients previously treated with imiquimod and have seen some remarkable responses. One memorable patient had documented circumferential HSIL, and we were unable to get him into the OR for 4 months. At surgery there was no documentable disease. Anecdotally, the vast majority of my patients have not experienced such an impressive response. This less favorable, and likely more generalizable, impression is supported in the literature; though, there certainly are responders which leaves many to feel it is worth having in the armamentarium [31]. To define its role more clearly as an adjunct to surgery, a trial with standardized surgical intervention would be necessary.

An initial study of topical 5-FU reported some early success, with 6 of the 11 patients experiencing a reduction of dysplasia on HRA [32]. Unfortunately almost ¾ of the patients experienced mild-to-moderate perianal pain and irritation. The benefits of this treatment approach over cautery destruction remain to be elucidated. I can envision a scenario where a topical medication such as 5-FU is added to a follow-up protocol following initial cautery destruction of extensive disease to minimize local recurrences. Yet, its use in conjunction with or as a replacement of TCA or IRC has not been explored.

Infrared Coagulation

Infrared coagulation (IRC) has proven to be an effective tool in the outpatient setting and has demonstrated ease of use in the hands of surgeons and primary care physicians alike [8, 12, 33]. IRC is used in this scenario as an office-based ablative device and has been typically touted to be associated with less pain compared to other destructive techniques. I have not found this to be true. Rather, I have found the claims to be difficult to substantiate once an adequate volume of experience is acquired. Destroying tissue in the anorectum generates pain no matter the technique. Managing the amount of tissue destruction and the depth of destruction is the most important operator-dependent factor. Managing patient expectations and providing adequate education and postoperative pain management instructions improves patient satisfaction. Like all techniques used to treat high-volume disease in high-risk patients, IRC has a reputation for high recurrence rates, but retreatment can eradicate HSIL [8, 12]. Recurrences may more accurately be characterized as persistence after an initial staged treatment that is appropriately focused on maintaining function while preventing cancer.

Vaccination

The advent of the quadrivalent vaccine has lent a new wrinkle to the discussion of both treatment as well as prevention and raises the specter that someday treatment of anal dysplasia and condylomata will be of historical interest only. Thus far, the vaccine has proven safe and effective in women, leading to decreased cervical infection and dysplasia rates [34–36]. Additionally, reports have demonstrated its safety and effectiveness in men in preventing anogenital HPV and external perianal condylomatous disease as well as preventing anal dysplasia in high-risk men who have sex with men (MSM) [37]. It also prevents HPV disease in HIV (+) children [38]. To date, vaccines have been largely untested in individuals over 26 years of age. Some have argued that they should be used even after exposure because the patient may not have been exposed to one of four subtypes in the quadrivalent vaccine and, therefore, would still receive benefit. I withhold a blanket recommendation and suggest it be discussed with each patient individually. My bias is it has no proven efficacy, and I tend not to recommend unless part of a trial.

Special Situations: The HIV (+) Patient

It is well known that HIV (+) men and women are at an increased risk for anal HSIL regardless of sexual practices [39, 40]. HIV positivity interferes with the response to the HPV, and persistent infection is more common. HIV (+) MSM are at the highest risk for development of anal cancer and appear to be at highest risk for progression of HSIL to cancer. HIV (−) men are at somewhat less risk but still significantly increased risk over the rest of the population [2]. Condylomatous disease may be a marker for more significant disease, as MSM have at least four serotypes present when tested. This data would support that HIV (+) and HIV (−) MSM should be evaluated with anal cytology and HRA. The initial cytology and HRA should be performed at an initial evaluation. The subsequent frequency of performing either or both tests is dictated by risk factors as outlined above.

Anal Cytology and Screening/ Surveillance Intervals

The frequency of anal cytology with or without HRA may be debated. More frequent anal Pap smears would seem to be indicated, while managing uncontrolled or previously untreated disease now under control much like more frequent colonoscopies are oftentimes recommended in patients with extensive polyps seen and treated on the first endoscopic examination. Once the anal dysplasia is cleared, again like colonic polyps or cervical dysplasia, the screening interval should be determined by the individual's risk factor assessment. We would not recommend the same colonoscopy frequency for a patient with a family cancer syndrome or a 20-year history of ulcerative colitis as we would for a patient with no risk factors. Likewise, HIV (+) MSM involved in high-risk behaviors warrant the most frequent evaluation, while a 20-year-old heterosexual with low-volume perianal condylomatous disease would warrant the least frequent surveillance, if any.

In the cervix, the benefit of Pap smears is actually found through the cumulative sensitivity of repeat testing. This is considered safe in large part due to the documented slow progression rate to cancer rates of 30–50 % in 30 years [28]. As stated, while the progression rate of anal HSIL to cancer is still undefined, it maybe be at a slower rate in the general population than the rate seen in the cervix and most likely varies significantly across patient populations with differing risk profiles [41]. The findings of higher than expected anal dysplasia rates in HIV (+) women and HIV (−) women suggests the progression rate is quite low (i.e., more remain in the dysplastic state without progressing to cancer) [42]. However, the incidence of anal cancer in MSM indicates that this group progresses at an alarming rate [21, 22] and should be screened accordingly. Further, very recent data would suggest an acceleration in both groups supporting the importance of close monitoring of this evolving topic.

While this may seem straightforward, in reality the addition of HRA to the monitoring protocol is equally problematic. If a provider has the ability to treat anal dysplasia in the office, then visualization in the office with HRA after an anal cytology might be beneficial. In those instances, if the provider noted a low volume of HSIL, he/she might biopsy and/or destroy the lesion at that visit. In other circumstances, the HSIL could be biopsied and treatment in the operating arranged. In yet other practice groups with low-risk individuals, with low-risk behaviors, where follow-up might not need to be as rigorous or in those practices where HRA is not available in the office, the cumulative sensitivity of anal cytology would seem to be acceptable. As with cervical disease, where an abnormal Pap smear is an indication for colposcopy, once the anal cytology is abnormal, the patient would need evaluation and treatment with HRA. We have documented progression to cancer in patients with known untreated HSIL, but we have not seen progression in patients under surveillance from completely normal Pap smears to cancer without interval abnormal Pap smears [9]. Therefore, in this practice setting, HRA may not be needed at all.

My bias is continued surveillance at an interval dictated by patient-risk factors appears indicated in MSM as is there does not appear to be a peak incidence of dysplasia at age 30 as is seen in women with cervical disease. Rather, in MSM with anal dysplasia, the disease evidence of HPV infection and dysplasia persists and incidence rates do not decrease raising the concern that this is associated with the continued increase in incidence of cancers seen in MSM [42].

Final Thoughts

Key Concept: While treatment recommendations may be variable, in general, HRA and targeted destruction of HSIL are effective means to control these lesions and minimize the chance of progression to malignancy.

A major challenge for those seeing patients with anal HSIL is who to treat. The management decisions are idiosyncratic and appear counterintuitive at times. For instance, low-risk patients with low-volume disease that is easily managed are often treated with ablative therapy, while high-risk patients with circumferential disease are observed. The argument supporting this decision is "we don't know the natural history of HSIL," "we don't know who will progress," and "if anal HSIL is so prevalent, then why don't we see more progress to cancer." I agree we don't know who will progress and do feel that the progression rate overall must be low. However, not knowing who will progress doesn't suggest we shouldn't treat. If this were the case, we shouldn't treat cervical dysplasia, colonic polyps, and ulcerative colitis with dysplasia, ductal carcinoma in situ, or Bowen's disease.

Take this scenario, for example. The traditional recommendations of many for the incidental finding of Bowen's disease in a hemorrhoidectomy specimen is reoperation with random biopsies and wide local excision of all disease based on intraoperative frozen sections [10]. One is left to ask, do we really know the natural history of untreated Bowen's disease? Is this more aggressive approach truly beneficial to the patient? I prefer to treat HSIL found incidentally after a hemorrhoidectomy in the operating room where I perform HRA and targeted destruction of all visualized disease, which is usually quite minimal. Furthermore, I do not feel compelled to enter an elderly but otherwise healthy 75-year-old patient successfully treated in this fashion into a surveillance program. Am I wrong not to follow these traditional recommendations? My own data suggest no, although this highlights our limitations of lacking high-level data to base decisions upon. The paper often cited for how we should treat Bowen's disease reports upon 47 patients [10]. The report out of my institution was based on 247 patients selected out of our patient population with circumferential disease – the worst-case scenario. In these patients, our progression rate, 1.2 %, was lower than reported in the literature for traditional treatment recommendations for Bowen's disease, which ranges from 2 to 6 % [43, 44].

Another common complaint is there is a lack of data to support HRA and targeted destruction. In reality, we now have multiple studies suggesting a lower rate of progression to cancer in patients who are treated with HRA and targeted destruction. Furthermore, we have data to support untreated HSIL progresses to cancer [9, 12, 13]. HRA with targeted treatment of HSIL is clearly an effective means to preventing progression to anal cancer in the patients who are at highest risk. If it works in these patients, it would seem that HRA and targeted destruction in lower-risk patients would be successful as well. Some of these patients are easy to get into the system as well. Women who are receiving anal Pap smears or Pap smears following appropriate guidelines would be easy to screen with anal cytology. Women have always had a higher rate of anal cancer than men, and therefore, the potential benefit seems clear. It would be easy to add an anal cytology to the surveillance plan.

Finally, it is interesting that many clinicians say "I don't do HRA, so I send them to someone who does" rather than learning how to perform HRA. Are those same physicians referring rectal cancers to centers with a robot or to surgeons who perform single-incision surgery? Or, as I believe is the case, are they learning this new technology? If so, where is the data for the benefit? Are they adopting technology before any long-term studies prove benefit? While I do believe patients should be referred to centers of excellence, I do not believe this to be the case for just HSIL and HRA. I do think it should apply equally to rectal cancers, colon cancers, inflammatory bowel disease, and complicated perianal diseases, but I do not hear physicians clamoring for this. Is the difference that industry is driving "the need" for robotic surgery and laparoscopic surgery and no driving industry exists for HRA? Is it the lack of billing codes that adequately reflect the increased training? While we may never know the answers to these latter questions, it is time that we, as providers caring for these patients, come full circle to learn the necessary skills to best manage this disease.

Summary Pearls

Anal cancer rates continue to increase and affect both men and women. HSIL, the precursor lesion, is readily identified with HRA. Lesions may be ablated with multiple agents – IRC, TCA, and electrocautery. Yes, pain will occur; however, the pain is equivalent to, or less than, that associated with a hemorrhoidectomy. You can easily learn HRA, and the tools necessary to practice HRA are readily available. The procedure can be performed in the office for low-volume disease or as an outpatient procedure in an operating room for those with high-volume disease or associated anal pathology. Treatment with HRA-directed ablation and follow-up anal cytology, digital rectal exams, and HRA is an effective method of controlling HSIL and decreasing the progression rate to anal cancer. Colorectal surgeons and providers caring for these patients should be comfortable performing HRA and offer this treatment within their regular practice.

References

1. Siegel R, Naishadham D, Jemal A. Cancer statistics, 2012. CA Cancer J Clin. 2012;62(1):10–29. Epub 2012/01/13.
2. Silverberg MJ, Lau B, Justice AC, Engels E, Gill MJ, Goedert JJ, et al. Risk of anal cancer in HIV-infected and HIV-uninfected individuals in North America. Clin Infect Dis. 2012;54(7):1026–34.
3. Darragh TM, Colgan TJ, Cox JT, Heller DS, Henry MR, Luff RD, et al. The Lower Anogenital Squamous Terminology Standardization Project for HPV-Associated Lesions: background and consensus recommendations from the College of American Pathologists and the American Society for Colposcopy and Cervical Pathology. Arch Pathol Lab Med. 2012;136(10):1266–97. Epub 2012/06/30.
4. Ferlitsch M, Reinhart K, Pramhas S, Wiener C, Gal O, Bannert C, et al. Sex-specific prevalence of adenomas, advanced adenomas, and colorectal cancer in individuals undergoing screening colonoscopy. JAMA. 2011;306(12):1352–8. Epub 2011/09/29.
5. Edge SB, American Joint Committee on Cancer. AJCC cancer staging manual. 7th ed. New York: Springer; 2010. xiv, 648 p.
6. Pineda CE, Berry JM, Jay N, Palefsky JM, Welton ML. High resolution anoscopy in the planned staged treatment of anal squamous intraepithelial lesions in HIV-negative patients. J Gastrointest Surg. 2007;11(11):1410–5; discussion 5–6. Epub 2007/08/22.
7. Jay N, Berry JM, Hogeboom CJ, Holly EA, Darragh TM, Palefsky JM. Colposcopic appearance of anal squamous intraepithelial lesions: relationship to histopathology. Dis Colon Rectum. 1997;40(8):919–28. Epub 1997/08/01.
8. Goldstone SE, Hundert JS, Huyett JW. Infrared coagulator ablation of high-grade anal squamous intraepithelial lesions in HIV-negative males who have sex with males. Dis Colon Rectum. 2007;50(5):565–75. Epub 2007/03/24.
9. Pineda CE, Berry JM, Jay N, Palefsky JM, Welton ML. High-resolution anoscopy targeted surgical destruction of anal high-grade squamous intraepithelial lesions: a ten-year experience. Dis Colon Rectum. 2008;51(6):829–35; discussion 35–7. Epub 2008/03/26.
10. Marchesa P, Fazio VW, Oliart S, Goldblum JR, Lavery IC. Perianal Bowen's disease: a clinicopathologic study of 47 patients. Dis Colon Rectum. 1997;40(11):1286–93.
11. Marks DK, Goldstone SE. Electrocautery ablation of high-grade anal squamous intraepithelial lesions in HIV-negative and HIV-positive men who have sex with men. J Acquir Immune Defic Syndr. 2012;59(3):259–65. Epub 2011/12/03.
12. Goldstone RN, Goldstone AB, Russ J, Goldstone SE. Long-term follow-up of infrared coagulator ablation of anal high-grade dysplasia in men who have sex with men. Dis Colon Rectum. 2011;54(10):1284–92. Epub 2011/09/10.
13. Berry JM, Jay N, Cranston RD, Darragh TM, Holly EA, Welton ML, Palefsky JM. Progression of high-grade anal squamous intraepithelial lesions to invasive anal cancer among HIV-positive men who have sex with men. Int J Cancer. 2013. doi: 10.1002/ijc.28431. [Epub ahead of print].
14. van Bree SH, Vlug MS, Bemelman WA, Hollmann MW, Ubbink DT, Zwinderman AH, et al. Faster recovery of gastrointestinal transit after laparoscopy and fast-track care in patients undergoing colonic surgery. Gastroenterology. 2011;141(3):872–80.e1–4. Epub 2011/06/28.
15. Veenhof AA, Vlug MS, van der Pas MH, Sietses C, van der Peet DL, de Lange-de Klerk ES, et al. Surgical stress response and postoperative immune function after laparoscopy or open surgery with fast track or standard perioperative care: a randomized trial. Ann Surg. 2012;255(2):216–21. Epub 2012/01/14.
16. Wu FP, Sietses C, von Blomberg BM, van Leeuwen PA, Meijer S, Cuesta MA. Systemic and peritoneal inflammatory response after laparoscopic or conventional colon resection in cancer patients: a prospective, randomized trial. Dis Colon Rectum. 2003;46(2):147–55. Epub 2003/02/11.
17. Basse L, Jakobsen DH, Bardram L, Billesbolle P, Lund C, Mogensen T, et al. Functional recovery after open versus laparoscopic colonic resection: a randomized, blinded study. Ann Surg. 2005;241(3):416–23. Epub 2005/02/25.
18. Kehlet H, Wilmore DW. Evidence-based surgical care and the evolution of fast-track surgery. Ann Surg. 2008;248(2):189–98.
19. Tyler JA, Fox JP, Desai MM, Perry WB, Glasgow SC. Outcomes and costs associated with robotic colectomy in the minimally invasive era. Dis Colon Rectum. 2013;56(4):458–66.
20. Chang GJ, Berry JM, Jay N, Palefsky JM, Welton ML. Surgical treatment of high-grade anal squamous intraepithelial lesions: a prospective study. Dis Colon Rectum. 2002;45(4):453–8. Epub 2002/05/15.
21. Frisch M. On the etiology of anal squamous carcinoma. Dan Med Bull. 2002;49(3):194–209. Epub 2002/09/20.
22. Cress RD, Holly EA. Incidence of anal cancer in California: increased incidence among men in San Francisco, 1973–1999. Prev Med. 2003;36(5):555–60. Epub 2003/04/12.
23. American Society of Colon and Rectal Surgeons, Beck DE. The ASCRS textbook of colon and rectal surgery. 2nd ed. New York: Springer; 2011. xxiv, 946 p.
24. Devaraj B, Cosman BC. Expectant management of anal squamous dysplasia in patients with HIV. Dis Colon Rectum. 2006;49(1):36–40. Epub 2005/11/12.
25. Scholefield JH, Castle MT, Watson NF. Malignant transformation of high-grade anal intraepithelial neoplasia. Br J Surg. 2005;92(9):1133–6. Epub 2005/07/27.
26. Litle VR, Leavenworth JD, Darragh TM, Kosinski LA, Moore 2nd DH, Smith-McCune KK, et al. Angiogenesis, proliferation, and apoptosis in anal high-grade squamous intraepithelial lesions. Dis Colon Rectum. 2000;43(3):346–52.
27. Machalek DA, Poynten M, Jin F, Fairley CK, Farnsworth A, Garland SM, et al. Anal human papillomavirus infection and associated neoplastic lesions in men who have sex with men: a systematic review and meta-analysis. Lancet Oncol. 2012;13(5):487–500. Epub 2012/03/27.
28. McCredie MR, Sharples KJ, Paul C, Baranyai J, Medley G, Jones RW, et al. Natural history of cervical neoplasia and risk of invasive cancer in women with cervical intraepithelial neoplasia 3: a retrospective cohort study. Lancet Oncol. 2008;9(5):425–34. Epub 2008/04/15.
29. Chin-Hong PV, Vittinghoff E, Cranston RD, Browne L, Buchbinder S, Colfax G, et al. Age-related prevalence of anal cancer precursors in homosexual men: the EXPLORE study. J Natl Cancer Inst. 2005;97(12):896–905. Epub 2005/06/16.
30. Pineda CE, Berry JM, Welton ML. High resolution anoscopy and targeted treatment of high-grade squamous intraepithelial lesions. Dis Colon Rectum. 2006;49(1):126. Epub 2005/10/14.
31. Mahto M, Nathan M, O'Mahony C. More than a decade on: review of the use of imiquimod in lower anogenital intraepithelial neoplasia. Int J STD AIDS. 2010;21(1):8–16. Epub 2009/12/24.
32. Snyder SM, Siekas L, Aboulafia DM. Initial experience with topical fluorouracil for treatment of HIV-associated anal intraepithelial

neoplasia. J Int Assoc Physicians AIDS Care (Chic). 2011;10(2):83–8. Epub 2011/01/27.

33. Weis SE, Vecino I, Pogoda JM, Susa JS. Treatment of high-grade anal intraepithelial neoplasia with infrared coagulation in a primary care population of HIV-infected men and women. Dis Colon Rectum. 2012;55(12):1236–43. Epub 2012/11/09.
34. Villa LL, Costa RL, Petta CA, Andrade RP, Ault KA, Giuliano AR, et al. Prophylactic quadrivalent human papillomavirus (types 6, 11, 16, and 18) L1 virus-like particle vaccine in young women: a randomised double-blind placebo-controlled multicentre phase II efficacy trial. Lancet Oncol. 2005;6(5):271–8. Epub 2005/05/03.
35. Garland SM, Hernandez-Avila M, Wheeler CM, Perez G, Harper DM, Leodolter S, et al. Quadrivalent vaccine against human papillomavirus to prevent anogenital diseases. N Engl J Med. 2007;356(19):1928–43. Epub 2007/05/15.
36. FUTURE II STUDY GROUP. Quadrivalent vaccine against human papilloma virus to prevent high grade cervical lesions. N Engl J Med 2007;356(19):1915–27. Epub 2007/05/15.
37. Palefsky JM, Giuliano AR, Goldstone S, Moreira Jr ED, Aranda C, Jessen H, et al. HPV vaccine against anal HPV infection and anal intraepithelial neoplasia. N Engl J Med. 2011;365(17):1576–85.
38. Centers for Disease C, Prevention. Recommendations on the use of quadrivalent human papillomavirus vaccine in males—Advisory Committee on Immunization Practices (ACIP), 2011. MMWR Morb Mortal Wkly Rep. 2011;60(50):1705–8.
39. Weis SE, Vecino I, Pogoda JM, Susa JS, Nevoit J, Radaford D, et al. Prevalence of anal intraepithelial neoplasia defined by anal cytology screening and high-resolution anoscopy in a primary care population of HIV-infected men and women. Dis Colon Rectum. 2011;54(4):433–41. Epub 2011/03/09.
40. Piketty C, Darragh TM, Da Costa M, Bruneval P, Heard I, Kazatchkine MD, et al. High prevalence of anal human papillomavirus infection and anal cancer precursors among HIV-infected persons in the absence of anal intercourse. Ann Intern Med. 2003;138(6):453–9. Epub 2003/03/18.
41. Tatti S, Suzuki V, Fleider L, Maldonado V, Caruso R, Tinnirello ML. Anal intraepithelial lesions in women with human papillomavirus-related disease. J Low Genit Tract Dis. 2012;16(4):454–9. Epub 2012/09/13.
42. Moscicki AB, Schiffman M, Burchell A, Albero G, Giuliano AR, Goodman MT, et al. Updating the natural history of human papillomavirus and anogenital cancers. Vaccine. 2012;30 Suppl 5: F24–33.
43. Cleary RK, Schaldenbrand JD, Fowler JJ, Schuler JM, Lampman RM. Perianal Bowen's disease and anal intraepithelial neoplasia: review of the literature. Dis Colon Rectum. 1999;42(7):945–51.
44. Marfing TE, Abel ME, Gallagher DM. Perianal Bowen's disease and associated malignancies. Results of a survey. Dis Colon Rectum. 1987;30(10):782–5.
45. Welton ML, Raju NL. Anal cancer. In: Beck DE, Roberts PL, Saclarides TJ, Senagore AJ, Stamos MJ, Wexner SD, editors. The ASCRS textbook of colon and rectal surgery. 2nd ed. New York: Springer; 2011. p. 337–57.

Chronic Anal Pain

23

Richard P. Billingham and Amir L. Bastawrous

Key Points

- Causes of discomfort in the anal area are common and diverse.
- Chronic anal pain must be differentiated from more common acute causes of anal pain.
- Common acute causes of anal pain include thrombosed external hemorrhoids, anal fissure, and perianal abscess/fistula.
- Chronic anal pain is less common than the acute problems mentioned, but may be identified and treated with a careful, systematic approach.
- The broad differential diagnosis for chronic anal pain should include less common causes including pelvic floor dysfunction, neurogenic, infectious, and neoplastic conditions.

Introduction

Pain in the anal area is a common disorder. It is often of short duration and is brought to the attention of a physician or other healthcare provider relatively soon after onset in some patients. Others languish due to ignorance, anxiety, and embarrassment. Patients may often ignore the pain. The discomfort is particularly disturbing to patients because the anus is a sensitive region and difficult for most individuals to visualize themselves. These conditions are generally readily diagnosed by the practitioner, in that they are easily seen or detectable on physical examination and often can be identified and cured. Any discussion of chronic anal pain must also detail acute anal disorders. These, if left undiagnosed or untreated, can become chronic and difficult to manage. So, before detailing chronic anal pain, we present a brief review of causes of acute anal pain.

R.P. Billingham, MD, FACS, FASCRS (✉)
A.L. Bastawrous, MD, MBA, FACS, FASCRS
Department of Colorectal Surgery, Swedish Colon and Rectal Clinic, Swedish Hospital Medical Center, Swedish Cancer Institute, 1101 Madison, Suite 510, Seattle, WA 98104, USA
e-mail: rbham@u.washington.edu; amir.bastawrous@swedish.org

Acute Anal Pain

Key Concept: *Common things occur commonly. Initially, ask about and look for a thrombosed external hemorrhoid, anal fissure, or abscess with acute anal pain.*

Most of the acute anal pain seen by physicians in this situation represents one of the three diagnoses: thrombosed external hemorrhoid, anal fissure, or abscess/fistula of the perianal or ischiorectal area. Often simply asking the proper questions and listening to the patient can make the diagnosis. The time course, relationship to bowel habits and associated symptoms usually make the diagnosis of these common complaints, often prior to even examining the patient. Generally, the combination of history and physical examination is enough to confirm the diagnosis.

Thrombosed External Hemorrhoid (Fig. 23.1)

Thrombosed external hemorrhoids will usually present acutely after a bout of straining, constipation, or diarrhea. The pain will be associated with a swelling that is painful to sit upon. The time course is usually 1 week or less for the pain if untreated and a few weeks for the clot to be absorbed. When symptomatic, office excision of the external hemorrhoid containing the clot—rather than making an incision through the external skin to enucleate the clot—gives both better short-term relief of pain and prevents recurrence at the site of that particular hemorrhoid. When there is hemorrhoidal crisis, with circumferential thrombosis of all or most of the external hemorrhoids, treatment should be performed in an operating room setting (Fig. 23.2).

S.R. Steele et al. (eds.), *Complexities in Colorectal Surgery*,
DOI 10.1007/978-1-4614-9022-7_23, © Springer Science+Business Media New York 2014

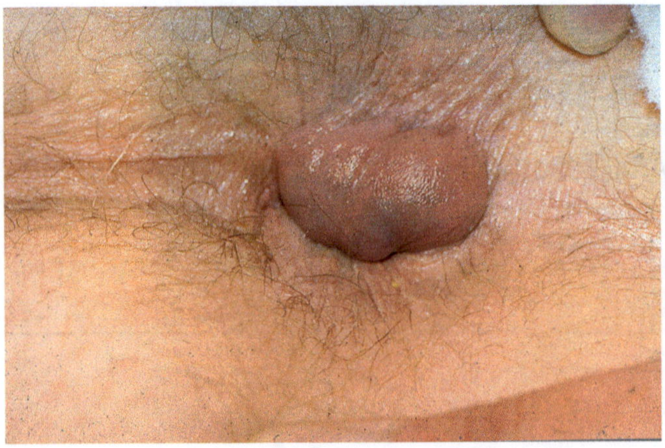

Fig. 23.1 Thrombosed external hemorrhoid

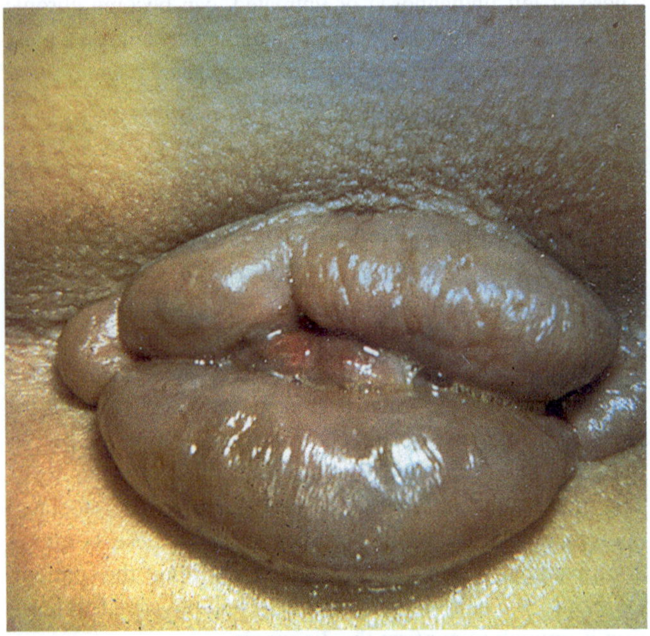

Fig. 23.2 "Hemorrhoidal crisis," with circumferential thrombosis of internal and external hemorrhoids

Anal Fissure (Fig. 23.3)

Acute pain that occurs after every bowel movement, particularly a bout of hard constipated stools, and is sometimes associated with spotting of blood, is typical of an anal fissure. Fissures are normally diagnosed clinically by their classic appearance involving visible internal anal sphincter fibers, rolled edges, sentinel pile, and hypertrophied internal papillae (when chronic, see Fig. 23.3). Acutely they may be seen as a superficial tear in the anoderm. Anal fissure pain can become chronic if not treated and may also be a result of associated sphincter spasm. The chronicity is typically not from the fissure being refractory in these situations but rather long lasting due to lack of treatment. Patients at times try to

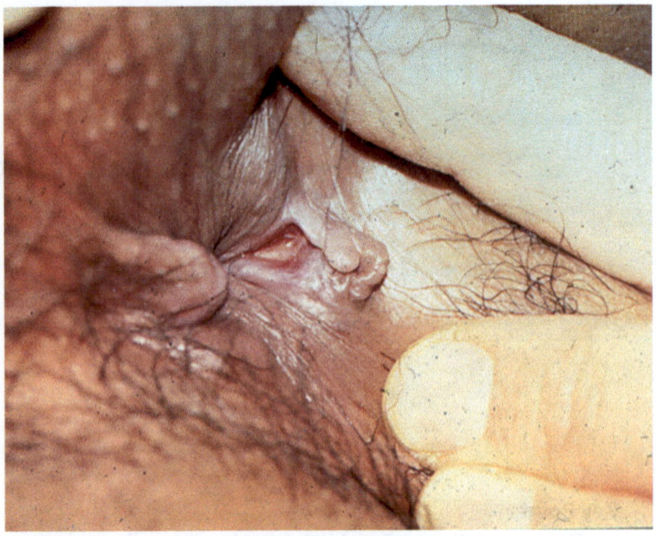

Fig. 23.3 Anal fissure and sentinel tag

self-medicate with over-the-counter remedies for many months without success. The gold standard treatment is lateral internal sphincterotomy. Most patients (and physicians) prefer to first try conservative measures (i.e., bulking agents, sitz baths, calcium channel blockers, glyceryl trinitrate, botulinum toxin) before sphincterotomy. Anal fissures, even after a competently performed lateral internal sphincterotomy, may occasionally persist as causes of pain if the fissure does not heal. Management options for persistent fissure include botulinum toxin injection, contralateral internal sphincterotomy, or cutaneous advancement flap down into the anal canal.

Anorectal Abscess/Fistula (Fig. 23.4)

Abscesses, which are commonly treated with antibiotics alone in the primary care arena or emergency department in the mistaken hope that they will resolve, invariably need surgical drainage if they don't drain spontaneously. For smaller, superficial perianal abscesses, drainage can generally easily be done in an office setting, using local anesthesia. It is our practice to remove an ellipse of skin overlying the abscess, to ensure a large enough opening to provide adequate drainage, and to delay premature cutaneous healing, which results in early recurrence of the abscess. The practices of "breaking up loculations," or "packing the wound so it will heal," are unnecessary and potentially detrimental by obstructing egress of purulence. It is sufficient to place a gauze pad over the wound. Larger abscesses, such as ischiorectal and/or horseshoe abscesses, are best treated in the operating room, using similar principles. Recurrence of abscess or persistence of drainage after operative treatment almost always indicates a fistula in ano. A fistula is itself rarely a cause of

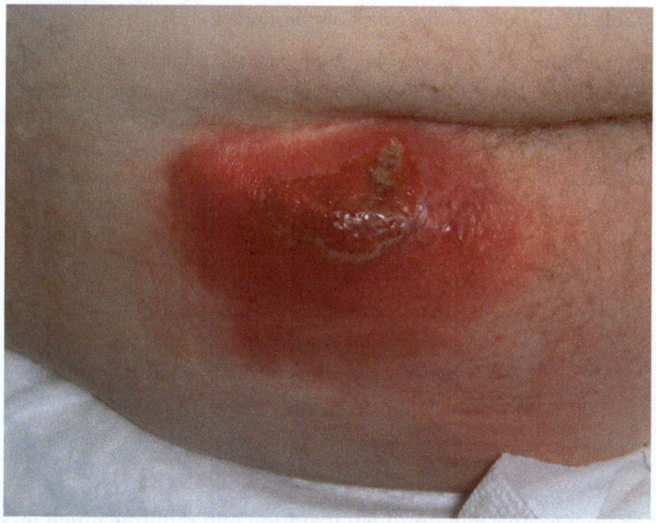

Fig. 23.4 Perianal abscess

anal pain. However, persistent drainage can cause pruritus which itself may be irritating and be thought of as chronic pain.

Acute or Chronic Anal Pain

Key Concept: Several other disease processes may present with acute or chronic anal pain; however, most are still easily diagnosed with a thorough history and clinical examination. Radiographic and endoscopic ancillary tests are required in select scenarios.

Less common conditions, which are less obvious than the above, but may produce either acute or chronic discomfort, include:

Anal Crohn's Disease (Fissures, Fistulae) (Fig. 23.5)

While even simple fistulae can sometimes cause pain, generally from undrained components of abscesses related to their origins, this is more likely to be the case with anal Crohn's disease and more complex fistulae. Furthermore, there may be pain from associated inflammation of the anus and rectum (proctitis). Evaluation is typically best performed with an examination under anesthesia, with emphasis on avoidance of fistulotomy, placement of setons through the known fistulae, and a careful search made for undrained areas, which can be opened and drained. Patients with anal Crohn's disease often have chronic anal pain related to unrelenting inflammation and irritation. Sphincter spasm is common as well. These patients are not usually candidates for sphincterotomy and may heal poorly from anal procedures.

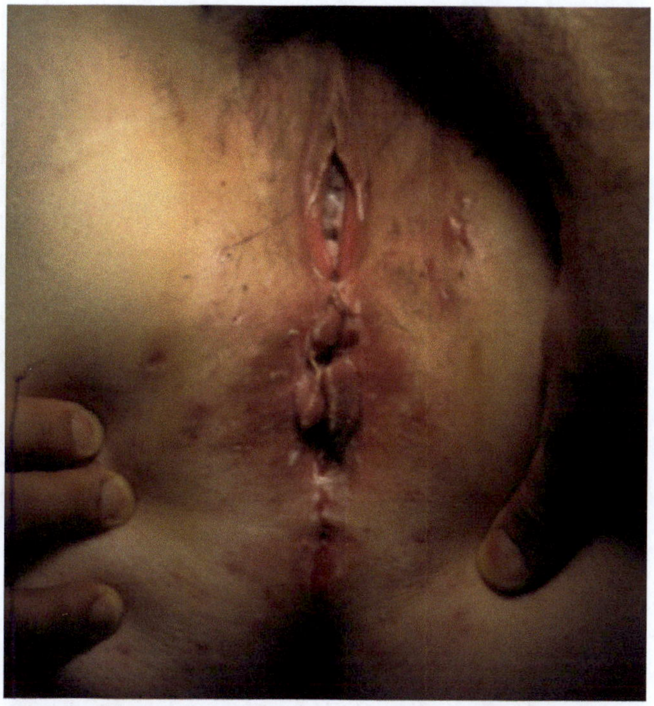

Fig. 23.5 Perianal Crohn's disease (Courtesy of W. Brian Sweeney, MD)

Hidradenitis Suppurativa (Fig. 23.6)

Hidradenitis suppurativa is a smoldering, uncomfortable cutaneous condition, arising from one or more of the sebaceous glands of the perineum. It is thought to represent a disorder of sebaceous gland metabolism, with similar lesions in the axillae and groins. When attempting to differentiate hidradenitis from other sources of perineal pathology, it is often helpful to perform a detailed examination of the skin adjacent to the anal verge. As this small circular area is devoid of hair and glands, disease in this location is not hidradenitis. Doxycycline, clindamycin, and Keflex are the most common antibiotics used, when given long term, for management of these lesions, while nonsteroidal anti-inflammatory drugs and immunosuppressants. For larger, more painful or nonresponsive lesions, conservative excision is often curative. At times, operative drainage of an acute cutaneous or deeper abscess is indicated [1].

Pruritus Ani (Fig. 23.7)

While the anus is a particularly sensitive region, discrimination of sensations is not always clear. Patients can report itching, burning, and pain symptoms interchangeably. Though the predominant symptom in pruritus ani is itching, pain can be reported, and in severe cases, tiny linear and radial ulcerations are typically seen on a bed of lichenified,

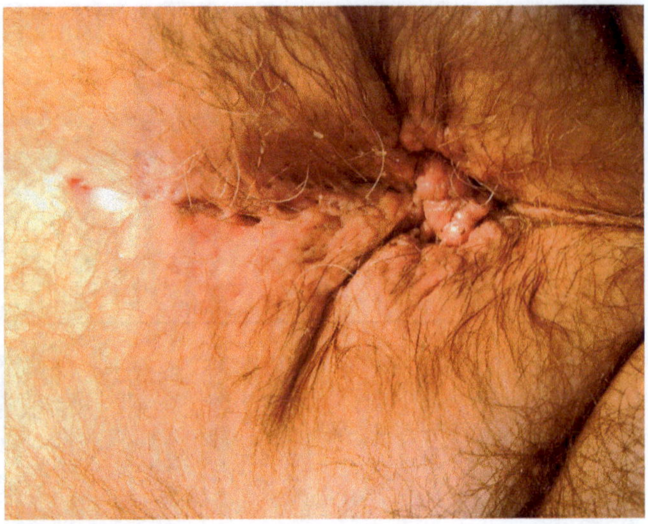

Fig. 23.6 Hidradenitis suppurativa

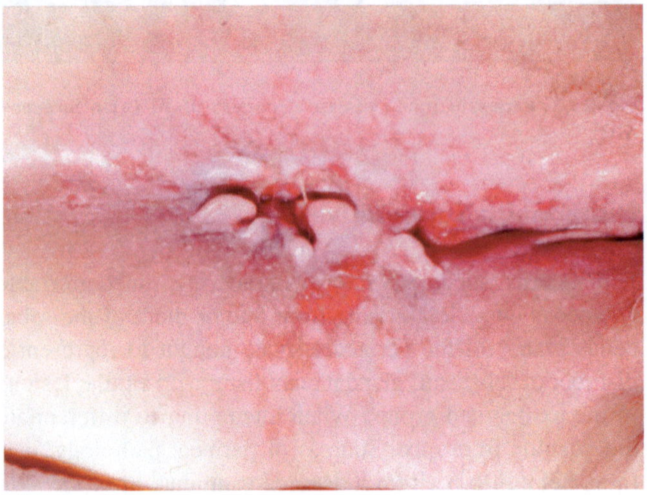

Fig. 23.7 Pruritus ani

chronically irritated skin. Pain from this source must be distinguished from anal fissures, ulcers of an infectious nature, or other common sources of anal pain as described above. Pruritus ani generally responds to discontinuation of chemical and mechanical irritants such as use of soaps or shampoos, salves, hemorrhoid creams or flushable wipes, excessive scrubbing, excessive wiping with dry toilet paper, and scratching. The latter—avoidance of scratching—is often the most difficult for patients, though absolutely required to stop the cycle of perpetual itching and irritation. In addition, efforts should be made to avoid perianal moisture, which is thought to perpetuate the process. Use of creams and ointments generally is counterproductive for this reason. Recommendations of cotton or cornstarch to keep the area drier during the day are often helpful. Also, if stools are loose and/or frequent, attention to normalizing these

Table 23.1 Initial management of pruritus ani

Diminish local trauma	Avoid soap, scrubbing, and scratching Use damp toilet paper to gently pat the anal area clean. Do not use "baby wipes," etc.
Diminish perianal moisture	1. Use a small amount of cotton, and/or some corn starch powder, applied to the anal area, and kept there all day to absorb moisture 2. Consider seepage of mucus or fecal matter as a possibly ongoing source of moisture. Possibilities include frequent stools, especially loose stools, diminished sphincter tone, or prolapsing hemorrhoidal or rectal mucosa. 3. Avoid creams, ointment, and other emollients which serve only to keep the area moist and are counterproductive

characteristics can diminish irritation and requires much less perianal cleaning after bowel movements. This can be achieved with decreasing excess water intake and/or increasing dry fiber in the diet, such as by using fiber tablets or wafers (Table 23.1).

There are a few rare patients who suffer from chronic irritation bordering on pain despite following the advised bowel and hygiene instructions. For pruritus symptoms which persist despite patients' strict adherence to these guidelines, consider biopsy to rule out other conditions such as lichen sclerosus et atrophicus, Bowen's or Paget's disease, or similar entities, which may require dermatologic referral and/or a different therapeutic strategy.

Retrorectal Tumors

Because of the rarity of these lesions, and consequentially the failure to consider these in the differential diagnosis, delays in diagnosis occur more commonly than not. While these are often palpable on deep digital examination, a CT or MRI is necessary to further characterize them as benign or malignant and to plan therapy even if palpable. In general, biopsy is not routinely required, and virtually all of these require resection. A more detailed discussion is presented in Bailey et al., *Colorectal Surgery* (Fig. 23.8) [2].

Bicycle Seat Issues

Serious cyclists may experience pain and/or numbness in the ischial tuberosities, perineum, or genitalia. It is worthwhile to inquire about this and other similar avocations that may require prolonged sitting in the evaluation of a patient with symptoms of this nature. The condition is usually related to pressure on perineal nerves. Numerous adjustments in seat design and position are available to prevent or treat such issues [3]. In addition, anti-chafing creams are routinely

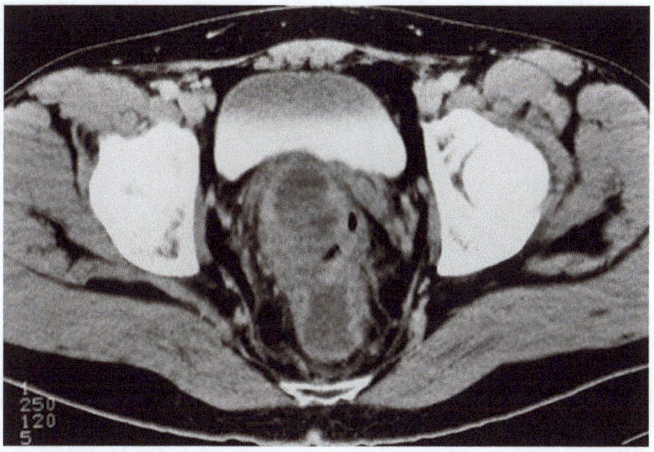

Fig. 23.8 Retrorectal tumor

helpful to avoid any accompanying skin breakdown and irritation that can be a source of constant irritation.

Prostatitis

Pain in the anterior rectum in the region of the prostate may be from inflammatory, neurological, or bacterial origin and may be acute or chronic. This may be associated with urinary symptoms and/or sexual dysfunction. This may lead to pelvic floor pain as well. Pain with palpation of the prostate is often diagnostic in the setting of normal anal and rectal tissues. A combination of alpha-blockers and antibiotics is generally used by urologists to treat the condition, to whom referral is recommended [4]. Patients sometimes say it feels like a dull ache in the pelvis or as if they are sitting on a saddle. The bacteriology will differ depending on the age group, with sexually transmitted organisms such as chlamydia predominating in younger men, while multiple bacteria including gram-negative rods are more common in older men. In either case, often a prolonged course of antibiotics is required to completely clear the infection and avoid chronic prostatitis that is hallmarked by chronic pain but minimal objective evidence of prostatic inflammation.

Constipation

Sometimes patients associate anorectal pain with large and/or dry bowel movements (dyschezia). Anal fissures are commonly associated with this symptom and should be sought, but overdistension of the sphincter mechanism alone, without the presence of a fissure, may be an issue for some. Attention to improving bowel consistency with bulk laxatives and/or osmotic laxatives may give effective long-term relief. Regardless of whether or not a fissure is seen, hypertonicity of the sphincter can often be felt on exam, and treatment is the same, regardless.

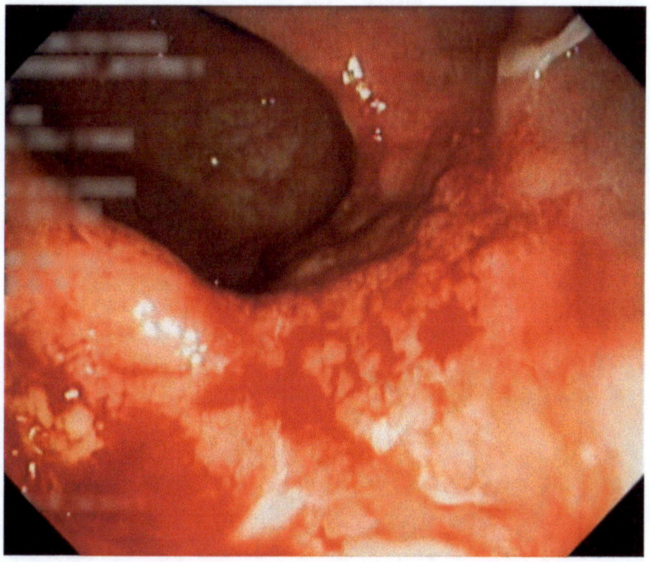

Fig. 23.9 Proctitis

Gynecological Sources

Gynecologic causes of pelvic pain, such as endometriosis, enterocele, rectocele, ovarian diseases, ectopic pregnancies, or fallopian tube abnormalities, typically do not cause anal pain. Rather, they result in deep-seated abdominal or pelvic pain, constipation, or defecation outlet dysfunction. Though they may be broadly included in the discussion of the differential diagnosis of anal pain, the reader is referred to one of several available gynecological textbooks where they are best addressed.

Proctitis/Pouchitis

Proctitis is inflammation of the rectum secondary to infections, postradiation, diversion, chemical irritation (corrosive or disinfectants), or inflammatory bowel diseases. Proctitis is usually associated with rectal bleeding, and diagnosis is generally readily made using office sigmoidoscopy (Fig. 23.9). By contrast, pouchitis occurs in 30–50 % of patients undergoing a restorative ileal pouch-anal anastomosis following total proctocolectomy for chronic ulcerative colitis (Fig. 23.10) [5]. Typically bacterial overgrowth in the pouch results in an inflammatory response. Inflammation can also occur in the remnant mucosa of the anus (i.e., "cuffitis"). Pouchitis and proctitis may be associated tenesmus, or with painful sensations in the pelvis, and is classically associated with a sharp rise in the number of bowel movements each

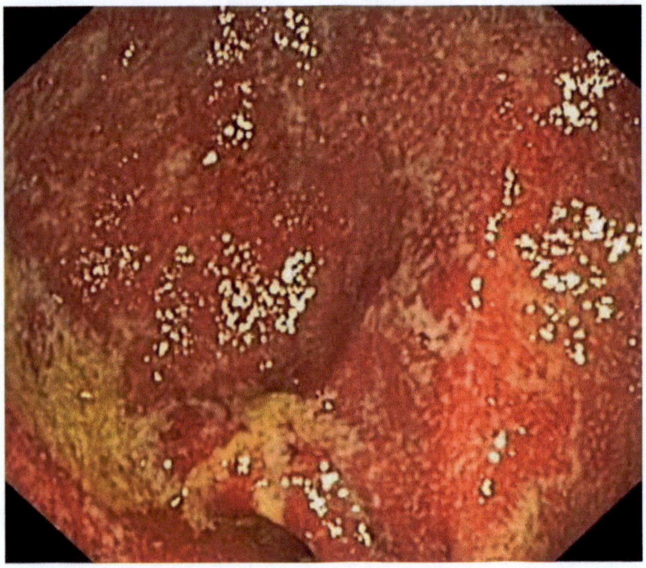

Fig. 23.10 Pouchitis (With permission from Science SourceÆ, registered trademark of Photo Researchers, Inc. Images and Text. Copyright © 2013 Photo Researchers, Inc. All Rights Reserved)

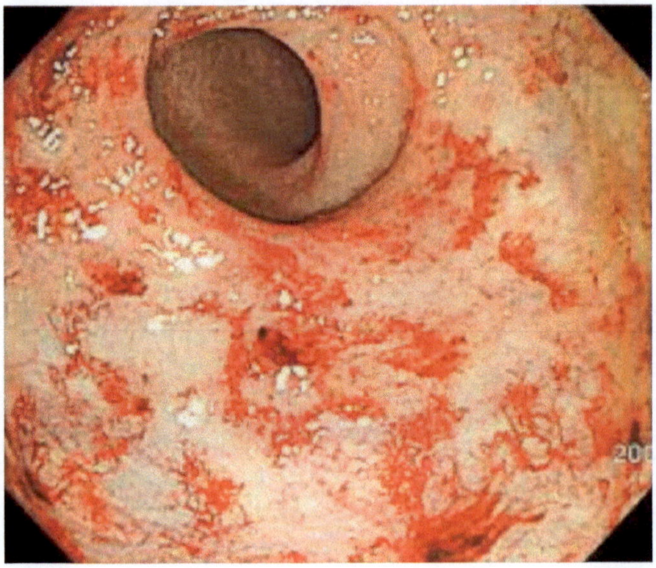

Fig. 23.11 Radiation proctitis

day. It is our experience that some patients develop pouchitis from overcompensating with antidiarrheals, in an effort to diminish the frequency of bowel movements below about 3/ day.

Treatment of pouchitis is generally with antibiotics (metronidazole or ciprofloxacin are the most commonly used). Probiotics are sometimes used in an effort to prevent pouchitis, but there are very limited data on the efficacy of this practice. Other more recalcitrant bouts of pouchitis require steroids, chronic cyclical courses of antibiotics, or even immunosuppressants or diversion. Proctitis is best managed by addressing the cause and may include anti-inflammatory agents or antibiotics as indicated given the underlying etiology. Proctitis resulting from radiation therapy is addressed in the section below.

Radiation

Radiation effects in the perianal area are occasionally painful and must be distinguished from pruritus ani, from dermatoses such as lichen sclerosus et atrophicus, and from Bowen's or Paget's diseases. Since the radiation to this area is usually given for anal or distal rectal, vulvar, and prostatic malignancies, the differential diagnosis should include a careful search for recurrence of these cancers. The radiation effects that cause pain include anoderm thinning, proctitis, sphincter injury, and stenosis. It is our practice to first attempt sucralfate suppositories (these can be made by compounding pharmacies). If bleeding persists, then dilute 10 % formalin placed topically. For more resistant sources of bleeding, laser therapy or argon beam coagulation are occasionally needed to destroy the damaged tissue (Fig. 23.11) [6].

Anorectal Stricture

Rectal and anal strictures can cause pain during defecation but are unlikely to be obscure sources of chronic anal pain, due to their easy detection by physical examination, and their association with defecation. The pain is usually related to tearing of narrowed anal canal anoderm or scar. While it is important to rule out any associated malignancy, treatment of benign strictures typically includes dilation and anoplasty.

Anal Cancer

When symptomatic, anal cancer is usually readily diagnosed by office examination. Anal canal cancers are generally associated with more pain than those that are located only on the perianal skin. Related conditions, such as Bowen's or Paget's disease, may also be considered but are generally associated with more itching and irritation than pain. With anal cancer, pain is usually related to associated ulceration and sphincter irritation/spasm related to infiltration (Fig. 23.12) [7]. Though beyond the scope of this chapter, management of anal cancer includes proper staging and typically multimodality chemoradiation therapy, though surgical resection may be indicated for very small early lesions and in the palliative setting.

Foreign Bodies

Sometimes, due to embarrassment on the part of the patient, a complaint of "chronic anorectal pain" will be the ostensible reason for a visit to the colon and rectal surgeon for a patient

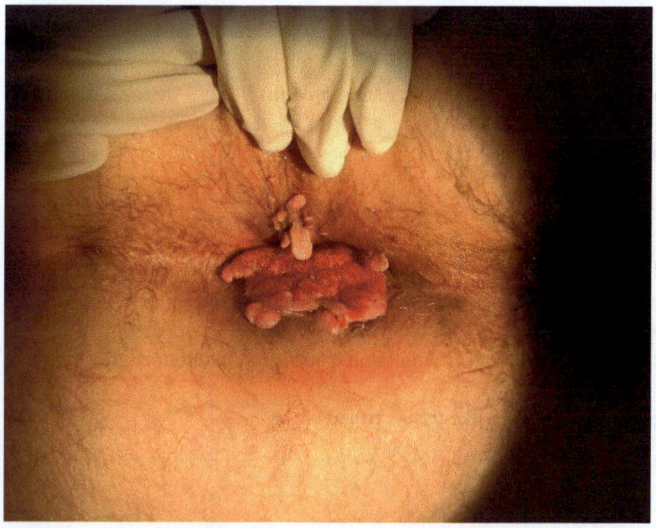

Fig. 23.12 Anal cancer

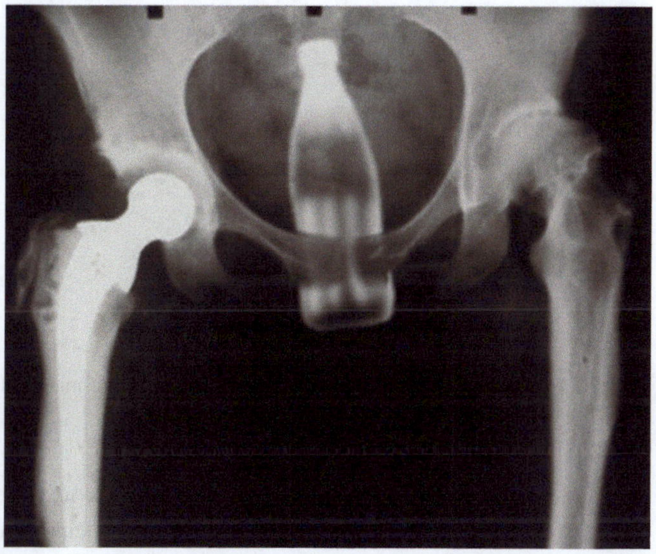

Fig. 23.13 Rectal foreign body

with a retained foreign body. Even if digital and anoscopic examinations are negative, rigid sigmoidoscopy and, if needed, a plain radiograph of the abdomen and pelvis are simple means to confirm or exclude this diagnosis from the differential. While this is never, by definition, chronic, the insult may have occurred a few days prior to presentation. The trauma with the insertion and (often) repeated attempts to remove it may result in further damage than initially suspected (Fig. 23.13) [8]. Management includes removal either in the outpatient or operating room settings, along with exclusion of an associated bowel perforation. Typically adequate sedation including an anorectal block is required for successful removal in the emergency department or clinic environment.

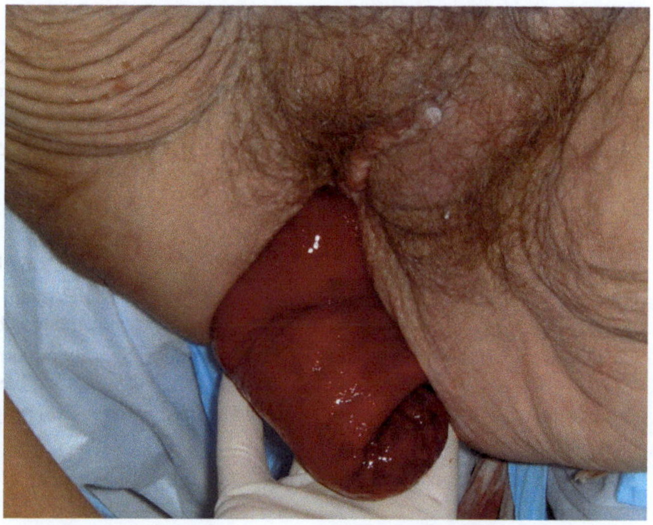

Fig. 23.14 Rectal prolapse

Rectal Prolapse

While classically not associated with acute sharp pain, patients with moderate degrees of rectal prolapse may note pain during and after defecation. Additionally, acute pain can occur with incarceration of the prolapsed rectum (Fig. 23.14) [9]. In the chronic setting, once the prolapsed rectum has been reduced, either spontaneously or manually, there may be minimal or no evidence of it on static examination in the prone jackknife or left lateral position. If the clinician is considering this in the differential diagnosis, a "toilet test" (with either simple straining or following enema administration) or video defecogram may be helpful in demonstrating this pathology.

Neurogenic Pain

While uncommon, disorders of the distal lumbar and sacral sensory nerves, whether from pressure or other entrapment, may give a key to ruptured discs, tumors, or congenital bony abnormalities. A neurologic exam looking for signs of weakness, sensory changes, or reflex abnormalities may be helpful in diagnosis. Radiological workup may include cross-sectional or MR imaging with appropriate referral as indicated.

Infectious Causes of Anal Pain (Table 23.2)

Gonorrhea

One of the many manifestations of gonorrhea can be anal pain. According to Gottesman and Gandhi, 50 % of males and 95 % of females are asymptomatic [10]. When symptoms do occur, they are usually attributable to proctitis, with

Table 23.2 Infectious causes of anal pain

Disease	Pathogen	Characteristics
Gonorrhea	*Neisseria gonorrhoeae*, gram (−) diplococcus in pairs and clusters	Pruritus, tenesmus, bloody mucopurulent discharge, proctitis
Chlamydia	*Chlamydia trachomatis*, obligate intracellular bacterium	Tenesmus, discharge, mild proctitis
LGV	*Chlamydia trachomatis*, serovars L1, L2, L3	Small shallow ulcers with rapid spontaneous healing
Syphilis	*Treponema pallidum*	Chancre, small clean-based eccentric ulcer, smooth firm borders with rolled edges
HSV	HSV 2, HSV 1 less common	Vesicles open, forming shallow ulcers that coalesce into multiple grouped lesions with erythematous base, single lesions/fissure can occur
Chancroid	*Haemophilus ducreyi*, gram (−) rod	Sharply circumscribed or irregular ulcer with ragged edges, no induration, gray/yellow exudates at base, multiple
Granuloma inguinale	*Calymmatobacterium granulomatis*	Extensive, progressive, granulation-like tissue, rolled edges

Adapted from Gottesman and Gandhi [10]

tenesmus, but occasionally severe anal pain is experienced (though the anal canal is usually not involved). Culture from within the rectum is generally reliable, but anal lubricants sometimes have antibacterial properties that may give a false-negative culture. For this reason, swabs can also be sent for DNA probe testing, using specialized specimen containers. Treatment typically includes oral cephalosporins or fluoroquinolones, and patients should be also treated for concomitant chlamydia and evaluated for other sexually transmitted diseases including HIV.

Herpes Simplex, Genitalis, and Zoster

Herpes simplex, including herpes zoster, is a common cause of perianal ulcers and pain. Inguinal lymphadenopathy, and even radiculopathy in the lumbosacral distribution, may also be present as a result of this virus. The perianal lesions may begin as pain alone, progressing to vesicles that rupture, causing shallow ulcers that take about 3 weeks to resolve spontaneously. Herpes can also affect the anal canal and rectal mucosa in some cases, with friability and ulcerations seen on anoscopy or sigmoidoscopy. Recurrences are common, at highly variable intervals, because of persistence of the viral genome in the ganglia of the sensory nerves supplying the anal and perianal area. HSV may also be associated with radiculopathy in the lumbosacral distribution, which can affect bladder function, cause impotence, and cause pain in the cutaneous distribution of these nerves, namely, the buttocks and thighs. Radiculopathic symptoms may still be present after disappearance of the cutaneous ulcerations. Treatment with oral acyclovir can often shorten the duration of symptoms by several days, but the drug does not prevent recurrence (Fig. 23.15) [10].

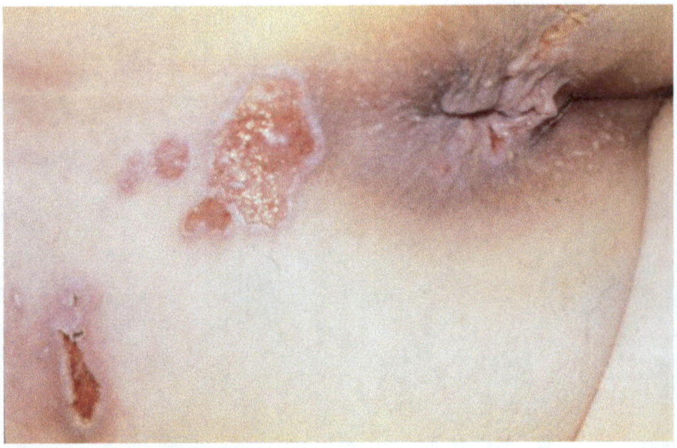

Fig. 23.15 Perianal herpes (With permission from Gottesman and Gandhi [10]. © Elsevier 2012)

Syphilis

Anal ulcers can be quite painful, mimicking the pain of anal fissure. However, such ulcers typically are not in the midline and may be multiple. In contrast, genital ulcers, or chancres, are typically not painful (Fig. 23.16). Treatment is usually successful with a single muscular injection of penicillin when detected in the early stages.

H. ducreyi (Chancroid)

Infection with this gram-negative coccobacillus results in genital and perianal ulcers, usually multiple and painful, occasionally associated with abscesses. Gram stain and culture on a chocolate agar are used for diagnosis. It is typically treated with azithromycin and a third-generation cephalosporin.

Chlamydia (LGV)

Lymphogranuloma venereum (LGV) results from infection with *Chlamydia trachomatis*. Following anorectal infection, a proctocolitis ensues where ulcers are usually not found in the anal canal but in the rectum. Rectal swabs for gram stain and culture are often unreliable. Sending such swabs for NAAT testing, in an appropriate specimen container, is more reliable.

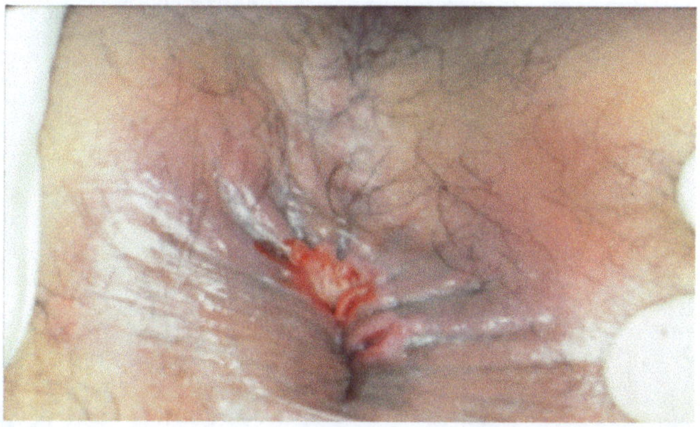

Fig. 23.16 Anal chancre from syphilis

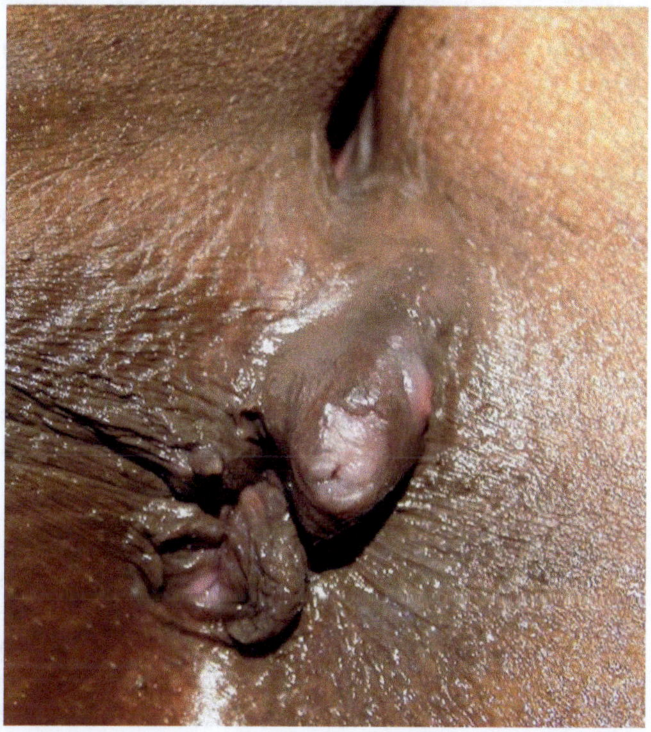

Fig. 23.17 Lymphogranuloma venereum (With permission from Dr. Pravin J. Gupta. http://drpravingupta.com/)

Gottesman and Gandhi point out that if a rectal gram stain shows polymorphonuclear leukocytes in the absence of visible gonococci, this constitutes presumptive evidence of *Chlamydia* (Fig. 23.17) [10]. Common treatment regimens include tetracycline, doxycycline, or erythromycin.

Chronic Anal Pain

Key Concept: Chronic anal pain can result from a variety of sources that include pelvic floor pathology and are oftentimes difficult to diagnose and less responsive to treatment. Multidisciplinary nonoperative therapies including biofeedback and stimulation are often useful to alleviate symptoms.

Chronic anal pain syndromes are those which are often more difficult to diagnose and treat and include levator syndrome, coccygodynia (which may often be a manifestation of levator syndrome), pudendal neuralgia, infectious diseases such as herpes zoster or syphilis, neurogenic pain, or other pain of unknown etiology.

Levator Spasm

Levator syndrome (also known as tension myalgia of the pelvic floor, proctalgia fugax, piriformis syndrome, puborectalis syndrome, or coccygodynia) is a vague, crampy intermittent pain around the lower rectal area. It defies localization, will sometimes develop after prolonged sitting, sometimes awaken patients at night, and is typically unpredictable in its frequency and intensity. It has been described as similar symptoms as urgency to have a bowel movement. The pain may last 10 min to an hour and resolves spontaneously (a variant of this pain, called "proctalgia fugax," is characterized by sudden sharp spasms in the anal muscle area, often lasting only a few seconds and disappearing). Interestingly, bowel movements tend to make this pain better (as opposed to the causes of acute pain listed above). A related diagnosis to levator ani syndrome is non-relaxing puborectalis. Patients may sometimes feel pain but mostly complain of constipation and inability to empty the rectum. This is also sometimes referred to as "anismus."

Diagnostic criteria for levator syndrome, as outlined by Wald in 1991 [11], are (1) chronic or recurrent episodes of rectal area pain or aching, (2) lasting 20 min or longer, (3) occurring for at least 3 months, and (4) in the absence of other causes. The diagnosis is "highly likely" if, on digital rectal examination, posterior traction on the levator muscle, particularly near its attachment to the coccyx, reproduces the discomfort or reveals "contracted levator muscles." The diagnosis can be made when the pain is reproduced with palpation of a lateral muscle cord, which is a portion of the levator ani in spasm. Even without this specific finding, the diagnosis is still "possible" if the symptoms meet the criteria listed above. A complete anorectal examination is necessary to look for, and exclude, other possible causes. Other tests, which may be appropriate in certain patients, include colonoscopy, CT, GI contrast studies, and sometimes even diagnostic laparoscopy. But typically, history and physical examination are sufficient.

Wexner and Jagelman [12] reported on a series of 19 patients with intractable pelvic pain. Paradoxical puborectalis contraction was frequently found, more often with EMG than on videodefecography. Grimaud et al. [13] noted that anal canal resting pressure was significantly higher than in controls and that half of such patients showed that the puborectalis muscle failed to relax on videodefecography.

Epidemiology

Thompson, in a series from the UK, (1981) [14], reported that 14 % of patients surveyed had such symptoms within the past 12 months; of these, 17 % of women reported this, while only 9 % of men did so. Wald [11] found that 6–7 % of the general population reported these symptoms but observed that only about 30 % ever consulted a physician about this problem. He also mentions that there appears to be no relationship between this syndrome and irritable bowel syndrome.

Management

One important step, after making the diagnosis, is reassurance of the patient that the condition, while annoying in various degrees, is not serious or life-threatening. Often such assurance assuages the anxiety, which usually accompanies this condition, and which may magnify the symptoms. Pharmacologic therapy, using anxiolytics or "muscle relaxants," is rarely helpful, either in treating individual episodes (which typically resolve before any oral medication could become effective) or in preventing the development of pain. Furthermore, the side effects of these medications are significant.

Vigorous digital massage of the muscle by the physician, in an office setting, was described by Thiele, but the muscle is generally too tender and painful, in this venue, to permit effectiveness [15]. Therefore, generally the first line of therapy is "electrogalvanic stimulation" (EGS; Fig. 23.18), a physical therapy technique used by therapists for many other skeletal muscular complaints. This was first reported by Sohn in 1982 [16]. EGS requires an intra-anal probe, a dedicated and interested physical therapist, and is commonly administered for 20–30 min at a session, for three sessions a week for 2 weeks. Salvati reported that 77 % of 90 patients so treated were relieved or improved [17]. In our own series, 60 % had good to excellent response, but over the longer term, only 25 % remained free of symptoms [18]. Hull's experience was that, of 52 patients, symptoms were relieved in only 19 %, partially relieved in 24 %, and 57 % of patients reported no relief [19]. Ger and Wexner found that 38 % of their patients reported good to excellent results [20].

For those for whom electrogalvanic stimulation is not available or is not effective, biofeedback has been recommended as another effective treatment. Grimaud reported a series in which all of his patients experienced relief after 8 weeks of once-weekly sessions, with only one relapsing patient after 2 months [13].

Other therapies with which success has been reported (often anecdotally) include acupuncture, injection of local anesthetic +/– steroids, levator massage under anesthesia (with or without the injection of botulinum toxin), inhalation of salbutamol (a beta-adrenergic), or even surgical division of the puborectalis muscle.

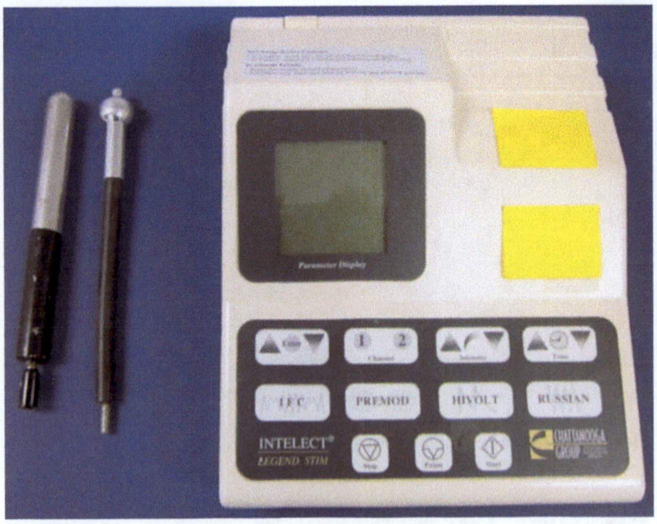

Fig. 23.18 Electrogalvanic stimulation (EGS) generator with anal probes

Coccygodynia

Coccygodynia, originally described by Simpson in 1859, is, in our experience, nearly always related to, and caused by, traction on the coccygeal periosteum by the tense levator muscle. Some have reported coccygeal hypermobility or "luxation" based on physical and radiologic exams and have recommended treatment with manipulation, injection, cryoanalgesia of posterior rami of lower sacral nerve roots (if the patient has responded to injection of these roots with a test dose of local anesthesia), or rarely, coccygectomy.

Pudendal Neuralgia

The sensory nerve from the anal canal and perianal area is the inferior rectal and perineal branches of the pudendal nerve [21]. Pudendal neuralgia, first described in 1988 by Amarenco et al. [22, 23], is an uncommon condition characterized by burning, pinching, or twisting sensations in the territory of the pudendal nerve, usually exacerbated by the sitting position and relieved by standing, and may be either unilateral or bilateral. This may be perceived in the perineum, vulvar, or anorectal areas. It is caused by compression of pudendal nerve within Alcock's canal at the border by the ischium and the obturator internus muscle. The pudendal nerve is a mixed sensory and motor nerve, arising from S2–S4. It supplies anal and urethral sphincters, pelvic floor muscles, and is a sensory nerve for the anal, perineal, and genital areas. It traverses the pelvic cavity, gluteal region, and perineum, where it divides to become the perineal nerve and the dorsal nerve of the penis or clitoris. The two most likely sites of compression are at the ischial spine in gluteal region or within the pudendal canal.

If symptoms are consistent with this diagnosis and other examinations and studies are negative, perineal electrophysiologic examination (looking for neurogenic

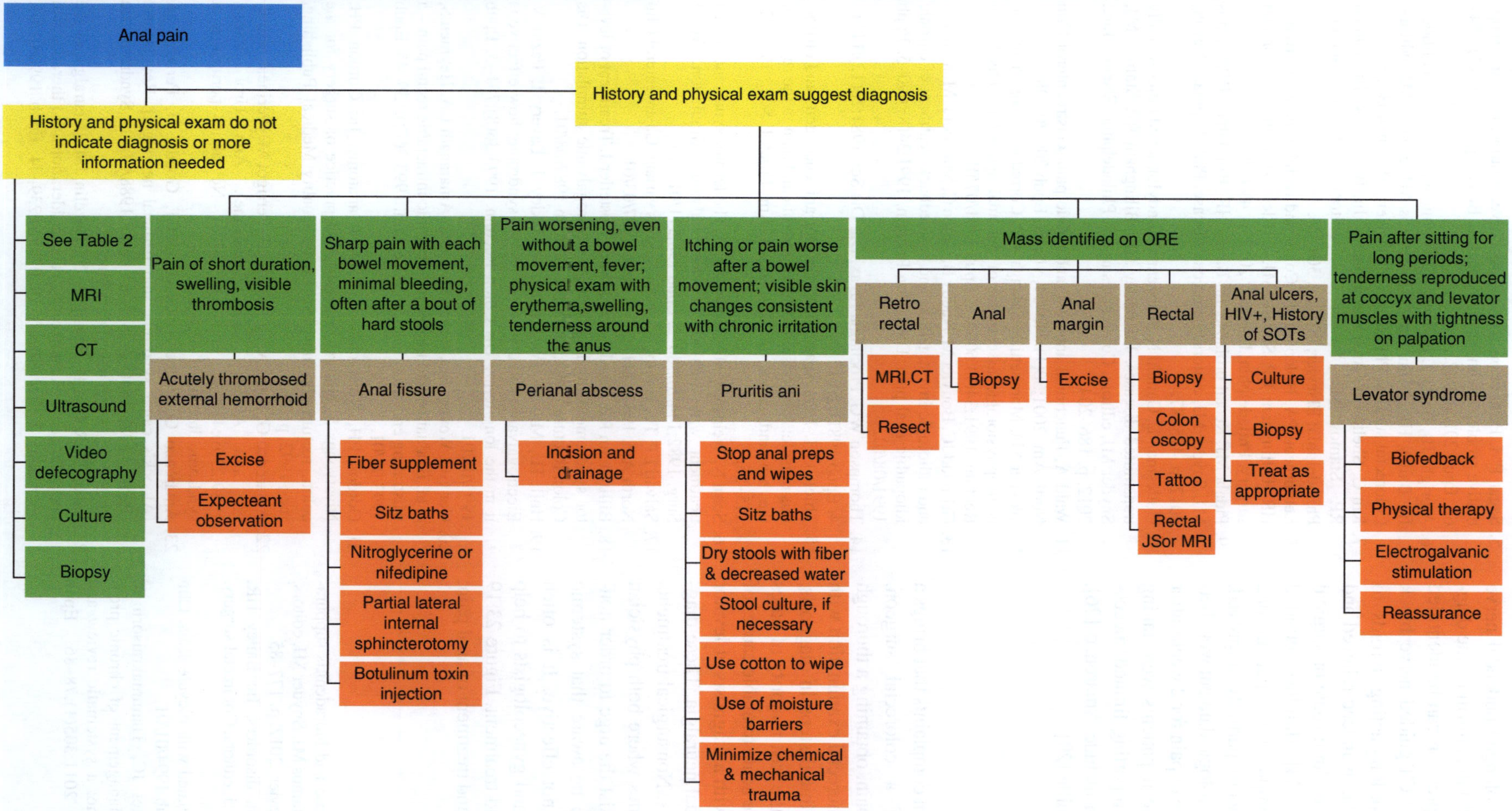

Fig. 23.19 Algorithm for the workup and treatment of anal pain

muscles within the pelvic floor or prolonged pudendal nerve terminal motor latency) is often helpful in confirming the diagnosis. The likely sites of nerve compression can be identified on CT, and one can do a diagnostic CT-guided nerve block using local anesthetic, with or without long-acting steroids, to see whether the pain is relieved. If pain is indeed relieved and returns, additional injection via the peridural route or surgical decompression can be considered [22–24]. Mauillion reported a series of 12 patients with such decompression: 4 patients had their pain totally relieved and 3 were partially improved. Results did not depend on electrophysiologic data but were better if they had complete disappearance of pain for 2 weeks after each of two nerve blocks and worse if patients were taking antidepressants [25]. Other authors reporting limited success with injection and/or decompression include Amarenco [26], Shafik [27], Bautrant [28], and Vancaille [29].

Summary Pearls

Anal pain is one of the most common complaints that brings a patient to seek the services of a colorectal surgeon. Distinguishing acute from chronic pain, obtaining a thorough history, and performing a detailed anorectal examination with anoscopy and proctoscopy are the initial steps in diagnosis. The etiology is easily identified in the vast majority of cases within minutes on the first visit. Once acute treatable causes of pain are ruled out you may be left with a diagnosis of levator syndrome, coccygodynia, or pudendal neuralgia. These diagnoses can be debilitating for patients. Nonsurgical treatments are most effective, but there are times where both physician and patient may feel frustrated. Resist the urge to order non-useful and unnecessary tests. Also be aware that systemic pharmacologic therapy is usually not effective. It is often important to work with urologists and gynecologists to help the patient through the diagnosis and treatment. Figure 23.19 shows an algorithm for the workup and treatment of anal pain.

References

1. Ford DH, Bailey HR. Pilonidal disease and hidradenitis suppurativa. In: Bailey HR, Billingham RP, Stamos MJ, Snyder MJ, editors. Colorectal surgery. Philadelphia: Elsevier; 2012. p. 177–85.
2. Cali Jr JR, Snyder MJ. Uncommon disorders. In: Bailey HR, Billingham RP, Stamos MJ, Snyder MJ, editors. Colorectal surgery. Philadelphia: Elsevier; 2012. p. 512–8.
3. Weiss BD. Clinical syndromes associated with bicycle seats. Clin Sports Med. 1994;13(1):175–86. Epub 1994/01/01.
4. Anothaisintawee T, Attia J, Nickel JC, Thammakraisorn S, Numthavaj P, McEvoy M, et al. Management of chronic prostatitis/chronic pelvic pain syndrome: a systematic review and network meta-analysis. JAMA. 2011;305(1):78–86. Epub 2011/01/06.
5. Sagar PM, Pemberton JH. Intraoperative, postoperative and reoperative problems with ileoanal pouches. Br J Surg. 2012;99(4):454–68. Epub 2012/02/07.
6. Albright JB, Beaty J. Radiation, ischemic and infectious colitides. In: Bailey HR, Billingham RP, Stamos MJ, Snyder MJ, editors. Colorectal surgery. Philadelphia: Elsevier; 2012. p. 403–25.
7. Kin C, Shelton A. Anal malignancies. In: Bailey HR, Billingham RP, Stamos MJ, Snyder MJ, editors. Colorectal surgery. Philadelphia: Elsevier; 2012. p. 308–25.
8. Letourneau PA, Holcomb JR. Colon and rectal trauma. In: Bailey HR, Billingham RP, Stamos MJ, Snyder MJ, editors. Colorectal surgery. Philadelphia: Elsevier; 2012. p. 499–508.
9. Pidala MJ. Rectal prolapse. In: Bailey HR, Billingham RP, Stamos MJ, Snyder MJ, editors. Colorectal disease. Philadelphia: Elsevier; 2012. p. 475–87.
10. Gottesman L, Gandhi N. Anogenital condyloma and other sexually transmitted diseases. In: Bailey HR, Bilingham RP, Stamos MJ, Snyder MJ, editors. Colorectal surgery. Philadelphia: Elsevier Inc.; 2012. p. 186–204.
11. Wald A. Functional anorectal and pelvic pain. Gastroenterol Clin North Am. 2001;30(1):243–51, viii–ix. Epub 2001/06/08.
12. Wexner SD, Marchetti F, Salanga VD, Corredor C, Jagelman DG. Neurophysiologic assessment of the anal sphincters. Dis Colon Rectum. 1991;34(7):606–12. Epub 1991/07/01.
13. Grimaud JC, Bouvier M, Naudy B, Guien C, Salducci J. Manometric and radiologic investigations and biofeedback treatment of chronic idiopathic anal pain. Dis Colon Rectum. 1991;34(8):690–5. Epub 1991/08/01.
14. Thompson WG. Proctalgia fugax. Dig Dis Sci. 1981;26(12):1121–4. Epub 1981/12/01.
15. Thiele GH. Tonic spasm of the levator ani, coccygeus and piriformis muscle: relationship to coccygodynia and pain in the region of the hip and down the leg. Trans Am Proctol Soc. 1936;37:145–55.
16. Sohn N, Weinstein MA, Robbins RD. The levator syndrome and its treatment with high-voltage electrogalvanic stimulation. Am J Surg. 1982;144(5):580–2. Epub 1982/11/01.
17. Salvati EP. The levator syndrome and its variant. Gastroenterol Clin North Am. 1987;16(1):71–8. Epub 1987/03/01.
18. Billingham RP, Isler JT, Friend WG, Hostetler J. Treatment of levator syndrome using high-voltage electrogalvanic stimulation. Dis Colon Rectum. 1987;30(8):584–7. Epub 1987/08/01.
19. Hull TL, Milsom JW, Church J, Oakley J, Lavery I, Fazio V. Electrogalvanic stimulation for levator syndrome: how effective is it in the long-term? Dis Colon Rectum. 1993;36(8):731–3. Epub 1993/08/01.
20. Ger GC, Wexner SD, Jorge JM, Lee E, Amaranath LA, Heymen S, et al. Evaluation and treatment of chronic intractable rectal pain – a frustrating endeavor. Dis Colon Rectum. 1993;36(2):139–45. Epub 1993/02/01.
21. Gordon PH, Nivatvongs S. Surgical anatomy. In: Gordon PH, Nivatvongs S, editors. Principles and practice of surgery for the colon, rectum and anus. St. Louis: Quality Medical Publishing, Inc.; 1992. p. 35–7.
22. Amarenco G, Savatovsky I, Budet C, Perrigot M. [Perineal neuralgia and Alcock's canal syndrome]. Ann Urol (Paris). 1989;23(6):488–92. Epub 1989/01/01. Nevralgies perineales et syndrome du canal d'Alcock.
23. Amarenco G, Lanoe Y, Ghnassia RT, Goudal H, Perrigot M. [Alcock's canal syndrome and perineal neuralgia]. Rev Neurol (Paris). 1988;144(8–9):523–6. Epub 1988/01/01. Syndrome du canal d'Alcock et nevralgie perineale.
24. Labat JJ, Robert R, Bensignor M, Buzelin JM. [Neuralgia of the pudendal nerve. Anatomo-clinical considerations and therapeutical approach]. J Urol (Paris). 1990;96(5):239–44. Epub 1990/01/01.

Les nevralgies du nerf pudendal (honteux interne). Considerations anatomo-cliniques et perspectives therapeutiques.
25. Mauillon J, Thoumas D, Leroi AM, Freger P, Michot F, Denis P. Results of pudendal nerve neurolysis-transposition in twelve patients suffering from pudendal neuralgia. Dis Colon Rectum. 1999;42(2):186–92. Epub 1999/04/22.
26. Amarenco G, Kerdraon J, Bouju P, Le Budet C, Cocquen AL, Bosc S, et al. [Treatments of perineal neuralgia caused by involvement of the pudendal nerve]. Rev Neurol (Paris). 1997;153(5):331–4. Epub 1997/06/01. Traitements des nevralgies perineales par atteinte du nerf pudendal. A propos de 170 cas.
27. Shafik A. Endoscopic pudendal canal decompression for the treatment of fecal incontinence due to pudendal canal syndrome. J Laparoendosc Adv Surg Tech A. 1997;7(4):227–34. Epub 1997/08/01.
28. Bautrant E, de Bisschop E, Vaini-Elies V, Massonnat J, Aleman I, Buntinx J, et al. [Modern algorithm for treating pudendal neuralgia: 212 cases and 104 decompressions]. J Gynecol Obstet Biol Reprod (Paris). 2003;32(8 Pt 1):705–12. Epub 2004/04/08. La prise en charge moderne des nevralgies pudendales. A partir d'une serie de 212 patientes et 104 interventions de decompression.
29. Vancaillie T, Eggermont J, Armstrong G, Jarvis S, Liu J, Beg N. Response to pudendal nerve block in women with pudendal neuralgia. Pain Med. 2012;13(4):596–603. Epub 2012/03/07.

Complex Pilonidal Disease and Acute and Chronic Perineal Wounds: Point – Counterpoint

24

Herand Abcarian and Guy Robert Orangio

Key Points

- Reconstruction of a complex perineal wound often requires a multidisciplinary team—enlist their input early and use their expertise.
- Flaps are very useful, especially in younger patients with pilonidal disease who do not have time or the support for chronic wound care and in large perineal defects.
- Healing by secondary intention still has a role in the place of chronic pilonidal wounds.
- The underlying disease process often governs the approach to large perineal wounds.
- Both nonoperative and operative approaches are needed for chronic open perineal wounds. Do not just rush back to surgery.

Surgical Management of Complex or Recurrent Pilonidal Sinus

Pilonidal sinus is an acquired disease, seen in the second decade of life with almost 4 to 1 greater ratio of men to women [1]. Herbert Mayo first described this disease in 1833, as a "hair-containing sinus" [2]. In 1880 Hodges introduced the term "pilonidal" which means "hair nest" [3]. Karydakis suggested that the disease is caused by loose hair becoming inserted into the skin, which leads to chronic inflammation and infection [4].

Patients with chronic pilonidal disease, complicated pilonidal sinus with multiple sinus tracts, and partially drained abscess cavities or recurrent pilonidal disease require surgical management. Midline pilonidal excision en bloc of the cyst and the sinus tracts is the most common operation performed. Excision down to the presacral fascia should be performed with complete excision of the cystic component of the pilonidal disease. The controversy is how to manage the post-excision wound in patients with complex pilonidal disease. Most of these patients have failed conservative measures and surgical treatment. In this setting, excision of the pilonidal disease is combined with flap closure and modification of the midline gluteal cleft. There are multiple flaps utilized: rhomboid flaps, Z-plasty, the Karydakis procedure, the Bascom cleft lift procedure, V–Y-plasty, gluteus maximus myocutaneous flaps, and skin grafting. The major disadvantages to the flap procedures are longer operative times, greater blood loss, and complications related directly to the flaps including infection, loss of flap, and scarring.

Pilonidal Cystectomy Combined with Fasciocutaneous Advancement Flap

Key Concept: Excision of a pilonidal cyst is bound to leave wound issues and often a disgruntled patient. Be familiar with the various flaps that are available for these complex wounds, as well as their intrinsic outcomes and challenges.

Historically the advancing flap was performed by Dr. Karydakis in Athens, Greece, in 1965. In 1992, he reported his results in 7,471 patients treated from 1966 to 1990, with over a 95 % follow-up ranging from 2 to 20 years. He had a

H. Abcarian, MD FACS
Division of Colon and Rectal Surgery,
Department of Surgery, University of Illinois at Chicago,
John H. Stroger Hospital of Cook County, 840 S. Wood Street,
MC 958, 518 E CSB, Chicago, IL 60612, USA
e-mail: abcarian@uic.edu

G.R. Orangio, MD, FACS, FASCRS (✉)
Division of Colon and Rectal Surgery, Department of Surgery,
Louisiana State University Health Science Center,
LSU School of Medicine, 1542 Tulane Ave, Room 734,
New Orleans, LA 70112, USA
e-mail: guyhd1950@gmail.com

Electronic supplementary material The online version of this chapter (doi: 10.1007/978-1-4614-9022-7_24) contains supplementary material, which is available to authorized users. Videos can also be accessed at http://www.springerimages.com/videos/978-1-4614-9021-0.

S.R. Steele et al. (eds.), *Complexities in Colorectal Surgery*,
DOI 10.1007/978-1-4614-9022-7_24, © Springer Science+Business Media New York 2014

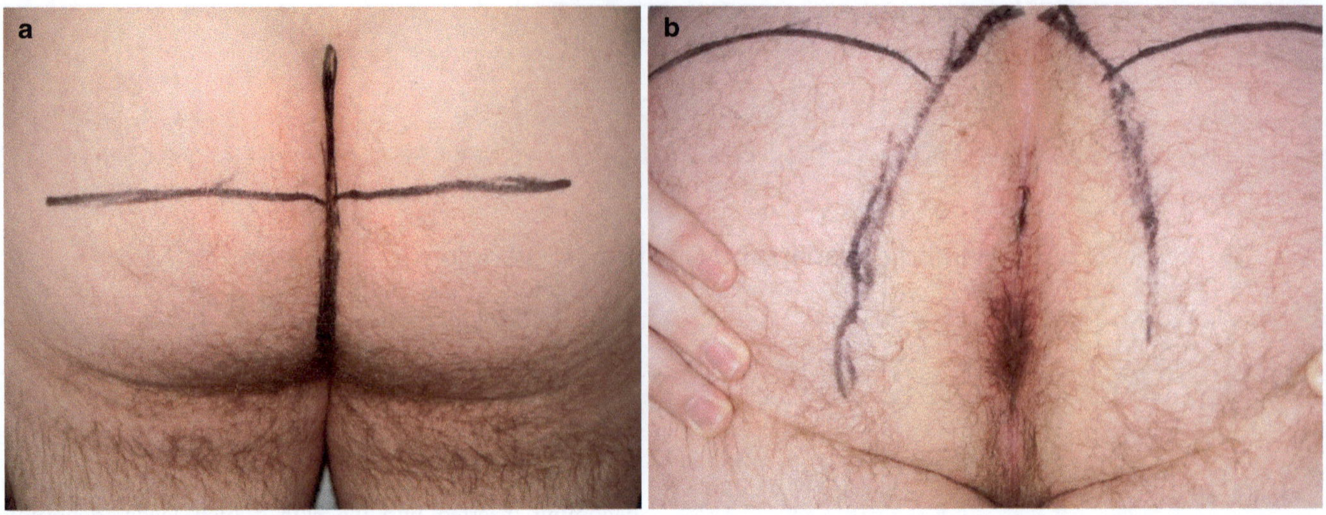

Fig. 24.1 (**a, b**) The Bascom cleft lift procedure. Compressing the buttocks together will allow marking of the diseased area and deep cleft that will require excision (Courtesy of Dr. Bascom)

remarkably low overall complication rate of 8.5 % and a 1 % recurrence rate [5]. The rhomboid or Limberg flap has also been shown to be effective by Urhan in 2002, where he reported 100 % healing in 102 patients treated with excision and flap closure [6]. The Bascom cleft lift procedure, described in 2002, is a technically challenging flap that undermines and obliterates the gluteal cleft in the area of disease [7]. The technique emphasizes identification of the deep cleft through a series of steps to indicate the diseased (and surrounding) area that needs to be resected to adequately remove the cleft (Fig. 24.1a, b). The V–Y (fasciocutaneous flap) advancement flap has been utilized since 1993 in patients with complex pilonidal disease [8]. In 2009, a series of 43 patients were treated with the V–Y advancement flap with one recurrence and a somewhat higher complication rate including 9.3 % infection, 7 % hematoma, and 16.3 % anesthesia over the flap. Unfortunately, over 90 % were dissatisfied with their scar [9]. The Z-plasty or flap has shown excellent results. In 2006, 144 patients were randomized to two groups comparing excision with open wound management (i.e., secondary intention) versus excision with Z-plasty. The Z-plasty had a statistically significant shorter wound healing, 15.4 days versus 41days ($P<0.001$), compared to conventional management [10]. In general, the utilization of the gluteus maximus myocutaneous flap is reserved for very recalcitrant pilonidal disease, with the first case report describing its use in 1984 [11].

You may find yourself saying "Okay, so what?" First, pilonidal disease is a common problem seen in a colorectal surgical practice. Most of the time, these patients are referred from internal medicine, family practice, dermatologists, and general surgeons for evaluation and treatment, in part, because of frustration with recurrent disease and also due to its chronic nature and/or the failure of either conservative and/or prior surgical therapy. Many patients have been treated with antibiotics, an in-office incision and drainage, or even pilonidal cystectomy. They are also just as frustrated because of the intermittent infections or chronic draining sinus that limits their activity, whether it is purulent or blood and foul odor. The majority of these patients are in the second decade of life: they are often now in college and have been dealing with pilonidal disease since high school, and it's not getting better. You, the true (or deemed) "colorectal specialist" are then confronted with a disgruntled patient and a benign disease that has become a social nuisance to them. I have a very long discussion with these patients (and their parents) about the different surgical approaches to this disease; many are familiar with these therapies—through family members, other patients, and in many cases online research. They usually want to schedule their surgery during spring or summer break, because they do not want to interrupt their education or externships for an operation.

My Approach (Dr. Orangio)

I recommend to these patients re-excision and the utilization of the VYAF, for several reasons: (1) they have a limited window for surgery and postoperative wound care; (2) they do not have the "privacy" or "facilities" or "personal" support to manage an open pilonidal wound that requires packing when they return to school; (3) they want minimal discomfort and the shortest recovery time. These patient criteria are the reason to offer this younger patient population and alternative to pilonidal cystectomy and secondary wound healing. They must be counseled about the "scarring" that remains post-VYAF because it is significant.

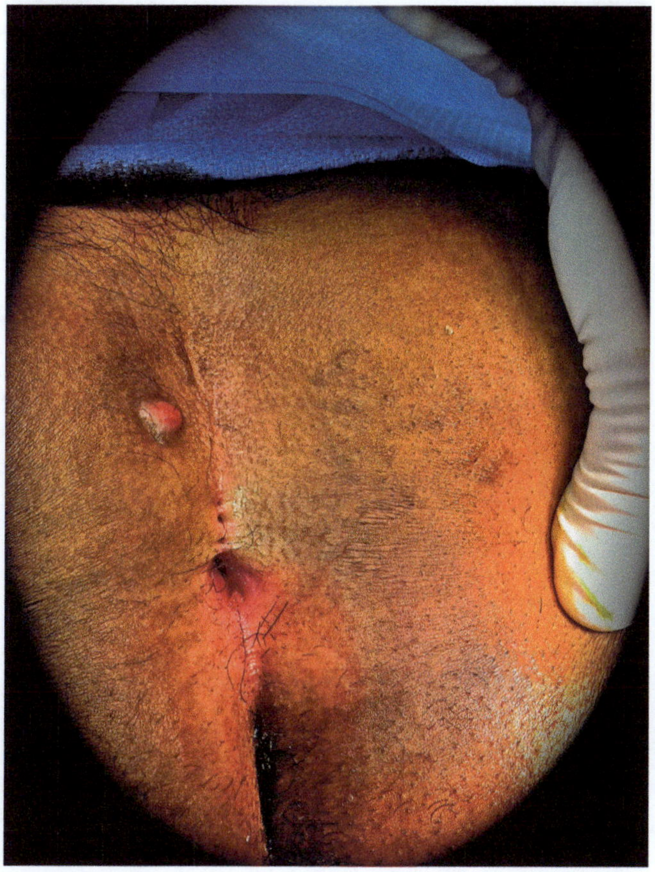

Fig. 24.2 Recurrent pilonidal disease with extensive midline tunneling and lateral tracts

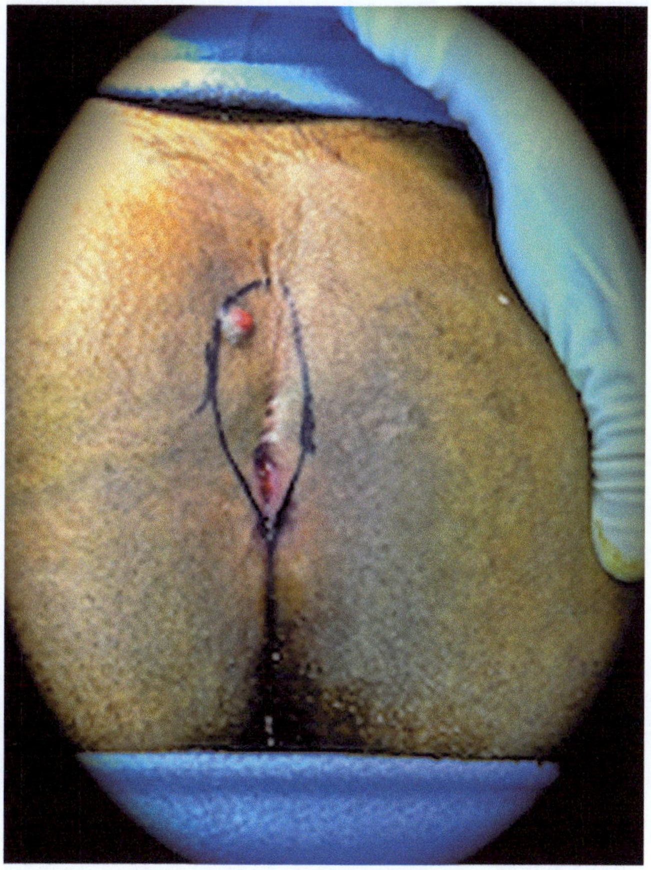

Fig. 24.3 Excision boundaries for recurrent pilonidal disease

A Case of Recurring Draining Sinuses

A 26-year-old male with a 10-year history of pilonidal disease presented with a previous incision and drainage of pilonidal abscesses and now with multiple residual draining pilonidal sinuses. My approach is to place all patients in the prone jackknife position and use general anesthesia with intravenous antibiotics (second- or third-generation cephalosporin). The gluteal cleft and gluteal areas are shaved bilaterally and prepped utilizing povidone. On examination, this patient has complex disease with multiple deep midline and lateral sinus tracts. I mark the excision site prior to beginning (Figs. 24.2 and 24.3).

An elliptical incision was performed with en bloc excision of all sinus tracts and scar, leaving a wound that is to the left of midline and down to the presacral fascia (Fig. 24.4). Although some surgeons prefer to keep the base of the ulcer in place, I feel this is a chronic wound and should be removed. The site for the V–Y advancement flap (VYAF) is marked and measured: 12 cm long and 10 cm wide (Fig. 24.5). The flap is dissected down to the level of the gluteal fascia, but not including the gluteal fascia. Then the medial and lateral portions of the flap are then dissected from the gluteal fascia leaving at least a 4–5 cm "vascular pedicle" (Figs. 24.6 and 24.7). It is important here not to cone in and ensure you are keeping your flap of equal and proper thickness to avoid any devascularized areas. Remember this will need to move, so adequate dissection and mobilization without compromising blood supply is key. With the vascular pedicle isolated, the VYAF can easily slide past the midline to allow for anchoring to the presacral fascia and to the contralateral wound margin, which is to the left of the midline. This will obliterate the infra-gluteal cleft and move the incision off of the midline to aid in healing (Figs. 24.8 and 24.9). Check the viability of the flap again. Ensure it is healthy at this stage or not under tension that you can still rather easily do something about. The margins of the wound and VYAF are approximated with subcuticular absorbable sutures and a "fluff" dressing is applied (Figs. 24.10, 24.11, and 24.12). I do not use drains, although some people like to use them to evacuate the fluid that may collect early on. The patient remains in the hospital for 24–48 h and is encouraged not to lie on their back and to sit up straight while sitting and eventually while driving. The patient is discharged and followed up in 10, 30, and 60 days postoperatively.

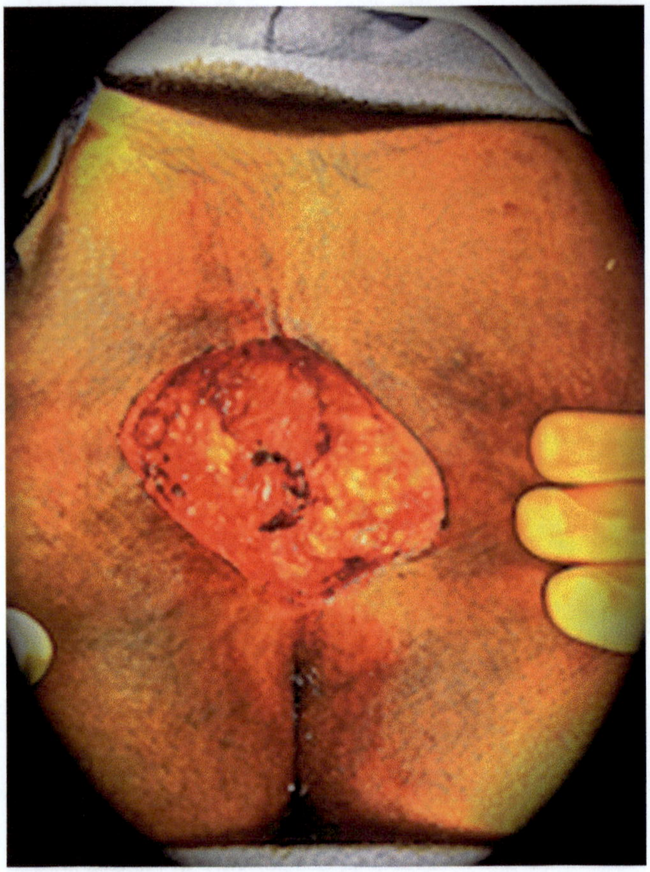

Fig. 24.4 Defect following excision of recurrent disease

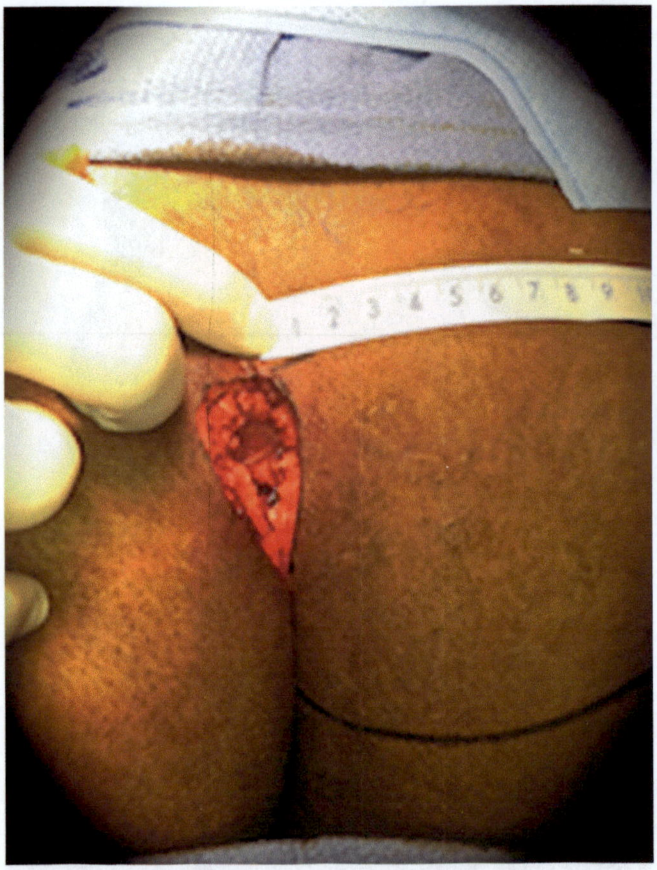

Fig. 24.5 Measuring out the dimensions for the V–Y advancement flap

Healing by Secondary Intention (Dr. Abcarian)

Key Concept: Healing by secondary intention has the benefit of lower recurrence rates but requires effort and time on both you and your patient for successful eventual healing.

Surgeons generally desire healing of all wounds in the earliest possible time. This is the basis of primary closure of all surgical wounds. The problem with pilonidal cyst closure by any surgical technique is its relatively high failure rate. Why do closures after pilonidal cystectomy fail? This conundrum has plagued surgeons throughout the years. In the pre-antibiotics era, Kleckner surveyed the then American Proctologic Society® in 1936 and found a recurrence rate of 33 % [12]. In 1977, Eftaiha and Abcarian reviewed all the available literature on the subject and reported a recurrence rate of 34 %. Conversely, excision of pilonidal cyst and allowing healing by secondary intention had a recurrence rate of 3 % [13]. So it seemed that all available surgical techniques of closure and use of antibiotics had made no significant reduction in recurrence rates.

In his 1963 textbook, Gabriel listed several criteria where he believed a pilonidal cystectomy wound should not be closed due to high failure rate. These included previous closures, free discharge of pus, hirsutism, secondary openings off the midline, and cysts greater than 7.5 cm (Fig. 24.13) [14]. Even now, it seems unlikely that wide excisions, undermining skin flaps and technically complicated plastic closure (Z-plasty, V–Y advancement flaps, etc.), will yield generally lasting results in the presence of the patient-/disease-related criteria spelled out by Gabriel decades ago.

Other causes of recurrence (and in many cases persistence) following both primary closure and healing by secondary intention of these wounds include (A) inadequate eradication of all the midline pits, which is the source of pilonidal infection. In the case illustrated in the earlier section of this chapter by Dr. Orangio, one can clearly see intact midline pits (Fig. 24.2, which should have been previously eradicated) in addition to midline draining abscess and secondary opening to the left of and posterior to the prior surgical incision. (B) The lateral (horizontal) tension on the intergluteal cleft with a longitudinal midline incision and closure that is essentially unavoidable. This mechanical factor must also play a role in the failure of flaps, even despite good mobilization. We can try to overcome this by instructing the patient to remain less active after a flap closure, but certainly absolute bed rest with the potential for deep vein thrombosis and life-threatening or lethal pulmonary embolism must be

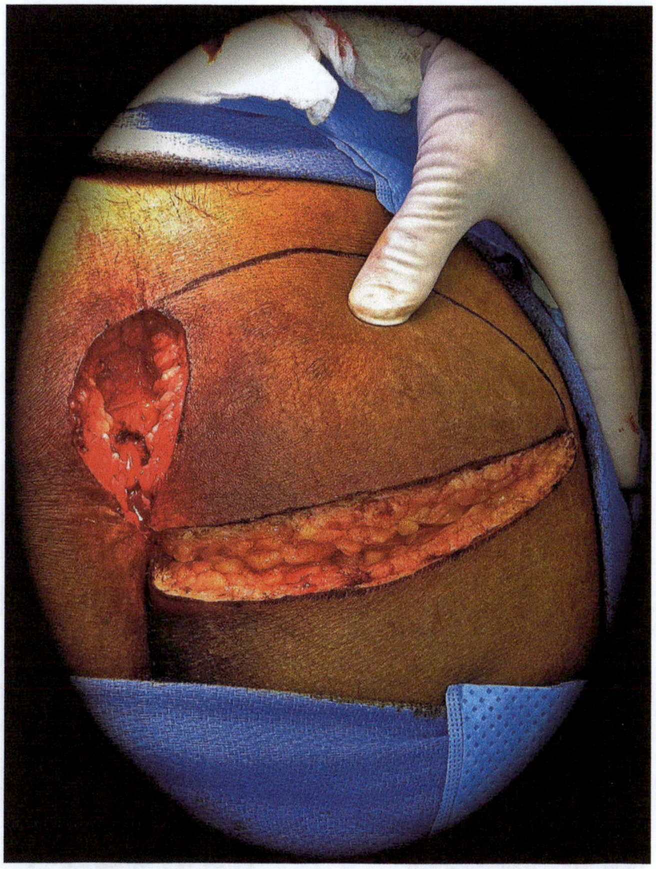

Fig. 24.6 Constructing the V–Y pedicle

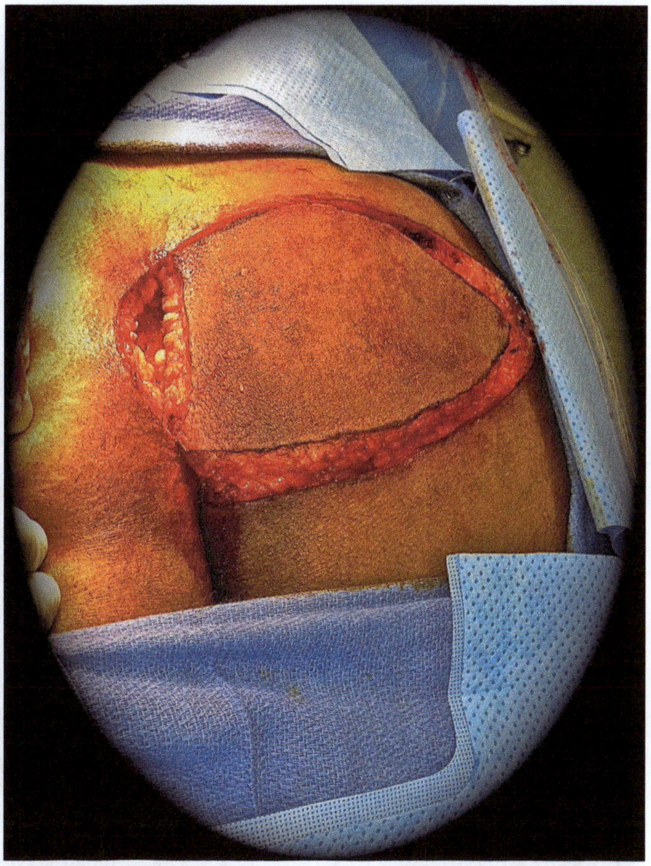

Fig. 24.7 Completed well-vascularized pedicle. Note the thickness of the pedicle

condemned. (C) The wide and deep dissection of tissues required for both excision and construction of flaps in the presence of infection that increases the risk of failure secondary to localized sepsis. This unfortunately cannot be overcome by a short course of broad-spectrum antibiotics. In fact, prolonged use of these antibiotics predisposes to an ever-increasing incidence of antibiotic-related complications such as *Clostridium difficile* colitis. (D) Finally, obesity makes the management and care of the open wound difficult.

So what is wrong with leaving the wound open after pilonidal cystectomy? These wounds, irrespective of size, cause very little pain and disability, and I have found it generally easy to care for (bathing and packing a coarse 4×4 gauze to separate the edge and keep the wound dry). Changing of the gauze three to four times daily will debride the open wound and prevent collection of infected discharge in the cleft. I've found that the best way to dry the wound after bathing is the use of a hair dryer on the cool setting. The anatomic distance of these wounds from the anus allows for painless bowel movements, and patients are uniformly happier than those having undergone excisional hemorrhoidectomy.

In many cases the correct operation has been done. The cyst is completely excised without deepening the excision down to the sacrococcygeal fascia. A small 3×4 cm cyst excised in total will leave a 4×5 cm defect, while carrying the excision down to the fascia opens up and expands the wound by 50–100 % of the original size [13]. In some cases there are lateral tracts or pockets of disease that may require additional excision; however, these can often close just fine with secondary intention (Figs. 24.14, 24.15, and 24.16).

Open wounds begin the "picture frame" shrinkage 2 weeks postoperatively and will need to be inspected on regular biweekly basis. The surgeon must take time to shave all edges of the open wound to prevent growth of hair into the wound during the healing process (Fig. 24.17). Also as the wound becomes shallower, the dressing gauze must be inserted into the wound to prevent patchy adherence of the wound edges. This is easy to instruct the patient because the only painful area is the skin surrounding the defect and not the depth of the wound. Small wounds ~3×4 cm typically heal in 4–6 weeks, while larger ones such as 4×6 cm may need up to 8–10 weeks for complete healing. Application of antibiotics, astringents, or anesthetic ointments is not helpful and may actually contribute to maceration of the wound by adding moisture.

In 1977 Rosenberg recommended reverse taping to pull the wound edges laterally and flatten the deep wound in very obese patients [15]. Although logically sound, it is difficult

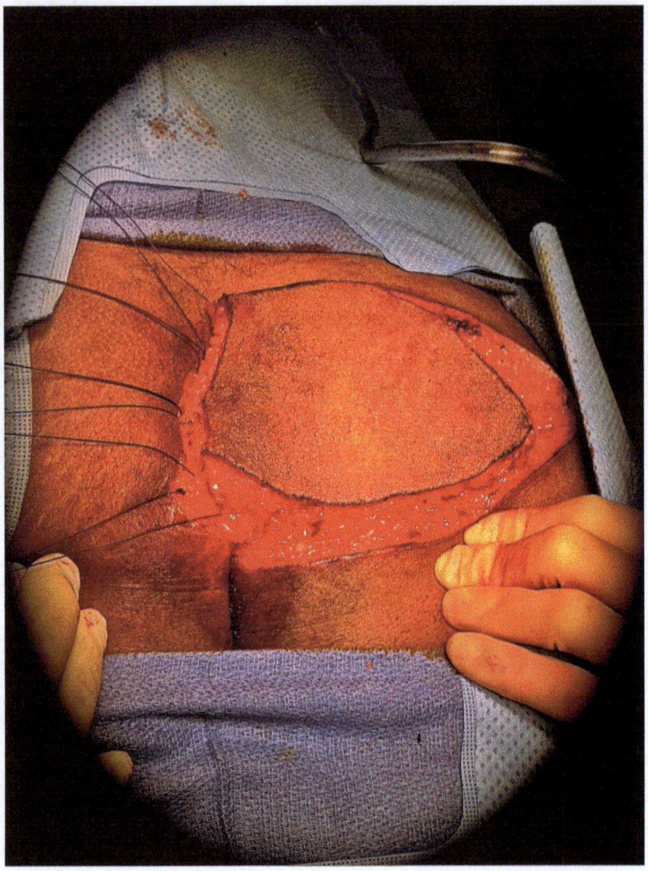

Fig. 24.8 Anchoring sutures in place

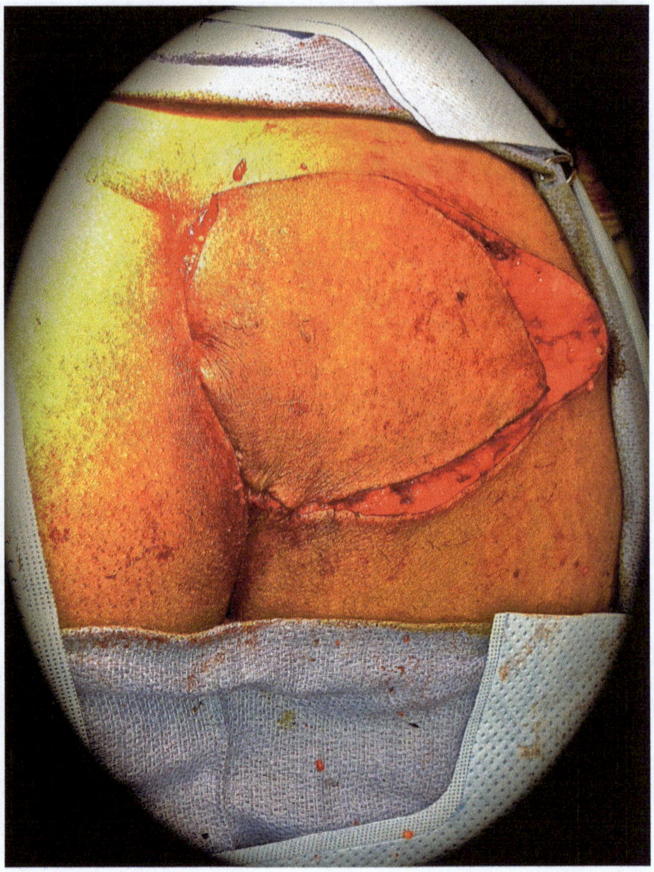

Fig. 24.9 Pedicle able to slide past the midline to obliterate the cleft

for the patient to tolerate the constant pulling sensation and interference of reverse taping with ambulation and daily activities. The current use of wound VAC® (LifeCell, New Jersey) has essentially made this technique obsolete. Yet, wound VACs are also cumbersome and need nursing or wound care professionals to change the foam pads at least every 48–72 h (especially in that location). Despite these drawbacks, with utilization of portable suction machines, this has allowed the patient to be able to ambulate and even return to work (Figs. 24.18 and 24.19).

In my opinion, the success rate of flaps represented in the literature is simply unbelievable (e.g., 100 % success rate of Limberg flaps in 102 patients presented by Urhan) [6]. In addition, the reported complication rates of V–Y-plasty are clearly unacceptable. If followed carefully and long enough, the 9.3 % infection rate and 7 % hematoma will inevitably grow with the number of recurrence/persistence of the disease [6].

My Approach (Dr. Abcarian)

If the purpose of the treatment of pilonidal sinus is an early return to duty (i.e., front line such as in the armed forces), I believe the Karydakis technique used on young military personnel offers the least complicated and most satisfactory procedure with low recurrence rate [5]. If not, I leave all pilonidal cystectomy wounds open, see the patient every 2 weeks, and shave the wound. Once healed, I recommend using depilatory cream to prevent hair growth in the vicinity of the healed wound once a month for an entire year. This plan has resulted in healing of an overwhelming majority of recurrent pilonidal cyst patients that have been referred to me throughout the years. I believe in the wisdom of Gabriel and his admonition of primary closure in infected, hairy, recurrent pilonidal with side branching to secondary openings off midline. I would only add obesity to his list.

Point: Counterpoint

Key Concept: There are many ways to approach the same disease process. You need to have a sound rationale behind what you do and never stop listening to (and learning from) other people's opinions and experiences.

Dr. Abcarian and Dr. Orangio

1. *Dr. Abcarian it appears that you essentially only utilize "healing by secondary intention" of pilonidal cystectomy wounds?*

   Abcarian: That is correct.

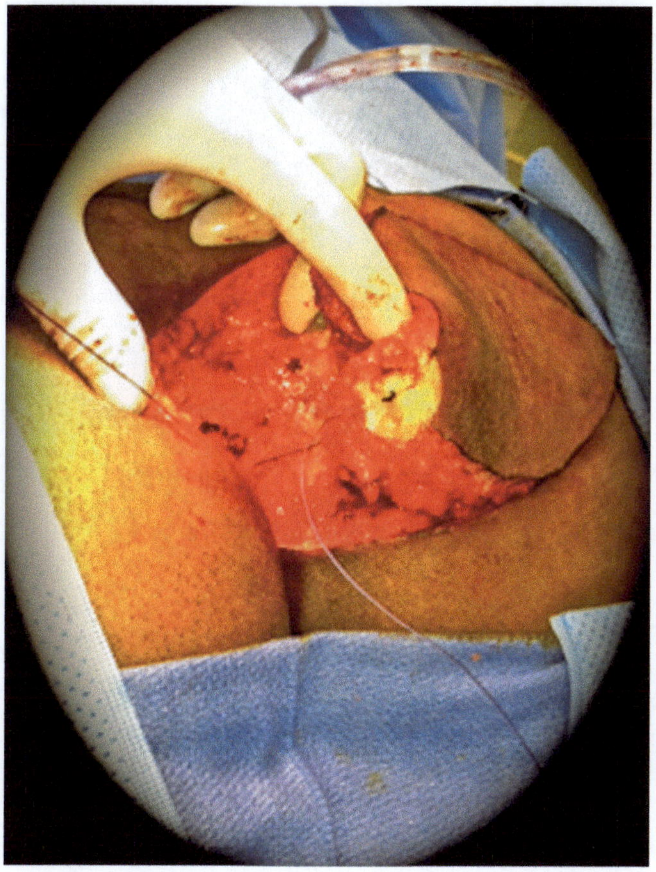

Fig. 24.10 Deep and subcuticular sutures in place on the flap

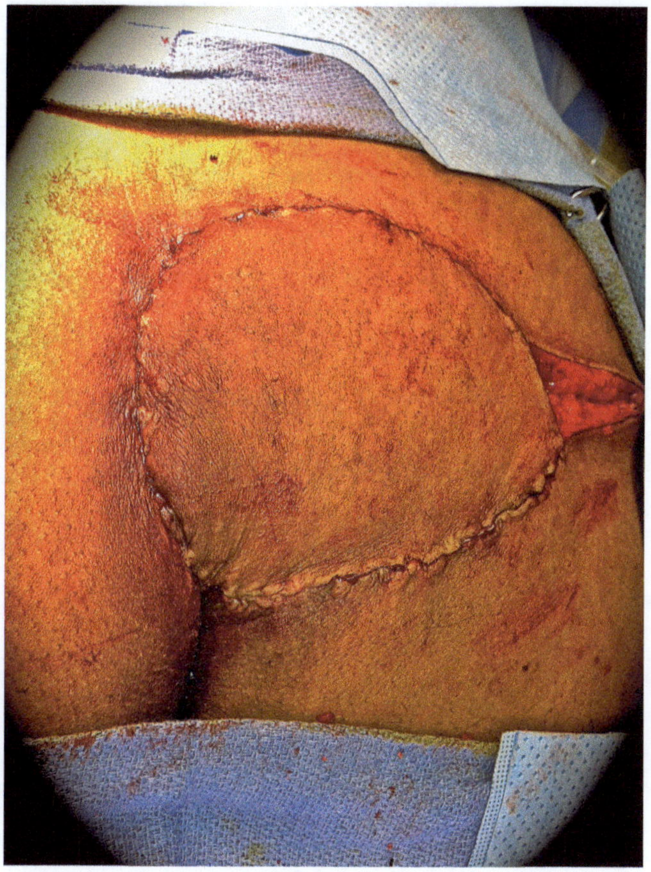

Fig. 24.11 Pedicle sutured in place leaving only the lateral defect

2. *I (Dr. Orangio) feel that for a subpopulation of patients with pilonidal disease who have failed "healing by secondary intention" or have recurrent pilonidal disease, the utilization of fasciocutaneous flaps should be included in the surgeon's armamentarium of options. The literature is quite supportive of this approach. Why do you disagree?*

   Abcarian: I have taken care of too many failed fasciocutaneous flaps in my 40 years of practice, and these are literally nightmares.

3. *Would you agree with me that recurrent pilonidal disease is secondary to inadequate primary excision?*

   Abcarian: In some cases yes, in others it is inadequate postoperative wound care by the patient and the surgeon.

4. *Why do you think that some patients have prolonged healing or even "nonhealing?" Do you feel this is because of poor compliance by the patient or not enough postoperative care by the primary surgeon?*

   Abcarian: Both. Some patients simply refuse instructions for home care (i.e., showering, shaving, and packing). Then there are surgeons who give a first postoperative appointment for 6 weeks after surgery.

5. *How do you manage the patient with a "nonhealing" wound, and at what point do you consider the process of healing with secondary intention a failure?*

   Abcarian: As long as the wound keeps getting smaller, the edges are shaved, and there is no patchy healing, I continue to examine and treat the wounds every 2 weeks.

6. *You mention Gabriel's textbook of 1963 discusses reasons for not utilizing a primary closure and tries to postulate that for those reasons fasciocutaneous flaps should not be used. Do you believe this is a valid criticism?*

   Abcarian: Hirsutism, recurrence after primary closure, cysts longer than 7.5 cm, side branching, and worse yet active discharge of pus—all should discourage anyone from a plastic closure of pilonidal wounds using flaps, whatever kind of flaps.

7. *In one section you seem to advocate the use of negative pressure wound dressing (VAC), could you explain to me why you would support this method over the utilization of any fasciocutaneous flaps?*

   Abcarian: Some deep wounds in obese patients are difficult to pack at home. It is possible though to place a VAC for3–4 weeks, allow the wound to shrink, and then care for it without need for VAC therapy. If VAC treatment fails, the patient is no worse off. One cannot say the same for failed fasciocutaneous flaps.

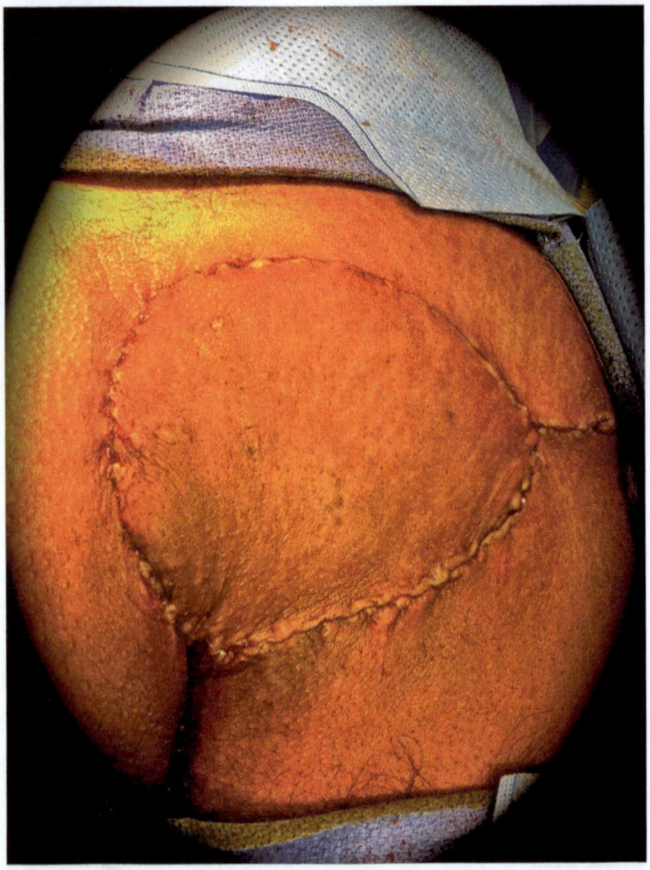

Fig. 24.12 Completed pedicle

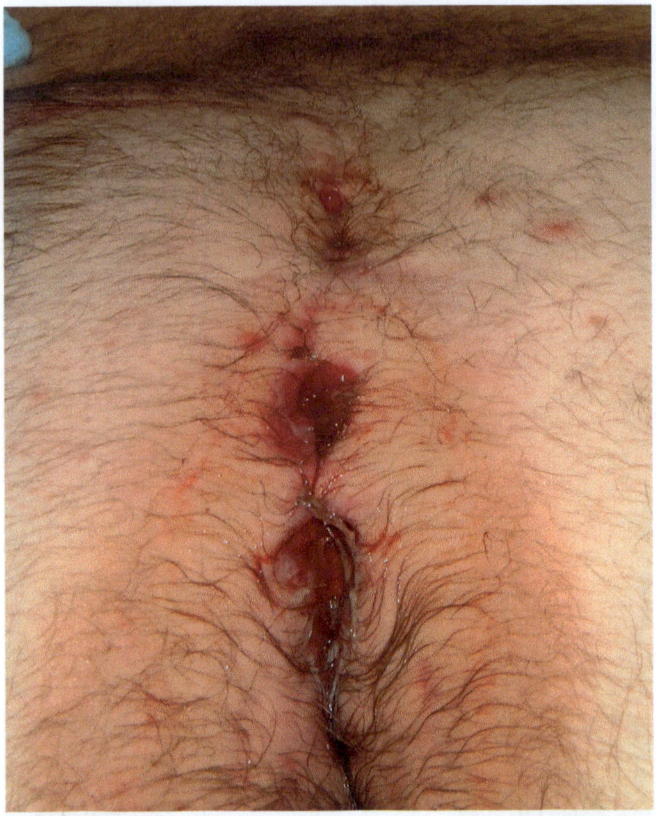

Fig. 24.13 Extensive pilonidal disease in a patient with multiple risk factors for recurrence

8. *Under what circumstances would you agree with myocutaneous flaps in pilonidal disease? There is some literature that does support its utilization in pilonidal disease.*

   Abcarian: Surgeons are creatures of habit. I do what has worked for me in 40 years of practice, which has included caring for many, many failed flaps of all kinds.
9. *Any closing comments about pilonidal wound management?*

   Abcarian: One is hard pressed to find an awful lot of downside with the excision of pilonidal cyst and allowing the wound to heal by secondary intention—except for the time it takes to heal. Having had a personal disastrous postoperative course with primary closure and the need for two additional operations to get this "simple" problem to heal taught me a valuable lesson. "Do not do onto others…."

   Thank you Dr. Abcarian

Management of the Perineal Wound

Key Concept: Perineal wound complications after abdominoperineal resection (APR) for low rectal cancer (LRC), anal canal cancer (ACC), and proctocolectomy (PC) for inflammatory bowel disease (IBD), especially Crohn's' Disease (CD), are a major cause of postoperative morbidity and mortality. Yet the disease process will often dictate your approach. Therefore, you need to have a stepwise approach that may utilize a multidisciplinary team to ensure adequate healing and avoid this complication, when possible.

Disease Process

Low Rectal Cancer and Anal Canal Cancer

Key Concept: These typically are large defects that often are not amenable to re-approximation and may require a multidisciplinary approach for closure.

In the era of multimodality therapy for anal canal cancer (ACC) and neoadjuvant therapy for low rectal cancer (LRC), the incidence of perineal wound complications has increased dramatically [16–18]. Both patient populations are given "sensitizing" doses of chemotherapy along with over 5,000 cGy of radiation for over 6 weeks and then subjected to APR. It should not be surprising to us that wound complications may result. In this cohort, primary closure of perineal wounds leads to postoperative wound complication in 10–40 % and up to as high as 80 % in patients who have failed primary chemoradiation for ACC and gone onto a

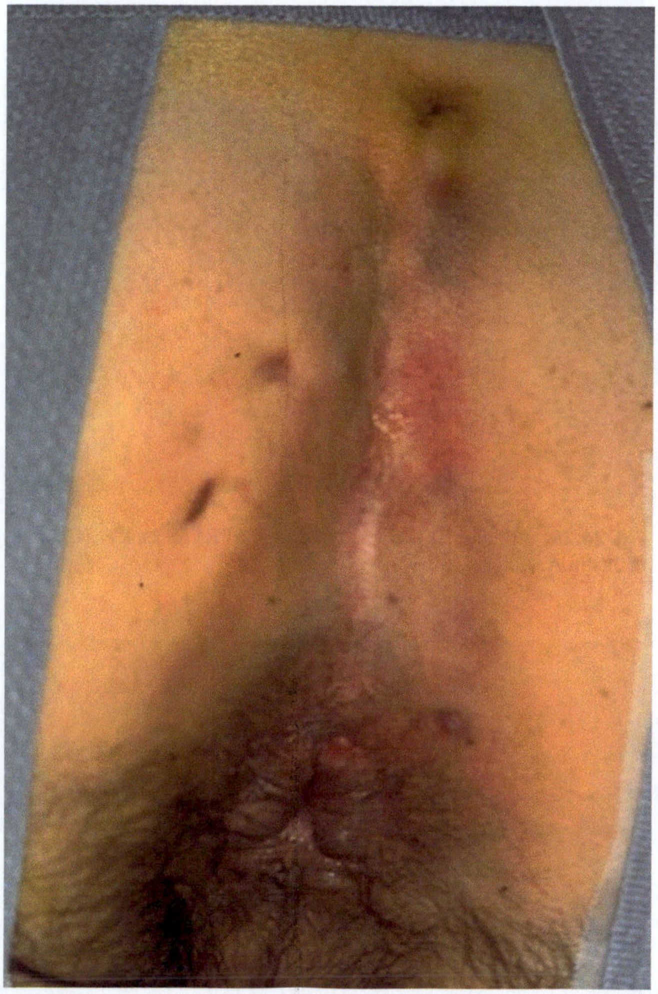

Fig. 24.14 Recurrent pilonidal disease (Courtesy of W. Brian Sweeney, MD)

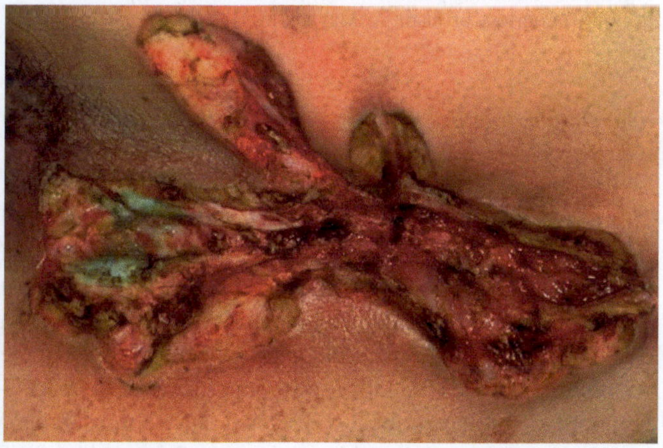

Fig. 24.15 Resulting wound after excision (Courtesy of W. Brian Sweeney, MD)

salvage APR [19, 20]. In either patient population, with extensive perineal disease or with vaginal/or vulvar involvement, they will require wider en bloc resections or even

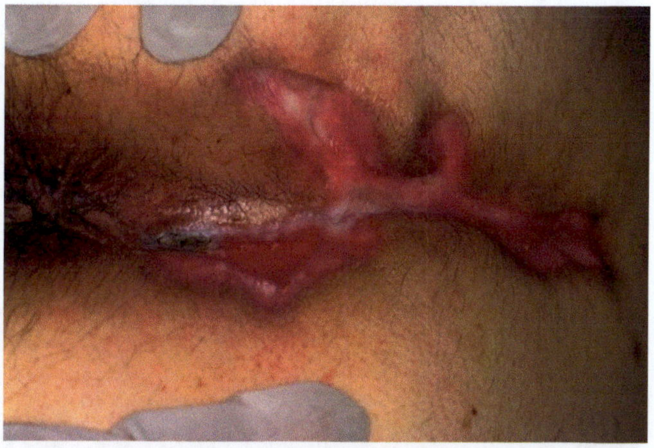

Fig. 24.16 Wound after near-complete closure with secondary intention (Courtesy of W. Brian Sweeney, MD)

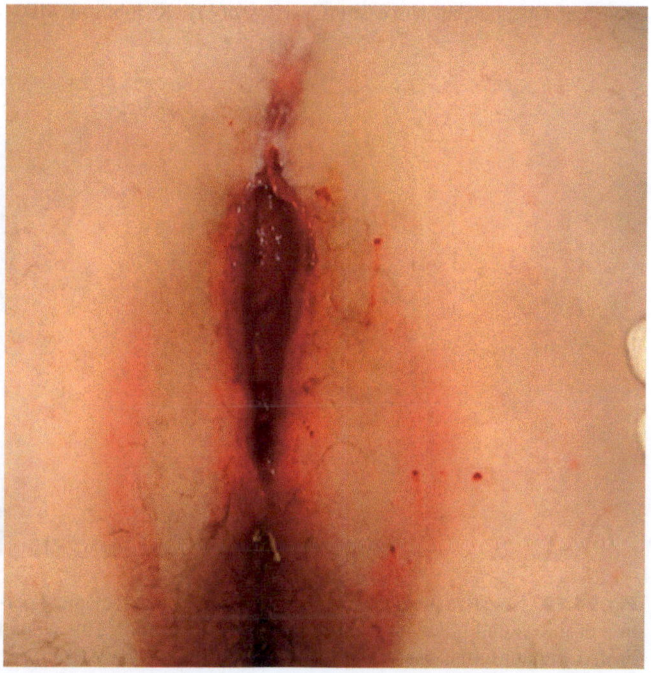

Fig. 24.17 The shaved wound after excision of the pilonidal disease

pelvic exenteration (Fig. 24.20). This population usually cannot have primary closure of the perineal wound.

The conduct of the APR is consistent for LRC and failed or recurrent ACC; the patient is in the modified perineal lithotomy position using adjustable stirrups. The abdominal portion (whether with laparotomy or laparoscopically) is conducted with meticulous dissection including high ligation of the major vessels (inferior mesenteric artery/vein), wide pelvic dissection of the rectum, and total mesorectal excision (TME). If able, I will use an omental interposition flap to fill the pelvis. The perineal portion can either be performed synchronously (my preference) or following repositioning in the prone position (Fig. 24.21). In either case, this involves wide

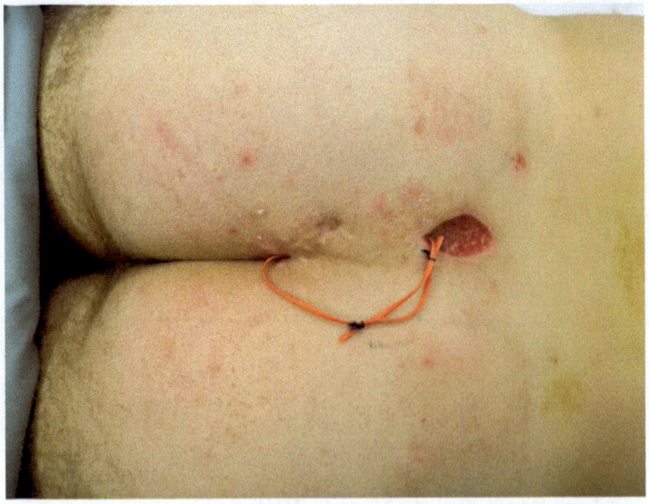

Fig. 24.18 Nonhealing pilonidal wound. Seton placed initially due to recurrent subcutaneous abscesses (Courtesy of Eric K. Johnson, MD)

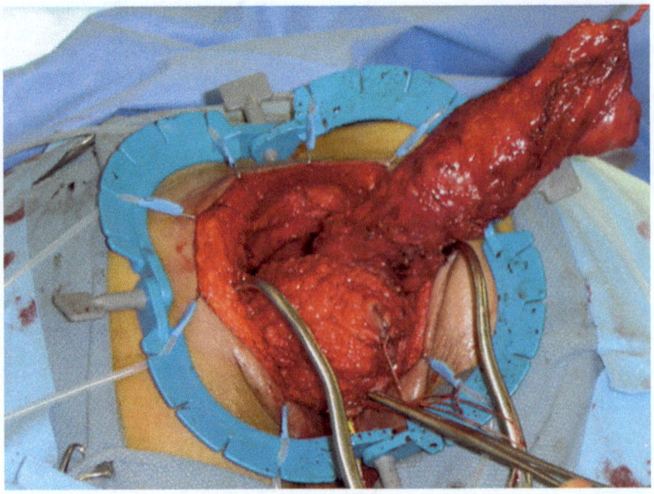

Fig. 24.20 Abdominal perineal resection (APR) for cancer (Courtesy of Justin A. Maykel, MD)

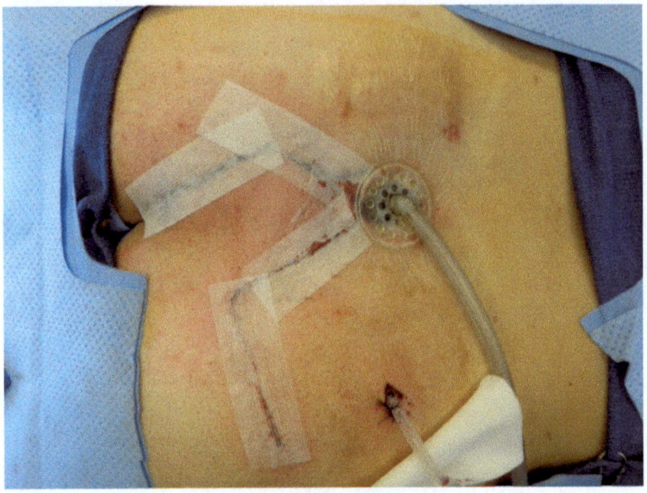

Fig. 24.19 Negative pressure suction device in place in the apical portion of the wound following nonhealing with flap closure. This wound healed without further incident (Courtesy of Eric K. Johnson, MD)

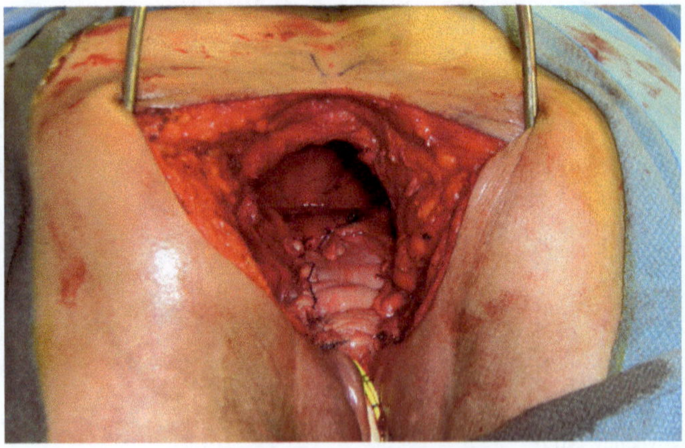

Fig. 24.21 Resulting perineal defect demonstrating the posterior vaginectomy (Courtesy of Justin A. Maykel, MD)

excision of the pelvic floor, detachment of the levator muscles from their bony attachments, and loose approximation of skin and subcutaneous tissue using interrupted absorbable sutures [17, 21, 22]. In select cases, a multidisciplinary approach (especially plastic surgery) will be required to aid in the construction of flaps for final pelvic floor reconstruction (Fig. 24.22). Drains, if needed, can be placed from the transabdominal or transperineal approach. With this method, the technical goal is to attempt primary closure of the perineal wound with undue tension and the least amount of morbidity.

Inflammatory Bowel Disease (IBD)

Key Concept: The extent of the inflammation (especially with CD) will determine your extent of resection. Preserve muscle and surrounding tissue, when possible, to aid in achieving a well-vascularized, tension-free closure.

Patients with either ulcerative colitis (UC) or Crohn's Disease (CD) who require proctocolectomy (PC) and end ileostomy have been a technical challenge and conundrum to surgeons for decades. The management of the perineal wound has been especially problematic for both the surgeon and the patient alike. The options have been (1) to leave the wound open and pack, with or without closure of the peritoneum; (2) close the perineal wound and place a transabdominal drain, again with or without closure of the peritoneum; and (3) perform an intersphincteric proctectomy to help preserve some of the surrounding muscle and tissue to aid in wound healing [23–28]. One of the most significant technical advancements has been the endoanal proctectomy [29, 30]. In 1977, Abcarian discussed that in patients with CD and the "watering can" anus composed of several fistulas,

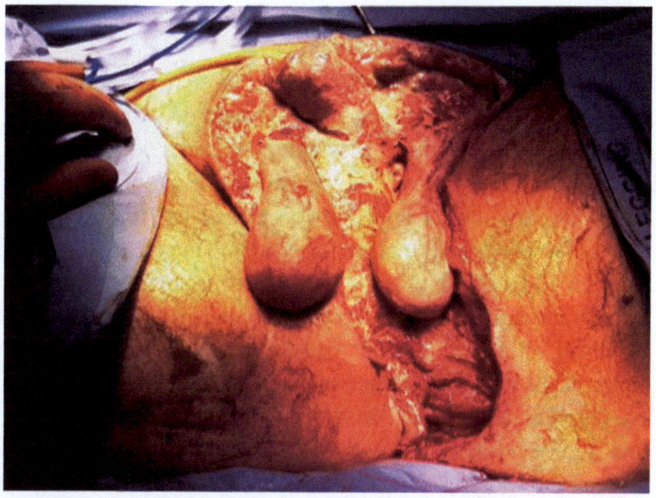

Fig. 24.22 Fournier's gangrene (Courtesy of W. Brian Sweeney, MD)

the extent of the APR was determined by the extent of the perianal disease and the overall activity of the disease [23, 24]. Abcarian advocated the endoanal proctectomy, with "coring out" of the fistula tracts to reduce the size of the excision. The recommendation of performing a two-stage procedure, whereby a total colectomy with ostomy is initially performed, and following a period to allow the perineal disease to "quiet down" return for the completion proctectomy, has shown conflicting results [25, 28]. On one hand, the overall healing of perineal wounds in patients with CD at 1 year is approximately 30 %. Contrast this in UC patients at 1 year, where it is ~89 %, and you can see how CD can be so challenging [24, 28]. The authors agree that in patients with CD who require a proctectomy, you should first determine the extent of active disease. If there is negligible disease with no active infection, an endoanal proctectomy and closure of the wound (with or without closure of the skin) is an acceptable approach. If there is active disease with active infection including draining fistulas, a more conservative approach to the perineal wound is appropriate. This may involve packing or placement of a negative pressure vacuum device.

We also agree that in patients with large superficial wounds resulting from excision of extensive bilateral hidradenitis suppurativa or post-wide debridement for synergistic bacterial infections (i.e., Fournier's gangrene, Fig. 24.22), these seldom result in nonhealing wounds. In both instances, the anal sphincters remain intact, and there is essentially no midline wound with constant lateral traction forces to contribute to nonhealing. In this case, grafting may be required due to the extent of debridement of the subcutaneous tissue and skin; however, there is typically no large perineal defect. This is in contrast with the post-APR (LRC/ACC) midline wound, which is often closed without any support from deeper tissues to anchor the closure.

Management of the Nonhealing Chronic Perineal Wounds

Key Concept: *Proper preoperative counseling regarding the possibility of chronic wound issues and early involvement of the wound care team are helpful in the management of these nonhealing perineal wounds.*

No matter the underlying disease that could be discussed regarding the complications of "failed" perineal wound—whether it is a wound infection, delayed healing >6 months, reoperation, dehiscence, abscess, ulcer, chronic sinus, or perineal hernia—they are all problems colorectal surgeons will face over their careers. Uniting them all, the management of any one of these complications is challenging and frustrating to everyone involved. The acute complications of infection, reoperation, dehiscence, or abscess formation are problems we have all dealt with likely several times and may require a multidisciplinary approach to their management. During the preoperative consultation regarding an abdominal or pelvic operation, the patient should understand not only about the potential for ostomy but also about the possibility of perineal wound complications. We often highlight that early involvement of the wound ostomy nursing (WON) team is invaluable to assist a patient in a life with an ostomy; however, we should also be utilizing their same early involvement for the management of the nonhealing perineal wound.

When approaching these wounds, my recommendation is you should take into consideration the following: disease process, work-up, and nonoperative therapy and operative therapy.

Disease Process

Key Concept: *Search for an underlying cause related to the patient's disease process to help guide your approach to figuring out why the wound won't heal.*

When confronted with the chronic open perineal wound (COPW), it is important to perform a few basic investigations. Post-APR for cancer, you should review their most recent CT or PET scan to ensure there is no recurrent disease. If negative, an examination under anesthesia with multiple biopsies to rule out recurrent cancer, in addition to cultures to assess the types of bacteria that have colonized the wound, should be performed. With the emergence of certain strains of virulent bacteria (i.e., VRE, MRSA), you may need to institute a prolonged course of directed antibiotic therapy prior to reconstruction. In patients with CD, you should also perform an examination under anesthesia and/or endoscopy to assess the underlying disease activity, and rule out presence of an abscess or fistula (from colon, small bowel, bladder, or vagina) to the perineum that could be causing persistent drainage resulting in chronic perineal "moisture" and chronic infection. Finally, occasionally retained rectal mucosa after a difficult pelvic dissection in either UC or CD will perpetuate purulent drainage and non healing. This will need to be removed.

Nonoperative Treatment

Key Concept: You do not always need to perform aggressive surgical revisions and flaps for chronic wounds. Sometimes you can start with the nonoperative "easy" things that may lead to closure.

Several tips are worth noting prior to going to the operating room. Aggressive debridement (chemical cauterization, wet-to-dry dressings, etc.) is important to remove all granulation tissue. Look also for retained foreign material (i.e., suture) that may be the source of a chronic wound. If there is an active fistula that must be addressed prior to any perineal reconstruction, especially in patients with CD, institute the appropriate directed medication or even surgical therapy to provide adequate closure or drainage. As stated previously, consider utilization of negative pressure wound care (NPWC/VAC) in patients with open perineal wounds for both the acute and chronic settings [31]. I (*GO*) have utilized these devices even during the acute phase, with open perineal wounds and extensive infection; though I agree with Dr. Abcarian that it is very difficult to "keep" a vacuum seal in this area. If your patient is immobile or has extensive pain with vacuum device dressing changes, consider the operating room or recovery unit with conscious sedation to allow for careful inspection of the wound and dressing change. I must admit that I have been impressed with the early results when utilized in a contaminated perineal wound. Remember that the patient is at higher risk of other complications because of their immobility, whether it is pneumonia, deep vein thrombosis, or pulmonary embolus, and should have the proper prophylaxis. I will also limit my utilization of the VAC wound therapy to 5–7 days. I have no experience with long-term home usage of this type of wound therapy for chronic perineal wounds; however, there is some literature that recommends utilization of VAC therapy following APR for cancer or pelvic exenteration [32]. Finally, only to mention the use of hyperbaric oxygen therapy, it has not shown any statistically significant benefit in the management of chronic perineal wounds in patients with CD [33], but I have little personal experience.

Operative Management

Key Concept: Anticipate the possibility of large perineal wounds occurring and get a multidisciplinary team available well in advance. It is better to not need them at all than to find yourself in a situation where you cannot close the wound and have not properly prepared.

In patients with a COPW, operative debridement of all granulation and scar tissue must be excised to the level of bleeding tissue. In some cases you may find a deep presacral infected space or sinus, and it has been resistant to conventional therapy, and a coccygectomy may be required. This will allow the tissue to collapse into the sinus tract or defect in order to facilitate closure. The use of myocutaneous flaps in both the acute and the chronic perineal wounds has led to a multidisciplinary approach to these patients: the primary surgeon, plastic reconstructive surgeon, and wound ostomy nurses. You need to each understand the other's role to ensure you do not "stray" into problems (i.e., too wide excision and understand the flap boundaries). Plastic surgery will usually mark the patient prior to the surgery, which will aid in avoiding this error. The three most common myocutaneous flaps utilized are the vertical rectus abdominis flap (VRAM), gracilis muscle flaps (GM), and the inferior gluteal artery flap (IGAF) [34–38]. These myocutaneous flaps have been associated with a reduced length of hospital stay and a low perineal wound complication rate [34–37]. Unfortunately the VRAM flap has not been shown to be suitable for laparoscopic APR, with a failure rate of 2–10 % and overall complication rates of 15–22 % [39, 40].

Most surgeons can predict in advance a large wound at completion of major operations and the need for "coverage." Female patients with extensive perineal disease involving the posterior vagina and/or the vulva and who had neoadjuvant therapy for LRC or patients with ACC who failed therapy or developed recurrent disease and an APR with posterior vaginectomy with or without vulvectomy are candidates for myocutaneous flaps at the initial surgery (Fig. 24.23). Many

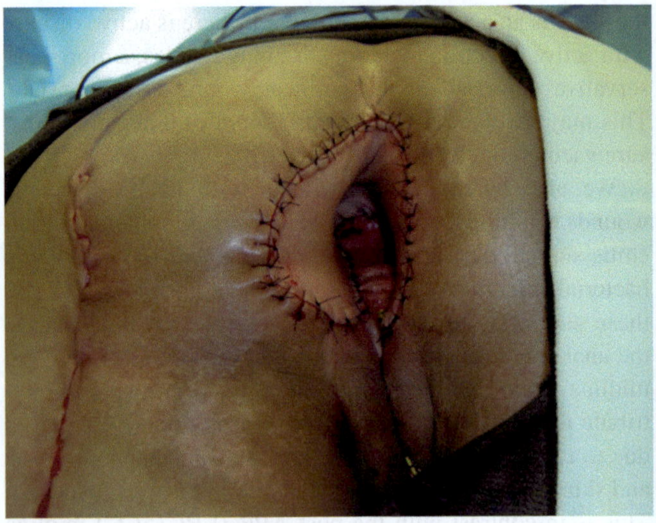

Fig. 24.23 Perineal reconstruction with a multidisciplinary approach (Courtesy of Justin A. Maykel, MD)

women will desire vaginal reconstruction because of the desire to remain sexually active postoperatively, and plastic surgery will be critical in helping plan this out accordingly.

In the situation when an APR is combined with a posterior vaginectomy, there is a residual wound that has been radiated, but reconstruction is still desired. The gracilis myocutaneous flap is especially suitable for this type of reconstruction. The well-vascularized muscle is placed in the defect, and the overlying vaginal mucosa and skin are tailored and sutured in place to form the posterior vaginal wall. In morbidly obese women with very deep, wide perineal wounds, bilateral gracilis myocutaneous flaps may also be utilized. Of note, the same flap may be used in a male patient by transferring the gracilis muscle to fill the defect and the attached skin to close the cutaneous defect.

Depending on size (both depth and width), location, and complexity of the perineal wound, it is occasionally possible to use omental pedicle flaps in combination with gracilis muscle or myocutaneous flaps: gluteus maximus or VRAM flaps. Using the VRAM flap requires a well-vascularized rectus abdominis, and it is important that one rectus muscle is kept intact and you do not utilize both rectus muscles. In general, one side is usually a site for the stoma. For example, if a patient had a diverting colostomy in the LLQ and subsequently a coloanal pull-through procedure (coloanal anastomosis) is done, this typically requires a proximal stoma to protect the anastomosis. You should then ensure that the ileostomy is brought out through the LLQ site in order to maintain the vascularity of the right rectus abdominis muscle.

In the case of a pelvic exenteration needing VRAM flap for perineal wounds, both the colostomy and urostomy should be placed on the left side and maintain the right rectus intact for VRAM flap. We (*GO/HA*) both agree about the increased possibility of a peristomal hernia and the need to relocate the ostomy to the contralateral side or same side along the rectus abdominis, if needed. However, with the advent of biologic material, there is less concern regarding inability to close the abdomen or repair peristomal hernias.

Finally, it is important to note that if the muscle transfer procedures fail, the result will inevitably be a larger wound that typically requires prolonged wound care. In many cases, this often means reverting back to wet-to-dry dressings or negative pressure therapy. You should remember, however, that long before wound VAC therapy and the multidisciplinary closures came into play, Dr. Abcarian reported on perianal wound healing after proctectomy and proctocolectomy. Large wounds left open using wet-to-dry dressing healed in 12–16 weeks in almost all cases [25]. So a visit to "back to the future" may be required if all else fails.

For smaller nonhealing chronic perineal wounds, and those associated with anal stenosis or other perianal processes, a sliding flap anoplasty may be required for healing (Video 24.1). Results are generally good, though care is needed to avoid one that is superficial, poorly mobilized, narrow based, and has inadequate blood supply. This is doomed to fail from the beginning and will simply leave you with a more complex wound than you or your patient will care for and one that is extremely difficult to manage.

Summary Pearls

There is no doubt that you will be faced with this unfortunate situation of dealing with chronic nonhealing pilonidal and perineal wounds if you are practicing colorectal surgery long enough. Hopefully the tips and tricks we talked about here will be useful and also point out that there are different approaches to these wounds. Have realistic expectations, and ensure your patients and their families do as well. Most importantly, do not keep trying the same thing over and over again if it is failing. Never miss out on an opportunity to talk with someone else or have another colleague examine the patient when things are not going well. You likely will be glad you did.

References

1. Dwight RW, Maloy JK. Pilonidal sinus; experience with 449 cases. N Engl J Med. 1953;249(23):926–30.
2. Mayo OH. Observations on injuries and disease of rectum. London: Burgess and Hill; 1833. p. 45–6 (Quoted from da Silva JH. Pilonidal cyst: cause and treatment. Dis Colon Rectum 2000;43:1146–56).
3. Hodge RM. Pilonidal sinus. Boston Med Surg J. 1880;103:485–6 (Quoted from da Silva JH. Pilonidal cyst: cause and treatment. Dis Colon Rectum. 2000;43:1146–56).
4. Karydakis GE. New approach to the problem of pilonidal sinus. Lancet. 1973;2(7843):1414–5.
5. Karydakis GE. Easy and successful treatment of pilonidal sinus after explanation of its causative process. Aust N Z J Surg. 1992;62(5):45–7.
6. Urhan MK, Kucukel F, Topgul K, Ozer I, Sari S. Rhomboid excision and Limberg flap for managing pilonidal sinus: results of 102 cases. Dis Colon Rectum. 2002;45(5):656–9.
7. Bascom J, Bascom T. Failed pilonidal surgery-new paradigm and new operation leading to cures. Arch Surg. 2002;137:114650.
8. Vijay P, Khatri MD, Espinosa MD, Amin AK. Management of recurrent pilonidal sinus by simple V-Y fasciocutaneous flap. Dis Colon Rectum. 1994;37:1232–5.
9. Eryilmaz R, Okan I, Coskun A, Bas G, Sahim M. Surgical treatment of complicated pilonidal sinus with a fasciocutaneous V-Y advancement flap. Dis Colon Rectum. 2009;52(12):2036–40.
10. Fazeli MS, Adel MG, Lebaschi AH. Comparison of outcomes in Z-plasty and delayed healing by secondary intention of the wound after excision of sacral pilonidal sinus: results of a randomized, clinical trial. Dis Colon Rectum. 2006;49:1831–6.
11. Perez-Gurri JA, Temple WJ, Ketcham AS. Gluteus maximus myocutaneous flap for the treatment of recalcitrant pilonidal disease. Dis Colon Rectum. 1984;47:262–4.
12. Kleckner MS. Pilonidal sinus: its surgical management. Trans Am Proctol Soc. 1936;36:166.
13. Eftaiha M, Abcarian H. The dilemma of pilonidal disease: surgical treatment. Dis Colon Rectum. 1977;20(4):279–96.

14. Gabriel WB. The principles and practice of rectal surgery. Springfield: Thomas; 1948.
15. Rosenberg L. The dilemma of pilonidal disease: reverse bandaging for cure of reluctant pilonidal wound. Dis Colon Rectum. 1977;20(4):290–1.
16. Bullard KM, Trudel JL, Baxter NN, Rothenberger DA. Primary perineal wound closure after preoperative radiotherapy and abdominoperineal resection has a high incidence of wound failure. Dis Colon Rectum. 2005;48:438–43.
17. Gazzaz GE, Kiran RP, Lavery I. Wound complications in rectal cancer patients undergoing primary closure of the perineal wound after abdominoperineal resection. Dis Colon Rectum. 2009;52: 1962–6.
18. Christian CK, Kwaan MR, Betensky RA, Breen EM, Zinner MJ, Bleday R. Risk factors for perineal wound complications following abdominoperineal resection. Dis Colon Rectum. 2005;48:43–8.
19. Nilsson PJ, Svensson C, Goldman S, Glimelius B. Salvage abdominoperineal resection in anal epidermoid cancer. Br J Surg. 2002; 89:1425–9.
20. Papacontantinou H, Bullard K, Rotherenberger D, Madoff R. Salvage APR after failed Nigro protocol: modest success, major morbidity (meeting abstract). Dis Colon Rectum. 2003;46:A63.
21. Page CP, Carlton Jr PK, Beck DW. Closure of pelvic and perineal wounds after removal of the rectum and anus. Dis Colon Rectum. 1980;23:2–9.
22. De Broux E, Parc Y, Rondelli F, Dehni N, Tiret E, Parc R. Sutured perineal omentoplasty after abdominoperineal resection for adenocarcinoma of the lower rectum. Dis Colon Rectum. 2005;48: 476–82.
23. De Dombal FT, Burton I, Goligher JC. The early and late results of surgical treatment for Crohn's disease. Br J Surg. 1971;58:805.
24. Corman ML, Veidenheimer MC, Coller JA, Ross VH. Perineal wound healing after proctectomy for inflammatory bowel disease. Dis Colon Rectum. 1978;21(3):155–9.
25. Abcarian H, Eftaliha M. Management of the perineal wound after proctocolectomy. Dis Colon Rectum. 1978;21:287–91.
26. Alpsan K, Singh A, Ahmad A. Clinical comparison of perineal wound management. Dis Colon Rectum. 1980;23(8):564–6.
27. Lubbers Evert JC. Healing of the perineal wound after proctectomy for nonmalignant conditions. Dis Colon Rectum. 1982;25(4): 351–7.
28. Oakley JR, Fazio VW, Jagelman DG, Lavery IC, Weakley FL, Easley K. Management of the perineal wound after rectal excision for ulcerative colitis. Dis Colon Rectum. 1985;28(12):885–8.
29. Turnbull RB, Fazio V. Advances in the surgical technique of ulcerative colitis surgery: endoanal proctectomy and two-directional myotomy ileostomy. Surg Annu. 1975;7:315–29.
30. Lyttle JA, Parks AG. Intersphincteric excision of the rectum. Br J Surg. 1977;62:413–6.
31. Schaffzin DM, Douglas JM, Stahl TJ, Smith LE. Vacuum-assisted closure of complex perineal wounds. Dis Colon Rectum. 2004;47:1745–8.
32. Cresti S, Ouaissi M, Sielezneff I, Jean-Batiste C, Pirro N, Berthet B, Consentino B, Sastre B. Advantage of vacuum assisted closure on healing of wound associated with omentoplasty after abdominoperineal excision: a case report. World J Surg Oncol. 2008;6:136.
33. Colombel JF, Mathieu D, Bouault JM, Lesage X, Zavadil P, Quandalle P, Cortot A. Hyperbaric oxygenation in severe perineal Crohn's disease. Dis Colon Rectum. 1995;38:609–14.
34. Chan S, Miller M, Ng R, Ross D, Roblin P, Carapeti E, Williams AB, George ML. Use of myocutaneous flaps for perineal closure following abdominoperineal excision of the rectum for adenocarcinoma. Colorectal Dis. 2009;12:555–60.
35. Hainsworth A, Al Akash M, Roblin P, Mohanna P, Ross D, George ML. Perineal reconstruction after abdominoperineal excision using inferior gluteal artery perforator flaps. Br J Surg. 2012;99:584–8.
36. Buchel EW, Finical S, Johnson C. Pelvic reconstruction using rectus abdominis musculocutaneous flaps. Ann Plast Surg. 2004;52: 22–6.
37. Chessin DB, Hatley J, Cohen AM, et al. Rectus flap reconstruction decreases perineal wound complications after pelvic chemoradiation: a cohort study. Ann Surg Oncol. 2005;12:14–110.
38. Lefevre JH, Parc Y, Kemeis S, et al. Abdomino-perineal resection for anal cancer: impact of vertical rectus abdominis myocutaneous flap on survival, recurrence, morbidity and wound healing. Ann Surg. 2009;250:707–11.
39. Nelson RA, Butler CE. Surgical outcomes of VRAM versus thigh flaps for immediate reconstruction of pelvis and perineal cancer resection defects. Plast Reconstr Surg. 2009;183:175–83.
40. Scheuffler O, Farhadi J, Kovach SJ, et al. Anatomical basis and clinical application of infragluteal perforator flap. Plast Reconstr Surg. 2006;118:1389–400.

Part V

Special Situations

Considerations in the Elderly

25

Joshua I.S. Bleier and Robert D. Fry

Key Points

- Preoperative risk assessment is based on identifying key cardiac and other comorbid risk factors.
- Management of common anorectal problems is different in the elderly because of the likelihood of relative sphincter dysfunction.
- Certain abdominal diagnoses are more common in the elderly and appropriate management is based on prompt diagnosis and effective management.
- Colonoscopy screening guidelines are null after age 85.
- Informed consent is more complex in the elderly, and patient autonomy, competency, and support systems must be considered.
- Laparoscopic surgery is safe and appropriate for select colorectal operations in the elderly.

Introduction

Key Concept: George Burns once said, "You can't help getting older, but you don't have to get old." Aging is most often defined objectively by years since birth, but subjectively, physiologically, and medically, it is more often a function of "how old you feel."

To a large degree, management of colorectal issues, whether benign or malignant, are pathology-driven. In most instances, colon cancers that are resectable should be resected; metastatic disease is an indication for adjuvant therapy; multiply recurrent attacks of diverticulitis indicate resection; mixed hemorrhoids refractory to the best conservative management may require hemorrhoidectomy; hematochezia or a change in bowel habits require endoscopic evaluation; screening colonoscopy reduces the risk of colon cancer; and low rectal cancers that don't involve the sphincters may be treated by sphincter-sparing operations, including colo-anal anastomoses. However, you as the surgeon know that indications are only part of the decision process. Pathology alone may provide the *indication* for surgery, but not necessarily the *decision* for it. Patient factors must be taken into consideration. Every assessment of the potential surgical patient takes into account fitness for surgery, as well the assessment of tolerating the outcome. But where does age play into this equation? Age is a nonspecific factor that may provide predictive information about how well a patient will tolerate a procedure. In general, the older the patient, the more comorbidities, the higher the risk for healing problems, the worse the baseline continence and sphincter function, and the higher the risk for cardiovascular disease. Chronological age is indisputable, but physiologic age is variable. Consider the unfortunate condition of progeria, in which children succumb to the physiologic maladies of advanced age such as heart attack, stroke, and atherosclerotic disease – and rarely live past the age of 13. Now contrast that with the 100-year-old man who completed a marathon in Toronto in 2011 (although it took him 8 h to do it!). The concept of physiologic age supersedes that of chronologic age in the assessment of the elderly patient. Determination of the physiologic age of the patient is an amalgam of all of the

J.I.S. Bleier, MD, FACS, FASCRS (✉)
Division of Colon and Rectal Surgery, Department of Surgery, Pennsylvania Hospital/Hospital of the University of Pennsylvania, University of Pennsylvania, 8th and Walnut, 20th Floor, Philadelphia, PA 19106, USA
e-mail: joshua.bleier@uphs.upenn.edu

R.D. Fry, MD, FACS, FASCRS
Division of Colon and Rectal Surgery, Department of Surgery, Pennsylvania Hospital, University of Pennsylvania, 8th and Walnut, 20th Floor, Philadelphia, PA 19106, USA
e-mail: robert.fry@uphs.upenn.edu

Electronic supplementary material The online version of this chapter (doi: 10.1007/978-1-4614-9022-7_25) contains supplementary material, which is available to authorized users. Videos can also be accessed at http://www.springerimages.com/videos/978-1-4614-9021-0.

S.R. Steele et al. (eds.), *Complexities in Colorectal Surgery*,
DOI 10.1007/978-1-4614-9022-7_25, © Springer Science+Business Media New York 2014

physiologic parameters that will be affected by the operation and its recovery. Prior dogma dictating age alone as a relative contraindication to surgery has been replaced by determination of fitness, a proxy for physiologic age. Advances in perioperative management have demonstrated that mere chronological age does not directly determine fitness and the ability to recover from surgery; it merely informs us of the increased possible risks, and overall fitness for intervention is determined by factors that are projected to be affected by the surgery. In this chapter, we will deal with these issues and the factors that affect them.

Evaluation for Surgery: Determination of Cardiovascular and Physiologic Risk Stratification

Key Concept: Rather than relying on age, use a systems-based evaluation to determine a perioperative risk profile for your patient.

The World Health Organization has broadly defined "elderly" as any patient who is eligible for pension benefits. However, given the varied standards across the world, anyone over the age of 50 may be loosely defined as "elderly." In the USA, this definition is likely inappropriate, as the retirement age is 65, and health risks do not substantially increase in the 6th decade of life. Nevertheless, most screening standards do change in the age group over 50. After 50, it is recommended that all patients receive a preoperative chest X-ray and laboratory work. There is no mandatory age indicating the requirement for preoperative cardiovascular testing; rather, this decision is the responsibility of the operating surgeon.

Preoperative Risk Assessment

Key Concept: Appropriate preoperative risk assessment is the surgeon's responsibility when planning for surgery of any kind. This is even more important in the elderly patient given the increased incidence of significant comorbidities associated with age.

The most recent American Heart Association guidelines [1] help to delineate the approach to risk stratification. An appropriate history and physical examination provides information that will identify risk factors. The initial decision process should be aimed at identifying any cardiac condition that would increase the risk of an adverse cardiac event in the perioperative period. In general, any patient with active cardiac disease, such as unstable coronary syndrome, decompensated or worsening congestive heart failure (CHF), significant arrhythmia, or significant valvular disease should receive cardiology evaluation and baseline cardiac testing (Table 25.1) [1].

Table 25.1 Active cardiac conditions for which the patient should undergo evaluation and treatment before noncardiac surgery

Condition	Examples
Unstable coronary syndromes	Unstable or severe angina (CCS class III or IV)[a]
	Recent MI[b]
Decompensated heart failure (NYHA functional class IV; worsening or new-onset HF)	
Significant arrhythmias	High-grade AV block
	Mobitz II AV block
	Third-degree AV block
	Symptomatic ventricular arrhythmias
	Supraventricular arrhythmias (including atrial fibrillation) with uncontrolled ventricular rate (HR > 100 bpm at rest)
	Symptomatic bradycardia
	Newly recognized ventricular tachycardia
Severe valvular disease	Sever aortic stenosis (mean pressure gradient greater than 40 mmHg, aortic valve area < 1.0 cm^2, or symptomatic)
	Symptomatic mitral stenosis (progressive dyspnea on exertion, exertional presyncope, or HF)

Adapted with permission from Fleisher et al. [1] © American College of Cardiology

CCS Canadian Cardiovascular Society, *HF* heart failure, *HR* heart rate, *MI* myocardial infarction, *NYHA* New York Heart Association

[a]May include stable angina in patients who are unusually sedentary

[b]The American College of Cardiology National Database Library defines recent MI as more than 7 days but less than or equal to 1 month (within 30 days)

In the absence of serious comorbidities, a rough assessment of exercise tolerance may be all that is needed to determine if further testing should be pursued. This is especially true when taken in context of the type of surgery you are performing. Anorectal surgery is considered a low-risk operation, regardless of anesthetic technique, and elective abdominal operations are considered intermediate risk operations. Age, as a sole criterion, defines only the need for EKG and chest X-ray for patients over 50. Advanced age alone is not an indication for further cardiac testing. In fact, for patients with good exercise tolerance (>4 METS) (Table 25.2) [2], further testing for any elective procedure is usually unnecessary.

Other significant clinical risk factors should be assessed. A history of ischemic heart disease, compensated or prior CHF, diabetes mellitus, renal insufficiency, or cerebrovascular disease all represent significant comorbidities that may require preoperative evaluation.

Exercise tolerance is an excellent overall assessment of fitness. In the setting of good exercise tolerance, even with

Table 25.2 Estimated energy requirements for various activities

Metabolic equivalent (MET)	Activity
1 MET	Eat, dress, use the toilet
	Walk indoors around the house
	Walk a block or 2 on level ground at 2–3 mph?
4 MET	Do light housework (dusting, washing dishes)
	Climb a flight of stairs or walk up a hill?
	Walk on level ground at 4 mph?
	Run a short distance
	Do heavy housework (scrubbing floors, lifting/moving furniture)
	Participate in moderate recreational activities (golf, bowling, dancing, double tennis, baseball or football catch)
>10 METS	Participate in strenuous sports (swimming, single tennis, football, basketball, skiing)

Adapted with permission from Fleisher et al. [1] © American College of Cardiology

multiple clinical risk factors described above, intermediate risk surgery can often be undertaken with acceptable risk. Perioperative heart rate control with beta-blockade should be considered mandatory in anyone with any of the above risk factors, since this has been shown to reduce cardiac morbidity and mortality [3].

When a patient has some of these other significant comorbidities, specific workup may be indicated as per the AHA guidelines [2]:

Pulmonary Disease

The presence of restrictive or obstructive pulmonary disease significantly increases the risk of perioperative pulmonary complications. In these cases, preoperative pulmonary testing to determine volume and diffusion capacity, response to bronchodilators, and a baseline blood gas will help guide postoperative therapy.

Diabetes Mellitus

This is the most common metabolic disease associated with advanced age and is often associated with coronary disease. The presence of insulin-dependent DM increases the risk of perioperative myocardial ischemia and heart failure. Careful attention (both intraoperatively and postoperatively) to glucose management with insulin infusions and tight glycemic control has been found to significantly reduce postoperative wound infection in CABG patients, and this paradigm can be applied to major abdominal surgery.

Renal Failure

Renal failure is associated with an increased risk of perioperative cardiac morbidity [4]. In addition, preoperative levels of creatinine >1.5–2 mg/dl is associated with an increased risk of postoperative renal failure, cardiac complications, and increased mortality.

Hematologic Disorders

Preoperative anemia can impose cardiac stress, worsen ischemia, and exacerbate preexisting CHF. In one study looking at patients undergoing prostate and major vascular surgery, a hematocrit <28 % was associated with an increased risk of perioperative ischemia and postoperative complications.

Anorectal Problems

Key Concept: In any patient with anorectal complaints, baseline function of the sphincter complex should be taken in to account when considering surgical options.

Examining and documenting sphincter tone and determining whether alterations in continence are present are imperative when evaluating older patients with anorectal complaints. Laurberg showed that in the elderly, there is significantly decreased baseline sphincter tone [5], decreased rectal sensation and distensibility, and increased perineal laxity in women [6]. Unfortunately, there has been no data showing any consistently reproducible predictive factors for postoperative changes in continence based on preoperative examination or physiologic testing.

Yet, there are some major points you should keep in mind when evaluating older patients with anorectal complaints:

(a) When considering hemorrhoidectomy in the elderly, as with younger patients, initial management should be conservative when possible.
(b) In the elderly, anorectal complaints are often centered on mucus seepage and soilage. Though dietary changes, bowel management (i.e., fiber, Imodium), and skin protection are successful first-line treatments, in most cases, patients with prolapse or large hemorrhoids will likely benefit from surgery.
(c) In our experience, the best predictor of postoperative function after surgery is preoperative function.
(d) A careful history, with special attention to bowel habits and continence, is crucial. If preoperative soilage or seepage is the major complaint, it is important to ascertain whether this is due to mucosal prolapse or true sphincter dysfunction.

Fecal Incontinence (FI)

Key Concept: FI occurs much more commonly than thought. While a full evaluation is helpful, most often by simply focusing on medical management in the elderly patient, you will provide the most benefit.

Fecal incontinence (FI) is a socially disabling disorder, which is far more prevalent in the elderly. Estimates at the rate of FI ranged from 2 to 17 % in a community setting, but these are likely underreported. A more recent HMO-population based study found reported rates of FI as high as 36 %. In the elderly, rates of FI are significantly higher, especially in the nursing home setting, where rates range from 33 % to as high as 65 % [7].

Management of FI depends on the etiology. A complete history, focusing on the details of bowel habits, diet and medication, as well as prior anorectal surgical and obstetric history, will often elucidate the etiology of the disorder and guide treatment. In the elderly, the differential diagnosis is quite long, including cognitive and neurologic diseases, chronic constipation with overflow, senescent physiologic changes, rectal prolapse, or iatrogenic or obstetric injury. Treatment is almost always geared towards the underlying condition, and optimization of bowel habits is crucially important in this population. It is also important to protect the perineal skin, as seepage of intestinal contents can often lead to severe maceration and breakdown if not properly attended too.

Rectal Prolapse

Key Concept: Procidentia, or true rectal prolapse, when encountered as an etiology for FI, is probably best treated surgically with a perineal approach.

Oftentimes, patients with FI will have diminished sphincter control due to long-standing (and previously unreported and undiagnosed) full-thickness rectal prolapse (Fig. 25.1). We advocate a perineal proctectomy in the elderly as this is well tolerated and avoids the morbidity of an abdominal operation (Fig. 25.2). In patients with significant comorbidities, it can even be performed under a spinal anesthetic or in the left lateral decubitus position to minimize intraoperative complications.

Sacral Nerve Stimulation (SNS)

Key Concept: SNS has an evolving role in FI for failed medical management and with its good preliminary results and trial period to confirm efficacy, may soon be a first-line treatment modality in this cohort.

Ultimately, symptoms of FI should be managed conservatively when possible. Considerations for surgery in the elderly have changed significantly in recent times. Historically, once conservative measures and biofeedback fail, and the patient was considered a suitable candidate for surgery, few options remained. Often, in men with profound FI, in the absence of a sphincter injury, fecal diversion remained the only option. In women with known sphincter injuries, sphincteroplasty was an option. However, this is a significantly morbid procedure

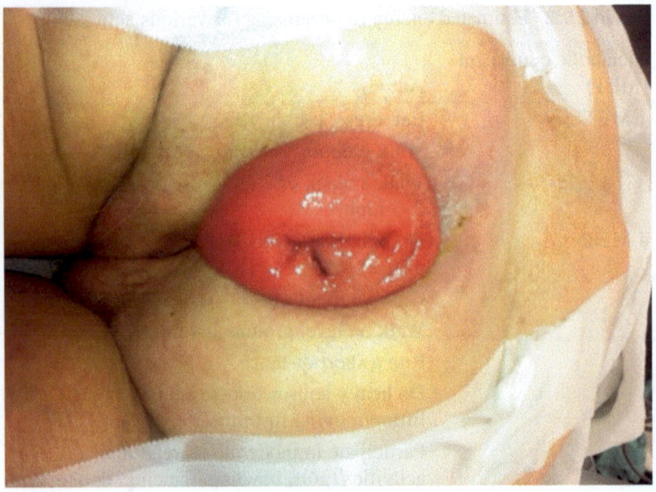

Fig. 25.1 Full-thickness rectal prolapse

with a difficult recovery and has fairly poor long-term results. More recently, the paradigm has undergone a significant shift. Sacral nerve stimulation, a modality that has had a decade of known efficacy in urinary incontinence, was recently approved for use by the FDA for fecal incontinence (Fig. 25.3). The indication included fecal incontinence in the presence of known sphincter injuries of up to 60°. Although the efficacy of SNS in treating FI has been known since it has been used for urinary incontinence for more than a decade, it was not until 2011 when the FDA finally approved FI as an independent indication for treatment. The initial studies showed significant success rates, defined as at least a 50 % reduction in fecal incontinence symptoms, in 60–100 % of patients. In the initial publication of the SNS study group, 133 patients underwent test simulation with a 90 % success rate. Even at 3 years of follow-up, 86 % of patients reported a greater than 50 % reduction in the number of incontinent episodes per week, and perfect continence was achieved in 40 % of the patients [8].

There are several advantages of this new approach – it is low risk, with a reported infection rate of less than 10 %, and no major morbidities reported. It works even in patients with sphincter defects, so that there is no further need to subject them to high risk of morbidity and poor long-term results with sphincteroplasty. Finally, because there is a test phase built into the implantation process, patients will know whether or not it works before they ever have a permanent implant placed. We suspect that this will have a long-term effect on the paradigm of treatment for fecal incontinence and that sacral nerve stimulation will become first-line therapy after conservative measures and behavioral modification have failed.

Ultimately, although not likely greeted warmly, you should always consider diversion as an option for patients nonresponsive to more conservative therapies that present with more severe leakage.

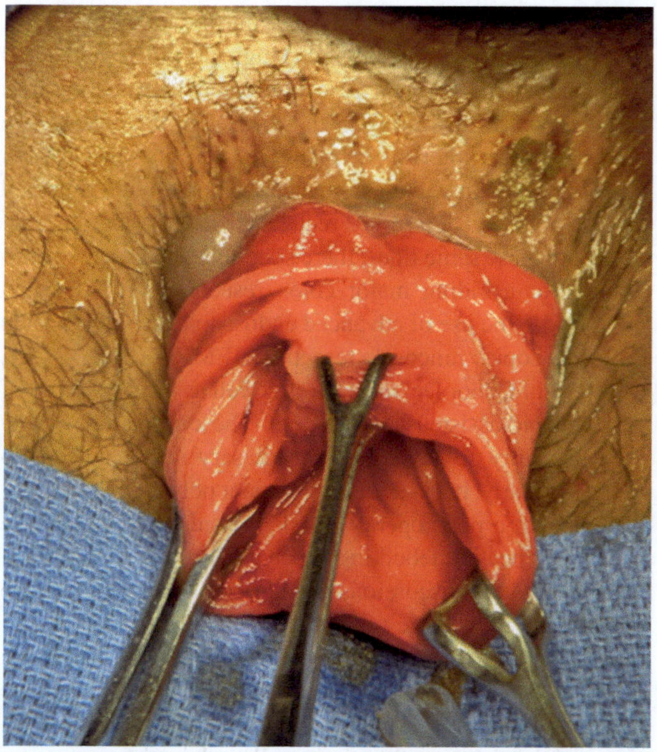

Fig. 25.2 Perineal approach to rectal prolapse

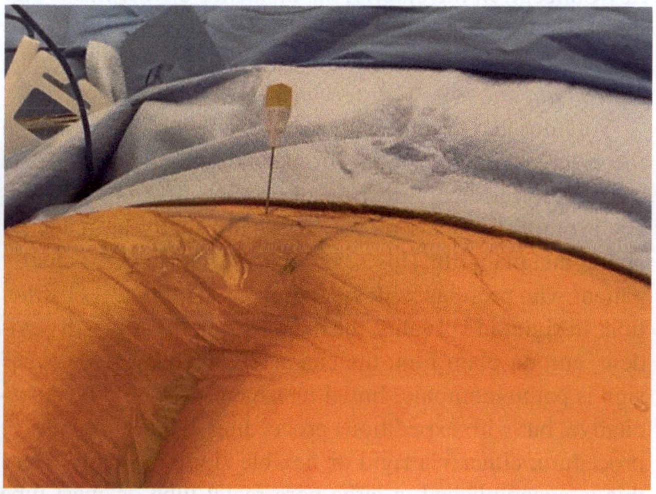

Fig. 25.3 Sacral nerve stimulation (SNS). Needle finding the correct sacral level

Abdominal Problems

Key Concept: With the increasing availability and expertise in minimally invasive approaches to more common colorectal disease processes, an abdominal approach can be performed with minimal morbidity, faster return to preoperative functional status, and improved quality of life.

Diverticulitis

Key Concept: Elderly patients without significant comorbidities can be managed similar to younger patients, including nonoperative treatment, though colostomy may often be the best option for those with poor baseline continence.

Recurrent diverticulitis has traditionally been treated with a dogmatic approach, based on few early data in the pre-interventional radiology era, without the benefit of modern antibiotics, critical care management, and advanced imaging techniques [9]. The last decade has seen a major paradigm shift in the management of recurrent diverticulitis. Newer approaches, based on the effectiveness of interventional radiology techniques and modern antibiotics, have demonstrated that in many cases, nonoperative management is appropriate. Newer reports have shown efficacy of innovative management with peritoneal lavage, as well as the safety of more prolonged antibiotic management for recurrent attacks. In the elderly, this may be important considering the significant morbidity associated with an abdominal operation. A review of patients treated by surgery demonstrated that if an emergent operation was done, it was usually required for the first attack [10]. In the elderly, the risk of mortality with emergent surgery for diverticulitis is significant. In octogenarians, the risk of mortality is increased up to sixfold [11, 12]. Complicated diverticulitis, especially an attack that requires either prolonged hospitalization for parenteral antibiotics or interventional radiologic drainage, is still an indication for elective surgery once the patient has recovered. This allows the surgeon the opportunity to optimize the patient for surgery based on the above-stated guidelines from the AHA. It is important for these patients to also have a preoperative colonoscopy to rule-out synchronous pathology. We still advocate operative intervention in the setting of recurrent attacks that are increasing in frequency or for symptoms that do not completely resolve. However, there is no set number of attacks that mandate intervention.

From a functional standpoint, although it is important to consider changes in bowel habits after resection, there should be little long-term significant effects on continence after sigmoid resection. It is important to ensure that the distal resection margin is at the proximal rectum to minimize the risk of recurrence. In elderly patients with compromised sphincter function or prior pelvic surgery, consideration should be given to fashioning a permanent colostomy. Given the higher incidence of significant comorbidities with advancing age, the use of diverting ileostomy after primary anastomosis should be considered, as this offers protection of a distal anastomosis and may avoid the significant morbidity of a second major abdominal operation needed to close a colostomy.

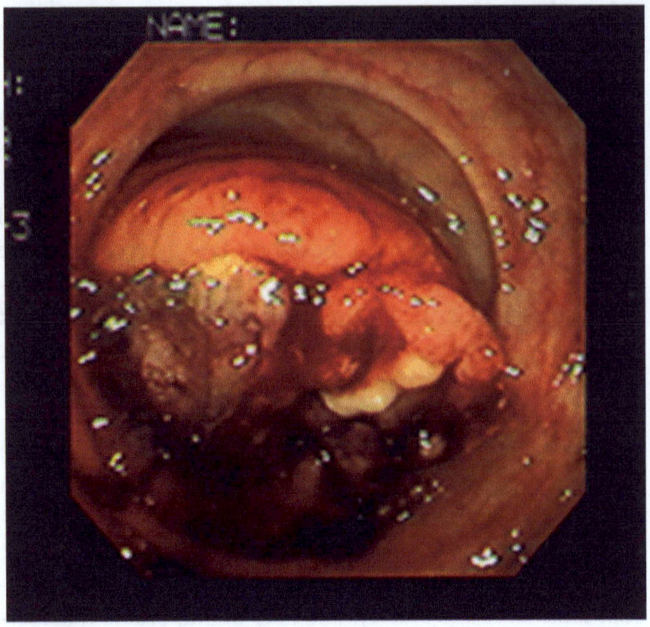

Fig. 25.4 Endoscopic view of an advanced rectal cancer (Courtesy of W. Brian Sweeny, MD)

Proctectomy for Malignancy

Key Concept: Considerations for proctectomy in the elderly must take into account the profound functional changes that accompany the operation. The appropriate indications for rectal resection for malignancy do not change based on age, but we must not place restoration of intestinal continuity as paramount.

In patients who have early rectal cancers, in whom primary operative therapy is indicated, strong consideration should be given to the wisdom of a low rectal anastomosis. The low anterior resection syndrome may result in significant alterations in bowel function, and in the elderly patient with borderline sphincter function, a low anastomosis may essentially create a perineal colostomy. In these cases, we recommend a permanent colostomy, as this will allow for more satisfactory bowel control. In the setting of locally advanced or node-positive malignancy (Fig. 25.4), the effect of radiation on the sphincter will dramatically increase the risk of postoperative continence disturbances. There is a well-established deleterious effect on sphincter function as a result of radiation [13], so alternative approaches should be considered. Local excision for early rectal malignancies may be a reasonable option with acceptable local and long-term recurrence rates. The use of transanal endoscopic microsurgery (TEM) has been shown to significantly increase the chance of cure after local resection alone in early rectal cancer [14]. It is becoming evident that some rectal cancers treated by chemoradiation will have a complete clinical response – and it becomes a matter of judgment as to whether such patients would benefit from further treatment [15]. When a resection will result in the high morbidity associated with abdominal perineal resection, more consideration is given to watchful waiting in these cases in the elderly. We wait with great interest the results of the recent ACOSOG Z6041 trial looking at neoadjuvant chemoradiation followed by transanal excision for T2 rectal cancers [16].

Along these same lines, there should be increased consideration for avoiding major colon resections for advanced polyps with the use of advanced endoscopic techniques such as endoscopic mucosal resection (EMR) (Video 25.1, Courtesy of Conor Delaney, MD) as well as the possibility of laparoscopic assisted-polypectomy. These modalities allow the possibility for avoiding unnecessary segmental colectomy. Similarly, in cases of large defiant polyps in the elderly patient with a poor operative risk, consideration should be given to repeated debulking procedures rather than radical resection. These discussions need to be fleshed out with the patient, and in the case of the elderly patient with the possibility of poor comprehension, it is important to make sure family is involved and to identify the appropriate healthcare proxy, so that all parties understand the reason for the decision and the risk-benefit ratio is well explained.

Volvulus

Key Concept: In the elderly, the incidence of volvulus is significantly increased, and appropriate and timely diagnosis and management can make a significant impact at minimizing complications and preserving function.

Volvulus can present with a wide variety of symptoms in the elderly patient, ranging from mild abdominal pain and constipation to abdominal distension, obstipation, and sepsis. Prompt diagnosis of volvulus can usually be made by abdominal plain film (Fig. 25.5a, b) or CT scan in the elderly patient who presents with symptoms of large bowel obstruction. In sigmoid volvulus, the diagnosis on CT is usually evident, and on plain film, the characteristic "bent inner-tube" sign is pathognomonic. Initial management should be resuscitative, but with expeditious proceeding to a decompressive procedure, either via rigid or flexible sigmoidoscopy. Once this is accomplished, a large-bore rectal tube or chest tube should be placed to prevent immediate recurrence. Once the large bowel has been decompressed, plans should be made for sigmoid resection at the same hospitalization. Effective decompression will give the surgeon time to perform risk assessment and medical optimization. At the time of operation, resection of the redundant sigmoid should be done expeditiously, with the decision for reanastomosis made with assessment of risk and quality of life issues.

Cecal volvulus is also more common in the elderly, although not as common as sigmoid volvulus. The diagnosis is made, either on CT scan, on plain film showing the characteristic "coffee-bean" sign. If the patient is stable,

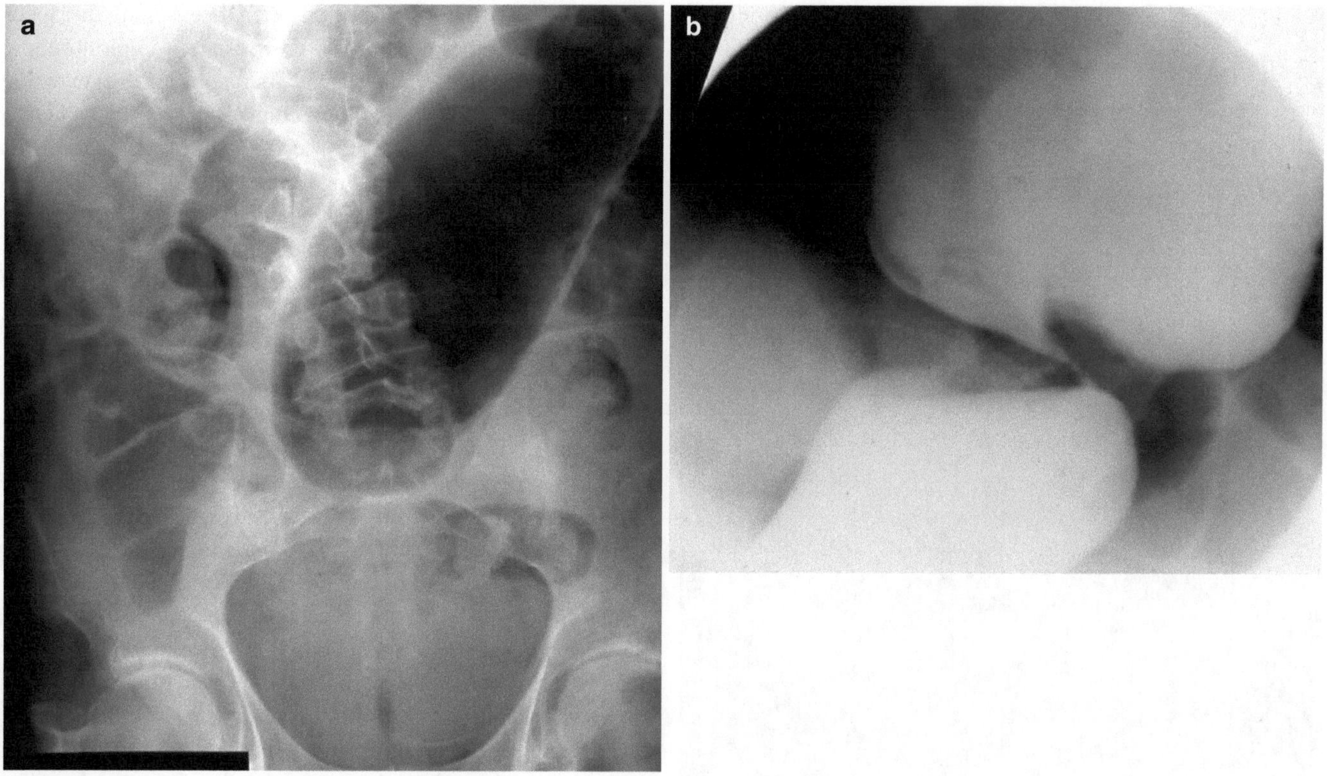

Fig. 25.5 (**a**) Cecal volvulus with the bowel pointing to the left upper quadrant. (**b**) Cecal volvulus with enteral contrast demonstrating the classic "bird's beak"

a preoperative colonoscopy should be performed since a distal obstructing lesion may precipitate volvulus. Additionally, colonoscopy may allow for transient detorsion of the volvulized segment.

Colonic Pseudo-obstruction (Ogilvie's Syndrome)

Key Concept: The incidence of colonic pseudo-obstruction is increased in the elderly and may complicate the postoperative course of elective or urgent orthopedic procedures. However, the need for surgical intervention should be rare with appropriate management.

When the diagnosis of Ogilvie's syndrome is suspected, initial management is aimed at correcting all metabolic disturbances and discontinuation of narcotic use. Distal mechanical obstruction MUST be ruled out. This is best accomplished by colonoscopy that can be both diagnostic and therapeutic in terms of colonic decompression. Other approaches are Gastrografin enema or as third-line option, CT scan (Fig. 25.6). Once mechanical obstruction is ruled out, several highly effective options exist. The most commonly used one is a peripherally acting acetylcholinesterase inhibitor such as neostigmine. Intravenous administration must be performed in a monitored setting because of the arrhythmogenic risk, but resolution of the pseudo-obstruction is usually immediate and dramatic. If this option isn't available or deemed too high a risk, then a spinal anesthetic and the resulting sympathetic blockade is almost as effective. Operative intervention is almost never needed.

Psychosocial Aspects

Key Concept: Unlike other patient cohorts, there is often a significant rate of associated cognitive, family, and psychosocial issues that may complicate the management of elderly patients and must be taken into consideration prior to proceeding with care.

When considering any surgical intervention in the elderly, consideration must be given to the issues of informed consent. Concomitant with the elderly is a significant rate of associated cognitive and psychosocial issues that complicate the issue of informed consent. It is important to determine the competency of the elderly patient in the setting of potentially life-altering and high-risk surgery. Issues such as the ability of an elderly person to care for themselves after surgery and the potential ramifications of a significant period of postoperative debilitation must be taken into account. Ultimately, the physician's responsibility is to inform the

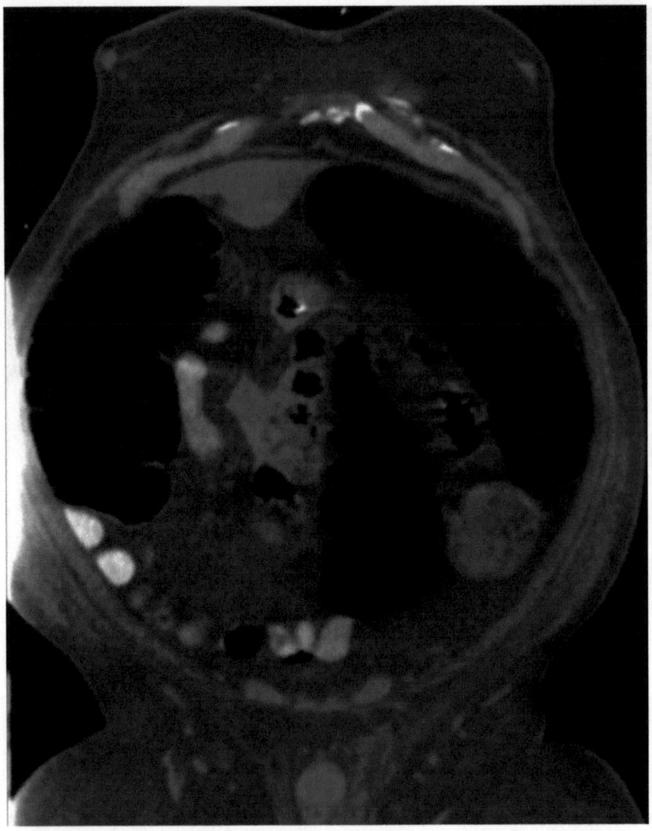

Fig. 25.6 CT scan for Ogilvie's syndrome demonstrating the distal decompression and large proximal dilation

competent patient of the various options and advocate for what is in the patient's best interest. However, the competent elderly adult has the right to choose, even if the choice may be against the recommendation of the surgeon. Whenever possible, the surgeon should make sure the patient's family or significant supporters are involved whenever there is a question of competence or the significant likelihood of disability in the postoperative period.

Controversies in Surgery in the Elderly

Key Concept: Recommendations regarding traditional screening modalities in the elderly may not apply.

Historically, surgeons assumed a strong "parental" role in decision making for their patients, serving a caretaker role. Traditionally, age alone was considered as a significant factor in the decision-making process. With the advent of newer, less morbid surgical techniques, advances in the effectiveness of critical care management, and with increasing life span, we have shifted away for this "age-ist" perspective. Chronologic age is no longer considered in isolation; rather, physiologic age and functional capacity are the significant determinants in surgical management.

Yet, age is still a consideration when determining therapeutic options in other scenarios. With respect to colonoscopic screening guidelines, in the 1995 version of the US Preventive Services Task Force (USPSTF) recommendations in the Guide to Clinical Preventive Services, second edition, screening was recommended for all adults age 50 or older. Interestingly, at that time, screening modalities included primarily fecal occult blood testing (FOBT) and flexible sigmoidoscopy. There was insufficient evidence to recommend for or against routine colonoscopic screening at that time. In the 2002 update to the USPSTSF recommendations, the recommendations for screening all adults above age 50 were reaffirmed, but now with colonoscopy as a primary screening modality [17]. By 2008, and now the most current version, the USPSTF "recommends against routine screening for colorectal cancer in adults 76–85 years of age." However, a caveat is given that colorectal cancer screening is supported in individual cases, usually based on a past history of colonic polyps or cancer, or a strong family history [17]. However, in people above 85 years of age, no screening is recommended. The recommendation for screening in higher-risk individuals, those with a family history or personal history of polyps or cancer, or inflammatory disease are varied and beyond the scope of this chapter. In general, there is no formal recommendation for screening after age 85 in any circumstance or if the patient is believed to have less than a 10-year life expectancy [18, 19].

Laparoscopic Surgery in the Elderly

Key Concept: Minimally invasive approaches to colorectal surgery have resulted in a paradigm shift in the management of patients and expectations, as well as improved outcomes.

It has been well established that laparoscopic approaches to benign abdominal disease result in decreased pain, shorter hospital stays, and improved cosmesis. In its use for colon cancer, we know that oncologic outcomes are equivalent. As such, laparoscopy has been established as first-line treatment, in general, in the absence of other contraindications. The definition of what a contraindication to laparoscopic surgery has undergone evolution, with significant comorbidity, obesity, and prior operations being absolute contraindications. Ironically, as our experience has grown, and we have seen the advantages of the minimally invasive approach, these original contraindications have now become primary *indications* for the MIS approach and can accentuate the advantages of laparoscopy. The use of laparoscopy in the elderly is no exception; multiple studies have validated the specific benefit of laparoscopy in this group. Frasson et al. looked a cohort of 535 patients undergoing elective laparoscopic or open colorectal surgery, 37.6 % of whom were over 70 years of age. A laparoscopic approach in the elderly group reduced the rate of postoperative morbidity

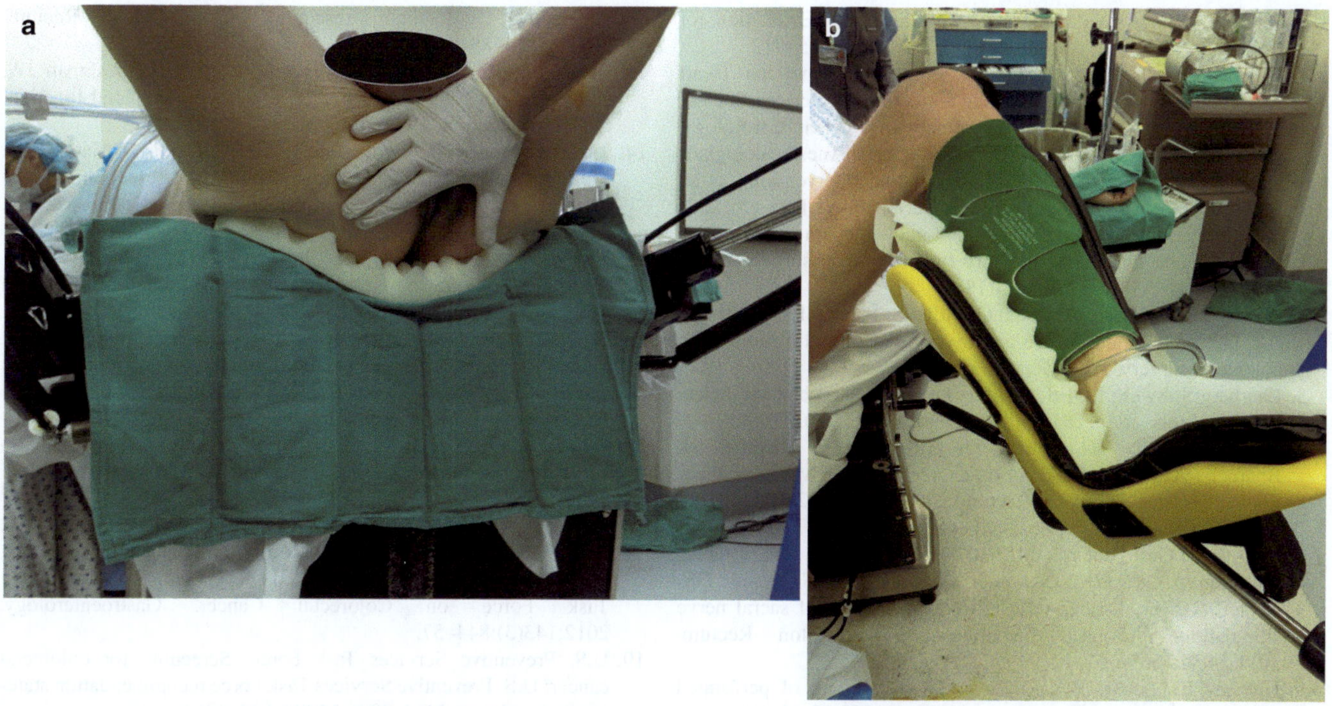

Fig. 25.7 (a, b) Additional padding over the sacrum and lower extremity

(20.2 vs. 37.5 %) as well as length of stay (LOS) (9.5 vs. 13 days). When compared to the younger cohort, these advantages were more pronounced in the elderly [20]. Stocchi et al. reported on 42 elderly patients undergoing laparoscopic colorectal surgery versus a case-matched set undergoing open colectomy. The laparoscopy group was associated with decreased postoperative morbidity, faster return of bowel function, decreased length of stay, and less pain [21]. The literature is replete with such studies, with the overall conclusion that laparoscopy is not only safe in the elderly but most likely associated with the same benefits enjoyed by the younger patients [22]. One important point you should remember, however, is that due to the frailty in older patients' skin and loss of subcutaneous fat, additional padding should be placed over bony prominences (Fig. 25.7a, b).

Summary Pearls

Management of the elderly patient with colorectal problems can be complex and may affect every aspect of your care: from diagnosis, informed consent, and considerations of cure versus function to the methods of operative technique and pre- and post-op surveillance. It is your job as a surgeon to do try to do what is best for your patients, treating them as individuals rather than as diagnoses. You must use our experience and judgment to inform your elderly patients and help them make the best decision possible, hopefully with the input of their loved ones and caretakers. Remember, in the modern surgical practice, chronologic age alone no longer is an absolute factor, rather you must determine the patient's physiologic age, which is really a proxy for their fitness for surgery. Maximizing successful and compassionate outcomes is an exercise in both technique and wisdom.

References

1. Fleisher LA, Beckman JA, Brown KA, Calkins H, Chaikof EL, Fleischmann KE, et al. ACC/AHA 2007 guidelines on perioperative cardiovascular evaluation and care for noncardiac surgery: executive summary: a report of the American College of Cardiology/American Heart Association Task Force on Practice Guidelines (Writing Committee to Revise the 2002 Guidelines on Perioperative Cardiovascular Evaluation for Noncardiac Surgery) Developed in Collaboration With the American Society of Echocardiography, American Society of Nuclear Cardiology, Heart Rhythm Society, Society of Cardiovascular Anesthesiologists, Society for Cardiovascular Angiography and Interventions, Society for Vascular Medicine and Biology, and Society for Vascular Surgery. J Am Coll Cardiol. 2007;50(17):1707–32.
2. American College of Cardiology/American Heart Association Task Force on Practice Guidelines (Writing Committee to Revise the 2002 Guidelines on Perioperative Cardiovascular Evaluation for Noncardiac Surgery), American Society of Echocardiography, American Society of Nuclear Cardiology, Heart Rhythm Society, Society of Cardiovascular Anesthesiologists, Society for Cardiovascular Angiography and Interventions, et al. ACC/AHA 2007 guidelines on perioperative cardiovascular evaluation and care for noncardiac surgery: executive summary: a report of the American College of Cardiology/American Heart Association Task Force on Practice Guidelines (Writing Committee to Revise the

2002 Guidelines on Perioperative Cardiovascular Evaluation for Noncardiac Surgery). Anesth Analg. 2008;106(3):685–712.
3. American College of Cardiology Foundation/American Heart Association Task Force on Practice Guidelines, American Society of Echocardiography, American Society of Nuclear Cardiology, Heart Rhythm Society, Society of Cardiovascular Anesthesiologists, Society for Cardiovascular Angiography and Interventions, et al. 2009 ACCF/AHA focused update on perioperative beta blockade incorporated into the ACC/AHA 2007 guidelines on perioperative cardiovascular evaluation and care for noncardiac surgery. J Am Coll Cardiol. 2009;54(22):e13–118.
4. Causey MW, Maykel JA, Hatch Q, Miller S, Steele SR. Identifying risk factors for renal failure and myocardial infarction following colorectal surgery. J Surg Res. 2011;170(1):32–7.
5. Laurberg S, Swash M. Effects of aging on the anorectal sphincters and their innervation. Dis Colon Rectum. 1989;32(9):737–42.
6. Fox JC, Fletcher JG, Zinsmeister AR, Seide B, Riederer SJ, Bharucha AE. Effect of aging on anorectal and pelvic floor functions in females. Dis Colon Rectum. 2006;49(11):1726–35.
7. Shah BJ, Chokhavatia S, Rose S. Fecal incontinence in the elderly: FAQ. Am J Gastroenterol. 2012;107(11):1635–46.
8. Mellgren A, Wexner SD, Coller JA, Devroede G, Lerew DR, Madoff RD, et al. Long-term efficacy and safety of sacral nerve stimulation for fecal incontinence. Dis Colon Rectum. 2011;54(9):1065–75.
9. Hinchey EJ, Schaal PG, Richards GK. Treatment of perforated diverticular disease of the colon. Adv Surg. 1978;12:85–109.
10. Eglinton T, Nguyen T, Raniga S, Dixon L, Dobbs B, Frizelle FA. Patterns of recurrence in patients with acute diverticulitis. Br J Surg. 2010;97(6):952–7.
11. Modini C, Romagnoli F, De Milito R, Romeo V, Petroni R, La Torre F, et al. Octogenarians: an increasing challenge for acute care and colorectal surgeons. An outcomes analysis of emergency colorectal surgery in the elderly. Colorectal Dis. 2012;14(6):e312–8.
12. Mamidanna R, Eid-Arimoku L, Almoudaris AM, Burns EM, Bottle A, Aylin P, et al. Poor 1-year survival in elderly patients undergoing nonelective colorectal resection. Dis Colon Rectum. 2012;55(7):788–96.
13. Birnbaum EH, Myerson RJ, Fry RD, Kodner IJ, Fleshman JW. Chronic effects of pelvic radiation therapy on anorectal function. Dis Colon Rectum. 1994;37(9):909–15.
14. Tsai BM, Finne CO, Nordenstam JF, Christoforidis D, Madoff RD, Mellgren A. Transanal endoscopic microsurgery resection of rectal tumors: outcomes and recommendations. Dis Colon Rectum. 2010;53(1):16–23.
15. Habr-Gama A, Perez RO, Sao Juliao GP, Proscurshim I, Gama-Rodrigues J. Nonoperative approaches to rectal cancer: a critical evaluation. Semin Radiat Oncol. 2011;21(3):234–9.
16. Garcia-Aguilar J, Shi Q, Thomas Jr CR, Chan E, Cataldo P, Marcet J, et al. A phase II trial of neoadjuvant chemoradiation and local excision for T2N0 rectal cancer: preliminary results of the ACOSOG Z6041 trial. Ann Surg Oncol. 2012;19(2):384–91.
17. U.S. Preventive Services Task Force. Screening for colorectal cancer: recommendation and rationale. Ann Intern Med. 2002;137(2):129–31.
18. Lieberman DA, Rex DK, Winawer SJ, Giardiello FM, Johnson DA, Levin TR. Guidelines for colonoscopy surveillance after screening and polypectomy: a consensus update by the US Multi-Society Task Force on Colorectal Cancer. Gastroenterology. 2012;143(3):844–57.
19. U.S. Preventive Services Task Force. Screening for colorectal cancer: U.S. Preventive Services Task Force recommendation statement. Ann Intern Med. 2008;149(9):627–37.
20. Frasson M, Braga M, Vignali A, Zuliani W, Di Carlo V. Benefits of laparoscopic colorectal resection are more pronounced in elderly patients. Dis Colon Rectum. 2008;51(3):296–300.
21. Stocchi L, Nelson H, Young-Fadok TM, Larson DR, Ilstrup DM. Safety and advantages of laparoscopic vs. open colectomy in the elderly: matched-control study. Dis Colon Rectum. 2000;43(3):326–32.
22. Mutch MG. Laparoscopic colectomy in the elderly: when is too old? Clin Colon Rectal Surg. 2006;19(1):33–9.

The Morbidly Obese Patient

26

Jonathan E. Efron and H. David Vargas

Key Points

- Obesity-related issues in surgery extend well beyond the operating room—prepare well ahead and have a plan for each phase.
- While BMI is helpful for stratifying patients, there are multiple ways to measure obesity.
- Even "easy" laparoscopic cases in the morbidly obese present technical challenges.
- Recognize the impact that obesity has on individual colorectal procedures and how you will approach them.

Introduction

Key concept: Obesity is quickly emerging as one of the largest healthcare issues facing all surgeons.

The obesity epidemic represents one of the greatest healthcare challenges of our generation. Obesity in America is now adding an astounding $190 billion to the annual national healthcare price tag, exceeding smoking as public health enemy number one when it comes to cost [1]. These patients comprise approximately one-third of our surgical practice requiring operative intervention for colorectal disease. Unfortunately in many cases, we still fail to grasp the extent of its reach. For example, obesity has not only been linked to the complications occurring in colorectal surgery but also has been shown to be a risk factor for colorectal cancer [2]. Furthermore, the novice surgeon may underestimate the complexity of the obese patient by simply focusing on the technical challenges imposed by physical characteristics. In contrast, the more mature and experienced surgeon hopefully will identify the increased risk posed by the comorbid conditions often associated with obesity, the ramifications for perioperative decision-making, and the impact on clinical outcomes. This chapter attempts to explore these issues and identify rational strategies for enhancing perioperative care and outcomes.

J.E. Efron, MD (✉)
Ravitch Division, Department of Surgery,
Johns Hopkins University, 1800 Orleans St,
Baltimore, MD 21287, USA
e-mail: jefron1@jhmi.edu

H.D. Vargas, MD
Department of Colon and Rectal Surgery,
Ochsner Clinic Foundation, 1514 Jefferson Highway,
New Orleans, LA 70121, USA
e-mail: dvargas@ochsner.org

Defining Obesity and Limitations of BMI

Key concept: Understand the utility as well as the limitations of BMI as it pertains to various categories of patients.

Many definitions exist for obesity. These include absolute weight, anthropometric measures, and, the most commonly used definition, the body mass index (BMI), which is a calculation based on weight and height. Currently, patients are considered obese if their BMI is greater than 30 and morbidly obese with a BMI greater than 40. While BMI serves as a useful snapshot to stratify patients, and correlate with estimated risk, it does not always give the complete picture. Body mass index as a metric alone possesses inherent limitations based on differences in adipose distribution, muscle mass, and differences across races and gender. For example, weight lifters and body builders have increased muscle mass and weight with little body fat; yet, calculations of BMI may classify such individuals as obese. With aging, loss of mean muscle mass and increases in adipose will render BMI inaccurate. Furthermore, racial disparities exist with BMI, as best exemplified in Asian Pacific races where BMI again fails to account for decreased lean muscle mass.

S.R. Steele et al. (eds.), *Complexities in Colorectal Surgery*,
DOI 10.1007/978-1-4614-9022-7_26, © Springer Science+Business Media New York 2014

Abdominal Obesity: Not All Obesity Is the Same

Key concept: Central obesity is more problematic as it relates to overall health than other types of obesity.

Central adipose distribution has been described by several different names—"abdominal obesity," "mesenteric obesity," "male pattern," or "android obesity." What is becoming apparent is that this central distribution best predicts comorbid conditions associated with obesity such as the metabolic syndrome. This syndrome is hallmarked by a cluster of conditions (not all need to be present depending on the definition) that include hypertension, hypertriglyceridemia, hyperglycemia (i.e., insulin resistance), hypercholesterolemia, microalbuminuria, and central obesity. Risk factors for metabolic syndrome include stress, obesity, endocrine disorders, sedentary lifestyle, older age, and select mental health and rheumatological disorders (i.e., schizophrenia, psoriasis). The syndrome, for which central obesity is a key component, increases the overall risk of cardiovascular morbidity and diabetes, though the clinical utility has been debated. Most important to colorectal surgeons, abdominal obesity may better determine the relative risk for postoperative morbidity.

From a technical standpoint, experienced surgeons often use the "eyeball test" and can subjectively distinguish the potential differences in degrees of difficulty when comparing a normal-sized patient with a morbidly obese one. If that is the case, then what is the ideal index for defining obesity? Anthropometric measurements such as waist circumference or waist-to-height ratios often represent a more pragmatic and clinically relevant method of defining obesity. There are, however, challenges in the task of consistently measuring abdominal girth. Furthermore, for surgeons, what is on the outside may or may not accurately reflect what is on the inside. CT scan imaging provides a novel alternative to measure adipose tissue. In fact, several authors have identified CT as a useful method to define mesenteric or central obesity and correlate it with outcomes and morbidity [3, 4].

This is not to say that BMI does not have value. Most of the current literature certainly relies primarily on this standard definition. Clearly, at a minimum this serves as a "screening" measure stratifying patients. However, how we define obesity and our tendency to focus on the "morbidly obese" underestimates the true challenge facing surgeons. Consider, for example, gender differences. A female with distribution of adipose primarily in the hips, buttocks, and thighs may, in fact, be easier to perform an abdominal operation than a male whose adipose is located primarily abdominally, even though her absolute BMI is higher. As a result, you must be cautious to avoid relying too heavily on BMI as a potential predictor of postoperative outcomes. Rather, choose to "screen" with BMI initially, and then identify specific distribution characteristics of the individual (i.e., fat distribution) when considering implications for surgery.

Preoperative Evaluation

Key concept: Identifying and managing the associated the medical morbidities commonly associated with obese patients helps prevent intraoperative and postoperative complications.

One of the first things to recognize is that obesity never occurs alone, and nearly every organ system can be affected. One or more comorbid medical conditions, including type 2 diabetes, coronary artery diseases, hypertension, joint problems, pulmonary issues, and stroke, are nearly always present or may manifest under stress [5]. Therefore, it is extremely important you take the time ahead of the operation to perform a thorough evaluation to deal with these in the elective setting (if possible). For those who present emergently, the degree of urgency will take precedence, but you can still institute preventative measures by identifying the scale of your patient's issues.

While Chap. 2 of this textbook provides a more comprehensive risk assessment for all patients, it is worth highlighting a few things as it pertains to the obese population. As with any patient, initial work-up includes a general history and physical examination. Your goals should be to both identify how to manage the disease you are presented with and also implement an appropriate time line. A perforated obstructing cancer requires immediate intervention, but identifying that the patient has pulmonary issues, underlying cardiac disease, or adrenal insufficiency may alter the way you manage them perioperatively. For elective operations, a standardized approach through a preoperative evaluation clinic is a meaningful method of assessing all high-risk surgical candidates. Obese, and particularly morbidly obese, patients should always be considered higher risk and evaluated through a standardized setting when possible [6]. Preoperative education and counseling helps to define goals of postoperative outcomes and expectations to minimize complications. In this arena you can discuss several things that may arise that are more common in obese patients. For example, it is imperative to inform the obese patient that they have a higher likelihood of needing to open the wound for a wound infection and will need to pack the wound postoperatively. For those with pulmonary issues, you should discuss the increased chance of needing to stay intubated for longer cases or the need for prolonged DVT chemoprophylaxis—even after discharge. It is also an opportunity to ensure that you have special wheelchairs, beds, and trapeze available to help your get out of bed, ambulate, and move around the hospital.

Systems-Based Evaluation and Prevention Tips

Pulmonary: Preoperative pulmonary evaluation should include an assessment of undiagnosed obstructive sleep apnea, for which the risk factor most closely associated is obesity [7]. Identifying these patients preoperatively is essential so that adequate postoperative management of the patient for the first 24 h is achieved. This postoperative care includes oxygenation monitoring and the use of continuous positive airway pressure (CPAP) management when sleeping or in the recovery unit, if required. While incentive spirometry and early ambulation are needed in all patients, it is critical in the obese, as atelectasis, pneumonia, and mucus plugging are all more common.

Cardiac: A thorough assessment of the obese patient's overall cardiac function is also mandatory. Hypertensive status, myocardial function, angina, and infarction history are some of the important factors to address. Diagnosing hypertension is based on the patient having elevated readings at two or more office visits and requires the patient to be seated for approximately 5 min with their feet on the ground. Remember, an appropriately sized arm cuff must be used, more applicable when measuring the pressure in an obese individual. A general physical examination is recommended for any operative candidate, but care should be taken in the obese to identify a nodular thyroid, identify a heart murmur or click, and listen for wheezing or rales on pulmonary examination. Look for signs of peripheral edema, venous stasis, or vascular insufficiency. These are all indications of congestive heart failure or poorly controlled cardiac function and require a more thorough cardiac examination.

When identified, hypertension requires correction prior to surgery with a goal of reaching a pressure less than 140/90 mmHg and even lower in those with concomitant renal disease or diabetes [8]. This goal may be achieved through lifestyle modifications or pharmacotherapy. Often there is no time to employ lifestyle modifications, but if possible, smoking cessation, weight loss, dietary changes, and increased physical exercise are all encouraged. In general, single drug therapy should be started and titrated; however, when the patient's pressure exceeds 160/100 mmHg, then combined drug therapy (typically utilizing a thiazide diuretic) is recommended [8]. When required, the patient's primary medical physician best manages initiation or manipulation of these medications.

Obesity and cardiovascular disease go hand in hand. The Framingham Heart Study identified obesity as an independent risk factor for sudden death, congestive heart failure, and coronary disease [9]. Central obesity, more commonly found in men, carries the highest cardiac risk in the obese population and carries the risk of the aforementioned metabolic syndrome [10]. The American College of Cardiology, in conjunction with the American Heart Association, has published specific guidelines on the preoperative cardiac evaluation of obese patients [11]. These are summarized in Table 26.1 and should be employed when planning elective surgery on an obese individual. If patients fall into the intermediate or high-risk category with respect to their cardiac risk, and are undergoing a laparotomy, further evaluation by a cardiologist is recommended.

Table 26.1 Preoperative risk stratification [10]

1. Identify those with active cardiac conditions/comorbidities suggestive of high risk and take steps to correct these conditions prior to elective surgery. They include: Stable or unstable angina Decompensated heart failure Recent MI (within 6 months) Decompensated heart failure Significant arrhythmia Severe valvular disease (specifically aortic or mitral stenosis)
2. Determine the severity of the surgery (inherent risk of the procedure) Low risk (<1 %) Endoscopic Superficial Intermediate risk (1–5 %) Peritoneal Thoracic Orthopedic High risk (>5 %) Major vascular Cytoreduction and HIPEC Select pelvic cases
3. For those undergoing intermediate- or high-risk surgery, proceed with assessment of their functional capacity: Assessment of metabolic equivalents (METs): based on treadmill test or patients ability to ambulate 4 blocks or two flights of stairs without symptoms. (a) >4 METs = those with adequate functional capacity as seen on treadmill or asymptomatic may proceed with surgery (b) For all others requiring further work-up (< 4METs): see Chap. 2 on perioperative risk assessment

Thromboembolic Disease: Obesity is also an independent risk factor for increasing the risk of deep vein thrombosis (DVT) or pulmonary embolism (PE) in patients undergoing abdominal surgery [12]. Many colorectal disorders such as cancer and inflammatory bowel disease also increase the risk of thromboembolic disease and are independent risk factors that are additive to an obese patient's risk of having a thromboembolic complications with colorectal surgery. Therefore, preoperative administration of subcutaneous heparin with the use of sequential stockings as per SCIP and ASCRS guidelines is highly recommended [13]. Care must be taken to ensure appropriate timing of the heparin and also of the adequate dose. Obese patients may require a higher dose of unfractionated heparin, depending on their weight. A Cochrane review comparing various strategies for preventing DVTs in colorectal surgery demonstrated no difference in outcomes when low molecular weight heparin was compared to unfractionated heparin; however, the addition of compression stockings to heparin appeared to provide greater protection from DVTs [14]. Currently, we recommend pneumatic compression stockings with an appropriate dose of unfractionated heparin preoperatively, during the hospital stay, and in some patients (i.e., prior DVT or excessive BMI), postoperatively for up to 30 days. Postoperative prophylaxis after discharge is controversial, but several large reviews have demonstrated a significant reduction in the incidence of DVTs and PE in those treated after discharge [15, 16].

Diabetes: Diabetes is an independent risk factor predicting postoperative morbidity [17]. While hemoglobin A1c levels provide a global assessment of a patient's overall glucose control, as it provides an indicator of the extent of hyperglycemia that has occurred during the life of a red blood cell (120 days), the perioperative stress may make even borderline insulin-resistant patients problematic to control. To facilitate adequate glucose control on the day of surgery, diabetic patients should be scheduled in the morning and the use half of their daily dose of insulin that morning. The patient also requires intraoperative monitoring and in some cases constant glucose monitoring with initiation of an insulin drip is required. Inadequate intraoperative glucose control (even in nondiabetics) has been shown to be associated with increased wound infections, operative re-interventions, and death [18]. However, correction of this proper insulin therapy lowers this risk to that of patients with normal blood glucose and is an important quality metric.

Laparoscopic Colectomy in the Obese Patient

Key concept: Even the straightforward laparoscopic cases in the obese patient present technical challenges that you need to prepare for and well versed with the technical nuisances to overcome them.

Laparoscopic colectomy offers improved postoperative outcomes compared to open in essentially every patient population, and this in no different in the obese patient. However, application of this technique in an obese patient clearly should be considered one of the most technically challenging laparoscopic operations, even for experienced surgeons. There are numerous reasons why this is difficult. Increased adipose of the retroperitoneum, mesentery, and omentum reduces peritoneal space and diminishes the "doming effect" of pneumoperitoneum, thus compromising video-scopic perspective. Additionally, mesenteric fat increases the volume of small bowel and mesentery to be retracted for exposure, while the overall thickness of the mesentery and its foreshortening makes vessel identification and division challenging. The omentum also poses a specific challenge for retraction due to its greater volume, weight, and adhesions. Unfortunately, the instrumentation that we use often adds to the complexity. The long thin miniature shaft and narrow end effectors used for grasping and dissection prove mechanically disadvantaged when attempting to manipulate the increased volume and weight of organs involved. Lastly, the use of gravity as the additional retractor in laparoscopic surgery poses significant issues in the morbidly obese. In order to adequately expose the operative field, extremes of body positioning with steep Trendelenburg and "reverse T" along with lateral tilt are needed. In reality, some of these are nearly impossible with the extremes of weight and poses hazards to peripheral nerves and even dislodgement of the patient (Fig. 26.1). Not surprisingly, the initial reports of laparoscopic colectomy often cited severe obesity as a relative contraindication to this technique.

As in any other operation, preparation for a laparoscopic colectomy in the obese patient remains paramount. First, you must mentally prepare and comprehend that these cases possess unique challenges that increase in complexity as BMI increases. Also, you must be realistic by considering your own laparoscopic experience and where you are on the learning curve. Identifying a complex operation involves consideration of patient characteristics such as obesity, severity of pathologic condition, urgency, prior abdominal operations, and type of colectomy planned. Conversion serves as a surrogate marker for the degree of technical difficulty of a procedure but also may be a marker for good judgment on your part. In a study of nearly 1,000 laparoscopic colectomies, the authors identified surgeon experience, left-sided resection, fistula and abscess, *and obesity* as risk factors for conversion. Furthermore, there is an exponentially greater risk of conversion (vs. simply cumulative) when multiple factors are present. For example, an obese patient requiring sigmoidectomy for diverticulitis complicated by colovesical fistula will be a daunting task for any surgeon but especially for the surgeon with limited laparoscopic experience. This is not to say that you should not attempt a diagnostic laparoscopy, proceed with initial dissection, and perform the operation laparoscopically to the extent you feel safe and comfortable. This is often a great objective, at any point along your learning curve. One effective strategy is to set a time limit and determine ahead of time that if you are not making progress by the end that you will convert. Another operative approach in the patient described above or other complicated left-sided resections is to focus on the splenic flexure and colon mobilization. After that is performed, the fistula and resection can be approached through a low midline or Pfannenstiel incision under direct vision. Remember, a splenic flexure takedown in a morbidly obese patient with a heavy, thick body wall that has to be retracted in the open setting is not easy either.

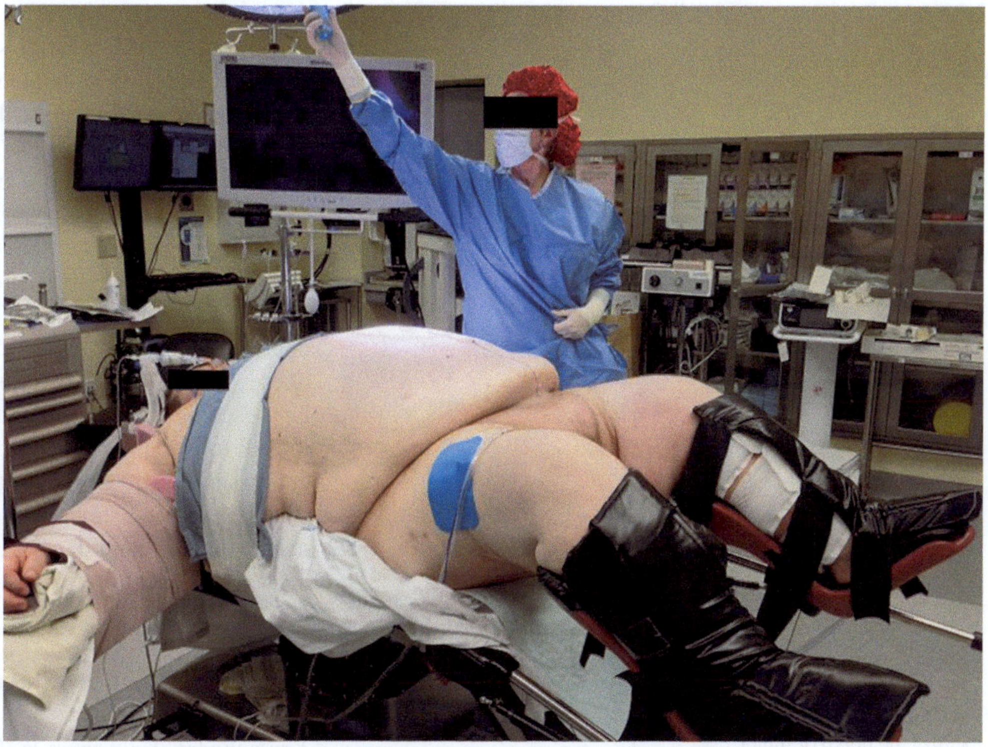

Fig. 26.1 Positioning a patient with massive obesity (BMI 80) for laparoscopic surgery (Courtesy of Justin A. Maykel, MD)

Lesion Localization

Key concept: Have a plan and backup plan in place with obese patients to ensure the proper identification of the pathology and corresponding boundaries of resection.

As highlighted above, scheduling the case early in the day, budgeting appropriate operative time, and ensuring you have adequate surgical assistance and technical support will reduce the burden of these complex cases. A clear operative plan must also be in order. It may seem intuitive, but the first specific task is the proper identification of the colonic pathology requiring resection. You have likely already heard the basics—check your CT, review the scope report, and tattoo the site of the pathology. However, in the obese patient it is not always that simple. Identifying a serosal tattoo can be a challenge, as a large omentum, enlarged appendices epiploica, and abundant retroperitoneal and mesenteric fat often obscure the mark. By now you recognize that any lesion described as being in the region of the hepatic flexure and proximal to the rectum should be expected to be particularly concerning in this regard. To preoperatively localize the lesion for operative planning, we place an endoscopic clip (Fig. 26.2) at the lesion as a backup plan (especially in obese patients) and perform plain radiography for segment localization. Alternatively, the metallic clip can be identified on CT. Admittedly, overlapping segments of colon, especially with a floppy transverse colon, could occur on plain radiography, although this has yet to have occurred in our experience. One helpful tip is that if the KUB is performed immediately after colonoscopy, the residual gas in the bowel provides a well-delineated outline of distinct bowel segments effectively and easier identification of the metallic clip. This enables you to go to the operating room with confidence in a clear operative plan.

This simple maneuver may allow you to position the patient supine for a right colectomy and avoid lithotomy positioning and the potential risks of DVT and peripheral nerve injury. Remember, positioning is a major component of operating on the morbidly obese, something we will address shortly. If nothing else, you can avoid searching for the tattoo prior to initiating dissection and mobilization, potentially reducing operative time. This is not to say we avoid a tattoo. Rather, the clip serves as a backup, and tattoo identification provides the ultimate intraoperative confirmation; therefore, we still find the tattoo of benefit. This also obviates the need for on-table colonoscopy to localize the lesion—another often discussed, but in practice, time-consuming and more difficult maneuver.

We routinely ask our institution's gastroenterologists to perform both a three-quadrant tattoo and endoscopic clip for lesions in the vicinity of the transverse colon, either flexure, or the descending colon. The difference in difficulty of a splenic flexure resection as opposed to sigmoid colectomy cannot be overstated in normal-sized patients. When you are dealing with the morbidly obese, this becomes magnified. Mid- or distal transverse colon lesions may be approached as an extended right colectomy versus variations of a left colectomy. Descending colon lesions pose similar challenges in

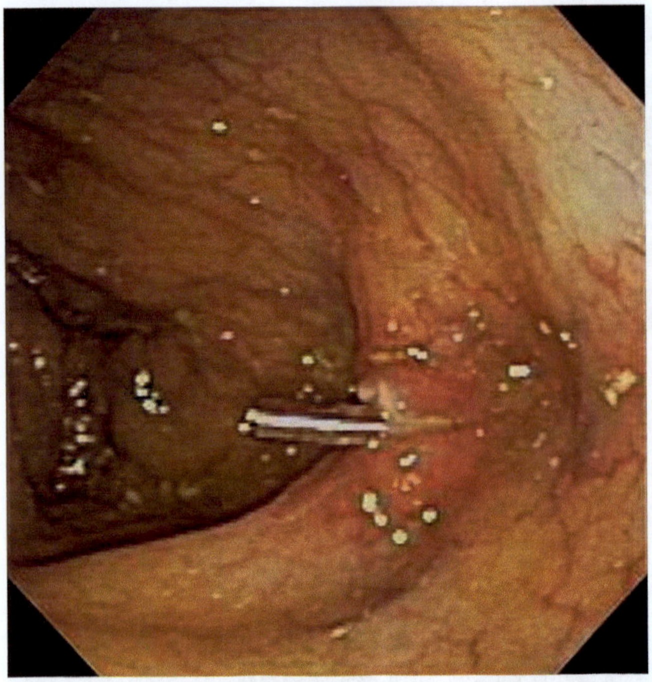

Fig. 26.2 Endoscopic photo of metal clip, useful to radiologically localize the polyp or tumor

terms of the extent of resection. Should you perform an extended left colectomy and potentially require consideration of transverse colon to rectal anastomosis? An ileal mesenteric window may be necessary to facilitate tension-free anastomosis, especially given the foreshortening of a thick mesentery in an obese patient. Another alternative to reach the pelvis with the mid-transverse colon is to fully mobilize the right colon and turn the right colon mesentery counterclockwise into the pelvis as a straight line. How often have you done that and what is the orientation of the right colon you are going use to bring down to avoid twisting or cutting off blood supply? These are often things we bring up on boards or in conference, but many of you may have never seen or tried these technical steps. The benefit of being able to think through this decision process prior to going to the operating room cannot be overstated. Thus, in the obese patient who already poses significant technical difficulties, being able to anticipate such operative decision-making prior to surgery enhances surgical performance.

The Value of Your Assistant

Key concept: Approaching your more complex cases in the obese patient with someone not facile in laparoscopic surgery, using the camera, or providing adequate exposure is a setup for failure from the beginning.

A standard laparoscopic resection in the obese patient will require a skilled surgical assistance. If you are at an institution with senior surgical residents or colorectal/minimally invasive fellows available, such an issue may not be germane. However, in a private institution, another attending or highly experienced surgical assistant should be present. Certainly, the feasibility of laparoscopic colectomy in the obese patient has been demonstrated. Delaney and colleagues compared laparoscopic colectomy in an obese cohort compared to a matched control group and found a similar length of stay and no increase in overall complications. However, not unexpectedly, they did show an increased operative time and higher conversion to open rate in the obese cohort [19]. Leroy and associates also reported on laparoscopic sigmoid colectomy in the obese patient where they described their consecutive series of 29 patients without conversion [20]. Utilizing a 5- or 6-port technique with excellent results, however, more pointedly illustrates the need for a team approach, with multiple skilled assistants, to achieve technical proficiency.

Patient Setup, Port Placement, and Exposure

Key concept: Your setup is the initial key to your success in the OR. While you may still struggle, problems at this stage will almost assuredly make things much more difficult.

By now you realize that the extremes of rotation allow you to maximize gravity's effect for providing exposure in laparoscopic colectomy (Fig. 26.3). This is much more difficult in the morbidly obese patient. The first step you need to focus on is properly positioning, padding, and securing the patient to the operating room table. Depending on your table, once your patient's weight approaches over 400 lb, you must ensure that the table meets the requirements for supporting them. To secure the patient, there are several systems available and different surgeons have their own preferences; yet all focus on avoiding slipping and causing any traction or pressure-related injury. We prefer to use 3-in. wide silk tape over a barrier towel across the patient's chest wrapped three times around the table. Others describe using beanbags, foam securing systems, IV bags at the shoulders (not recommended), arm sleds, and gel pads on the operating room table. Some even secure the bed sheet to the lowered foot of the bed. While it is important for you to find what works for you, consider this word of caution if you are a beanbag user. Because we rely on a fulcrum of downward movement of your graspers to raise the colon (especially with a medial approach), having your beanbag inflated high up on the patient's side will cause you to hit the beanbag and lose this ability. Curling it slightly back or avoiding this tight "high-riding cocoon" will avoid this common mistake. We also recommend a "dry run" before prepping and draping by having anesthesia put the patient in all 4 extremes of position and ensuring the patient is adequately secured. That way,

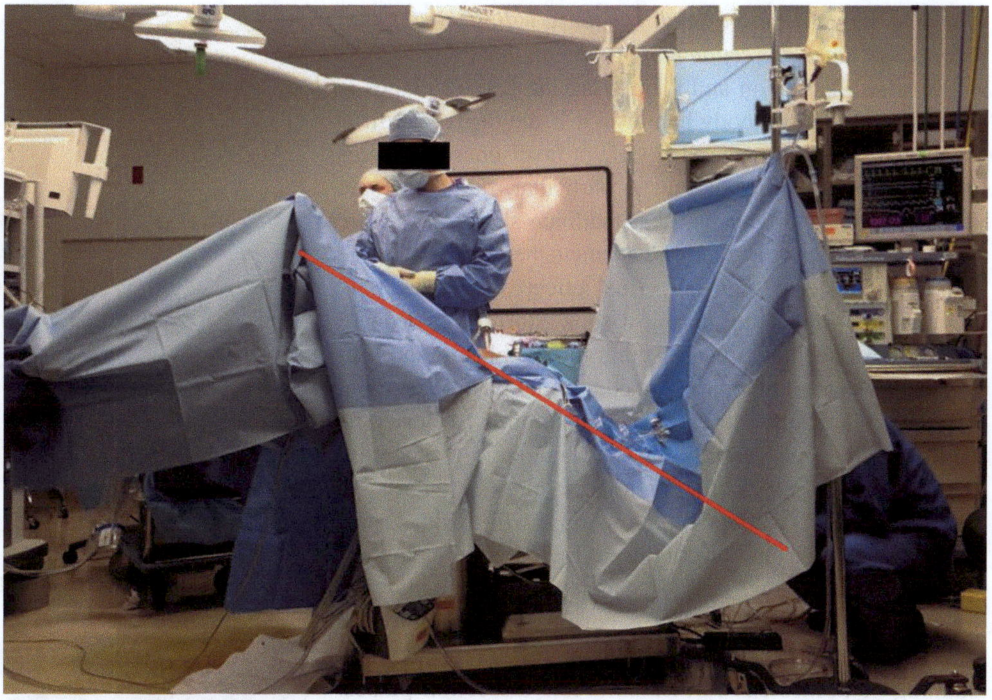

Fig. 26.3 OR positioning for laparoscopic colectomy showing steep Trendelenburg, a maneuver that helps with retraction and exposure. *Red line* indicates the patient's orientation in steep Trendelenberg

everyone in the operating room can see the patient does not fall and provides confidence during the case when the drapes are on and the operating room is dark and you ask for steeper positioning.

We recommend insertion of ureteral stents for patients with prior pelvic surgery, radiation, and other situations where ureteral anatomy may be altered. We also find stents helpful when fistulizing disease is present—either to the bladder or the vagina—or if large abscesses or phlegmons (either retroperitoneal or pelvic) complicate the intestinal disease. In our opinion, obesity in and of itself is not an indication for ureteral stent insertion. Identification of the ureter in a very large patient with excessive mesenteric and retroperitoneal fat can be daunting and cause a lot of heartache and prolonged operating room time. Stents may be one means by which critical steps of the operation can be facilitated.

We recommend using more ports than you are normally accustomed for additional graspers to provide retraction and aid in the dissection. Have them available ahead of time. Since these are "bariatric patients," you need to have bariatric length equipment—cameras, graspers, and staplers. Traditional ports that you are accustomed to using may not adequately reach through the body wall and longer trocars may be required. Regarding port placement, the principles of maximizing exposure to all parts of the abdomen by maintaining good ergonomics and triangulation still apply in the obese individual. Again, as you need to elevate the heavy colon and bulky mesentery, moving your ports a little more medially than normal will allow you to maintain the optimal fulcrum. When the ports are placed too lateral, you will often hit the bed with your grasper and not be able to manipulate the instruments freely. Remember, this is further exacerbated by the lack of working space in between the bowel and anterior abdominal wall with a standard pneumoperitoneum at 15 mmHg.

Exposure to the central mesentery is difficult as a result of bulky visceral fat. A medial-to-lateral approach may thus be difficult, or even not possible. Therefore, you should be skilled and prepared to employ the spectrum of colonic mobilization techniques: lateral to medial, superior or "top-down" starting at the transverse colon, and inferior to superior. Be flexible and be willing to switch to a different approach during the various steps of the operation to accommodate the patient's habitus and pathologic condition. In addition to placing additional ports, one way to handle the bulky omentum is to take down the falciform ligament. This will provide a broad space over the top of the liver and the anterior stomach to flip the omentum back up on itself. A small sponge pad placed through a 10 mm trocar or hand port can "stick" to the omentum and anterior abdominal wall, retracting the omentum away from the operative field. Opening the sponge (or rolling it) and using it as a barrier to hold back the creeping small bowel is often helpful as well.

Dissection Techniques

Key concept: *Gaining access to the correct plane and using precise sharp dissection will be helpful. Take care of all bleeding early as even small amounts will distort tissue planes and make dissection more problematic.*

Standard dissection and identifying the correct planes is similar regardless of body habitus—it is the degree of difficulty that varies. In general, I (HDV) favor energy devices for mobilizing the bowel and, in particular, find ultrasonic dissectors to have finer tips that facilitate sharp dissection. The key, ultimately, is to ensure adequate hemostasis. Tissue planes are distorted and the visual effect of "yellow out" (similar to "white out" during a snow storm) can lead to imprecise dissection, violating embryologic planes, and lead to small (or large) amounts of meddlesome bleeding. Avoid grasping on the fatty mesentery and attempting to elevate its bulk—it will likely tear and bleed. Atraumatic graspers on the bowel or epiploica utilizing a larger bite (i.e., similar to grasping a vein), while avoiding tearing, will avoid serosal or even full-thickness bowel injuries. Increased blood loss—another surrogate marker for technical difficulty—may not be measurably different, but it is our impression that obese patients have greater bleeding during mobilization and blood staining of tissues can further obfuscate dissection planes. Furthermore, due to differences in hemoglobin-related light absorption, this will result in decreased laparoscopic illumination and visualization.

The extent of mobilization should be considered. You should anticipate mesenteric shortening and the resulting possibility of encountering increased tension at your intended anastomosis site. This mandates a disciplined attention to ensuring complete mobilization of the colon to avoid this scenario. We have found several keys to help in this aspect. First, mobilize back to the root of the mesentery—while this is often a bit worrisome for the novice surgeon in a heavy patient with thick mesentery and ill-defined planes, it is needed to gain length. Next, completely mobilize the mesentery cranially and caudally, and always mobilize the flexures. Many surgeons selectively take down the flexures—in obese patients, this is the norm. The omentum can either be dissected off the colon or taken with specimen, the lesser sac needs to be entered, and you have to divide the retroperitoneal attachments to ensure a full flexure mobilization. Additionally, vessels are divided high to achieve full mobilization and to avoid ischemia at the distal end of the bowel. This proximal division reduces the number of vessels and volume of tissue to be divided, but requires precise, disciplined dissection with skeletonization of the named vessels to ensure adequate primary and collateral vascularization. I (HDV) prefer staplers for vessel division, due to the volume of tissue divided, though many surgeons successfully used energy devices alone. All these maneuvers typically provide enough mobility to the remaining bowel to effect a tension-free anastomosis. This is also crucial when bringing up a colostomy. Without adequate mobilization and preservation of blood supply, your patient may be left with a sunken or stenotic stoma (Fig. 26.4), an extremely difficult problem to deal with in this population.

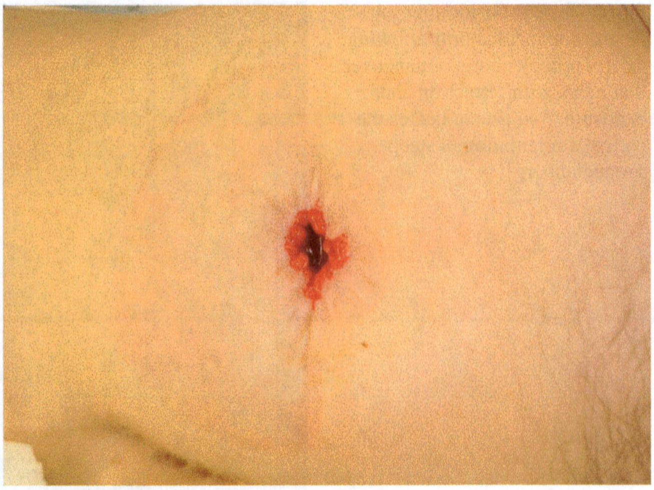

Fig. 26.4 Stenotic stoma as a result of ischemia created when devascularizing the bowel to allow reach through thick abdominal wall (Courtesy of Philip Y. Pearson, MD)

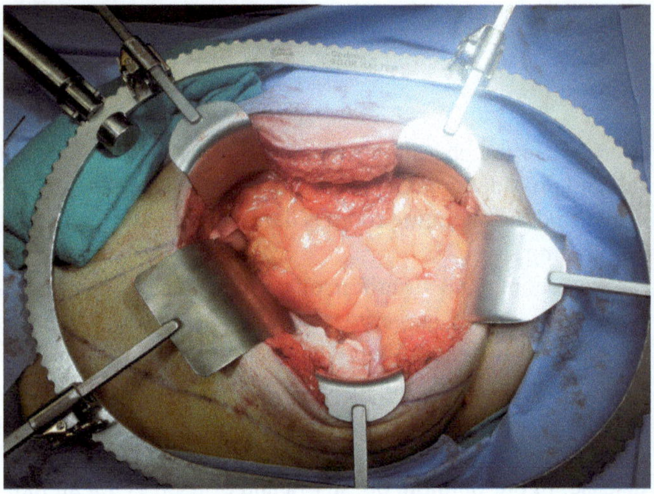

Fig. 26.5 Intraoperative photo of large sigmoid colon enveloped by massive visceral adipose tissue filling a relatively large incision

Regardless of the technique used, extracorporeal division of mesenteric vessels should be avoided. This will prove very difficult through a small laparoscopic incision, with limited ability to visualize and manipulate a large foreshortened colon and bulky mesentery that fills the small wound (Fig. 26.5). The mesentery will be placed on tension and risks avulsion and bleeding. Your best visualization will be laparoscopically, and you will have the best opportunity to do something should any problems arise. Avoid the temptation—divide the major vessels intracorporeally.

Specimen Extraction and Ideal Wound Placement

Key concept: Specimen extraction wounds should be midline, and expect larger incisions to accommodate the larger-sized specimen.

The size of the extraction site—already remarkably small given the body habitus—should not inhibit specimen extraction. Although all the reported sites can work (lateral, Pfannenstiel, lower quadrant), when faced with a difficult dilemma, the midline represents the shortest distance from the root of the mesentery to the abdominal wall. Invariably, small amounts of the mesentery must still be divided and complete extraction facilitates any extracorporeal dissection. Also, take into account that exteriorization of the right colon can be more difficult through a small incision, as classically both ends are brought out and divided extracorporeally. This results in a larger specimen that has to be brought through the wound. Consider dividing one end of the bowel intracorporeally or dividing through the incision prior to exteriorization. Be careful in both of these instances to maintain proper orientation of the mesentery and avoid the 180° twist.

Another aspect of right colectomy should be the cranial-caudal position of the midline wound. When choosing your incision site, ignore the umbilicus altogether. Exteriorization of the transverse colon will be difficult if your wound is positioned too low. In an obese patient, the umbilicus is often displaced caudally due to the size and weight of the pannus (Fig. 26.6) and actually is a poor anatomic landmark of the position of intraperitoneal organs. While an intracorporeal anastomosis in the obese patient can be performed [21], an extracorporeal anastomosis can be more easily performed by moving the incision cranially. Though the wound becomes more conspicuous, we cannot emphasize enough that cosmesis remains a secondary concern when attempting to perform a critical step of a complex operation for serious pathology in a challenging patient. The most pragmatic technical solution to such challenges will prove most reliable and reproducible. Use the midline and avoid being fooled by the umbilicus.

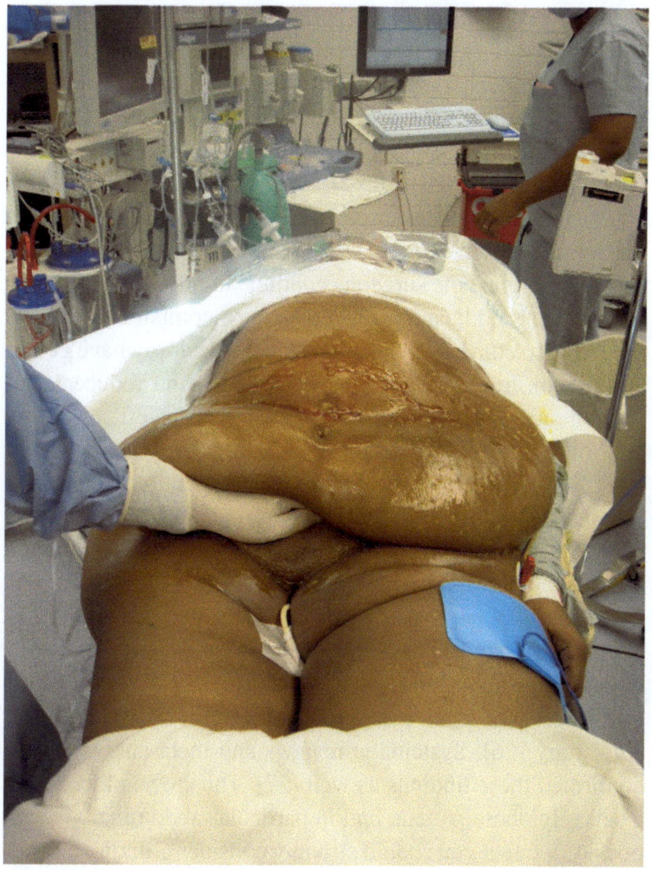

Fig. 26.6 Caudally positioned umbilicus in a patient with large pannus

The Role of Hand-Assisted Laparoscopic Colectomy in the Obese Patient

Key concept: Hand-assisted laparoscopic colectomy may provide another approach in obese patients to reduce the conversion rates and operative times, with similar other outcomes when compared to straight laparoscopy.

The literature comparing laparoscopic colectomy in obese (BMI > 30) to normal weight patients reveals increased operative time and increased conversions in the obese patient. Not surprisingly, there is a learning curve associated specifically with laparoscopic colectomy in the obese patient, further affirming the complexity of this undertaking. Sarli et al. found that after 80 cases, operative time and conversion decreased to similar levels witnessed in the nonobese patient [22]. This makes intuitive sense, as more experience with complex, difficult operations results in improved proficiency. Yet, it also drives home the point that the learning curve varies based on the indication and specific patient operated on. While the ASCRS consensus statement on laparoscopic colectomy for curable cancer recommends at least 20 baseline cases performed for benign disease or metastatic cancer [23], we recommend further preparatory experience when considering the added difficulty encountered with obese patients.

Hand-assisted laparoscopic colectomy (HALC) offers a technique that overcomes some the limitations of conventional laparoscopic surgery. Rather than attempting to retract with multiple miniature graspers, manual retraction proves atraumatic and efficient. In particular, manual retraction enables the surgeon to provide exposure where the planes of dissection are kept "flat" and linear. This allows a deliberate, continuous dissection over greater distances with limited adjustments in retraction and exposure. Hand assist also allows for dissection in a direction back towards the camera, again providing for greater versatility in mobilization options. Lastly, palpation enables surgeons (especially those early in their learning curve) to confirm vital structures when visual cues often can be misleading due to the previously mentioned "yellow out" phenomenon. Palpation takes a 2-dimensional laparoscopic experience and transforms it to a 3-dimensional one, which bolsters a surgeon's confidence in the precision of the dissection. Although some surgeons continue to question the merits of hand-assisted laparoscopic colectomy, comparative studies of HALC to conventional laparoscopic colectomy have generally demonstrated reduced operative times and reduced conversion rates [24]. Complex operations such as left colectomy and total abdominal colectomy, in particular, benefit from a hand-assisted technique with reduced operative times and conversion. Specific to obese patients, data examining HALC compared to straight laparoscopic in this population reported reduced operative times and reduced conversion, without any differences in pain, analgesic use, or length of stay [25]. Comparative studies have looked at long-term outcomes such as hernia formation and bowel obstruction and have not found any differences when compared to conventional laparoscopic colectomy [26]. Systematic reviews and meta-analyses have confirmed these findings as well [27]. Thus, when faced with a severely obese patient, and in particular abdominal/visceral obesity, we feel you should strongly consider utilizing a hand-assisted technique. We should point out, however, that whether your approach is hand-assisted or straight laparoscopic, the recommendations regarding the conduct of a laparoscopic colectomy for malignancy remain identical.

Technical Considerations

Key concept: Obesity has specific considerations for each procedure and/or colorectal disease process you may encounter. Understand how it may impact your individual patient and your management strategy.

Pelvic Dissection

Key concept: Obesity leads to distorted planes in the pelvis with difficulty identifying crucial structures.

When discussing pelvic dissections, we are primarily referring to operating on the rectum at a level below the sacral promontory. The diagnoses that lead to pelvic dissection include inflammatory bowel disease, cancer, and functional disorders such as rectal prolapse. The pelvis in obese patients (especially in the narrow male pelvis) can be extremely hostile. The anatomy is often distorted due to retroperitoneal fat that displaces structures such as the iliac arteries and the autonomic nerves anteriorly and medially. It is surprisingly easy to mistakenly enter the wrong plane of dissection and inadvertently injure any of these structures. We have found that initiating our pelvic dissection right at the sacral promontory helps prevent inadvertent vascular injury. Identifying the ureter is also challenging, as it may be located deep in the retroperitoneum and encased in adipose tissue. As stated before, consider placing ureteral catheters in morbidly obese patients as this may make identification of the ureters easier. If not, the most common location for identification remains the crossing at the iliac bifurcation. Do not hesitate to attempt to look both medially and laterally if you are unable to identify the ureter initially. We have even had to go proximally, adjacent to the kidney in certain cases and follow the ureter down into the pelvis. Never just assume the ureter is out of the way.

In the open approach, attempting to operate through a small incision in obese individuals often leads to inability to visualize critical structures because of encroachment of fat and loss of abdominal domain. These two factors make retracting very difficult. By extending the size of the incision for adequate visualization and retraction of abdominal structures, you can lower the risk of inadvertent injury of vital structures. Even by placing the patient in a head down position, and packing the small bowel off, this may not be enough in the obese patient. We have found that in the case of a proctectomy, proximal division and packing off the descending colon in the upper abdomen allow for the distal aspect to be used as a handle and frees up some space for dissection. The lower you go in the pelvis, you may need to use more than one pelvic retractor to displace excessive fat and tissue that may encroach on the dissection. We prefer a St. Marks retractor, though Wylie renal vein retractors are often useful due to their narrow profile and "lipped" end. Customized longer instruments may be needed for adequate retraction and exposure deep in the pelvis. This is particularly important when retracting the vagina to divide the rectum and perform a stapled anastomosis under direct vision to avoid an iatrogenic rectovaginal fistula. We are also more apt to place an EEA sizer in the vagina to aid in visualization of the posterior vaginal wall or cuff and help with upward retraction.

Ileal Pouch-Anal Anastomosis (IPAA) in the Obese Patient

Key concept: IPAA presents its own unique set of potential complications in the obese patient, but the traditional "pouch principles" of ensuring adequate length for the pouch to reach and proximal diversion are similar to the nonobese patient.

The most common operation performed for inflammatory bowel disease requiring a pelvic dissection is a restorative proctocolectomy with ileal pouch-anal anastomosis for ulcerative colitis. Controversy exists as to the increase risk found in the obese patient when performing an IPAA procedure. Kiran and associates examined their experience with IPAA operations in obese patients (BMI > 32.7) [28]. They found that obese patients had a significantly higher rate of wound infection, anastomotic separation, and bowel obstruction. Canedo et al. did not find significant difference in overall complications when comparing patients with a BMI higher than 30 to a control group [29]. One of the authors of this chapter (JE) found a significantly higher rate of pelvic sepsis and perioperative morbidity in the obese group (BMI ≥ 33.7) [30]. Integrity of the pouch-anal anastomosis is clearly dependent on multiple factors including nutritional status, medications, severity of disease, and technical competency. It is not surprising, therefore, that the literature would vary in associating obesity as an independent risk factor for pouch problems. It should be noted that the literature is fairly uniform in demonstrating that the majority of obese patients will have equivalent pouch function if the procedure is performed without significant pelvic septic complications. Only Wibmer and colleagues identified obesity as a risk factor for permanent ileostomy formation after ileal pouch-anal anastomosis [31]. Interestingly, a laparoscopic approach has been associated with a lower complications rate for IPAA, even when accounting for BMI [32].

There are several strategies when approaching obese patients who are requesting an IPAA. If the patient has severe disease and is on multiple immunosuppressants, performing a total abdominal colectomy with ileostomy initially is a fairly routine approach for most surgeons. This allows the patient an opportunity to restore their nutrition reserves and wean off all ulcerative colitis medications. Specifically to the obese population, this strategy also provides the incentive for the patient to lose excess weight prior to the proctectomy and IPAA formation. We must admit, however, in our experience such weight loss is often not often achieved. Adequate weight loss can be utilized as a potential "carrot," although patients with a BMI > 40 must clearly understand the risks associated with the surgery.

Getting the pouch to reach without tension may be challenging if the patient has a long torso, but standard mobilization maneuvers will often allow it to reach the anus. Given the available data that demonstrates higher pelvic sepsis rates, every effort should be made to divert the stool stream proximal to the pouch. In obese patients, the fatty mesentery and the thickness of the abdominal wall makes creating the loop ileostomy extremely difficult. Oftentimes a very proximal stoma is required to achieve diversion. While this will result in high output from the ileostomy, possibly even requiring long-term fluid supplementation or TPN, we feel it is required to avoid the sequela of pelvic sepsis in these obese patients. We do discuss the potential problems with the ileostomy (i.e., skin problems, pouching issues, high output) in our preoperative counseling and emphasize to the patient this is potentially a short-term tradeoff for the benefit of long-term good pouch function.

Another option for proximal diversion in the obese patient is the formation of an end-loop stoma. This requires division of the small intestine and careful division of the small bowel mesentery so the proximal end of the diverted stoma can be brought out as an end stoma. Care must be taken when dividing the mesentery of the small intestine so that you do not disrupt the blood supply distally to the ileal pouch. This stoma usually requires a laparotomy to close, as the distal end stays within the abdominal cavity, though not always. Despite this fact, it is still advisable to perform and end-loop stoma when no other option exists for proximal diversion to avoid the sequelae of pelvic sepsis.

Rectal Cancer in the Obese Patient

Key concept: Obesity has both technical and management implications for patients with rectal cancer. Ensure you discuss the potential impact regarding the need for open surgery, possibility of requiring an APR for distal lesions and overall worse outcomes.

Obesity has been shown to increase the conversion rate in laparoscopic surgery for rectal cancer. In a recent review of 490 patients who underwent laparoscopic surgery for rectal cancer, Denost et al. found that those patients with a BMI of greater than 30 had a 32 % conversion rate. However, the overall and cancer-specific survival, as well as the quality of the mesorectal resection did not differ between groups [33]. A general rule of thumb (especially early in your experience) is that large tumors in obese males should be considered for an open operation, despite the potential increase in wound complications.

With advances in technology, the hope is to decrease some of these risks and to improve outcomes. At present, there is minimal data published on robotic proctectomy for rectal cancer in obese patients. Baek et al. have retrospectively reviewed their experience utilizing the robot for rectal cancer and have found adequate lymph node yield, mesorectal quality, and comparable 5-year survival to open procedures [34]. No one has yet reported their experience specifically in obese individuals. Similar positioning and dissection tips as previously discussed are applicable here as well. This especially pertains to securing the patient to the table to avoid slippage, as the patient is normally in steep Trendelenburg for extended periods.

Distal tumors may be especially difficult to adequately resect without performing an abdominal-perineal resection in the obese patient. The anal canal is often long, the low rectum and perineum are difficult to adequately visualize, and a hand-sewn colo-anal anastomosis may be difficult (if not impossible) to perform. Your patients need to be informed of that possibility preoperatively. Some tips for handling the perineum when having to perform an APR or a hand-sewn colo-anal anastomosis include the following: (1) rolls of blankets or gelfoam bolsters should be placed under the sacral and lumbar spine, as this helps to elevate the perineum and gives improved exposure; (2) tape the patient's buttocks apart prior to prepping the perineum to provide better exposure; (3) place the legs in the steep modified lithotomy position when performing the perineal dissection to help retract some of the buttock tissue and open the space exposing the anus; (4) use long narrow vaginal retractors to help in retracting excess tissue during the perineal dissection; and (5) the prone position may provide better exposure for the perineal dissection and may require "flipping" the patient for this portion of the dissection.

There is debate as to whether or not obese individuals have worse oncological outcomes from rectal cancer surgery than nonobese patients. There is no definitive evidence to support this, but we do consider treating with neoadjuvant chemoradiation for distal tumors where the dissection is going to be difficult. Again this should be discussed with patient, weighing the risk of radiation therapy compared to the risk of local recurrence due to a difficult dissection resulting in positive margins.

Anorectal Surgery in the Obese Patient

Key concept: Exposure is the key to anorectal surgery in the obese patient.

Successful anorectal surgery with any patient is dependent upon positioning and exposure. While either the prone jackknife or the lithotomy position can provide adequate exposure to the anus, focus should be on taping the buttock cheeks apart with the use of benzoin to improve access. When in the prone jackknife position, appropriate padding at all pressure points, and even ensuring the pannus is adequately padded, is necessary. It is important to recognize this position reduces some loss of ventilatory capacity that occurs from the abdominal pressure on the diaphragm. In either position, sedation may also lead to collapse of the posterior pharynx and obstructed breathing that requires a nasal or oral airway. There are even special Allen stirrups made to accommodate obese individuals to avoid compression complications such as lower extremity ischemia or nerve injury.

The use of self-retaining retractors such as the Lonestar helps gain access to the anal canal by effacing redundant tissue near the anus. The use of larger anoscopes also helps facilitate exposure. We also prefer advanced bipolar vessel-sealing devices to help reduce bleeding and thereby facilitate visualization in a tight area. Unfortunately, obesity has been shown to independently affect the outcome of various anorectal operations (see below).

Anorectal Fistulas

Key concept: Adhere to standard principles when delineating and managing obese patients with anorectal fistulas.

Anorectal fistulas can be technically difficult in obese patient similar to nonobese patients. Occasionally with the size of the perianal subcutaneous fat, the tracts are deeper. In addition, in those patients with muscular or large buttocks, visualization of the proximal anal canal, and even the dentate line, can be more challenging. We prefer to position the patient in either the prone jackknife or modified lithotomy position based on the suspected location of the internal opening of the fistula. Those with posterior openings are performed in the modified lithotomy position, while those with anterior internal openings should be operated on in the prone jackknife position. The use of a Lonestar retractor or any other self-effacing anal retractor is advised.

Obesity has been shown to be a negative predictor for success in repair of complex anorectal fistulas. Schwandner examined the results from 220 patients who underwent endorectal advancement flap for complex perianal fistulas [35]. He found a both higher recurrence rate (14 % vs. 28 %) and reoperation rate for sepsis in the failure group in patients with a BMI greater than 30. Multivariate analysis identified obesity as an independent predictor of failure. At present, obesity has not been associated with worse outcomes (either recurrence or functional) in those patients undergoing fistulotomy for low-lying fistula tracts.

Sphincteroplasty

Key concept: Small technical maneuvers may help with visualization, but sphincteroplasty in obese and nonobese is associated with similar outcomes.

The technical aspects of sphincter repair in the obese patient are essentially no different. We have anecdotally noted that the Lonestar and Gelpi retractors may be more crucial to ensuring adequate exposure of the planes. In addition, the muscle is not that much deeper compared to normal-sized patients. Adequate lateral retraction of the buttocks is probably the most important factor to provide good visualization. In terms of outcomes, Nikiteas and colleagues identified obesity as a risk factor for poor outcomes following sphincter repair in women that had experienced delayed incontinence as a result of obstetric trauma [36]. Whether or not this translates to a modifiable issue (i.e., an earlier repair or subsequent weight loss leading to improved results) is less clear. In general, obesity has not been definitively shown to affect the outcome of overlapping sphincteroplasty.

Hemorrhoidectomy

Key concept: No definitive data has shown a difference in outcomes following hemorrhoidectomy in obese versus *non-obese patients.*

There are few differences in hemorrhoid surgery in the obese patient. We have found that exposure is usually better in the prone jackknife position, if the patient can tolerate it. If anesthesia has a concern about sedation in this position (i.e., if you prefer local with conscious sedation), we will leave the bed in the room to provide a quick "rollover" for any airway issues. In either position, we highly recommend taping apart the buttock cheeks and the using the previously described methods for retraction. We feel that the use of a vessel-sealing device significantly reduces blood loss and thereby improves visualization for hemorrhoidectomies. It also significantly decreases the length of the operation and we recommend its use in obese patients.

Summary Pearls

Obese patients present a unique challenge to surgeons managing colorectal disease. Expect difficulties with exposure for both the laparoscopic and open approaches, as well as routine anorectal procedures. Cases will generally be longer, and plan accordingly. You may notice increased conversions when compared to similar laparoscopic resection in a nonobese patient. Try to avoid this by planning well in advance where risk profile assessment and intervention can lead to improved outcomes. Do not underestimate the usefulness of a skilled assistant. Add additional ports, move the bed to enhance gravity effects for exposure, employ a variety of mobilization techniques and use an energy device to reduce meddlesome bleeding. Through it all, recognize that the learning curve associated with any procedure is magnified (and extended) when applying it to obese patients. Finally, be honest with your comfort and expertise level when dealing with this patient population to mitigate complications and improve outcomes.

References

1. Unger R. Obesity now costs Americans more in health care spending than smoking. Forbes, April 2013. p. 112–3.
2. Jafri SH, Mills G. Lifestyle modification in colorectal cancer patients: an integrative oncology approach. Future Oncol. 2013;9(2):207–18.
3. Balentine CJ, Marshall C, Robinson C, et al. Validating quantitative obesity measurements in colorectal cancer patients. J Surg Res. 2010;164(1):18–22.
4. Shimizu A, Tani M, Kawai M, Hirono S, Miyazawa M, Uchiyama K, Yamaue H. Influence of visceral obesity for postoperative pulmonary complications after pancreaticoduodenectomy. J Gastrointest Surg. 2011;15(8):1401–10.
5. US Department of Health and Human Services. The Surgeon General's call to action to prevent and decrease overweight and obesity 2001. Rockville: US Department of Health and Human Services, US Public Health Service, Office of the Surgeon General; 2001. Available at http://www.surgeongeneral.gov/topics/obesity/calltoaction/CalltoAction.pdf. Accessed July 2013.
6. Geiger TM, Muldoon R. Complications following colon and rectal surgery in the obese patient. Clin Colon Rectal Surg. 2011; 24(4):274–82.
7. Mannarino MR, DiFlilippo F, Pirro M. Obstructive sleep apnea syndrome. Eur J Intern Med. 2012;23(7):586–93.
8. Chobanian AV, Bakris GL, Black HR, et al. Seventh report of the joint national committee on prevention, detection, evaluation, and treatment of high blood pressure. Hypertension. 2003;42:1206–52.
9. Hubert HB, Feinler M, McNamara PM, et al. Obesity as an independent risk factor for cardiovascular disease: a 26 year follow-up of participants in the Framingham Heart Study. Circulation. 1983; 67(5):968–77.
10. Rexrode KM, Carey VJ, Hennekens CH, et al. Abdominal adiposity and coronary heart disease in women. JAMA. 1998;280:1843–8.
11. Fleisher LA, Beckman JA, Brown KA, Calkins H, Chaikof E, Fleischmann KE, et al. ACC/AHA 2007 guidelines on perioperative cardiovascular evaluation and care for noncardiac surgery: executive summary. A report of the American College of Cardiology/American Heart Association Task Force on Practice Guidelines (Writing Committee to Revise the 2002 Guidelines on Perioperative Cardiovascular Evaluation for Noncardiac Surgery). Circulation. 2007;116:1971–96.
12. Patel NM, Patel MS. Medical complications of obesity and optimization of patients for colorectal surgery. Clin Colon Rectal Surg. 2011;24(4):211–21.
13. Stahl TJ, Gregorcyk SG, Hyman NH, Buie WD, and the Standards Practice Task Force of the American Society of Colon and Rectal Surgeons. Practice parameters for the prevention of venous thrombosis. Dis Colon Rectum. 2006;49:1477–83.
14. Wille-Jørgensen P, Rasmussen MS, Andersen BR, Borly L. Heparins and mechanical methods for thromboprophylaxis in colorectal surgery. Cochrane Database Syst Rev. 2004;(1): CD001217. doi: 10.1002/14651858.CD001217.
15. Flemming FJ, Kim MJ, Salloum RM, et al. How much do we need to worry about venous thromboembolism after hospital discharge? A study of colorectal surgery patients using the National Surgical Quality Improvement Program database. Dis Colon Rectum. 2010;53:1355–60.
16. Rasmussen MS, Jørgensen LN, Wille-Jørgensen P. Prolonged thromboprophylaxis with low molecular weight heparin for abdominal or pelvic surgery. Cochrane Database Syst Rev. 2009;(1): CD004318.
17. Gavin LA. Perioperative management of the diabetic patient. Endocrinol Metab Clin North Am. 1992;21:457–75.
18. Kwon S, Thompson R, Dellinger P, Yanez D, Farrohki E, Flum D. Importance of perioperative glycemic control in general surgery: a report from the Surgical Care and Outcomes Assessment Program. Ann Surg. 2013;257(1):8–14.
19. Delaney CP, Pokala N, Senagore AJ, et al. Is laparoscopic colectomy applicable to patients with body mass index >30? A case-matched comparative study with open colectomy. Dis Colon Rectum. 2005;48(5):975–81.

20. Leroy J, Ananian P, Rubino F, Claudon B, Mutter D, Marescaux J. The impact of obesity on technical feasibility and postoperative outcomes of laparoscopic left colectomy. Ann Surg. 2005;241(1): 69–76.
21. Blumberg D. Laparoscopic colectomy performed using a completely intracorporeal technique is associated with similar outcome in obese and thin patients. Surg Laparosc Endosc Percutan Tech. 2009;19(1):57–61.
22. Sarli L, Rollo A, Cecchini S, Regina G, Sansebastiano G, Marchesi F, Veronesi L, Ferro M, Roncoroni L. Impact of obesity on laparoscopic-assisted left colectomy in different stages of the learning curve. Surg Laparosc Endosc Percutan Tech. 2009;19(2): 114–7.
23. ASCRS Position Statement. Laparoscopy colectomy for curable cancer. Available at http://www.fascrs.org/physicians/position_statements/laparoscopic_colectomy/. Accessed July 2013.
24. Marcello PW, Fleshman JW, Milsom JW, et al. Hand-assisted laparoscopic vs. laparoscopic colorectal surgery: a multicenter, prospective, randomized trial. Dis Colon Rectum. 2008;51(6): 818-26.
25. Heneghan HM, Martin ST, Kiran RP, Khoury W, Stocchi L, Remzi FH, Vogel JD. Laparoscopic colorectal surgery for obese patients: decreased conversions with the hand-assisted technique. J Gastrointest Surg. 2013;17(3):548–54.
26. Makino T, Shukla PJ, Rubino F, Milsom JW. The impact of obesity on perioperative outcomes after laparoscopic colorectal resection. Ann Surg. 2012;255(2):228–36.
27. Aalbers AG, Doeksen A, Van Berge Henegouwen MI, Bemelman WA. Hand-assisted laparoscopic versus open approach in colorectal surgery: a systematic review. Colorectal Dis. 2010;12(4): 287–95.
28. Kiran RP, Remzi FH, Fazio VW, et al. Complications and functional results after ileoanal pouch formation in obese patients. J Gastrointest Surg. 2008;12(4):668–74.
29. Canedo JA, Pinto RA, McLemore EC, Rosen L, Wexner SD. Restorative proctectomy with ileal-pouch anal anastomosis in obese patients. Dis Colon Rectum. 2010;53(7):1030–4.
30. Efron JE, Uriburu JP, Wexner SD, et al. Restorative proctocolectomy with ileal pouch anal anastomosis in obese patients. Obes Surg. 2001;11(3):246–51.
31. Wibmer AG, Kroesen AJ, Grone J, et al. Predictors of permanent ileostomy after restorative proctocolectomy. Br J Surg. 2010; 97(10):1561–6.
32. Causey MW, Stoddard D, Johnson EK, et al. Laparoscopy impacts outcomes favorably following colectomy for ulcerative colitis: a critical analysis of the ACS-NSQIP database. Surg Endosc. 2013;27(2):603–9.
33. Denost Q, Quintane L, Buscail E, Martenot M, Laurent C, Rullier E. Short and long term impact of body mass index on laparoscopic rectal cancer surgery. Colorectal Dis. 2013;15(4):463–9.
34. Baek JH, McKenzie S, Garcia-Aguilar J, Pigazzi A. Oncologic outcomes of robotic-assisted total mesorectal excision for the treatment of rectal cancer. Ann Surg. 2010;251(5):882–6.
35. Schwandner O. Obesity is a negative predictor of success after surgery for complex anal fistula. BMC Gastroenterol. 2011;11:61.
36. Nikiteas N, Korsgen S, Kumar D, Keighley MR. Audit of sphincter repair. Factors associated with poor outcome. Dis Colon Rectum. 1996;39(10):1164–70.

The Pediatric Patient

27

Tiffany Tanner, Nathan P. Zwintscher, Robert A. Cusick, and Kenneth S. Azarow

Key Points

- Children have many of the same common anorectal disorders as adults. While many are treated similarly, perianal abscesses and fistula-in-ano are often treated differently in children.
- Constipation is a significant problem in childhood that typically can be treated successfully with medication and lifestyle modifications; however, it may be a chronic condition in a significant percentage of patients.
- Look for more extensive associated defects in children with fecal incontinence that may require more extensive evaluation. The initial approach is most often medical.
- Inflammatory bowel disease in children may have a more aggressive course.
- Polyps in children occur in the setting of genetic predispositions and should be evaluated accordingly.

T. Tanner, MD
Department of Surgery, University of Nebraska Medical Center, 983280 Nebraska Medical Center, Omaha, NE 68198, USA
e-mail: ttanner@unmc.edu

N.P. Zwintscher, MD
Department of Surgery, Madigan Healthcare System, 9040 Jackson Ave, Tacoma, WA 98431, USA
e-mail: npzwintscher@gmail.com

R.A. Cusick, MD (✉)
Department of Pediatric Surgery, Children's Hospital and Medical Center, Omaha and University of Nebraska Medical Center, 8200 Dodge Street, Omaha, NE 68114, USA
e-mail: rcusick@childrensomaha.org

K.S. Azarow, MD (✉)
Division of Pediatric Surgery, Department of Surgery, Oregon Health Science University, Doernbecher Children's Hospital, Portland, OR, USA

Oregon Health Science University, Doernbecher Children's Hospital, 3181 S.W. Sam Jackson Park Road, Portland, OR 97239, USA
e-mail: azarow@ohsu.edu

Introduction

In many parts of the United States and world, pediatric patients are cared for by pediatric specialists, with those requiring surgery managed primarily by pediatric surgeons. Furthermore, to speak to the uniqueness of colorectal disease in this population, subspecialty training in pediatric colorectal surgery after completion of a pediatric surgery fellowship has begun to emerge. Yet, other locations do not have this situation, and patients with common colorectal problems will still be referred to general surgeons, colorectal surgeons, and general pediatric surgeons. In many cases, "classic" surgical training either does not apply or needs to be modified to account for growth, development, or a different natural history of disease in this population. It is our intent that this chapter be used as a guide to assist all those who are faced with management decisions for these patients both in and out of the operating room.

Anorectal Disease

Key Concept: Common anorectal complaints seen in adult patients also occur in pediatric patients. In many cases, these are managed the same way, with the most common exception of anorectal abscess and fistula.

Perianal Abscess and Fistula-in-Ano

Key Concept: Perianal abscesses should be approached in a stepwise fashion beginning with aspiration and antibiotics, with incision and drainage reserved for recurrent or more severe cases. Many fistulas will spontaneously close without surgical intervention (especially in infants), and immediate operative therapy should be avoided. Primary surgical treatment of a fistula-in-ano should be reserved for older children and failures to spontaneously resolve.

It is said that "the abscess is the parent of fistula-in-ano," and both are typically diseases of the same origin, arising

S.R. Steele et al. (eds.), *Complexities in Colorectal Surgery*,
DOI 10.1007/978-1-4614-9022-7_27, © Springer Science+Business Media New York 2014

from abnormal crypt of Morgagni. In children, distinctions between the two entities are not even made [1, 2]. Overall, abscess and fistula-in-ano occur not uncommonly in children, with an estimated rate of 0.5–4.3 % [3]. While males are predominately affected in children under 2 years of age (12:1), the ratio becomes less extreme (2–3:1) for those older [4]. For those under 2 years, a congenital etiology has been hypothesized, suggesting that the gender difference may be explained by an androgen excess or androgen-sensitive glands in utero, causing a formation of abnormal glands [2, 5]. Other postulated theories include entrapment of migratory cells from the urogenital sinus during development of the perineum, anal crypt infections, anal fissure, or dermal infections [5–7]. These may account, in part, for some of the rationale why we treat them differently than adults.

Perianal abscess and fistula-in-ano most commonly occur laterally (i.e., 3 and 9 o'clock) [2, 6, 7]. Interestingly, cultures taken from the abscesses vary between genders, with females growing a predominance of skin flora (i.e., *Streptococcus*, *Staphylococcus aureus*) and males having mostly enteric flora (i.e., *E. coli*, *Klebsiella*, *Enterococcus*, *Proteus*) [2]. Although the presence of mixed enteric organisms in the aspirate is suggestive of a fistula, there has been no statically significant correlation between its presence and the type of organisms in culture [4]. Of note, there has been a significant increase in the incidence of methicillin-resistant *Staphylococcus aureus* (MRSA) in both the hospital and community settings, and this also holds true in the genital area [8]. In 2008, MRSA was found to be the most common organism in superficial genitourinary abscesses in children [9]. In their single institution study, Woods showed that nearly half of all MRSA abscesses were found in the genital area [10]. Furthermore, they showed that hospital wide, the rise in MRSA infections was predominantly in children 1–3 years of age (male>female) [10]. You need to keep this in mind when choosing antibiotics or encountering recurrent or recalcitrant disease.

Unfortunately, there is no straightforward recommendation for therapy. In fact, the treatment of abscess and fistula is widely debated in the literature [11] and ranges from antibiotics alone to aggressively probing for a fistula and performing a fistulotomy or fistulectomy, when present. The controversy is, in part, likely due to the wide range of concomitant and resultant fistula formation (~20–85 %) [2, 3]· and finding the balance between over- and undertreatment. Those that propose a nonoperative management strategy advocate a detailed hygiene plan, sitz baths, and antibiotics [3]. They cite the fact that surgical drainage of an abscess results in an ~40 % rate of development of fistula-in-ano versus an ~6 % rate with nonsurgical drainage [3]. Admittedly, this may have been secondary to ~10 % of their population being immunocompromised and wanting to avoid a perineal wound. However, even in this subset, nonoperative management resulted in no subsequent fistula formation or need for operative intervention [3].

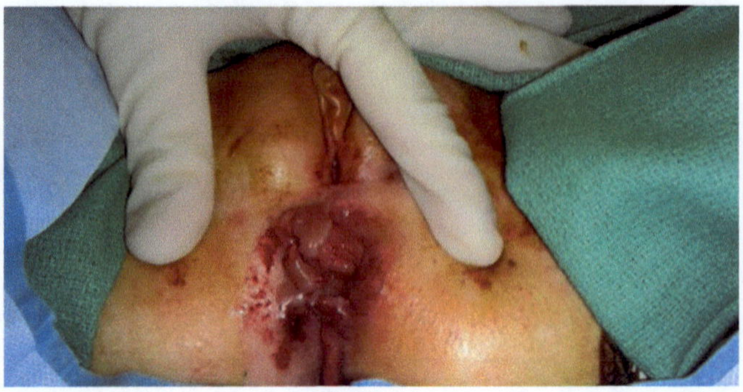

Fig. 27.1 Perineal Crohn's disease in an 8-year-old male showing multiple fistulas

Others advocate the similar use of local hygiene and sitz baths for an early-stage perianal abscess but call for a progressive stepwise approach—starting with antibiotics and finally aspiration drainage with an 18-gauge needle [7]. If there is no resolution of the collection within 24 h, a formal incision and drainage (I&D) is performed along with fistulectomy for patients with concomitant fistulas (~11 %) [7]. Of note, in one series, patients treated with needle aspiration had a 20 % failure rate requiring escalation of care [7], highlighting the need for close follow-up evaluation. Afsarlar noted their recurrence rate of a perianal abscess was 30 %, regardless of whether it spontaneously drained or was I&D'd and with or without antibiotics [2]. Antibiotics have, however, been reported to decrease the rate of fistula development by ~12.5–50 %, regardless of the antibiotics used [2, 3, 6, 7]. Others have also reported no difference in fistula rates (~20–38 %) between spontaneous and surgical drainage [2]. Even those treated with observation alone (no antibiotics) have been associated with fistula resolution rates of 17–80 % within 1 year [2, 6].

For children <2 years old, only 15–25 % will have a concomitant fistula at the time of their primary surgery [4, 11]. In this same cohort that undergoes I&D, ~6–15 % will ultimately develop a fistula [4, 11]. This is in contrast to children over 8 years, where reported recurrence rates approach 50 % and abscess to fistula progression is ~25 % [4]. Important to note, a significant portion of children over 8 years that develop fistula recurrences are eventually diagnosed with inflammatory bowel disease (Fig. 27.1), and you should work them up appropriately [4, 11]. It is not surprising, therefore, that immunosuppressive agents such as tacrolimus have been associated with successful fistula resolution without the need for operative intervention [4].

Hemorrhoids

Key Concept: *Hemorrhoids are normally from constipation and should almost always be treated nonoperatively.*

Hemorrhoids are extremely uncommon in children, with the prevalence increasing in older kids and teens [12].

Symptoms are similar to adults including bleeding, prolapse, itching, pain, blood-streaked stools, and a bulge or dilated venous plexus at the anal orifice. Treatment in children is usually conservative with diet modification, increased liquid intake, and sitz baths. Laxatives can also be helpful, and glycerin suppositories work well for younger children. The vast majority of hemorrhoids resolve with medical treatment for constipation alone. Operative intervention is reserved for the rare failure and consists of the procedures as adults [12].

Anal Fissure

Key Concept: Anal fissure presentation and treatment is similar to adults.

While anal fissures can occur at any age, they most commonly present around 2 years old [12]. Symptoms are similar to adults, with rectal pain, bleeding, streaked stools, as well as crying with defecation. The lesions in infants may be found anywhere, although they are more common in the posterior midline. Females, similar to adults, more commonly have anterior midline fissures [12]. If the lesions are off the midline or are multiple, consider a workup for Crohn's disease or a culture and/or biopsy to exclude malignancy, tuberculosis, venereal disease, or immunodeficiency in the appropriate setting. Recognize, however, that most anal fissures are secondary to constipation and will heal spontaneously with a simple focus on maintaining adequate fluid intake along with a proper bowel regimen, and that more intensive will only be required in a small subset of patients. Similar to adults, glyceryl trinitrate 2 % (GTN) has been associated with improvements in fissure healing and symptom relief compared with lidocaine or placebo in both the short term (10 days) and at 8 weeks [12]. Healing rates have been up to 84 %, with symptomatic relief reported in 91–94 % with GTN [12–15]. Botulinum toxin can also be used for resolution of anal fissure, though most data consists of case reports. Keshtgar showed in their study that 4 children who underwent treatment for anal fissure with transcutaneous botulinum toxin had resolution of their lesion [16]. Finally, successful use of lateral subcutaneous sphincterotomy has also been described in children, with a complete resolution of all fissures in small series [12, 17].

Our approach is as follows: Asymptomatic lesions are likely to resolve and should be managed expectantly with dietary and fluid management. If intervention is necessary, an initial trial of topical therapy (lidocaine, GTN) should be used. Recurrences can be treated medically (GTN is not used or botulinum toxin), with surgery reserved for continued failures. You should remember that any surgical intervention involving a small child or infant should be done so with the *most extreme caution*, as incontinence and anal stenosis are reported in up to 30 % [12].

Rectal Prolapse

Key Concept: Rectal prolapse in children is most commonly secondary to constipation, and the majority will resolve with treatment directed towards proper bowel habits. Surgery should be reserved only for refractory cases with severe symptoms.

Rectal prolapse is a common problem in children, with a peak incidence in the first year of life and most occurrences taking place under 4 years old around the time of toilet training [18–20]. Prolapse in this cohort is a symptom of an underlying condition, usually constipation, but can also be caused by increased abdominal pressure (i.e., chronic cough), acute or chronic diarrhea, parasites, neoplastic disease of the rectum, malnutrition, cystic fibrosis, or pelvic floor weakness [12]. While the exact etiology is unknown, the rectosigmoid in children with prolapse tends to be ~1.5-fold longer than their normal counterparts [21].

Most cases are mild and typically resolve spontaneously shortly after the rectum prolapses [18, 19]. You should use manual reduction prior to the onset of edema for an acute prolapse that does not reduce on its own. Firm steady pressure may be necessary to decrease the swelling and allow reduction. Importantly, perform a digital examination to ensure the reduction is complete, and exclude any distal source of pathology. Another helpful tip in children is to approximate the buttocks with adhesive tape for several hours to reduce recurrence [18]. Roughly 90 % of rectal prolapse cases in children under the age of 4 will resolve with these simple steps alone and rarely continues after 6 years old [18]. Parents should be instructed to use stool softeners and/or laxatives, while avoiding prolonged straining and ensuring the use of a proper toilet size for their child to prevent recurrent episodes. We also tell parents to promptly reduce a prolapse if it were to reoccur and to bring the child in for reevaluation.

Children over 4 years of age are more likely to have neurologic (i.e., spinal cord lesions) or muscular defects and require intervention. You should also consider screening for cystic fibrosis (CF), as up to 11 % of children with rectal prolapse will have CF [22]. Indications for surgery include failure of conservative measures, continued prolapse after 1 year despite nonoperative therapy, greater than 2 episodes requiring manual reduction, or chronic pain, bleeding, and perianal excoriation from the recurrent prolapse [18]. The simplest, most benign, and still efficacious, intervention is sclerosing injections. Several different agents have been used with efficacy rates ranging from 83 to 100 %, depending on the sclerosant (i.e., 30 % saline, 5 % phenol in almond oil, ethanol 70 %) and number of treatments [23–28]. However, this should be used with caution, as reported complications include temporary fecal incontinence, temporary limping, bleeding, perirectal inflammation, urinary retention, necrosis of the rectal mucosa, and abscess formation [23, 28].

Both perineal and abdominal approaches are available for refractory cases; however, similar to adults, no single operation has been shown to have significantly better results [20, 22]. Although the Thiersch procedure is not used much in adults anymore, it may be ideal for select children with prolapse secondary to weak pelvic floor muscles or those associated with cystic fibrosis [18]. A less invasive procedure somewhat unique to children (and not used extensively anymore) is linear cauterization, which has a reported success rate up to 94 % [29]. Some institutions also advocate a combination of these techniques, with linear cauterization used in conjunction with sclerotherapy injection and a Thiersch procedure [20].

Although you may not have much experience in any of these, other procedures you may hear include posterior sagittal transsphincteric rectopexy, Ekehorn's rectosacropexy (placing a U-shaped suture through the rectal ampulla and tying the suture outside at the sacrococcygeal junction), and a transcoccygeal rectopexy with puborectalis plication. Success and recurrence rates remain highly variable in limited series [30–32]. More commonly used procedures in adults, such as the Altemeier perineal proctosigmoidectomy, have also been associated with good results in the pediatric population.

Laparoscopic approaches such as suture rectopexy, posterior mesh rectopexy, and resection of the sigmoid colon with or without rectopexy have also been associated with good outcomes in children [21]. Recurrence rates are ~5 %, with failures perhaps higher in children with cystic fibrosis [33]. In general, we do not use prosthetic mesh initially in the pediatric population. Adding a sigmoid resection with rectopexy in children has been also controversial, although it has been shown to be safe, eliminates the risk of volvulus, and has a low morbidity and low recurrence rate [21]. Finally, similar to adults, the addition of a resection is preferred in those with intractable constipation and prolonged transit studies.

Constipation

Key Concept: Similar to adults, constipation therapy should be guided by a thorough history and physical examination, with initial dietary, fluid, and nonoperative management. Select diagnoses with severe nonresponsive symptoms may be considered for operative intervention.

Constipation is a common problem in childhood, affecting 7–30 % of children [34]. You should remember that constipation is a symptom rather than a diagnosis, manifesting with painful defecation, difficulty with passage of stools, or decreased stool frequency [35]. It is a major problem, responsible for ~3 % of visits to outpatient clinics and up to 20 % of pediatric gastroenterological complaints [35]. When not treated adequately, constipation can lead to psychological problems, low self-esteem, withdrawal, and social isolation [36–38].

Table 27.1 Rome III criteria for pediatric functional constipation

Two or fewer defecations per week
At least one episode of fecal incontinence per week
Stool retentive posturing
Painful or hard bowel movements
Large diameter stools that could obstruct the toilet
Presence of large fecal mass in the abdomen or rectum

With permission from Mugie et al. [38]. Copyright © 2011 Nature Publishing Group

Table 27.2 Features suggestive of organic causes of constipation [38]

Organic causes
History: delayed passage of meconium (>48 h after birth), early onset of symptoms (<6 months of age), bilious vomiting, bloody stools, ribbon like stools, delayed or abnormal development, no withholding, no response to conventional treatment, and extraintestinal symptoms (fever, fatigue, eczema, bladder disease, neurological disturbances, oral ulcerations)
Physical exam: failure to thrive, fever, absent cremasteric reflex, abdominal distension, abnormal position of anus, perianal fistula, absent anal wink, tuft of hair on spine, deep sacral dimple, decreased lower extremity strength/tone/reflex, asymmetry of the lumbosacral region or flattening of the gluteal muscles/lower limb, spina bifida, and explosive diarrhea after rectal exam
Sexual abuse
History: smear feces
Physical exam: extreme fear during anal inspection or rectal examination, anal scars, fissures, and hematomas

With permission from Burgers and Di Lorenzo [39]

Evaluation

Key Concept: History and physical examination guide most of the evaluation, with ancillary testing used mostly for directed findings, difficult cases, or those who have nonresponsive severe constipation.

Functional constipation is the underlying reason in more than 95 % of children [39], with the diagnosis confirmed by having two or more of the symptoms listed in Table 27.1 [38]. A thorough history and physical examination is typically sufficient to rule out most pathological causes, and extensive additional testing prior to medical and dietary treatment is unnecessary (Table 27.2) [38]. Similar to adults, a comprehensive history should include the frequency and character of the stools, withholding behavior, timing of incontinence, straining, and pain with defecation. Children who present with constipation under 6 months of age, especially who have delayed passage of meconium greater than 48 h after birth, or those who present with abdominal distention and refusal to feed are concerning symptoms for

Table 27.3 Causes of constipation in children

Idiopathic constipation (most common)
Dietary
Inadequate fluid/fiber intake
High milk intake
Dietary protein allergy
Cow's milk allergy
Anal/rectal disorders
Anal stenosis, anterior ectopic anus
Anal fissure (acute, chronic)
Perianal group A streptococcal infection
Eosinophilic proctitis
Megarectum
Neurogenic abnormalities
Sacral dysgenesis (anorectal anomaly)
Myelomeningocele (spina bifida)
Spinal cord abnormalities/trauma
Static encephalopathy
Tethered cord
Hirschsprung's disease
Intestinal neuronal dysplasia
Cerebral palsy
Endocrine and metabolic disorders
Hypothyroidism
Hypercalcaemia
Renal tubular acidosis
Diabetes mellitus
Hypokalemia
Vitamin D intoxication
Medications
Opioids
Anticholinergic agents
Antidepressants
Phenytoin
Phenothiazine
Abnormal defecation dynamics
Fear and withholding habit
Pelvic floor muscle dyssynergia
Other
Anorexia nervosa
Sexual abuse
Scleroderma
Cystic fibrosis
Celiac disease

With permission from Keshtgar et al. [35] © 2004 by W.B. Saunders

Hirschsprung's disease, anal stenosis, or ectopic anus (Table 27.3) [35, 39]. Other concerning symptoms that should prompt you to consider a more extensive workup are accompanying urinary tract infections, weight loss, neuromuscular development, and psychological or behavioral problems (Table 27.2) [39].

In addition to a complete abdominal and perineal examination, differences in the examination for pediatric patients should involve looking for other signs of congenital syndrome anomalies (i.e., VACTERL) and ensure there is fecal impaction or anal stenosis [13]. A fecal mass either found in the abdomen or rectum is present in 30–70 % of children with constipation [16]. Investigations for children may include a basic metabolic panel to exclude electrolyte imbalance and thyroid or celiac panels to work up patients with severe unremitting constipation. You should note that most laboratory investigations rarely uncover an underlying disease [35, 38]. Plain abdominal x-rays are seldom helpful to assess fecal retention, and actually correlate poorly between symptoms and pathology, leaving more open to misinterpretation [39, 40]. For children over 12 months of age, anorectal manometry can be extremely valuable when Hirschsprung's disease is in the differential diagnosis. Failure of relaxation of the internal sphincter is an absolute indication for rectal biopsy and has a high positive predictive value for the absence of ganglion cells [35]. Furthermore, in any infant or other patient in whom Hirschsprung's disease is suggested, a rectal biopsy is the gold standard for diagnosis. You should remember that short-segment Hirschsprung's disease may manifest later in childhood (or even adult life) with constipation, and work up those select patients accordingly. While ultrasound has been suggested to look at fecal load in the colon, it really is not very useful. This is similar to the colon transit studies, where some authors feel it is helpful [37]. One could argue that in children with normal transit time, surgery is not typically indicated [41]. Others suggest it aids in determining the point at which normal peristalsis is lost [39, 42]. However, we rarely find it useful in the primary workup for constipation. Finally, though the indication for endoscopy for primary constipation symptoms is rare, high-risk or concerning symptoms should direct the need accordingly.

Treatment

Key Concept: Use medical management and dietary changes as first-line therapy—they will work most of the time.

Years of experience and expert opinion guide most of constipation management. We find that the most useful first step is often helping the patient and family to understand the problem and enlist their cooperation and compliance in what is often a trial and error period [36, 38]. Interestingly, there is an association between not only low-fiber intake and constipation but also a positive family history, obesity, and low levels of parental education with an increased prevalence of childhood constipation [38, 43]. The American Academy of Pediatricians suggests a balanced diet that includes whole grains, fruits, and vegetables as the first-line treatment of constipation; however, when comparing fiber supplementation to placebo, there was no significant difference in defecation frequency or resolution of symptoms [36]. We feel there is very little downside, so we agree with this initial approach, along with ensuring adequate fluid intake and physical activity [44]. Children with a developmental age of at least 4 years should also be instructed to have dedicated toilet time for 5–10 min after each meal (three times per day) to encourage regular toileting [45].

If you encounter children who have severe constipation marred by fecal impaction and/or overflow incontinence, disimpaction can be accomplished using either oral or rectal therapies [44–48]: high-dose PEG 3350 (1.5/g/kg/day, max dose of 100 g/day) orally for outpatient use and milk of molasses enemas (mixed 1: 10 mL/kg with maximum of 500 mL) followed with maintenance PEG 3350 have been compared with relatively similar results beyond the first day [47]. In general, enemas relieve symptoms faster than the oral treatment, but either approach is feasible. Other authors have shown that PEG with electrolytes is more effective than suppositories, rectal enemas, or even manual evacuation [49]. If you would like to avoid rectal therapy or if oral disimpaction fails, you may need to take the child to the operating room for disimpaction under general sedation.

Maintenance treatment must be initiated immediately and may be necessary for several months. You should discontinue this treatment only after there are regular bowel movements for several weeks without effort and the child is toilet trained [34, 44]. Tailored therapy is best and you can choose from a variety of laxatives. Unlike adults, laxatives cannot be assumed to work in a similar manner in children due to the fact that the etiology for childhood constipation is typically different than that of their adult counterparts [36, 38]. PEG with electrolytes is our preferred agent and has been shown to be more effective in achieving treatment success compared to other laxatives (lactulose and milk of magnesia) [50–52]. There is also evidence suggesting that mineral oil is efficacious, though chronic use should be avoided, as it has been associated with vitamin deficiencies [52]. Other agents such as probiotics may be helpful in the treatment of functional constipation, but there is very little data available, and we withhold recommendation. Behavioral therapy alone or biofeedback should not be the sole treatment of constipation in children; however, there is some evidence that behavioral intervention plus laxative therapy improves continence in this age group [38, 44].

Surgery: Sphincter Procedures, Antegrade Continence Enema, and Stoma

Key Concept: Several surgeries somewhat unique to children are available for symptomatic severe constipation that is nonresponsive to medical management.

Surgical options for constipation depend in large part on the underlying etiology. Procedures include anal dilation, intra-sphincteric injection of botulinum toxin, antegrade continence enema (ACE), excision of colon and/or megarectum and diversion, and reconstructive proctocolectomy [35, 53]. While (as previously stated) transit studies and total colonic manometry don't play a major role in the initial evaluation of constipation, we do use them prior to performing a definitive surgery. We find its major use is to ensure the distal-most segment of the colon or remaining rectum will have a functional motility pattern that will effectively allow for the passage of stool [42]. We also recommend a period of inpatient or close home observation to document objective evidence in order to help identify misreporting and exaggerating symptoms and thus avoiding unnecessary operations [53].

Anal dilation and myomectomy of the internal anal sphincter have been performed with the thought that children with constipation have hypertrophy of their internal anal sphincter, and anal dilation would decrease sphincter tone and allow for painless defecation [35]. Unfortunately two double-blinded randomized controlled trials have shown that anal dilation does not benefit children with chronic constipation [35], and we do not generally advocate its use. Myomectomy of the internal anal sphincter has been associated with weakening of the sphincter in subsequent years, and again, we are not strong proponents. Botulinum toxin sphincter injection has reported rates of symptom resolution in up to 94 %, without the long-term problems [16]. While this is generally well tolerated, ~20 % may require repeat injection [16].

Antegrade enemas are a therapeutic option for children who have intractable constipation or fecal incontinence and have failed either (a) a maximal medical management or (b) a sphincter procedure [35, 38, 53, 54]. Originally described by Malone in 1990 [54], subsequent modifications include an appendicostomy placed in an open or laparoscopic fashion, the cecum or rectum reconstructed to create a continent conduit, or a percutaneous cecostomy tube or button placed laparoscopically or open (Fig. 27.2) [35, 54]. The concept remains the same: to deliver antegrade enemas to clean out the entire colon to reduce soiling, with reported success rates of 52–92 % [53]. Each procedure has their own complications including stenosis, prolapse, skin infections, granulation tissue formation, leakage, and prostheses dislodgment [16, 19]. Results do not seem to differ in the complications or outcomes between a right and left ACE [55]. Ultimately, most children with idiopathic constipation can progress to a point they use no oral medications, and the stoma can be no longer used or taken down.

Patients with Hirschsprung's disease should be managed by the appropriate surgical therapy, which is most often a pull-through procedure that can be performed open or laparoscopically (Figs. 27.3, 27.4, and 27.5) and is one or several stages. One rare, but obviously significant, complication you may see is in children with chronic

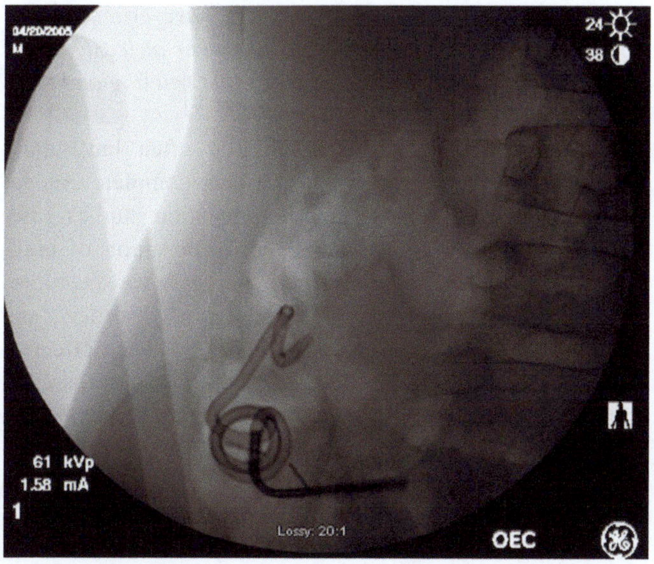

Fig. 27.2 Plain film of an antegrade cecostomy tube in place

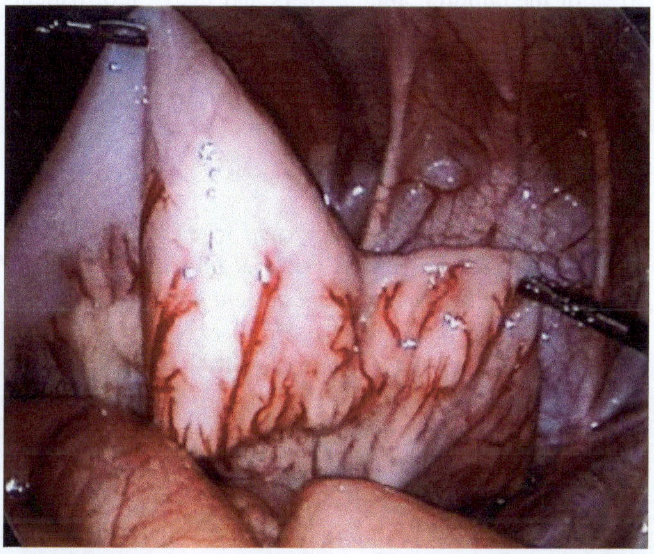

Fig. 27.3 Abdominal view at the beginning of laparoscopic-assisted pull-through procedure. The transition from dilated/normal sigmoid colon (*right* on the image) to contracted/aganglionic colon (*left* on the image). We will typically perform a few submucosal biopsies to confirm the presence of ganglion cells (Courtesy of David Gourlay, MD)

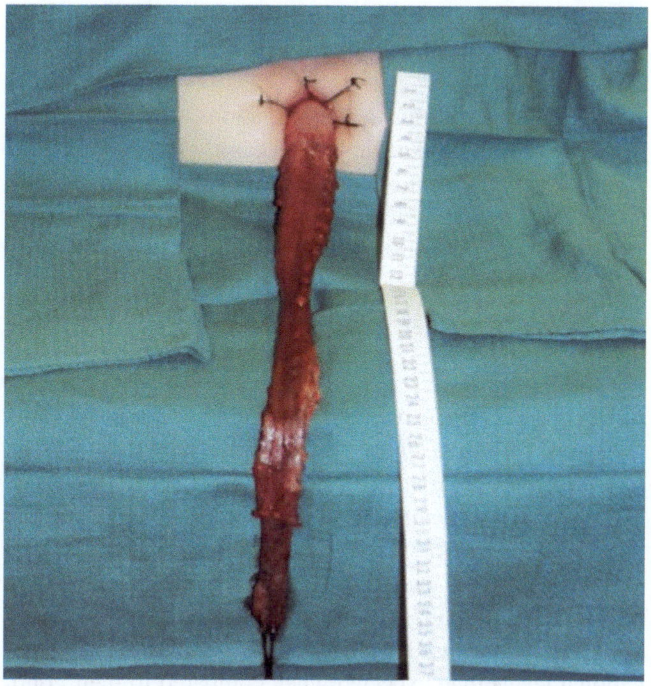

Fig. 27.4 Mobilized aganglionic sigmoid-rectum pulled through the anus. We have determined the level where ganglion cells are present (pictured here close to the anus). After transecting the aganglionic segment, a hand-sewn coloanal anastomosis is performed above the dentate line (Courtesy of David, Gourlay, MD)

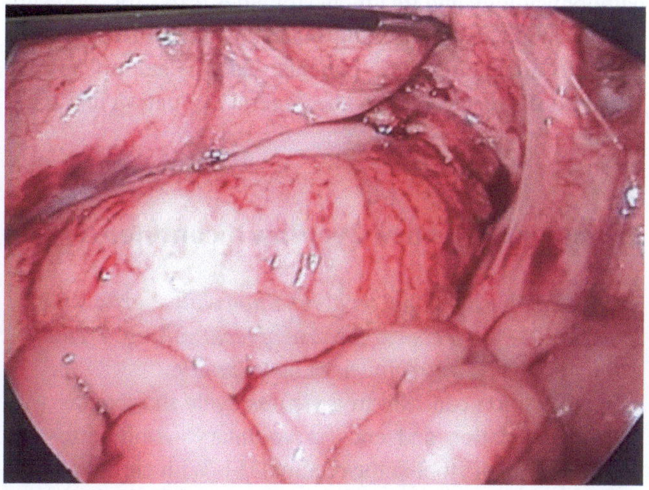

Fig. 27.5 Abdominal view of the completed pull-through (Courtesy of David Gourlay, MD)

constipation; a small percentage may develop dilation of the rectum and sigmoid (megarectum). Resection of the dilated segments may be performed in the most extreme cases that have failed all other options, including ACE [53, 57]. Unfortunately, this rarely results in a complete or immediate cure, as children can still have fecal incontinence or constipation and may still need further resection [38]. Yet, almost all will be able to reduce their laxative need, and roughly half will be able to eliminate their laxative requirement altogether [56]. Finally, when combined with the physiological manometric data, the need for permanent stomas secondary to failure for these procedures can be reduced [20].

For those patients with severe problems that are nonresponsive and significantly affect their quality of life, a stoma can be performed. In this case, we prefer to use a temporary diverting loop ileostomy in hopes the child will wish to consider alternative treatments [16]. Finally, there are case reports of a restorative proctocolectomy performed in this final group with generally good results; however, we have little experience with this and feel it should not be undertaken lightly [57].

It is important to manage expectations accordingly. You should let all parties known that 1 year after the commencement for the treatment of constipation, the problem can persist in 50 % of children with another 50 % of those children still suffering from constipation 5 years later [34, 58].

Incontinence

Key Concept: Fecal incontinence in children encompasses both encopresis (the expulsion of a normal bowel movement in inappropriate places in someone 4 years or older developmentally) and soiling (involuntary leakage of small amounts of stool), with the difference arising from the quantity of feces lost.

Kids with fecal incontinence have significant social consequences (like adults) such as restriction of social activities, as well as an increase in behavioral problems, and lower educational levels than expected when compared to their continent counterparts [59–62]. There are five main groups of children with fecal incontinence: constipation with fecal retention and overflow incontinence, functional non-retentive fecal soiling, anorectal malformations, spinal problems, and sphincter damage or dysfunction [59, 60]. The pathophysiology and treatment strategies differ for each subgroup. While we understand that you may not be the one primarily managing these patients, we will attempt to give you a brief overview and some general evaluation and management tips.

Functional Retentive Overflow Incontinence

Key Concept: Functional fecal retention with overflow incontinence is the most common cause of fecal soiling. Treatment should be aimed at treatment of constipation.

Constipation can lead to a vicious cycle that begins with painful defecation and ends in voluntary withholding and accumulation of stool in the rectum [16]. With chronicity, the rectum may become dilated, and sensation is gradually lost; therefore, when the softer stool arrives from the more proximal colon, it cannot be accommodated and leaks around the bolus of hard stool [46]. Because of the lack of sensation, this passage of soft stool is not sensed until the incontinence has occurred. This functional problem is typically self-limiting but requires aggressive treatment of constipation [59, 60].

Functional Non-retentive Fecal Soiling

Key Concept: This is a subgroup of patients who lack a history or physical exam findings consistent with constipation or functional fecal retention, but who have evacuation of large bowel movements in their underwear at least once a week. Treatment should be aimed at toilet training and positive feedback.

Confounding things, these children often have daily bowel movements in the toilet with near complete evacuation of stool and normal colonic transition studies [59]. Historically this was considered a manifestation of emotional disturbances in school-aged children; however, studies have not shown any serious psychological disorders, and treatment with psychotherapy alone has not been effective [63]. Treatment for these children should involve parental education and encourage defecation 5 min after each meal, a rewards system, and usage of a diary with avoidance of accusatory toilet training and guilt [59]. Laxatives have been shown to worsen outcomes, and functional non-retentive fecal soiling should be treated differently from retentive soiling [64]. Involvement of a mental health professional may be beneficial [59]. Resolution of the symptoms occurs in only 30 % of the children after 2 years and in 70 % of patients after 4 years with the problem persisting into young adulthood in up to 22 % of the population [65].

Anorectal Malformations

Key Concept: These patients present with a wide range in abnormalities, depending on the level of malformation and associated defects, with the management and outcomes often contingent on the malformation. However, a trial at medical therapy is still warranted in this group.

These malformations can be subdivided into three categories: [1] low anomalies, when the rectum has descended below the level of the puborectalis—typically without a fistula to the genitourinary tract and either with or without a cutaneous perineal fistula; [2] intermediate anomalies located at or just below the puborectalis muscle—often having a fistulous connection to the distal genitourinary tract; and [3] high anomalies with the rectum ending above the puborectalis (which may or may not be developed)—with a fistula to the urinary tract or vagina with no perineal opening (Fig. 27.6) [59]. Dependent upon the degree of pelvic floor development, there is great variation in the functional outcomes after repair of these malformations [60]. Generally, lower malformations have good functional outcomes, although they still suffer from occasional incontinence, constipation, an inability to control flatus, or sexual dysfunction [59]· Patients with lower defects mostly have voluntary bowel movements; however, up to 30 % can still experience soiling. Contrast this with patients with high anomalies, where 30 % may experience voluntary bowel movements and up to 90 % experience soiling [59, 66]. Major advances in pediatric surgery in recent decades have allowed for improved anatomic reconstruction primarily due to the

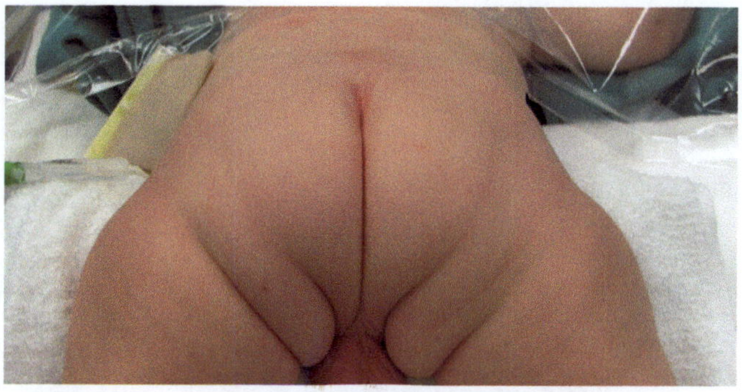

Fig. 27.6 Imperforate anus in an infant with no external opening

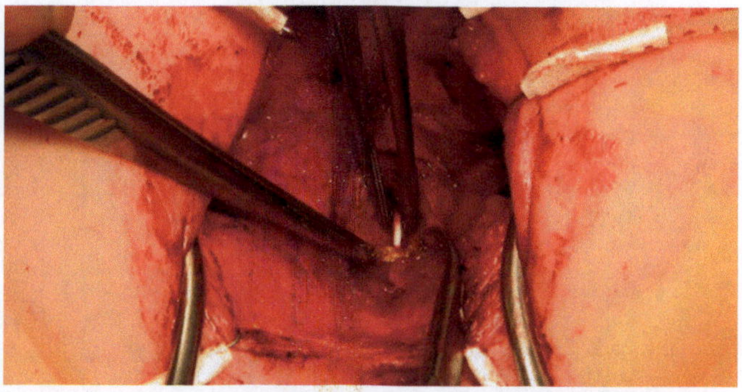

Fig. 27.7 PSARP procedure demonstrating the recto-urethral fistula and catheter in the urethral opening

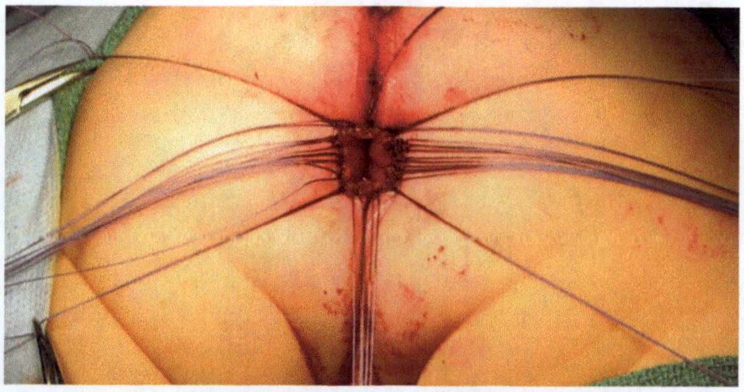

Fig. 27.8 Completed imperforate anus anastomosis with restoration of intestinal continuity to the perineum

posterior sagittal anorectoplasty (PSARP) for higher anorectal anomalies (Figs. 27.7 and 27.8) [59, 67]. These patients have improved outcomes, with up to half of patients experiencing full continence and only ~20 % having frequent soiling [59, 67], although they may still suffer from severe problems with constipation [66].

Remember that three elements are necessary for continence: functional sphincters, normal rectosigmoid motility, and intact sensation [59, 66]. Children with anorectal malformations who have subsequent defecation disorders should undergo both colonic and anorectal manometric testing to tailor their treatment [68]. It's not surprising that patients who have a functional internal anal sphincter have higher anal resting tone and better outcomes in continence [69]. However, presence of severe sacral defects is one of the most important negative prognostic factors for continence [59]. These patients (i.e., incontinence from anorectal malformations with minor defects) are ideal for biofeedback, as they are more likely to respond. On the downside, this is time consuming, requires full cooperation from patients, and may not be helpful in patients with hypoplastic sphincters [70]. Therefore, medical treatment should first be used to modify the consistency of stool, with antidiarrheals for loose stools and enemas for those patients that have constipation and overflow incontinence [59, 60]. The enemas may be given retrograde or in an antegrade fashion via an ACE, which tends to be more effective than retrograde enemas [59, 60]. Many patients undergo a second surgery for their incontinence; however, long-term outcomes are no better and may be worse than those who only had one reconstruction [71].

In patients where the anal canal is not surrounded by the sphincter complex, a PSARP has been advocated. The long-term outcomes are variable in this cohort, with a small group of patients having complete resolution of their symptoms and most patients still relying on other measures for continence [72]. These patients may also get fecal soiling due to intractable constipation and overflow incontinence. They may also have a resulting megarectum either from distal obstruction or inadequate treatment of constipation. Although invasive, resection of this dilated portion of bowel can lead to improvement of symptoms of constipation and overflow incontinence. This should be considered only in children who have a functional internal anal sphincter, good anal sphincter tone, and no signs of neuropathy [73].

Spinal Pathology

Key Concept: The degree of bowel functional disorders from spinal pathology depends on the level of the defect. Although medical therapy is again a good first-line therapy, many will require a surgical procedure.

The most common causes of neuropathic bowel in children are spina bifida and myelomeningocele. The most common type of spina bifida affects the lumbosacral region causing bowel and bladder dysfunction [59]. Typical anal changes for these patients are poor voluntary sphincter function, poor colonic motility (specifically the left colon), and poor anorectal sensation [60]. However, the involuntary internal sphincter function is usually spared [60]. More than 50 % of patients with myelodysplasia suffer from fecal incontinence [60]. High lesions affect voluntary sphincter function, sensation, and colonic motility, and these patients are prone to fecal retention [60]. In patients with lower lesions, the functional problem is that patients cannot control their bowel emptying and stools evacuate spontaneously without warning; however, patients can rectally stimulate themselves or strain and have some degree of defecation control [60]. Dietary changes and toilet routines should be established; however, enemas are frequently necessary in these patients, and many of these patients can benefit from an ACE procedure [60].

Sphincter Damage

Key Concept: The age of the patient, degree of the defect, and presence of any associated nerve damage will determine the need for surgery and eventual outcome.

Partial sphincter injuries are often expected to scar and heal spontaneously, while other more serious defects will require reconstruction of the sphincters. For example, patients who have undergone a pull-through for Hirschsprung's disease have incontinence rates reported as high as 50 % [74]. This is primarily due to the partial sphincterotomy incorporated into some of the pull-through procedures, as well as the large degree of sphincter stretching in others. It is important to note that these are not necessarily the final outcomes, especially in the infant population. The incidence of incontinence decreases with age, and many have complete resolution by the time adulthood is reached [75]. Therefore, patients with continence problems after a pull-through operation can usually be treated conservatively at first. However, if severe problems persist in the bowel, we prefer retrograde or antegrade enemas [59].

Fecal incontinence associated with mild or moderate perineal trauma should raise concern for sexual abuse and should prompt a thorough workup including psychotherapists to prevent further physiological or psychological injury (if present) [59]. Finally, penetrating trauma or impalement injury can cause severe sphincter damage and should undergo immediate primary repair and protecting colostomy when necessary (Fig. 27.9a, b) [59, 76].

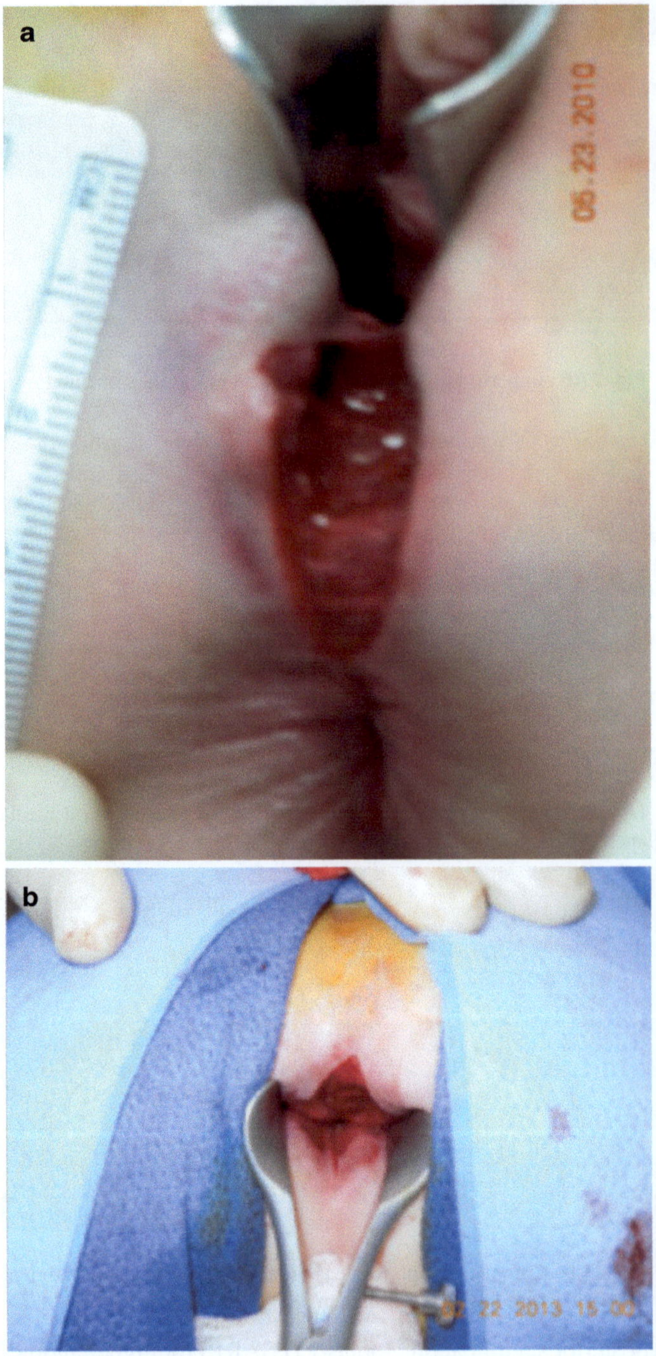

Fig. 27.9 (**a**, **b**) Traumatic sphincter injury

Inflammatory Bowel Disease (IBD)

Key Concept: Treatment of IBD in children follows many of the same principles as adults.

Similar to adults, treatment of IBD in kids is focused on modulating the immune response, suppressing inflammation, preserving bowel mucosa and intestinal length. This may be particularly true in children with Crohn's disease (CD), due to repeated patterns of flares and remission, thus yielding a high risk for complications and an overall malabsorptive state over a longer period of time. In children, this malabsorptive state can rapidly result in malnutrition and poor overall growth [77, 78]. Indeed, growth itself (i.e., bone age) can be used as a marker of disease [77].

IBD can affect children in any age group, although the average age at diagnosis is 12.5 years. Twenty percent of children with IBD are diagnosed before age 10, and <5 % are diagnosed prior to the age of 5 [79]. Unfortunately, a definitive diagnosis of IBD in the pediatric population can be more challenging than in adults. Furthermore, up to 15 % will have the final diagnosis of CD or ulcerative colitis (UC) changed during the course of the disease [80]. This is a factor that needs to be heavily considered prior to performing any rectal reconstructions after total colectomy and proctectomy in children.

In children, both CD and UC present with varying degrees of abdominal pain, diarrhea, rectal bleeding, weight loss, anemia, as well as derangements in growth, nutritional status, and psychosocial development [81, 82]. The lives of children with IBD are also impacted in less obvious ways, such as the ability to participate in recess or organized sports. Children with UC and CD have an impaired aerobic and anaerobic exercise capacity [83]. Furthermore, in light of obesity rates nearing 33 % in American children, 20 % of patients with CD are classified as obese or overweight, whereas the rates in children with UC approached that of the general population [84, 85].

Anorectal Crohn's Disease

Key Concept: Patients who are diagnosed with CD before the age of 6 tend to progress along a more benign course. In contrast, children presenting between the ages of 6 and 17 have more aggressive disease and an increased propensity for developing abscesses and perianal fistulas.

Pediatric perianal CD can have a varying course [86]; and anywhere from 10 to 47 % of newly diagnosed Crohn's patients will present with perianal disease at the time of initial diagnosis [87, 88]. Ultimately, upwards of 60 % of children may have perianal disease including skin tags, fissures, fistulas, and abscesses (Fig. 27.1) [88, 89]. While the majority of children will eventually have some manifestation of perianal CD, most will resolve with medical therapy alone [87]. In contrast to adults, in a study of 325 children, only 12 % required an operation for the anorectal component of their disease [88]. Medical treatment of perianal CD varies widely, with agents such as metronidazole, alone or in addition to 6-mercaptopurine (6-MP), demonstrating benefit [88, 90]. The combination of azathioprine and 6-MP for at least 6 months has demonstrated a 40 % fistula closure rate, 67 % improvement in perianal drainage, and overall improved disease activity indices [91]. Infliximab has also had some success in decreasing the signs and symptoms of perianal disease in those children with moderate to severe CD [92]. When using infliximab, you should ensure that there are no undrained abscesses, as an ongoing infection is a contraindication to its use. Topical tacrolimus has also been shown to be effective in treating IBD-related fistula-in-ano, with the same caveat that there is not an underlying deep space infection [4]. Consequently, pelvic MRI has been shown to be a useful imaging adjunct in defining or ruling out underlying pelvic abscesses in children, as well as the extent and location of fistulas [93]. Endoscopic ultrasound is also useful in defining fistulizing perianal CD and can provide important anatomical information prior to any attempted surgical therapy [94]. If simple fistulas do not resolve with medical therapy alone, a fistulotomy or seton may be used depending on the extent of muscle involved. Extensive, complex fistulas likely will need both medical optimization and seton placement [90].

Fortunately, most perianal disease in children follows a generally benign course and will not become extensive [88, 89, 95, 96]. However, a minority will progress to develop very complicated fistulas, while others go on to become highly destructive perianal disease (HDPD). In a retrospective review of 350 pediatric patients, 8 had complicated fistulas such as recto-urethro-perineal, rectovaginal, rectolabial, and perineal fistulas. In that same study, six developed HDPD with deep perineal ulcerations, undermining of the perineum, and perirectal tissue with a significant exudate. Worth noting, two children progressed so far as fecal incontinence [89]. As you can see, perianal CD can be quite difficult to treat and may not respond well to any treatment. Their course is hallmarked by repeated abscesses requiring multiple incisions and drainages, setons, and extensive trials with medical therapy, and even fecal diversion may be necessary [96, 97].

Crohn's Colitis

Key Concept: Don't be fooled by Crohn's colitis in children. Ensure the proper diagnosis between CD and UC in young patients presenting with colitis prior to embarking on extensive, irreversible, surgical therapy.

Pediatric patients presenting with IBD prior to age 5 are more likely to present with isolated colonic Crohn's disease or Crohn's colitis, adding to the confusion over a proper diagnosis [86]. Crohn's colitis can be more difficult to distinguish from UC in children than in adults, yet the importance of the diagnosis distinction is no less important. Growth failure is more common in children with Crohn's colitis than their counterparts with UC, as is the presence of perianal disease [98]. In one study of 70 children, 13 % had their diagnosis changed from UC to CD or IC *after* colectomy [99]. Performing an ileal pouch anal anastomosis (IPAA) in the setting of CD will certainly lead to more complications [100, 101]. Similar to adults, these can include chronic pouchitis, pouch fistulas, and even pouch failure [101]. Perianal disease is also associated with worse outcomes after IPAA [101]. For these reasons, the diagnosis of Crohn's colitis is a contraindication to IPAA, and if a colectomy is warranted for separate clinic reasons, an ileorectal anastomosis would be the suggested non-diverting alternative [102]. Finally, while a child with Crohn's colitis may experience temporary benefit or remission from a colectomy, the disease is very likely to recur within the small intestine [98].

Ileocolic Crohn's Disease

Key Concept: Resection or stricturoplasty for isolated ileocolic disease appears to have equivalent outcomes.

Although CD can affect any part of the gastrointestinal tract in children, the most common location remains the terminal ileum and right colon [99, 103]. With isolated active disease there is some controversy as to the proper treatment. In 11 pediatric patients who underwent resection of their isolated disease at the terminal ileum and right colon, zero had evidence of recurrence at a mean of 2.6-year follow-up (maximum 7 years) [104]. Others have reported no difference in relapse or recurrence following resection of the disease versus stricturoplasty [105]. In a separate study of 130 children, it was found that those who had surgery within 3 years of their initial diagnosis derived a protective benefit from the need for later immunosuppression. They also tended to catch up in height and weight better [106]. While it is difficult what to make of these findings, for those children that ultimately do need surgery for CD, the open, laparoscopic, and laparoscopic-assisted approaches have all been proven to be safe [107–109].

Chronic Ulcerative Colitis

Key Concept: UC in children presents with an aggressive nature more often than in adults, with over one-third eventually requiring a colectomy.

While CD in children tends to present quite similarly to adults, pediatric UC generally has a much "more severe phenotype" than UC in adults [110]. Children present with more extensive and widespread disease and have higher rates of acute exacerbation [110–112]. Remarkably, upwards of 80 % will present with a pancolitis [103]. In a population comparison study, the pediatric adolescent patients with UC incurred the highest total hospital costs compared to other age groups, largely secondary to their number of inpatient hospitalizations [113].

Further highlighting this issue, 45 % of children with UC will become steroid dependent, and more than 30 % of children will fail steroid management [110, 111]. An average of 30–40 % of pediatric UC patients will ultimately need a colectomy; however, ranges from 10 to 60 % have been reported [111, 114, 115]. The most common reason children with chronic UC undergo surgery is for refractory bleeding [99]. In the elective setting, a total proctocolectomy with ileal pouch anal anastomosis can be performed. One must be cautious of children on infliximab, as the complication rate is nearly twice that as compared to children not on infliximab. It is recommended to wait at least 8 weeks after the last dose of infliximab or perform a colectomy with end ileostomy as the first operation [116]. A 3-stage operation would also be the recommended course in the setting of an acute exacerbation that required an urgent operation and even more so in the setting of high-dose steroid therapy [117].

Short of performing an emergent operation, a few points regarding their evaluation and course are worth mentioning. First, while not all laboratory tests are useful in pediatric UC, in two-thirds of children with UC, either CRP or ESR will be reflective of their disease. More importantly, if one of the tests does reflect disease severity, then it is likely to continue to predict disease severity throughout the entire clinical course [118]. Next, to aid in assessing the severity of chronic UC, the Pediatric Ulcerative Colitis Activity Index (PUCAI) was created. It correlates with the oft-used Mayo score in adults. The score ranges from 0 to 85 and includes points for abdominal pain, rectal bleeding, consistency of stools, number of stools per day, nocturnal stools, and activity level [119]. In general, a PUCAI score less than 10 indicates remission, 10–34 mild disease, 35–64 moderate, and greater than 65 points severe disease [111]. If the score remains greater than 45 on day 3 of treatment of an acute exacerbation, then steroids will likely fail, and alternate medical therapy should be initiated [120]. If the score is greater than 70 on day 5 of treatment, then both alternate medical and surgical therapies should be considered [120]. A clinically significant response to treatment is usually indicated by a drop in the PUCAI score of at least 20 points [111].

Ulcerative Colitis Emergencies

Key Concept: Children with UC present for emergent surgery just like adults with free perforation, fulminant colitis, toxic megacolon, and massive hemorrhage. In the emergent setting, the procedure of choice is a subtotal colectomy with end ileostomy.

Emergent subtotal colectomy and end ileostomy for UC in children allow for all the advantages seen in adults [121]. Removal of the majority of disease, shorter operative time without pouch creation, and allowance for subsequent medical optimization prior to a definitive or restorative operation have all been demonstrated in children as well [122]. Fortunately, it is rare for pediatric patients to require a colectomy in the urgent or emergent setting. Reported rates have varied between 1.5 and 13 % [123–125].

Polyposis Syndromes

Key Concept: Polyps in children occur in the setting of familial and genetic syndromes and should be worked up accordingly.

Intestinal polyps are less prevalent in children than adults. The most common presenting complaints are abdominal pain and gastrointestinal bleeding [126]. Of the inherited polyposis syndromes, familial adenomatous polyposis (FAP) is most common and affects about 1 child in every 10,000 [127]. In children with FAP, polyps will usually begin to appear at the age of 16 and will progress to hundreds to thousands of polyps. The average age of transformation to colorectal cancer is 39 years [127]. Children with FAP should begin colonoscopic screening by age 10. Once adenomas are discovered, a total proctocolectomy with ileal pouch anal anastomosis should be performed. In small children, it is important to note that a stapled anastomosis is almost always technically impossible due to the size of the pelvis and of the ileal and anal lumens. In this setting, we prefer a mucosectomy and hand-sewn anastomosis. Alternatively, a primary ileorectal anastomosis is an acceptable alternative, provided endoscopic control and surveillance of the residual rectum continues routinely [128]. At the time the first adenoma is found, upper endoscopy screening should begin as well [127]. Some would argue that upper gastrointestinal tract screening should actually start at the same time as the first colonoscopy, though there are some differing views on this matter [129]. We prefer to identify the exact genetic mutation, as children with a mutation in the adenomatous polyposis coli (APC) gene at codon 1309 should be referred for colectomy earlier, as these children present with a more aggressive disease [130]. Additionally, in families with known FAP, the risk of hepatoblastoma is up to 800 times that of the general population. In these families hepatoblastoma screening should begin at birth with an abdominal ultrasound and alpha-fetoprotein (AFP) levels [127].

The incidence of juvenile polyposis syndrome (JPS) is less than that of FAP, reportedly occurring in ~1:100,000 children. Like FAP, JPS is autosomal dominant. Typically patients will develop in the range of 50–100 colonic polyps. Screening with upper and lower endoscopy should begin by age 15 [127]. Repeat surveillance has been recommended every 1–2 years for symptomatic patients and every 3 years for those at risk for JPS [127, 131, 132]. We feel juvenile polyps should be biopsied as the colorectal cancer risk in JPS is approximately 50 % [127, 133]. Once adenomatous changes are seen on the final pathology of a juvenile polyp in a child with JPS, a referral for a proctocolectomy should be made [126, 133].

Finally, Peutz-Jeghers syndrome (PJS) presents with hamartomatous polyps and mucocutaneous pigmented skin lesions of the mouth and lips (Fig. 27.10) [127]. It occurs in 1 out 200,000 children. Abdominal pain is a common complaint, often secondary to intussusception with the polyps as the lead point [127]. Colonoscopic surveillance should begin when symptoms develop or in the early teen years. Upper endoscopy should start by age 10 [127]. Capsule endoscopy is also gaining ground for small bowel surveillance. Large polyps and those that will potentially lead to symptoms can then be resected prior to causing problems (Figs. 27.11 and 27.12) [134]. The risk of malignancy with PJS is generally outside of the gastrointestinal tract [131].

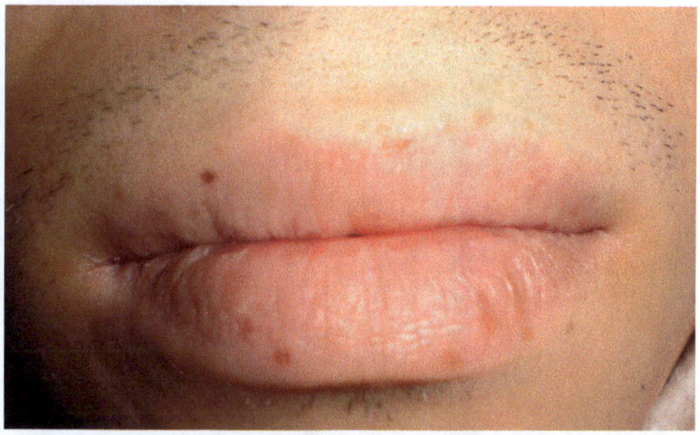

Fig. 27.10 Mucocutaneous pigmentation in a patient with Peutz-Jeghers syndrome (Courtesy of Phillip Y. Pearson, MD)

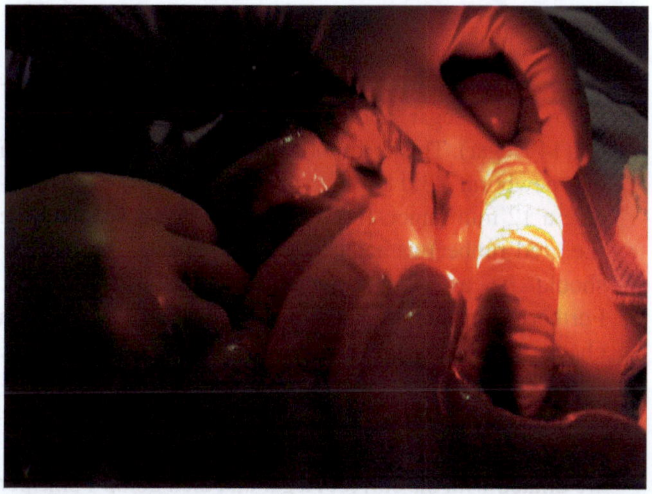

Fig. 27.11 Transillumination of the bowel during intraoperative small bowel endoscopy in a patient with Peutz-Jeghers syndrome (Courtesy of Phillip Y. Pearson, MD)

Summary Pearls

Again, while we recognize you may not treat, or even evaluate, many children with colorectal disease, our goal was and is to provide you with some baseline information and tips and tricks to think about when encountering these patients. As such, here are a final few thoughts that may serve you well when dealing with children.

Examination

1. If you care for infants, you should know the size of your fingers—both in terms of length and especially in terms of Hegar dilator size (i.e., mm in diameter). The average

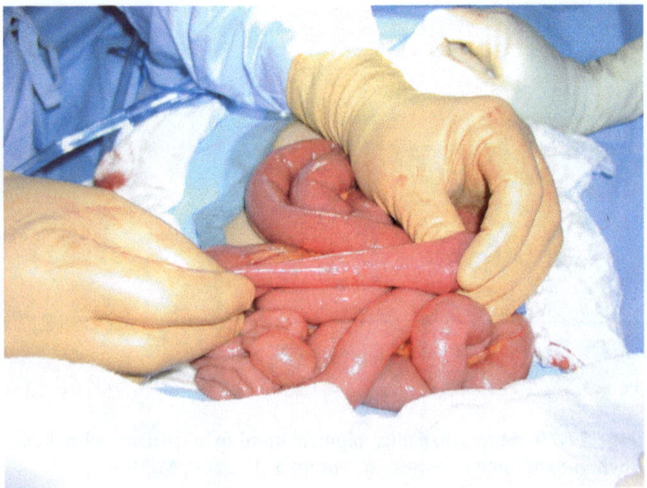

Fig. 27.12 Small bowel polyp in a patient with Peutz-Jeghers syndrome (Courtesy of Phillip Y. Pearson)

surgeon has a fifth finger of approximately 12 mm diameter (i.e., 12 Hegar) and an index finger of 14 mm diameter (14 Hegar). This is important because in the evaluation of a newborn, a 3.0 kg infant should normally accommodate a 12 mm finger. Below 2.5 kg, either a soft flexible (i.e., red rubber) catheter or the appropriate-sized Hegar should be used to evacuate the anus and rectum. Furthermore, after any anal or rectal procedure, there is a chance that a repair could stricture down as it heals. Almost all of these strictures are amenable to serial dilations over time. The protocol usually involves an examination at 2–3 weeks postoperatively. If a stricture is present, we dilated with the correct Hegar and then go up 1 size per week until an adequate lumen has been established.

2. In infant females with constipation, the examination should also include the urethra and the vagina. A Crede's maneuver, i.e., place pressure on the bladder, can help demonstrate the urethra. The relationship between the anus and the vagina should next be noted. A more anteriorly located anus, especially if stenotic, is a common cause of constipation in infant girls. The anus may even be within the fourchette of the vagina (external to the hymen). This would require a PSARP for repair. Remember, one of the most severe mistakes you can make is to confuse a persistent cloaca for an imperforate anus alone.

Preoperatively and Intraoperatively

1. An effective means to bowel prep a child is by using polyethylene glycol solution with electrolytes at 20–25 mL/kg/h until clear. Often infants need rectal stimulation to initiate stooling during the prep but should then continue on their own.
2. The best thing to use intraoperatively for identifying the sphincter complex is electrical stimulation. If a proprietary electric stimulator is unavailable (such as the Peña stimulator), you can use a nerve stimulator with one lead as the alligator is clamped to a 2-G needle grounded in the gluteus maximus. Your other lead (to test the adequacy of sphincter contraction) is used by clamping a 21-G needle and probing for the complex. It is important that you hold the needle on its plastic hub by a small hemostat to avoid conduction up to you. The center of the sphincter complex is located and marked in this way.
3. When performing surgery in the perineum of small children and infants, a protected needle tip cautery is the instrument of choice for precise dissection. It allows for hemostasis while protecting the working end from leaning against normal tissue not intended to be cauterized. It also minimizes spread of the current. Retraction of the anal opening to gain access to the rectal mucosa is accomplished in either of 2 ways: by suturing the anus open or by using a self-retaining retractor with sharp hooks that attach to the anal opening (i.e., Lone Star).
4. A difficult anastomosis within the anal canal can be made simpler by dissection more proximally which serves to initially prolapse the rectum and anus, perform an extracorporeal anastomosis, and allow it to retract back in. Dissection for approximately 3 cm above the dentate line is necessary in order to achieve adequate prolapse of the rectum and allow this to happen. In this manner, access to the peritoneal cavity can be accomplished as well as completing whatever procedure is being performed in an extracorporeal fashion.

Postoperatively

1. Infants are obligate nasal breathers; therefore, orogastric tubes are preferred to nasogastric tubes for infants when they are required.
2. Phosphate enemas should be avoided in infants and small children to avoid electrolyte shifts. Normal saline enemas are preferred. The volume of the colon on average is 20 mL/kg, and this is the volume that should be used to clean out an entire colon that is filled with stool.
3. If a full enema is not required to initiate stooling, a glycerine suppository is well tolerated by infants.

Conclusion

It is common for many of you to experience a certain degree of angst when asked to evaluate an infant or child. This is common, especially when this may be on an infrequent basis. Remember, similar to many of your other patients (just in a smaller package): do no harm, preserve long-term function when possible, and decide what has to be done right then and what can wait for more experienced hands.

References

1. Eisenhammer S. Internal anal sphincter and anorectal abscess. Surg Gynecol Obstet. 1956;103:501–6.
2. Afsarlar CE, et al. Perianal abscess and fistula-in-ano in children: clinical characteristic, management and outcome. Pediatr Surg Int. 2011;27:1063–8.
3. Christison-Lagay ER, et al. Nonoperative management of perianal abscess in infants is associate with decreased risk for fistula formation. Pediatrics. 2007;120:e548–52.
4. Niyogi A, Agarwal T, Broadhurst J, Abel RM. Management of perianal abscess and fistula-in-ano in children. Eur J Pediatr Surg. 2010;20:35–9.
5. Al-Salem AH, Laing W, Talwalker V. Fistula- in-ano in infancy and childhood. J Pediatr Surg. 1994;29:436–8.
6. Watanabe Y, Todani T, Yamamoto S. Conservative management of fistula in ano in infants. Pediatr Surg Int. 1998;13:274–6.
7. Serour F, Gorenstein A. Characteristics of perianal abscess and fistula-in-ano in healthy children. World J Surg. 2006;30: 467–72.
8. Karamatsu ML, Thorp AW, Brown L. Changes in community-associated methicillin-resistant staphylococcus aureus skin and soft tissue infections presenting to pediatric emergency department. Pediatr Emerg Care. 2012;28:131–5.
9. Alt AL, Routh JC, Ashley RA, Boyce TG, Kramer SA. Superficial genitourinary abscesses in children: emergence of methicillin resistant Staphylococcus aureus. J Urol. 2008;180:1472–5.
10. Woods DL, Amrute KV. Trends of genital and nongenital community-acquired methicillin-resistant Staphylococcus aureus infections in urban pediatric population. J Low Genit Tract Dis. 2012;0:1–6.
11. Buddicom E, Jamieson A, Beasley S, King S. Perianal abscess in children: aiming for optimal management. ANZ J Surg. 2012; 82:60–2.
12. Stites T, Lund DP. Common anorectal problems. Semin Pediatr Surg. 2007;16:71–8.
13. Kenny SE, Irvine T, Driver CP, et al. Double blinded randomised controlled trial of topical glyceryl trinitrate in anal fissure. Arch Dis Child. 2001;85:404–7.
14. Tander B, Guven A, Demirbag S, et al. A prospective, randomized, double-blinded, placebo-controlled trial of glyceryl-trinitrate ointment in the treatment of children with anal fissure. J Pediatr Surg. 1999;34:1810–2.
15. Sonmez K, Demirogullari B, Ekingen G, et al. Randomized, placebo controlled treatment of anal fissure by lidocaine, EMLA, and GTN in children. J Pediatr Surg. 2002;37:1313–6.
16. Keshtgar AS, Ward HC, Clayden GS. Transcutaneous needle-free injection of botulinum toxin: a novel treatment of childhood constipation and anal fissure. J Pediatr Surg. 2009;44:1791–8.
17. Cohen A, Dehn T. Lateral subcutaneous sphincterotomy for treatment of anal fissure in children. Br J Surg. 1995;82: 1341–2.
18. Siafakas C, Vottler TP, Andersen JM. Rectal prolapse in pediatrics. Clin Pediatr. 1999;38(2):63–72.
19. Laituri CA, Garey CL, Fraser JD, et al. 15-Year experience in the treatment of rectal prolapse in children. J Pediatr Surg. 2010;45: 1607–9.
20. Flum AS, Golladay ES, Teitelbaum DH. Recurrent rectal prolapse following primary surgical treatment. Pediatr Surg Int. 2010;26:427–31.
21. Ismail M, Gabr K, Shalaby R. Laparoscopic management of persistent complete rectal prolapse in children. J Pediatr Surg. 2010;45: 533–9.
22. Antao B, Bradley V, Roberts JP, Shawis R. Management of rectal prolapse in children. Dis Colon Rectum. 2005;48:1620–5.
23. Chan WK, Kay SM, Laberge J, Gallucci JG, Bensoussan AL, Yazbeck S. Injection sclerotherapy in the treatment of rectal prolapse in infants and children. J Pediatr Surg. 1998;33:225–58.
24. Kay N, Zachary RB. The treatment of rectal prolapse in children with injections of 30 percent saline solutions. J Pediatr Surg. 1970;5:334–7.
25. Dutta BN, Das AK. Treatment of prolapse rectum in children with injections of sclerosing agents. J Indian Med Assoc. 1977;69: 275–6.
26. Wyllie GG. The injection treatment of rectal prolapse. J Pediatr Surg. 1979;14:62–4.
27. Malyshev YI, Gulin VA. Our experience with the treatment of rectal prolapse in infants and children. Am J Proctol. 1973;24: 470–2.
28. Bahador A, Foroutan HR, Hosseini S, Davani S. Effect of submucosal alcohol injection on prolonged rectal prolapse in infants and children. J Indian Assoc Pediatr Surg. 2008;13(1):11–3.
29. High DW, Hertzler JH, Phillippart AI, Benson CD. Linear cauterization for the treatment of rectal prolapse in infants and children. Surg Gynecol Obstet. 1982;154:400–2.
30. Sanders S, Vural O, Unal M. Management of rectal prolapse in children: Ekehorn's rectosacropexy. Pediatr Surg Int. 1999;15:111–4.
31. Pena A, Hong A. The posterior sagittal trans-sphincteric and trans-rectal approach. Tech Coloproctol. 2003;7:35–44.
32. Ashcraft KW, Garred JL, Holder TM, Amoury RA, Sharp RJ, Murphy JP. Rectal prolapse: 17-year experience with the posterior repair and suspension. J Pediatr Surg. 1990;25:992–5.
33. Puri B. Rectal prolapse in children: laparoscopic suture rectopexy is a suitable alternative. J Indian Assoc Pediatr Surg. 2010;15:47–9.
34. Coccorullo P, Quitadamo P, Martinelli M, Staiano A. Novel and alternative therapies for childhood constipation. J Pediatr Gastroenterol Nutr. 2009;48:S104–6.
35. Keshtgar AS, Ward HC, Clayden GS. Diagnosis and management of children with intractable constipation. Semin Pediatr Surg. 2004;13:300–9.
36. Pijpers MM, Tabbers MM, Benninga MA, Berger MY. Current recommended treatments of childhood constipation are not evidence based: a systematic literature review on the effect of laxative treatment and dietary measures. Arch Dis Child. 2009;94: 117–31.
37. Berger MY, Tabbers MM, Kurver MJ, Boluyt N, Benninga MA. Value of abdominal radiography, colonic transit time and rectal ultrasound scanning in the diagnosis of idiopathic constipation in children: a systematic review. J Pediatr. 2012;161:44–50.
38. Mugie SM, Di Lorenzo C, Benninga MA. Constipation in childhood. Nature reviews. Gastroenterol Hepatol. 2011;8:502–11.
39. Burgers R, Di Lorenzo C. Diagnostic testing in constipation: is it necessary. J Pediatr Gastroenterol Nutr. 2011;53 Suppl 2: S49–51.
40. Giramonti KM, Kogan BA, Agboola OO, Ribons L, Dangman B. The association of constipation with childhood urinary tract infections. J Pediatr Urol. 2005;1:273–8.
41. Di Lorenzo C, Flores C, Reddy AF, Hyman PE. Use of colonic manometry to differentiate causes of intractable constipation in children. J Pediatr. 1992;120:690–5.
42. Martin MJ, Steele SR, Noel JM, et al. Total colonic manometry in the surgical evaluation of functional colonic obstruction. J Pediatr Surg. 2004;39(3):352–9.
43. Kranz S, Brauchla M, Slavin JL, Miller KB. What do we know about dietary fiber intake in children and health? The effects of fiber intake on constipation, obesity, and diabetes in children. Am Soc Nutr Adv Nutr. 2012;3:47–53.
44. Gordon J, Blakely K, Blannin J, et al. Constipation in children and young people. Diagnosis and management of idiopathic childhood constipation in primary and secondary care. National Collaborating

Center of Women's and Children's Health commissioned by the National Institute for Health and Care Excellence (NICE) Guidelines; 2010. http://www.nice.org.uk/nicemedia/live/12993/48741/48741.pdf. Accessed 17 January 2014.

45. Giannetti E, Sciorio E, Staiano A. Treatment of constipation: where do we go? J Pediatr Gastroenterol Nutr. 2011;53:S53–5.
46. Ali SR, Ahmed S, Qadir M, Humayun KN. Fecal incontinence and constipation in children: a clinical conundrum. Oman Med J. 2011; 26:376–8.
47. Miller MK, Dowd MD, Friesen CA, Walsh-Kelly CM. A randomized trial of enema versus polyethylene glycol 3350 for fecal disimpaction in children presenting to an emergency department. Pediatr Emerg Care. 2012;28:115–9.
48. Bekkali NH, et al. Rectal fecal impaction treatment in childhood constipation: enemas versus high doses oral PEG. Pediatrics. 2009;124:e1108–15.
49. Guest JF, et al. Clinical and economic impact of using macrogol 3350 plus electrolytes in an outpatient setting compared to enemas and suppositories and manual evacuation to treat paediatric faecal impaction based on actual clinical practice in England and Wales. Curr Med Res Opin. 2007;23:2213–25.
50. Nurko S, et al. PEG 3350 in the treatment of childhood constipation: a multicenter, double-blinded, placebo-controlled trial. J Pediatr. 2008;153:254–61.
51. Thompson MA, et al. Polyethylene glycol 3350 plus electrolytes for chronic constipation in children: a double blinded, placebo controlled, crossover study. Arch Dis Child. 2007;92:996–1000.
52. Gordon M, Naidoo K, Akobeng AK, Thomas AG. Osmotic and stimulant laxatives for the management of childhood constipation (Review). Cochrane Database Syst Rev. 2012;(7):CD009118.
53. Clayden GS, Adeyinka T, Kufeji D, Keshtgar AS. Surgical management of severe chronic constipation. Arch Dis Child. 2010;95:859–60.
54. Wong AL, Kravarusic D, Wong SL. Impact of cecostomy and antegrade colonic enemas on management of fecal incontinence and constipation ten years of experience in pediatric population. J Pediatr Surg. 2008;43:1445–51.
55. Kim HY, Jung SE, Lee SC, Park KW, Kim WK. Is the outcome of the left colon antegrade continence enema better than that of the right antegrade continence enema? J Pediatr Surg. 2009;44:783–7.
56. Levitt MA, Martin CA, Falcone Jr RA, Pena A. Transanal rectosigmoid resection for severe intractable idiopathic constipation. J Pediatr Surg. 2009;44:1285–91.
57. Asipu D, Jaffray B. Treatment of severe childhood constipation with restorative proctocolectomy. Arch Dis Child. 2009;95: 867–70.
58. Jaffray B. What happens to children with idiopathic constipation who receive an antegrade continent enema? An actuarial analysis of 80 consecutive cases. J Pediatr Surg. 2009;44:404–7.
59. Di Lorenzo C, Benninga MA. Pathophysiology of pediatric fecal incontinence. Gastroenterology. 2004;126(Suppl):S33–40.
60. Rintala RJ. Fecal incontinence in anorectal malformations, neuropathy, and miscellaneous conditions. Semin Pediatr Surg. 2002;11(2):75–82.
61. Bai Y, Yuan Z, Wang W, Zhao Y, Wang H, Wang W. Quality of life for children with fecal incontinence after surgically corrected anorectal malformation. J Pediatr Surg. 2000;35:462–4.
62. Hassink EA, Rieu PN, Brugman AT, et al. Quality of life after operatively corrected high anorectal malformation. A long-term follow-up-study in patients 18 years of age or older. J Pediatr Surg. 1994;29:773–6.
63. Brazzelli M, Griffiths P. Behavioural and cognitive interventions with or without other treatments for defaecation disorders in children. Cochrane Database Syst Rev. 2001;(4):CD002240.
64. van Ginkel R, Benninga MA, Blommaart PJ, van der Plas RN, Boeckxstaens GE, Buller HA. Lack of benefit of laxatives as adjunctive therapy for functional nonretentive fecal soiling in children. Journal of Pediatrics. 2000;137:808–13.
65. Benninga MA, Taminiau JA. Diagnosis and treatment efficacy of functional non-retentive fecal soiling in childhood. J Pediatr Gastroenterol Nutr. 2001;32 suppl 1:S41–3.
66. Levitt MA, Pena A. Outcomes from the correction of anorectal malformations. Curr Opin Pediatr. 2005;17:394–401.
67. Rintala RJ, Lindahi HG. Fecal continence in patients having undergone posterior sagittal anorectoplasty procedure for a high anorectal malformation improves at adolescence, as constipation disappears. J Pediatr Surg. 2001;36:1218–21.
68. Heikene JB, Werlin SL, Di Lorenzo C, Hyman PE, Cocjin J, Flores AF, et al. Colonic motility in children with repaired imperforate anus. Dig Dis Sci. 1999;44:1288–92.
69. Rintala R, Lindahl H. Is normal bowel function possible after repair of intermediate and high anorectal malformations. J Pediatr Surg. 1995;30:491–5.
70. Iwai N, Nagashima M, Shimotake T, Iwata G. Biofeedback therapy for fecal incontinence after surgery for anorectal malformations: preliminary results. J Pediatr Surg. 1993;28:863–6.
71. Hassink EA, Rieu PN, Severijnen RS, et al. Are adults content or continent after repair for high anal atresia? A long-term follow-up study in patients 18 years of age or older. Ann Surg. 1993;218: 196–200.
72. Pena A. Posterior sagittal anorectoplasty as a second operation for the treatment of fecal incontinence. J Pediatr Surg. 1983;18: 762–72.
73. Keshtgar AS, Ward HC, Richards C, Clayden GS. Outcome of excision of megarectum in children with anorectal malformation. J Pediatr Surg. 2007;42:227–33.
74. Tsuji H, Spitz I, Kiely EM, et al. Management and long-term follow-up of infants with total colonic aganglionosis. J Pediatr Surg. 1999;34:158–61.
75. Heikkinen M, Rintala R, Louhimo I. Bowel function and quality of life in adult patients with operated Hirschsprung's disease. Pediatr Surg Int. 1995;10:342–4.
76. Reinberg O, Yazbeck S. Major perineal trauma in children. J Pediatr Surg. 1989;24:982–4.
77. Gupta N, Lustig RH, Kohn MA, et al. Determination of bone age in pediatric patients with Crohn's disease should become part of routine care. Inflamm Bowel Dis. 2013;19(1):61–5.
78. Mallon DP, Suskind DL. Nutrition in pediatric inflammatory bowel disease. Nutr Clin Pract. 2010;25:335–9.
79. Glick SR, Carvalho RS. Inflammatory bowel disease. Pediatr Rev. 2010;32:14–24.
80. Mamula P, Telega GW, Markowitz JE, et al. Inflammatory bowel disease in children 5 years of age and younger. Am J Gastroenterol. 2002;97:2005–10.
81. Motil KJ, Grand RJ. Ulcerative colitis and Crohn disease in children. Pediatr Rev. 1987;9:109–20.
82. Bradley GM, Oliva-Hemker M. Pediatric ulcerative colitis: current treatment approaches including role of Infliximab. Biologics. 2012;6:125–34.
83. Ploeger HE, Takken T, Wilk B, et al. Exercise capacity in pediatric patients with inflammatory bowel disease. J Pediatr. 2011;158: 814–9.
84. Daniels SR, Jacobson MS, McCrindle BW, et al. American heart association childhood obesity research summit: executive summary. Circulation. 2009;119:2114–23.
85. Long MD, Crandall WV, Leibowitz IH, et al. Prevalence and epidemiology of overweight and obesity in children with inflammatory bowel disease. Inflamm Bowel Dis. 2011;17:2162–8.
86. Gupta N, Bostrom AG, Kirschner BS, et al. Presentation and disease course in early- compared to later-onset pediatric Crohn's disease. Am J Gastroenterol. 2008;103:2092–8.
87. Keljo DJ, Markowitz J, Langton C, et al. Course and treatment of perianal disease in children newly diagnosed with Crohn's disease. Inflamm Bowel Dis. 2009;15:383–7.
88. Palder SB, Shandling B, Bilik R, et al. Perianal complications of pediatric Crohn's disease. J Pediatr Surg. 1991;26:513–5.

89. Markowitz J, Grancher K, Rosa J, et al. Highly destructive perianal disease in children with Crohn's disease. J Pediatr Gastroenterol Nutr. 1995;21:149–53.
90. Stein BL, Gordon PH. Perianal inflammatory conditions in inflammatory bowel disease. Curr Opin Gen Surg. 1993:141–6.
91. Jeshion WC, Larsen KL, Jawad AF, et al. Azathioprine and 6-mercaptopurine for the treatment of perianal Crohn's disease in children. J Clin Gastroenterol. 2000;30:294–8.
92. Crandall W, Hyams J, Kugathasan S, et al. Infliximab therapy in children with concurrent perianal Crohn disease: observations from REACH. J Pediatr Gastroenterol Nutr. 2009;49:183–90.
93. Essary B, Kim J, Anupindi S, et al. Pelvic MRI in children with Crohn disease and suspected perianal involvement. Pediatr Radiol. 2007;37:201–8.
94. Rosen MJ, Moulton DE, Koyama T, et al. Endoscopic ultrasound to guide the combined medical and surgical management of pediatric perianal Crohn's disease. Inflamm Bowel Dis. 2010;16:461–8.
95. Markowitz J, Daum F, Aiges H, et al. Perianal disease in children and adolescents with Crohn's disease. Gastroenterology. 1984;86:829–33.
96. Shetty AK, Udall Jr J, Schmidt-Sommerfeld E. Highly destructive perianal Crohn's disease. J Natl Med Assoc. 1998;90:491–2.
97. Tolia V. Perianal Crohn's disease in children and adolescents. Am J Gastroenterol. 1996;91:922–6.
98. Ament ME. Inflammatory disease of the colon: ulcerative colitis and Crohn's colitis. J Pediatr. 1975;86:322–34.
99. Mortellaro VE, Green J, Islam S, et al. Occurrence of Crohn's disease in children after total colectomy for ulcerative colitis. J Surg Res. 2011;170:38–40.
100. Le Q, Melmed G, Dubinsky M, et al. Surgical outcome of ileal pouch-anal anastomosis when used intentionally for well-defined Crohn's disease. Inflamm Bowel Dis. 2013;19(1):30–6.
101. Alexander F, Sarigol S, DiFiore J, et al. Fate of the pouch in 151 pediatric patients after ileal pouch anal anastomosis. J Pediatr Surg. 2003;38:78–82.
102. Alexander F. Complications of ileal pouch anal anastomosis. Semin Pediatr Surg. 2007;16:200–4.
103. Sawczenko A, Sandhu BK. Presenting features of inflammatory bowel disease in Great Britain and Ireland. Arch Dis Child. 2003;88:995–1000.
104. Coran AG, Klein MD, Sarahan TM. The surgical management of terminal ileal and right colon Crohn's disease in children. J Pediatr Surg. 1983;18:592–4.
105. Romeo E, Jasonni V, Caldaro T, et al. Strictureplasty and intestinal resection: different options in complicated pediatric-onset Crohn disease. J Pediatr Surg. 2012;47:944–8.
106. Boualit M, Salleron J, Turck D, et al. Long-term outcome after first intestinal resection in pediatric-onset Crohn's disease: a population-based study. Inflamm Bowel Dis. 2013;19(1):7–14.
107. Bonnard A, Fouquet V, Berrebi D, et al. Crohn's disease in children. Preliminary experience with a laparoscopic approach. Eur J Pediatr Surg. 2006;16:90–3.
108. Diamond IR, Langer JC. Laparoscopic-assisted versus open ileocolic resection for adolescent Crohn disease. J Pediatr Gastroenterol Nutr. 2001;33:543–7.
109. Dutta S, Rothenberg SS, Chang J, et al. Total intracorporeal laparoscopic resection of Crohn's disease. J Pediatr Surg. 2003;38:717–9.
110. Turner D, Griffiths AM. Acute severe ulcerative colitis in children: a systematic review. Inflamm Bowel Dis. 2011;17:440–9.
111. Turner D, Levine A, Escher JC, et al. Management of pediatric ulcerative colitis: Joint ECCO and ESPGHAN Evidence-based Consensus Guidelines. J Pediatr Gastroenterol Nutr. 2010;55:340–61.
112. Langholz E, Munkholm P, Krasilnikoff PA, et al. Inflammatory bowel diseases with onset in childhood. Clinical features, morbidity, and mortality in a regional cohort. Scand J Gastroenterol. 1997;32:139–47.
113. Bickston SJ, Waters HC, Dabbous O, et al. Administrative claims analysis of all-cause annual costs of care and resource utilization by age category for ulcerative colitis patients. J Manag Care Pharm. 2008;14:352–62.
114. Mattei P, Rombeau JL. Surgical treatment of ulcerative colitis. In: Mamula P, Markowitz JE, Baldassano RN, editors. Pediatric inflammatory bowel disease. New York: Springer; 2008.
115. Turner D, Walsh CM, Benchimol EI, et al. Severe paediatric ulcerative colitis: incidence, outcomes and optimal timing for second-line therapy. Gut. 2008;57:331–8.
116. Kennedy R, Potter DD, Moir C, et al. Pediatric chronic ulcerative colitis: does infliximab increase post-ileal pouch anal anastomosis complications? J Pediatr Surg. 2012;47:199–203.
117. Turner D, Travis SP, Griffiths AM, et al. Consensus for managing acute severe ulcerative colitis in children: a systematic review and joint statement from ECCO, ESPGHAN, and the Porto IBD Working Group of ESPGHAN. Am J Gastroenterol. 2011;106:574–88.
118. Turner D, Mack DR, Hyams J, et al. C-reactive protein (CRP), erythrocyte sedimentation rate (ESR) or both? A systematic evaluation in pediatric ulcerative colitis. J Crohns Colitis. 2011;5:423–9.
119. Turner D, Otley AR, Mack D, et al. Development, validation, and evaluation of a pediatric ulcerative colitis activity index: a prospective multicenter study. Gastroenterology. 2007;133:423–32.
120. Turner D, Mack D, Leleiko N, et al. Severe pediatric ulcerative colitis: a prospective multicenter study of outcomes and predictors of response. Gastroenterology. 2010;138:2282–91.
121. Binderow SR, Wexner SD. Current surgical therapy for mucosal ulcerative colitis. Dis Colon Rectum. 1994;37:610–24.
122. Cima RR. Timing and indications for colectomy in chronic ulcerative colitis: surgical consideration. Dig Dis. 2010;28:501–7.
123. Patton D, Gupta N, Wojcicki JM, et al. Postoperative outcome of colectomy for pediatric patients with ulcerative colitis. J Pediatr Gastroenterol Nutr. 2010;51:151–4.
124. Travis SP, Stange EF, Lemann M, et al. European evidence-based consensus on the management of ulcerative colitis: current management. J Crohns Colitis. 2008;2:24–62.
125. Hyman NH, Cataldo P, Osler T. Urgent subtotal colectomy for severe inflammatory bowel disease. Dis Colon Rectum. 2005;48:70–3.
126. Adolph VR, Bernabe K. Polyps in children. Clin Colon Rectal Surg. 2008;21:280–5.
127. Barnard J. Screening and surveillance recommendations for pediatric gastrointestinal polyposis syndromes. J Pediatr Gastroenterol Nutr. 2009;48 Suppl 2:S75–8.
128. Booij KA, Mathus-Vliegen EM, Taminiau JA, et al. Evaluation of 28 years of surgical treatment of children and young adults with familial adenomatous polyposis. J Pediatr Surg. 2010;45:525–32.
129. Attard TM, Cuffari C, Tajouri T, et al. Multicenter experience with upper gastrointestinal polyps in pediatric patients with familial adenomatous polyposis. Am J Gastroenterol. 2004;99:681–6.
130. Attard TM, Tajouri T, Peterson KD, et al. Familial adenomatous polyposis in children younger than age ten years: a multidisciplinary clinic experience. Dis Colon Rectum. 2008;51:207–12.
131. Corredor J, Wambach J, Barnard J. Gastrointestinal polyps in children: advances in molecular genetics, diagnosis, and management. J Pediatr. 2001;138:621–8.
132. Brosens LA, van Hattem A, Hylind LM, et al. Risk of colorectal cancer in juvenile polyposis. Gut. 2007;56:965–7.
133. Heiss KF, Schaffner D, Ricketts RR, et al. Malignant risk in juvenile polyposis coli: increasing documentation in the pediatric age group. J Pediatr Surg. 1993;28:1188–93.
134. Gastineau S, Viala J, Caldari D, et al. Contribution of capsule endoscopy to Peutz-Jeghers syndrome management in children. Dig Liver Dis. 2012;44:839–43.

Functional Problems Following Colorectal Surgery

28

Lillias Holmes Maguire, Stanley Goldberg, and Liliana Bordeianou

Key Points

- Functional complications are increasingly common following colorectal surgery as new paradigms and techniques more frequently preserve intestinal continuity.
- Conservative treatment includes medications and dietary changes to alter stool consistency and intestinal transit time.
- Surgical treatment options are available for patients with appropriate anatomy and comorbidity and escalate from gel injection and sacral nerve stimulation to artificial bowel sphincters and permanent fecal diversion.

Introduction

Key Concept: Increased performance of in-continuity management has led to increasing concern for functional outcomes

Over the past decades, the progress in colorectal surgery techniques has meant that many more patients are avoiding fecal diversion. Avoiding the creation of an ostomy provides the patient with many benefits—both mental and physical. However, postoperative recovery of satisfactory bowel function remains a great long-term challenge to patients and to their physicians.

The surgeon must also consider the functional outcomes, along with the risks and benefits of appropriate operative therapy, in patients contemplating reconstructive surgery. Every patient deserves clear preoperative counseling and accurate expectations in regard to his bowel function after surgery. Patients need to understand their risk of dealing with problems such as diarrhea, incontinence, urgency, frequency, constipation, and evacuation difficulties over both the short and long term. While sparing the sphincter may be possible, your ability to appropriately anticipate and implement the correct approach to solving these functional postoperative problems can often have an even greater impact on your colorectal patient's quality of life.

Scope of the Problem

Key Concept: Postoperative functional problems are not limited to low anastomoses but span the spectrum of colorectal procedures.

L.H. Maguire, MD
Division of Gastrointestinal Surgery, Massachusetts General Hospital, 55 Fruit St., Boston, MA 02114, USA
e-mail: lhmaguire@partners.org

S. Goldberg, MD
Division of Colorectal Surgery, Department of Surgery, University of Minnesota, 6363 France Avenue South, Suite 212, Minneapolis, MN 55435, USA
e-mail: drstanandlu@aol.com

L. Bordeianou, MD, MPH (✉)
Department of Surgery, Massachusetts General Hospital and Harvard Medical School, 15 Parkman Street, WAC-4-460, Boston, MA, USA
e-mail: lbordeianou@partners.org

Electronic supplementary material The online version of this chapter (doi: 10.1007/978-1-4614-9022-7_28) contains supplementary material, which is available to authorized users. Videos can also be accessed at http://www.springerimages.com/videos/978-1-4614-9021-0.

S.R. Steele et al. (eds.), *Complexities in Colorectal Surgery*,
DOI 10.1007/978-1-4614-9022-7_28, © Springer Science+Business Media New York 2014

Colectomy

Key Concept: Bowel function and the bowel function-related quality of life after colectomy are influenced by the location, surgical technique, and the extent of resection.

Although proctectomy poses a greater challenge to normal function, patients undergoing partial colectomy may also experience alteration in bowel habits. Increased stool frequency and fecal incontinence are more frequently observed following left- versus right-sided segmental colectomy [1]. In patients undergoing subtotal colectomy, the rates of bowel dysfunction are even higher. At an average of 5.5 years after operation, not surprisingly, patients reported significantly higher overall quality of life after segmental versus subtotal or total colectomy [2]. Compared to patients who underwent segmental resections, patients with ileorectal or ileosigmoid anastomoses reported significantly increased stool frequency and restriction in preoperative activities. Interestingly, and rarely mentioned, while no difference in incontinence was found between groups, 16 % of patients reported weekly daytime fecal incontinence after segmental colectomy.

Surgical technique also influences postoperative functional outcomes. Increased short-term fecal incontinence was noted in patients after laparoscopic left hemicolectomy for malignancy as compared to those undergoing the same procedure for diverticulitis [3]. The authors suspected this finding might be secondary to damage to thoracolumbar sympathetic nerves during high ligation of the inferior mesenteric artery (IMA) during cancer operations. A randomized trial of IMA-preserving versus IMA-sparing laparoscopic sigmoidectomy for diverticular disease supported this hypothesis; fewer defecatory problems and improved quality of life were reported in the IMA-preserving arm [4]. The appropriateness of high versus low tie of the IMA remains a matter for debate in oncologic operations [5], but seldom in the literature is this level correlated back to function. Furthermore, even in patients who undergo surgery for diverticulitis and have low IMA ligation, rates of postoperative fecal incontinence, urgency, and obstructed defecation are increased when compared to those of the general population [6]. This is not to suggest you should avoid an appropriate level of vascular ligation in the setting of malignancy; rather, it highlights the importance of discussing more realistic functional outcomes your patients can expect.

Proctectomy

Rectal Cancer

Key Concept: Functional outcomes following proctectomy and reconstruction for rectal cancer are dependent on many factors including tumor location, neoadjuvant and adjuvant radiotherapy, prior surgery, pelvic nerve injury, and type of rectal reconstruction performed.

Changing paradigms in the treatment of rectal cancer have legitimized sphincter-sparing techniques for rectal cancer and generated new procedures for rectal resection, such as intersphincteric resection, and reconstruction, such as coloplasty and colonic J-pouch. Adoption of total mesorectal excision (TME) has reduced local recurrence rates and radial margin positivity and the adoption of minimally invasive techniques has allowed for improved visualization of pelvic anatomy. These combined approaches, along with neoadjuvant chemoradiation therapy, have improved oncologic outcomes and resulted in more patients avoiding permanent stomas. Whether avoiding a stoma represents real quality of life improvement is debated [7], but regardless, more post-proctectomy rectal cancer patients face the challenge of attaining satisfactory bowel function.

Changing oncologic approaches mean the creation of lower anastomoses than previously performed. While TME provides the appropriate en bloc resection, it essentially mandates an anastomosis at the pelvic floor. Intersphincteric resection (ISR) is a surgical option for patients with very low rectal cancers that allows restoration of continuity in patients that would have historically undergone an APR (Video 28.1). Despite stoma avoidance, resection of the internal sphincter again poses a challenge to bowel-related quality of life. Data on postoperative function are widely distributed. In the 14 studies reporting functional outcomes, the average postoperative Wexner scores ranged from 2.8 to 12 [8], and only an average of 51 % (range 35–67 %) reported perfect continence [9]. Retrospective comparison of patients after ISR versus standard coloanal anastomosis demonstrated comparable overall quality of life between the patient groups and similar bowel function in terms of stool frequency and urgency; yet only 53 % demonstrated good continence after ISR compared to 81 % after traditional coloanal anastomosis [10].

After resection, rectal reconstruction with proximal colon can be attempted with a straight coloanal anastomosis via stapled or hand-sewn techniques. Alternatively, an attempt at recreation of the rectal reservoir can be created using a colonic J-pouch, coloplasty, or end-to-side anastomosis. One prospective, randomized comparison between these coloplasty, J-pouch, and straight anastomosis demonstrated a superior functional outcome with the J-pouch compared to coloplasty and straight anastomosis, without difference in the overall quality of life [11]. Regardless of technique all patients experienced gradually decreasing stool frequency and improving continence over the 24-month duration of the study. Notably, at the end of the 2-year observation, 55–76 % of patients were using pads for fecal soiling regardless of restorative technique [11]. A systematic review of 16 randomized controlled trials maintained these conclusions, upholding the functional superiority of the J-pouch relative to the straight anastomosis but suggested further study for coloplasty and end-to-side anastomosis [12].

Regardless of reconstructive technique, the vast majority of patients can be expected to develop altered bowel function postoperatively, grouped under the title of "low anterior resection syndrome" (LARS). LARS includes a spectrum of multiple symptoms including incontinence, increased stool frequency, and clustering or fragmentation of stools, tenesmus, and anorectal pain. Symptoms may be limited to bowel function or associated with urinary and sexual dysfunction. Severity, and consequently, impact on quality of life is variable. Patients report symptoms of urgency, incontinence, and difficult evacuation at rates of 12–45, 10–71, and 16–74 %, respectively [13]. While many will experience some improvement over time, symptoms can persist as late as 15 years postoperatively, and perhaps longer [14]. Multiple factors contribute to the development and severity of LARS including a diminished reservoir, internal anal sphincter damage, and loss of anorectal sensation [15]. Shorter intestinal length and resection of the rectal reservoir leads to a higher, liquid stool volume being delivered to a smaller capacity neorectum. Resultant immediate and persistent reductions in urgent volume, maximal tolerable volume, and rectal compliance are evident on anorectal manometry [16]. Several other mechanisms may contribute to the development of LARS. Damage to the sphincter complex may occur intraoperatively—directly during stapler insertion or dilation or indirectly to its innervation. Sympathetic nerves to the internal anal sphincter are at risk during high ligation of the IMA, and parasympathetic nerves may be compromised in the attempt to achieve wide lateral margins. Lower sphincter pressures in response to rectal distension are associated with greater symptom severity [17]. Resection and nerve damage frequently abolish the rectoanal inhibitory reflex (RAIR), contributing to incontinence, although return of function is common after several months to 1 year [18]. In summary, multiple potential insults to bowel physiology contribute to the constellation of symptoms seen in LARS. Patients requiring proctectomy for rectal cancer should be provided realistic expectations regarding their postoperative bowel function.

Ulcerative Colitis and Familial Cancer Syndromes

Key Concept: Surgical therapy for UC and FAP includes total proctocolectomy with ileal pouch construction. Factors such as loss of colonic water resorption, lack of rectal reservoir, and resection of the anal-transition zone (ATZ) during mucosectomy all contribute to functional problems despite generally high patient satisfaction.

Ileal pouch-anal anastomosis (IPAA) has replaced end ileostomy as the standard option for patients with familial adenomatous polyposis and inflammatory bowel disease (IBD) patients requiring total colectomy and proctectomy. This procedure restores intestinal continuity and leaves the sphincter mechanism intact. However, it is technically challenging, prone to early and late postoperative complications, and not without functional significance. The semiliquid quality of ileal stool makes full continence challenging and bowel movements frequent. Recent long-term retrospective review of 3,707 patients after IPAA revealed, even at 10 years postoperatively, an average of six to nine bowel movements per day, 15–26 % daytime use of pads, and 29–53 % rate of seepage. Furthermore, other factors such as the development of pelvic sepsis have been associated with long-term functional problems. In a review of 3,234 patients undergoing IPAA, 200 (6.2 %) developed pelvic sepsis, with corresponding higher rates of hemorrhage, leak, wound infection, and fistula (all $P<0.001$). Moreover, the development of sepsis resulted in higher rates of incontinence, worse quality of life, and ultimately greater pouch failure (19.5 % vs. 4 %, $P<0.001$) [19]. Despite these high rates, patients had high quality of life scores and >90 % were pleased with their decision to have IPAA [20]. These results are similar to those from other high-volume centers with long-term follow-up [21, 22].

Anorectal Procedures

Key Concept: The most common functional problems following anorectal surgery include seepage, anal pain, and incontinence. Due to the wide range of procedures and preexisting functional variation among patients, rates of functional problems specifically attributable to anorectal surgery are difficult to determine.

Compared to proctectomy and colectomy, functional outcomes after anorectal procedures are relatively less studied and are unique to each procedure. The frequent preoperative presence of evacuation disorders, constipation, and incontinence must also be taken into account and contribute to the wide variation in postoperative functional problems reported in the literature. A retrospective study of 111 patients undergoing a variety of anorectal procedures for multiple different diagnoses found no change in pre- and postoperative continence and an overall improvement in quality of life [23]. However, some anorectal procedures are at high risk for postoperative functional impairments, particularly when sphincter tissue is transected or compromised during the procedure, as in anal fistulotomy (Fig. 28.1a, b). While incontinence after anal fistula surgery is typically temporary and mostly with gas or liquid stool, more significant problems can occur—with as rates up to 45 % of patients at one high-volume center [24]. Newer procedures for anal fistula that avoid sphincterotomy have been developed. Bioprosthetic plugs and sealants have been devised with variable success rates. A relatively new procedure for anal fistula, ligation of the intersphincteric fistula tract (LIFT), also provides an approach to fistula surgery that avoids sphincter compromise (Figs. 28.2, 28.3, and 28.4). Recently, a retrospective study of 38 patients over 26 months revealed no incontinence [25].

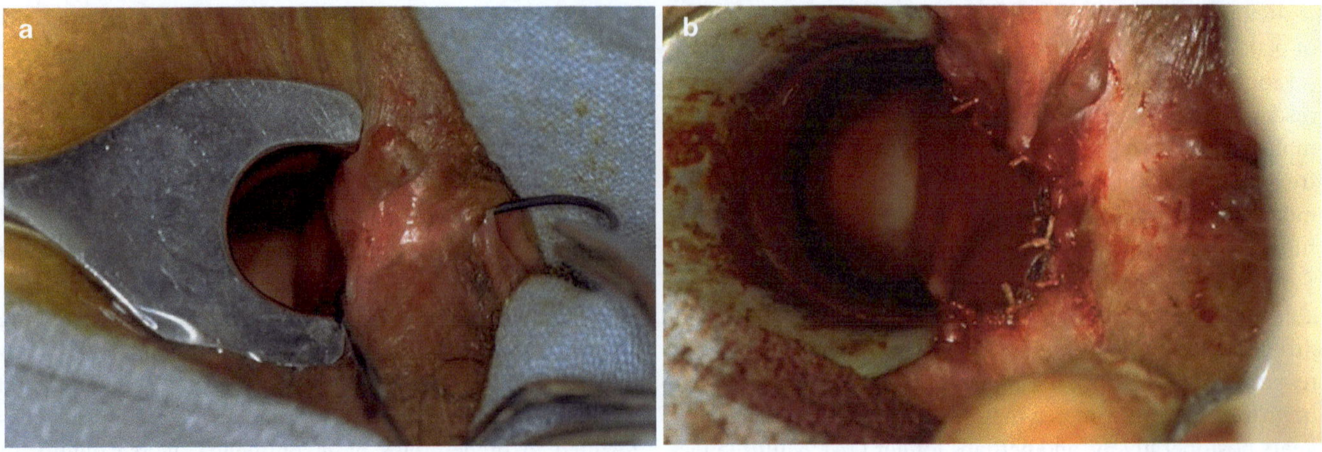

Fig. 28.1 (**a**) Fistula with seton in place (Courtesy of W. Brian Sweeney, MD). (**b**) Fistulotomy with marsupialization of the tract (Courtesy of W. Brian Sweeney, MD)

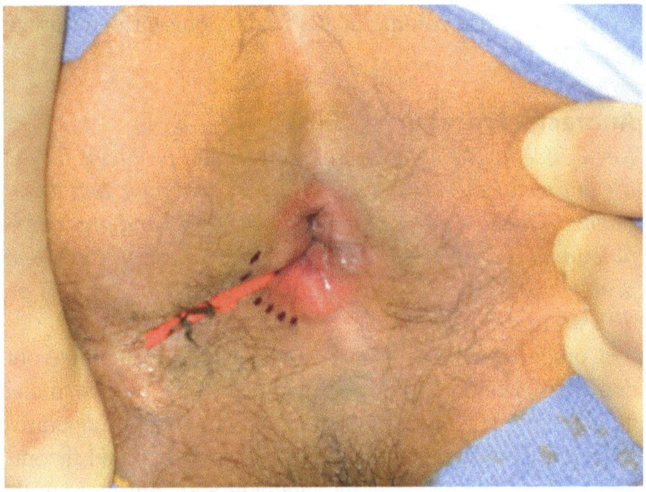

Fig. 28.2 Seton in place in a fistula in ano

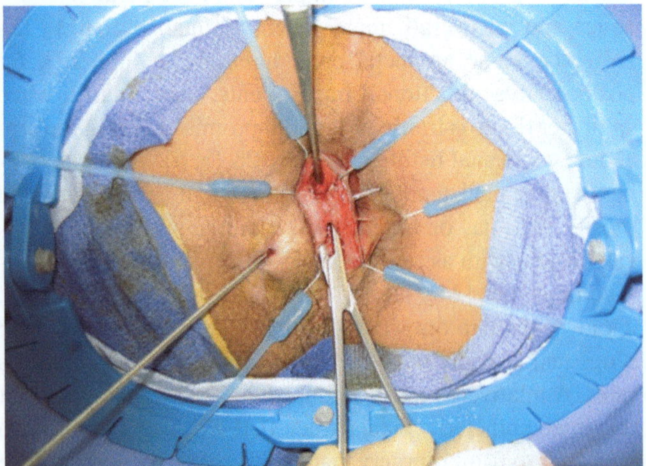

Fig. 28.3 Fistula tract dissected out in the intersphincteric space

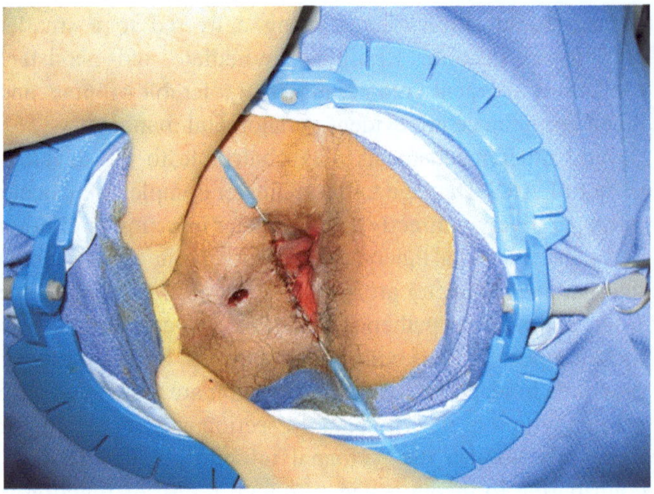

Fig. 28.4 Closure of the fistula tract

The novelty of these procedures limits the data available on postoperative success and function, but early studies seem promising. Similar reports of altered function typically consisting of seepage, chronic pain, and even tenesmus (along with worsening quality of life) have been described for hemorrhoidectomy, lateral internal sphincterotomy, pilonidal surgery, and fulguration, among others [26].

Transanal endoscopic microsurgery (TEM) has been accepted as an alternative to surgery for the treatment of early rectal cancers with improved functional results being an important motivating factor (see Video 14.1). Patients undergoing TEM were assessed over 60 months of follow-up and found to have early worsening of continence, urgency, and quality of life with a return to baseline or better over the course of the follow-up [27]. Overall, risks of altered bowel function after anorectal surgery must be individualized to the patient, procedure, surgeon, and underlying disease.

Prolapse Surgery

Key Concept: Functional outcomes following correction of rectal prolapse depend on both the procedure performed (rectopexy, resection-rectopexy, perineal procedures) and the preoperative condition of the patient (i.e., constipation vs. incontinence).

More than 100 different operations have been described for prolapse; therefore, it is not surprising to see rates of functional problems following prolapse repair to be widely variable. While several different mechanisms contribute to normal defecation, abdominal prolapse procedures risk damage to nerves controlling defecation, while perineal procedures remove the rectum with resultant loss of its intrinsic capacitance and reservoir. Additionally, some patients preoperatively suffer severe alterations to anorectal physiology that may prove recalcitrant to surgical improvement. A prospective analysis of 86 patients over 36 months of follow-up after ventral rectopexy demonstrated improvement in continence in 68 % of patients. However, the authors noted that 50 % of patients remained incontinent postoperatively. Older patients with longer duration of prolapse and worse preoperative continence scores were more likely to be incontinent postoperatively [28]. Perineal operations remain a viable option for debilitated patients with rectal prolapse, but data on functional outcome are variable. In one study, 6-month follow-up after Altemeier procedure, i.e., perineal rectosigmoidectomy, revealed that 62 % of patients demonstrated improvement in continence, although 25 % remained incontinent [29]. In contrast, only 28 % of patients had improved continence after Altemeier procedure in long-term follow-up of 93 patients, and several had deterioration or *de novo* incontinence [30]. Prospective trials of perineal versus abdominal approaches to rectal prolapse are forthcoming and may improve the surgeon's expectations for postoperative functional outcomes.

Management

Key Concept: The approach to functional problems following colorectal surgery should initially be on the exclusion of a potentially reversible technical error, followed by symptom-based therapy directed towards the patient's individual symptom complex.

We start the treatment of any patient with defecatory dysfunction after surgery by excluding a technical error. Once healed from surgery, the patient should undergo a flexible sigmoidoscopy (for a high anastomosis) or a digital rectal exam (for a low anastomosis) to exclude an anastomotic stricture or proctitis/colitis. If a stricture is found, it should be dilated and the symptoms should then be reassessed post dilatation. In absence of stricture, the treatment can focus on amelioration of symptoms, as described below.

Table 28.1 OTC agents for symptom management

Name	Dose	Mechanism
Loperamide (*Imodium*)	4–8 mg/day	Opioid agonist—peripheral
Diphenoxylate/atropine (*Lomotil*)	5 mg 4 times/day	Opioid agonist
Tincture of opium	6 mg 4 times/day	Opioid agonist
Bismuth (*Pepto-Bismol, Kaopectate*)	524 mg as needed, up to 8 doses/24 h	Antisecretory, antimicrobial, antiinflammatory
Psyllium (*Metamucil, Konsyl, Reguloid*)	No standard	Soluble fiber, bulking agent

Diarrhea

Key Concept: Most diarrheas can be treated with medical therapy alone through bulking and motility-slowing agents. Excluding/identifying any underlying infection and accounting for any anatomical changes (i.e., short bowel, TI resection) will also aid in the selection of the appropriate medical therapy.

The treatment of diarrhea following colorectal surgery focuses on dietary changes and medications (Table 28.1). These symptoms range in frequency depending on the operation, but the best literature on the topic stems from patients treated with IPAA. Postoperative patients with IPAA make frequent dietary changes to control stool frequency and consistency. In a survey of 64 postoperative patients, the vast majority identified specific food triggers of increased stool frequency, decreased consistency, and perineal irritation; 61 of 64 surveyed obeyed a strict dietary regimen [31]. Dietary restrictions were also found in patients following pelvic radiotherapy, with elimination of raw vegetables seeming to be the most helpful measure [32]. Long-term dietary restrictions, in combination with bacterial overgrowth and functional alteration of the terminal ileum, can yield important nutritional deficiencies, specifically vitamin B_{12}, iron, vitamin E, and fat malabsorption [33]. The presence of anemia or other signs and symptoms of malnutrition should prompt investigation and oral supplementation.

The staple of medical treatment for diarrhea following colorectal resections, independent of the size of resection, is therapy designed to reduce gastrointestinal transit time and alter stool consistency. Many patients remain dependent on these agents over the long term. Few of these therapies have any experimental data in any patient population with chronic diarrhea, much less postsurgical patients. Opiates such as loperamide, tincture of opium, and diphenoxylate function to reduce GI propulsion. Loperamide has its effect only in the intestinal muscle, whereas others have the potential for central nervous system activity and are controlled substances.

Intraluminal bulking agents such as fiber supplementation and psyllium may provide improved stool consistency to some patients. Bismuth has some utility in nonspecific chronic diarrhea and may provide relief to some patients.

Development of new drugs has been limited. Serotonin receptor antagonists were found to be associated with ischemic colitis and calmodulin therapies demonstrated no superiority to loperamide [34]. Octreotide, which has been found of utility in other forms of chronic diarrhea, was tested in a small randomized, placebo-controlled trial. It demonstrated no improvement in bowel frequency in patients with post-IPAA diarrhea and a potential increase in painful tenesmus, causing two patients to withdraw from the study [35].

One potential new therapy is probiotic bacterial cultures. Probiotics are postulated to improve gastrointestinal symptoms by modifying the immunologic, digestive, or nutritional functions of commensal gut bacteria. Treatment with probiotics in multiple formulations has been studied in a variety of gastrointestinal conditions. Utility has been demonstrated in infectious diarrhea and antibiotic-associated diarrhea, but study data have been less convincing in IBD and irritable bowel syndrome [36]. In the postoperative setting, 67 patients with IPAA due to UC or FAP demonstrated improvement in abdominal cramping, leakage, need for pad use, and involuntary defecation following a 4-week intervention with live *Lactobacilli* and *Bifidobacteria* [37]. Mucosal inflammation, scored by endoscopy, was also decreased by the intervention in UC patients. Larger, controlled trials are needed before utility can be shown conclusively.

Ileal resection or disease results in spillover of bile acids into the colon, interfering with electrolyte and water absorption and frequently causing diarrhea. Cholestyramine, colestipol, and colesevelam, bile acid sequestrants, prevent the outpouring of water and electrolytes. In a single-blind prospective trial, cholestyramine reduced stool frequency and volume in patients with ileal resections <100 cm. It demonstrated no improvement in patients with >100 cm resected [38]. IPAA also disrupts the ileum and interferes with enterohepatic circulation, as demonstrated by elevated postprandial serum levels of unconjugated bile acids [39] and abnormal 75Se homotaurocholate uptake in patients following IPAA [40]. Pouchitis, stasis, and bacterial overgrowth may all worsen this condition [41]. Although its role in diarrhea for patients after colectomy or IPAA is not well established, cholestyramine may provide relief to some patients suffering from diarrhea and has demonstrated efficacy in alleviated perianal skin irritation following IPAA [42]. Additionally, any suggestion of pouchitis (i.e., abrupt increase in watery stools, fever, pelvic pain) should prompt an endoscopic evaluation of the pouch, biopsy, and likely empiric treatment with antibiotics such as Flagyl and/or Floxin.

To summarize, our algorithm for the treatment of diarrhea is to always perform a colonoscopy or a flexible sigmoidoscopy first to evaluate the colon and exclude ischemic or inflammatory colitis or an anastomotic stricture. All patients are tested for *Clostridium difficile* colitis before initiating drug therapy. Whenever possible, patients are asked to stop all antibiotics to make sure the diarrhea is not antibiotic induced. They are then started on a probiotic. All patients after right-sided colectomy or small bowel resections are started on cholestyramine. In the absence of improvement with probiotics and cholestyramine, when appropriate, we then start a fiber supplement, such as Metamucil® (Procter & Gamble) or Benefiber® (Novartis). The patients are asked to start with half the dosage listed on the medicine box and are informed to expect bloating and distention as they adjust to the supplement. In 10 days, the patients are asked to escalate to the dose suggested on the box. Any fiber supplement brand is adequate and we ask the patient to choose the one that he prefers. If fiber fails, we escalate to loperamide. We instruct the patients to take as many as eight loperamide tablets per day to achieve 2–3 formed bowel movements daily. If fiber and loperamide fail, we continue with fiber supplementation and switch to Lomotil (diphenoxylate/atropine). Finally, we reserve prescriptions for diluted tincture of opium (DTO) for desperate cases.

Fecal Incontinence

Key Concept: The treatment of the patient reporting complaints of anal leakage of mucus, gas, liquid, or stool should always start with identification of the underlying cause of their incontinence.

The most common cause of incontinence is not sphincter insufficiency, but diarrhea. Thus, in the patients reporting diarrhea, we always start with its treatment, as described above. In those who continue to have leakage despite adequate regulation of bowel frequency and consistency with bulking agents (fiber) and constipation agents (i.e., Loperamide), we consider a prescription of amitriptyline, which can be added at a dose of 10–25 mg at night as tolerated. Amitriptyline is a tricyclic antidepressant agent that was studied in an open label trial of patients with fecal incontinence and was found to decrease incontinence scores [43]. Seventy-two percent of patients who were treated with the drug in the study reported full remission with a sustained improvement at 6 months.

In patients who continue to do poorly, we proceed with a thorough work-up aimed at excluding fecal obstruction and subsequent overflow incontinence. To start with, we perform a flexible sigmoidoscopy or a colonoscopy to exclude an anastomotic stricture. Once a stricture is excluded, we proceed with anorectal manometry testing to assess for any evidence of a paradoxical contraction of the puborectalis. In the patients who are found to have signs suggestive of this condition, we proceed with treating fecal incontinence with a daily glycerin suppository and a weekly tap water enema. This treatment has been shown to be effective in at least one-third of the patients with this condition [44].

Finally, when all medical therapy fails, we consider surgical therapies that escalate depending on the patient's interest in proceeding with further treatments and their disease severity, as well as the remaining anatomy and the underlying diagnosis. For example, the patient who has not received pelvic radiation and who does not have Crohn's disease may be a candidate for receiving a submucosal injection of Solesta® gel (Salix Pharmaceuticals Inc., Raleigh, NC) into their anal sphincter. The gel, which was recently approved by the FDA, has been shown to have a 60 % response rate at a 6-month follow-up, which was nearly twice the improvement rate seen in the placebo group [45].

In the patients who cannot have direct anal sphincter injections, sacral nerve stimulation (SNS) (Medtronic Interstim®, St. Paul, MN) is another great potential option that was also recently approved by FDA in the US. Its only drawback (besides its high price) is the fact that the device is not MRI compatible. The device is only planted, however, after a 2–3 weeks trial of stimulation. Eighty percent of the patients who do well during the stimulation phase can expect a 50 % reduction in the frequency and the severity of their fecal incontinence. Forty percent can expect complete continence [46].

Those who remain incontinent following medical therapy and minimal invasive treatments with either Solesta® or SNS, or both, could consider implantation of an artificial bowel sphincter (ABS), a hidden mini stoma, to perform Malone antegrade colonic enemas (MACE) or a permanent ostomy. I reserve the option of ABS only for the patient who has a colon and has solid bowel movements. Furthermore, the patient's perineum needs to allow for a safe implantation (i.e., no Crohn's, radiation, diabetes, immunodeficiency). Similarly, the MACE procedure is only feasible in a patient who has a colon that could then be irrigated to empty. The patients without a colon who fail SNS are unfortunately only candidates for an ileostomy.

Constipation/Obstructed Defecation

Key Concept: *Recognize the presence of obstructed defecation in patients with pre- or postoperative anorectal complaints as these will need to be addressed but may prevent unnecessary surgical re-intervention.*

Patients with obstructed defecation syndrome (ODS) present with inadequate rectal emptying, straining, and the need to manipulate the perineum or vagina to facilitate defecation. Occasionally, these patients may also have a component of overflow incontinence with rectal seeping, anal irritation, and pruritus. Many will also present to the clinician for hemorrhoids or anal fissures. A subsequent hemorrhoidectomy in such a patient would improve the appearance of the anus, but not the patient's function. Difficult defecation will most likely continue in the postoperative setting and symptoms may escalate, especially if a postoperative stricture develops. Similarly, patients with anal fissures in the setting of ODS are very likely to suffer recurrence after their initial therapy. Recognition of ODS can prevent unnecessary surgery and the need for recurrent interventions.

In patients with symptoms suggestive of ODS, we begin with anorectal manometry and EMG. We diagnose ODS if high anal pressures and paradoxical contractions of the puborectalis are seen on EMG (Fig. 28.5). In the presence of these findings, the patient is asked to initiate a fiber supplement. If still unable to empty well, we teach the patient to self-administer daily tap water enemas. If these maneuvers fail, we arrange for pelvic floor muscle retraining with EMG-guided biofeedback. The goal of the therapy is to teach the patient to relax, rather than constrict, his pelvic floor musculature while attempting to defecate [47–49].

Patients who fail medical management undergo defecography. The test diagnoses intrarectal and rectoanal intussusception, enterocele, rectocele, and full-thickness rectal prolapse (Figs. 28.6 and 28.7). When these findings are present, we consider surgical correction. In general, we prefer to perform a stapled transanal rectal resection (STARR) procedure (Fig. 28.8) on patients without prior pelvic surgery who have isolated recto-rectal or rectoanal intussusception with or without a rectocele. Patients with concomitant enteroceles and large intussusception or full-thickness prolapse are advised to have a ventral rectopexy [50].

Medical therapy and biofeedback are appropriate for patients after any colorectal procedure, but the surgical procedures mentioned above only apply to the patients without a prior proctectomy.

Key Concept: *In patients with ODS after proctectomy for rectal cancer, ODS could be due to tumor recurrence, anastomotic stricture, or to poor rectal compliance.*

The patients suffering from ODS who have a history of resection for rectal cancer should undergo a colonoscopy and rectal MRI or PET scan to exclude tumor recurrence. Finally, strictures at the coloanal or colorectal anastomosis should be dilated, when present. In those without stricture or recurrence, anorectal physiology testing should be performed. Compliance testing should always be performed as part of physiologic investigation. Decreased rectal compliance and rectal hypersensitivity are common in these patients and is usually detected via decreased maximum tolerated volume on manometry. When poor compliance is present, sensitivity retraining with a balloon is much more helpful during biofeedback than simple EMG-guided therapy. Finally, when ODS is combined with overflow incontinence or frank incontinence,

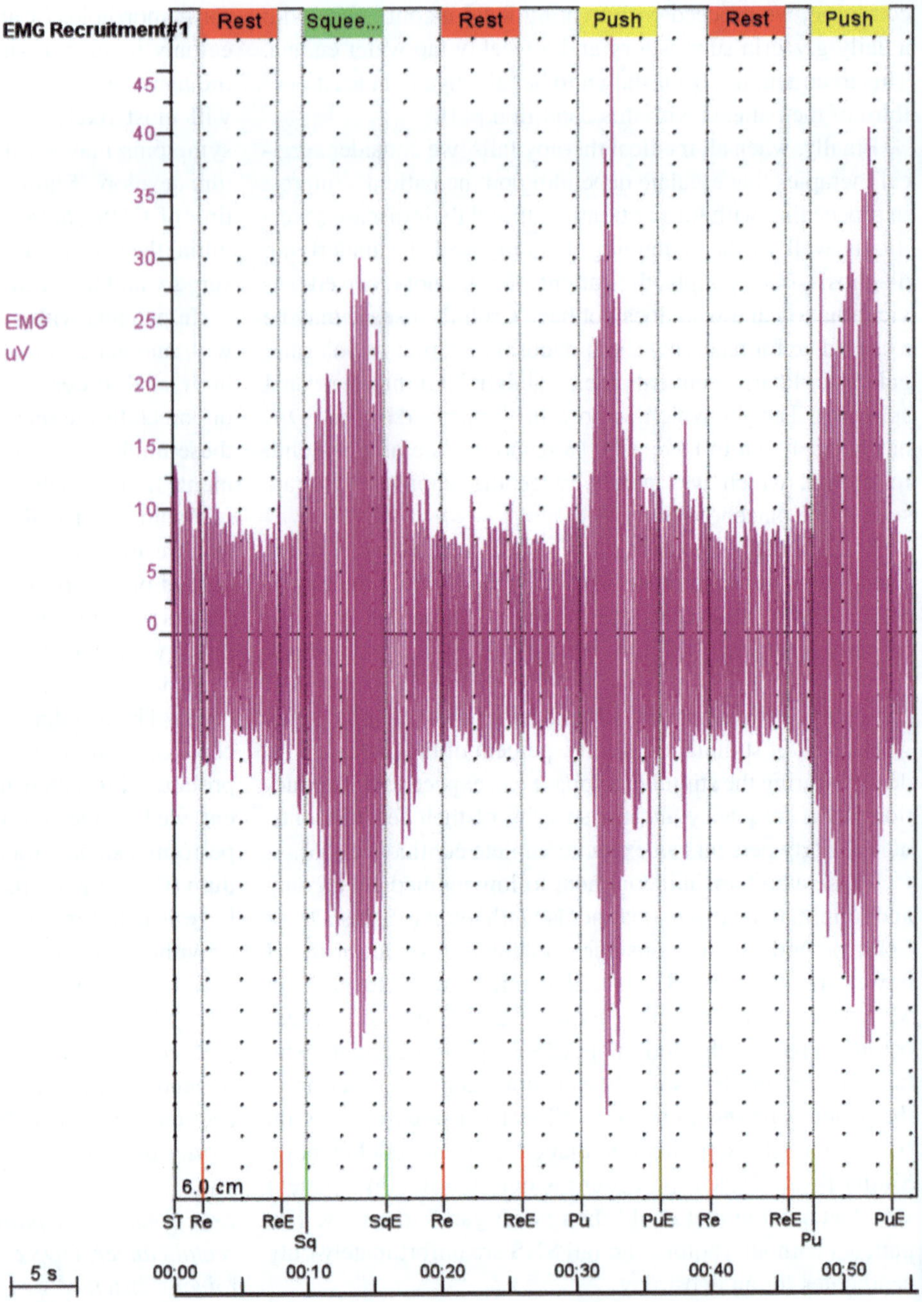

Fig. 28.5 Electromyography (*EMG*) with paradoxical contraction of anal sphincter at attempt to defecate

sacral nerve stimulation (SNS) could be considered as a possible option. SNS has been found to improve both fecal incontinence as well as rectal emptying [51]. However, SNS implantation needs to be weighed against the potential need for pelvic MRI as the device is not MRI compatible.

Key Concept: ODS in the patient with an ileoanal J-pouch could be due to pouchitis, stricture, cuffitis, or pouch intussusception.

ODS after J-pouch creation constitutes a special challenge. The cause of ODS can be far more complex. Evaluation of these patients should always start with a pouchoscopy to exclude pouchitis, development of Crohn's disease, or a stricture at the ileoanal anastomosis or ileostomy closure site. In addition, an honest assessment of the residual rectal cuff is important. Many patients with ODS after a J-pouch may have a long, noncompliant rectal cuff to blame for their symptoms. In these patients, steroid application to the cuff to treat "cuffitis" may help, as well as a generous anal dilatation to allow for a 22–24 Hagar dilator.

Finally, a subgroup of ileoanal J-pouch patients may have a floppy, intussuscepting rectal pouch or pouch that is too large to empty. In both cases, a pouch revision to a size that accommodates about 1,525 mL when distended with or

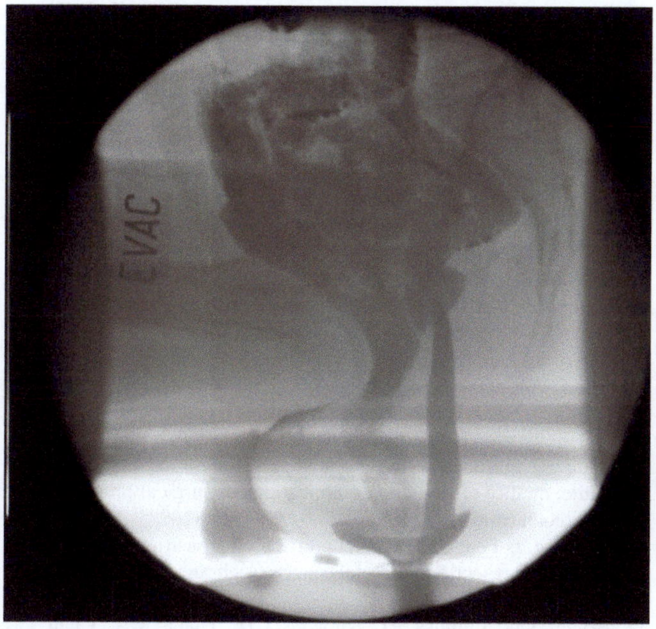

Fig. 28.6 Defecography with intussusception and enterocele

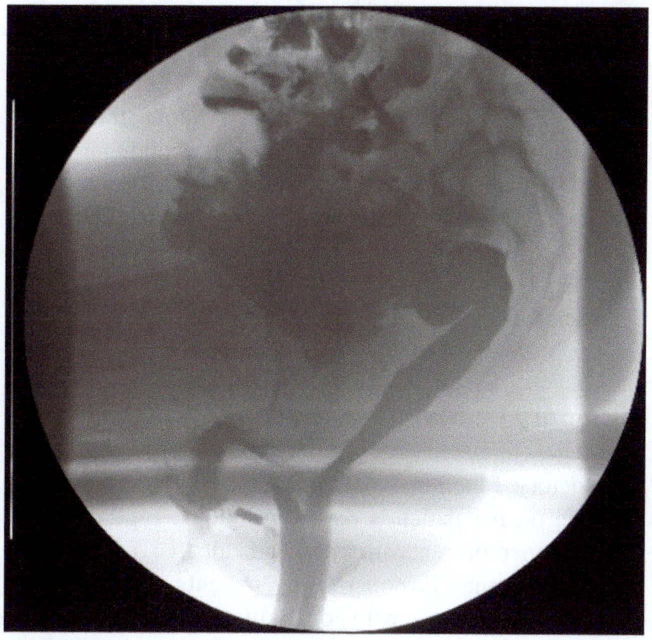

Fig. 28.7 Defecography with isolated intraanal intussusception/early rectal prolapse

Fig. 28.8 Stapled transanal rectal resection

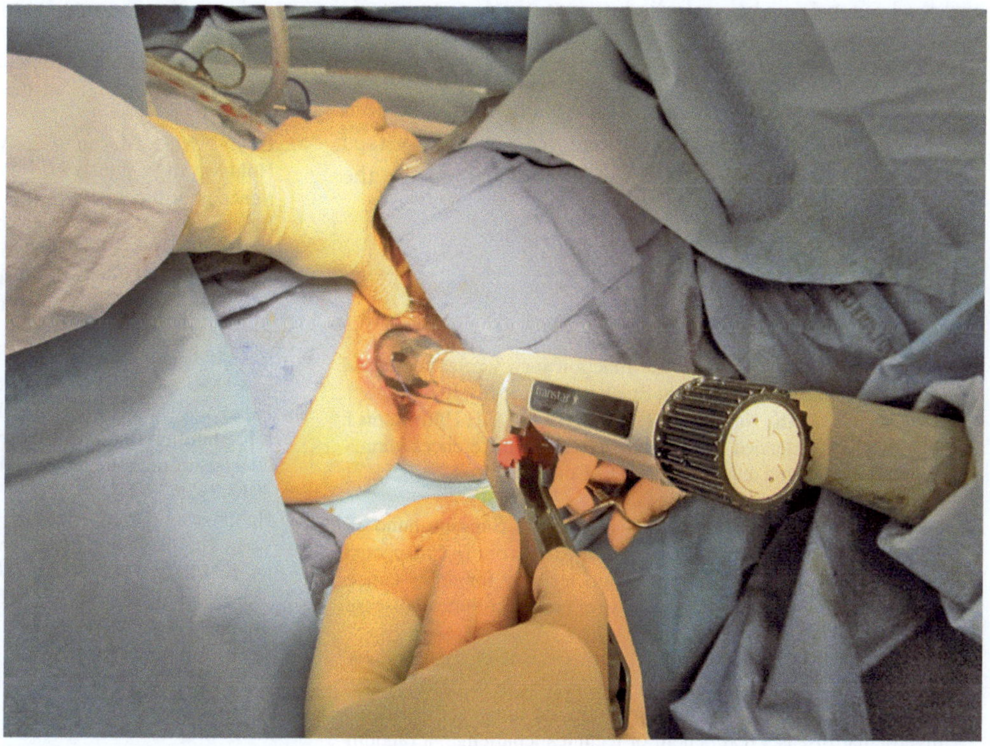

without a pouch suspension to the sacral promontory can prevent further intussusception and encourage better emptying. In patients with a normal size pouch and isolated intussusception, the pouch revision could be done transanally. However, in the majority of patients, an abdominal procedure is needed, and its risk needs to be carefully considered along with the potential benefit that it could confer.

If surgery is not appropriate, medical management with fiber and tap water enemas as described earlier could be considered.

Summary Pearls

Satisfactory functional outcome after colorectal surgery depends on the patient's pathophysiology, type of resection, manner of reconstruction, and degree of injury to nerves and tissues. Postoperatively, patients frequently have altered bowel function with potentially significant effects on health, recovery, and quality of life. The appropriate therapy for postoperative functional problems includes a range of escalating treatments from dietary changes and medications to surgery. Although few medical treatments have emerged recently or been studied prospectively, new surgical options have been developed including submucosal gel injection, sacral nerve stimulation, and artificial sphincters. Selecting the appropriate therapy for each unique patient and problem is an evolving challenge you will likely face and need to have a stepwise logical approach to ensure the best outcomes.

References

1. Ho YH, Low D, Goh HS. Bowel function survey after segmental colorectal resections. Dis Colon Rectum. 1996;39(3):307–10.
2. You YN, Chua HK, Nelson H, Hassan I, Barnes SA, Harrington J. Segmental vs. extended colectomy: measurable differences in morbidity, function, and quality of life. Dis Colon Rectum. 2008;51(7):1036–43.
3. Sarli L, Pavlidis C, Cinieri FG, Regina G, Sansebastiano G, Veronesi L, Ferro M, Morari S, Violi V, Roncoroni L. Prospective comparison of laparoscopic left hemicolectomy for colon cancer with laparoscopic left hemicolectomy for benign colorectal disease. World J Surg. 2006;30(3):446–52.
4. Masoni L, Mari FS, Nigri G, Favi F, Gasparrini M, Dall'oglio A, Pindozzi F, Pancaldi A, Brescia A. Preservation of the inferior mesenteric artery via laparoscopic sigmoid colectomy performed for diverticular disease: real benefit or technical challenge: a randomized controlled clinical trial. Surg Endosc. 2013;27(1):199–206.
5. Cirocchi R, Trastulli S, Farinella E, Desiderio J, Vettoretto N, Parisi A, Boselli C, Noya G. High tie versus low tie of the inferior mesenteric artery in colorectal cancer: a RCT is needed. Surg Oncol. 2012;21(3):e111–23.
6. Levack MM, Savitt LR, Berger DL, Shellito PC, Hodin RA, Rattner DW, Goldberg SM, Bordeianou L. Sigmoidectomy syndrome? Patients' perspectives on the functional outcomes following surgery for diverticulitis. Dis Colon Rectum. 2012;55(1):10–7.
7. Digennaro R, Tondo M, Cuccia F, Giannini I, Pezzolla F, Rinaldi M, Scala D, Romano G, Altomare DF. Coloanal anastomosis or abdominoperineal resection for very low rectal cancer: what will benefit, the surgeon's pride or the patient's quality of life? Int J Colorectal Dis. 2013;28:949–57.
8. Akagi Y, Kinugasa T, Shirouzu K. Intersphincteric resection for very low rectal cancer: a systematic review. Surg Today. 2013;43:838–47.
9. Martin ST, Heneghan HM, Winter DC. Systematic review of outcomes after intersphincteric resection for low rectal cancer. Br J Surg. 2012;99(5):603–12.
10. Bretagnol F, Rullier E, Laurent C, Zerbib F, Gontier R, Saric J. Comparison of functional results and quality of life between intersphincteric resection and conventional coloanal anastomosis for low rectal cancer. Dis Colon Rectum. 2004;47(6):832–8.
11. Fazio VW, Zutshi M, Remzi FH, Parc Y, Ruppert R, Fürst A, Celebrezze Jr J, Galanduik S, Orangio G, Hyman N, Bokey L, Tiret E, Kirchdorfer B, Medich D, Tietze M, Hull T, Hammel J. A randomized multicenter trial to compare long-term functional outcome, quality of life, and complications of surgical procedures for low rectal cancers. Ann Surg. 2007;246(3):481–8.
12. Brown CJ, Fenech DS, McLeod RS. Reconstructive techniques after rectal resection for rectal cancer. Cochrane Database Syst Rev. 2008;(2):CD006040.
13. Bryant CL, Lunniss PJ, Knowles CH, Thaha MA, Chan CL. Anterior resection syndrome. Lancet Oncol. 2012;13(9):e403–8.
14. Lundby L, Krogh K, Jensen VJ, Gandrup P, Qvist N, Overgaard J, Laurberg S. Long-term anorectal dysfunction after postoperative radiotherapy for rectal cancer. Dis Colon Rectum. 2005;48(7):1343–9.
15. Brown SR, Seow-Choen F. Preservation of rectal function after low anterior resection with formation of a neorectum. Semin Surg Oncol. 2000;19(4):376–85.
16. Lee SJ, Park YS. Serial evaluation of anorectal function following low anterior resection of the rectum. Int J Colorectal Dis. 1998;13(5–6):241–6.
17. Lewis WG, Martin IG, Williamson ME, Stephenson BM, Holdsworth PJ, Finan PJ, Johnston D. Why do some patients experience poor functional results after anterior resection of the rectum for carcinoma? Dis Colon Rectum. 1995;38(3):259–63.
18. O'Riordain MG, Molloy RG, Gillen P, Horgan A, Kirwan WO. Rectoanal inhibitory reflex following low stapled anterior resection of the rectum. Dis Colon Rectum. 1992;35(9):874–8.
19. Kelly JM, Fazio VW, Remzi FH, Shen B, Kiran RP. Pelvic sepsis after IPAA adversely affects function of the pouch and quality of life. Dis Colon Rectum. 2012;55(4):387–92.
20. Fazio VW, Kiran RP, Remzi FH, Coffey JC, Heneghan HM, Kirat HT, Manilich E, Shen B, Martin ST. Ileal pouch anal anastomosis: analysis of outcome and quality of life in 3707 patients. Ann Surg. 2013;257:679–85.
21. Hahnloser D, Pemberton JH, Wolff BG, et al. Results at up to 20 years after ileal pouch-anal anastomosis for chronic ulcerative colitis. Br J Surg. 2007;94:333–40.
22. Marcello PW, Roberts PL, Schoetz Jr DJ, et al. Long-term results of the ileoanal pouch procedure. Arch Surg. 1993;128:500–3.
23. Grucela A, Gurland B, Kiran RP. Functional outcomes and quality of life after anorectal surgery. Am Surg. 2012;78(9):952–6.
24. Garcia-Aguilar J, Belmonte C, Wong WD, Goldberg SM, Madoff RD. Anal fistula surgery. Factors associated with recurrence and incontinence. Dis Colon Rectum. 1996;39(7):723–9.
25. Liu WY, Aboulian A, Kaji AH, Kumar RR. Long-term results of ligation of intersphincteric fistula tract (LIFT) for fistula-in-ano. Dis Colon Rectum. 2013;56(3):343–7.
26. Steele SR. Anorectal disease. Surg Clin North Am. 2010;90(1):1–217.
27. Allaix ME, Rebecchi F, Giaccone C, Mistrangelo M, Morino M. Long-term functional results and quality of life after transanal endoscopic microsurgery. Br J Surg. 2011;98(11):1635–43.

28. Cunin D, Siproudhis L, Desfourneaux V, Bouteloup PY, Meunier B, Ropert A, Berkelmans I, Bretagne JF, Boudjema K, Bouguen G. Incontinence in full-thickness rectal prolapse: low level of improvement after laparoscopic rectopexy. Colorectal Dis. 2013;15:470–6.
29. Ris F, Colin JF, Chilcott M, Remue C, Jamart J, Kartheuser A. Altemeier's procedure for rectal prolapse: analysis of long-term outcome in 60 patients. Colorectal Dis. 2012;14(9):1106–11.
30. Altomare DF, Binda G, Ganio E, De Nardi P, Giamundo P, Pescatori M, Rectal Prolapse Study Group. Long-term outcome of Altemeier's procedure for rectal prolapse. Dis Colon Rectum. 2009;52(4): 698–703.
31. Coffey JC, Winter DC, Neary P, Murphy A, Redmond HP, Kirwan WO. Quality of life after ileal pouch–anal anastomosis: an evaluation of diet and other factors using the Cleveland Global Quality of Life instrument. Dis Colon Rectum. 2002;4:30–8.
32. Gami B, Harrington K, Blake P, Dearnaley D, Tait D, Davies J, Norman AR, Andreyev HJ. How patients manage gastrointestinal symptoms after pelvic radiotherapy. Aliment Pharmacol Ther. 2003;18(10):987.
33. Buckman SA, Heise CP. Nutrition considerations surrounding restorative proctocolectomy. Nutr Clin Pract. 2010;25(3):250–6.
34. Kent AJ, Banks MR. Pharmacological management of diarrhea. Gastroenterol Clin North Am. 2010;39(3):495–507.
35. Van Assche G, Ferrante M, Vermeire S, Noman M, Rans K, Van der Biest L, Penninckx F, Wolthuis A, Rutgeerts P, D'Hoore A. Octreotide for the treatment of diarrhoea in patients with ileal pouch anal anastomosis: a placebo-controlled crossover study. Colorectal Dis. 2012;14(4):e181–6.
36. Ciorba MA. A gastroenterologist's guide to probiotics. Clin Gastroenterol Hepatol. 2012;10(9):960–8.
37. Laake KO, Bjørneklett A, Aamodt G, Aabakken L, Jacobsen M, Bakka A, Vatn MH. Outcome of four weeks' intervention with probiotics on symptoms and endoscopic appearance after surgical reconstruction with a J-configurated ileal-pouch-anal-anastomosis in ulcerative colitis. Scand J Gastroenterol. 2005;40(1):43–51.
38. Hofmann AF, Poley JR. Cholestyramine treatment of diarrhea associated with ileal resection. N Engl J Med. 1969;281(8):397–402.
39. Salemans JM, Nagengast FM, Tangerman A, Van Schaik A, de Haan AF, Jansen JB. Postprandial conjugated and unconjugated serum bile acid levels after proctocolectomy with ileal pouch-anal anastomosis. Scand J Gastroenterol. 1993;28(9):786–90.
40. Fiorentini MT, Locatelli L, Ceccopieri B, et al. Physiology of ileoanal anastomosis with ileal reservoir for ulcerative colitis and adenomatosis coli. Dis Colon Rectum. 1987;30:267–72.
41. Khanna R, Shen B. Adverse metabolic sequelae following restorative proctocolectomy with an ileal pouch. Gastroenterol Hepatol (N Y). 2012;8(5):322–6.
42. Møller P, Lohmann M, Brynitz S. Cholestyramine ointment in the treatment of perianal skin irritation following ileoanal anastomosis. Dis Colon Rectum. 1987;30(2):106–7.
43. Santoro GA, Eitan BZ, Pryde A, Bartolo DC. Open study of low-dose amitriptyline in the treatment of patients with idiopathic fecal incontinence. Dis Colon Rectum. 2000;43(12):1676–81.
44. Chassagne P, Jego A, Gloc P, Capet C, Trivalle C, Doucet J, Denis P, Bercoff E. Does treatment of constipation improve faecal incontinence in institutionalized elderly patients? Age Ageing. 2000; 29(2):159–64.
45. Graf W, Mellgren A, Matzel KE, Hull T, Johansson C, Bernstein M, NASHA Dx Study Group. Efficacy of dextranomer in stabilised hyaluronic acid for treatment of faecal incontinence: a randomised, sham-controlled trial. Lancet. 2011;377(9770):997–1003.
46. Wexner SD, Coller JA, Devroede G, Hull T, McCallum R, Chan M, Ayscue JM, Shobeiri AS, Margolin D, England M, Kaufman H, Snape WJ, Mutlu E, Chua H, Pettit P, Nagle D, Madoff RD, Lerew DR, Mellgren A. Sacral nerve stimulation for fecal incontinence: results of a 120-patient prospective multicenter study. Ann Surg. 2010;251(3):441–9.
47. Gilliland R, Heymen S, Altomare DF, Park UC, Vickers D, Wexner SD. Outcome and predictors of success of biofeedback for constipation. Br J Surg. 1997;84(8):1123–6.
48. Chiarioni G, Salandini L, Whitehead WE. Biofeedback benefits only patients with outlet dysfunction, not patients with isolated slow transit constipation. Gastroenterology. 2005;129(1):86–97.
49. Hwang YH, Person B, Choi JS, Nam YS, Singh JJ, Weiss EG, Nogueras JJ, Wexner SD. Biofeedback therapy for rectal intussusception. Tech Coloproctol. 2006;10(1):11–5; discussion 15–6.
50. D'Hoore A, Cadoni R, Penninckx F. Long-term outcome of laparoscopic ventral rectopexy for total rectal prolapse. Br J Surg. 2004;91(11):1500–5.
51. Thomas GP, Dudding TC, Rahbour G, Nicholls RJ, Vaizey CJ. Sacral nerve stimulation for constipation. Br J Surg. 2013;100(2): 174–81.

Short Bowel Syndrome

29

Ilun Yang and Robin P. Boushey

Key Points

- Recognizing patients who are at risk for short bowel syndrome and practicing bowel economy during surgery are crucial.
- Knowledge of residual intestinal anatomy is essential for determining prognosis and management.
- Patients with short bowel syndrome should be managed by a multidisciplinary team of healthcare professionals with the required expertise.
- A combination of intestinal rehabilitation and surgical strategies is often required to achieve independence from parenteral nutrition.

Introduction

Key Concept: Symptoms related to short bowel syndrome are not only secondary to the length of the remaining bowel but also due to the amount of functioning residual bowel and other anatomic considerations (i.e., presence or absence of the ileocecal valve).

Short bowel syndrome (SBS) is a spectrum of malabsorption that can follow extensive resection of the small intestine. It usually occurs when there is less than 200 cm of residual small bowel; however, several factors other than small intestinal length, as discussed below, contribute to determining the degree of malabsorption [1]. SBS is the most common cause of intestinal failure, in which an individual's functioning gut mass is insufficient for maintaining adequate nutrition and hydration without enteral or intravenous supplementation [2]. In adults, etiologies leading to SBS include mesenteric ischemia, Crohn's disease, volvulus, trauma, radiation enteritis, and tumors (e.g., desmoid) [3–5]. With its range of clinical manifestations, SBS can dramatically impact quality of life and is associated with significant morbidity and mortality.

The presentation and management of SBS depend on factors including anatomy of the remaining bowel, intestinal adaptation, and underlying etiology. This chapter will review these issues and discuss the medical and surgical management of this condition and its complications.

Pathophysiology

Key Concept: Several physiological and anatomical factors play a role in the development (or avoidance) of short bowel syndrome.

Small Intestinal Resection

Key Concept: The degree of malabsorption and type of fluid, electrolyte, and nutritional deficiencies experienced will depend on the location and function of bowel resected.

The extent of small bowel resection is a central determinant of outcome in SBS. The implications of losing a particular length of intestine depend on its location and corresponding absorptive functions. Normally, the jejunum is the primary site of absorption for macronutrients such as carbohydrates, fat, and protein. Following jejunal resection, the remaining small intestine is able to compensate through adaptive changes such as increased absorptive surface area and upregulated digestive enzymes [6]. In contrast, the sequelae following ileal resection can be more problematic due to the ileum's unique functions. The ileum reabsorbs the vast majority of bile salts and returns it to the liver via the enterohepatic circulation. Ileal resection may result in watery diarrhea due to the

I. Yang, MD, FRCSC
Department of Surgery, McMaster University, Hamilton, ON, Canada

R.P. Boushey, BSc, MD, PhD, CIP, FRCSC (✉)
Department of Surgery, The Ottawa Hospital, Ottawa, ON, Canada
e-mail: rboushey@ottawahospital.on.ca

S.R. Steele et al. (eds.), *Complexities in Colorectal Surgery*,
DOI 10.1007/978-1-4614-9022-7_29, © Springer Science+Business Media New York 2014

passage of unabsorbed bile salts into the colon and the increased colonic secretion of water and electrolytes. The ileum is also the predominant absorptive site of the intrinsic factor-vitamin B_{12} complex [7]. Consequently, a terminal ileal resection of more than 60 cm is associated with vitamin B_{12} malabsorption [8]. Loss of more than 100 cm of ileum results in bile salt deficiency, poor absorption of fat-soluble vitamins, and steatorrhea secondary to fat malabsorption [9].

The site of bowel resection also influences absorption related to the loss of control mechanisms for gastric emptying and intestinal transit. Rapid gastric emptying can be detrimental for nutrient absorption due to inadequate mixing of gastric and pancreatobiliary secretions. Likewise, decreased intestinal transit time may worsen malabsorption if the bowel's capacity to assimilate nutrients is exceeded. In normal physiology, as unabsorbed macronutrients arrive at a segment of intestine, an inhibitory feedback mechanism is activated to slow gastric emptying and gut transit. This "brake" system is present throughout the small and large bowel; however, the ileal brake is more potent than the jejunal brake [10]. In addition, the cells that release the GI hormones thought to mediate the ileal brake (e.g., peptide YY, glucagon-like peptides, and neurotensin) are found in the terminal ileum [11, 12]. Consequently, rapid gastric emptying and intestinal transit are common following ileal resection, particularly in patients with a jejunostomy as they also lack the benefit of a colonic brake.

The jejunum and ileum also differ in their ability to absorb water and electrolytes. In the jejunum, sodium absorption is primarily mediated by flow along osmotic pressure gradients; in contrast, the ileum has an efficient active transport mechanism for absorbing sodium [13]. Furthermore, the jejunal epithelium is more permeable to passive shifts of fluid and electrolytes due to its lack of tight intercellular junctions [14]. Hence, the overall absorption process occurs more efficiently at the ileum, which is particularly important following meals of high osmolarity. These factors explain the dramatic losses in fluid and electrolytes that can be seen following ileal resection, particularly in the absence of a colon in continuity.

Loss of the Ileocecal Valve

Key Concept: While debatable, the presence of an intact, functioning ileocecal valve can lessen short bowel syndrome symptoms.

The impact of ileocecal valve (ICV) resection on outcomes in SBS has been debated. In the pediatric surgery literature, several studies have demonstrated shorter duration of parenteral nutrition dependence with the presence of an intact ICV, while others have failed to show an effect [15–17]. The presence of the ICV may be beneficial as a potential barrier to retrograde entry of colonic bacteria and resultant small bowel bacterial overgrowth [18]. An increased bacterial load contributes to malabsorption of macronutrients, vitamin B_{12}, and bile salts [19]. However, one study suggested that the ICV's protective effect against bacterial overgrowth may be insignificant in the face of a short residual small bowel and intestinal dysmotility [20]. Similarly, intestinal transit time has been shown to be largely uninfluenced by the presence or absence of the ICV [21]. Overall, it is likely that the extent of bowel resected concomitantly, rather than the loss of the ICV itself, accounts mainly for the resultant malabsorption.

Loss of the Colon

Key Concept: The colon's ability to absorb water and sodium, as well as undergo adaptation to cover other losses, plays a key role with extensive small bowel resection.

The presence of a colon in continuity has important benefits in SBS. In normal physiology, the large intestine absorbs approximately 90 % of the water and sodium contained in the ileal effluent [22]. The organ also contributes to the body's energy stores by absorbing short-chain fatty acids (SCFA) derived from carbohydrate fermentation. Following small bowel resection, these absorptive capabilities of the colon proportionately become even more crucial. The colonic mucosa undergoes adaptive morphological changes such as increased absorptive surface [23]. Unabsorbed carbohydrates from the shortened small bowel are salvaged by the large bowel to provide a significant source of energy [24]. Similar to the small intestinal "brake" described above, a feedback mechanism to slow gastrointestinal transit also exists in the colon [12]. With the colon in continuity, 50–70 cm of remaining small bowel may be sufficient to prevent dependence on parenteral nutrition; in the colon's absence, at least 100 cm of residual bowel is needed [25, 26]. The extent of colectomy has also been shown to correlate with functional outcomes such as severity of diarrhea following ileal resection [27]. On the other hand, the presence of an intact colon increases the risk of certain complications such as hyperoxaluria and D-lactic acidosis (see Clinical Manifestations below).

Etiology-Specific Considerations

Crohn's Disease

Key Concept: Crohn's disease may lead to SBS due to underlying inflammation or repeated resections that lead to malabsorption.

SBS occurs in 5–10 % of patients with Crohn's disease, typically as a result of multiple bowel resections over time [28]. Additional risk factors for developing SBS include those with early age at diagnosis, ileocolonic disease at initial presentation, and a history of unplanned laparotomies for intra-abdominal sepsis [29, 30]. As Crohn's disease is most frequently found in the ileocecal region, the terminal ileum and ileocecal valve are commonly resected, leading to the respective sequelae of malabsorption described above. If the residual bowel is involved with Crohn's disease, then its absorptive function and adaptive capacity would likely be compromised [31]. One also needs to be mindful of the presence of enteroenteral or enterocolic fistulas that may bypass a segment of bowel and decrease overall absorption.

The concern regarding the development of SBS highlights the importance of a collaborative multidisciplinary approach to managing Crohn's disease. Optimization of medical treatment may reduce the need for resection, and surgery should ideally be reserved for treating specific complications. Resection margins should be conservatively chosen and need only to be grossly normal to minimize recurrence [32]. For symptomatic small bowel stenosis, stricturoplasty should be favored over resection [33]. For colonic disease, in the absence of neoplasm or pancolitis associated with severe anorectal disease, segmental colectomy is the preferred option to preserve as much colon as possible for absorption.

Mesenteric Ischemia

Key Concept: Severe mesenteric ischemia (i.e., thrombotic, embolic, nonocclusive, and venous) may acutely lead to frankly necrotic bowel requiring extensive resection. When possible, every attempt should be made to salvage as much viable bowel as possible.

In contrast to the setting of Crohn's disease, SBS related to mesenteric ischemia is more likely to result from a single massive bowel resection rather than repeated resections over time [34]. In a review by Thompson [34] of 95 patients with SBS, among those who survived the initial 30 days postoperatively, patients following a single massive resection were more likely to require long-term parenteral nutrition than those who had repeated resections and similar residual bowel length. Mesenteric ischemia is the most common cause (25 %) of intestinal failure in adults [31]. Early diagnosis and treatment in acute mesenteric ischemia are essential to maximize bowel salvage. Fluid resuscitation and, if required, β-adrenergic agonists should be initiated to optimize perfusion [35]. Anticoagulation therapy is instituted when appropriate, depending on the etiology of ischemia [36]. For acute arterial insufficiency, prompt surgical intervention is critical to successful management. Appropriate expertise should be available for surgical options including bypass, embolectomy, and thrombectomy. Careful assessment of bowel viability is performed, using methods such as evaluation of bowel appearance and peristalsis, Doppler assessment at the antimesenteric border, and Wood lamp examination following intravenous fluorescein [37]. While frankly necrotic bowel should be resected, overaggressive resection of "borderline" segments should be avoided. Instead, a second-look laparotomy after 24–48 h should be performed to reassess viability.

Radiation Enteritis

Key Concept: Radiation therapy can result in various inherent and secondary manifestations, with repeated surgical resection for its complications being the primary cause of SBS.

Intestinal injury due to external radiation therapy (XRT) for abdominal and pelvic malignancies accounts for approximately 20 % of patients with SBS [38, 39]. In addition to surgical interventions for radiation-related complications, radiation damage to intact bowel can also result in reduced functional gut mass.

Obstruction secondary to stricture is the most common complication of radiation enteritis that requires surgery [40]. Depending on intraoperative findings that may include a "frozen abdomen," surgical options include resection, bypass, and ostomy formation. Stricturoplasty has been utilized successfully in this setting, for selected patients with strictures within long intestinal segments and limited residual bowel [41]. Other complications of radiation enteritis that may require surgery include fistula and perforation. In general, principles of management include eradicating sepsis, optimizing nutritional status, and maximizing functional in-continuity bowel length [42]. One study described the use of hyperbaric oxygen to treat XRT-induced intestinal injury and reported a 58 % response rate in improved obstructive symptoms and fistula closure [43].

Clinical Manifestations

Key Concept: The clinical presentation of patients with short bowel syndrome is largely determined by the anatomy of their remaining GI tract, though diarrhea, malnutrition, weight loss, and dehydration are very common.

In general, patients can be considered as having one of three configurations of residual bowel: (1) "jejunum-colon," a jejunocolic anastomosis following a jejunoileal resection; (2) "jejunoileum," jejunum anastomosed to >10 cm of terminal ileum with an intact colon following a predominantly jejunal resection; and (3) "jejunostomy," an end stoma following resection of jejunum, ileum, and colon [5].

In the early postoperative period, jejunum-colon patients may experience diarrhea and steatorrhea, but otherwise often appear well. In the ensuing months, however, they gradually experience increasing difficulties with malnutrition and weight loss [5]. For jejunoileum patients, the preservation of their terminal ileum and colon typically allows these individuals to avoid significant problems with absorption; long-term enteral or parenteral nutritional supplementation is rarely needed. Exceptions arise when a substantial portion of the remaining bowel is involved with underlying pathology such as Crohn's disease or radiation enteritis, thus compromising residual absorptive function. Patients with a jejunostomy, beginning in the immediate postoperative period, almost uniformly have significant issues with maintaining hydration, due to high stomal output of water and sodium. This may result in signs and symptoms such as thirst, oliguria, and hypotension.

Changes in mental status, such as confusion and slurred speech, may be observed in patients with short bowel. Potential causes include deficiencies in thiamine and magnesium, as well as impaired ammonia detoxification due to inadequate amino acids which require small bowel for synthesis [44]. Specific to patients with an intact colon, mental status changes can also result from D-lactic acidosis [45]. As unabsorbed carbohydrate reaches the colon, it is fermented by anaerobes to produce D-lactic acid. The absorption of this metabolite can lead to severe metabolic acidosis and clinical manifestations such as confusion, ataxia, and ophthalmoplegia.

"Stones" are a more common manifestation in patients with short bowel syndrome. In a review of 84 patients with less than 200 cm of residual small bowel, the prevalence of asymptomatic gallstones was 44 %, and this was uninfluenced by the presence or absence of an intact colon [26]. The formation of gallstones in SBS patients likely relates to biliary stasis and resultant biliary sludge; in addition, bile acid depletion following ileal resection results in increased cholesterol concentration in bile. The risk of developing complications related to gallstones is higher in patients who require long-term total parenteral nutrition (TPN) [46]. There is also an increased incidence of renal stones among SBS patients, especially those with their colon in continuity. The pathogenesis primarily relates to hyperoxaluria. Malabsorbed fatty acids in the colon precipitate with intraluminal calcium, thus leaving more soluble oxalate to be absorbed [26]. This problem is compounded by an increase in colonic permeability to oxalate that is induced by the presence of unabsorbed bile salts [47]. Consequently, a quarter of jejunum-colon patients will develop symptomatic nephrolithiasis [26]. Meanwhile, all patients with SBS are potentially more susceptible to renal stones due to other factors such as dehydration and reduced urine volume.

Diagnosis and Assessment

Key Concept: The diagnosis of SBS is usually obvious based on clinical findings of malabsorption in the context of extensive intestinal loss. Intraoperatively, the ***remaining*** *length and type of bowel should be determined in order to anticipate the likely consequences of resection.*

Knowledge of the residual bowel length is much more useful than that of the resected length, given the wide variation among "normal" bowel lengths (302–846 cm in two studies of intraoperative measurements) [48, 49]. If measurements from the time of surgery are unavailable, then radiological studies may be used; one study demonstrated good correlation between radiographic and intraoperative measurements in the setting of a short (<200 cm) intestine [50]. Another method of estimating residual bowel length involves the measurement of citrulline, an amino acid that is not incorporated into protein and is produced by small bowel enterocytes [51]. Multiple studies have consistently demonstrated a strong positive correlation between plasma citrulline levels and remnant small bowel length [52–54]. Of further clinical relevance, citrulline measurement can be prognostic for SBS patients in whom bowel adaptation is mostly complete. In a study of 57 patients for whom at least 2 years have elapsed since bowel resection, a plasma citrulline level of <20 μmol/L was highly suggestive of permanent intestinal failure, with a positive predictive value of 95 % and negative predictive value of 86 % [52].

Medical Management

Key Concept: A multidisciplinary approach to management (preferably by specialized centers) is typically required to optimize outcomes in SBS patients, with reliance on several classes of medical therapy to achieve symptomatic control.

The overarching goal in managing short bowel syndrome is to allow the patient to resume as normal a lifestyle as possible. This requires collaborative efforts and input from gastroenterologists, surgeons, dieticians, nurses, pharmacists, and social workers. Given the number of anatomical, etiological, and patient-related factors that influence this condition, management of each patient with SBS is highly individualized. Common elements of medical treatment include parenteral and enteral nutritional supplementation, as well as pharmacologic agents and therapies to increase absorption, decrease secretion, and enhance intestinal adaption.

The concept of intestinal rehabilitation in short bowel syndrome refers to the use of nutritional and pharmacologic methods to optimize remnant intestinal function and maximize the chances of independence from parenteral nutrition [55]. The approach is invariably multidisciplinary, and it can be protocolled to improve therapeutic accuracy and consistency of care [56]. There is evidence to support the argument that intestinal failure patients requiring home parenteral nutrition should be primarily followed by specialized centers of excellence where comprehensive bowel rehabilitation programs exist [55, 57].

Parenteral Nutrition

Key Concept: Despite the multitude of potential complications associated with its use, parenteral nutrition is a life-saving intervention for many patients with SBS, and a significant percentage of patients can eventually be weaned off parenteral nutrition completely.

Total parenteral nutrition (TPN) is often the first form of alimentary support initiated following massive bowel resection, and in most instances it is continued for at least 7–10 days. Parenteral nutrition can be used to provide macronutrients and energy required for intestinal adaptation and to prevent deficiencies in vitamins and minerals [3, 5]. To replace water and electrolyte losses during the immediate postoperative period, usually both parenteral nutrition and supplemental intravenous fluid are needed. Sodium, potassium, and magnesium are commonly deficient in this context, and their serum levels should be closely monitored to help guide the composition of parenteral solutions.

In general, patients require approximately 25–35 kcal/kg/day; parenterally, this is delivered with a combination of dextrose, lipids, and amino acids. Fat should account for 20–30 % of the total energy requirement, and protein should be provided at 1.0–1.5 g/kg/day [1]. Intravenous lipid emulsion, traditionally derived from soybean oils, is thought to contribute to parenteral nutrition-associated liver disease (PNALD) [58]. Several groups have recently suggested the use of fish oil-based lipid emulsions to mitigate and reverse cholestasis [59–61]. While these early reports have demonstrated encouraging results with fish oil, further studies are required to better define its safety and efficacy.

Some patients may require parenteral supplementation of certain vitamins, depending on their remnant bowel anatomy and amount of enteral intake. Water-soluble vitamin deficiencies are rare in SBS except in patients with a proximal jejunostomy. To maintain normal thiamine levels, 3 mg of thiamine hydrochloride may be included in TPN solutions [62]. Vitamin B_{12} deficiency should be anticipated following resection of more than 60 cm of ileum, and subcutaneous injections of 200 μg monthly may be required [7, 8]. As well, supplementation of fat-soluble vitamins is often needed after loss of ileum due to impaired absorption of fat and bile acids [9]. Trace metals can also be replaced parenterally when enteral intake is unable to match gastrointestinal losses. In particular, zinc and selenium deficiencies may arise in the setting of severe diarrhea [63, 64].

Home parenteral nutrition is the mainstay of therapy for the majority of patients with chronic intestinal failure [57]. Its successful implementation requires a multidisciplinary effort that extends beyond hospital discharge with home care support until patient self-management is achieved. While in hospital, patients and their caregivers should receive education regarding preparation and administration of parenteral solutions, catheter care, and signs and symptoms of potential complications [1].

Parenteral nutrition is usually tapered as enteral feeding is successfully advanced. Depending on the amount and function of a patient's residual bowel, complete or partial transition to enteral intake may be possible. Tolerance of enteral and oral nutrition can continue to improve over the first few years after resection, as the remnant intestine's absorptive function is enhanced through adaptation [55]. Overall, up to half of patients who initially require home parenteral nutrition are able to achieve independence from it [65, 66].

Complications Associated with Long-Term Parenteral Nutrition

Key Concept: The long-term use of parenteral nutrition is associated with several potentially life-threatening complications. Their repeated occurrences often curtail continued delivery of parenteral nutrition and account for significant mortality among patients with chronic intestinal failure.

Parenteral nutrition is not without a wide array of morbidity and mortality [65, 67]. A range of liver pathologies have been associated with chronic parenteral nutrition, including cholestasis, steatosis, steatohepatitis, fibrosis, and cirrhosis [68]. Cholestatic liver disease is particularly common among SBS patients due to other contributory factors such as lack of enteral intake and recurrent sepsis related to bacterial overgrowth or indwelling catheter [31]. In one study of 90 patients with intestinal failure receiving home parenteral nutrition, chronic cholestasis occurred in 65 % of patients after a median of 6 months, and complicated liver disease (extensive portal fibrosis or cirrhosis) was demonstrated in 50 % of patients at 6 years [69]. To reduce to the risk of these complications, the study's authors suggested limiting the intake of ω-6 rich lipid emulsions to less than 1 g/kg/day [69]. Excessive dextrose feeding should also be avoided [70]. Other strategies to prevent liver disease include optimizing the patient's enteral intake and preventing sepsis of any etiology [58]. As mentioned previously, the use of fish-oil-based lipid emulsions have also shown some promise in this regard [59–61]. The use of ursodeoxycholic acid can also be considered, as there is limited evidence for its benefit in treating cholestasis [71, 72].

Sepsis related to the indwelling venous feeding catheter is a significant cause of mortality among patients on chronic parenteral nutrition. A French study involving 124 adults with nonmalignant SBS found that 5 of the 32 deaths (16 %) among patients with permanent intestinal failure were directly attributable to catheter-related sepsis [39]. However, with proper line care technique, the incidence of line sepsis can be as low as 0.26 episodes per patient year [73]. A local infection at the catheter's exit site will often respond to intravenous antibiotic therapy with empiric coverage for *S. aureus*, though the choice of antimicrobial agents may require subsequent adjustment based on culture and sensitivity results [1]. Lack of response to antibiotic therapy, evidence of infection along the subcutaneous tunnel tract, or septicemia in an unstable patient will mandate removal of the catheter [1, 57].

Thrombosis of the catheter is a relatively rare event, occurring at an incidence of 0.07 episodes per catheter year in patients receiving home parenteral nutrition [74]. Venous access occlusion accounts for approximately one quarter of all catheter removals [75]. Furthermore, catheter-related venous thrombosis may be complicated by SVC syndrome and pulmonary embolus [74, 76]. It is not uncommon for catheter-related sepsis to precede thrombosis, and the former's presence should raise the index of clinical suspicion for the latter and prompt consideration of prophylactic anticoagulation with either warfarin or heparin [57, 77]. Treatment for confirmed venous thrombosis usually consists of at least 6 months of anticoagulation with low-molecular-weight heparin [57].

Other complications that have been described in patients requiring chronic parenteral nutrition include renal dysfunction, metabolic bone disease, and cognitive deficits [67, 78].

Enteral Nutrition and Oral Diet

Key Concept: Whenever possible, enteral intake should be provided preferentially over parenteral nutrition as the former has several clear advantages. The composition should be individualized based on the residual anatomy.

There is no question that the enteral route is preferred in this setting, as the advantages are clear. Chief among these is the dependence of intestinal adaption upon exposure of the bowel to luminal nutrients [79]. As these nutrients come in contact with bowel epithelium, adaptive hyperplasia of the intestinal mucosa is induced [80]. In addition, enteral nutrition increases the secretion of trophic gastrointestinal hormones that stimulate adaptation [79]. In contrast to the plethora of potential complications associated with long-term parenteral nutrition, enteral feeding is relatively safe. As well, the administration of enteral nutrition is significantly less labor intensive.

Following massive bowel resection, the introduction of enteral nutrition is usually delayed until the patient is hemodynamically stable. Initially, enteral feeding may be continuously infused via nasogastric tube, gastrostomy, or jejunostomy; this mode of delivery tends to be better tolerated than bolus feeds. As the patient's overall condition improves, gradual transition to oral diet can take place. There is evidence to suggest that continuous tube feeding (exclusively or in conjunction with oral feeding) increases absorption of lipids, proteins, and energy compared with oral feeding alone [81]. Therefore, even patients who are tolerating an oral diet may benefit from tube feeding supplementation as it can reduce or obviate dependence on parenteral nutrition.

The composition of enteral and oral feedings should be individualized based on the patient's remnant intestinal anatomy, comorbid conditions, and susceptibility to certain complications. In general, patients with an intact colon should be given a high-carbohydrate diet to take advantage of SCFA production via fermentation, an additional source of energy [24]. If concerns arise regarding D-lactic acidosis (see above), mono- and oligosaccharides should be restricted in favor of polysaccharides; in addition, thiamine supplementation and broad-spectrum antibiotics are indicated [5]. While there were early advocates for restricting dietary fat to reduce diarrhea, triglycerides are valuable nutrients as they are relatively energy-dense – 9.0 kcal/g compared to 4.0 kcal/g for carbohydrates – and, in the case of long-chain fatty acids, particularly effective stimulators of intestinal adaptation [2, 82]. Therefore, a normal fat content is recommended for patients with retained colon. The diet for these individuals should be low in oxalate content to prevent nephrolithiasis [5].

Compared to jejunum-colon patients, individuals with a jejunostomy face greater challenges with respect to salt and water depletion. Large amounts of stomal losses are exacerbated by enteral feeding, and careful attention must be given to the composition of fluid intake. Patients should drink glucose-saline replacement solutions while limiting their oral intake of hypotonic fluids – such as water, tea, coffee, or juices – to less than 500 ml daily [5]. Non-elemental diets tend to be favored over peptide-based diets for macronutrient delivery as the former have lower osmolarity while providing comparable absorption [83]. The diet of jejunostomy patients should also contain a normal amount of fat. Increased dietary fat leads to proportionately increased fat absorption along the remaining jejunum without significantly higher stomal effluent volumes [84].

Transition to oral diet should take place gradually for patients with short bowel syndrome. Small and frequent meals are better tolerated and absorbed. However, in order to compensate for the malabsorbed portion of their dietary intake, patients should be encouraged to eventually consume more food overall than the amount to which they had previously become accustomed [85].

Pharmacologic Agents

Key Concept: Commonly used drug therapies in short bowel syndrome constitute several different classes but act by either mitigating secretory losses or slowing gut transit.

H2 blockers and proton pump inhibitors reduce gastric acid secretion, and both medication classes have been shown to decrease stomal effluent volumes in SBS patients [86–88]. They also prevent peptic ulceration and esophagitis that may result from transient hypergastrinemia and gastric hypersecretion in SBS [31, 89]. It should be noted, however, that these drugs neither alter macronutrient absorption nor reduce the need for parenteral support [5]. Octreotide has similarly been shown to reduce intestinal fluid losses secondary to diarrhea or high stomal output [90, 91]. In addition to decreasing gastric and pancreatic secretions, octreotide also delays gastric emptying and intestinal transit [92]. However, experimental models have demonstrated octreotide to exert inhibitory effects on intestinal adaptation, a potentially significant downside to its use in short bowel syndrome [93, 94].

Loperamide is an antimotility agent with proven efficacy in reducing water and sodium losses from an ileostomy [95, 96]. Typical doses are 4–16 mg/day, but much higher doses may be required as the drug's pharmacokinetics depend upon the enterohepatic circulation which is often disrupted following massive bowel resection [3, 5]. Codeine has similar effects in decreasing diarrhea, but there is evidence to suggest that it impairs fat absorption [95, 97]. With any medication that is administered orally to patients with short bowel, there needs to be vigilance to ensure that it is being adequately absorbed as opposed to emerging undigested in stomal output or stool [5].

Cholestyramine can improve secretory diarrhea following ileal resection by binding unabsorbed bile salts [98]. It should be given at a dose of 4 g prior to meals, up to three times daily [4]. However, this drug should not be used in patients who have had more than 100 cm of ileum resected; such extensive resection depletes the bile salt pool and renders cholestyramine ineffective, and the drug may actually worsen steatorrhea and cause fat-soluble vitamin deficiency [1, 2, 99].

Growth Factors

Key Concept: The use of growth factors is an emerging class of therapy for SBS with still widely variable results. While promising, they are most commonly used in specialized centers or still under investigation.

An increasingly active area of research involves the potential of several growth factors to enhance intestinal adaptation and improve absorption in patients with short bowel syndrome. The current depth of evidence varies among these novel therapies, and some of these medications have been incorporated into intestinal rehabilitation programs at specialized centers.

The application of growth hormone in the treatment of SBS was first suggested by early animal model studies that demonstrated the substance's positive effect on mucosal hyperplasia after extensive bowel resection [100, 101]. Similarly, the amino acid glutamine, the primary fuel of enterocytes, was shown to exert trophic effects on bowel and stimulate nutrient absorption [102, 103]. By instituting regimens that included growth hormone, glutamine, and dietary fiber, some centers have produced case series data showing enhanced absorptive capacity and weaning from parenteral nutrition [104, 105]. However, the combination of growth hormone plus glutamine failed to improve nutrient absorption compared to placebo in two randomized controlled studies [106, 107]. The benefit of growth hormone alone in SBS has also been investigated in two randomized placebo-controlled trials; one of the studies demonstrated modestly increased absorptive capacity with growth hormone while the other detected no difference [108, 109]. Similarly, glutamine alone has not been found to be beneficial compared to placebo [110]. Nevertheless, these trials are uniformly small in sample size, and the role and efficacy of these substances in treating SBS remain controversial.

Glucagon-like peptide-2 (GLP-2) is a naturally occurring polypeptide synthesized by enteroendocrine L-cells located primarily in the terminal ileum and colon [67]. Secreted in response to enteral nutrition, GLP-2 promotes bowel mucosal growth, enhances absorptive capacity, and stimulates mesenteric blood flow [80, 111, 112]. Accordingly, jejunostomy patients without an intact colon, who are known to have relatively little capacity for intestinal adaptation, have been shown to exhibit markedly impaired GLP-2 activity following meals [113]. It follows, therefore, that GLP-2 therapy may have a clinically significant impact on bowel adaptation and absorptive function in patients with SBS. In a small, non-placebo-controlled study of SBS patients, GLP-2 treatment reduced fecal wet weight but did not significantly change energy absorption or mucosal morphology [114]. Teduglutide, a long-acting analogue of GLP-2, was similarly shown in an open-label phase 2 study to increase wet weight absorption [115]. In this study, the drug's benefit was seen even in patients with an intact colon and near-normal endogenous GLP-2 levels, a finding which suggests that supraphysiological doses of teduglutide may be advantageous. In a recent multicenter, randomized, placebo-controlled trial, 83 parenteral nutrition-dependent SBS patients were assigned to receive one of placebo, 0.05 mg/kg/day teduglutide, or 0.10 mg/kg/day teduglutide [116]. The study's primary efficacy end point was a graded response score (GRS) that accounted for reduction in parenteral requirements and duration of response. The GRS was significantly better in the 0.05 mg/kg/day teduglutide compared to placebo, while no statistically significant benefit was seen with the 0.10 mg/kg/day dose. Ad hoc analysis attributed the latter result to a trend toward higher baseline parenteral volume in the 0.10 mg/kg/day group. Three teduglutide-treated patients were completely weaned off parenteral support. The study also confirmed teduglutide's intestinotrophic effect through serum citrulline measurements, which increased with both low- and high-dose treatment, but not with placebo. Interestingly, there is also some literature that suggests teduglutide, which has anti-inflammatory properties, may induce remission and mucosal healing in patients with Crohn's disease [117]. Whether this may translate to demonstrable efficacy of teduglutide in Crohn's-related SBS is just one of many questions surrounding this therapy that require further study.

Several other growth factors have received attention for their potential role in the treatment of short bowel syndrome. Transforming growth factor-α, a polypeptide found in epithelium along the gastrointestinal tract, has been shown to improve intestinal adaptation in animal models of SBS [118, 119]. Hepatocyte growth factor, when administered in rats following massive small bowel resection, enhanced intestinal epithelial cell function and mucosal mass beyond the normal adaptive response [120]. Studies of other growth factors including interleukin-11, insulin-like growth factor, and keratinocyte growth factor also demonstrated positive effects [121–123]. The intestinotrophic effects of these peptides have yet to be demonstrated in humans.

Surgical Management

Key Concept: Surgery for SBS aims to improve the patient's quality of life by increasing residual absorptive function and reducing overall morbidity and complications.

Surgical options for SBS include small bowel transplantation and a variety of non-transplant procedures. The choice and timing of these interventions depend on the patient's remnant intestinal anatomy, comorbid conditions, and response to medical management.

Restoration of Intestinal Continuity

Key Concept: Never miss out on an opportunity to restore intestinal continuity if enough residual bowel remains.

For patients with an end stoma and residual distal bowel, intestinal continuity should be reestablished when possible. This intervention restores the absorptive functions and hormonal "braking" mechanisms of the previously diverted bowel and prolongs intestinal transit [124]. The resulting improvement in overall absorption may be sufficient to allow weaning off parenteral nutrition [67]. When large bowel is brought back into continuity, one should be cognizant of the corresponding increase in the patient's susceptibility to complications such as nephrolithiasis and D-lactic acidosis.

With respect to timing, reoperation should be deferred until the patient is hemodynamically stable and medically optimized. Further waiting may be prudent to avoid difficult adhesions and minimize surgical morbidity. Any intra-abdominal sepsis should be resolved preoperatively, if possible. Many underlying etiologies in SBS predispose to stricture formation, and distal obstruction must be ruled out prior to restoring intestinal continuity.

Procedures to Slow Intestinal Transit

Key Concept: For patients who have failed medical therapy and have maximized adaptation, surgical procedures aimed at slowing intestinal transit can improve absorption as fluids and nutrients remain in contact with bowel mucosa for longer periods of time.

In general, these slowing procedures should be considered only for patients whose residual bowel is already in continuity and maximally adapted [125]. Of these individuals, the subset with relatively ample intestinal length, but with lack of response to medical therapy, is most likely to benefit from this surgical strategy [67].

Among this group of procedures, segmental reversal of small bowel has been most extensively evaluated and appears to be the most effective [125]. The technique involves separating a segment of small bowel from the adjacent intestine while leaving its blood supply intact and subsequently reanastomosing the segment in the opposite direction of normal intestinal flow. To avoid complete volvulus of the mesentery, each of the proximal and distal parts of the bowel can be rotated 90° so that the mesentery of the reversed segment only needs to be rotated 180° [126]. The ideal length of reversed segment appears to be approximately 10–15 cm; if the antiperistaltic segment is too long, bowel obstruction can result [127]. The location of the reversed segment should be chosen as distally as possible to decrease the symptoms of obstruction [31]. While results vary throughout the literature, adult series have generally shown a favorable response to segmental reversal in approximately 70 % of the patients [124].

Other techniques to slow intestinal transit include colonic interposition, creation of intestinal valves to produce a partial obstruction, and implantation of reversed electrical pacing devices [128–130]. Published experience is very limited for these procedures, and they should only be employed by highly experienced surgeons in the absence of more proven alternatives.

Procedures to Lengthen Residual Bowel

Key Concept: Intestinal lengthening surgery should be considered for patients with dilated and severely shortened bowel that precludes independence from parenteral nutrition despite optimal adaptation and medical treatment.

These techniques create additional length by exploiting the compensatory dilatation of the residual bowel that normally occurs following extensive bowel resection [124]. The operations also taper the bowel, which results in improved

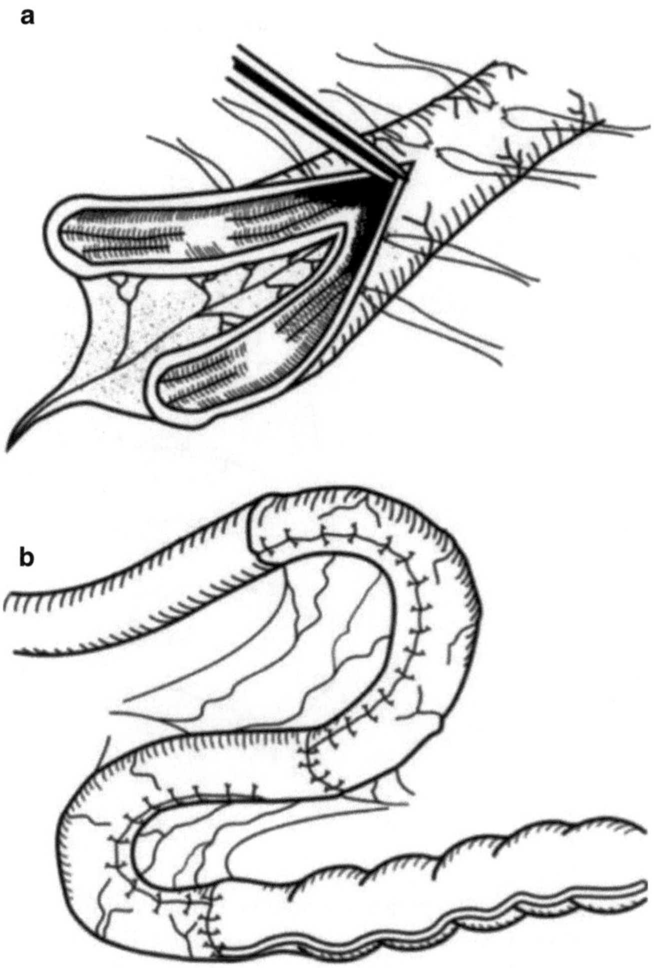

Fig. 29.1 The Bianchi longitudinal intestinal lengthening procedure (Reprinted from Bianchi [160], (**a**) The bowel and its mesentery are divided longitudinally to yield two vascularized halves of the bowel wall. (**b**) End-to-end anastomosis of the newly formed bowel loops results in a longer but narrower segment of bowel compared to the original loop. © Elsevier 2006)

motility and reduced bacterial overgrowth. It should be noted that patients with advanced liver disease are poor candidates for lengthening and should be referred for intestinal transplantation instead [131].

The Bianchi longitudinal intestinal lengthening procedure involves separating the two layers of small bowel mesentery, each layer containing blood vessels that enter one side of the bowel wall (Fig. 29.1) [132]. The dilated bowel is then divided longitudinally between the mesenteric layers to form two parallel lumens. End-to-end anastomosis of these two newly formed bowel loops creates an intestinal segment that is longer but narrower than the original segment [125]. Over time, the absorptive surface area may increase as the lengthened segment dilates [124]. The reported experience with the Bianchi procedure predominantly consists of case series data in the pediatric literature [133]. In two larger series, the majority of patients who underwent the procedure were successfully weaned off parenteral nutrition [131, 134].

A more recent addition to the intestinal lengthening armamentarium is the serial transverse enteroplasty (STEP) [135]. The technique involves the partial transection of dilated bowel using a linear cutting stapler, which is applied sequentially from alternating and opposite directions, in transverse fashion (Fig. 29.2). The goal is to produce a zigzag pattern of lengthened bowel with a diameter of approximately 2 cm. In contrast to the Bianchi procedure, STEP can be employed for recurrent bowel dilatation after previous lengthening [133]. Published results with this technique have been promising. A multicenter registry of 21 SBS patients undergoing STEP reported that the percentage of total calories tolerated enterally increased from 31 to 67 % at a median follow-up of 12.6 months [136]. A single-institution experience that included 34 STEP and 43 Bianchi procedures demonstrated a trend toward a higher rate of weaning from parenteral nutrition in patients who underwent STEP (60 % vs. 55 %) [131]. Long-term outcomes after STEP were reported in a single-center series of 12 pediatric patients; while 2 patients subsequently received liver-intestinal transplants and 2 others died of liver failure, 7 of the remaining 8 patients were weaned off parenteral nutrition by 4 years post-STEP [137].

Other Non-transplant Procedures

Key Concept: Dilation and adaption of the bowel can be helpful but also can lead to complications that may need to be addressed with other surgical procedures.

As alluded to previously, dilatation of the intestinal remnant normally occurs as an adaptive response following resection in order to slow intestinal transit and increase mucosal absorptive area [124]. However, this compensatory process can lead to pathologic consequences such as dysmotility, bacterial overgrowth, and impairment of absorptive function. For such scenarios in patients with moderately shortened bowel, plication of the bowel wall and tapering enteroplasty may be beneficial [67, 127].

Small Bowel Transplantation

Key Concept: Small bowel transplantation is a viable therapeutic option for intestinal failure as improvements have occurred in immunosuppressive agents. While select patients are typically in the end stage who have failed parenteral nutrition, there is controversy regarding the need to expand this to more patients earlier in their SBS course.

Historically, transplantation of the small intestine was believed to be associated with seemingly insurmountable challenges related to the organ's immunogenicity and colonization with microorganisms [138]. Earlier efforts were

Fig. 29.2 The serial transverse enteroplasty (STEP) procedure (Reprinted from Javid et al. [161] © Elsevier 2005)

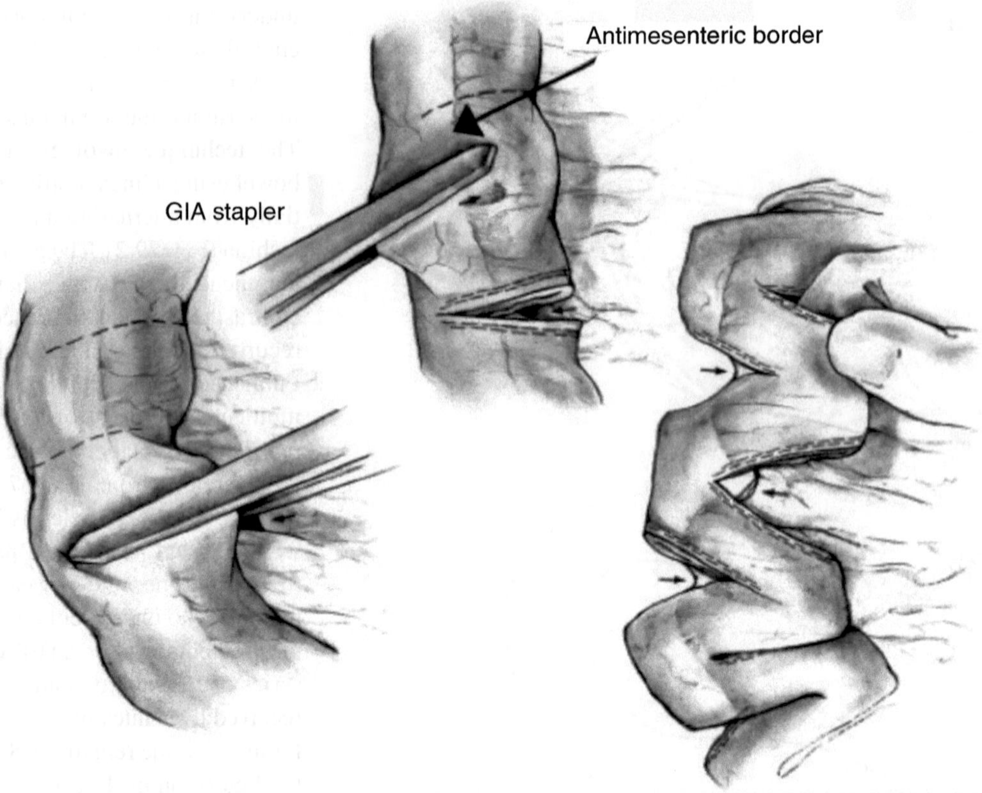

associated with very high rates of morbidity and mortality related to rejection, graft loss, and bacterial translocation leading to sepsis. More recently, refinement of surgical technique in addition to enhanced immunosuppressive and other perioperative strategies has significantly improved outcomes [138, 139]. Therefore, small bowel transplantation has become firmly established as a viable therapeutic option for intestinal failure. Depending on the extent of liver disease and other abdominal pathology, a combined liver-intestine or multivisceral graft may be indicated [139]. Recent data from high-volume intestinal transplant centers demonstrate 1-year patient and graft survival rates that exceed 80 and 70 %, respectively [140–142]. While long-term survival has also dramatically improved in recent decades, they still fall short of outcomes seen with other abdominal organ transplants [143]. The Pittsburgh group reported their series of intestinal and multivisceral transplants divided into time periods; for the 322 transplants performed during the study's latest era (between 2001 and 2008), 5-year patient and graft survival rates were 68 and 53 %, respectively [142]. There are ongoing efforts to develop novel strategies to overcome late graft loss and its sequelae [142, 144].

Traditionally, intestinal transplantation has been reserved for patients with permanent intestinal failure who can no longer be maintained on total parenteral nutrition therapy [145]. Specifically, patients should be considered for transplantation if they have impending or overt liver failure, repeated loss of central venous access due to thrombosis, recurrent episodes of catheter-related sepsis, or frequent dehydration despite intravenous supplementation [146]. For these patients, prompt referral to a transplant center for evaluation is imperative for optimizing outcome [147, 148]. Early transplantation, as defined by less than 12 months of prior parenteral nutrition therapy, has been shown to be associated with better survival [142]. As clinical outcomes of intestinal transplantation continue to improve, some experts have advocated for the restrictive indications to be broadened [149]. Indeed, there has been increasing debate regarding the role of "preemptive" transplantation in patients who are at high risk of developing parenteral nutrition failure; this may apply to patients with ultrashort small intestine (<50 cm), primary motility disorders, chronic obstruction, and radiation injury [144, 149]. The poor prognosis associated with parenteral nutrition failure supports early consideration of transplantation [149]. Furthermore, there are multiple studies that demonstrate improved quality of life indicators following transplantation [143, 149]. As well, intestinal transplantation has been shown to be cost-effective for managing intestinal failure as long as graft function is maintained for at least 2–3 years after surgery [150].

Future Directions

Key Concept: We remain hampered by a widespread lack of effective options for severe SBS, although emerging technology is in the investigative phase to give patients additional hope.

Despite its recent advances, small intestinal transplantation continues to be limited by issues such as donor availability, graft rejection, and adverse effects related to immunosuppression. As a potential solution to overcome these difficulties, tissue-engineered small intestine has been studied in animal models [151, 152]. The technology makes use of biomaterials such as small intestinal submucosa to generate new tissue and takes advantage of the regenerative ability of intestinal epithelium [153]. While normal structural components have been successfully generated, peristaltic motion of the intestine has yet to be recreated [133]. As well, it may be difficult to procure the necessary neonatal intestinal organelles in humans and to scale up the size of the tissue-engineered intestine to clinically useful dimensions [153]. Nevertheless, if this technology were to become feasible in the future, it has the potential to dramatically alter the management of short bowel syndrome.

Outcomes

Key Concept: The prognosis of patients with short bowel syndrome is determined by their remnant intestinal anatomy and underlying disease and modulated by their response to medical and surgical treatments.

Overall, patients who are dependent on home parenteral nutrition (HPN) have higher mortality than their age-matched counterparts in the general population [154]. A French group recently reported their results over a 25-year period including 268 consecutive adult SBS patients who required HPN [66]. Survival was 94, 70, and 52 % at 1, 5, and 10 years, respectively. Complications related to SBS and HPN combined accounted for only 26 % of the mortality. The study also found the probabilities of a patient remaining dependent on HPN were 74, 64, and 48 % at 1, 2, and 5 years, respectively. Factors significantly associated with HPN dependence at 5 years included remnant small intestinal length of less than 75 cm, less than 4/7 of colon remaining, and postoperative citrulline concentration of less than 20 μmol/L. Comparable results have been reported by other centers regarding the prognosis of HPN-dependent patients, including 5-year survival rates ranging between 60 and 78 % [65, 155, 156].

There have been few studies addressing quality of life (QOL) of patients on HPN. Jeppesen et al. used two validated (QOL) questionnaires on 49 HPN-dependent patients and 36 patients who did not receive HPN but had anatomical or functional short bowel [157]. Compared to the latter group, the former was found to have a poorer quality of life that was comparable to that reported for dialysis-dependent patients with chronic renal failure. Another research demonstrated that lowest QOL scores are more common during the first year on HPN, particularly if the patient was previously well [158]. Quality of life then gradually improves under its plateaus after 4–5 years on HPN. A US study found low quality of life in patients requiring long-term HPN to be associated with length of time on total parenteral nutrition, lack of family supports, and financial difficulties [159]. With respect to intestinal transplantation, there is increasing evidence that it results in improved quality of life measures [144]. In a comparison of QOL measures between 79 adult transplant survivors and 79 HPN patients, Abu-Elmagd et al. reported superior results with transplantation across several psychological, emotional, and social domains [143].

Summary Pearls

You will be confronted with patients with SBS, and they may be some of the most challenging that you will encounter. It is important to remember that the management of the patient with short bowel syndrome is guided by a thorough understanding of the remnant intestinal anatomy and physiology as well as the underlying disease (Fig. 29.3). These factors will largely determine the patient's clinical manifestation, which may range from mild malabsorption correctable with dietary modifications to intestinal failure requiring complex bowel rehabilitation and surgical strategies. As outcomes in published series consistently correlate with residual length of small intestine, it is worthwhile during the initial resection operation to preserve as much of it as possible. Similarly, an intact colon is valuable as it can compensate for the lost absorptive function, and its presence is associated with independence from home parenteral nutrition.

A multidisciplinary approach is essential for the optimal care of these complex patients. In particular, individuals who are dependent on home parenteral nutrition should be managed by a center with appropriate expertise and resources. This is likely to optimize intestinal rehabilitation, reduce complications associated with long-term parenteral nutrition, and facilitate access to specialized medical and surgical therapies. For nutritional support, you should use the enteral route whenever possible; the presence of luminal nutrients is necessary for intestinal adaption, a process which may continue for several years following resection. Antisecretory and antimotility medications may be useful adjuncts for reducing water and salt losses. Among the growth factors, GLP-2 and its analogue, teduglutide, are promising intestinotrophic agents that can augment a bowel rehabilitation regimen.

In the absence of contraindications to surgery, you should attempt to restore intestinal continuity. For patients whose

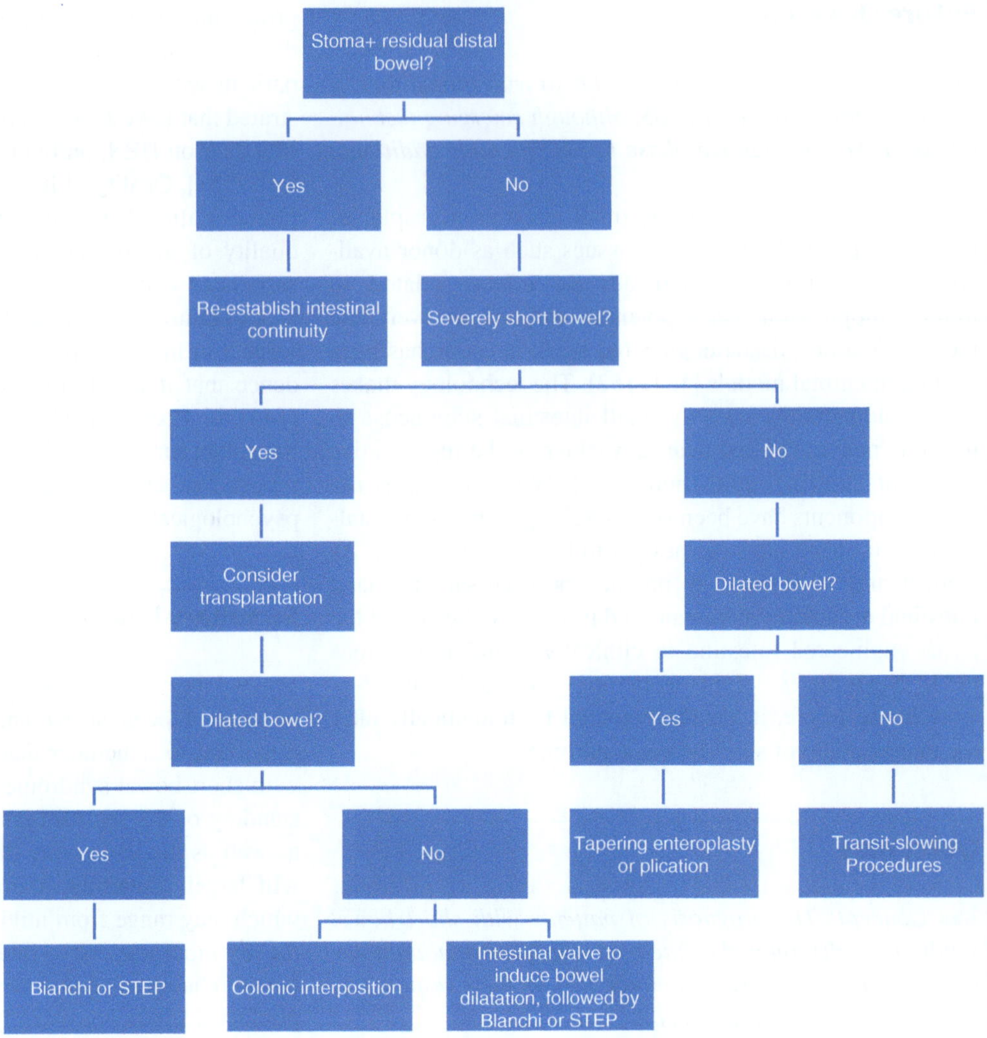

Fig. 29.3 Algorithm for surgical management of short bowel syndrome

bowel is already in continuity, but cannot wean off parenteral nutrition despite seemingly adequate intestinal length, segmental reversal of small bowel should be considered to slow transit. On the other hand, for patients who are clearly limited by a very short bowel that is dilated, either the Bianchi procedure or STEP may be appropriate. Of these two bowel-lengthening operations, STEP is likely easier to perform and can be used as a repeat procedure. Finally, intestinal transplantation has evolved over recent years to offer improved survival and quality of life outcomes. Most importantly, for SBS patients with adverse risk factors for failing parenteral nutrition or if you do not feel comfortable or have the resources to care for these patients, referral for evaluation regarding transplantation should be considered early in their course.

References

1. Buchman A, Scolapio J, Fryer J. AGA technical review on short bowel syndrome and intestinal transplantation. Gastroenterology. 2003;124:1111–34.
2. Jeejeebhoy KN. Management of short bowel syndrome: avoidance of total parenteral nutrition. Gastroenterology. 2006;130(2 Suppl 1):S60–6.
3. Buchman AL. Etiology and initial management of short bowel syndrome. Gastroenterology. 2006;130(2 Suppl 1):S5–15.
4. Westergaard H. Short bowel syndrome. Semin Gastrointest Dis. 2002;13(4):210–20.
5. Nightingale J, Woodward JM. Guidelines for management of patients with a short bowel. Gut. 2006;55 Suppl 4:iv1–12.
6. Longshore S, Wakeman D, McMellen M, Warner B. Bowel resection induced intestinal adaptation: progress from bench to bedside. Minerva Pediatr. 2009;61(3):239–51.
7. Jeejeebhoy KN. Short bowel syndrome: a nutritional and medical approach. CMAJ. 2002;166(10):1297–302.
8. Thompson W, Wrathell E. The relation between ileal resection and vitamin B12 absorption. Can J Surg. 1977;20(5):461.
9. Hofmann AF. Bile acid malabsorption caused by ileal resection. Arch Intern Med. 1972;130(4):597–605.
10. Lin H, Zhao X, Wang L. Intestinal transit is more potently inhibited by fat in the distal (ileal brake) than in the proximal (jejunal brake) gut. Dig Dis Sci. 1997;42(1):19–25.
11. Stanley S, Wynne K, Bloom S. Gastrointestinal satiety signals III. Glucagon-like peptide 1, oxyntomodulin, peptide YY, and pancreatic polypeptide. Am J Physiol Gastrointest Liver Physiol. 2004;286:G693–7.

12. Nightingale J, Kamm M, van der Sijp J, Ghatei M, Bloom S, Lennard-Jones J. Gastrointestinal hormones in short bowel syndrome. Peptide YY may be the "colonic brake" to gastric emptying. Gut. 1996;39:267–72.
13. Fordtran J, Rector F, Carter N. The mechanisms of sodium absorption in the human small intestine. J Clin Invest. 1968;47(4): 884–900.
14. Davis G, Santa Ana C, Morawski S, Fordtran J. Permeability characteristics of human jejunum, ileum, proximal colon and distal colon: results of potential difference measurements and unidirectional fluxes. Gastroenterology. 1982;83(4):844–50.
15. Chaet M, Farrell M, Ziegler M, Warner B. Intensive nutritional support and remedial surgical intervention for extreme short bowel syndrome. J Pediatr Gastroenterol Nutr. 1994;19(3):295–8.
16. Sondheimer J, Cadnapaphornchai M, Sontag M, Zerbe G. Predicting the duration of dependence on parenteral nutrition after neonatal intestinal resection. J Pediatr. 1998;132:80–4.
17. Andorsky D, Lund D, Lillehei C, Jaksic T, DiCanzio J, Richardson D, et al. Nutritional and other postoperative management of neonates with short bowel syndrome correlates with clinical outcomes. J Pediatr. 2001;139:27–33.
18. Dibaise JK, Young RJ, Vanderhoof JA. Enteric microbial flora, bacterial overgrowth, and short-bowel syndrome. Clin Gastroenterol Hepatology. 2006;4(1):11–20.
19. Vanderhoof J, Young R, Murray N, Kaufman S. Treatment strategies for small bowel bacterial overgrowth in short bowel syndrome. J Pediatr Gastroenterol Nutr. 1998;27(2):155–60.
20. Kaufman S, Loseke C, Lupo J, Young R, Murray N, Pinch L, et al. Influence of bacterial overgrowth and intestinal inflammation on duration of parenteral nutrition in children with short bowel syndrome. J Pediatr. 1997;131:356–61.
21. Fich A, Steadman C, Phillips S, Camilleri M, Brown M, Haddad A, et al. Ileocolonic transit does not change after right hemicolectomy. Gastroenterology. 1992;103(3):794–9.
22. Fry R, Mahmoud N, Maron D, Ross H, Rombeau J. Colon and rectum. In: Townsend C, Beauchamp R, Evers B, Mattox K, editors. Sabiston textbook of surgery. 18th ed. Philadelphia: Saunders, Elsevier; 2007.
23. Joly F, Mayeur C, Messing B, Lavergne-Slove A, Cazals-Hatem D, Noordine M-L, et al. Morphological adaptation with preserved proliferation/transporter content in the colon of patients with short bowel syndrome. Am J Physiol Gastrointest Liver Physiol. 2009;297(1):G116–23.
24. Royall D, Wolever T, Jeejeebhoy K. Evidence for colonic conservation of malabsorbed carbohydrate in short bowel syndrome. Am J Gastroenterol. 1992;87(6):751–6.
25. Gouttebel MC, Saint-Aubert B, Astre C, Joyeux H. Total parenteral nutrition needs in different types of short bowel syndrome. Dig Dis Sci. 1986;31(7):718–23.
26. Nightingale JM, Lennard-Jones JE, Gertner DJ, Wood SR, Bartram CI. Colonic preservation reduces need for parenteral therapy, increases incidence of renal stones, but does not change high prevalence of gall stones in patients with a short bowel. Gut. 1992;33(11):1493–7.
27. Mitchell JE, Breuer RI, Zuckerman L, Berlin J, Schilli R, Dunn JK. The colon influences ileal resection diarrhea. Dig Dis Sci. 1980; 25(1):33–41.
28. Thompson J. Short bowel syndrome and Crohn's disease. J Gastrointest Surg. 2003;7(8):1069–72.
29. Polito J, Childs B, Mellits E, Tokayer A, Harris M, Bayless T. Crohn's disease: influence of age at diagnosis and site and clinical type of disease. Gastroenterology. 1996;111(3):580–6.
30. Agwunobi A, Carlson G, Anderson I, Irving M, Scott N. Mechanisms of intestinal failure in Crohn's disease. Dis Colon Rectum. 2001;44(12):1834–7.
31. Donohoe CL, Reynolds JV. Short bowel syndrome. Surgeon. 2010;8(5):270–9. Elsevier Ltd.
32. Kotanagi H, Kramer K, Fazio VW, Petras RE. Do microscopic abnormalities at resection margins correlate with increased anastomotic recurrence in Crohn's disease? Retrospective analysis of 100 cases. Dis Colon Rectum. 1991;34(10):909–16.
33. Yamamoto T, Fazio VW, Tekkis PP. Safety and efficacy of strictureplasty for Crohn's disease: a systematic review and meta-analysis. Dis Colon Rectum. 2007;50(11):1968–86.
34. Thompson JS. Comparison of massive vs. repeated resection leading to short bowel syndrome. J Gastrointest Surg. 2000;4(1): 101–4.
35. Falkensammer J, Oldenburg WA. Surgical and medical management of mesenteric ischemia. Curr Treat Options Cardiovasc Med. 2006;8:137–43.
36. Sise MJ. Mesenteric ischemia: the whole spectrum. Scand J Surg. 2010;99(2):106–10.
37. Ballard JL, Stone WM, Hallett JW, Pairolero PC, Cherry KJ. A critical analysis of adjuvant techniques used to assess bowel viability in acute mesenteric ischemia. Am Surg. 1993; 59(5):309–11.
38. Thompson JS. Inflammatory disease and outcome of short bowel syndrome. Am J Surg. 2000;180(6):551–5.
39. Messing B, Crenn P, Beau P, Christine M, Ruault B, Rambaud JC, et al. Long-term survival and parenteral nutrition dependence in adult patients with the short bowel syndrome. Gastroenterology. 1999;117:1043–50.
40. Boland E, Thompson J, Rochling F, Sudan D. A 25-year experience with postresection short-bowel syndrome secondary to radiation therapy. Am J Surg. 2010;200:690–3. Elsevier Inc.
41. Dietz D, Remzi F, Fazio V. Strictureplasty for obstructing small-bowel lesions in diffuse radiation enteritis-successful outcome in five patients. Dis Colon Rectum. 2001;44(12): 1772–7.
42. Girvent M, Carlson GL, Shaffer J, Irving M, Scott NA. Intestinal failure after surgery for complicated radiation enteritis. Ann R Coll Surg Engl. 2000;82:198–201.
43. Marshall GT, Thirlby RC, Bredfeldt JE, Hampson NB. Treatment of gastrointestinal radiation injury with hyperbaric oxygen. Undersea Hyperb Med. 2007;34:35–42.
44. Yokoyama K, Ogura Y, Kawabata M, Hinoshita F, Suzuki Y, Hara S, et al. Hyperammonemia in a patient with short bowel syndrome and chronic renal failure. Nephron. 1996;72:693–5.
45. Mayne A, Handy D, Preece M, George R, Booth I. Dietary management of D-lactic acidosis in short bowel syndrome. Arch Dis Child. 1990;65:229–31.
46. Dray X, Joly F, Reijasse D, Attar A, Alves A, Panis Y, et al. Incidence, risk factors, and complications of cholelithiasis in patients with home parenteral nutrition. J Am Coll Surg. 2007; 204(1):13–21.
47. Dobbins J, Binder H. Effect of bile salts and fatty acids on the colonic absorption of oxalate. Gastroenterology. 1976;70: 1096–100.
48. Backman L, Hallberg D. Small intestinal length. An intraoperative study in obesity. Acta Chir Scand. 1974;140:57–63.
49. Slater G, Aufses A. Small bowel length in Crohn's disease. Am J Gastroenterol. 1991;8:1037–40.
50. Nightingale J, Bartram C, Lennard-Jones J. Length of residual small bowel after partial resection: correlation between radiographic and surgical measurements. Gastrointest Radiol. 1991;16:305–6.
51. Crenn P, Messing B, Cynober L. Citrulline as a biomarker of intestinal failure due to enterocyte mass reduction. Clin Nutr. 2008; 27(3):328–39.
52. Crenn P, Coudray-Lucas C, Thuillier F, Cynober L, Messing B. Postabsorptive plasma citrulline concentration is a marker of absorptive enterocyte mass and intestinal failure in humans. Gastroenterology. 2000;119:1496–505.
53. Jianfeng G, Weiming Z, Ning L, Fangnan L, Li T, Nan L, et al. Serum citrulline is a simple quantitative marker for small intestinal

enterocytes mass and absorption function in short bowel patients. J Surg Res. 2005;127(2):177–82.
54. Luo M, Fernandez-Estivariz C, Manatunga A, Bazargan N, Gu L, Jones D, et al. Are plasma citrulline and glutamine biomarkers of intestinal absorptive function in patients with short bowel syndrome? J Parenter Enteral Nutr. 2007;31:1–7.
55. Ziegler T, Leader L. Parenteral nutrition: transient or permanent therapy in intestinal failure? Gastroenterology. 2006;130:S37–42.
56. Sigalet D, Boctor D, Brindle M, Lam V, Robertson M. Elements of successful intestinal rehabilitation. J Pediatr Surg [Internet]. 2011;46(1):150–6. Available from: http://www.ncbi.nlm.nih.gov/pubmed/21238657. Cited 20 Sep 2012. Elsevier Inc.
57. Messing B, Joly F. Guidelines for management of home parenteral support in adult chronic intestinal failure patients. Gastroenterology. 2006;130(2 Suppl 1):S43–51.
58. Goulet O, Joly F, Corriol O, Colomb-Jung V. Some new insights in intestinal failure-associated liver disease. Curr Opin Organ Transplant. 2009;14(3):256–61.
59. Ekema G, Falchetti D, Boroni G, Tanca AR, Altana C, Righetti L, et al. Reversal of severe parenteral nutrition-associated liver disease in an infant with short bowel syndrome using parenteral fish oil (omega-3 fatty acids). J Pediatr Surg. 2008;43(6):1191–5.
60. Gura KM, Lee S, Valim C, Zhou J, Kim S, Modi BP, et al. Safety and efficacy of a fish-oil-based fat emulsion in the treatment of parenteral nutrition-associated liver disease. Pediatrics. 2008;121(3): e678–86.
61. Mertes N, Grimm H, Fürst P, Stehle P. Safety and efficacy of a new parenteral lipid emulsion (SMOFlipid) in surgical patients: a randomized, double-blind, multicenter study. Ann Nutr Metab. 2006;50(3):253–9.
62. Schiano T, Klang M, Quesada E, Scott F, Tao Y, Shike M. Thiamine status in patients receiving long-term home parenteral nutrition. Am J Gastroenterol. 1996;91(12):2555–9.
63. Wolman S, Anderson G, Marliss E, Jeejeebhoy K. Zinc in total parenteral nutrition: requirements and metabolic effects. Gastroenterology. 1979;76:458–67.
64. Lane H, Lotspeich C, Moore C, Ballard J, Dudrick S, Warren D. The effect of selenium supplementation on selenium status of patients receiving chronic total parenteral nutrition. J Parenter Enteral Nutr. 1987;11:177–82.
65. Vantini I, Benini L, Bonfante F, Talamini G, Sembenini C, Chiarioni G, et al. Survival rate and prognostic factors in patients with intestinal failure. Dig Liver Dis. 2004;36:46–55.
66. Amiot A, Messing B, Corcos O, Panis Y, Joly F. Determinants of home parenteral nutrition dependence and survival of 268 patients with non-malignant short bowel syndrome. Clin Nutr. 2012;23:1–7. Elsevier Ltd.
67. Bines JE. Intestinal failure: a new era in clinical management. J Gastroenterol Hepatol. 2009;24 Suppl 3:S86–92.
68. Briones E, Iber F. Liver and biliary tract changes associated with total parenteral nutrition: pathogenesis and prevention. J Am Coll Nutr. 1995;14:219–28.
69. Cavicchi M, Beau P, Crenn P, Degott C, Messing B. Prevalence of liver disease and contributing factors in patients receiving home parenteral nutrition for permanent intestinal failure. Ann Intern Med. 2000;132(7):525–32.
70. Lowry S, Brennan M. Abnormal liver function during parenteral nutrition: relation to infusion excess. J Surg Res. 1979;26:300.
71. Lindor K, Burnes J. Ursodeoxycholic acid for the treatment of home parenteral nutrition-associated cholestasis. Gastroenterology. 1991;101:250–3.
72. Spagnuolo M, Iorio R, Vegnente A, Guarino A. Ursodeoxycholic acid for treatment of cholestasis in children on long-term total parenteral nutrition: a pilot study. Gastroenterology. 1996;111:716–9.
73. Buchman A, Moukarzel A, Goodson B, Herzog F, Pollack P, Reyen L, et al. Catheter-related infections associated with home parenteral nutrition and predictive factors for the need for catheter removal in their treatment. J Parenter Enteral Nutr. 1994; 18:297–302.
74. Buchman A, Misra S, Moukarzel A, Ament M. Catheter thrombosis and superior/inferior vena cava syndrome are rare complications of long term parenteral nutrition. Clin Nutr. 1994;13(6):356–60.
75. Moukarzel A, Haddad I, Ament M, Buchman A, Reyen L, Maggioni A, et al. 230 patient years of experience with home long-term parenteral nutrition in childhood: natural history and life of central venous catheters. J Pediatr Surg. 1994;29(10):1323–7.
76. Leiby J, Purcell H, Demaria J, Kraut E, Sagone A, Metz E. Pulmonary embolism as a result of Hickman catheter-related thrombosis. Am J Med. 1989;86:228–31.
77. Gould J, Carloss H, Skinner W. Groshong catheter-associated subclavian venous thrombosis. Am J Med. 1993;95:419–23.
78. Buchman A, Sohel M, Brown M, Jenden D, Ahn C, Roch M, et al. Verbal and visual memory improve after choline supplementation in long-term total parenteral nutrition: a pilot study. J Parenter Enteral Nutr. 2001;25:30–5.
79. DiBaise JK, Young RJ, Vanderhoof JA. Intestinal rehabilitation and the short bowel syndrome: part 1. Am J Gastroenterol. 2004; 99(7):1386–95.
80. Drucker D, Erlich P, Asa S, Brubaker P. Induction of intestinal epithelial proliferation by glucagon-like peptide 2. Proc Natl Acad Sci U S A. 1996;93(15):7911–26.
81. Joly F, Dray X, Corcos O, Barbot L, Kapel N, Messing B. Tube feeding improves intestinal absorption in short bowel syndrome patients. Gastroenterology. 2009;136(3):824–31. AGA Institute American Gastroenterological Association.
82. Vanderhoof J. Short bowel syndrome. Neonatal Gastroenterol. 1996;23:377–86.
83. McIntyre P, Fitchew M, Lennard-Jones J. Patients with a jejunostomy do not need a special diet. Gastroenterology. 1986;91:25–33.
84. Lennard-Jones J. Review article: practical management of the short bowel. Aliment Pharmacol Ther. 1994;8:563–77.
85. Cosnes J, Lamy P, Beaugerie L, Le Quintrec M, Gendre J, Le Quintrec Y. Adaptive hyperphagia in patients with postsurgical malabsorption. Gastroenterology. 1990;99(6):1814–9.
86. Aly A, Barany F, Kollberg B, Monsen U, Wisen O, Johansson C. Effect of an H2-receptor blocking agent on diarrhoeas after extensive small bowel resection in Crohn's disease. Acta Med Scand. 1980;207:119–22.
87. Jacobsen O, Ladefoged K, Stage J, Jarnum S. Effects of cimetidine on jejunostomy effluents in patients with severe short-bowel syndrome. Scand J Gastroenterol. 1986;21(7):824–8.
88. Jeppesen P, Staun M, Tjellesen L, Mortensen P. Effect of intravenous ranitidine and omeprazole on intestinal absorption of water, sodium, and macronutrients in patients with intestinal resection. Gut. 1998;43:763–9.
89. Williams N, Evans P, King R. Gastric acid secretion and gastrin production in the short bowel syndrome. Gut. 1985;26(9):914–9.
90. Cooper J, Williams N, King R, Barker M. Effects of a long-acting somatostatin analogue in patients with severe ileostomy diarrhoea. Br J Surg. 1986;73(2):128–31.
91. Kusuhara K, Kusunoki M, Okamoto T, Sakanoue Y, Utsunomiya J. Reduction of the effluent volume in high-output ileostomy patients by a somatostatin analogue, SMS 201–995. Int J Colorectal Dis. 1992;7(4):202–5.
92. Rodrigues C, Lennard-Jones J, Thompson D, Farthing M. The effects of octreotide, soy polysaccharide, codeine and loperamide on nutrient, fluid and electrolyte absorption in the short-bowel syndrome. Aliment Pharmacol Ther. 1989;3(2):159–69.
93. Sukhotnik I, Khateeb K, Krausz MM, Sabo E, Siplovich L, Coran AG, et al. Sandostatin impairs postresection intestinal adaptation in a rat model of short bowel syndrome. Dig Dis Sci. 2002;47(9): 2095–102.

94. Hodin RA, Saldinger P, Meng S. Small bowel adaptation: counter regulatory effects of epidermal growth factor and somatostatin on the program of early gene expression. Surgery. 1995;118(2):206–10.
95. King R, Norton T, Hill G. A double-blind crossover study of the effect of loperamide hydrochloride and codeine phosphate on ileostomy output. Aust N Z J Surg. 1982;52(2):121–4.
96. Tytgat G, Huibregtse K. Loperamide and ileostomy output – placebo-controlled double-blind crossover study. BMJ. 1975;2:667–8.
97. Newton C. Effect of codeine phosphate, Lomotil, and Isogel on ileostomy function. Gut. 1978;19(5):377–83.
98. Hofmann A, Poley J. Role of bile acid malabsorption in the pathogenesis of diarrhoea and steatorrhoea in patients with ileal resection. I. Response to cholestyramine or replacement of dietary long chain triglyceride by medium chain triglycerides. Gastroenterology. 1972;62:918–34.
99. Compston J, Horton L. Oral 25-hydroxyvitamin D3 in treatment of osteomalacia associated with ileal resection and cholestyramine. Gastroenterology. 1978;74:900–2.
100. Hart M, Phares C, Erdman S, Grandjean C, Park J, Vanderhoof J. Augmentation of postresection mucosal hyperplasia by plerocercoid growth factor (PGF) – analog of human growth hormone. Dig Dis Sci. 1987;32(11):1275–80.
101. Shulman D, Hu C, Duckett G, Lavallee-Grey M. Effects of short-term growth hormone therapy in rats undergoing 75% small intestinal resection. J Pediatr Gastroenterol Nutr. 1992;14:3–11.
102. Tamada H, Nezu R, Matsuo Y, Imamura I, Takagi Y, Okada A. Alanyl glutamine-enriched total parenteral nutrition restores intestinal adaptation after either proximal or distal massive resection in rats. J Parenter Enteral Nutr. 1993;17(3):236–42.
103. Gardemann A, Watanabe Y, Grosse V, Hesse S, Jungermann K. Increases in intestinal glucose absorption and hepatic glucose uptake elicited by luminal but not vascular glutamine in the jointly perfused small intestine and liver of the rat. Biochem J. 1992;283:759–65.
104. Byrne TA, Morrissey TB, Nattakom TV, Ziegler TR, Wilmore DW. Growth hormone, glutamine, and a modified diet enhance nutrient absorption in patients with severe short bowel syndrome. JPEN J Parenter Enteral Nutr. 1995;19(4):296–302.
105. Weiming Z, Ning L, Jieshou L. Effect of recombinant human growth hormone and enteral nutrition on short bowel syndrome. J Parenter Enteral Nutr. 2004;28(6):377.
106. Scolapio J, Camilleri M, Fleming C, Oenning L, Burton D, Sebo T, et al. Effect of growth hormone, glutamine, and diet on adaptation in short-bowel syndrome: a randomized, controlled study. Gastroenterology. 1997;113(4):1074.
107. Szkudlarek J, Jeppesen P, Mortensen P. Effect of high dose growth hormone with glutamine and no change in diet on intestinal absorption in short bowel patients: a randomised, double blind, crossover, placebo controlled study. Gut. 2000;47(2):199.
108. Seguy D, Vahedi K, Kapel N, Souberbielle J, Messing B. Low-dose growth hormone in adult home parenteral nutrition-dependent short bowel syndrome patients: a positive study. Gastroenterology. 2003;124(2):293.
109. Ellegard L, Bosaeus I, Nordgren S, Bengtsson B. Low-dose recombinant human growth hormone increases body weight and lean body mass in patients with short bowel syndrome. Ann Surg. 1997;225(1):88–96.
110. Scolapio J, McGreevy K, Tennyson G, Burnett O. Effect of glutamine in short-bowel syndrome. Clin Nutr. 2001;20(4):319.
111. Meier J, Nauck M, Pott A, Heinze K, Goetze O, Bulut K, et al. Glucagon-like peptide 2 stimulates glucagon secretion, enhances lipid absorption, and inhibits gastric acid secretion in humans. Gastroenterology. 2006;130(1):44–54.
112. Guan X, Karpen H, Stephens J, Bukowski J, Niu S, Zhang G, et al. GLP-2 receptor localizes to enteric neurons and endocrine cells expressing vasoactive peptides and mediates increased blood flow. Gastroenterology. 2006;130(1):150–64.
113. Jeppesen P, Hartmann B, Hansen B, Thulesen J, Holst J, Mortensen P. Impaired meal stimulated glucagon-like peptide 2 response in ileal resected short bowel patients with intestinal failure. Gut. 1999;45(4):559–63.
114. Jeppesen P, Lund P, Gottschalck I, Nielsen H, Holst J, Mortensen J, et al. Short bowel patients treated for two years with glucagon-like peptide 2: effects on intestinal morphology and absorption, renal function, bone and body composition, and muscle function. Gastroenterol Res Pract. 2009;616054:12.
115. Jeppesen P, Sanguinetti E, Buchman A, Howard L, Scolapio J, Ziegler T, et al. Teduglutide (ALX-0600), a dipeptidyl peptidase IV resistant glucagon-like peptide 2 analogue, improves intestinal function in short bowel syndrome patients. Gut. 2005;54(9):1224–31.
116. Jeppesen P, Gilroy R, Pertkiewicz M, Allard J, Messing B, O'Keefe S. Randomised placebo-controlled trial of teduglutide in reducing parenteral nutrition and/or intravenous fluid requirements in patients with short bowel syndrome. Gut. 2011;60(7):902–14.
117. Buchman AL, Katz S, Fang JC, Bernstein CN, Abou-Assi SG, Teduglutide Study Group. Teduglutide, a novel mucosally active analog of glucagon-like peptide-2 (GLP-2) for the treatment of moderate to severe Crohn's disease. Inflamm Bowel Dis. 2010;16(6):962–73.
118. Sukhotnik I, Yakirevich E, Coran AG, Siplovich L, Krausz M, Hirsh M, et al. Effect of transforming growth factor-α on intestinal adaptation in a rat model of short bowel syndrome. J Surg Res. 2002;108(2):235–42.
119. Falcone R, Stern L, Kemp C, Erwin C, Warner B. Intestinal adaptation occurs independent of transforming growth factor-alpha. J Pediatr Surg. 2000;35(2):365–70.
120. Kato Y, Yu D, Schwartz M. Enhancement of intestinal adaptation by hepatocyte growth factor. J Pediatr Surg. 1998;33(2):235.
121. Alavi K, Prasad R, Lundgren K, Schwartz M. Interleukin-11 enhances small intestine absorptive function and mucosal mass after intestinal adaptation. J Pediatr Surg. 2000;35(2):371.
122. Ziegler T, Mantell M, Chow J, Rombeau J, Smith R. Intestinal adaptation after extensive small bowel resection: differential changes in growth and insulin-like growth factor system messenger ribonucleic acids in jejunum and ileum. Endocrinology. 1998;139(7):3119–26.
123. Yang H, Wildhaber B, Teitelbaum D. 2003 Harry M. Vars Research Award. Keratinocyte growth factor improves epithelial function after massive small bowel resection. JPEN J Parenter Enteral Nutr. 2003;27(3):198.
124. Wales PW. Surgical therapy for short bowel syndrome. Pediatr Surg Int. 2004;20:647–57.
125. Carlson G. Surgical management of intestinal failure. Proc Nutr Soc. 2003;62(3):711–8.
126. Panis Y, Messing B, Rivet P, Coffin B, Hautefeuille P, Matuchansky C, et al. Segmental reversal of the small bowel as an alternative to intestinal transplantation in patients with short bowel syndrome. Ann Surg. 1997;225(4):401–7.
127. Barksdale EM, Stanford A. The surgical management of short bowel syndrome. Curr Gastroenterol Rep. 2002;4(3):229–37.
128. Brolin R. Colon interposition for extreme short bowel syndrome: a case report. Surgery. 1986;100(3):576–80.
129. Thompson J, Langnas A, Pinch L, Kaufman S, Quigley E, Vanderhoof J. Surgical approach to short bowel syndrome. Experience in a population of 160 patients. Ann Surg. 1995;222(4):600–5.

130. Devine R, Kelly K. Surgical therapy of the short bowel syndrome. Gastroenteol Clin N Am. 1989;18(3):603–18.
131. Sudan D, Thompson J, Botha J, Grant W, Antonson D, Raynor S, et al. Comparison of intestinal lengthening procedures for patients with short bowel syndrome. Ann Surg. 2007;246(4):593–601; discussion 601–4.
132. Bianchi A. Intestinal loop lengthening – a technique for increasing small intestinal length. J Pediatr Surg. 1980;15:145–51.
133. Sudan D. Advances in the nontransplant medical and surgical management of intestinal failure. Curr Opin Organ Transplant. 2009;14:274–9.
134. Reinshagen K, Kabs C, Wirth H, Hable N, Brade J, Zahn K, et al. Long-term outcome in patients with short bowel syndrome after longitudinal intestinal lengthening and tailoring. J Pediatr Gastroenterol Nutr. 2008;47:573–8.
135. Kim HB, Fauza D, Garza J, Oh J-T, Nurko S, Jaksic T. Serial transverse enteroplasty (STEP): a novel bowel lengthening procedure. J Pediatr Surg. 2003;38(3):425–9.
136. Modi BP, Javid PJ, Jaksic T, Piper H, Langer M, Duggan C, et al. First report of the international serial transverse enteroplasty data registry: indications, efficacy, and complications. J Am Coll Surg. 2007;204(3):365–71.
137. Oliveira C, de Silva N, Wales PW. Five-year outcomes after serial transverse enteroplasty in children with short bowel syndrome. J Pediatr Surg. 2012;47(5):931–7. Elsevier B.V.
138. Abu-Elmagd K. Intestinal transplantation for short bowel syndrome and gastrointestinal failure: current consensus, rewarding outcomes, and practical guidelines. Gastroenterology. 2006;130: S132–7.
139. Tzakis AG, Kato T, Levi DM, DeFaria W, Selvaggi G, Weppler D, et al. 100 multivisceral transplants at a single center. Ann Surg. 2005;242:480–93.
140. Fishbein TM, Kaufman SS, Florman SS, Gondolesi GE, Schiano T, Kim-Schluger L, et al. Isolated intestinal transplantation: proof of clinical efficacy. Transplantation. 2003;76(4):636–40.
141. Nishida S, Levi D, Kato T, Nery JR, Mittal N, Hadjis N, et al. Ninety-five cases of intestinal transplantation at the University of Miami. J Gastrointest Surg. 2002;6(2):233–9.
142. Abu-Elmagd KM, Costa G, Bond GJ, Soltys K, Sindhi R, Wu T, et al. Five hundred intestinal and multivisceral transplantations at a single center: major advances with new challenges. Ann Surg. 2009;250(4):567–81.
143. Abu-Elmagd KM, Kosmach-Park B, Costa G, Zenati M, Martin L, Koritsky DA. Long-term survival, nutritional autonomy, and quality of life after intestinal and multivisceral transplantation. Ann Surg. 2012;256(3):494–508.
144. Fishbein TM. Intestinal transplantation. N Engl J Med. 2009;361(10):998–1008.
145. Fishbein TM, Matsumoto CS. Intestinal replacement therapy: timing and indications for referral of patients to an intestinal rehabilitation and transplant program. Gastroenterology. 2006;130: S147–51.
146. Vianna RM, Mangus RS. Present prospects and future perspectives of intestinal and multivisceral transplantation. Curr Opin Clin Nutr Metab Care. 2009;12(3):281–6.
147. Fecteau A, Atkinson P, Grant D. Early referral is essential for successful pediatric small bowel transplantation: the Canadian experience. J Pediatr Surg. 2001;36:681–4.
148. DeLegge M, Alsolaiman MM, Barbour E, Bassas S, Siddiqi MF, Moore NM. Short bowel syndrome: parenteral nutrition versus intestinal transplantation. Where are we today? Dig Dis Sci. 2007;52(4):876–92.
149. O'Keefe SJD, Emerling M, Koritsky D, Martin D, Stamos J, Kandil H, et al. Nutrition and quality of life following small intestinal transplantation. Am J Gastroenterol. 2007;102(5):1093–100.
150. Sudan D. Cost and quality of life after intestinal transplantation. Gastroenterology. 2006;130:S158–62.
151. Grikscheit TC, Siddique A, Ochoa ER, Srinivasan A, Alsberg E, Hodin RA, et al. Tissue-engineered small intestine improves recovery after massive small bowel resection. Ann Surg. 2004; 240(5):748–54.
152. Gupta A, Dixit A, Sales KM, Winslet MC, Seifalian AM. Tissue engineering of small intestine – current status. Biomacromolecules. 2006;7(10):2701–9.
153. Dunn J. Is the tissue-engineered intestine clinically viable? Nat Clin Pract Gastroenterol Hepatol. 2008;5(7):366–7.
154. Howard L, Heaphey L, Fleming CR, Lininger L, Steiger E. Four years of North American registry home parenteral nutrition outcome data and their implications for patient management. J Parenter Enteral Nutr. 1991;15(4):384–93.
155. Lloyd DA, Vega R, Bassett P, Forbes A, Gabe SM. Survival and dependence on home parenteral nutrition: experience over a 25-year period in a UK referral centre. Aliment Pharmacol Ther. 2006;24(8):1231–40.
156. Scolapio JS, Fleming CR, Kelly DG, Wick DM, Zinsmeister AR. Survival of home parenteral nutrition-treated patients: 20 years of experience at the Mayo Clinic. Mayo Clin Proc. 1999;74(3): 217–22. Mayo Foundation for Medical Education and Research.
157. Jeppesen PB, Langholz E, Mortensen PB. Quality of life in patients receiving home parenteral nutrition. Gut. 1999; 44(6):844–52.
158. Richards D, Carlson G. Quality of life assessment and cost effectiveness. In: Nightingale J, editor. Intestinal failure. London: Greenwich Medical Media Limited; 2001. p. 447–57.
159. Smith CE. Quality of life in long-term total parenteral nutrition patients and their family caregivers. J Parenter Enteral Nutr. 1993;17:501–6.
160. Bianchi A. From the cradle to enteral autonomy: the role of autologous gastrointestinal reconstruction. Gastroenterology. 2006;130:S141.
161. Javid PJ, Kim HB, Duggan CP, Jaksic T. Serial transverse enteroplasty is associated with successful short-term outcomes in infants with short bowel syndrome. J Pediatr Surg. 2005; 40:1020.

The Intraoperative Consult

30

H. Randolph Bailey and Terah C. Isaacson

Key Points

- Careful assessment and good operative exposure are key steps in preparing for any operation.
- Do not compromise known surgical principles or sound judgment in order to satisfy a requesting physician.
- Most of the situations that you will encounter will be similar to something you have seen in the past; use your experience and build upon it.

Initial Mindset

Key concept: Gather your thoughts and as much information about the patient as quickly as possible, then rely on your past experiences and sound judgment.

The busy schedules of surgeons rarely afford a free moment, and, in fact, the call for assistance from a colleague in the operating room often comes when you are the most involved in the care of your own patients. When you receive the phone call for an intraoperative consultation, you must make a determination as to how to deal with your own schedule. It is important to understand the immediacy of the need for your help. At times, an injury may have occurred during a gynecological procedure that can be addressed in an hour or two at the end of that procedure. In the case of significant bleeding or an unstable patient, a more immediate need is required and you must notify (apologize to) your patients accordingly.

Between the time of the call from the consulting surgeon and your arrival in the operating room, a lot of potential scenarios can go quickly through your mind. By calling upon similar situations that you have encountered in the past, you may develop a plan of management with multiple alternatives. It is important to rapidly obtain as much information as possible. These include demographic information, indication for the operation, prior surgical history, type of operation, and the circumstances surrounding the need for consultation. You should try and obtain the patient's imaging and endoscopic history to better understand the current situation. A quick review of recent images may give you an idea about previous surgeries and additional pathology that may warrant consideration. All of these details will allow you to start to visualize the expected operative findings, associated complexity, as well as the possibilities of anatomic variations. In the case where minimal or no history is available, approach the patient with consideration of their age, body habitus, and assessment by the requesting physician and anesthesiologist of their current state of health.

Another very important consideration is your prior relationship with the consulting surgeon and your thoughts on his/her judgment and technical abilities. Your experience as a specialist has likely put you in a position where you have seen many of these challenges before, so try to replay in your mind those experiences and what made the outcomes successful.

Initial Evaluation

Upon entering the operating suite, the situation must be rapidly assessed. This includes obtaining information from the anesthesiologist on the stability and ASA status of the patient and type of antibiotics given and when. If bowel resection was not a planned procedure, it must be confirmed that the patient has received coverage of enteric gram (–) bacilli,

H.R. Bailey, MD, FACS (✉)
Division of Colon and Rectal Surgery,
The University of Texas Health Science Center,
Houston Methodist, 6550 Fannin St, Suite 2307,
Houston, TX 77030, USA
e-mail: hrbailey@swbell.net

T.C. Isaacson, MD
Division of Colon and Rectal Surgery,
Houston Methodist, 6550 Fannin St, Suite 2307,
Houston, TX 77030, USA
e-mail: cterah@gmail.com

S.R. Steele et al. (eds.), *Complexities in Colorectal Surgery*,
DOI 10.1007/978-1-4614-9022-7_30, © Springer Science+Business Media New York 2014

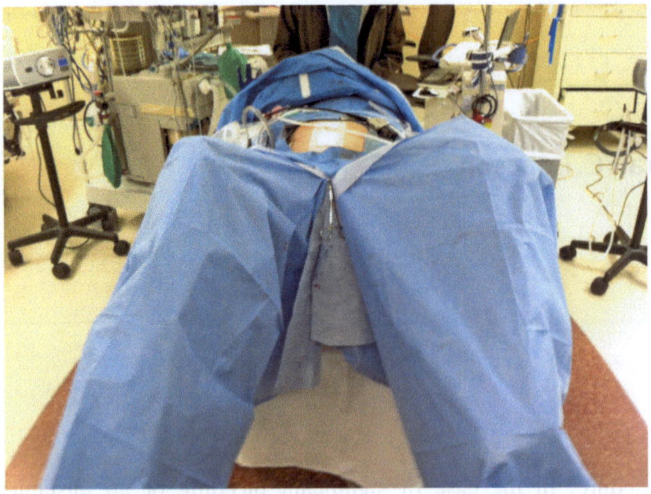

Fig. 30.1 Draping technique to facilitate exposure to the perineum

Enterococcus and anaerobes. Timing must also be considered, and another dose of "bowel appropriate" antibiotics may be indicated depending on the initial antibiotic choice and its timing [1].

Positioning

Key concept: Don't be afraid to change the patient's position to help accomplish what you need to do.

Evaluate the position of the patient. Depending on the reason for the consultation, it may be useful to move the patient from supine to low lithotomy position. This can frequently be done without contaminating the abdominal incision and is relatively easy to accomplish if *you* help the staff with positioning. You must identify the location of the patient on the operating table and make sure that all connections including those for self-retaining retractors are free prior to moving the patient down on the table. Stirrups or low lithotomy boots can be placed on the sides of the table, legs put into position, and the sterile drape cut down the middle. Sterile leggings can then be placed over the drape and will allow for excellent exposure to the anus, rectum, or pelvis if needed (Fig. 30.1). The low lithotomy position allows for endoscopic evaluation of the rectum (and possibly the entire colon), placement of ureteral stents, transanal insertion of stapling devices for an anastomosis, and anastomotic testing.

Initial Survey

A survey of the available instrumentation, possible endoscopic or radiologic needs, and additional available staff should be addressed with the operating room personnel. In years past, when I traveled to multiple hospitals, I used to carry a set of "special" instruments in my car. The basic operating instruments are now available in most hospitals. In the cases of endometriosis that cannot be differentiated from rectal cancer or other situations requiring identification or localization of lesions, rigid proctosigmoidoscopy or flexible sigmoidoscopy can be very helpful. To gain a better understanding of the anatomy and allow planning your approach, you may even consider doing these procedures prior to scrubbing. Rarely is radiology necessary beyond confirming instrument and sponge counts. You may find the need for ureteral stents to be placed. The lithotomy position facilitates stent placement. If you are not in a hospital where you work frequently, asking the consulting surgeon for their choice of urologist may be wise.

Examination

Key concept: Don't just focus on the problem at hand, but the entire situation. Establish roles early.

Once at the patient's side, look first at the problem for which you are consulted. Next, evaluate the rest of the abdominal viscera including the extent of adhesions and the magnitude of any injury present. The length of the remaining small bowel and its accessibility are important. After appraising the situation and the interventions required, you must determine whether you will assume control of the case or "assist" the requesting physician. If the consulting surgeon needs assistance with adhesiolysis for improved exposure of their operative field, I normally act only as a consultant and return the operation to the primary surgeon for completion. If, on the other hand, there is a significant bowel injury or a need for bowel resection, then I would assume primary control of the operation and often the postoperative care. Again, this has a lot to do with my prior relationships with the primary surgeon.

Exposure/Operative Procedure

Key concept: You should be familiar with several methods to extend your incision and provide adequate exposure.

After deciding what needs to be done, you must determine if the exposure is adequate to perform the indicated procedures. The beauty of a midline incision is that it can be extended as needed. If you have a Pfannenstiel incision and need greater exposure, it can be enlarged by conversion to a Cherney incision. This involves extending the fascial incision to the pubic tubercles laterally and dividing the tendonous attachments of the rectus abdominis muscles to the pubic crest [2]. Additionally, the Maylard incision divides the rectus muscle to facilitate improved exposure, but is limited to the lower part of the peritoneal cavity (Fig. 30.2a–d). If the

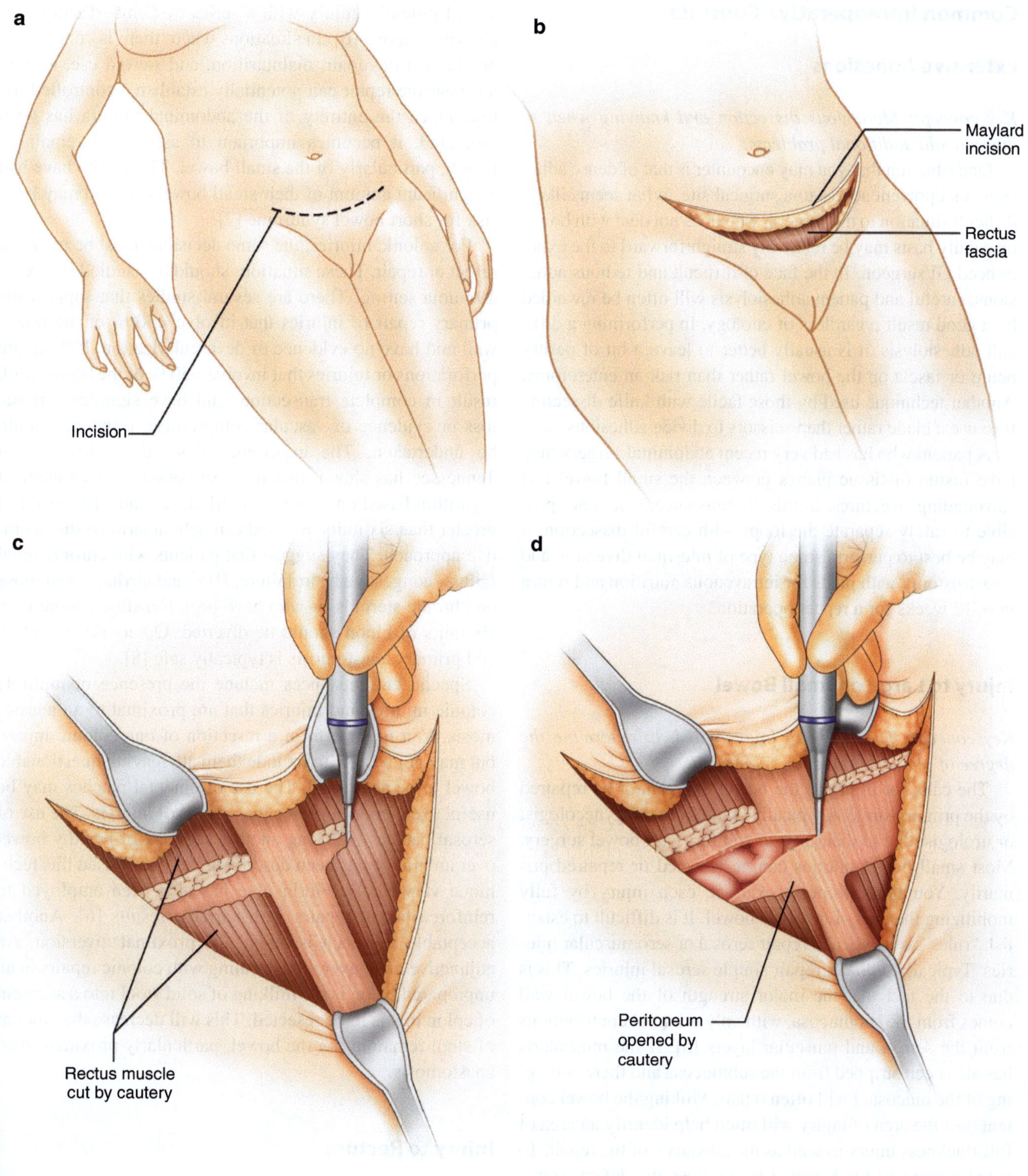

Fig. 30.2 (a–d) Maylard incision technique

upper abdomen requires significant attention that cannot be reached through the lower incision, it may be necessary to convert to a midline incision extending up as high as necessary. This is referred to as an "inverted T" incision and may provide good exposure for the entire abdomen [3]. Another approach is the "hockey-stick" incision. This is created by a vertical incision at the lateral aspect of the lower transverse incision. It is made lateral to the rectus muscle, which is usually divided. The incision can be extended upward to the costal margin, if needed, for further exposure [4].

Common Intraoperative Consults

Extensive Adhesions

Key concept: Meticulous dissection and knowing when to divert avoid additional problems.

One situation that you may encounter is that of dense adhesions that prevent access to a surgical site. What seems like a difficult situation to the surgeon who does not deal with bowel on a daily basis may be relatively straightforward to the experienced GI surgeon. In the face of difficult and tedious adhesions, careful and patient adhesiolysis will often be rewarded by a good result regardless of etiology. In performing a difficult adhesiolysis, it is usually better to leave a bit of peritoneum or fascia on the bowel rather than risk an enterotomy. Another technique used by those facile with knife dissection is to use a blade rather than scissors to divide adhesions.

A patient who has had very recent abdominal surgery may have fusion of tissue planes between the small bowel and surrounding structures. In this circumstance, if it is not possible to safely separate the loops with careful dissection, it may be best to perform some type of intestinal diversion and a gastrostomy with plans for intravenous nutrition and return in 6–12 weeks for a repeat operation.

Injury to Large or Small Bowel

Key concept: The extent of injury will help determine the degree of repair or resection required.

The calls for injury to the bowel that cannot be repaired by the primary surgeon typically come from the gynecologist or urologist due to their lack of comfort with bowel surgery. Most small bowel injuries can be resected or repaired primarily. You must properly examine each injury by fully mobilizing the area of involved bowel. It is difficult to establish "rules" as to when to repair serosal or seromuscular injuries. Typically, I do not repair simple serosal injuries. This is due to the fact that the major strength of the bowel wall comes from the submucosa, with only minimal contributions from the serosa and muscular layers [5]. If the muscularis has also been stripped from the submucosa and there is bulging of the mucosa, I will often repair. Milking the bowel content past the area of injury will often help identify an area of full-thickness injury as well as the adequacy of the repair. To avoid narrowing the bowel, I try to close the defects transversely with interrupted Lembert sutures. I then return at the end of the procedure and carefully inspect the repair for evidence of ischemia. If it looks questionable or ischemic, I would favor segmental resection. With electrosurgical injuries, it can be difficult to evaluate the depth or extent of the thermal damage and the potential exists for delayed perforation. The simplest and safest approach is imbrication of the site of potential injury with a series of Lembert sutures as described above [6]. In situations where there is concern for breakdown of repair, malnutrition, and steroid use, a drain left near the repair can potentially establish a controlled fistula. Once the entirety of the abdominal viscera has been evaluated, it becomes important to assess the remaining length, particularly of the small bowel. Those who have had a significant amount of their small bowel resected may be at risk for short bowel syndrome [7].

For colonic injuries, the same decisions must be made, to resect or repair. These situations should be handled similar to a trauma setting. There are several studies that support the primary repair of injuries that involve <50 % of the bowel wall and have no evidence of devascularization. If there are perforations or injuries that involve >50 % of the bowel wall, result in complete transection, and have significant tissue loss or evidence of vascular compromise, resection should be undertaken. The experience from the University of Tennessee has shown that in these patients a management algorithm based on patient comorbidities and transfusion of greater than six units of blood can help determine the operative approach. They suggest that patients with chronic renal failure, congestive heart failure, HIV, and cirrhosis and those on chronic steroids or who have been transfused more than six units of blood should be diverted. Otherwise, resection and primary anastomosis is typically safe [8].

Special circumstances include the presence of multiple colonic injuries and injuries that are proximal to an anastomosis. You may perform a resection of one colonic injury, but may not be able to include them all, leaving questionable bowel to be addressed. The use of omental patches may be useful to cover or reinforce these types of injuries. The use of serosal patches (suturing another segment of healthy bowel over an injury) has been described, but I have used this technique very rarely. Fibrin glue has also been employed to reinforce bowel repairs with variable results [6]. Another acceptable approach is repair and proximal diversion. An adjunctive maneuver when dealing with colonic repairs in an unprepared colon is the milking of solid stool into a segment of colon that is to be resected. This will decrease the amount of stool remaining in the bowel, particularly proximal to an anastomosis.

Injury to Rectum

Key concept: While diversion plays a larger role with rectal injuries, factors such as the location of the injury, patient's clinical status, tissue health, and degree of contamination are extremely important in decision-making.

Rectal injuries are among the more common reasons for intraoperative consultation. Whether or not the patient has had pelvic radiation, dates of administration and the dose

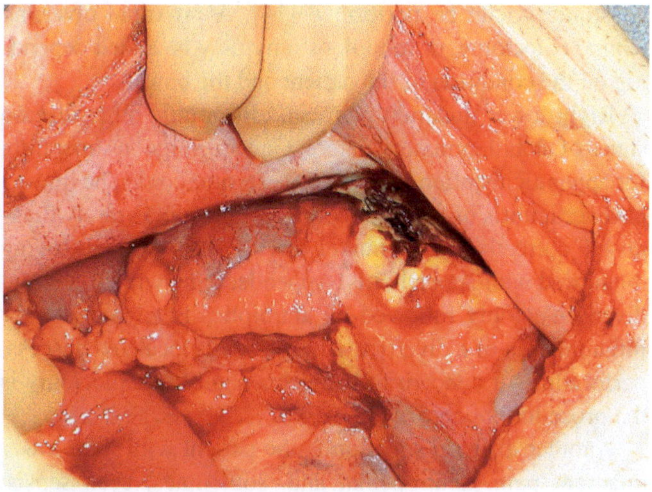

Fig. 30.3 Rectosigmoid perforation from a prior colonic stent (Courtesy of Philip Y. Pearson, MD)

given are important details for safe operative decision-making. The timing of the radiation is at least as important as the dosage. Beyond 8–12 weeks, intimal fibrosis and thickening may lead to a decrease in blood flow to and impaired healing of the radiated segment of bowel. Performing a proximal diversion or bringing in well-vascularized tissue to buttress the repair of radiated bowel should be considered. Possibilities for such reinforcement include an omental pedicle or muscle flaps such as gracilis or rectus abdominis. These can also be valuable techniques to use in patients who have an injury to the rectum during a hysterectomy. Interposing tissue such as the omentum between the rectal repair and fresh vaginal cuff may reduce the incidence of postoperative rectovaginal fistula formation.

As in colon injuries, much of the decision-making in rectal injuries is similar to that in the treatment of trauma. The mechanism of injury is of importance whether it be sharp, avulsion, or thermal (Fig. 30.3). The amount of contamination, the stability of the patient, and whether the injury is intraperitoneal or extraperitoneal are also of consideration. If a bowel injury is nondestructive and in the upper one-third of the rectum (intraperitoneal), these can safely be managed with primary repair and selective diversion depending on the circumstances of the consult. In the lower two-thirds of the rectum (extraperitoneal), injuries should be debrided to healthy tissue and repaired; if possible, a presacral drain (brought out through the abdominal wall) and diversion should be considered [9]. If the patient is unstable, has received several transfusions, or is medically unfit, diversion should be very strongly considered. Additionally, I may have a lower threshold to divert in a consulting situation than I would in an operation where I am the primary surgeon. This holds true because you may or may not know every clinical aspect of the case and you want to do the safest thing possible. The patient may have issues with incontinence that no one has addressed, and creating a low colorectal anastomosis may exacerbate this.

Mass

Key concept: In the absence of obstruction, obtaining issue and returning at a future time with more information and discussion with the patient are often beneficial.

The operating surgeon may encounter a mass either by palpation of the colon during routine exploration or in an extraluminal location with involvement of the bowel. In the initial evaluation of the mass, the degree of obstruction that is present must be determined. If obstruction is not an issue or malignancy can be ruled out (as in endometriosis), it may be best to return at another time after proper bowel evaluation and after obtaining informed consent from the patient. If obstruction is present in the colon and it has not been prepped, the risk of contamination and anastomotic problems should be considered. At this time, my preference remains in favor of bowel preparation for elective cases. In the consulting situation, if the patient has not been prepped, I am willing to do anastomoses without bowel preparation in light of the data that have shown no increased complications. A Cochrane Review performed in 2011 showed no statistically significant evidence that patients benefit from mechanical bowel preparation nor the use of rectal enemas [10]. In addition, one study showed that the liquid stool present in patients that had bowel preps caused a significantly higher rate of spillage and therefore could lead to a higher rate of infection [11]. As mentioned previously, solid stool can be maneuvered into the portion to be removed to decrease the amount of stool burden proximal to your anastomosis. It must be remembered that the data regarding colonic resection and bowel preparation do not apply to situations where the bowel is obstructed. The intestine proximal to an obstruction is typically dilated and congested, and I feel that anastomosis to such a segment of bowel is dangerous. If the bowel is resected back to healthy small bowel, an anastomosis can still be considered. A bypass may also be considered if the mass is unable to be removed.

If the mass is extraluminal and not causing obstruction, biopsy should be performed to determine the nature of the problem as well as to determine the presence of possible malignancy. Removal can be considered if the risks do not seem excessive. In addition to adenocarcinoma, other less frequent findings on biopsy include endometriosis (which will be discussed later), carcinoid, desmoid, lymphoma, and necrotic tissue (such as a lymph node). Carcinoid frequently involves the appendix or terminal ileum. Resection is frequently safe and advisable for carcinoid tumors. Remember that ileal carcinoids are often multiple, so careful examination of the adjacent bowel is advisable. Desmoid tumors are seen most frequently in patients with familial adenomatous polyposis and can involve the mesentery or the abdominal wall. My general approach to desmoids would be not to resect. Smaller lesions on the abdominal wall may be safely removed, but with nonobstructing smaller lesions involving the mesentery, the first line of therapy is often medical with sulindac and anti-estrogens. Larger desmoids may be difficult to remove safely due to the involvement of mesenteric vessels and often result in significant portions of bowel being resected. These are best treated with chemotherapy [12].

Isolated gastrointestinal lymphomas rarely cause obstruction or perforation due to their pliable nature and most often present with acute abdominal pain. They should be resected for potential cure, staging information, and avoidance of complications. A recent review of primary small bowel and colonic lymphoma showed that small bowel lymphoma did benefit from postoperative chemotherapy. Colorectal lymphoma on the other hand did not show a significant difference with chemotherapy or surgery alone as most required surgery for complications or diagnosis [13]. Necrotic lymph node tissue may need to be debrided, but does not need to be resected to clear margins. This may be an indication for a drain.

Colonic Inflammation

Key concept: Many inflammatory conditions can be treated medically, while perforations should be repaired at the time.

These consultations usually arise in the setting of pelvic surgery, typically gynecological or urologic procedures. They may also arise in the setting of right lower quadrant pain and immunosuppression. The sigmoid or descending colon may be noted to have inflammation or be adhered significantly to structures of interest to the requesting surgeon. It is important to note that inflammation of the colon in the face of diverticulosis may be related to a variety of colitides that may best be treated medically. Therefore, inflammation of the colon, by itself, is not an indication for resection. Purulence is often encountered. Most of these patients have been asymptomatic as far as episodes of acute diverticulitis are concerned. A detailed history, if available, is helpful in these situations. This is often not readily available, and discussions with family members may or may not yield any additional clinical information.

In general, simply following sound surgical principles applies. A perforation associated with diverticular disease can be identified with air insufflation by inserting a rigid proctoscope and examining the air-filled bowel with saline in the pelvis. If no air leak is identified and there is minimal to no contamination, often times the diverticulitis can be observed with appropriate antibiotic coverage. This may be combined with intra-abdominal drains depending on the comfort level of the operating surgeon. In the face of perforation without gross contamination, a resection with primary anastomosis can be performed [14]. A proximal diverting stoma, colostomy, or loop ileostomy may be added depending on the condition of the patient and the bowel.

Right lower quadrant pain can also mimic other disease states of an inflammatory nature. General surgeons operating for appendicitis often encounter these situations. The finding of diverticulitis of the right colon or appendix is rarely diagnosed correctly preoperatively, with most patients being diagnosed with appendicitis. Appendectomy with or without diverticulectomy followed by antibiotics is appropriate for inflammation of a diverticulum. If there is localized abscess, perforation, or concern for cancer, a right hemicolectomy is the procedure of choice [15].

Another difficult situation is the patient with right lower quadrant pain, neutropenia, and, sometimes, even sepsis. Oftentimes in neutropenic enterocolitis, the most difficult decision is when to take the patient to the operating room, and if you are being consulted intraoperatively, this decision has already been made. Most literature is based on retrospective case series, but do show a trend toward improved outcomes with surgery. Most authors recommend a right hemicolectomy as the mucosal injury can be more extensive than the serosal surface reveals. An end ileostomy with mucous fistula would be the safest approach in this situation involving immunosuppression and potential sepsis [16].

Cancer and Polyps

Key concept: Proper lesion location and adherence to oncologic principles such as en bloc resection is imperative. Other situations may be best handled by closing the patient and obtaining appropriate staging information.

Several issues can arise in operations for malignant processes of the colon and rectum. A common intraoperative consult is the call for assistance in locating a mass. In the colon, this can occur if the lesion was not tattooed or the endoscopist experienced looping of the scope resulting in inaccurate localization. The difficulty in identifying distal lesions of the large bowel may be the variation that can occur with measurements obtained by flexible versus rigid instruments. If the operating surgeon did not confirm the location prior to the abdominal operation, the first step is to place the patient into low lithotomy and examine thoroughly with a finger, rigid proctoscope, or even a flexible sigmoidoscope or colonoscope depending on the likely location of the mass. If the operation is being done laparoscopically, it may be prudent to convert to a hand-assisted or open technique. Intraoperative colonoscopy may be difficult in a laparoscopic procedure due to massive distention of the colon. In a hand-assisted operation, it may be possible to pass the scope through the colon with minimal insufflation. Then, short segments of the colon can be insufflated and decompressed with the aid of the intra-abdominal hand. CO_2 insufflation has been described, but may be difficult to setup unless you have worked out the details of the technique in advance. Also, the CO_2 absorbs more rapidly than room air, but still may keep the bowel distended making resection more difficult. Methodical palpation of the colon can also aid in locating the mass. Once the lesion is identified, you may have finished your consultation. If, on the other hand, the lesion is not identified even after these maneuvers, it may be prudent to close the patient and reevaluate at a later date.

Another circumstance which may arise is the cancer that is located much lower in the rectum than the operating surgeon expected, and he/she is not comfortable performing the resection at that level. This becomes a situation in which (unless you are consulted by your partner or someone in your rounding group) you must become the primary surgeon and decision-maker. Standard principles for resection of rectal cancer should apply, and the need for neoadjuvant therapy should be considered. It may be best to close the abdomen and refer the patient for neoadjuvant therapy if this has not been done. This decision should be made before mobilizing the rectum since a second attempt at mobilization is much more difficult and dangerous. If the staging of the rectal tumor is not clear, intraoperative ultrasound can be performed to assist in determining if the patient would be a candidate for such therapy. This may be a situation where you may wish to discuss the case with the family prior to going forward with any intervention and fully discuss the risks and benefits of the indicated procedure.

Another common issue that arises is the presence of cancer in other organs that unexpectedly appears to be invading the large or small bowel. This can occur with urologists when operating on the bladder or prostate as well as with gynecologists operating for pelvic tumors (Fig. 30.4). Less common is for a right colon cancer to invade either the duodenum or pancreas (or vice versa). It is key to understand the typical behavior of the primary cancer, the type of preoperative therapy that has been given, and the expected outcome of therapy. If the surgery is for palliation and resection of the bowel would involve major vessels or other substantial morbidity, it may be prudent to opt instead for a bypass procedure or diversion. If the patient is healthy and the resection is for cure in a field that has not been radiated, an en bloc resection of the primary tumor and adjacent organs should be the goal. These situations will be widely variable, but using your best surgical judgment and following sound surgical principles will achieve the best results.

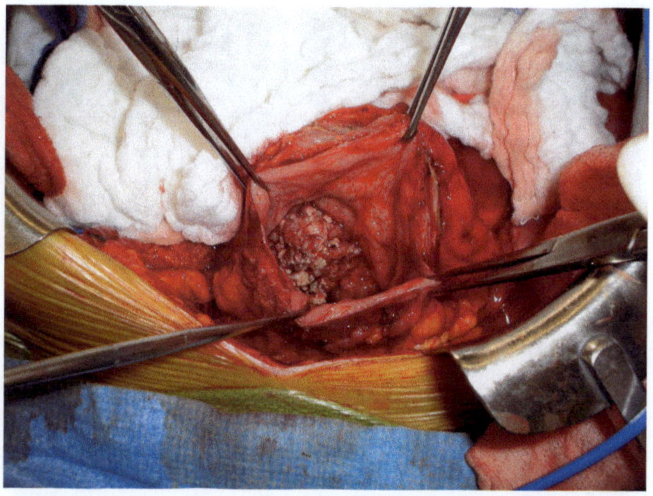

Fig. 30.4 Rectosigmoid cancer invading the bladder (Courtesy of Philip Y. Pearson, MD)

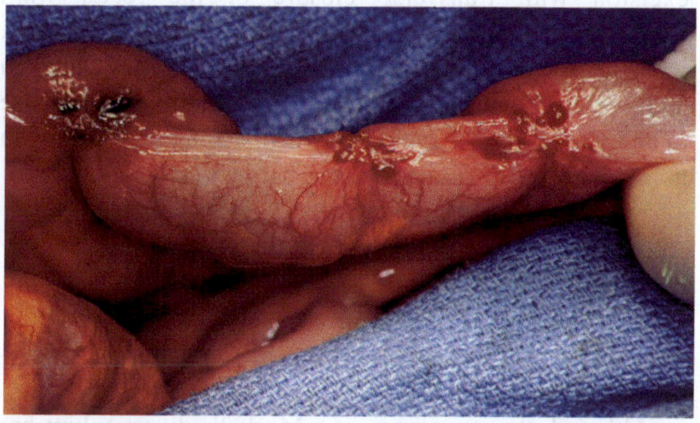

Fig. 30.5 Endometriosis implants on the small bowel and cecum

Endometriosis

Key concept: Resect all visible disease with a disc excision or segmental resection when possible.

As colorectal surgeons, we work closely with gynecologists and especially those with an interest in endometriosis. It is not uncommon to be asked to evaluate a lesion that cannot be differentiated from bowel malignancy. Endometriosis can appear as small, pigmented peritoneal nodules or firm fibrotic masses of the bowel that mimic cancer (Fig. 30.5). It rarely invades into the mucosa, but can present as a partial obstruction due to mass effect or scarring. It has been shown that aggressive management of gastrointestinal endometriosis is safe and produces good long-term outcomes for patients in terms of reduction of symptoms and ability to conceive [17]. Our recommended approach is to attempt to resect all visible and palpable disease. This is typically done in conjunction with the gynecologist who will manage the ovarian and peritoneal implants. Bowel involvement can be managed with either disc excision or segmental resection. Unless the peritoneal implants on the bowel are very small and superficial, we do not favor partial-thickness excision. The technique is frequently bloody and may leave disease behind. For extensive cul-de-sac disease, low anterior resection can be performed safely [17]. Smaller rectal lesions may be removed by disc

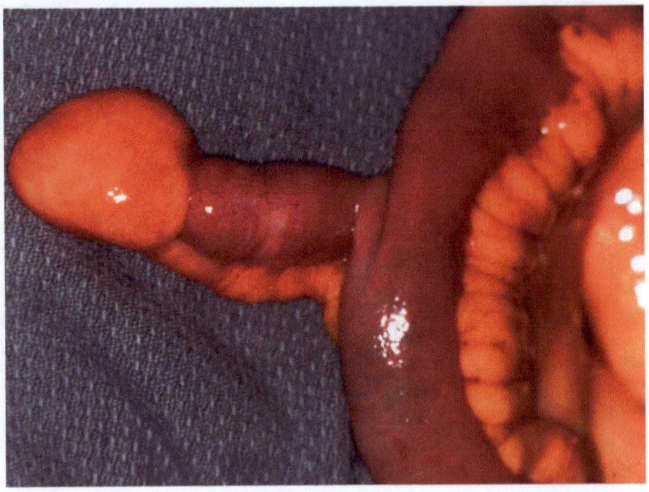

Fig. 30.6 Meckel's diverticulum (Courtesy of W. Brian Sweeney, MD)

excision with transverse closure of the rectal wall. Depending on the expertise of the consulting gynecologist, if the disease is extensive, biopsy of a lesion may be taken and a referral made to a gynecologist with greater expertise in endometriosis. Treatment may involve medical therapy in combination with further elective surgery [18].

Meckel's Diverticulum

Key concept: While debatable, resection of a Meckel's diverticulum is often warranted.

Although the prevalence of a Meckel's diverticulum has been shown to be lower than originally thought, at just 1.23 %, the surgical management of this often incidental finding has recently been challenged [19]. The findings associated with a diverticulum can range from an asymptomatic, incidental discovery to that of bleeding, obstruction, and even tumor involving the diverticulum (Fig. 30.6). The most recent literature supports its removal as it has been shown that the incidence of ileal cancer is higher in patients with a Meckel's diverticulum than in those who do not have a diverticulum [20].

Presacral Bleeding

Key concept: You should be familiar with several methods to aid in hemostasis for severe pelvic bleeding.

This situation may be one that you also encounter in your own patients. Presacral bleeding can be life threatening and lead to substantial morbidity if measures are not taken to quickly and effectively manage the situation. Several techniques exist to help with hemostasis, but the more commonly employed methods of electrocautery and suture ligation have the potential of making the bleeding worse. This is a situation where packing and appropriate preparation of the operative team is a crucial first step. Once blood products are available and the operative and anesthesia teams are prepared and perhaps the incision are enlarged to improve exposure, slow removal of the packs will allow for visualization of the area in question. Sterile thumbtacks have been shown to be an effective method to control bleeding. These are pushed through the usually thin bony table of the sacrum directly over the site of bleeding. Muscle "welding" has also been shown in small case series to be a safe, readily available, and highly effective technique. This method involves taking a 2×2 cm piece of free rectus muscle and compressing it against the area of sacral bleeding with a forceps. Electrocautery is then applied to the muscle to create a coagulum that occludes the venous bleeding [21, 22]. Several new hemostatic agents are also available. In cases of massive ongoing bleeding, packing the pelvis and transferring the patient to an ICU for correction of coagulopathy can be an invaluable maneuver. Re-exploration 24–48 h later usually reveals that the bleeding has ceased.

Ischemic Bowel

Key concept: Clinical evaluation and adjunctive tests aid in assessing the viability of bowel to determine if resection is warranted.

During the course of difficult dissection, a blood vessel feeding the bowel may be injured requiring ligation for control. You may be called to evaluate the viability of a segment of bowel and give your opinion on management. Initial evaluation should include looking at the color of the serosal surface, the presence of bowel peristalsis, and pulsation or bleeding from the marginal arteries. These observations can often be misleading, and other methods to determine if resection is in order and how much to resect may be needed. Additional techniques described include the use of fluorescence or Doppler ultrasound. Fluorescence encompasses two techniques, that of perfusion fluorometry and laser fluorescence angiography (LFA). Both involve injecting sodium fluorescein or indocyanine green intravenously and then evaluating the bowel with either a Wood's lamp or laser light. A single study reports that the use of intraoperative LFA reduced the risk of revision due to anastomotic leakage by 60 % in patients undergoing elective colorectal surgery regardless of their age (and by 64 % in patients above the age of 70) [23]. The technique is, however, not widely available. We have no personal experience with LFA. The use of Doppler ultrasound to detect signals on the antimesenteric portion of the bowel can be helpful. Doppler ultrasound was evaluated in a recent series of 200 patients undergoing colorectal resections and showed only 1 % incidence of anastomotic insufficiency [24, 25]. Often, the equipment available will determine the method employed.

If, after all of these interventions, you are still unable to determine if the bowel is viable, temporary closure and re-evaluation in 12–24 h may allow better definition of nonviable bowel. For ostomies that appear ischemic, resection back to healthy bleeding tissue is required as these rarely improve after leaving the operating room.

Vaginal Delivery Complications

Key concept: Early repair may aid in repair of sphincter injuries following childbirth.

During vaginal deliveries, third- and fourth-degree injuries involve the anal sphincter complex. Colorectal surgeons have the detailed knowledge of the anatomy of the anal canal, but rarely see the injuries acutely. This lends itself to a multidisciplinary approach [26]. You may be called for these consultations when the obstetrician has found a deformity with which he/she is uncomfortable dealing. It is my personal preference to be called early about these injuries involving the sphincters and rectal wall because I think that the tissues are healthier and that the planes are easier to identify. Contrary to my preference for dealing with the injuries acutely, it has been shown that if the repairs are done within 72 h or at 14 days, there are not any differences in the long-term functional outcome [27]. There are typically two types of injuries. There are lacerations that involve only the sphincter muscles, and there are traumatic disruptions that lead to complete avulsion of the rectovaginal septum resulting in a traumatic cloaca. For the simpler sphincter injuries, two approaches have been identified: end-to-end repair and overlapping repair. These are performed with interrupted sutures approximating the ends of the muscle in four quadrants or overlapping the sphincter mechanism. Studies have not shown any difference in long-term outcomes with either repair [28]. It has been shown that the incidence of fecal incontinence is higher in women if the internal sphincter is not repaired [29]. If we are called to the delivery suite, I make a point of demonstrating the IS to the obstetrician (and residents) as I repair it separately. The internal sphincter (IS) is typically identified as (white) muscle tissue beneath the mucosa and separate from the external sphincter. I repair the IS with interrupted Vicryl suture. My management of the anterior external sphincter is repair in an end-to-end fashion with interrupted PDS sutures. Overlapping is certainly acceptable. In the acute situation, it is rarely necessary to do much mobilization. The tissues are often quite lax in the puerperal perineum. Other considerations are the importance of bowel-specific antibiotics and performing the repair under optimal circumstances. The latter often requires moving the patient to an operating room with proper lighting, stirrups, and instruments. For the traumatic cloaca, some believe that it is best to allow these patients to heal over a 3- to 6-month period and then come back for repair once the inflammation has resolved and the tissues soften [30]. Again, I believe the tissues are easier to identify and work with at an earlier time frame. In addition, women with the cloaca-type injury are often miserable during the period of waiting. An enema program using a cone-tip irrigator (used for colostomy irrigation) or even fecal diversion may make their existence more tolerable.

Endoscopic Complications

Key concept: Endoscopic complications can often be treated endoscopically, though operative intervention may be required.

Complications of endoscopy include hemorrhage, perforation, and uncommon problems such as a snare imbedded into a polyp that cannot be removed. Bleeding can often be controlled with electrocautery, but this needs to be used with caution given the potential for ischemia and necrosis with delayed perforation. Additional methods include the placement of clips over the vessel and submucosal injection of epinephrine. Tattooing the area of bleeding, to allow rapid localization, can be invaluable if operative control becomes necessary. Bleeding that does not respond to local endoscopic techniques may require angiography with embolization. Perforation may be identified during the endoscopy by direct visualization of intra-abdominal contents. Tears can be noted in the mucosa which allow escape of air into the submucosa, creating the appearance of "bubbles." If the perforation is full thickness, placement of a clip for temporary control of contamination may be a useful technique. If the tear is not full thickness, you may observe the patient clinically. Localized perforations with minimal free air and localized peritoneal tenderness may be treated similarly to diverticulitis with antibiotics and careful observation. Due to bowel preparation prior to the colonoscopy, free perforation is usually associated with minimal contamination. It frequently requires operative intervention, but can usually be managed by primary closure, with or without resection. If bleeding or perforation occurs after polypectomy, it may be prudent to try to determine the histology of the polyp. If operation is necessary, it may be reasonable to perform an oncologic resection. Occasionally, an electrosurgical snare may become imbedded in a polyp and not cut completely through and be unable to be withdrawn. In my experience, this may occur with large submucosal lipomas that have very different conduction properties than "normal" polyps (Fig. 30.7). If additional pressure on the snare or use of short bursts of "cutting" current does not succeed in removal, it may be best to cut through the snare and leave it in the colon. This can be accomplished by using another instrument to push the snare out of the chan-

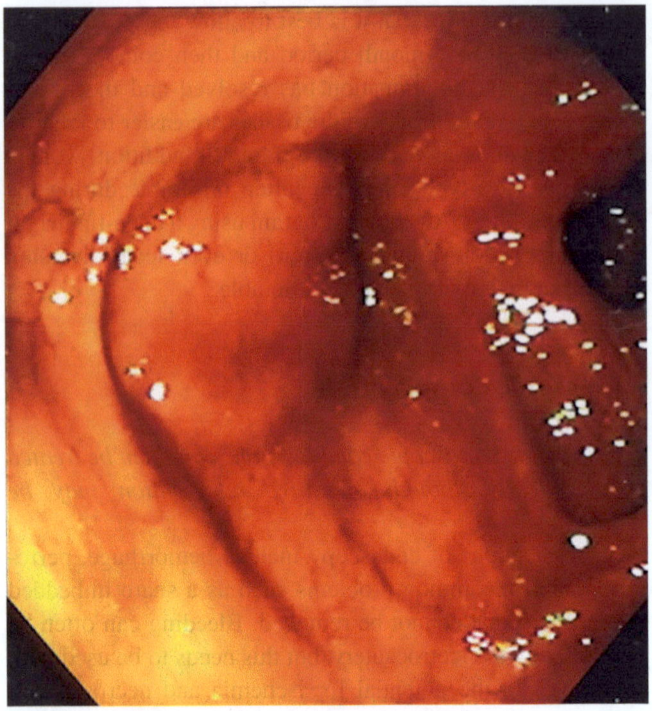

Fig. 30.7 Submucosal mass (i.e., lipoma) seen on endoscopy (Courtesy of Philip Y. Pearson, MD)

nel as the scope is removed. The plastic sheath can then usually be removed leaving only the wire. The patient can be observed in the hospital with a tug on the wire once or twice a day. After a few days, the wire will dislodge and be removed. The lesson to be learned from this type of experience is not to try to remove large lipomas with the snare!

Patients with Inflammatory Bowel Disease

Key concept: Resection is often required for patients with Crohn's disease. Pay attention to the status of any secondarily involved organs as they may require intervention.

The diagnosis of right lower quadrant pain often leads to an appendectomy, but the findings can be unexpected and result in a consultation with a colorectal surgeon. If an appendix is noted to be normal, but the terminal ileum is noted to be inflamed, the decision about how to proceed centers on the appearance of the colon. If the appendico-cecal junction is normal, an appendectomy should be performed and the patient referred for postoperative medical management of presumed Crohn's disease. If the colon is inflamed as well, there are two options. If the disease is limited and the patient is not extremely ill, there may be a role for closure and medical treatment. If the patient has extensive disease and is experiencing significant clinical symptoms, resection of this area is indicated (Fig. 30.8). In terms of the configuration of the

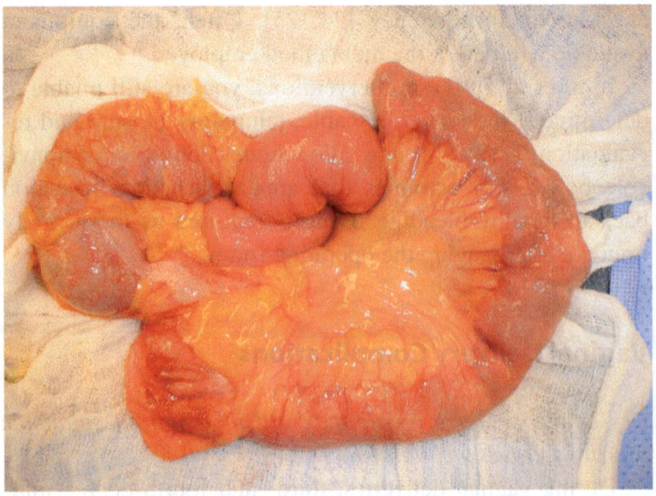

Fig. 30.8 Crohn's stricture at the terminal ileum (left lower portion of picture; Courtesy of Philip Y. Pearson, MD)

anastomosis, it has been shown in a randomized trial that there were no differences in leak or complication rates with a side-to-side stapled versus a hand-sewn end-to-end anastomosis [31]. Most would agree that with abnormally thickened bowel, hand-sewn techniques are safer than staplers. In addition, the configuration of the anastomosis has not been shown to influence peri-anastomotic recurrence [32].

Crohn's disease can also involve other areas of the colon, such as the sigmoid colon, through fistulous communication. Operative conduct depends on the degree of inflammation in the bystander organ. If the amount of inflammation is minimal, disc excision of the fistulous communication with primary closure can be done. Segmental resection of the ileal or ileocecal disease then follows. If there is significant inflammation of the sigmoid, a double resection to reach grossly normal appearing (and feeling) tissue at the resection margins may be required.

Intraoperative Conditions

Laparoscopic Approach Desired

Some surgeons focus on the initial approach of their surgery, be it laparoscopic or robotic, and may be concerned about giving the patient a significant incision. This is an issue that has to be discussed early in the consultation. If I feel that I cannot do what is necessary without making a larger incision, I would offer the surgeon the opportunity to get another consultant. It may also be important to discuss the issue of making a larger incision with the patient's family. They know the patient well, and there may be ramifications if they wake up with an incision larger than expected. It is best to include as many people possible in this discussion.

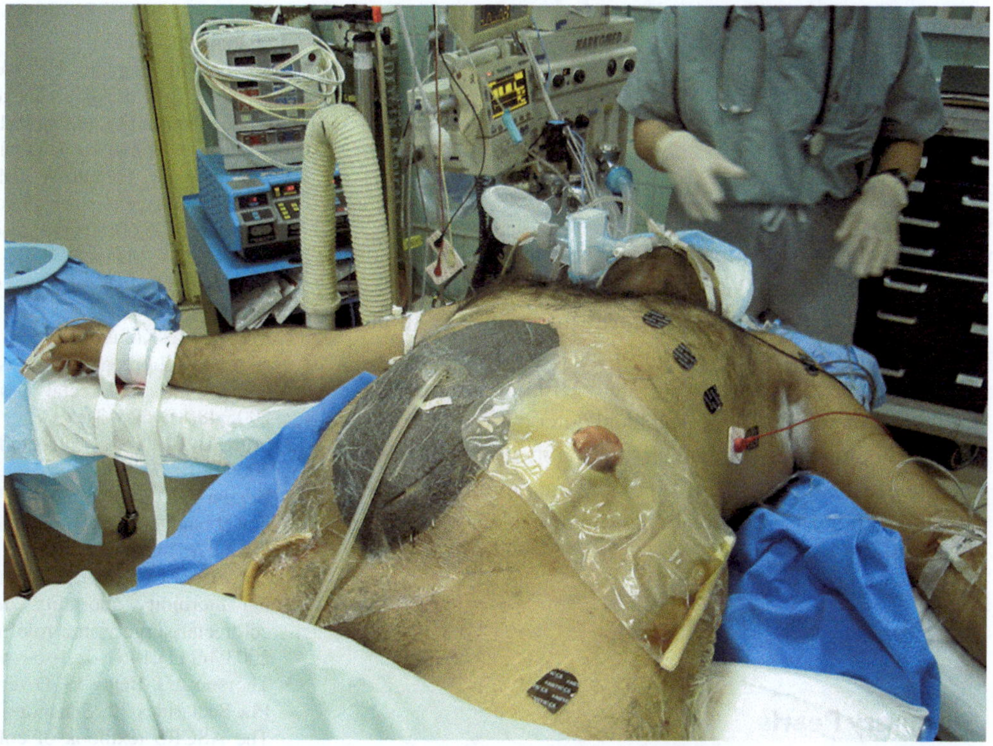

Fig. 30.9 Temporary closure of an open abdomen with a negative pressure device (Courtesy of Matthew J. Martin, MD)

Not Marked for a Stoma

Key concept: Plan ahead when considering a stoma and do whatever maneuvers you can to place it in the best possible location.

If you have any concern that a stoma may be required, this is something that you should mention early on in your consultation. If the requesting surgeon thinks you should be able to avoid a stoma altogether and you disagree, a similar discussion as mentioned previously should be undertaken. Discussion with the family is also of extreme importance. If the decision is made to proceed and the patient has not been marked preoperatively, attention to aspects of creating a proper stoma should be followed. Inspection of the abdomen should be undertaken to avoid scars, skin creases, and other disorders of the skin including psoriasis. Although difficult, it is possible to sit the patient upright on the operating table to observe the abdominal creases. This becomes especially important in an obese patient to avoid the stoma being hidden below a large pannus or in a valley. Stomas should be placed through the rectus sheath to reduce the incidence of hernia formation [33]. Siting a stoma in the umbilicus is another alternative described by Raza and colleagues [34].

Damage Control: How Do You Bail?

There will be situations where the pathology encountered is so complex, the patient is not doing well, or the bowel has become too edematous and you will need to make a decision to control the situation as best possible. If there are multiple areas of injured bowel, these will typically need to be resected or closed to prevent further contamination. The "damage control" approach used in trauma may be applicable. The injured intestine can be removed and the ends closed with staples or umbilical tape, leaving the bowel in discontinuity for return when the patient is stable. The abdomen can be closed quickly using a negative pressure device and the "open abdomen" technique (Fig. 30.9). Additional methods of managing intestinal injury are exteriorization or tube drainage. Injuries can be brought up through the incision, or a tube can be placed into the bowel and brought out through the abdominal wall.

Communication with Family

The intraoperative consult frequently leads to other issues outside the operating room. Due to the fact that the operative consent likely did not encompass the procedure you were called to perform, informed consent must be addressed. Unless the patient is unstable or my role primarily involves adhesiolysis, I attempt to breakout and meet with the patient's family. I explain the situation, what my plans are, and the risks of the proposed operation. At this juncture it is important to focus on doing the right thing for the patient. Once the case is complete and you know the extent of what you needed to do and the implications of the unplanned operation, you can address further concerns. They may have questions about what happened and if this was a mistake. This is also true when talking with the patient. It is important to try and give the consulting surgeon as much credit as is reasonable and still be honest with the patient and family. Be courteous to the consulting surgeon as you are now on a team taking care of the patient.

Legal Issues and Documentation

In terms of documentation and legal issues, the previous discussion still holds. Clearly explain the circumstances surrounding your consultation. Give the primary surgeon recognition for the observation of an issue that was out of his/her scope of practice, and state without judgment the findings. Sometimes a less than ideal outcome is due to either something that you do which does not succeed or your inability to fix the problem. When the outcome is poor, continue to be honest, and explain the situation clearly accepting responsibility for some of the outcome when appropriate. Above all else, do the safe thing for the patient regardless of the concerns of the primary surgeon.

Summary Pearls

The ability to properly manage consultations that occur during another surgeon's case makes you an invaluable resource. There are many unusual and unique circumstances that can present, but with proper identification of the problem and adherence to the surgical principles you have learned, most can be appropriately and safely managed. Communication with the requesting surgeon and the family is very important and will help achieve the best outcome for the patient.

References

1. Bratzler DW, Hunt DR. The Surgical Infection Prevention and Surgical Care Improvement Projects: national initiatives to improve outcomes for patients having surgery. Clin Infect Dis. 2006;43: 322–30.
2. Burch JC, Horace TL, Bradley CF. A clinical evaluation of Cherney's incision. Ann Surg. 1948;127(5):830–5.
3. Karakousis CP. Surgical treatment of locally progressive stage IIIB carcinoma of the cervix: use of the inverted "T" incision. Eur J Obstet Gynecol Reprod Biol. 2004;115(2):216–8.
4. Nanni G, Tondolo V, Citterio F, Romagnoli J, Borgetti M, Boldrini G, et al. Comparison of oblique versus hockey-stick surgical incision for kidney transplantation. Transplant Proc. 2005;37(6): 2479–81.
5. Egorov VI, Schastlivtsev IV, Prut EV, Baranov AO, Turusov RA. Mechanical properties of the human gastrointestinal tract. J Biomech. 2002;35(10):1417–25.
6. Box GN, Lee HJ, Abraham JB, Deane LA, Santos RJ, Elchico ER, et al. Evaluation of the outcomes of electrosurgical induced bowel injury treated with tissue glue/sealant versus sutured repair in a rabbit model. J Endourol. 2009;23(3):535–40.
7. O'Keefe SJ, Buchman AL, Fishbein TM, Jeejeebhoy KN, Jeppesen PB, Shaffer J. Short bowel syndrome and intestinal failure: consensus definitions and overview. Clin Gastroenterol Hepatol. 2006;4(1):6–10.
8. Sharpe JP, Magnotti LJ, Weinberg JA, Parks NA, Maish GO, Shahan CP, et al. Adherence to a simplified management algorithm reduces morbidity and mortality after penetrating colon injuries: a 15-year experience. J Am Coll Surg. 2012;214(4):591–7.
9. Weinberg JA, Fabian TC, Magnotti LJ, et al. Penetrating rectal trauma: management by anatomic distinction improves outcome. J Trauma. 2006;60:508–13; discussion 513–14.
10. Güenaga KF, Matos D, Wille-Jørgensen P. Mechanical bowel preparation for elective colorectal surgery. Cochrane Database Syst Rev. 2011;(9):CD001544.
11. Mahajna A, Krausz M, Rosin D, Shabtai M, Hershko D, Ayalon A, et al. Bowel preparation is associated with spillage of bowel contents in colorectal surgery. Dis Colon Rectum. 2005;48(8):1626–31.
12. Sturt NJ, Clark SK. Current ideas in desmoid tumours. Fam Cancer. 2006;5(3):275–85.
13. Beaton C, Davies M, Beynon J. The management of primary small bowel and colon lymphoma – a review. Int J Colorectal Dis. 2012;27(5):555–63.
14. Zorcolo L, Covotta L, Carlomagno N, Bartolo DC. Toward lowering morbidity, mortality, and stoma formation in emergency colorectal surgery: the role of specialization. Dis Colon Rectum. 2003;46(11):1461–7; discussion 1467–8.
15. Thorson AG, Beaty JS. Diverticular disease. In: Beck DE, Roberts PL, Saclarides TJ, Senagore TJ, Stamos MJ, Wexner SD, editors. The ASCRS textbook of colon and rectal surgery. 2nd ed. New York: Springer; 2011. p. 375–93.
16. Machado NO. Neutropenic enterocolitis: a continuing medical and surgical challenge. N Am J Med Sci. 2010;2(7):293–300.
17. Bailey HR, Ott MT, Hartendorp P. Aggressive surgical management for advanced colorectal endometriosis. Dis Colon Rectum. 1994;37(8):747–53.
18. Yap C, Furness S, Farquhar C. Pre and post operative medical therapy for endometriosis surgery. Cochrane Database Syst Rev. 2004;(3):CD003678.
19. Zani A, Eaton S, Rees CM, et al. Incidentally detected Meckel diverticulum: to resect or not to resect? Ann Surg. 2008;247(2):276–81.
20. Thirunavukarasu P, Sathaiah M, Sukumar S, Bartels CJ, Zeh 3rd H, Lee KK, et al. Meckel's diverticulum – a high-risk region for malignancy in the ileum. Insights from a population-based epidemiological study and implications in surgical management. Ann Surg. 2011;253(2):223–30.
21. Nivatvongs S, Fang DT. The use of thumbtacks to stop massive presacral hemorrhage. Dis Colon Rectum. 1986;29(9): 589–90.
22. Harrison JL, Hooks VH, Pearl RK, Cheape JD, Lawrence MA, Orsay CP. Muscle fragment welding for control of massive presacral bleeding during rectal mobilization: a review of eight cases. Dis Colon Rectum. 2003;46(8):1115–7.
23. Kudszus S, Roesel C, Schachtrupp A, Höer JJ. Intraoperative laser fluorescence angiography in colorectal surgery: a noninvasive analysis to reduce the rate of anastomotic leakage. Langenbecks Arch Surg. 2010;395(8):1025–30.
24. Ambrosetti P, Robert J, Mathey P, Rohner A. Left-sided colon and colorectal anastomoses: Doppler ultrasound as an aid to assess bowel vascularization. A prospective evaluation of 200 consecutive elective cases. Int J Colorectal Dis. 1994;9(4):211–4.
25. Urbanavičius L, Pattyn P, de Putte DV, Venskutonis D. How to assess intestinal viability during surgery: a review of techniques. World J Gastrointest Surg. 2011;3(5):59–69.
26. Cook TA, Keane D, Mortensen NJ. Is there a role for the colorectal team in the management of acute severe third-degree vaginal tears? Colorectal Dis. 1999;1:263–6.

27. Soerensen MM, Bek KM, Buntzen S, Højberg KE, Laurberg S. Long-term outcome of delayed primary or early secondary reconstruction of the anal sphincter after obstetrical injury. Dis Colon Rectum. 2008;51(3):312–7.
28. Farrell SA. Overlapping compared with end-to-end repair of third and fourth-degree obstetric anal sphincter tears. Curr Opin Obstet Gynecol. 2011;23(5):386–90.
29. Siddighi S, et al. Effects of an educational workshop on performance of 4th degree perineal laceration repair, Obstet Gynecol. 2007;109:289–94.
30. Venkatesh KS, Ramanujam P. Surgical treatment of traumatic cloaca. Dis Colon Rectum. 1996;39(7):811–6.
31. McLeod RS, Wolff BG, Ross S, Parkes R, Investigators of the CAST Trial. Recurrence of Crohn's disease after ileocolic resection is not affected by anastomotic type: results of a multi-center, randomized, controlled trial. Dis Colon Rectum. 2009;52:919–27.
32. Simillis C, Purkayastha S, Yamamoto T, Strong SA, Darzi AW, Tekkis PP. A meta-analysis comparing conventional end-to-end anastomosis vs. other anastomotic configurations after resection in Crohn's disease. Dis Colon Rectum. 2007;50:1674–87.
33. Sands LR, Marchetti F. Intestinal stomas. In: Beck DE, Roberts PL, Saclarides TJ, Senagore TJ, Stamos MJ, Wexner SD, editors. The ASCRS textbook of colon and rectal surgery. 2nd ed. New York: Springer; 2011. p. 517–33.
34. Raza SD, Portin BA, Bernhoft WH. Umbilical colostomy: a better intestinal stoma. Dis Colon Rectum. 1977;20(3):223–30.

Laparoscopic Complications

31

Joongho Shin and Sang W. Lee

Key Points

- Understanding anatomy, tissue planes, the steps of the operation, and how to prevent potential complications associated with laparoscopic colectomy is critical.
- Having a consistent, systematic approach is essential in avoiding complications during laparoscopic colectomy.
- In re-operative laparoscopic colectomy, early proactive conversion is likely to result in favorable outcome. Reactive conversion in response to intraoperative complications should be avoided.

Introduction

Key Concept: Whether you are early in your learning curve or performing more complex cases laparoscopically, you need to be aware of the potential complications and how to manage them.

Now that we have multiple large randomized controlled clinical trials clearly demonstrating equivalent oncologic and superior perioperative outcomes after laparoscopic colectomies, more colectomies are being performed laparoscopically [1, 2]. Despite proven benefits of laparoscopic colectomy, only about 20–30 % of all elective colon resections are being performed laparoscopically in the United States [3]. Although multiple factors contribute to this tepid gain, a steep learning curve remains as one of the most important factors.

As "novice" laparoscopic colon surgeons embark on mastering the skills of laparoscopic colon surgery, it is crucial that they are cognizant of common complications associated with a laparoscopic approach. It is not only important to immediately recognize complications and appropriately treat them when they do occur, but also it is imperative to have a consistent and systematic approach to each case in order to avoid them.

In this chapter, we will review most commonly encountered, as well as unique, complications, which are associated with laparoscopic colon surgery. In addition, we will outline a systematic approach that focuses on steps to avoid common pitfalls that can lead to potential complications.

Tips to Avoiding Complications at the Beginning

Positioning

Key Concept: Ideal positioning provides an optimal surgical access while minimizing a risk of injury to the patients.

Our preference is to place all patients in the modified lithotomy position with both arms tucked to the sides. This provides an excellent access, which allows surgeons to work in line with the pathology and avoids any confusion among OR staff members about positioning. By resting both arms to the sides of the patients, crush injury to digits can occur during replacement of the leg section of the table. We use a combination of a Kerlix bandage roll, an arm board, and a protective wrap (pediatric diapers) around the hands and wrists to protect fingers and to avoid hyperextension of the wrist (Fig. 31.1). According to American Society of Anesthesiologist Closed Claim Project database, perioperative nerve-related injuries are one of the most common

J. Shin, MD
Department of Surgery, New York-Presbyterian/Weill Cornell Medical Center, New York, NY, USA
e-mail: jos9071@med.cornell.edu

S.W. Lee, MD, FACS, FASCRS (✉)
Department of Surgery, Division of Colon and Rectal Surgery, Weill Cornell Medical College, 525 East 68th Street, 172, New York, NY 10065, USA
e-mail: sal2013@med.cornell.edu

Electronic supplementary material The online version of this chapter (doi: 10.1007/978-1-4614-9022-7_31) contains supplementary material, which is available to authorized users. Videos can also be accessed at http://www.springerimages.com/videos/978-1-4614-9021-0.

S.R. Steele et al. (eds.), *Complexities in Colorectal Surgery*,
DOI 10.1007/978-1-4614-9022-7_31, © Springer Science+Business Media New York 2014

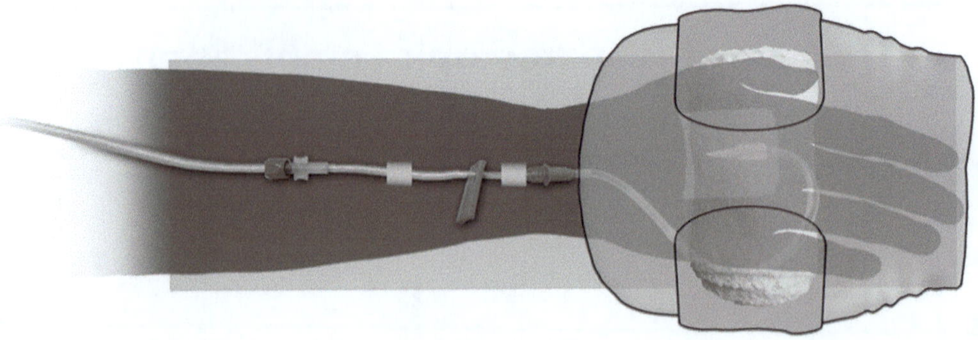

Fig. 31.1 Protecting hands with Kerlix roll and diaper

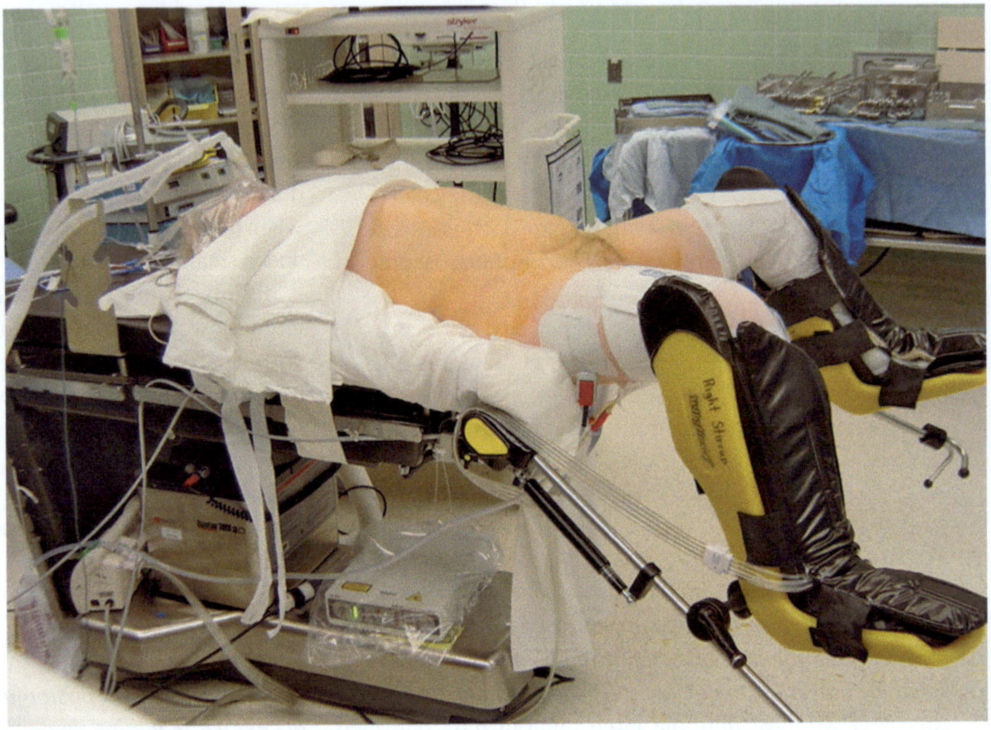

Fig. 31.2 Patient positioning. Notice the padding and the degree of flexion at the hip

complications related to positioning [4]. Careful positioning and padding can prevent injuries to upper extremities caused by stretching or compression.

The angle between the body and the thighs of the patients should be kept at near 180°, in order to avoid clashing of instruments with patient's thighs when working in the upper quadrants of the abdomen (Fig. 31.2). Care should be taken to avoid hyperextension of the legs at the hips, which can lead to damage to the sciatic and obturator nerves. This is best avoided by lowering both legs to the appropriate level without hyperextending them before draping the patients; a blind positioning of the legs after draping can potentially cause injury.

Dealing with the Small Bowel

Key Concept: Gravity is your friend in keeping the small bowel out of the way and often requires steep changes in position.

Gaining an adequate exposure away from the small intestines can be a challenge. In general, the working quadrant of the abdomen should be positioned higher than the other quadrants, so that the small intestines fall away from the operative field (Fig. 31.3). Although extreme positioning with routine use of a beanbag and tapes can be helpful, this time-consuming and cumbersome practice is not necessary, though admittedly up to individual surgeon preference. More

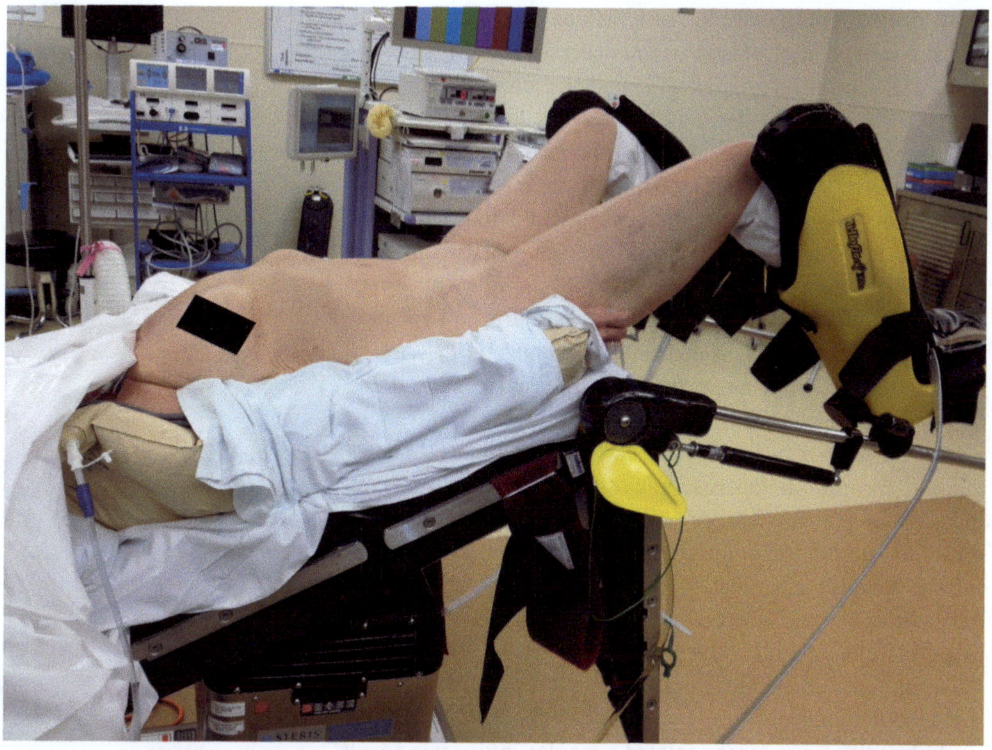

Fig. 31.3 Steep positioning will allow gravity to move the small bowel out of the way when working in the pelvis

often, a commonly available gel pad placed on the operating room table provides enough support and traction to keep the patients from sliding in almost all instances. The use of shoulder braces, which can cause brachial nerve injury, should be avoided. In cases where gravity and positioning are not enough, placing an additional retractor, a moist gauze pad placed through a larger trocar, a moist laparotomy pad, or a radiologically tagged surgical towel placed through a hand-access incision can be helpful in retracting the small intestines away from the field [5].

Trocar- and Instrument-Related Injuries

Key Concept: Not only can poor trocar placement lead to a more difficult operation, but trocar and instrument-related injuries (though rare) can lead to overt or missed injuries to almost all intra-abdominal structures with devastating consequences.

Trocar-related injuries might occur regardless of the type of entry method used. Overall, the incidence of bowel injury during laparoscopy is relatively small (0.13 %). According to a meta-analysis performed by Van der Voort and colleagues [6], the most common site of bowel injury caused by trocar insertion is the small intestines (55 %) followed by the colon (38 %). Small bowel injury during laparoscopic surgery may happen in several ways: (1) Veress needle injury, (2) thermal injury, (3) crush injury, or (4) laceration by laparoscopic instrument or ports. Thermal injury can occur by either lateral thermal spread or stray currents generating heat along the path between the active and the ground electrodes (Video 31.1). Lateral thermal spread is less of a concern for bipolar energy device. In a study using porcine muscles, only the monopolar energy device increased the temperature of the tissue higher than the safe level of 42 °C when measured 1 cm away from the tip of the instruments on 5–15 s applications [7]. More importantly, for all different types of energy devices (monopolar, bipolar, ultrasonic), the tip remained above the safe temperature (42 °C) for several seconds. After 5-s application at highest settings, it took monopolar diathermy, ultrasonic, and bipolar device, 35, 10, and 5 s, respectively, for tips to cool down below the safe working temperature. In general, it is a safe practice to minimize the use of monopolar diathermy in laparoscopic colectomy and to not touch any surrounding tissues with energy devices immediately after prolonged energy activation. Inadvertent currents can spread by either insulation failure or by direct coupling [8]. Direct coupling occurs when an energy device touches another metallic instrument. To avoid and detect inadvertent energy device-induced thermal injury, it is important to keep the entire length of the instrument in laparoscopic view during energy application whenever it is possible. Additionally, use of plastic trocars (versus older metal trocars) will minimize the risk of capacitive coupling.

A crush injury to the small intestines happens when a laparoscopic instrument, such as a bowel grasper, forcibly pulls in a loop of the small intestines into a trocar. In order to avoid this type of injury, the instrument should only be removed after a confirmation that the jaw of instrument is empty and closed. A penetrating injury to the small intestines can occur during a blind insertion of a sharp laparoscopic instrument. Laparoscopic instruments should be inserted in the ventral direction away from the internal organs under direct visualization. The instrument should not be advanced if any amount of resistance is encountered. Finally, one of the most common laparoscopic instrument injuries is an inadvertent serosal tear or wall injury from grasping the bowel too hard or tearing the bowel while "running" or moving the bowel. Unfortunately, this is often a missed injury as the instrument and affected bowel are off screen. To minimize this, you should always keep both instruments in plain view, along with gentle handling of the bowel with atraumatic bowel graspers.

Although rare, a trocar-related vascular injury can result in a fatal complication. In a review of 696,502 laparoscopic procedures [9], Azevedo et al., found the incidence of major vessel injury to be 0.006 %. In order to avoid a major vessel injury during closed entry, precaution and vigilance need to be maintained at all times. The patient should be in a flat supine position rather than the Trendelenburg position, as the latter decreases the distance between the sacral promontory and the abdominal wall, leading to an increase in the risk of major vessel injury. One of the ways to avoid potential complications related to Veress needle insertion is to limit its use in re-operative cases. An insertion technique which has worked very well for us is a technique in which we create a negative intraperitoneal pressure by pulling up on the stalk of umbilicus with a Kocher clamp while inserting a Veress needle through the base of the umbilicus, the thinnest portion of the abdominal wall. It is important to keep the stopcock of a Veress needle open to air during insertion, so that a rush of air into negatively pressured peritoneal cavity will cause the small intestines to fall away from the abdominal wall immediately upon entry (Fig. 31.4).

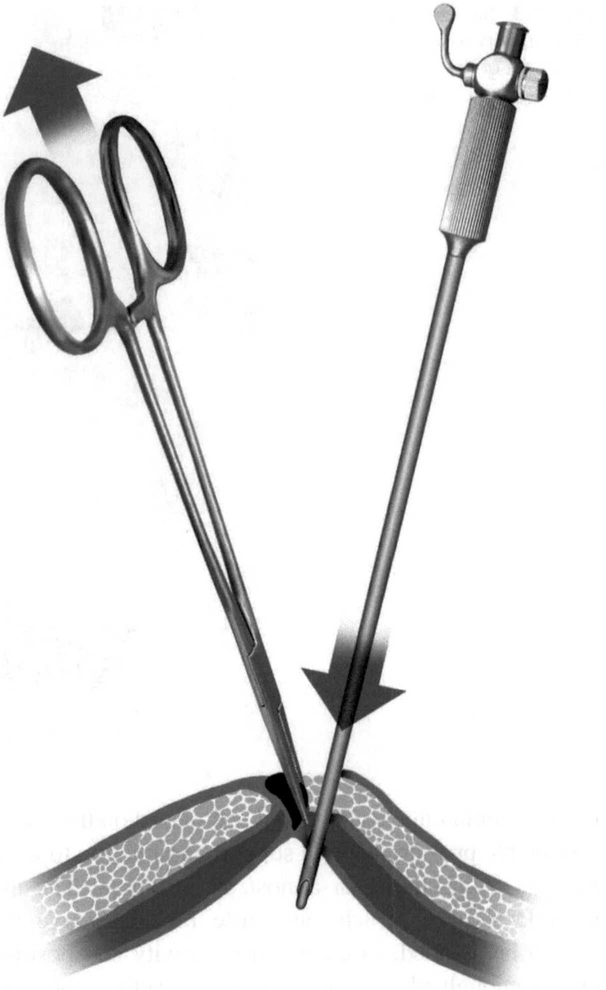

Fig. 31.4 Veress needle enters the thinnest portion of the abdominal wall, while negative pressure is being created by pulling up the umbilical stalk with Kocher clamp

Unique Complications: Right Colectomy

Key Concept: Right colectomy poses the potential for unique complications including damage to the duodenum, ileocolic/middle colic vessels, and right ureter. A systematic approach, knowledge of the pertinent anatomy, and achieving the correct plane of dissection from the start will keep you out of trouble.

Exposure

Obtaining an adequate exposure is a prerequisite to avoid complications in any types of surgery. To achieve this during laparoscopic right colectomy, the patient is placed in the Trendelenburg position with the right side of the patient tilted up. The transverse colon along with the greater omentum is retracted in the cephalad direction. Loops of the terminal ileum are gently swept into the pelvis, and the rest of small bowel is allowed to fall to the patient's left side. In difficult cases, use of moist gauze placed through a trocar can be helpful in retracting.

Identifying the Correct Dissection Plane

Embryologically, the colon starts as a midline structure. As the fetus develops, the colon rotates and fuses laterally to the retroperitoneum. The "white line" of Toldt

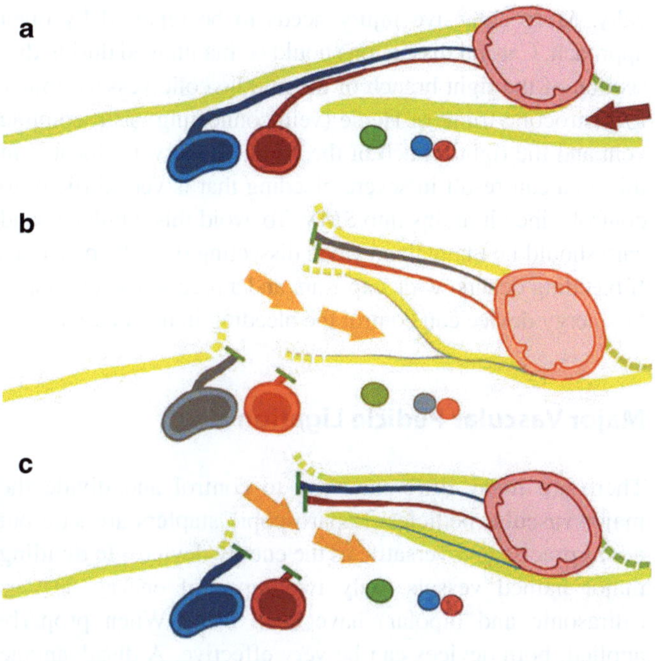

Fig. 31.5 (**a**) Entering correct plane from lateral to medial approach. (**b**) Entering correct plane from medial-to-lateral approach. (**c**) Entering wrong plane from medial-to-lateral approach by dissecting too deep into retroperitoneum

represents the most lateral fusion line between the colon and the retroperitoneum. The mobilization of the colon during the resection essentially reverses the fusion process that took place during embryologic development by surgically separating the two planes. In one sense, it is more natural to perform this dissection using the lateral to medial approach. By incising just medial to the Toldt fascia, the potential space between the colon and the retroperitoneum is accessed directly (Fig. 31.5a). During this approach, a dissection should not be carried out lateral to the Toldt fascia as this will likely lead to entry deep into the retroperitoneum and potential injuries to the retroperitoneal structures.

During the medial-to-lateral dissection, the major vessels are usually divided first (Fig. 31.5b). Because the major (ileocolic, IMA) vessels are located medial to the embryologic fusion plane, there is a natural tendency to delve into the retroperitoneum (Fig. 31.5c). This can result in unnecessary bleeding and/or injury to retroperitoneal structures such as the ureter or the duodenum. To avoid getting into the wrong plane, the right colon and its mesentery should be tented upward with strong retraction while bluntly separating the retroperitoneum away. This upward tension is best achieved by bowel grasper with its jaw open wide (Fig. 31.6). The correct plane is usually one superficial layer above the perceived plane. The mantra "the purple goes down" well describes the process of separating the colon mesentery away from the retroperitoneum (Fig. 31.7).

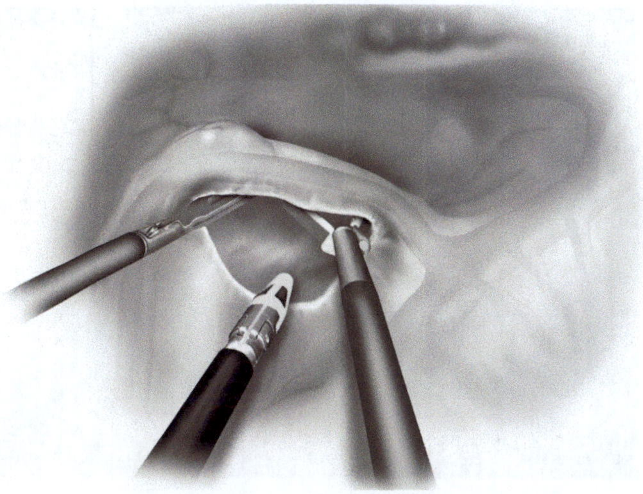

Fig. 31.6 Strong upward tension of colon mesentery using bowel grasper with its jaw open allows surgeon to see the interface better

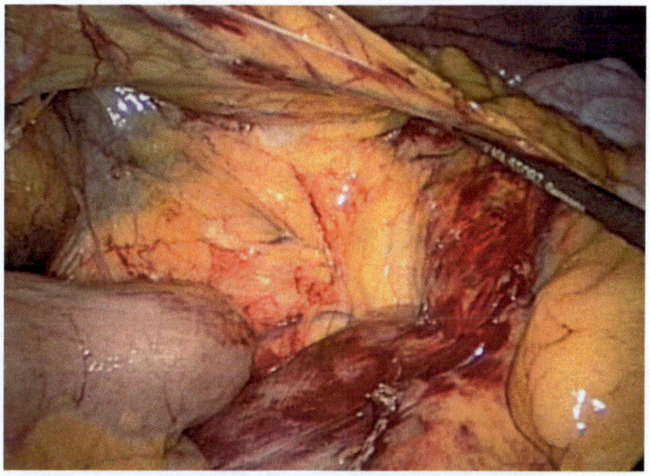

Fig. 31.7 "Purple goes down." Medial approach to a right colon demonstrates the yellow undersurface of the right colon mesentery and "purple" retroperitoneal fascia left down

Identifying/Handling the Duodenum

Identification of the duodenum is the key step in performing a laparoscopic right colectomy. The relationship between the ileocolic vessels and the duodenum is constant in all patients. The ileocolic artery is the first branching artery off of the superior mesenteric artery below the duodenal sweep. A gentle anterolateral retraction of the mesentery near the ileocolic junction will tent up the ileocolic vessels. A wide mesenteric window is then created below the ileocolic vessels. The duodenum must be identified before ligating the ileocolic pedicle in all cases (Fig. 31.8). One of the most common mistakes that can be made early in the experience is to create a window too distally away from the duodenum. If

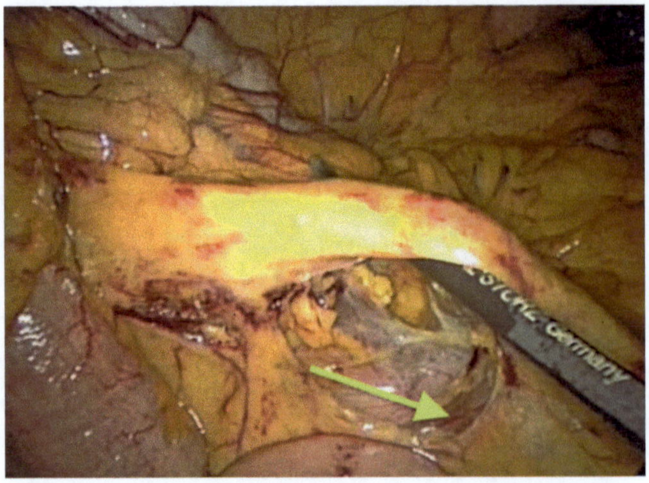

Fig. 31.8 Defining the duodenum on a right colectomy. The ileocolic pedicle is elevated with the duodenum under the proximal vessel (*arrow*)

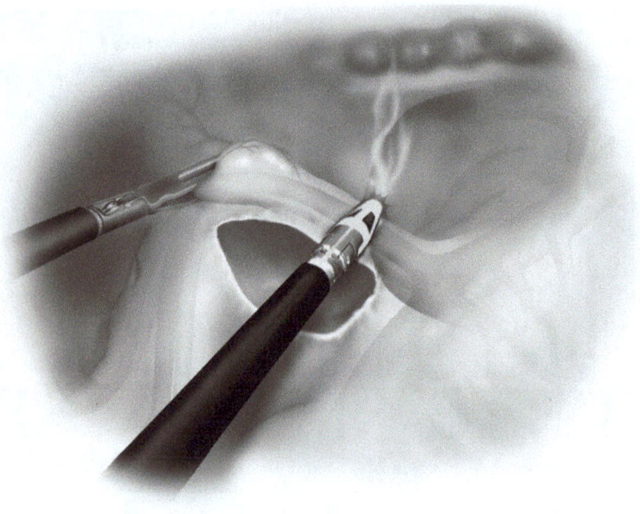

Fig. 31.9 Thermal injury to duodenum can occur during ligation of ileocolic vessels if the duodenum is not safely dissected away and the tip of a bipolar device is not clearly visualized

one has a difficulty identifying the duodenum, more proximal dissection should be carried out.

In dissecting the duodenum away from the mesocolon, one must be mindful of two potential complications: (1) injury to the duodenum and (2) avulsion of the gastrocolic trunk of Henle. Thermal injury to the duodenum can happen if the tip of energy device is too close to the duodenum while dividing ileocolic or middle colic pedicle (Fig. 31.9). It is imperative to visualize the entire length of the active blade. A blunt injury to the duodenum can also result from aggressive dissection of the middle colic vessels. Therefore, direct manipulation of the duodenum should be minimized. If the injury should occur, it needs to be immediately recognized and repaired. Small or partial thickness injury can be suture repaired laparoscopically. More extensive injury needs to be repaired by open approach. Careful dissection should be maintained during dissection of the right branch of the middle colic vessels. Injury to gastrocolic trunk of Henle (vein connecting gastroepiploic vein and the right branch of the middle colic vein) located in this area can result in severe bleeding that is very difficult to control, since it drains into SMV. To avoid this, vigilance and care should be maintained when dissecting over the pancreas. If bleeding occurs, wide exposure and a precise use of a bipolar energy device can control the bleeding in most cases.

Major Vascular Pedicle Ligation

There are many different ways to control and divide the major vascular pedicles. Laparoscopic staplers are safe but not as precise and versatile as the energy devices. In dividing major named vessels, only two types of energy devices (ultrasonic and bipolar) have been used. When properly applied, both devices can be very effective. A disadvantage associated with an ultrasonic device is that it usually does not allow the user to control when the vessels are transected (Video 31.2, Courtesy of David Longcope, MD). On the other hand, a bipolar energy device allows multiple application of the sealing using the energy, and the vessels are only transected when the surgeon decides it. Bipolar energy devices are not effective in sealing calcified vessels. A vessel loop should be made available in the OR for all laparoscopic colon cases (Video 31.3).

The Right Ureter

The right gonadal vessels and the ureter are typically located safely away from the dissection plane during laparoscopic right colectomy and therefore they do not need to be identified routinely. The potential injury to the right ureter may occur while incising the base of the terminal ileal mesentery from the retroperitoneum (Video 31.4). It is useful to look for the ureter coursing over the iliac bifurcation before starting dissection in this area. A thorough dissection from the medial side prior to and strong ventral and cephalad retraction of the terminal ileum during the detachment of the ileal mesentery can help avoid this complication.

Unique Complication: Sigmoidectomy

Key Concept: Similar to a right colectomy, a sigmoid colectomy has certain structures at higher risk of injury. Proper identification of the left ureter, avoidance of splenic injury, and handling the IMA/IMV and middle colic vessels are key aspects to a safe dissection.

Exposure/Mobilization of the Left Kidney

Patients are placed in the Trendelenburg position with the left side of the patient tilted up. The transverse colon along with the greater omentum is placed in the cephalad direction over the liver. Loops of the terminal ileum are allowed to fall to the patient's right side. As described previously, it is common to get too deep into the retroperitoneum during medial-to-lateral approach. It is essential to maintain the correct dissection plane in order to minimize the risk of injury to the ureter and gonadal vessels. From a lateral approach, it is important to follow the correct plane (i.e., stay more medial) during the cephalad dissection toward the splenic flexure, as it is often a natural tendency to stray too lateral and find yourself behind the left kidney.

Identifying the Ureter

Several retrospective studies have shown that laparoscopic colectomy has higher incidence of ureteral injury compared to open colectomy [10, 11]. In a study that reviewed incidence of ureteral injury from laparoscopic vs. open colectomy in a single institution between 2005 and 2010 [11], the incidence of injury from laparoscopic colectomy was 0.66 % (7/1,060) compared to open, 0.15 % (7/4,669; $p=0.007$). As shown in open surgery, preoperative ureteral stenting did not decrease the rate of injury but facilitated identification of injury. It remains to be seen whether the incidence will decrease as surgical community becomes more experienced with the procedure. Regardless, ureteral injury results in high morbidity, and every effort should be made to avoid it. Early identification of urinary tract injuries is critical in minimizing morbidity and preserving renal function. Although routine use of ureteral stent is not recommended, placement in select patients who are at high risk for ureter injury such as prior history of pelvic surgery, history of infectious or inflammatory colitis, or large tumor is reasonable.

Identification of the left ureter is *the key step* in performing a laparoscopic sigmoidectomy. The inferior mesenteric pedicle should not be divided until the left ureter is clearly identified and dissected away from the mesentery. When performing medial-to-lateral dissection during laparoscopic sigmoidectomy, it is important to create a wide enough window dorsal to the inferior mesenteric artery into the retroperitoneum so that the left ureter and the gonadal vessel can be identified. At this level, the left ureter is located medial to the gonadal vessels. If the left ureter cannot be identified through this window, one should consider a possibility that the dissection plane is too deep and the ureter and the gonadal vessels are still attached to colon mesentery. This is likely to be the case if you see the bare psoas muscle or iliac vessels. An alternative to this approach is to create a window proximally, between IMA and IMV near their origins. One must be aware that the left ureter is located lateral to the gonadal vessels at this level (Fig. 31.10). In sigmoidectomy for diverticulitis, where retroperitoneal inflammation makes identification of the ureter difficult, this approach can be useful, since the proximal ureter should be free of inflammatory process. Another option is to find the ureter by mobilizing the colon from lateral to medially. If all attempts fail, the case should be converted to either hand assisted or open. In hand-assisted cases, the left ureter can be dissected directly through the hand-access incision. If all of these fail, the case needs to be converted to open procedure or consideration of an intraoperative stent placement to facilitate identification.

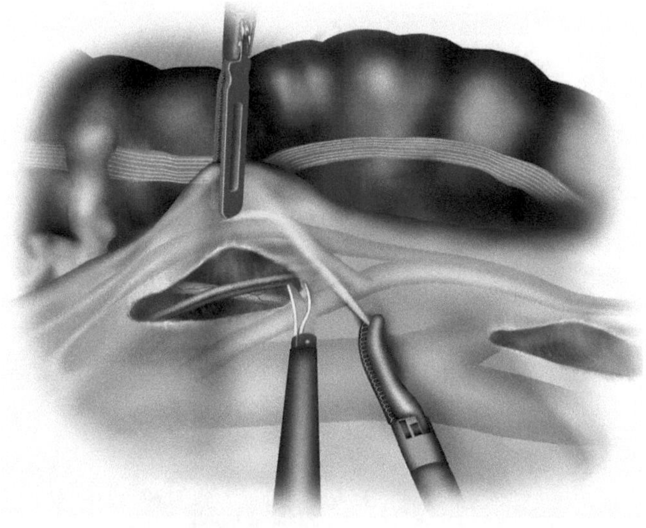

Fig. 31.10 Alternative mesenteric window between IMV and IMA near its origin. Note that ureter runs lateral to gonadal vessel in this area

Splenic Flexure

We use so called the "omega" maneuver to take down splenic flexure. We start the dissection by detaching the greater omentum from the distal transverse colon and getting into the lesser sac. It is advisable to start this dissection near the mid-transverse colon where the anterior and posterior leaflets of the greater omentum are fused together. In obese patients with fatty omentum, sometimes it may be necessary to divide the gastrocolic ligament and the omentum just inferior to stomach in order to access lesser sac more reliably. Once you are in the lesser sac, it is important to triangulate the tissues (Fig. 31.11) in order to avoid causing inadvertent thermal injury to transverse colon. The greater omentum and the colon should be retracted dorsally and laterally away from each other, while the camera is directed down from a plane above the horizon to obtain a full view of the course of the colon distal to the dissection field. Short application of bipolar energy is preferred. Blunt dissection in this area, especially near the spleen, should be avoided, as bleeding from torn omental vessel or capsular tear can significantly impede and delay the operation.

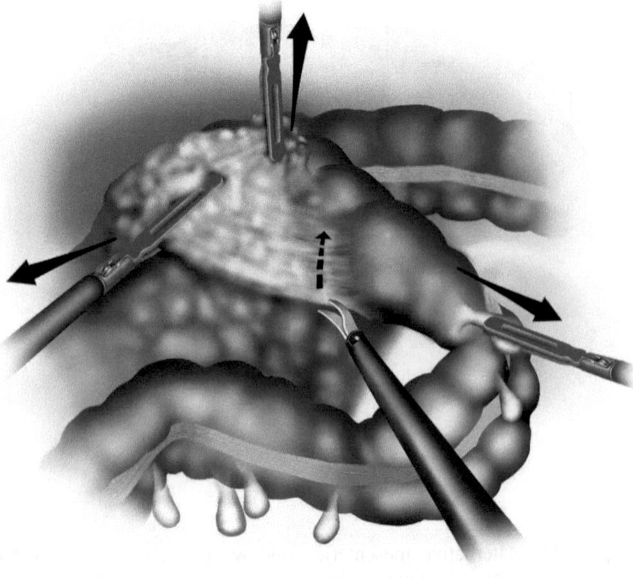

Fig. 31.11 Triangulation of tissues prevents inadvertent thermal injury to the transverse colon while taking down splenic flexure

Once the dissection along the transverse colon is carried out as far distally as possible, an approach from lateral aspect of the left colon is commenced. The Gerota's fascia is dissected and retroperitoneal attachment between the Gerota's fascia and descending colon is sharply divided using an energy device. The Gerota's fascia over the left kidney is intimately associated with the splenic flexure of the colon. During splenic flexure mobilization, it is therefore possible to inadvertently mobilize the left kidney along with proximal left colon. The best way to avoid this is to dissect and separate the Gerota's fascia away from the colon mesentery as much as possible during medial-to-lateral dissection prior to lateral mobilization the flexure. The Gerota's fascia should be dissected as far laterally as possible toward the Toldt fascia and toward the splenic flexure from the medial approach.

It is also important to stay as close to the colon as possible when dividing the lateral attachments of the proximal left colon near the splenic flexure. As you approach the spleen, anterior and caudal traction of splenic flexure exposes splenocolic ligament, which is divided using an energy device (Video 31.5).

Redo Operation and Conversion

Key Concept: A laparoscopic approach to recurrent operations should be undertaken with caution, focusing on correct tissue planes and a willingness to add additional ports or conversion as needed. Remember, conversion does not equate to failure and often indicates a wise surgeon.

Re-operative surgery is common, but can be technically challenging. Although history of previous surgery is not a contraindication to laparoscopy, it should not be attempted until adequate technical proficiency is achieved. Patients who undergo a successful laparoscopy can expect the usual short-term benefits associated with laparoscopy, although conversion rates are significantly higher in re-operative laparoscopic surgery. Key components to a successful re-operative laparoscopic surgery consist of having a clear understanding of pathophysiology and a detailed knowledge of prior surgical procedures. It is important to obtain and review previous operative and medical records. In patients who had previous colon resections, it is essential to know which of the named mesenteric vessels were taken during the previous operations so that a potential segmental ischemia of the colon can be avoided. In select patients, additional imaging may be helpful.

Forty percent of bowel injuries during laparoscopy occur during initial entry into the abdomen. Although there are no prospective randomized trials comparing different techniques of access methods, it is prudent to enter the abdomen using the open Hasson technique away from the previous incisions. Upon entry, a careful inspection for potential damages to the small intestines adherent to abdominal wall must be carried out. After a quick initial survey of the extent and type of adhesions, a decision to convert should be entertained early in the operation. The adhesions between the small intestines and the abdominal wall are much easier to deal with laparoscopically than either extensive inter-loop intestinal adhesions or adhesions to pelvic structures. Early conversion should be considered in patients with either extensive inter-loop or pelvic adhesions, especially when they are impeding progress, though if away from the disease process should be left alone.

Regardless of surgeon's level of skill and experience, the possibility of conversion to open approach is unavoidable. Conversion should be considered as a solution to overcome the limitation of laparoscopic surgery rather than complication and more often than not reflects good surgical judgment [12].

There has been a significant controversy over whether conversion to the open approach during laparoscopic colectomy has negative impact on patient outcomes. Multiple studies have shown that patient who were converted during laparoscopic colectomies, when compared with those who had successful laparoscopic colectomies, had longer operative time, increased blood loss, higher wound infection rate, and longer length of stay [13, 14]. What is alarming is that some studies suggest that converted patients may do worse than the open-surgery patients. Hewett and colleagues recently reported results from an Australasian randomized study comparing laparoscopic with open surgery for cancer. In this study, converted patients had longer operative time, longer hospitalization, and higher infection rate than laparoscopic *or* open patients [15]. Other studies point to no worse outcome [16]. One reason for the discrepancy in reported outcomes is a lack of standard definition of conversion. Another more important and clinically more relevant factor is recognition that not all conversions are equal. Belizon and colleagues reported that clinical impact of conversion depends on whether the case is converted early (<30 min) or late [12]. After initial laparoscopic assessment of risk for conversion, early proactive conversion is likely to result in favorable outcome. In contrast, reactive conversion undertaken late in the operation in response to intraoperative complications, such as enterotomy or bleeding, is likely to result in poorer outcomes. Unfortunately, most studies do not differentiate between the two types of conversions, and selection bias likely plays a large role in the outcomes of these studies.

An important learning principle is that early conversion based on initial laparoscopic intraoperative findings may be critical in avoiding complications in patients who are at an already high risk of conversion. For example, studies have shown that laparoscopic colectomies for sigmoid diverticulitis are more likely to convert [12]. Several studies have shown that hand-assisted laparoscopic colectomy is associated with significantly lower conversion rate and, as a result, lower postoperative complication rates when compared with "straight" laparoscopy [17, 18]. Advantages associated with hand-assisted laparoscopy were more dramatic when dealing with complicated diverticulitis with either abscess or fistulae. An argument for routine use of hand-assisted laparoscopic surgery for certain indications, such as sigmoid diverticulitis, is strong, although this is certainly open for debate.

Our approach to re-operative laparoscopy is as follows. We enter the abdomen using the open technique away from the previous incisions and lateral to rectus sheath. After an initial inspection, we quickly decide whether to proceed laparoscopically or not. If we do decide to proceed laparoscopically, the abdominal wall in the area of planned ports is cleared and all the ports are inserted. We then separate the greater omentum from the intestines. This will allow the transverse colon and the greater omentum to be retracted in the cephalad direction away from the operative field. Next, we separate the small intestines from the colon by taking down adhesions sharply. It is prudent to set aside a fixed amount of time after which conversion should be considered. If no significant surgical progress has been made during that time, there should not be any hesitation in converting to an alternate approach.

Not all cases have to be converted to open. In straight laparoscopic cases, you can consider converting to HALS or place additional ports. For example, if you encounter locally invasive sigmoid cancer, or dense inter-loop adhesions in lower abdomen, HALS gives you an option of interchanging hand-assisted laparoscopy with open approach.

Summary Pearls

Laparoscopic colon surgery is associated with many short-term outcome advantages when compared with open surgery. In expert hands, it is safe and may offer less potential for complications. Unfortunately complications are unavoidable regardless of skill levels. We should be aware of both common and unique complications that are associated with laparoscopic colorectal surgery. It is crucial to recognize them immediately and deal with them as quickly as possible. In this chapter we described some of the strategies to avoid these complications. Having a consistent and systematic surgical approach is essential in avoiding or minimizing complications in any type of surgery. Although controversial, conversion in certain situations can lead to increase in complications. Reactive conversion late in the procedure in response to an unexpected injury is likely to lead to poorer outcomes. In contrast, early proactive conversion in patients who are at high risk for conversion likely will minimize the risk of complications. In either situation, it is important that you remember it is the patient who takes all the risks and your job as a minimally invasive surgeon is to minimize or avoid them altogether.

References

1. Group COoSTS. A comparison of laparoscopically assisted and open colectomy for colon cancer. N Engl J Med. 2004;350(20):2050–9. PubMed PMID: 15141043.
2. Green BL, Marshall HC, Collinson F, Quirke P, Guillou P, Jayne DG, et al. Long-term follow-up of the Medical Research Council CLASICC trial of conventional versus laparoscopically assisted resection in colorectal cancer. Br J Surg. 2013;100:75–82.
3. Carmichael JC, Masoomi H, Mills S, Stamos MJ, Nguyen NT. Utilization of laparoscopy in colorectal surgery for cancer at academic medical centers: does site of surgery affect rate of laparoscopy? Am Surg. 2011;77(10):1300–4.
4. Olivar H, Sharar SR, Stephens LS, Posner KL, Domino KB. Similar liability for trauma and nontrauma surgical anesthesia: a closed claims analysis. Anesth Analg. 2012;115(5):1196–203.
5. Nakajima K, Milsom JW, Margolin DA, Szilagy EJ. Use of the surgical towel in colorectal hand-assisted laparoscopic surgery (HALS). Surg Endosc. 2004;18(3):552–3.
6. van der Voort M, Heijnsdijk EA, Gouma DJ. Bowel injury as a complication of laparoscopy. Br J Surg. 2004;91(10):1253–8.
7. Sutton PA, Awad S, Perkins AC, Lobo DN. Comparison of lateral thermal spread using monopolar and bipolar diathermy, the Harmonic Scalpel and the Ligasure. Br J Surg. 2010;97(3):428–33.
8. Milsom JW, Bohm B, Nakajima K. Surgical energy source. Laparoscopic colorectal surgery. 2nd ed. New York: Springer; 2006. p. 30–48.
9. Azevedo JL, Azevedo OC, Miyahira SA, Miguel GP, Becker OM, Hypólito OH, et al. Injuries caused by Veress needle insertion for creation of pneumoperitoneum: a systematic literature review. Surg Endosc. 2009;23(7):1428–32.
10. Parpala-Spårman T, Paananen I, Santala M, Ohtonen P, Hellström P. Increasing numbers of ureteric injuries after the introduction of laparoscopic surgery. Scand J Urol Nephrol. 2008;42(5):422–7.

11. Palaniappa NC, Telem DA, Ranasinghe NE, Divino CM. Incidence of iatrogenic ureteral injury after laparoscopic colectomy. Arch Surg. 2012;147(3):267–71.
12. Belizon A, Sardinha CT, Sher ME. Converted laparoscopic colectomy: what are the consequences? Surg Endosc. 2006;20(6):947–51.
13. Gervaz P, Pikarsky A, Utech M, Secic M, Efron J, Belin B, et al. Converted laparoscopic colorectal surgery. Surg Endosc. 2001;15(8):827–32.
14. Gonzalez R, Smith CD, Mason E, Duncan T, Wilson R, Miller J, et al. Consequences of conversion in laparoscopic colorectal surgery. Dis Colon Rectum. 2006;49(2):197–204.
15. Hewett PJ, Allardyce RA, Bagshaw PF, Frampton CM, Frizelle FA, Rieger NA, et al. Short-term outcomes of the Australasian randomized clinical study comparing laparoscopic and conventional open surgical treatments for colon cancer: the ALCCaS trial. Ann Surg. 2008;248(5):728–38.
16. Casillas S, Delaney CP, Senagore AJ, Brady K, Fazio VW. Does conversion of a laparoscopic colectomy adversely affect patient outcome? Dis Colon Rectum. 2004;47(10):1680–5.
17. Lee SW, Yoo J, Dujovny N, Sonoda T, Milsom JW. Laparoscopic vs. hand-assisted laparoscopic sigmoidectomy for diverticulitis. Dis Colon Rectum. 2006;49(4):464–9.
18. Marcello PW, Fleshman JW, Milsom JW, Read TE, Arnell TD, Birnbaum EH, et al. Hand-assisted laparoscopic vs. laparoscopic colorectal surgery: a multicenter, prospective, randomized trial. Dis Colon Rectum. 2008;51(6):818–26.

Laparoscopy, Robotics, and Endoscopy

32

Deborah S. Keller and Conor P. Delaney

Key Points

- Incorporating emerging technologies into practice is critical to the advancement of skills but needs to be weighed against the true (not perceived) benefits they offer the patient.
- Laparoscopy offers continued benefits for colorectal surgery, even when compared to newer technologies.
- The learning curve for new techniques is individualized, variable, and has a direct impact on outcomes.
- Cost should be a major consideration when deciding on which approach to undertake for colorectal disease.

Laparoscopy: Introducing Technology in Colorectal Surgery

Key Concept: Laparoscopy is a safe and effective technique that optimizes patient outcomes. Health-care efficiencies continue to improve with increased incorporation of laparoscopy. For inexperienced minimally invasive surgeons or in difficult cases, hand-assisted laparoscopy may offer a bridge to laparoscopic surgery with comparable patient benefits.

Colorectal surgery has embraced technology as a means to improve efficiency and patient outcomes. Over the last 20 years, there has been a gradual evolution from conventional open to laparoscopic colorectal surgery (LC). The expanded use of laparoscopy has been the most successful technological advance in improving early postoperative outcomes and reducing health-care costs in colorectal surgery. Although there were initial concerns about the oncological safety of LC [1, 2], the landmark Clinical Outcomes of Surgical Therapy (COST) Trial demonstrated the safety, oncologic equivalency, and apparent benefits in secondary endpoints [i.e., return of bowel function, length of stay (LOS), pain] for the laparoscopic group [3]. Subsequently, multiple randomized controlled trials and a Cochrane Review further affirmed the oncologic equivalence, safety, reductions in pain and postoperative ileus, preservation of normal pulmonary function, improved cosmesis, shorter LOS, and better quality of life with LC versus open colorectal surgery (OC) [4–10]. When viewed in a broader sense, LC is associated with better resource utilization through lower rates of complications, readmissions, intensive care unit need, and post-discharge nursing facilities when compared to conventional OC [11].

The transition to laparoscopic rectal resection (LRR) has been slower for the colorectal field to integrate. The safety of LRR for rectal cancer was less clearly defined initially, as early controlled trials concentrated on the oncologic safety of *colon* cancer [3, 5]. Initial concerns over proper oncologic margins, local recurrence, sexual dysfunction, and appropriate training measures hindered widespread acceptance, even to this day [12]. Data such as the UK MRC-CLASICC Trial Group has expanded the safety profile of LRR, finding no difference in overall survival, disease-free survival, local recurrence, wound recurrence, or quality of life between the laparoscopic and open approaches [13, 14]. Further trials [15–25] and meta-analyses [26–28] affirmed the equivalent oncological outcomes for LRR in the treatment of primary rectal cancer. The randomized comparison of open versus laparo-

D.S. Keller, MD
Division of Colorectal Surgery, Department of Surgery, University Hospitals Case Medical Center, Case Western Reserve University, Cleveland, OH, USA

C.P. Delaney, MD, MCh, PhD, FRCSI, FACS, FASCRS (✉)
Division of Colorectal Surgery, Department of Surgery, University Hospitals Case Medical Center, Case Western Reserve University, 11100 Euclid Avenue, 7 Lakeside, Cleveland, OH 44106, USA
e-mail: conor.delaney@uhhospitals.org

Electronic supplementary material The online version of this chapter (doi: 10.1007/978-1-4614-9022-7_32) contains supplementary material, which is available to authorized users. Videos can also be accessed at http://www.springerimages.com/videos/978-1-4614-9021-0.

S.R. Steele et al. (eds.), *Complexities in Colorectal Surgery*,
DOI 10.1007/978-1-4614-9022-7_32,

scopic surgery for mid and low rectal cancer after neoadjuvant chemoradiotherapy (COREAN) trial found laparoscopic surgery after preoperative chemoradiotherapy for mid or low rectal cancer is not only safe and oncologically equivalent to open resection but also associated with improved short-term benefits, including earlier recovery of bowel function, better physical functioning, and fewer micturition, gastrointestinal, and defecation problems [19].

Despite the proven advantages, the integration of laparoscopic technology into clinical practice has been slow. The steep learning curve is a major factor limiting widespread use [29–32]. Previous studies suggested LC requires at least 50 cases to gain proficiency [33–35], with a minimum of 20 laparoscopic colon cancer operations required for inclusion into clinical trials [3, 36]. In rectal cases, the narrow confines of the bony pelvis, standard practice of autonomic nerve-sparing total mesorectal excision (TME), and limited angulation of current stapling technology make laparoscopic surgery even more challenging [37].

Hand-Assisted Laparoscopic Surgery (HALS)

Key Concept: *Hand-assisted laparoscopic surgery (HALS) has been proposed as a technology that might help bridge or speed the laparoscopic learning curve, with equivalent results to traditional straight laparoscopic colectomy.*

With HALS, a sleeve appliance is used to maintain pneumoperitoneum, while the operator's hand is inserted through a small incision into the abdomen. As with standard laparoscopic surgery, the surgeon visualizes the operative field with a video monitor but has the advantage of his assisting hand, allowing tactile feedback and assistance in retraction, palpation, and dissection (Video 32.1a and b) [38]. HALS may be useful for surgeons exclusively trained in open surgery, as the tactile feedback and hand-eye coordination may allow this technique to be easier to master [39, 40]. A randomized trial comparing surgeon performance, technical skills, and operative error in a HALS versus straight laparoscopic colectomy simulator model found better performances with the HALS approach, suggesting the HALS procedure may be technically easier to perform [41]. HALS can also be effective in reoperative patients with a higher likelihood of conversion. In a comprehensive review of nearly 1,000 minimal access colectomies performed over a 3-year period, the authors found that, in their hands, HALS substantially reduced operative time and conversion rates compared to conventional LC and increased the number of minimal access colectomies performed [42]. Thus, HALS may bridge the technical divide between minimal laparoscopic and open procedures, expanding minimally invasive colorectal surgery for those less proficient in straight laparoscopy.

Laparoscopy is appropriate for the majority of benign colorectal and malignant colon procedures. Reported contraindications include hemodynamic instability, inability to tolerate pneumoperitoneum, labile cardiac status, ascites, cirrhosis, portal hypertension, intraperitoneal mesh, peritonitis, and mechanical bowel obstruction. With increasing experience, the absolute contraindications are diminishing – with past absolutes like malignant disease, obesity, pregnancy, and previous abdominal operations now mostly relative to the surgeon's experience. *Laparoscopic resection for rectal cancer* has proven feasible, and oncologic outcomes are promising from the initial studies, but still not oncologically equivalent. While ongoing trials are attempting to clarify the role of LRR for cancer, the continued implementation of LRR using meticulous oncologic techniques by experienced surgeons for select patients is appropriate [43]. Both SAGES and ASCRS recognize that LRR is an alternative to traditional resection of benign disease involving the rectum and encourage the development of properly designed studies to evaluate the safety, efficacy, and benefits of this approach. Nevertheless, initial outcomes have been promising.

Future Direction: Robotic Technology

Key Concept: *Robotic technology holds promise in improved mechanics with reduced conversion rates, but further experience and long-term data are needed to define patient outcomes and evaluate financial implications.*

Robotics is the current emerging technologic trend in surgery. Since achieving market dominance in prostate surgery, beneficial outcomes have been suggested for robotic technology in colorectal surgery [44, 45]. The application of robotic technology offers new possibilities for performing procedures remotely, and some consider it may help overcome the limitations of laparoscopic surgery [46]. Robotics has the advantage of wristed, powered instruments, and 3-D HD vision that delivers highly accurate depth perception (Fig. 32.1). Even though laparoscopic 3-D camera systems are now available, these systems lack the stable view offered by the robotic system and may be associated with side effects of headaches, dizziness, and nausea [47]. The robot is presumed to be more ergonomic for performing routine segmental colectomies via single incision, by crossing the robotic instruments and reassigning control of the arms in a more natural fashion [48]. While prospective data are awaited, retrospective case series support that robotic technology may offer increased precision and accuracy of anatomical dissection over conventional laparoscopic surgery [49], thereby facilitating more complex procedures (see Video 28.1). Furthermore, robotic technology may have a smaller learning curve compared to laparoscopic colorectal surgery, requiring only 20–40 cases to be competent in the technique; however, the evidence is inconclusive thus far [50].

Authors of some early robotic colectomy trials have suggested clinical benefits. Robotics may also afford better nerve function after TME. A nonrandomized review of

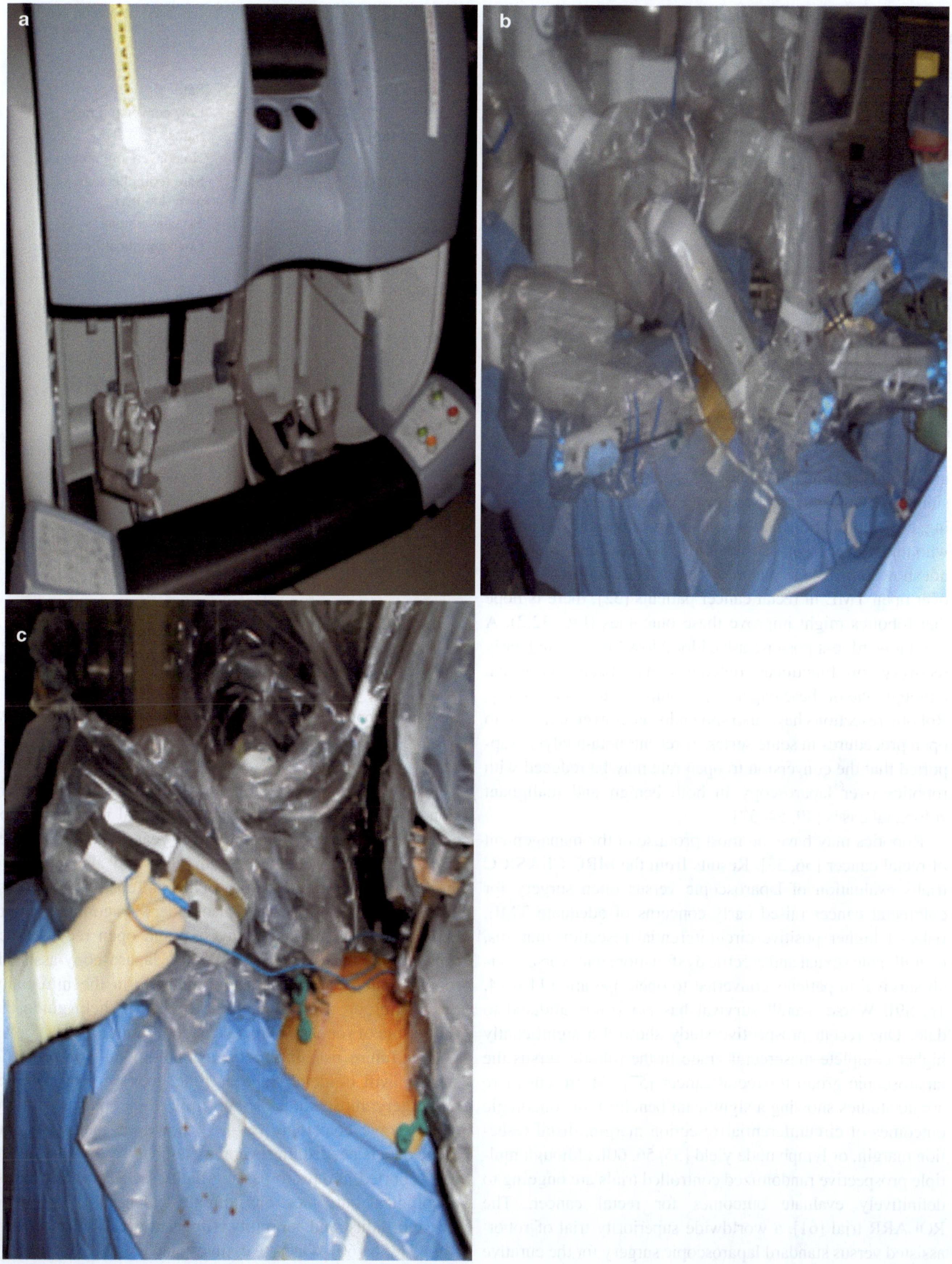

Fig. 32.1 Robotic technology. (**a**) The robotic console, (**b**) proper robotic arm positioning, (**c**) Robotic instrumentation placed with aid of bedside assistant

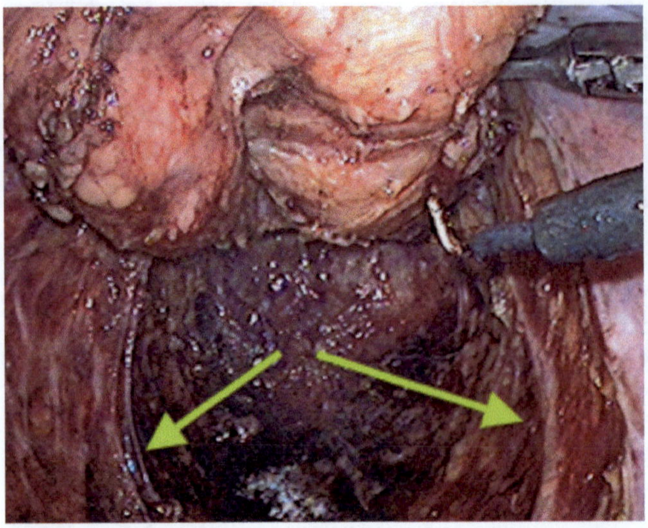

Fig. 32.2 Pelvic hypogastric nerves (*arrows*) seen on laparoscopy (Courtesy Matthew Mutch, MD)

urogenital function after robot-assisted total mesorectal excision for rectal cancer showed faster recovery of normal voiding, erectile function, and sexual desire compared to patients who underwent laparoscopic TME [51]. As laparoscopy did not show improved sexual and urinary dysfunction outcomes over open TME in rectal cancer patients [52], there is hope that robotics might improve these outcomes (Fig. 32.2). A trend toward less postoperative blood loss [49, 53] and early recovery of functional outcomes has been described, although one of these papers was compared to open surgery. Robotic resections have also shown lower conversion rates to open procedures in some series. A recent meta-analysis supported that the conversion to open rate may be reduced with robotics over laparoscopy in both benign and malignant colorectal cases [49, 54–57].

Robotics may have the most promise in the management of rectal cancer [56, 58]. Results from the MRC-CLASICC trial's evaluation of laparoscopic versus open surgery for colorectal cancer raised early concerns of adequate TME, risks of higher positive circumferential resection margins, overall male sexual and erectile dysfunction, and worse overall survival in patients converted to open operation [13, 14, 18, 59]. Worse overall survival has not been validated to date. One recent prospective study showed a significantly higher complete mesorectal grade in the robotic versus the laparoscopic group for rectal cancer [57]. At present there are no studies showing a significant benefit in the oncologic outcomes of circumferential resection margin, distal resection margin, or lymph node yield [55, 56, 60], although multiple prospective randomized controlled trials are ongoing to definitively evaluate outcomes for rectal cancer. The ROLARR trial [61], a worldwide superiority trial of robot-assisted versus standard laparoscopic surgery for the curative treatment of rectal cancer, is currently underway. The ROLARR trial is investigating differences in rate of conversion to open operation, rate of pathological involvement of circumferential resection margin, 3-year local recurrence, disease-free and overall survival rates, and also operative morbidity and mortality, quality of life, and cost-effectiveness. The ACOSOG Z6051 trial is also underway, comparing outcomes between minimally invasive and open rectal resection, including pure laparoscopic, laparoscopy-assisted, robot-assisted, or hand-assisted methods in the minimally invasive group. Results of these trials will help guide the future role of robotics in rectal cancer (Table 32.1).

Table 32.1 Early outcomes from robot-assisted colorectal surgery

Author	*N*	Conclusion
Diverticulitis		
Zimmern [62]	16	Safe
		Low conversion rate
Abodeely [63]	22	Safe
		No conversion, no leaks
Ragupathi [64]	24	Safe (complicated diverticulitis)
		No conversions
		Low complication rate
Rectal prolapse		
de Hoog [65]	20	Safe
		High recurrence rate
Zimmern [62]	8	Safe
Abodeely [63]	10	Safe
Bokhari [66]	5	Safe
Right hemicolectomy		
de Souza [67]	40 (vs. lap)	Safe
		Outcomes comparable to lap
		Higher cost with robotics
		Longer procedure time with robotics
Luca [68]	33 (vs. open)	Oncologic outcomes similar
		Increased EBL with open
		Reduced LOS with robotics
		Higher cost with robotics
		Longer op time with robotics

From Complications, Considerations, and Consequences of Colorectal Surgery: Unique Complications of Robotic Surgery (Courtesy of Sonia Ramamoorthy MD and Vincent Obias, MD)
Lap laparoscopic, *LN* lymph node, *EBL* estimated blood loss, *LOS* length of stay

The future use of robotic technology in non-prostatic surgery will be determined as time goes on. For colorectal surgery, most studies show similar outcomes to straight laparoscopic colectomy [69–71]; however, long-term outcome data is needed. In several meta-analyses, no advantage was reported in days to passing flatus, LOS, complications, oncological outcomes, anastomotic leakage, or postoperative morbidity and mortality, suggesting equivalent safety [49, 54–56, 60]. Operative times and costs are routinely increased by robotics. Although robotic colorectal surgery may facilitate a reduction in conversion to open surgery, the trials currently in process will help elucidate this finding. Similarly, prospective data are required to support the ability of the robot to improve nerve function and mesorectal grade after TME. The cost implications of any improvements will require evaluation. Overall, robotic surgery for colon and rectal cancer appears feasible and safe; however, the current literature only evaluates short-term outcomes, and data on local recurrence and survival is awaited.

Other issues related to the immature technology deserve attention. The costs are immense with no proven benefit to justify the additional expenditure at present. At a price of more than $1.7 million per robot, $125,000 in annual maintenance costs, and up to $2,000 per case for the cost of single-use instruments, robotic surgery is the most expensive approach. Barbash and colleagues reported if robot-assisted surgeries completely replace conventional surgeries, as is the trend in prostatectomy, an additional $1.5 billion in additional health-care costs would be generated annually – more than $2.5 billion when including the amortized costs of the robots [72]. A recent *Journal of the American Medical Association* study evaluated the uptake of robotically assisted hysterectomy, costs, and complications compared to the laparoscopic approach [73]. In reviewing nearly 265,000 women who underwent hysterectomy between 2007 and 2010 for benign gynecologic disorders, the authors found robotically assisted hysterectomy dramatically increased from 0.5 to 9.5 %. The robotic cases added an average of $2,189 per procedure, compared to traditional laparoscopic surgery, without any significant benefit in outcomes or complications. Looking at the growth trend, the authors found using robotics for all routine hysterectomies would add an unnecessary $1 to $1.9 billion in unnecessary health-care costs each year [73].

Aggressive marketing may be a factor for the continued growth. Both industry reports and the American College of Gynecologists president noted many patients are learning about the claimed advantages of robotic surgery from widespread marketing hype and an aggressive salesforce [74, 75]. To examine if hospitals are misleading patients about the benefits of robotic surgery to increase patient volume, Jin et al. performed a systematic analysis of 400 US hospital websites. The authors found 41 % described robotic surgery; of those, 78 % used manufacturer-provided stock images, and 33 % linked directly to the manufacturer's website. Unsupported claims of clinical advantages (86 %) and improved cancer control (32 %) were also found, while no sites mentioned risks of robotic surgery. The authors concluded hospitals overestimate benefits, underestimate risks, and are strongly influenced by the robotic system manufacturer [76].

A learning curve is always present when any new technology is introduced, during which an increase in complication rates can be expected. With robotics, there is no expert consensus on how much training is needed despite rapidly expanding use [72]. Expectantly, major complication data and legal issues are mounting. A series of liability cases against Intuitive Surgical have begun litigation, exposing the company's failure in its commitments to properly train surgeons to use the da Vinci robotic surgery suite safely [74]. With these issues, investor anxiety is growing. An industrial research report on Intuitive Surgical questioned the company's stock price and market position given the lack of clinical evidence of superior surgical outcomes and gathering storm of legal liability from failure to adequately disclose risks leading to surgical complications [77].

These factors have culminated in the American College of Gynecologists President James T. Breeden's statement against the routine use of robotics. Dr. Breeden highlighted an absence of strong evidence that robotic hysterectomy is even as good as, and far more costly than, minimally invasive surgical techniques for routine surgical care. Aggressive direct-to-consumer marketing may mislead the public into believing that they are the best choice. Patients should be advised that robotic surgery should be reserved for complex, specific conditions [75].

Single-Incision Laparoscopy Surgery

Key Concept: Single-incision laparoscopic colectomy provides the potential for improved cosmesis, postoperative pain, and recovery time at the drawback of higher costs, operating time, and technical skill required.

Single-incision laparoscopic surgery (SILS) was introduced to further the enhanced outcomes of traditional laparoscopy. SILS was first reported in 1999 for cholecystectomy [78] then extended to laparoscopic colectomy in 2008 by Remzi et al. [79] and Bucher et al. [80]. SILS uses a single port within the umbilicus with three or more working channels incorporated in the single port. Straight or articulating instruments are used via a fixed platform or small low-profile adjacently placed trans-fascial trocars, theoretically allowing intracorporeal triangulation of parallel instruments (Video 32.2, Courtesy of Virgilio George, MD). Studies have proven SILS is feasible and safe [81–86]. From early reports, SILS has similar postoperative outcomes and complications to traditional laparoscopic surgery. Operative time, conversions, estimated blood loss, surgical site infection, and hospital readmissions were all similar [87]. Although some reports noted longer operative times, the results are generally comparable with conventional LC. SILS even has demonstrated benefits over traditional laparoscopic surgery, including better cosmesis, reduced pain, and faster recovery [88]. The cosmetic benefit of a single incision is a major draw. The potential advantages of a small skin incision include not only better cosmetic result but also a lower rate of port-site-related complications (Fig. 32.3) [89].

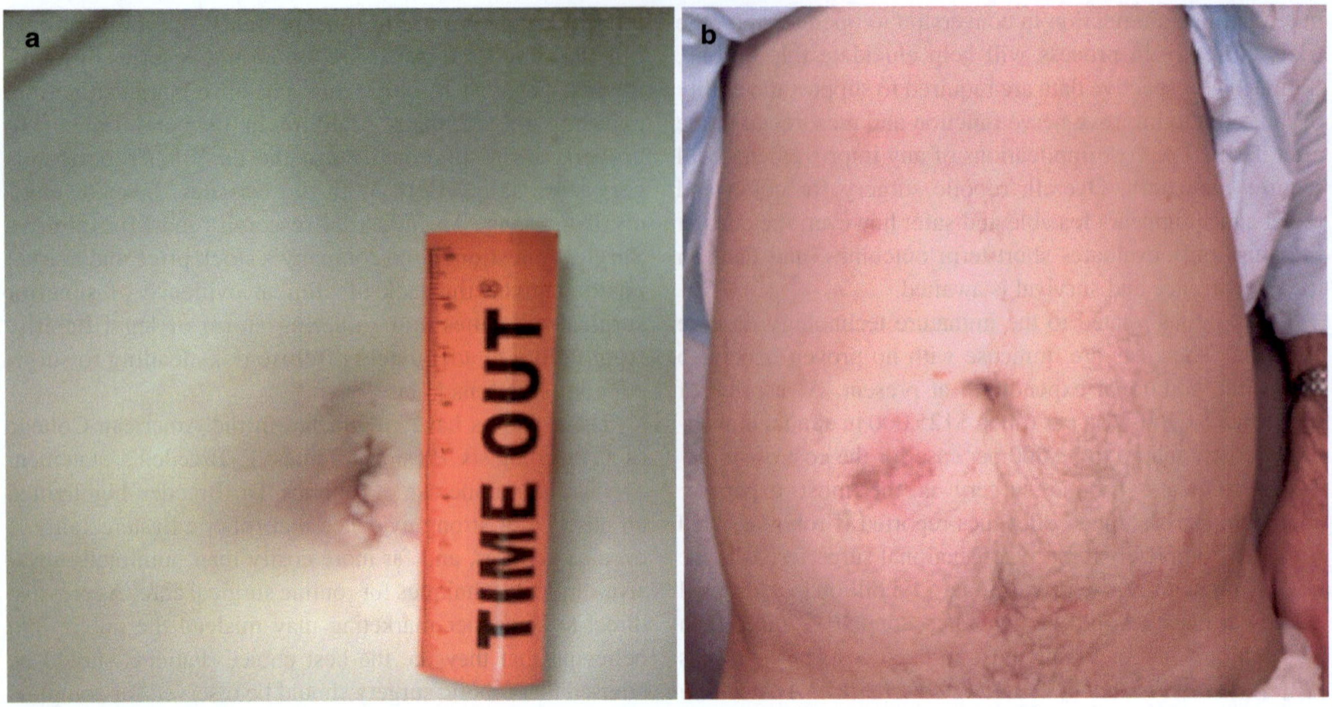

Fig. 32.3 Cosmetic comparison for total colectomy through (**a**) SILS and (**b**) traditional laparoscopic approach

Another reported advantage of a single incision is less postoperative pain than conventional LC [87, 90]. The reduction in pain translated to lower total narcotic use was in the immediate postoperative period, with lower pain scores reported up to postoperative day 2. SILS has also shown a significantly shorter length of stay (LOS); studies have demonstrated LOS more than 1 day shorter for SILS compared to multi-post-laparoscopy (Table 32.2) [81, 87].

Despite the benefits, some issues exist with SILS. The proximity of the trocars at a fixed position, restricted freedom of the hands, and *clashing of the instruments* is somewhat contradictory to the traditional teaching of instrument triangulation in laparoscopy [91]. The problems in exposure and the risk of "*crowding*" *while maneuvering laparoscopic instruments* add to the difficulty in the SILS technique [92] (Video 32.3, Courtesy of Virgilio George, MD). An additional learning curve is involved for the technique, extra incisions are sometimes required [82, 93], and there is a minor increase in cost over laparoscopic surgery [84, 94]. SILS may also make teaching more difficult. Previous studies have demonstrated unique requirements of SILS, with skill sets and ergonomic demands which cannot be directly adapted from existing LAP experience [95]. Thus, the implementation of an evidence- and competency-based SILS curriculum is necessary to ensure appropriate training of future SILS surgeons. Currently, resident training modes are in development for SILS, and the attending may be performing more of the case, at the expense of resident education. Many of these issues can be improved with operator ascension up the learning curve and refinement of the SILS technology. Robotic-utilizing surgeons feel that robotics may also reduce the negativities of SILS such as loss of triangulation and poor visualization and further advance the technology.

Evolving Endoscopic Techniques

Endoscopic Mucosal Resection (EMR)

Key Concept: *EMR provides en bloc or piecemeal removal of premalignant and early colorectal lesions typically <20 mm that may have otherwise required resection.*

Advanced endoscopic technology has been introduced to allow for treatment of colorectal tumors without the morbidity of a surgical resection. These endoscopic techniques have permitted more aggressive and successful polypectomy, including en bloc removal of otherwise unresectable lesions [96]. *Endoscopic mucosal resection* (EMR) is an option for endoscopic polypectomy of colorectal polyps without stalks. EMR differs from standard snare polypectomy by the use of submucosal solution injection, which allows for the complete resection of the mucosa through the mid to deep submucosa [97]. EMR is useful for the removal of adenomas that are too large for standard snare polypectomy and essentially allows removal of colonic lesions in a minimally invasive way that would otherwise require surgical colectomy (see Video 25.1) [98]. Although not an absolute contraindication, it is typically more difficult to remove tumors >20 mm

Table 32.2 Published reports of single-incision colectomy

Author	Year	Patients	BMI	Mean OR time (min)	LOS (d)	Incision length (cm)	R/L
Bucher [80]	2008	1	N/A	158	N/A	3	1/0
Remzi [79]	2008	1	35	115	4	3.5	1/0
Rieger	2009	7	24.3	89	5.4	3.1	6/1
Geisler	2009	1	24	172	4	2	TPC
Merchant [91]	2009	1	N/A	N/A	3	2.5	1/0
Remzi	2009	1	25.8	198	3	3	0/1
Bucher	2009	1	26	213[a]	N/A	2	0/1
Law	2009	1	N/A	180	3	3	0/1
Chambers [88]	2009	6	N/A	82	1.9	2.5	[b]2/1
Leroy	2009	1	21	90	4	2	0/1
Bucher	2010	1	22	125	2	2	0/1
Adair [83]	2010	17	26.2	139	5	3	17/0
Gandhi	2010	24	28.5	143	2.7	3.8	19/5
Papaconstantinou [81]	2011	29	30	128.8	3.4	4.9	29/0
Chen [85]	2011	18	23.3	175	5	4	18/0
Fichera	2011	10	21.9	139	5.1	–	TPC
McNally	2011	27	27	114	3	–	14/8[c]
Wu	2011	27	–	180	7	4.1	8/18[d]
Ross	2011	39	25.6	120	4.4	4.2	30/9
Ramos-Valadez	2012	20	27.7	159.2	3.2	3.3	0/20
Walters	2012	100	26	105	4		100/0

N/A not available, *TPC* total proctocolectomy, *BMI* body mass index, *R* right-sided surgery, *L* left-sided surgery, *LOS* length of stay, *min* minutes, *d* days
[a]Concomitant cholecystectomy
[b]In addition: 2 TPC and 1 abdominal colectomy with ileorectal anastomosis
[c]In addition, 5 SILS transverse colectomies
[d]In addition, 1 TPC

by en bloc resection using EMR, with reported success rates of ~30 %; thus, decisions should be made on an individual basis [99–101]. Piecemeal excision (while limiting the full extent of final pathological analysis) can also be used to facilitate removal of larger lesions to a large extent in experienced hands [102].

To perform EMR, the lesion is oriented to maximize the influence of gravity, then a submucosal injection creates a fluid "cushion" between the mucosa and muscularis propria to elevate the lesion into the lumen. Following the injection lift, a snare is deployed to fully remove the lesion with a 2–3 mm margin of normal mucosa [102]. Because the plane of resection during EMR is typically the middle to deep submucosal layer, compared with standard polypectomy, which normally provides resection at a mucosal level, EMR offers the advantage of providing en bloc resection specimens.

Outcomes for EMR are very good for experienced providers. A meta-analysis and systematic review of successful en bloc resections of large colorectal polyps by EMR found complete cure rates improved from 44.19 to 69.17 %, concluding EMR is an effective technique and offers an alternative to surgery [103]. An Australian study of EMR in 174 patients with difficult polyps reported a 95 % procedural success, 90 % avoided the need for surgery, no perforations, and significant cost savings compared to surgical resection [104]. The most frequently reported major complications – perforation (0–5 %) and bleeding (0.5–6 %) – may require surgical management, and removal of large sessile lesions is technically demanding, often requiring a lengthy procedure time to retrieve fragments of lesions and may require multiple endoscopic sessions for complete ablation of a large adenoma [98].

Endoscopic Submucosal Dissection (ESD)

Key Concept: *ESD provides an improved ability for en bloc resection over EMR and is a better option for larger superficial colorectal tumors; however, it is technically demanding and has a higher rate of complications.*

Endoscopic submucosal dissection (ESD) was developed to overcome the limitations of conventional EMR. ESD is primarily used in Japan and in select centers in Europe and the USA to resect larger polyps and selected invasive tumors and aid in achieving higher rates of en bloc resection of superficial tumors than EMR. ESD is a complicated technique for treating large superficial colorectal tumors because it provides a higher en bloc resection rate and is less invasive than surgical resection. Others have proposed that this technique is suitable for all large polyps, early colorectal cancer, and those lesions that cannot be accessed by transanal or TEMS routes and wish to avoid major resection. ESD can be considered in lesions that have a higher rate of submucosal infiltration and require detailed histopathologic diagnosis by en bloc resection or when fibrosis has developed on the submucosal layer from biopsy and EMR is difficult because of non-lifting signs [105].

The technique of ESD involves an endoscope with a single channel, along with a high-frequency generator (Video 32.4, Courtesy of Peter Marcello, MD). After identification of a lesion, a mixture of 1 % hyaluronic acid solution and 10 % glycerin solution is injected around the lesions to elevate the submucosa [106]. The border of the tumor is initially marked by indigo carmine dye with 1 cm margins. Following a mucosal incision, a partial or circumferential incision is made with injection of hyaluronic acid solution into the submucosa, and the dissection is carried down to the deep submucosa. This process is continued around the tumor until the entire lesion is resected en bloc [107]. The en bloc excision with ESD has a number of theoretical advantages, including more accurate histologic assessment, reduced recurrence, decreased endoscopic surveillance requirements, and potential surveillance cost savings [102]. For laterally spreading rectal tumors, ESD is becoming more prevalent, although transanal endoscopic microsurgery is still frequently used [108]. ESD also has the additional advantages of minimal invasiveness and avoidance of anesthesia [109]. Successful en bloc resection has been reported in up to 85–89 % of cases, with piecemeal resection in the remaining 10–15 % [100, 105, 110–112]. However, there are risks with this new technology. ESD is still associated with higher perforation rate, longer procedure times, and increased technical difficulty [113]. The thinner colorectal wall and winding nature of the colon make colorectal ESD an especially difficult operative technique [114]. Further, residual disease has been reported in 2–3 % with ESD [115]. The application of colorectal ESD needs to be further evaluated, with improvements in technology in the technical skill, and surgical devices are required before widespread use.

Endoscopic techniques have evolved to the point where they can be applied to full-thickness resection of polyps, reducing risk compared to surgical resection and accelerating patient recovery. The *Tissue Apposition System* (*TAS*) was developed to facilitate this approach (Video 32.5). TAS is a novel endoscopic suturing system that enables endoluminal full-thickness closure [96]. The polypectomy site is closed under laparoscopic observation to avoid injury to surrounding structures. In a feasibility study, TAS was demonstrated to be safe under laparoscopic guidance [96]. Initial studies have shown no long-term complications and normal healed mucosa with the sutures and anchoring devices in place at follow-up colonoscopy [116]. TAS may increase the number of patients whose difficult polyps can be removed endoscopically, avoiding the need for a surgical resection in select patients. Based on early results, TAS sets the future direction in minimizing surgery for endoscopically unresectable colonic polyps. These endoscopic technological advances are improving lesion assessment and standardization, and new methods and techniques are being developed to enhance procedural safety and efficacy.

Combining Laparoscopy and Endoscopy

Key Concept: Combining colonoscopy with laparoscopy allows removal of select previously inaccessible polyps without the morbidity of a surgical resection. Additionally, a standard resection can be performed at that time given advanced pathology, technical problems, or an inability to perform endoscopic removal.

Adding the laparoscopic approach to endoscopically unresectable polyps enriches the therapeutic spectrum. Due to location or size, some polyps are deemed unsafe or technically impossible to treat endoscopically and require colectomy. The perceived risk of iatrogenic injury including hemorrhage and colonic perforation may prevent an attempt at polypectomy [117]. In such cases, where standard polypectomy via the colonoscope is considered not technically possible, patients may be referred for colonic resection. However, there is significant morbidity associated with a surgical resection, including wound infection, anastomotic leak, ileus, and death [3, 5, 10, 18, 118]. By combining laparoscopic mobilization of the bowel with colonoscopic polypectomy – *combined laparoscopic and endoscopic resection* (*CLER*) – previously inaccessible polyps could be snared, and laparotomy with enterotomy or bowel resection can be avoided (Fig. 32.4; Video 32.6). Franklin et al. reported on a series of 110 patients undergoing colonoscopic polypectomy following laparoscopic mobilization of the colon [119]. Smaller studies have also demonstrated the feasibility of CLER technique for small series of unresectable polyps [120–124]. A 10-year review of CLER for noninvasive or benign colorectal polyps found low rates of conversion (5 %), major post-operative complications, and intraoperative complications (1 %). However, follow-up colonoscopy revealed metachronous adenomas in more than one-third of patients [125]. The authors concluded that CLER is an efficient, safe, and minimally invasive alternative to open resection for selected patients with difficult polyps. Further experience and results of large-scale trials are needed before applying CLER more broadly. Above all, it is imperative to have the polyp assessed by an experienced endoscopist before embarking on a CLER as this may save the patient from undergoing general anesthesia. The majority of polyps are still possible to remove by standard endoscopic techniques.

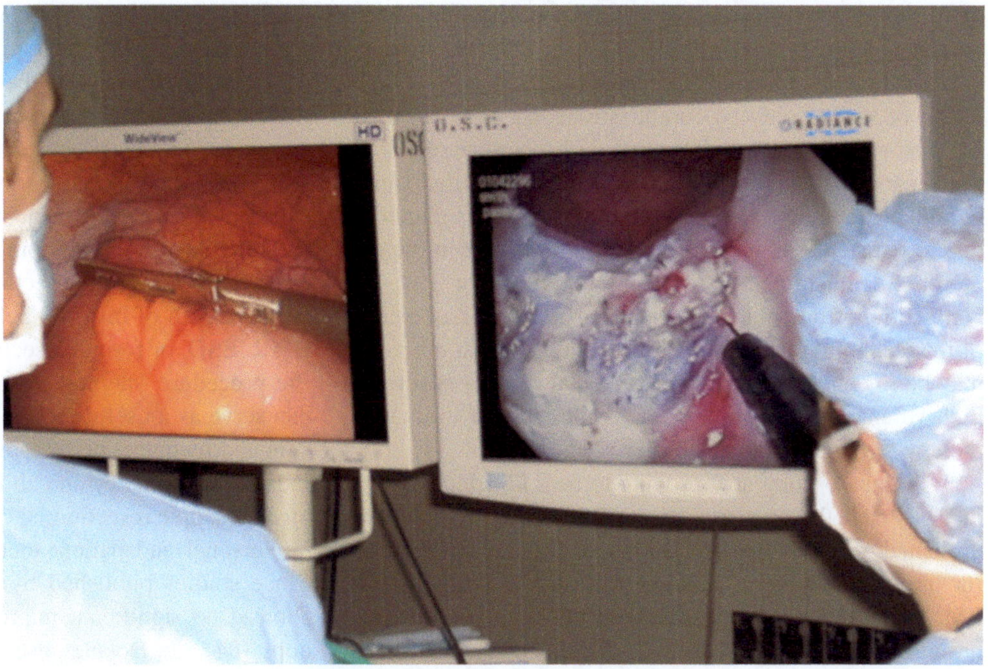

Fig. 32.4 Combined laparoscopic and endoscopic resection procedure

The Cost of New Technology

Key Concept: *There is a balance on the cost of acquisition, learning, and maintenance of new technology with the potential benefits that each surgeon must consider.*

It is increasingly necessary to consider the cost of new technology with the need for the new innovations, especially given the ongoing health-care crisis in the USA. It is well known that health-care costs are rising at an unsustainable rate, as evidenced by expenditures in the USA nearing $2.6 trillion in 2010, over ten times the $256 billion spent in 1980 [126]. Projections show that this trend is continuing, with National Health Expenditures doubling from 2.6 to 5.2 trillion and accounting for 20 % of the gross domestic product by 2020 [127]. In an era of increasing health-care costs, decreasing reimbursements, and low operating margins, cost-efficiency will become an essential for financial survival for patients, employers, providers, and payers alike. Surgical interventions are a prime target for cost-effectiveness, as they are associated with significant equipment costs and increased costs and lower reimbursement associated with complications. If there is a measurable patient benefit and the possibility to become more efficient with the technology (either through experience or direct equipment costs), the benefits will eventually outweigh the costs. Laparoscopic colorectal surgery is the ideal model when considering balancing costs versus technology. LC has evolved into a cost-effective technology. Compared to OC, the laparoscopic method is associated with higher operating room costs [128–131]; however, the initial higher operating room and equipment cost is generally offset by shorter LOS and improvements in patient quality of life [6, 7, 11, 128, 130, 132, 133]. Moreover, laparoscopy has facilitated the application of enhanced recovery pathways in colorectal surgery [134, 135], along with their associated improved resource utilization [11, 136]. These potential benefits may outweigh the increased costs at the time of surgery. As LC has increased in use and efficiency, cost improvements and lower overall direct costs have resulted [7, 136]. While cost efficiencies had been less clear for LRR, a recent model reported a cost-benefit of $4,283 for both laparoscopic colon and rectal cancer resections [137].

One of the major concerns about robotic surgery is its cost. Those in favor of robotics emphasize that robotics is a technology that is still relatively new. Whereas much of the reported early experience of laparoscopy demonstrated higher costs when compared to open, that has changed over time. Furthermore, despite the cost-efficiency of laparoscopy in colon resections, a recent 2009 Inpatient Sample shows that only 35 % of colectomies performed in the USA were done laparoscopically [138]. In cases where the difficulty of performing laparoscopic surgery prevents its use, robotic technology is another minimally invasive option. The reduction in conversion to open rates that may be provided through robotics may justify its cost, although a 5 % reduction in conversion rate, then the additional cost per conversion saved would equal 20 times the additional cost of a single robotic case – generally estimated as about $2,500 per case in most series. Currently, the increase in cost for robotics ranges from acquisition, maintenance, and operative time [46, 49, 60, 69, 72]. These additional costs are borne by the health-care facility, without any increase in reimbursement or incremental advantage related to reduction in length of stay or reduced complications, benefits that made LC cost-effective when compared with open surgery [71]. The financial feasibility of robotic colorectal surgery may require incremental admission volume for other diagnoses due to reduced length of stay [139], a reduction in the cost of robot acquisition and reusable equipment, or increased competition from manufacturers and wider dissemination of the technology [50]. The best practice for cost-efficiency may be to concentrate robotic colorectal surgery at selected high-volume centers while it undergoes further evaluation, thereby trying to optimize efficiency and quality.

With laparoscopy now proving to be cost-effective in its maturity and the cost analysis of robotics currently being evaluated, we must keep in mind these arguments apply also for the other emerging technologies such as SILS, CLER, ESD, and EMR. On the upside, SILS improves cosmesis and has reported other advantages. On the downside, SILS technology utilizes new single-port access devices and can potentially increase operative times, cost, and make learning curves more complicated for trainees. In addition, while ESD and EMR may avoid a formal resection, patients undergoing ESD and EMR have an increased need for multiple follow-up colonoscopies, which can increase health-care costs as well. Emerging technologies give modern medicine an exciting opportunity to improve patient outcomes but can increase cost – especially direct costs. By integrating cost-effective technology into practice, we have the opportunity to improve both patient and financial outcomes.

Summary Pearls, Patient Selection, and Personal Preferences

Key Concept: While the concept of new technology is exciting, careful consideration of the patient and their pathology is necessary to choose the appropriate technology. Each surgeon must develop their own preferences for new technology based on their training and personal experience.

Careful planning is needed to decide when to use ESD or EMR versus CLER or a formal resection. En bloc excision using EMR is limited to lesions 20 mm or smaller, with minimal invasion to the submucosa, more than one-third of the luminal diameter, and no invasion to lymphatic channels or vessels. As it is difficult to perform en bloc EMR resection for lesions larger than 20 mm, piecemeal EMR becomes the least invasive and least costly option for these lesions [102].

In our hands, ESD is reserved for polyps that fail EMR, or are not suitable for EMR because of scarring or location. Based on polyp anatomy and location, a decision is then made to perform ESD or CLER. This is done in the operating room, so that if during intraoperative endoscopy a decision is made that the polyp cannot be removed, a laparoscopic colectomy is performed at the same time. We have not used ESD for cancers and prefer to perform a laparoscopic segmental colectomy in those cases, as our morbidity rates are low [136]. The inability to raise the base of a polyp after submucosal injection can indicate the presence of cancer invading deep into the submucosa and that patient should be referred for surgical resection [140]. Having the ability to predict depth of invasion helps to decide whether to pursue EMR, ESD, or formal resection remains somewhat difficult. Pre-procedure staging with endoscopic ultrasound (EUS) can serve as a useful tool by determining the depth of invasion and by detecting the presence of lymph nodes that may indicate malignancy and ability to perform (or not perform) an endoscopic resection.

Personal and patient factors influence the use of SILS. Since studies published by Drs. Champagne and Delaney showed no significant improvement over standard laparoscopy [84], Dr. Delaney uses SILS in a selected fashion and primarily to educate residents. In contrast, many surgeons are proponents of SILS – they and their patients appreciate the improved cosmesis and reduction in postoperative pain. Surgeons that endorse SILS tend to use both laparoscopic and robotic SILS in their practice, finding SILS to be easier with the robot.

The application and indications for CLER are still under development. Dr. Delaney does not often use CLER. If the gastroenterologist performing the colonoscopy feels he or she can get to a lesion endoscopically with help, Dr. Delaney will use a CLER approach. Otherwise, if a lesion is not amenable to endoscopic polypectomy, he offers a formal resection; the option of CLER is discussed but only performed if the patient insists. In his experience, a large percentage of these unresectable lesions are invasive cancer, and a formal colectomy is needed anyway. Further, the morbidity of a segmental colectomy is favorable versus attempting CLER. Dr. Delaney performs EMR preferentially for all cases, including rectal polyps, saving patients the anesthesia required for ESD, CLER, or resection. In 30–50 % of cases referred by outside gastroenterologists for resection, he removes the polyps endoscopically.

The use of robotics is a hotly debated topic. Dr. Delaney does not use robotics since the initial paper he published in 2003 [70], as well as a series of patients he did since that time. In his opinion, the cost of this technology is not justified for abdominal or rectal resections, and there is no tangible benefit realized over traditional laparoscopy. In an opposing view, other surgeons are strong supporters of robotics. They find it offers improved surgeon ergonomics and a superior approach in pelvic dissections, SILS, and high BMI patients that would not be possible with traditional laparoscopy. These surgeons consider that robotics is a natural evolution of minimally invasive surgery and that the technology will be more widely accepted when there is more robotic competition and choices. This increased market competition will hopefully drive the cost of robotic technology down, as it did in laparoscopy.

Conclusion

The future of technology in colorectal surgery is exciting. New technology innovation in health care is an important driver of growth. With the current state of health care, it behooves us to strategically incorporate new innovations to streamline the delivery of quality health care and optimize patient outcomes. Successful integration of technology requires patience along the learning curve and careful patient selection to match the appropriate technology to the patient and disease process. Using the integration of laparoscopy as a model, the benefits have the potential to outweigh early technical difficulties and inefficiencies. Incorporating new technology will facilitate meeting meaningful use requirements and connecting with physicians, payers, and the community. Furthermore, wisely investing in new technology allows measuring incremental improvement in clinical outcomes for patients and use of health-care resources.

References

1. Akle CA. Early parietal recurrence of adenocarcinoma of the colon after laparoscopic colectomy. Port site metastasis after laparoscopic colorectal surgery for cure of malignancy. Br J Surg. 1996;83(3):427.
2. Jenkins NL, Roth JS, Johnson JO, Pofahl WE. Laparoscopic colorectal surgery: indications and techniques. Curr Surg. 2005;62(3):319–23.
3. Clinical Outcomes of Surgical Therapy Study Group. A comparison of laparoscopically assisted and open colectomy for colon cancer. N Engl J Med. 2004;350(20):2050–9.
4. Bonjer HJ, Hop WC, Nelson H, Sargent DJ, Lacy AM, Castells A, et al. Laparoscopically assisted vs open colectomy for colon cancer: a meta-analysis. Arch Surg. 2007;142(3):298–303.
5. Lacy AM, Garcia-Valdecasas JC, Delgado S, Castells A, Taura P, Pique JM, et al. Laparoscopy-assisted colectomy versus open colectomy for treatment of non-metastatic colon cancer: a randomised trial. Lancet. 2002;359(9325):2224–9.
6. Schwenk W, Haase O, Neudecker J, Muller JM. Short term benefits for laparoscopic colorectal resection. Cochrane Database Syst Rev. 2005;(3):CD003145.
7. Delaney CP, Kiran RP, Senagore AJ, Brady K, Fazio VW. Case-matched comparison of clinical and financial outcome after laparoscopic or open colorectal surgery. Ann Surg. 2003;238(1):67–72.
8. Delaney CP, Marcello PW, Sonoda T, Wise P, Bauer J, Techner L. Gastrointestinal recovery after laparoscopic colectomy: results of a prospective, observational, multicenter study. Surg Endosc. 2010;24(3):653–61.
9. Champagne BJ, Delaney CP. Laparoscopic approaches to rectal cancer. Clin Colon Rectal Surg. 2007;20(3):237–48.
10. Veldkamp R, Kuhry E, Hop WC, Jeekel J, Kazemier G, Bonjer HJ, et al. Laparoscopic surgery versus open surgery for colon cancer: short-term outcomes of a randomised trial. Lancet Oncol. 2005;6(7):477–84.
11. Delaney CP, Chang E, Senagore AJ, Broder M. Clinical outcomes and resource utilization associated with laparoscopic and open colectomy using a large national database. Ann Surg. 2008;247(5):819–24.
12. Champagne BJ, Makhija R. Minimally invasive surgery for rectal cancer: are we there yet? World J Gastroenterol. 2011;17(7):862–6.
13. Jayne DG, Guillou PJ, Thorpe H, Quirke P, Copeland J, Smith AM, et al. Randomized trial of laparoscopic-assisted resection of colorectal carcinoma: 3-year results of the UK MRC CLASICC Trial Group. J Clin Oncol. 2007;25(21):3061–8.
14. Jayne DG, Thorpe HC, Copeland J, Quirke P, Brown JM, Guillou PJ. Five-year follow-up of the Medical Research Council CLASICC trial of laparoscopically assisted versus open surgery for colorectal cancer. Br J Surg. 2010;97(11):1638–45.
15. Aziz O, Constantinides V, Tekkis PP, Athanasiou T, Purkayastha S, Paraskeva P, et al. Laparoscopic versus open surgery for rectal cancer: a meta-analysis. Ann Surg Oncol. 2006;13(3):413–24.
16. Baik SH, Gincherman M, Mutch MG, Birnbaum EH, Fleshman JW. Laparoscopic vs open resection for patients with rectal cancer: comparison of perioperative outcomes and long-term survival. Dis Colon Rectum. 2011;54(1):6–14.
17. Gao F, Cao YF, Chen LS. Meta-analysis of short-term outcomes after laparoscopic resection for rectal cancer. Int J Colorectal Dis. 2006;21(7):652–6.
18. Guillou PJ, Quirke P, Thorpe H, Walker J, Jayne DG, Smith AM, et al. Short-term endpoints of conventional versus laparoscopic-assisted surgery in patients with colorectal cancer (MRC CLASICC trial): multicentre, randomised controlled trial. Lancet. 2005;365(9472):1718–26.
19. Kang SB, Park JW, Jeong SY, Nam BH, Choi HS, Kim DW, et al. Open versus laparoscopic surgery for mid or low rectal cancer after neoadjuvant chemoradiotherapy (COREAN trial): short-term outcomes of an open-label randomised controlled trial. Lancet Oncol. 2010;11(7):637–45.
20. Laurent C, Leblanc F, Gineste C, Saric J, Rullier E. Laparoscopic approach in surgical treatment of rectal cancer. Br J Surg. 2007;94(12):1555–61.
21. Lelong B, Bege T, Esterni B, Guiramand J, Turrini O, Moutardier V, et al. Short-term outcome after laparoscopic or open restorative mesorectal excision for rectal cancer: a comparative cohort study. Dis Colon Rectum. 2007;50(2):176–83.
22. Leung KL, Lai PB, Ho RL, Meng WC, Yiu RY, Lee JF, et al. Systemic cytokine response after laparoscopic-assisted resection of rectosigmoid carcinoma: a prospective randomized trial. Ann Surg. 2000;231(4):506–11.
23. Lujan J, Valero G, Hernandez Q, Sanchez A, Frutos MD, Parrilla P. Randomized clinical trial comparing laparoscopic and open surgery in patients with rectal cancer. Br J Surg. 2009;96(9):982–9.
24. Ng SS, Leung KL, Lee JF, Yiu RY, Li JC, Teoh AY, et al. Laparoscopic-assisted versus open abdominoperineal resection for low rectal cancer: a prospective randomized trial. Ann Surg Oncol. 2008;15(9):2418–25.
25. Ng SS, Leung KL, Lee JF, Yiu RY, Li JC, Hon SS. Long-term morbidity and oncologic outcomes of laparoscopic-assisted anterior resection for upper rectal cancer: ten-year results of a prospective, randomized trial. Dis Colon Rectum. 2009;52(4):558–66.
26. Anderson C, Uman G, Pigazzi A. Oncologic outcomes of laparoscopic surgery for rectal cancer: a systematic review and meta-analysis of the literature. Eur J Surg Oncol. 2008;34(10):1135–42.
27. Huang MJ, Liang JL, Wang H, Kang L, Deng YH, Wang JP. Laparoscopic-assisted versus open surgery for rectal cancer: a meta-analysis of randomized controlled trials on oncologic adequacy of resection and long-term oncologic outcomes. Int J Colorectal Dis. 2011;26(4):415–21.
28. Ohtani H, Tamamori Y, Azuma T, Mori Y, Nishiguchi Y, Maeda K, et al. A meta-analysis of the short- and long-term results of randomized controlled trials that compared laparoscopy-assisted and con-

ventional open surgery for rectal cancer. J Gastrointest Surg. 2011;15(8):1375–85.

29. Choi DH, Jeong WK, Lim SW, Chung TS, Park JI, Lim SB, et al. Learning curves for laparoscopic sigmoidectomy used to manage curable sigmoid colon cancer: single-institute, three-surgeon experience. Surg Endosc. 2009;23(3):622–8.
30. Pandey S, Slawik S, Cross K, Soulsby R, Pullyblank AM, Dixon AR. Laparoscopic appendicectomy: a training model for laparoscopic right hemicolectomy? Colorectal Dis. 2007;9(6):536–9.
31. Tekkis PP, Senagore AJ, Delaney CP. Conversion rates in laparoscopic colorectal surgery: a predictive model with, 1253 patients. Surg Endosc. 2005;19(1):47–54.
32. Wexner SD, Cohen SM. Port site metastases after laparoscopic colorectal surgery for cure of malignancy. Br J Surg. 1995;82(3): 295–8.
33. Akiyoshi T, Kuroyanagi H, Ueno M, Oya M, Fujimoto Y, Konishi T, et al. Learning curve for standardized laparoscopic surgery for colorectal cancer under supervision: a single-center experience. Surg Endosc. 2011;25(5):1409–14.
34. Li JC, Hon SS, Ng SS, Lee JF, Yiu RY, Leung KL. The learning curve for laparoscopic colectomy: experience of a surgical fellow in an university colorectal unit. Surg Endosc. 2009;23(7):1603–8.
35. Park IJ, Choi GS, Lim KH, Kang BM, Jun SH. Multidimensional analysis of the learning curve for laparoscopic colorectal surgery: lessons from 1,000 cases of laparoscopic colorectal surgery. Surg Endosc. 2009;23(4):839–46.
36. Nelson H, Petrelli N, Carlin A, Couture J, Fleshman J, Guillem J, et al. Guidelines 2000 for colon and rectal cancer surgery. J Natl Cancer Inst. 2001;93(8):583–96.
37. Row D, Weiser MR. An update on laparoscopic resection for rectal cancer. Cancer Control. 2010;17(1):16–24.
38. Kavic MS. Hand-assisted laparoscopic surgery–HALS. JSLS. 2001;5(2):101–3.
39. Hand-assisted laparoscopic surgery vs standard laparoscopic surgery for colorectal disease: a prospective randomized trial. HALS Study Group. Surg Endosc. 2000;14(10):896–901.
40. Meijer DW, Bannenberg JJ, Jakimowicz JJ. Hand-assisted laparoscopic surgery: an overview. Surg Endosc. 2000;14(10):891–5.
41. Leblanc F, Delaney CP, Neary PC, Rose J, Augestad KM, Senagore AJ, et al. Assessment of comparative skills between hand-assisted and straight laparoscopic colorectal training on an augmented reality simulator. Dis Colon Rectum. 2010;53(9):1323–7.
42. Cima RR, Pattana-arun J, Larson DW, Dozois EJ, Wolff BG, Pemberton JH. Experience with 969 minimal access colectomies: the role of hand-assisted laparoscopy in expanding minimally invasive surgery for complex colectomies. J Am Coll Surg. 2008;206(5):946–50; discussion 950–2.
43. Asgeirsson T, Delaney CP. Laparoscopic proctectomy: oncologic considerations. Surg Laparosc Endosc Percutan Tech. 2012;22(3): 175–9.
44. Alasari S, Min BS. Robotic colorectal surgery: a systematic review. ISRN Surg. 2012;2012:293894.
45. Baik SH. Robotic colorectal surgery. Yonsei Med J. 2008;49(6):891–6.
46. Abbou CC, Hoznek A, Salomon L, Olsson LE, Lobontiu A, Saint F, et al. Laparoscopic radical prostatectomy with a remote controlled robot. J Urol. 2001;165(6 Pt 1):1964–6.
47. Kong SH, Oh BM, Yoon H, Ahn HS, Lee HJ, Chung SG, et al. Comparison of two- and three-dimensional camera systems in laparoscopic performance: a novel 3D system with one camera. Surg Endosc. 2010;24(5):1132–43.
48. Ostrowitz MB, Eschete D, Zemon H, DeNoto G. Robotic-assisted single-incision right colectomy: early experience. Int J Med Robot. 2009;5(4):465–70.
49. Park SY, Choi GS, Park JS, Kim HJ, Ryuk JP. Short-term clinical outcome of robot-assisted intersphincteric resection for low rectal cancer: a retrospective comparison with conventional laparoscopy. Surg Endosc. 2013;27:48–55.
50. Ahmed K, Ibrahim A, Wang TT, Khan N, Challacombe B, Khan MS, et al. Assessing the cost effectiveness of robotics in urological surgery – a systematic review. BJU Int. 2012;110:1544–56.
51. Kim JY, Kim NK, Lee KY, Hur H, Min BS, Kim JH. A comparative study of voiding and sexual function after total mesorectal excision with autonomic nerve preservation for rectal cancer: laparoscopic versus robotic surgery. Ann Surg Oncol. 2012;19(8): 2485–93.
52. Morino M, Parini U, Allaix ME, Monasterolo G, Brachet Contul R, Garrone C. Male sexual and urinary function after laparoscopic total mesorectal excision. Surg Endosc. 2009;23(6):1233–40.
53. Yang Y, Wang F, Zhang P, Shi C, Zou Y, Qin H, et al. Robot-assisted versus conventional laparoscopic surgery for colorectal disease, focusing on rectal cancer: a meta-analysis. Ann Surg Oncol. 2012; 19:3727–36.
54. Ortiz-Oshiro E, Sanchez-Egido I, Moreno-Sierra J, Perez CF, Diaz JS, Fernandez-Represa JA. Robotic assistance may reduce conversion to open in rectal carcinoma laparoscopic surgery: systematic review and meta-analysis. Int J Med Robot. 2012;8:360–70.
55. Memon S, Heriot AG, Murphy DG, Bressel M, Lynch AC. Robotic versus laparoscopic proctectomy for rectal cancer: a meta-analysis. Ann Surg Oncol. 2012;19(7):2095–101.
56. Trastulli S, Farinella E, Cirocchi R, Cavaliere D, Avenia N, Sciannameo F, et al. Robotic resection compared with laparoscopic rectal resection for cancer: systematic review and meta-analysis of short-term outcome. Colorectal Dis. 2012;14(4):e134–56.
57. Baik SH, Kwon HY, Kim JS, Hur H, Sohn SK, Cho CH, et al. Robotic versus laparoscopic low anterior resection of rectal cancer: short-term outcome of a prospective comparative study. Ann Surg Oncol. 2009;16(6):1480–7.
58. Kim KY, Hwang DW, Park YK, Lee HS. A single surgeon's experience with 54 consecutive cases of multivisceral resection for locally advanced primary colorectal cancer: can the laparoscopic approach be performed safely? Surg Endosc. 2012;26(2):493–500.
59. Jayne DG, Brown JM, Thorpe H, Walker J, Quirke P, Guillou PJ. Bladder and sexual function following resection for rectal cancer in a randomized clinical trial of laparoscopic versus open technique. Br J Surg. 2005;92(9):1124–32.
60. Lin S, Jiang HG, Chen ZH, Zhou SY, Liu XS, Yu JR. Meta-analysis of robotic and laparoscopic surgery for treatment of rectal cancer. World J Gastroenterol. 2011;17(47):5214–20.
61. Collinson FJ, Jayne DG, Pigazzi A, Tsang C, Barrie JM, Edlin R, et al. An international, multicentre, prospective, randomised, controlled, unblinded, parallel-group trial of robotic-assisted versus standard laparoscopic surgery for the curative treatment of rectal cancer. Int J Colorectal Dis. 2012;27(2):233–41.
62. Zimmern A, Prasad L, Desouza A, Marecik S, Park J, Abcarian H. Robotic colon and rectal surgery: a series of 131 cases. World J Surg. 2010;34:1954–58.
63. Abodeely A, Lagares-Garcia JA, Duron V, Vrees M. Safety and learning curve in robotic colorectal surgery. Robot Surg 2010;4(3):161–5.
64. Ragupathi M, Ramos-Valadez DI, Patel CB, Haas EM. Robotic-assisted laparoscopic surgery for recurrent diverticulitis: experience in consecutive cases and a review of the literature. Surg Endosc. 2011;25:199–206.
65. de Hoog DE, Heemskerk J, Nieman FH, van Gemert WG, Baeten CG, Bouvy ND. Recurrence and functional results after open versus conventional laparoscopic versus robot-assisted laparoscopic rectopexy for rectal prolapse: a case-control study. Int J Colorectal Dis. 2009;24:1201–6.
66. Bokhari MB, Patel CB, Ramos-Valadez DI, Ragupathi M, Haas EM. Learning curve for robotic-assisted laparoscopic colorectal surgery. Surg Endosc. 2011;25:855–60.
67. de Souza AL, Prasad LM, Park JJ, Marecik SJ, Blumetti J, Abcarian H. Robotic assistance in right hemicolectomy: is there a role? Dis Colon Rectum 2010;53(7):1000–6.

68. Luca F, Ghezzi TL, Valvo M et al. Surgical and pathological outcomes after right hemicolectomy: case-matched study comparing robotic and open surgery. Int J Med Robot. 2011 May 11. doi: 10.1002/rcs.398. [Epub ahead of print].
69. D'Annibale A, Morpurgo E, Fiscon V, Trevisan P, Sovernigo G, Orsini C, et al. Robotic and laparoscopic surgery for treatment of colorectal diseases. Dis Colon Rectum. 2004;47(12):2162–8.
70. Delaney CP, Lynch AC, Senagore AJ, Fazio VW. Comparison of robotically performed and traditional laparoscopic colorectal surgery. Dis Colon Rectum. 2003;46(12):1633–9.
71. Delaney CP, Senagore AJ, Ponsky L. Robot-assisted surgery and health care costs. N Engl J Med. 2010;363(22):2175; author reply 2176.
72. Barbash GI, Glied SA. New technology and health care costs–the case of robot-assisted surgery. N Engl J Med. 2010;363(8):701–4.
73. Wright JD, Ananth CV, Lewin SN, Burke WM, Lu YS, Neugut AI, et al. Robotically assisted vs laparoscopic hysterectomy among women with benign gynecologic disease. JAMA. 2013; 309(7):689–98.
74. Citron intuitive surgical's bad day in court: trial proceeds in three weeks. 2013. Available Online at http://www.citronresearch.com/wp-content/uploads/2013/03/Intuitive-Surgical-Taylor-case-update-final.pdf.
75. Breeden JT. Statement on robotic surgery by the American College of Obstetricians and Gynecologists. 2013. Available Online at http://www.acog.org/About_ACOG/News_Room/News_Releases/2013/Statement_on_Robotic_Surgery.
76. Jin LX, Ibrahim AM, Newman NA, Makarov DV, Pronovost PJ, Makary MA. Robotic surgery claims on United States hospital websites. J Healthc Qual. 2011;33(6):48–52.
77. Citron research reports on intuitive surgical: has the halo been broken on intuitive surgical? 2012. Available Online at http://www.citronresearch.com/wp-content/uploads/2012/12/isrg-final1.pdf.
78. Piskun G, Rajpal S. Transumbilical laparoscopic cholecystectomy utilizes no incisions outside the umbilicus. J Laparoendosc Adv Surg Tech A. 1999;9(4):361–4.
79. Remzi FH, Kirat HT, Kaouk JH, Geisler DP. Single-port laparoscopy in colorectal surgery. Colorectal Dis. 2008;10(8):823–6.
80. Bucher P, Pugin F, Morel P. Single port access laparoscopic right hemicolectomy. Int J Colorectal Dis. 2008;23(10):1013–6.
81. Papaconstantinou HT, Sharp N, Thomas JS. Single-incision laparoscopic right colectomy: a case-matched comparison with standard laparoscopic and hand-assisted laparoscopic techniques. J Am Coll Surg. 2011;213(1):72–80; discussion 80–2.
82. Kim SJ, Ryu GO, Choi BJ, Kim JG, Lee KJ, Lee SC, et al. The short-term outcomes of conventional and single-port laparoscopic surgery for colorectal cancer. Ann Surg. 2011;254(6):933–40.
83. Adair J, Gromski MA, Lim RB, Nagle D. Single-incision laparoscopic right colectomy: experience with 17 consecutive cases and comparison with multiport laparoscopic right colectomy. Dis Colon Rectum. 2010;53(11):1549–54.
84. Champagne BJ, Papaconstantinou HT, Parmar SS, Nagle DA, Young-Fadok TM, Lee EC, et al. Single-incision versus standard multiport laparoscopic colectomy: a multicenter, case-controlled comparison. Ann Surg. 2012;255(1):66–9.
85. Chen WT, Chang SC, Chiang HC, Lo WY, Jeng LB, Wu C, et al. Single-incision laparoscopic versus conventional laparoscopic right hemicolectomy: a comparison of short-term surgical results. Surg Endosc. 2011;25(6):1887–92.
86. Huscher CG, Mingoli A, Sgarzini G, Mereu A, Binda B, Brachini G, et al. Standard laparoscopic versus single-incision laparoscopic colectomy for cancer: early results of a randomized prospective study. Am J Surg. 2012;204(1):115–20.
87. Vasilakis V, Clark CE, Liasis L, Papaconstantinou HT. Noncosmetic benefits of single-incision laparoscopic sigmoid colectomy for diverticular disease: A case-matched comparison with multiport laparoscopic technique. J Surg Res. 2013;180:201–7.
88. Chambers WM, Bicsak M, Lamparelli M, Dixon AR. Single-incision laparoscopic surgery (SILS) in complex colorectal surgery: a technique offering potential and not just cosmesis. Colorectal Dis. 2011;13(4):393–8.
89. Bulut O, Nielsen CB, Jespersen N. Single-port access laparoscopic surgery for rectal cancer: initial experience with 10 cases. Dis Colon Rectum. 2011;54(7):803–9.
90. Poon JT, Cheung CW, Fan JK, Lo OS, Law WL. Single-incision versus conventional laparoscopic colectomy for colonic neoplasm: a randomized, controlled trial. Surg Endosc. 2012;26(10): 2729–34.
91. Merchant AM, Cook MW, White BC, Davis SS, Sweeney JF, Lin E. Transumbilical Gelport access technique for performing single incision laparoscopic surgery (SILS). J Gastrointest Surg. 2009; 13(1):159–62.
92. Gaujoux S, Bretagnol F, Ferron M, Panis Y. Single-incision laparoscopic colonic surgery. Colorectal Dis. 2011;13(9):1066–71.
93. Champagne BJ, Lee EC, Leblanc F, Stein SL, Delaney CP. Single-incision vs straight laparoscopic segmental colectomy: a case-controlled study. Dis Colon Rectum. 2011;54(2):183–6.
94. Park JS, Choi GS, Park SY, Kim HJ, Ryuk JP. Randomized clinical trial of robot-assisted versus standard laparoscopic right colectomy. Br J Surg. 2012;99(9):1219–26.
95. Pucher PH, Sodergren MH, Singh P, Darzi A, Parakseva P. Have we learned from lessons of the past? A systematic review of training for single incision laparoscopic surgery. Surg Endosc. 2013;27:1478–84.
96. Delaney CP, Champagne BJ, Marks JM, Sanuk L, Ermlich B, Chak A. Tissue apposition system: new technology to minimize surgery for endoscopically unresectable colonic polyps. Surg Endosc. 2010;24(12):3113–8.
97. Nelson DB, Block KP, Bosco JJ, Burdick JS, Curtis WD, Faigel DO, et al. Endoscopic mucosal resection: May 2000. Gastrointest Endosc. 2000;52(6 Pt 1):860–3.
98. Repici A, Pellicano R, Strangio G, Danese S, Fagoonee S, Malesci A. Endoscopic mucosal resection for early colorectal neoplasia: pathologic basis, procedures, and outcomes. Dis Colon Rectum. 2009;52(8):1502–15.
99. Iishi H, Tatsuta M, Iseki K, Narahara H, Uedo N, Sakai N, et al. Endoscopic piecemeal resection with submucosal saline injection of large sessile colorectal polyps. Gastrointest Endosc. 2000;51(6):697–700.
100. Saito Y, Fukuzawa M, Matsuda T, Fukunaga S, Sakamoto T, Uraoka T, et al. Clinical outcome of endoscopic submucosal dissection versus endoscopic mucosal resection of large colorectal tumors as determined by curative resection. Surg Endosc. 2010;24(2):343–52.
101. Tanaka S, Haruma K, Oka S, Takahashi R, Kunihiro M, Kitadai Y, et al. Clinicopathologic features and endoscopic treatment of superficially spreading colorectal neoplasms larger than 20 mm. Gastrointest Endosc. 2001;54(1):62–6.
102. Holt BA, Bourke MJ. Wide field endoscopic resection for advanced colonic mucosal neoplasia: current status and future directions. Clin Gastroenterol Hepatol. 2012;10(9):969–79.
103. Puli SR, Kakugawa Y, Gotoda T, Antillon D, Saito Y, Antillon MR. Meta-analysis and systematic review of colorectal endoscopic mucosal resection. World J Gastroenterol. 2009;15(34):4273–7.
104. Swan MP, Bourke MJ, Alexander S, Moss A, Williams SJ. Large refractory colonic polyps: is it time to change our practice? A prospective study of the clinical and economic impact of a tertiary referral colonic mucosal resection and polypectomy service (with videos). Gastrointest Endosc. 2009;70(6):1128–36.
105. Tanaka S, Oka S, Kaneko I, Hirata M, Mouri R, Kanao H, et al. Endoscopic submucosal dissection for colorectal neoplasia: possibility of standardization. Gastrointest Endosc. 2007;66(1):100–7.
106. Yamamoto H, Kawata H, Sunada K, Sasaki A, Nakazawa K, Miyata T, et al. Successful en-bloc resection of large superficial tumors in the stomach and colon using sodium hyaluronate and small-caliber-tip transparent hood. Endoscopy. 2003;35(8):690–4.

107. Steele SR. ASCRS core subject update 2011. Endoscopy/Polyps. Available Online at: http://www.fascrs.org/physicians/education/core_subjects/2011/Endoscopy. Accessed October 2013.
108. Chang DK. Current status of colorectal endoscopic submucosal dissection in Korea. Clin Endosc. 2012;45(3):288–9.
109. Park SU, Min YW, Shin JU, Choi JH, Kim YH, Kim JJ, et al. Endoscopic submucosal dissection or transanal endoscopic microsurgery for nonpolypoid rectal high grade dysplasia and submucosa-invading rectal cancer. Endoscopy. 2012;44:1031–6.
110. Fujishiro M, Yahagi N, Kakushima N, Kodashima S, Muraki Y, Ono S, et al. Outcomes of endoscopic submucosal dissection for colorectal epithelial neoplasms in 200 consecutive cases. Clin Gastroenterol Hepatol. 2007;5(6):678–83. quiz 645.
111. Tamegai Y, Saito Y, Masaki N, Hinohara C, Oshima T, Kogure E, et al. Endoscopic submucosal dissection: a safe technique for colorectal tumors. Endoscopy. 2007;39(5):418–22.
112. Yoshida N, Naito Y, Sakai K, Sumida Y, Kanemasa K, Inoue K, et al. Outcome of endoscopic submucosal dissection for colorectal tumors in elderly people. Int J Colorectal Dis. 2010;25(4):455–61.
113. Lee BI. Indications, knives, and electric current: what's the best? Clin Endosc. 2012;45(3):285–7.
114. Huang C, Huang RX, Xiang P, Qiu ZJ. Current research status of endoscopic submucosal dissection for colorectal neoplasms. Clin Invest Med. 2012;35(4):E158.
115. Oka S, Tanaka S, Kanao H, Ishikawa H, Watanabe T, Igarashi M, et al. Current status in the occurrence of postoperative bleeding, perforation and residual/local recurrence during colonoscopic treatment in Japan. Dig Endosc. 2010;22(4):376–80.
116. Agrawal D, Chak A, Champagne BJ, Marks JM, Delaney CP. Endoscopic mucosal resection with full-thickness closure for difficult polyps: a prospective clinical trial. Gastrointest Endosc. 2010;71(6):1082–8.
117. Wood JJ, Lord AC, Wheeler JM, Borley NR. Laparo-endoscopic resection for extensive and inaccessible colorectal polyps: a feasible and safe procedure. Ann R Coll Surg Engl. 2011;93(3):241–5.
118. Tekkis PP, Poloniecki JD, Thompson MR, Stamatakis JD. Operative mortality in colorectal cancer: prospective national study. BMJ. 2003;327(7425):1196–201.
119. Franklin MEJ, Leyva-Alvizo A, Abrego-Medina D, Glass JL, Trevino J, Arellano PP, et al. Laparoscopically monitored colonoscopic polypectomy: an established form of endoluminal therapy for colorectal polyps. Surg Endosc. 2007;21(9):1650–3.
120. Hensman C, Luck AJ, Hewett PJ. Laparoscopic-assisted colonoscopic polypectomy: technique and preliminary experience. Surg Endosc. 1999;13(3):231–2.
121. Mal F, Perniceni T, Levard H, Boudet MJ, Levy P, Gayet B. Colonic polyps considered unresectable by endoscopy. Removal by combinations of laparoscopy and endoscopy in 65 patients. Gastroenterol Clin Biol. 1998;22(4):425–30.
122. Smedh K, Skullman S, Kald A, Anderberg B, Nystrom P. Laparoscopic bowel mobilization combined with intraoperative colonoscopic polypectomy in patients with an inaccessible polyp of the colon. Surg Endosc. 1997;11(6):643–4.
123. Winter H, Lang RA, Spelsberg FW, Jauch KW, Huttl TP. Laparoscopic colonoscopic rendezvous procedures for the treatment of polyps and early stage carcinomas of the colon. Int J Colorectal Dis. 2007;22(11):1377–81.
124. Grunhagen DJ, van Ierland MC, Doornebosch PG, Bruijninckx MM, Winograd R, de Graaf EJ. Laparoscopic-monitored colonoscopic polypectomy: a multimodality method to avoid segmental colon resection. Colorectal Dis. 2011;13(11):1280–4.
125. Wilhelm D, von Delius S, Weber L, Meining A, Schneider A, Friess H, et al. Combined laparoscopic-endoscopic resections of colorectal polyps: 10-year experience and follow-up. Surg Endosc. 2009;23(4):688–93.
126. Keehan SP, Cuckler GA, Sisko AM, Madison AJ, Smith SD, Lizonitz JM, et al. National health expenditure projections: modest annual growth until coverage expands and economic growth accelerates. Health Aff (Millwood). 2012;31(7):1600–12.
127. Davis K. Toward a high performance health system: the Commonwealth Fund's new commission. Health Aff (Millwood). 2005;24(5):1356–60.
128. Klarenbeek BR, Bergamaschi R, Veenhof AA, van der Peet DL, van den Broek WT, de Lange ES, et al. Laparoscopic versus open sigmoid resection for diverticular disease: follow-up assessment of the randomized control Sigma trial. Surg Endosc. 2011;25(4):1121–6.
129. Shabbir A, Roslani AC, Wong KS, Tsang CB, Wong HB, Cheong WK. Is laparoscopic colectomy as cost beneficial as open colectomy? ANZ J Surg. 2009;79(4):265–70.
130. Musser DJ, Boorse RC, Madera F, Reed 3rd JF. Laparoscopic colectomy: at what cost? Surg Laparosc Endosc. 1994;4(1):1–5.
131. Hayes JL, Hansen P. Is laparoscopic colectomy for cancer cost-effective relative to open colectomy? ANZ J Surg. 2007;77(9):782–6.
132. Abraham NS, Young JM, Solomon MJ. Meta-analysis of short-term outcomes after laparoscopic resection for colorectal cancer. Br J Surg. 2004;91(9):1111–24.
133. Braga M, Frasson M, Zuliani W, Vignali A, Pecorelli N, Di Carlo V. Randomized clinical trial of laparoscopic versus open left colonic resection. Br J Surg. 2010;97(8):1180–6.
134. Spanjersberg WR, Reurings J, Keus F, van Laarhoven CJ. Fast track surgery versus conventional recovery strategies for colorectal surgery. Cochrane Database Syst Rev. 2011;(2):CD007635.
135. Vlug MS, Wind J, Hollmann MW, Ubbink DT, Cense HA, Engel AF, et al. Laparoscopy in combination with fast track multimodal management is the best perioperative strategy in patients undergoing colonic surgery: a randomized clinical trial (LAFA-study). Ann Surg. 2011;254(6):868–75.
136. Delaney CP, Brady K, Woconish D, Parmar SP, Champagne BJ. Towards optimizing perioperative colorectal care: outcomes for 1,000 consecutive laparoscopic colon procedures using enhanced recovery pathways. Am J Surg. 2012;203(3):353–5; discussion 355–6.
137. Jensen CC, Prasad LM, Abcarian H. Cost-effectiveness of laparoscopic vs open resection for colon and rectal cancer. Dis Colon Rectum. 2012;55(10):1017–23.
138. Fox J, Gross CP, Longo W, Reddy V. Laparoscopic colectomy for the treatment of cancer has been widely adopted in the United States. Dis Colon Rectum. 2012;55(5):501–8.
139. Leddy LS, Lendvay TS, Satava RM. Robotic surgery: applications and cost effectiveness. Open Access Surg. 2010;3:99–107.
140. Uno Y, Munakata A. The non-lifting sign of invasive colon cancer. Gastrointest Endosc. 1994;40(4):485–9.

Technical Aspects

33

Bradley Davis and Janice F. Rafferty

Key Points

- While several anastomotic techniques are utilized, adhering to the traditional principles of proper tissue handling, ensuring adequate blood supply, and avoiding tension remain essential to optimizing outcomes.
- Methods for creating adequate length for a technically sound left-sided bowel anastomosis include proper mobilization of the splenic flexure and mesentery, division of the inferior mesenteric vein near the ligament of Treitz, ligation of the inferior mesenteric artery, and rectal mobilization (when applicable).
- You should have a stepwise and thorough algorithm for troubleshooting the difficult anastomosis.
- With more operations being performed through minimally invasive approaches, laparoscopic techniques for mobilizing the colon and maintaining optimal visualization are vital to minimizing complications.
- Leak testing is a critical component to left-sided anastomoses, and you should understand what to do with a positive leak test or incomplete donuts.

Introduction

The practice of surgery requires a broad, yet flexible skill set that allows a surgeon to adapt to increasingly complex procedures. Every operative case represents an opportunity to be challenged mentally and technically. Furthermore, every surgeon is faced with the fundamental question at some point in their career: what will it take to get this patient off of the table? Whether it is a hostile reoperative abdomen (see Video 33.1, Courtesy of Amir Bastawrous, MD) or a stapler misfire on a low rectal cancer, there are situations in the operating room that are low frequency but high acuity that require an optimal breadth and depth of skills and sound decision-making. In this chapter, we specifically review these infrequent technical challenges and offer an approach that has been successful in our practice. Although there will not always be randomized controlled trials to show us the way, when there is experience in the literature, we will attempt to bring it to light. Unfortunately, this is frequently the case when confronted with these situations, and we must rely on our experience, that of others, and the small amount of available evidence to guide our management.

Intestinal Anastomosis

Stapled Versus Hand Sewn and Single Versus Double Layer

Key Concept: *The success of a technically perfect anastomosis is not dependent on whether the bowel is stapled or hand sewn (single or double layer).*

Numerous studies have attempted to define the characteristics of the perfect anastomosis, and while the technique has largely been standardized, there remains an ever-present risk of failure with significant consequences to the patient. In modern surgical practice, the choice of suture or staples (and how to use them) has been shown to make little difference in anastomotic success or failure. In reality, few studies have ever shown superiority of one over the other. The most recent Cochrane review [1], published in 2012, was an update of a previous meta-analysis [2] and analyzed the results of 1,233 patients undergoing colorectal resec-

B. Davis, MD • J.F. Rafferty, MD (✉)
Division of Colon and Rectal Surgery, Department of Surgery, University of Cincinnati, Cincinnati, OH, USA
e-mail: davisbd@ucmail.uc.edu; janice.rafferty@uc.edu

Electronic supplementary material The online version of this chapter (doi: 10.1007/978-1-4614-9022-7_33) contains supplementary material, which is available to authorized users. Videos can also be accessed at http://www.springerimages.com/videos/978-1-4614-9021-0.

S.R. Steele et al. (eds.), *Complexities in Colorectal Surgery*,
DOI 10.1007/978-1-4614-9022-7_33, © Springer Science+Business Media New York 2014

tions and anastomosis. The authors found that suturing and stapling were equivalent for all relevant parameters for anastomotic construction, including anastomotic leak rates, both clinically and radiographically. The choice of one hand-sewn technique over another has not been shown to be superior, and in fact, the state of art for intestinal suturing has really remained unchanged since Antoine Lembert first described the inverted suture for intestinal anastomosis [3].

The choice of a single or double layer of suture has also been the basis of a randomized trial by Burch et al. who concluded that a single continuous layer of bowel apposition is quicker and has no adverse outcomes when compared to a double layer of interrupted suture [4]. While this study excluded anastomoses to the rectum, other investigators have demonstrated the reliability of the single-layer technique (even in rectal cases) with a low rate of complications [5, 6]. The choice of suture material has also been extensively reviewed, and while monofilament suture produces less of an inflammatory response, there is no evidence that this or any other specific property of suture impacts the success of an intestinal anastomosis [7–11].

Right-Sided and Small Bowel Resections

Key Concept: There is a small amount of data to suggest that a side-to-side anastomosis is associated with lower leak rates and improved outcomes compared to an end-to-end one in right-sided and small bowel locations. Special consideration should be given to proper orientation and dealing with the resultant mesenteric defect.

Small bowel and right-sided colon resections and anastomoses share many of the same technical concerns and are grouped together for the purposes of this review. The collateral blood supply is robust and tension across an anastomosis should never be a problem. Few studies have specifically looked at the differences between the configuration of the anastomosis, with the exception of ileocolic resections for Crohn's disease (CD) and loop ileostomy closures. The two most common choices are end to end (usually hand sewn) or side to side (usually stapled). Didolkar et al. randomized cancer patients to either a stapled or hand-sewn anastomosis and reported their results stratified by configuration [12]. The performance of a side-to-side anastomosis was comparable to an end-to-end one, although the overall numbers were small. A larger study by Kracht et al. randomized patients undergoing a right colon resection to one of five groups based on the configuration and technique of the anastomosis. Group 1 ($n=84$) were reconstructed end to end with an interrupted suturing technique, group 2 ($n=77$) with an end-to-end continuous suturing technique, group 3 ($n=82$) with a side-to-side interrupted suturing technique, group 4 ($n=91$) with a side-to-side continuous suturing technique, and, lastly, group 5 ($n=106$) with a stapled side-to-side anastomosis [13]. The sutured anastomosis groups were all comparable with respect to postoperative complications, and the anatomic configuration of the anastomosis did not influence leak rates. They did observe a lower leak rate for stapled anastomoses compared to the hand sewn, but this observation has been refuted in larger studies [14–16]. Several authors have suggested that a side-to-side anastomosis is associated with lower leak rates and fewer recurrences than one fashioned end to end in Crohn's disease, but the mechanics of why this would occur are not well understood [14, 17–19]. Recurrence rates are likely comparable endoscopically, although the larger lumen associated with the stapled side-to-side anastomosis may prevent symptomatic recurrence due to strictures. Balik et al. examined the outcomes of 225 patients having a loop ileostomy closure with either an end-to-end or side-to-side configuration and found a statistically significant difference in return of gastrointestinal function and hospital stay favoring the side-to-side group [20]. Leung et al. did not find this difference, demonstrating that the two techniques were comparable with ileostomy closures [21].

Surgeons are typically very specific in their approach with stapled anastomoses and their preferences in dealing with crossing staple lines. Some prefer to use different staplers (i.e., a "TA" stapler for the transverse portion), some hand sew the transverse portion to avoid crossing staple lines altogether, others over-sew the entire staple line, while a single crotch stitch is the ideal method for many surgeons. Yet, very little data is available to support one method over the other. In a canine model of stapled side-to-side anastomosis, offsetting the staple lines resulted in fewer complications [22], an observation that may be due to the reduction in blood flow associated with intersecting staple lines [23]. The bursting pressure of side-to-side stapled anastomosis was also improved in a porcine model when a crotch stitch was used to reinforce the enteroenterostomy [24]. Large-scale data examining these subtle technical nuisances is in reality limited, with most surgeons relying on the method they were taught in training or evolved over time based on prior successes (or failures).

We routinely perform small bowel and right-sided anastomosis using the side-to-side four-stapled technique. The enterectomy (vertical) staple line should be oriented mesenteric to antimesenteric (Fig. 33.1a) so that the enteroenterostomy staple line can be oriented along the antimesenteric side of the bowel wall. After making a small enterotomy on the antimesenteric corner of the staple line, an enteroenterostomy is created using a linear cutting stapler—taking great care to avoid incorporating the mesentery (Fig. 33.1b). The staple lines should be assessed for hemostasis, as this can be a source of postoperative hematochezia, particularly if a mesenteric vessel is incorporated into the staple line. The subsequent enterotomy (transverse portion) can be closed

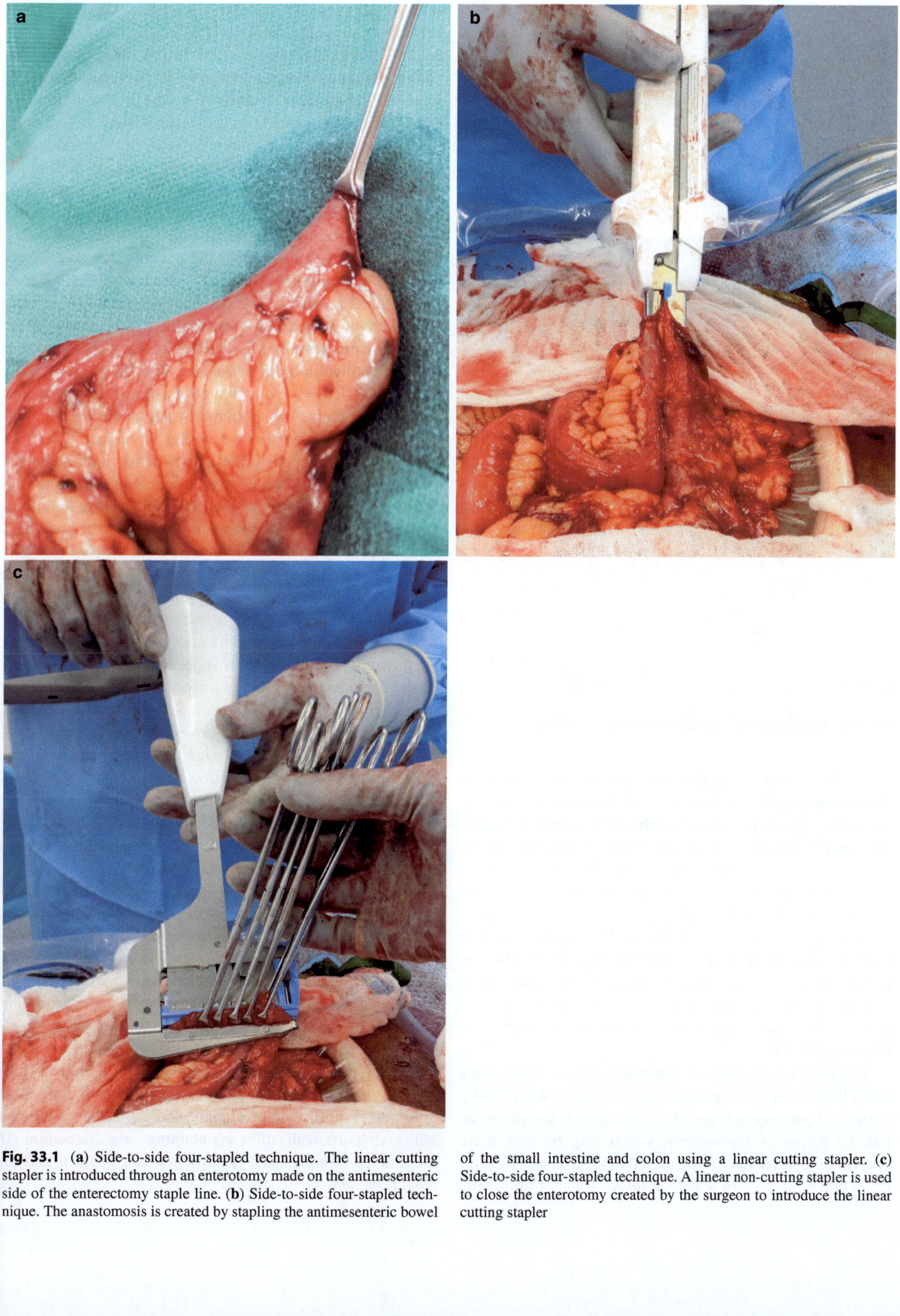

Fig. 33.1 (**a**) Side-to-side four-stapled technique. The linear cutting stapler is introduced through an enterotomy made on the antimesenteric side of the enterectomy staple line. (**b**) Side-to-side four-stapled technique. The anastomosis is created by stapling the antimesenteric bowel of the small intestine and colon using a linear cutting stapler. (**c**) Side-to-side four-stapled technique. A linear non-cutting stapler is used to close the enterotomy created by the surgeon to introduce the linear cutting stapler

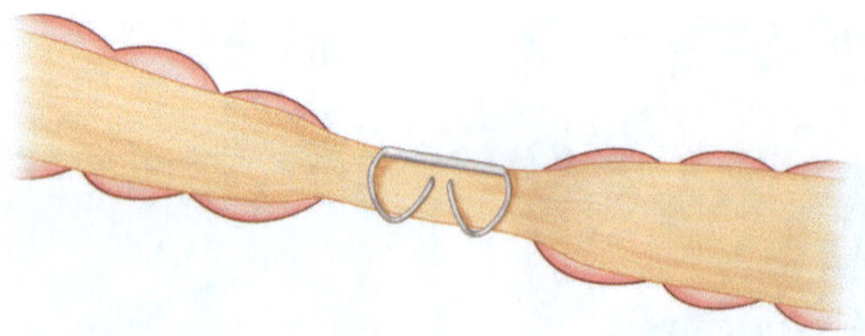

Fig. 33.2 Ideal "B"-shaped staple configuration

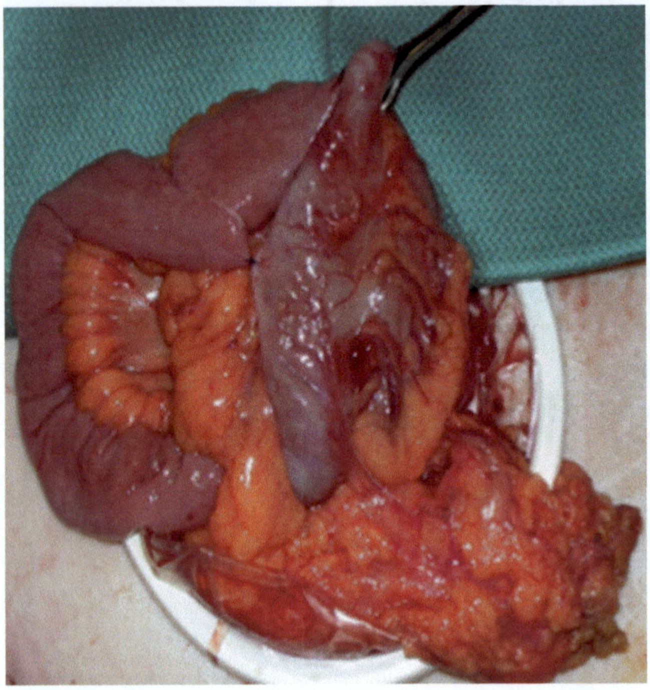

Fig. 33.3 Right colon anastomosis with mesentery closed

with either sutures or staples in such a way as to offset the staple lines (Fig. 33.1c). The choice of staple length is largely one of the surgeon preferences, although a wide lumen anastomosis (75 mm) may result in fewer symptomatic recurrences in patients with Crohn's disease [25]. The choice of staple height should be based on the thickness of tissue, as ischemia can result if the final staple height is too short [26]. Conversely, the staples may not be able to deform into their final "B" shape if the tissue is too thick (Fig. 33.2). This can be mitigated by compressing the tissue in the stapler prior to deployment, which has been shown in animal models to decrease the incidence of staple deformation and staple line bleeding [27, 28].

The decision to close the mesenteric defect following a small bowel resection or right colon anastomosis is mostly a personal preference (Fig. 33.3). The goal is to prevent an internal hernia postoperatively, which may be seen more often after laparoscopic colon resection [29]. This is theoretically due to the lack of adhesion formation after minimally invasive surgery and the ease with which the bowel may herniate through the mesenteric defect. Retrospective studies offer some insight into this infrequent complication. Cabot and colleagues reported on 530 consecutive patients who had laparoscopic right colon resection and found a 0.8 % incidence of small bowel obstruction due to herniation through an unclosed mesenteric defect [30]. No randomized head-to-head comparison of closure versus no closure of the mesenteric defect exists, though a higher complication rate with mesenteric closure has been reported in a retrospective review of patients undergoing a large bowel resection [31]. In this series by Causey et al., 133 patients had a colectomy (right, 36 %; sigmoid colon, 33 %; and left, 11 %); 52 % of the mesenteric defects were closed. Postoperative complications were attributed to the mesenteric defect in 6 % of the patients; with closure of the mesentery, the only significant factor identified in multivariate analysis (OR = 5.5; 95 % CI 1.069–28.524, $P=0.041$). While this study is by no means definitive, it points out the flaws of assuming that all complications can be avoided by closing the defect. There are no doubt pros and cons of both approaches, and the choice is likely a result of an individual surgeon's training and experience. Those of us who choose not to close the defect fear compromising the mesenteric blood flow or creating a smaller mesenteric defect that may be more prone to incarcerate should a hernia occur. If the mesentery is closed, care should be taken to avoid the intestinal blood supply as this can result in a hematoma or worse—anastomotic ischemia. If a hematoma develops, it can usually be managed with simple pressure applied by gently squeezing the leaf of the mesentery between the operator's fingers for a few minutes with the goal of controlling the bleeding and limiting the size of the hematoma. It is probably not necessary to open the peritoneum as this will result in further bleeding and control will be more difficult. Suture ligation of the hematoma should also be used with caution, and typically avoided. The risk is that sutures used to ligate mesenteric bleeding could compromise the blood supply to an anastomosis that has already been fashioned and will be difficult to assess.

When performing a right colectomy laparoscopically, it is important that the orientation of the mesentery and the anastomosis is confirmed prior to closing the fascia as it is possible to twist the ileal side 360° after transection (Fig. 33.4). This is more likely to occur with laparoscopy when performing an extracorporeal anastomosis through a small midline incision. We avoid this twist by starting at the ligated vascular pedicle and following the cut edge of both the small bowel and colonic mesentery completely to the bowel wall. We then place atraumatic graspers on both ends only after these are confirmed to be straight and use Babcock clamps with extracorporealization maintaining this orientation. If there is any concern, the laparoscope can confirm that no twist is present.

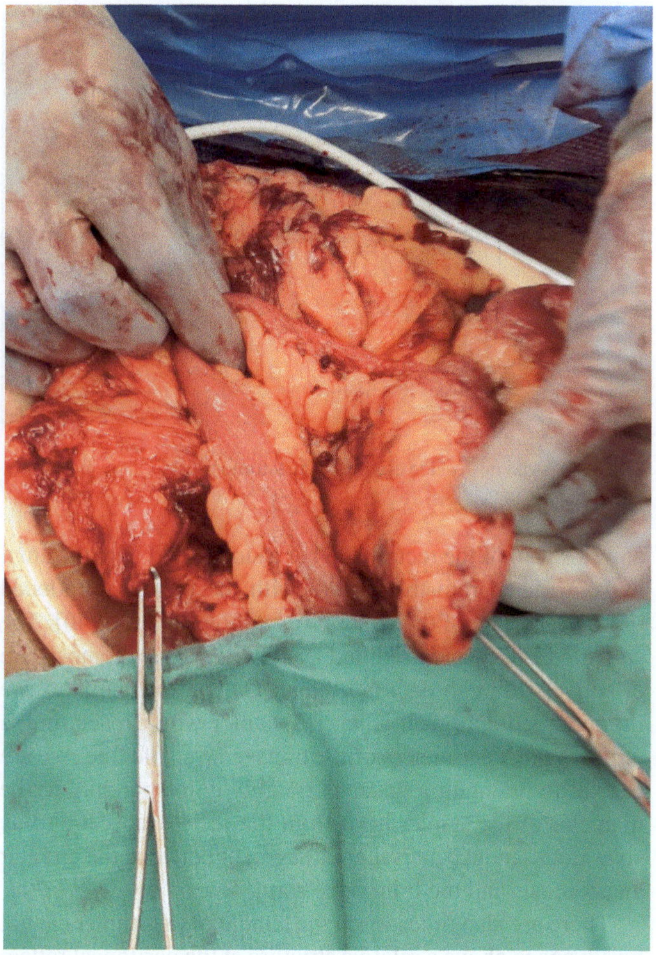

Fig. 33.4 The ileal mesentery is mobile and could be easily twisted 360°. This is readily apparent in this picture and obvious—however, through a small laparoscopic incision, it may not be evident without reevaluating with the camera

Left-Sided and Rectal Resection

Key Concept: *Left-sided and rectal anastomoses have their own unique set of requirements for success and potential complications. Being familiar with single versus double stapled, hand sewn, and end to end versus modified end to side will allow several options in the face of difficulties.*

Left colon and rectal resections with anastomosis represent a higher degree of complexity, as reliance on stapling, collateral blood supply and mesenteric length are all critical to a safe anastomosis. All staplers have a certain incidence of failure, but the consequence of device failure when stapling low in the pelvis can be much more significant. Mechanical staplers have been in use for decades, but new products continue to come to the operating room as well as ongoing modifications of old devices. In some instances, these new products represent a significant leap forward and offer surgeons opportunities to do things that previously were not possible, while others attempt to improve upon technology that is already effective. Adoption of these devices requires a clear understanding of the advantages and performance characteristics of each and mandates a thoughtful approach to incorporation into practice.

Regardless of the manufacturer, all of these devices have a failure rate, and more importantly, when device failure occurs, the surgeon must have a plan to salvage the anastomosis. The exact incidence of failure is difficult to establish, but in 2007, Mardestein et al. reported on 1,188 stapler misfires reported to the FDA during a 12-month period [32]. Of the misfires, 588 occurred during colorectal procedures with failure to form staples and inability to remove the stapler as the most common problem. From these adverse events, 266 occurred during rectal resections and 80 were considered major, resulting in 23 unplanned permanent ostomies. Stapler misfire during a laparoscopic procedure was associated with a 43 % conversion rate. This high rate of conversion to open surgery following stapler misfire was confirmed by Pandya et al. in their analysis of 200 consecutive laparoscopic colectomies [33].

It is unknown how many of these failures were surgeon related, but it is imperative that everyone involved in the case has intimate familiarity with the proper use of the device. The primary surgeon may not be the person deploying the stapler, and errors can occur when there is an assumption that a co-surgeon or assistant knows how to properly deploy a given stapler. In our operating room, the surgery resident is often responsible for deploying the stapler, and it is not unusual for him or her to be doing so for the first time. We have avoided this situation by focused education on the proper use of the various staplers prior to the operating room for trainees. This information can also be included into the time out or preoperative briefing procedure so that proper orientation can occur.

We routinely employ a double-stapled technique when performing a rectal anastomosis by transecting the rectum with a linear stapler distally and placing the purse-string suture on the proximal side to secure the anvil of the circular stapler. The handle of the end-to-end anastomotic stapler is then advanced through the anus to the top of the rectum and the spike deployed usually adjacent or through the transverse staple line. The anvil and spike are then united and compressed either manually or to a predetermined height, depending on the stapler manufacturer and tissue thickness. Once deployed, the anvil is extracted through the lumen of the newly created anastomosis along with rings of tissue incorporated into the head of the device. While little evidence exists to support one staple diameter over another, it is our practice to use the largest stapler that will safely fit into the conduit and negotiate the rectal stump. For most adults this is usually 29 mm; and we rarely use the 33-mm or 25-mm diameter stapler. There is some evidence to suggest that when stapling an ileal pouch to the anus, symptomatic strictures occur more frequently when a 29-mm stapler is used compared to a 33 mm [34]. Others have suggested that stenosis is a function of mechanical circular stapling regardless of the diameter [35]. We have not seen this in our practice and maintain like others that symptomatic stenosis is rare following stapled end-to-end anastomoses [36, 37] or side-to-end anastomosis, especially when careful attention to preservation of blood supply is maintained.

The double-stapled technique can be modified by placing a purse string on both the proximal and distal side and using the circular stapler to create the anastomosis—the single-stapled technique. This can prove difficult in the setting of a low rectal anastomosis, and studies have shown that there is no clinical difference between the two techniques [38].

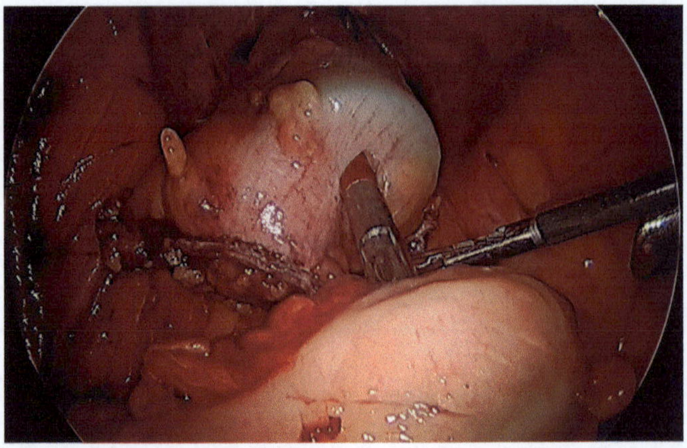

Fig. 33.5 An end-to-side colorectal anastomosis

The Mechanical Stapler

Key Concept: Preparing the rectum prior to introducing the stapler may avoid difficulties with reaching the apex of the rectal stump. Additionally, having an algorithm for the "stuck" stapler will allow rapid identification of the cause and determine the optimal next step.

One of the most common and frustrating stapler complications occurs when the handle of the end-to-end stapler won't reach to the top of the rectal stump. There are a number of reasons this might occur, and most times can be prevented. First, it is important to ask yourself if your distal transection line is as low as you think it is (or need it to be). In some cases of a rectosigmoid anastomosis, a knuckle of sigmoid colon may give the false appearance that you are at the level of the extraperitoneal rectum, when in fact distal sigmoid remains. Barring this, there are several other instances where this can occur. Inspissated mucous in a chronically diverted rectal stump may physically prevent the stapler from reaching the top, and a preoperative endoscopic evaluation of the Hartmann stump can help clear these remnants and prevent this problem. This can also be prevented with preoperative or intraoperative rectal irrigation using a rigid proctoscope. If the rectum is soft and there is no mucous or other debris obstructing the stapler, a well-lubricated sizer can be used to gently dilate the lumen of the rectum starting small and working up to the larger sizes (29 or 33 mm). If the sizer will not reach the top of the rectum, it is unlikely that the stapler ever will. Care should be taken to avoid inadvertently pushing the sizer through the staple line. Occasionally, insufflation of the rectum with air (with a rigid proctoscope or flexible endoscope) or lubricant will distend the top of the rectum sufficiently to allow passage of the stapler. If nothing works and a hand-sewn anastomosis is not possible or desirable, then a stapled end-to-side anastomosis can be performed (Fig. 33.5 and Video 33.2). This can be done by bringing the spike of the end-to-end stapler through the anterior wall of the rectum [39] or a side to end with the anvil purse stringed into the rectum with the handle introduced through the side of the conduit (usually left colon) [40]. The so-called Baker and modified Baker type of anastomosis are effective, although data is limited. Our preference is to use the modified approach when the stapler won't reach, but is within a few centimeters of the transverse staple line. We are careful to maintain a distance roughly corresponding to the diameter of the stapler head from the rectal transection line so as not to induce an ischemic segment between the circular anastomosis and the transverse staple line.

There are also times when the handle of the stapler cannot be advanced above a relative stricture at the peritoneal reflection; this stricture can be caused by conditions such as perforated diverticulitis, which causes fibrosis of the peritoneum in the cul de sac. This fibrosis can prevent the stapler from traversing the second rectal valve. Forcing the stapler in this situation can cause a laceration, or worse a perforation, of the rectal stump. The laceration may not be readily apparent if it is located in the posterior aspect of the rectal wall and into the mesorectum. If a laceration or perforation occurs, then the surgeon should consider resecting the rectum below this point and performing the anastomosis at this level. Instead of forcing the stapler in this situation, it is our practice to abandon the stapled technique in favor of a hand-sewn end-to-end anastomosis.

Another less common scenario occurs when the stapler becomes stuck, a situation that occurs more frequently in our experience with an end-to-end anastomotic device. After deploying the stapler and creating the anastomosis, it is recommended that the anvil be opened, usually a full turn of the handle in an effort to release the newly formed anastomosis from the head of the device. Opening the device too much can result in the anvil separating from the head, causing it to lodge in the proximal side of the anastomosis. If this occurs, an endoscope can be used to retrieve the anvil [41] while allowing the surgeon an opportunity to inspect the anastomosis and determine its integrity. If the stapler can't be removed, the surgeon must assess the situation to determine if the stapler has properly deployed. If the knife blade has failed to create the lumen, it won't be possible to remove the stapler and no amount of manipulation will dislodge it. The outside of the anastomosis should be inspected (if possible) to determine if the staples have deployed and deformed appropriately as failure to do so will indicate a catastrophic stapler failure and a need to redo the anastomosis—a situation that when low in the pelvis may prove difficult or impossible. One approach in this situation is to mobilize further to gain additional proximal length and attempt a hand-sewn coloanal. If the staples have deployed but the stapler cannot be removed, it is possible to slide a red rubber catheter into the rectum along the stapler handle and insufflate with air, which can help determine if a lumen has been created and possibly facilitate dislodging the circular staple line from the head of the stapler. Kyzer et al. reported difficulty extracting the stapler in 3 out of 215 stapled end-to-end anastomosis and described a technique of placing stay sutures around the anastomosis in an effort to lift it out of the stapler head [36]. If all else fails, the stapler may need to be removed by dividing the bowel above and below the anastomosis and pulling the head and tissue of the failed anastomosis through the rectum. If there is enough length distally, a second attempt at a stapled end-to-end anastomosis can be made versus a hand-sewn anastomosis or (worse case) diversion.

The Anastomotic Donut and Leak Testing

Key Concept: All left-sided anastomosis should undergo leak testing!

Complications of the circular stapler can also include incomplete anastomotic donuts (i.e., rings), a situation that may imply inadequate tissue incorporation (Fig. 33.6). An air leak test will confirm the presence or absence of an incomplete anastomosis. If the donuts are incomplete but there is no air leak, it is our practice to treat the anastomosis as if it were intact. However, the finding of incomplete donuts is part of the decision-making process regarding the potential need for proximal diversion.

We routinely perform an air leak test on all left-sided anastomoses regardless of the donut integrity or whether the anastomosis was stapled or sewn in an effort to identify and prevent anastomotic leaks [42–44]. This practice is supported by the work of Ricciardi et al. who reviewed the outcomes of 825 left-sided resections and found evidence that 8 % of those tested were positive for an air leak [44]. Postoperative leaks occurred in 7.7 % of anastomoses that tested positive, in 3.8 % of those that tested negative, and in 8.1 % of those that were not tested ($P<0.03$). Furthermore, this simple maneuver can provide insight as to potential outcomes

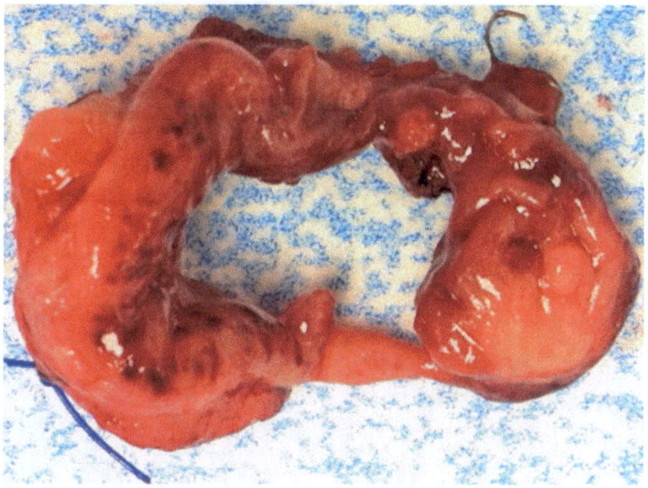

Fig. 33.6 An incomplete anastomotic donut with no serosa or mucosa noted on the inferior aspect

based on how this situation is handled. The authors found the anastomotic leak rate was 12.1 % when an anastomosis that was initially positive for an air leak was suture repaired so that they were air tight, compared to 0 % when they were completely redone or were diverted proximally (P=NS). Beard et al. performed a randomized trial of 145 patients undergoing left-sided and rectal resections to intraoperative air leak testing or nothing. In the test group, 25 % of anastomoses leaked air and were repaired. Clinically, relevant anastomotic leaks occurred in 4 % of the test group and in 14 % in the no test group ($P=0.043$) [42]. While these benefits have not been uniformly demonstrated [45], no authors have shown that air leak testing is harmful, and likely never will. Given the potential benefit and the ease of performing this test, surgeons should consider it a routine part of their practice for left-sided and rectal resections. While some surgeons advocate air leak testing of right-sided anastomosis, we do not routinely do this.

Offodile et al. reported a 19 % incidence of technical errors associated with 349 circular stapler deployments which included a positive air leak test ($n=19$), difficulties inserting or extracting the stapler ($n=18$), incomplete or thin donuts ($n=13$), tissue damage ($n=10$), and others ($n=7$). Technical errors associated with the circular stapler were associated with a higher incidence of proximal diversion (34 % vs. 17 %, $P<0.0003$) and conversion to open in laparoscopic cases (22 % vs. 13 %, $P<0.045$), in part due to the level of the anastomosis. Overall, there was no difference with regard to leaks, reoperation, suture line strictures, and hospital stay—likely a reflection of proper surgical judgment following the initial difficulties [46].

Complications associated with the linear stapler can also occur, and in our experience, the most common complication is failure of the device to deploy and deform the staples. This can represent a true device failure or be the result

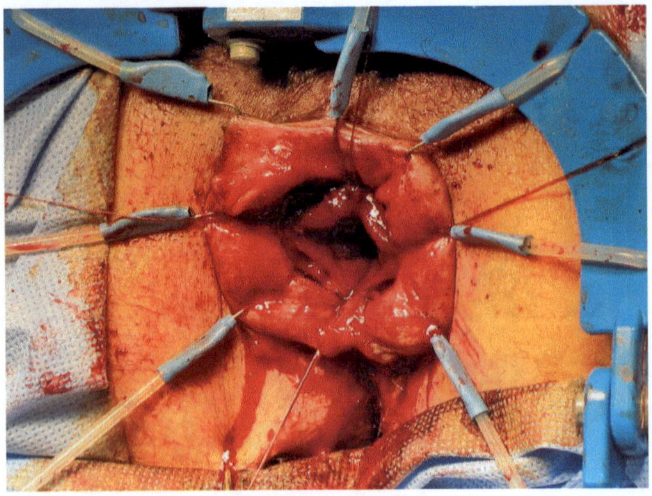

Fig. 33.7 Hand-sewn coloanal anastomosis

of surgeon failure to deploy the stapler properly prior to transecting the bowel. The end result is the same—a distal rectal stump that is gaping. One obvious indication that this has occurred is the amount of bleeding that ensues, often the first clue especially when this occurs deep in the pelvis. In this instance, the surgeon can either attempt to get a stapler across the rectum a second time, assuming enough length, or convert the anastomosis to a double purse-string technique by attempting to place a purse string on the rectal stump. Both are quite difficult, especially in a narrow pelvis. This can be attempted transabdominally or transanally. To facilitate a transanal approach, a Lone Star (Lone Star Medical Products®, Stafford, TX, USA) can be used to evert the anal canal (Fig. 33.7), and an anal retractor can be inserted such as a Hill-Ferguson or Sawyer. The purse string in this instance can be tied on the anal side leaving a small aperture to introduce the anvil, or the sutures can be passed into the abdomen and tied down around the spike of the stapler after it is brought up through the anus. A linear stapler that won't release after firing represents a mechanical failure and usually cannot be salvaged. In this instance, it will need to be released by cutting the bowel distally.

Gaining Enough Length

Key Concept: You need to be familiar and comfortable with each of the several methods used to gain additional length for left-sided and rectal anastomoses to avoid tension.

Another critical aspect of a successful colorectal anastomosis is ensuring adequate length of the conduit so that there is no tension. The choice of proximal transection will depend largely on the pathology and the condition of the bowel, as it is imperative that the two ends be healthy. Length can be achieved by completely mobilizing the attachments of the left colon to the retroperitoneum and flexure. The other critical aspect to obtaining adequate bowel length is mobilizing the mesentery, which will tether the left colon into the abdomen unless it is freed. There are several decisions the surgeon will need to make starting with the most important—where to divide the bowel both distally and proximally. For diverticular disease, the entire sigmoid should be removed along with any proximal colon that is inflamed or hypertrophied. In this regard, it is critical to review the most recent CT findings to ensure that any proximal inflammation is resected to mitigate the risk of recurrence. The distal transection line should always be to the top of the rectum, identified where the taenia coli splay on the anterior surface. If the disease is isolated to the sigmoid, it is not always necessary to mobilize the splenic flexure, and studies reviewing the selective approach to mobilizing the flexure have been favorable [47–50]. Key points are that the conduit be free of disease and of adequate length. When the flexure must be mobilized, several techniques are available to accomplish what can be a very difficult and variable surgical procedure. All techniques can be done either laparoscopically or open, although we find a medial to lateral approach starting underneath the inferior mesenteric artery (IMA) to be difficult to do open as it is an awkward place to see without the aid of a 30° laparoscope.

In general, if we are performing an open procedure, the dissection is performed lateral to medial. During the first step, the omentum is dissected off of the transverse colon by dividing the gastrocolic ligament, entering the lesser sac. One error in this situation is to try and mobilize the flexure through a small midline incision. This creates a situation whereby the surgeon and the assistant are not able to adequately see the field at the same time, increasing the risk of injuries to the colon, spleen, and mesentery. A nice rule of thumb is that the midline incision should extend above the umbilicus and the retractors should be set so that there is maximal pull on the left subcostal retractor. It will be necessary to reset the retractors for adequate pelvic exposure, as it is rare that retraction that allows visualization of the splenic flexure will also allow optimal visualization of the pelvis. If the field is too small, then the surgeon is often left in the dark, literally, and a headlamp can facilitate illumination of the left upper quadrant. With the surgeon retracting medially and inferiorly, the assistant divides the peritoneal attachments. If the assistant is not able to visualize the plane, consider moving him or her between the patient's legs so that they can get a more natural look at the anatomy. Another option in a tough dissection is to get into the lesser sac along the greater curve of the stomach leaving the omentum on the colon. This may help release the flexure and open up the space particularly if the flexure is very high or in the hilum of the spleen. It is important to avoid excessive traction on the spleen as this may result in splenic injury (see Video 31.5). In a review of 975,825 patients who underwent colorectal resection during a 2-year period, Masoomi et al. reported a rate of splenic injury of 0.96 %, of which 85 % were treated with complete splenectomy (splenorrhaphy, 13 %; partial splenectomy, 1.7 %) [51]. The most common procedure associated with splenic injury was transverse colectomy (3.4 %). Using multivariate regression analysis, the investigators found that transverse colectomy (adjusted odds ratio [AOR], 5.30), left colectomy (AOR, 5.08), total colectomy (AOR, 2.85), open operation (AOR, 2.68), malignant tumor (AOR, 2.11), diverticulitis (AOR, 1.93), teaching hospital (AOR, 1.73), male sex (AOR 1.20), peripheral vascular disease (AOR, 1.14), and emergent admission (AOR, 1.06) were associated with a higher risk of splenic injury. Excessive traction and poor visualization can also result in an inadvertent colotomy. If this occurs, spillage should be controlled with a temporary mass closure suture and the flexure mobilization completed. This will allow better assessment of the injury and a more definitive repair. It is usually not necessary to resect the injury unless the blood supply was also compromised. If the IMA has been ligated along with the marginal blood supply, then the entire conduit may become ischemic and resection will likely be necessary. This is a catastrophic complication, often making it extremely difficult to have more proximal colon reach the pelvis, and should be avoided by appropriate visualization through an adequate incision with good lighting.

When approaching the flexure laparoscopically, a medial to lateral dissection is preferred; it is possible to mobilize the left colon all the way to the flexure so that only a thin layer of peritoneum remains for the lateral dissection [52]. Another option is to start by entering the retroperitoneum at the inferior mesenteric vein (IMV) and proceed medially from there. This will lead the surgeon to the area under the splenic flexure and can be used alone or in conjunction with the more traditional approach. Care should be taken to avoid inadvertently dissecting underneath the pancreas when using this approach.

Once the left colon and splenic flexure are fully mobilized, additional length for tension-free low colorectal anastomosis will be gained by appropriate mobilization of the mesentery. If a cancer resection is being performed, it is desirable to ligate the inferior mesenteric artery (IMA) at its origin, regardless of reach, to ensure an adequate nodal harvest. There is some controversy regarding the necessity of ligating the IMA flush to the aorta (high tie) when compared to preservation of the left colic branch (low tie). The oncological necessity of a high tie is predicated on the fact that lymph nodes (LN) at the origin of the IMA can harbor malignant cells and recurrences following low tie are more frequent [53]. The impact of the high tie may be more important for advanced carcinomas [54], and the effect of radiation may mitigate this benefit further. The oncologic benefits of a high tie have not been uniformly seen [55]. Taking the IMA flush on the aorta and mobilizing the left colon mesentery just lateral to the ligament of Treitz will offer the most length but may cause the conduit to become ischemic in the absence of adequate collateral circulation. If the descending or transverse colon is to be used as the proximal half of the anastomosis, the marginal blood supply should be adequate, but must be carefully preserved. The marginal blood supply originating from the middle colic artery may not be adequate if the sigmoid colon is to be used as the proximal half of the anastomosis, as the conduit will likely be too long [56, 57]. If it is necessary to use the sigmoid colon as part of the colorectal or coloanal anastomosis, then the left colic artery should be preserved [58, 59]. The surgeon will have to decide if length is achieved more adequately by keeping the conduit long (preserving the sigmoid colon) or fully mobilizing the mesentery (dividing the left colic). While the safety of using the sigmoid colon as the proximal conduit in rectal resections has been demonstrated [60], there are certain risks that come with its use. Hall et al. measured the tissue oxygen tension ($pt0_2$) of the left colon before and after ligation of the IMA in 62 patients undergoing anterior resection [61]. Baseline data demonstrated that the $pt0_2$ varied significantly between the sigmoid, the descending, and transverse colon. After the IMA was ligated, the $pt0_2$ was significantly reduced in the sigmoid colon when compared to the left or transverse colon. This difference was observed regardless of a high or low tie. This data suggests that it is the site of colon transection and not the site of arterial ligation that impacts the integrity of the anastomotic blood supply.

To gain additional length, the inferior mesenteric vein (IMV) must be ligated adjacent to the IMA, and a second time at the inferior border of the pancreas just lateral to the ligament of Treitz. Ligating the vein twice while carefully preserving the marginal artery at the splenic flexure will add several centimeters to the length of the conduit while preserving arterial blood supply. A common error in an effort to gain length is to divide the colonic mesentery up toward the splenic flexure of the colon, with the end result cutting off the blood supply to the distal conduit, which is now based on the middle colic artery. If the marginal blood supply is compromised due to inadvertent injury while mobilizing the flexure or wandering too close the mesenteric border during ligation of the mesentery, the conduit will become ischemic and very likely unusable.

In the final analysis, the importance of a tension-free anastomosis cannot be overemphasized. In reality, you will often need to employ a combination of lengthening maneuvers. Interestingly, while the importance of avoiding tension to help ensure the integrity of an anastomosis is uniformly accepted, the degree of "acceptable" tension has been poorly studied, as most experimental models of leaks rely on the assessment of bursting pressure and not stretch [62]. An exception is the study by Shikata and colleagues who characterized the blood flow of various intestinal segments before and after the application of a tensile force following anastomosis. They used an experimental canine model and found that the effects of tension on the submucosal blood flow were much better tolerated in the small bowel when compared to the colon [63]. This data helps to corroborate the clinical assertion that an anastomosis under tension is more likely to fail as it is less likely that a small bowel resection and anastomosis, given the laxity of the small bowel mesentery, will leak when compared to a left-sided colonic resection that is more likely to be on stretch. Common sense would also indicate an anastomosis that is taut is in danger of failing for the additional reasons of mechanical forces that attempt to pull the newly anastomosed bowel away from each other [64].

Once the anastomosis has been performed, there may be a great deal of laxity between the proximal and distal bowel (ileocolic) or there may not be any (coloanal). In most cases, it comes down to your intraoperative assessment as the primary surgeon to determine if the anastomosis will fail. As a general rule, if the cut edge of the mesentery traversing the pelvic brim is too tight to allow a finger (or open laparoscopic 5-mm grasper) to easily slip underneath, the anastomosis is at risk since the blood supply is under tension—even if the bowel ends appear to approximate easily without tension. Every effort should then be made to lengthen the mesentery, even if this has already been attempted, as often reassessment will identify a small adhesion to release. In general, if the mesentery is lax, there is likely no tension at the anastomosis.

There are unfortunately times when despite fully mobilizing both the mesentery and the left colon, the conduit simply won't reach the pelvis. This can be due to a number of factors, but is usually associated with a short fatty mesentery. You then find yourself in a situation where gaining length means dividing more mesentery (often the transverse mesocolon), which results in ischemia to the conduit and the need for more length. There are limited options when this occurs—perform a total colectomy and an ileorectal anastomosis or rotate the right colon 180° around the ileocolic pedicle in an effort to preserve the ileocecal valve. The latter option referred to as the Deloyers procedure [65] has proven successful, although a comparison to an ileorectal anastomosis have not been reported. Presumably, the simplicity of an ileorectal anastomosis in cases where the entire rectum is preserved would outweigh the benefits of preserving the right colon. However, if part of the rectum has been resected, then the functional results of an ileorectal are likely to be poor, and the Deloyers procedure would obviate the need for a permanent ostomy. The blood supply for this procedure is dependent on the ileocolic artery, and all mesenteric attachments of the ascending colon should be divided being careful to preserve the marginal vessel adjacent to the right colon. The colonic segment is then rotated clockwise and anastomosed to the rectum. A window in the ileal mesentery has also been described, but is not necessary with the colon will be situated anterior to the small bowel. Manceau et al. described their experience with this procedure in 48 consecutive cases [66] with a median follow-up of 26 months. There were no anastomotic leaks in this series, although 65 % of the patients had a temporary diverting ileostomy. One patient required a permanent stoma due to poor functional results, and 23 % of patient routinely used loperamide, with a median number of three bowel movements in a day. In those cases where only a few centimeters would allow less tension on the anastomosis, distal mobilization of the rectum to elevate it out of the pelvic hollow can also be a useful maneuver.

Mesenteric length can also be problematic when creating an ileoanal anastomosis; and several maneuvers have been described to obtain pouch length. The length of each arm of the J pouch is typically 15–20 cm and is measured from the cut ileum at the ileocecal valve. However, the apex of the ileum when folded at this distance may not easily reach the anus, and a more proximal apex may reach more easily, at the cost of reservoir size. In these cases, it is important to not be too dogmatic about length of pouch and choose a location that is most likely to reach the anus as long as the resultant pouch will serve as an adequate reservoir. Over time, the pouch will normally dilate and function appropriately. To gauge for adequate length, once the tip of the J pouch has been located, it should be able to reach just beyond the pubic symphysis. For those situations where this does not occur, the first and easiest step to obtain mesenteric length is to completely mobilize the cut edge of the ileal mesentery up to the level of the duodenum in the right upper quadrant. Next, the surgeon can score the peritoneum in several locations along the superior mesenteric artery (SMA). Importantly, both the anterior and posterior leafs should be divided. This will result in a modest increase in length. If the ileocolic pedicle has been preserved, it may now need to be divided if it is tethering the ileum near the duodenum. Conversely, it can be used as the main blood supply at the pouch that is tethered by the superior mesenteric artery; in this case, the SMA can in fact be divided—although this should be done so with *extreme* caution after exhausting all other options for length. Should you feel this is necessary, we encourage initial placement of a "bulldog" atraumatic vascular clamp to ensure the entire small bowel does not become ischemic with this maneuver. It is better to create an ostomy than proceed. A less risky maneuver is to create windows in the ileal mesentery by dividing the proximal arcades individually (Fig. 33.8), a maneuver that can be facilitated by transilluminating the mesentery with the OR lights or the headlight. A single window will give several centimeters of length and should be situated at the point of maximal tension. A second arcade can be taken if necessary, but the risk of ischemia

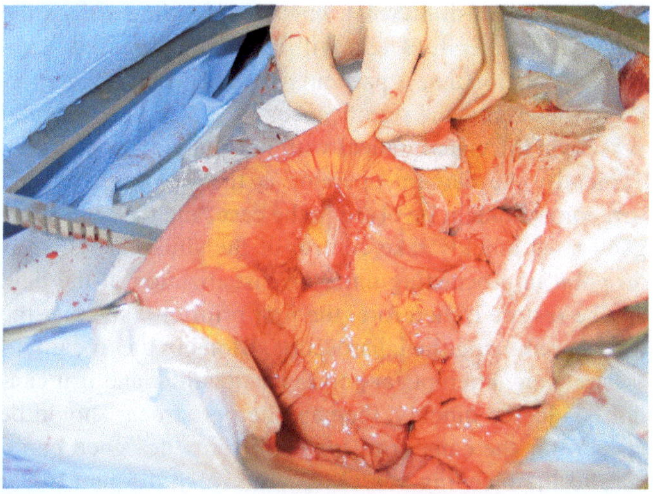

Fig. 33.8 Mesenteric window

to the tip of the J pouch exists. Regardless of the maneuvers used to lengthen the mesentery, it is imperative that they be done before making the pouch, as there is very little that can be done to gain length to a mesentery that is no longer accessible.

Size Mismatch

Key Concept: *A side-to-end anastomosis or Cheatle slit can mitigate size mismatches at the anastomosis.*

The issue of size mismatch as it pertains to colorectal surgery has mostly been mitigated through the use of mechanical staplers. A side-to-side anastomosis can be performed on varying diameters of both small and large bowel and is a frequent finding when resecting ileal strictures that are chronic. When the descending colon is found to be too large in diameter or too thick walled to technically accommodate a purse string, consider placing the anvil with the spike into the proximal descending colon, then stapling the end of the colon closed. Bring the spike and neck of the anvil out along the antimesenteric side of the colon several cm proximal to the transverse stapled closure, and perform a side-to-end colorectal anastomosis. If an end-to-end sutured anastomosis is preferred and there is a discrepancy in the diameter of the bowel, a Cheatle slit can be performed by making a longitudinal incision along the antimesenteric border of the bowel. This situation may also arise when closing a colostomy and performing a colorectal anastomosis in a patient who has been diverted for a prolonged period of time. In this instance, the rectum may have a small diameter that will not safely accept the handle of a circular stapler. A Cheatle slit along the anterior wall of the rectum will functionally increase its diameter so that a hand-sewn anastomosis can be performed.

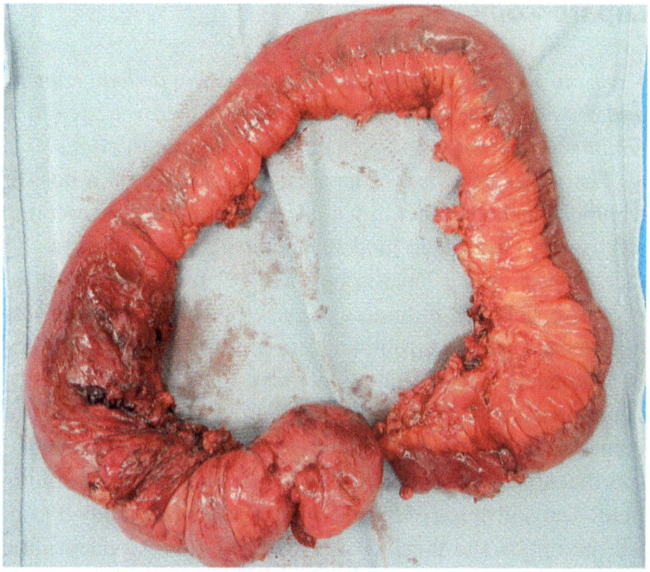

Fig. 33.9 Thickened Crohn's mesentery

Miscellaneous Technical Challenges

Difficult Crohn's Disease Mesentery

Key Concept: *The mesentery in a Crohn's patient is often best resected with the use of serial clamps and suture ligation.*

Safe division of the mesenteric blood supply that lies within a markedly thickened, indurated mesentery can be quite difficult. The rule of thumb for the site of bowel resection relies on the condition of the mesentery; one should resect to grossly normal mesentery in the small bowel in an effort to find an un-inflamed margin. Unfortunately, the intervening mesentery is often very thick, yet quite fragile (Fig. 33.9). In our experience, the use of energy devices to divide the mesentery in this setting is to be discouraged, as it is not effective. Retraction of a mesenteric vessel into a thickened mesentery has led many surgeons into a dire situation, where the blood supply to the entire small bowel is at risk. Perhaps a more effective way to control this hostile mesentery is to employ Kocher clamps on either side; the tooth at the end of the clamp will effectively capture the tissue without slippage. Leave a few millimeters more tissue on the side staying in than on the specimen side, and suture ligate the tissue in the Kocher. We find a heavy braided suture placed in a figure-of-eight fashion to be effective. The technique for securing the knot requires extreme caution and a light touch while firmly securing the knot in tissue that often fractures. When possible, stay close to the mesenteric border of the bowel when ligating the blood supply, keeping in mind that the main arcade can be located just a few millimeters away in the foreshortened mesentery.

Laparoscopy

Key Concept: The importance of maintaining a clean camera and optimal view when using a minimally invasive approach cannot be overemphasized to minimizing complications.

The widespread use of laparoscopy has created a host of technical challenges not observed in open surgery for colorectal disease. One of the fundamental challenges surgeons will face in performing laparoscopy will be maintaining a clear operative field. To minimize the risk of postoperative trocar hernias and pain, we routinely use a 5-mm laparoscope that unfortunately will not allow as much light to illuminate the abdominal cavity. Fogging of the laparoscopic lens, splatter of irrigation fluid, blood, and bodily fluids are among those factors that affect a surgeon's ability to maintain a clear operating field. Aerosolization of fat and other debris will quickly diminish the optics and preclude safe visualization. Condensation on the lens due to temperature discrepancies will also degrade the optics and is perhaps the most common reason a surgeon will remove the laparoscope during surgery. Several commercial products exist to help mitigate the detrimental effects of smoke and condensation on the tip of the laparoscope, and a thorough evaluation of these technologies is appropriate for all surgeons considering laparoscopy as part of their colorectal practice. The most commonly used product is the fog reduction/elimination device (FRED, US Surgical, North Haven, CT) which consists of less than 15 % isopropyl alcohol, 2 % surfactant, and more than 85 % water [67]. Advantages include ease of use, widespread availability, and low cost, while the main disadvantage is the need to remove the laparoscope and the cooling that occurs upon removal of the laparoscope—leading to further condensation and worsening view. A newer product, which we have begun to use with great success, is the DHELP [68] (Defogging Heated Endoscopic Light Protector, New Wave Surgical, Coral Springs, FL), a compact device that both heats the tip of the laparoscope and applies defogging solution at the same time. While it is still necessary to remove the laparoscope to utilize this device, we have found the warming that occurs greatly eliminates the need for repeat cleanings. Another effective strategy to maintain the laparoscopic image is the use of heated insufflation tubing, which can also be used to humidify the gas as it enters the abdomen. This has also been shown to reduce postoperative hypothermia in clinical trials [69]. The suction-irrigator can be used effectively in short bursts to keep the operative field free of smoke, especially when working in the narrow confines of the pelvis. We routinely use a laparoscopic suction-irrigator as a retractor on the rectum applying short bursts of suction during cautery or energy use in coordination with the assistant. This requires some practice, as too much suction will result in collapse of the operative field from loss of pneumoperitoneum. Setting the gas flow rate to 40 L/min and attaching the insufflation tubing to the largest trocar available can help mitigate this problem.

On rare occasions when pulsatile bleeding strikes the camera, the operative field will be totally obscured—creating a situation that is particularly unnerving. It is important to determine the significance of the bleeding (omental vessel vs. IMA) and to deal with it as quickly as possible. Typically, the camera operator is the least experienced surgeon or student involved in the case, and the senior surgeon must quickly take control of the situation. There is no point in proceeding until the visualization of the field can be restored; therefore, the first priority is to clear the lens by removing the laparoscope. Blood in the trocar will frustrate any attempts at good visualization, and if it cannot be cleared quickly, then an alternate trocar should be chosen for the camera as long as it provides good exposure to the bleeding vessel. Alternatively, a 5-mm trocar can be upsized to accommodate a 10-mm laparoscope, which will be less temperamental in the face of blood and debris. Once the operative view has been restored, an assessment of the bleeding can be made and dealt with appropriately. Our preferred method of dealing with this type of bleeding is a 3-0 PDS ENDOLOOP™ (Ethicon, Cincinnati, OH), and when necessary, an additional 5-mm trocar can be inserted to provide a point of entry. Never allow the lack of an additional 5-mm or 10-mm trocar to result in a conversion, advice that is often lost in the stress of the situation.

Serosal and Thermal Injuries

Key Concept: Serosal and thermal injuries should be managed in the same way laparoscopically as in an open procedure.

A relatively common scenario during laparoscopy is an inadvertent serosal or thermal injury that certainly occurs during open surgery but is often easier to deal with in that setting. It is our practice to repair all serosal injuries irrespective of laparoscopy using a 3-0 Vicryl Lembert suture. In our experience, it is important to repair these as soon as they are recognized, as they can be difficult to relocate after even a few minutes. This is particularly true during a laparoscopic case where inspecting the entire bowel can be much more labor-intensive than in open surgery. The utility of over-sewing serosal injuries is not well studied, but animal models have failed to identify any benefit [70]. It is likely that very superficial injuries occur frequently and go unrepaired without detriment to the patient, but in the absence of demonstrable harm, we suggest repairing recognized serosal injuries for fear of delayed intestinal perforation and leaks. It is also important to recognize thermal injuries, which can occur during use of electrosurgical devices, bipolar and ultrasonic energy devices. It is estimated that such injuries occur between 0.6 and 3 times per every 1,000 cases [71]. More concerning, in a survey of the membership of the American College of Surgeons, 18 % had personally experienced complications related to electrosurgical injuries [72]. Electrothermal injury may result from direct application, insulation failure, direct coupling, and capacitive coupling. Direct application is the probably the most common and easiest to recognize (see Video 31.1). It is important to immediately evaluate the injury and decide if it necessitates repair. Finding the injury at a later time will prove difficult irrespective of laparoscopy. The decision to over-sew these injuries will depend on the operator's judgment as to whether the bowel wall integrity has been compromised. Coagulation burns are deeper than those caused by a blended or cutting current [73], and injuries that blanch white have usually gotten hot enough to cause protein denaturation, but may not result in full-thickness injury. As a rule, if the injury is a result of a very short burst of energy and there is minimal tissue change, no further intervention is required. If, however, the injury is the result of sustained burst of energy or occurs out of the direct field of view, as can occur during laparoscopy, it should be repaired. The best way to avoid these injuries is to use cautery sparingly and avoid instruments that don't have an insulated tip—as such, our preferred cautery device is an insulated spatula and not the end of the scissor tips or a Maryland clamp. When using radiofrequency or bipolar energy, it is critical to avoid contact with the bowel right after deployment and be very careful when removing these devices as an injury can occur from the heated jaws as they pass off the field of view. Equipment should be inspected before each case to ensure that the insulation is intact and worn instruments should be discarded. The risk of a break may be increased when using a 5-mm insulated instrument through a 10-mm sleeve or by repeated use of disposable equipment. Direct coupling comes from unintended contact of a non-insulated instrument (e.g., laparoscope, metal grasper forceps) within the abdomen. Electric current will flow from the active electrode into the secondary conductor and energize it. Capacitive coupling occurs when electric current is transferred from one conductor (the active electrode) through intact insulation and into adjacent conductive materials (e.g., bowel) without direct contact and is perhaps the most difficult injury to diagnose. You must keep thermal injury in mind when managing a postoperative patient who is not doing well, as these injuries tend to occur much earlier than would be expected of an anastomotic complication.

The Misplaced Needle

Key Concept: Avoid this situation by using swedged on needles, following the needle from introduction to exit with the camera, and use fluoroscopy should a needle be misplaced.

Another potentially difficult situation that occurs primarily with laparoscopy is the loss of a needle in the abdomen. This can occur for many reasons, but is largely preventable. The surgeon must first ensure that any suture being used in a laparoscopic case is swedged on and not controlled release, which should be confirmed before any suture is introduced into the abdomen. With nursing turnover in the operating room and in the fog of a difficult case, it is possible that a controlled release needle will be inadvertently handed to the surgeon, particularly in cases where laparoscopic suturing is not routine. It is also good practice to always follow the needle and suture with the camera as it is being extracted as it may catch on the trocar and release even if swedged on. If the camera operator is diligent, this can often be visualized and the needle quickly recovered. If the needle is lost, the most effective way to locate it is with fluoroscopy, and the quicker this is called for, the faster the needle will be retrieved. Use of plain abdominal films is of little value. It is not acceptable to leave a lost needle in the abdomen of a patient, and if necessary, the procedure should be converted to open.

Colon and Rectal Injuries

Key Concept: Management of these injuries will depend on the condition of the patient and degree of injury to the bowel.

Inadvertent colotomies or rectal injuries can occur during any abdominal surgery, and the decision to resect or repair will depend on the extent of the injury and the blood supply to the bowel. Small defects that are well vascularized can be repaired in most cases, absent superimposed radiation injury. A single or double layer of suture will often suffice. Rectal injuries that occur during surgeries for prostatic disease or gynecologic procedures should be assessed in a similar fashion. The overall condition of the patient and the bowel will determine if a primary repair will suffice without proximal diversion. Joniau et al. reported an incidence of rectal injury during prostatectomy in 0.7 % [74] of cases, and Yildirim and colleagues reported successful repair of seven rectal injuries concomitant with prostatectomy without postoperative complications and without fecal diversion [75]. During a difficult rectal mobilization, it is often advisable to perform an air leak test prior to the anastomosis to exclude a missed injury, which may prove difficult to visualize afterwards.

Summary Pearls

Inevitably, things go wrong in surgery, no matter how diligent or talented you are or how "straightforward" the case seems to be. The best defense is no doubt a great offense; in other words, have a deep understanding of the technology you are using, an assessment of every team member's level of comfort with each device, and couple that with a broad experience and ingenuity to attempt to minimize complications from occurring. It is not unusual for an assistant or scrub nurse to be assembling or using a device for the first time, and often, errors may occur simply due to this lack of familiarity. Fortunately, these events are infrequent. However, as a result, the operator may have little experience in dealing with them when they do arise. Discussing device failures or unusual complications that occur in the operating room with colleagues is one way to disseminate the knowledge learned. These attributes and actions encompass the professional backbone of the exceptional surgeon. Yet despite excellent intentions, technical challenges will confront the busy abdominal surgeon every day. When they arise, it is not the time to lose focus or become angry or frustrated. Rather, quite the opposite, you must have complete awareness that your next move is often your best opportunity to salvage the situation. In this chapter, we delved into some of the most common, yet most vexing, challenges met during the course of a colorectal operation. Our hope is we were able to provide you with what we hope are clinical pearls that may be a solution to a difficult intraoperative situation you may soon face.

References

1. Neutzling CB, et al. Stapled versus handsewn methods for colorectal anastomosis surgery. Cochrane Database Syst Rev. 2012;2:CD003144.
2. Lustosa SA, et al. Stapled versus handsewn methods for colorectal anastomosis surgery. Cochrane Database Syst Rev. 2001;(3):CD003144.
3. Ballantyne GH. Intestinal suturing. Review of the experimental foundations for traditional doctrines. Dis Colon Rectum. 1983;26(12):836–43. Review. PubMed PMID: 6357675.
4. Burch JM, et al. Single-layer continuous versus two-layer interrupted intestinal anastomosis: a prospective randomized trial. Ann Surg. 2000;231(6):832–7.
5. Sarin S, Lightwood RG. Continuous single-layer gastrointestinal anastomosis: a prospective audit. Br J Surg. 1989;76(5):493–5.
6. Law WL, et al. Single-layer continuous colon and rectal anastomosis using monofilament absorbable suture (Maxon): study of 500 cases. Dis Colon Rectum. 1999;42(6):736–40.
7. Hastings JC, et al. Effect of suture materials on healing wounds of the stomach and colon. Surg Gynecol Obstet. 1975;140(5):701–7.
8. Trimpi HD, et al. Advances in intestinal anastomosis: experimental study and an analysis of 984 patients. Dis Colon Rectum. 1977;20(2):107–17.
9. Munday C, McGinn FP. A comparison of polyglycolic acid and catgut sutures in rat colonic anastomoses. Br J Surg. 1976;63(11):870–2.
10. Lord MG, Broughton AC, Williams HT. A morphologic study on the effect of suturing the submucosa of the large intestine. Surg Gynecol Obstet. 1978;146(2):211–6.
11. Koruda MJ, Rolandelli RH. Experimental studies on the healing of colonic anastomoses. J Surg Res. 1990;48(5):504–15.
12. Didolkar MS, et al. A prospective randomized study of sutured versus stapled bowel anastomoses in patients with cancer. Cancer. 1986;57(3):456–60.
13. Kracht M, et al. Ileocolonic anastomosis after right hemicolectomy for carcinoma: stapled or hand-sewn? A prospective, multicenter, randomized trial. Int J Colorectal Dis. 1993;8(1):29–33.
14. Choy PY, et al. Stapled versus handsewn methods for ileocolic anastomoses. Cochrane Database Syst Rev. 2011;9, CD004320.
15. Suturing or stapling in gastrointestinal surgery: a prospective randomized study. West of Scotland and Highland Anastomosis Study Group. Br J Surg. 1991;78(3):337–41.
16. Docherty JG, et al. Comparison of manually constructed and stapled anastomoses in colorectal surgery. West of Scotland and Highland Anastomosis Study Group. Ann Surg. 1995;221(2):176–84.
17. Simillis C, et al. A meta-analysis comparing conventional end-to-end anastomosis vs. other anastomotic configurations after resection in Crohn's disease. Dis Colon Rectum. 2007; 50(10):1674–87.
18. Resegotti A, et al. Side-to-side stapled anastomosis strongly reduces anastomotic leak rates in Crohn's disease surgery. Dis Colon Rectum. 2005;48(3):464–8.
19. Yamamoto T, et al. Stapled functional end-to-end anastomosis versus sutured end-to-end anastomosis after ileocolonic resection in Crohn disease. Scand J Gastroenterol. 1999;34(7):708–13.
20. Balik E, et al. Revisiting stapled and handsewn loop ileostomy closures: a large retrospective series. Clinics (Sao Paulo). 2011;66(11):1935–41.
21. Leung TT, et al. Comparison of stapled versus handsewn loop ileostomy closure: a meta-analysis. J Gastrointest Surg. 2008;12(5):939–44.
22. Ritchey ML, Lally KP, Ostericher R. Comparison of different techniques of stapled bowel anastomoses in a canine model. Arch Surg. 1993;128(12):1365–7.
23. Zilling T, Walther BS. Are intersecting staple lines a hazard in intestinal anastomosis? Dis Colon Rectum. 1992;35(9):892–6.
24. Goto T, et al. Evaluation of the mechanical strength and patency of functional end-to-end anastomoses. Surg Endosc. 2007;21(9):1508–11.
25. Munoz-Juarez M, et al. Wide-lumen stapled anastomosis vs. conventional end-to-end anastomosis in the treatment of Crohn's disease. Dis Colon Rectum. 2001;44(1):20–5.
26. Chung RS. Blood flow in colonic anastomoses. Effect of stapling and suturing. Ann Surg. 1987;206(3):335–9.
27. Nakayama S, et al. The importance of precompression time for secure stapling with a linear stapler. Surg Endosc. 2011;25(7):2382–6.
28. Morita K, et al. Effects of the time interval between clamping and linear stapling for resection of porcine small intestine. Surg Endosc. 2008;22(3):750–6.
29. Saklani A, et al. Internal herniation following laparoscopic left hemicolectomy: an underreported event. J Laparoendosc Adv Surg Tech A. 2012;22(5):496–500.
30. Cabot JC, et al. Long-term consequences of not closing the mesenteric defect after laparoscopic right colectomy. Dis Colon Rectum. 2010;53(3):289–92.
31. Causey MW, Oguntoye M, Steele SR. Incidence of complications following colectomy with mesenteric closure versus no mesenteric closure: does it really matter? J Surg Res. 2011;171(2):571–5.
32. Marderstein E, Trunzo J, Stulberg J, Champagne B, Reynolds H, Delaney CP. Analysis of stapler misfire during colorectal surgical procedures using a National Event Report Database. 2007. Available from: http://www.casesurgery.com/research/Abstract08WEB.pdf.
33. Pandya S, et al. Laparoscopic colectomy: indications for conversion to laparotomy. Arch Surg. 1999;134(5):471–5.
34. Kirat HT, et al. Influence of stapler size used at ileal pouch-anal anastomosis on anastomotic leak, stricture, long-term functional outcomes, and quality of life. Am J Surg. 2010;200(1):68–72.
35. Polese L, et al. Risk factors for colorectal anastomotic stenoses and their impact on quality of life: what are the lessons to learn? Colorectal Dis. 2012;14(3):e124–8.

36. Kyzer S, Gordon PH. Experience with the use of the circular stapler in rectal surgery. Dis Colon Rectum. 1992;35(7):696–706.
37. Detry RJ, et al. Use of the circular stapler in 1000 consecutive colorectal anastomoses: experience of one surgical team. Surgery. 1995;117(2):140–5.
38. Moore JW, Chapuis PH, Bokey EL. Morbidity and mortality after single- and double-stapled colorectal anastomoses in patients with carcinoma of the rectum. Aust N Z J Surg. 1996;66(12):820–3.
39. Yamamoto H, et al. Feasibility of end-to-anterior wall anastomosis in conversion of the double-stapling technique during laparoscopically assisted surgery. Surg Endosc. 2010;24(9):2178–81.
40. Nakada I, et al. Abdominal stapled side-to-end anastomosis (Baker type) in low and high anterior resection: experiences and results in 69 consecutive patients at a regional general hospital in Japan. Colorectal Dis. 2004;6(3):165–70.
41. Levine RA, Kadro O. When staplers misfire: endoscopic rescue of low pelvic anastomoses. Tech Coloproctol. 2010;14(4): 349–51.
42. Beard JD, et al. Intraoperative air testing of colorectal anastomoses: a prospective, randomized trial. Br J Surg. 1990;77(10): 1095–7.
43. Yalin R, et al. Importance of testing stapled rectal anastomoses with air. Eur J Surg. 1993;159(1):49–51.
44. Ricciardi R, et al. Anastomotic leak testing after colorectal resection: what are the data? Arch Surg. 2009;144(5):407–11; discussion 411–2.
45. Schmidt O, Merkel S, Hohenberger W. Anastomotic leakage after low rectal stapler anastomosis: significance of intraoperative anastomotic testing. Eur J Surg Oncol. 2003;29(3):239–43.
46. Offodile 2nd AC, et al. High incidence of technical errors involving the EEA circular stapler: a single institution experience. J Am Coll Surg. 2010;210(3):331–5.
47. Brennan DJ, et al. Routine mobilization of the splenic flexure is not necessary during anterior resection for rectal cancer. Dis Colon Rectum. 2007;50(3):302–7; discussion 307.
48. Park JS, et al. Laparoscopic versus open resection without splenic flexure mobilization for the treatment of rectum and sigmoid cancer: a study from a single institution that selectively used splenic flexure mobilization. Surg Laparosc Endosc Percutan Tech. 2009;19(1):62–8.
49. Chand M, Miskovic D, Parvaiz AC. Is splenic flexure mobilization necessary in laparoscopic anterior resection? Dis Colon Rectum. 2012;55(11):1195–7.
50. Marsden MR, et al. The selective use of splenic flexure mobilization is safe in both laparoscopic and open anterior resections. Colorectal Dis. 2012;14(10):1255–61.
51. Masoomi H, et al. Predictive factors of splenic injury in colorectal surgery: data from the Nationwide Inpatient Sample, 2006–2008. Arch Surg. 2012;147(4):324–9.
52. Kim HJ, Kim CH, Lim SW, Huh JW, Kim YJ, Kim HR. An extended medial to lateral approach to mobilize the splenic flexure during laparoscopic low anterior resection. Colorectal disease: the official journal of the Association of Coloproctology of Great Britain and Ireland. 2012. Epub 2012/10/16. doi: 10.1111/codi.12056. PubMed PMID: 23061515.
53. Kanemitsu Y, et al. Survival benefit of high ligation of the inferior mesenteric artery in sigmoid colon or rectal cancer surgery. Br J Surg. 2006;93(5):609–15.
54. Chin CC, et al. The oncologic benefit of high ligation of the inferior mesenteric artery in the surgical treatment of rectal or sigmoid colon cancer. Int J Colorectal Dis. 2008;23(8):783–8.
55. Titu LV, Tweedle E, Rooney PS. High tie of the inferior mesenteric artery in curative surgery for left colonic and rectal cancers: a systematic review. Dig Surg. 2008;25(2):148–57.
56. Rutegard M, et al. High tie in anterior resection for rectal cancer confers no increased risk of anastomotic leakage. Br J Surg. 2012;99(1):127–32.
57. Karanjia ND, et al. Leakage from stapled low anastomosis after total mesorectal excision for carcinoma of the rectum. Br J Surg. 1994;81(8):1224–6.
58. Lange MM, et al. Level of arterial ligation in rectal cancer surgery: low tie preferred over high tie. A review. Dis Colon Rectum. 2008;51(7):1139–45.
59. Buunen M, et al. Level of arterial ligation in total mesorectal excision (TME): an anatomical study. Int J Colorectal Dis. 2009;24(11):1317–20.
60. Kim J, Choi DJ, Kim SH. Laparoscopic rectal resection without splenic flexure mobilization: a prospective study assessing anastomotic safety. Hepatogastroenterology. 2009;56(94–95):1354–8.
61. Hall NR, et al. High tie of the inferior mesenteric artery in distal colorectal resections–a safe vascular procedure. Int J Colorectal Dis. 1995;10(1):29–32.
62. Nelsen TS, Anders CJ. Dynamic aspects of small intestinal rupture with special consideration of anastomotic strength. Arch Surg. 1966;93(2):309–14.
63. Shikata J, Shida T. Effects of tension on local blood flow in experimental intestinal anastomoses. J Surg Res. 1986;40(2):105–11.
64. Howes EL, Sooy JW, Samuel HC. The healing of wounds as determined by their tensile strength. JAMA. 1929;92(1):42–5.
65. Deloyers L. Suspension of the right colon permits without exception preservation of the anal sphincter after extensive colectomy of the transverse and left colon (including rectum). Technic -indications- immediate and late results. Lyon Chir. 1964;60:404–13.
66. Manceau G, et al. Right colon to rectal anastomosis (Deloyers procedure) as a salvage technique for low colorectal or coloanal anastomosis: postoperative and long-term outcomes. Dis Colon Rectum. 2012;55(3):363–8.
67. Material Safety Data Sheet: FRED™ Anti-Fog Solution. North Haven, C.U.S.S. Material Safety Data Sheet: FRED™ Anti-Fog Solution. North Haven: United States Surgical. 2004. Available from: http://www.autosuture.com/imageServer.aspx?contentID=6591&contenttype=application/pdf.
68. DHELP. Visualization challenges and solutions in laparoscopic surgery 2010. Available from: http://www.newwavesurgical.com/sites/default/files/imce-uploads/value_analysis_final_9.7.2012.pdf.
69. Ott DE, et al. Reduction of laparoscopic-induced hypothermia, postoperative pain and recovery room length of stay by preconditioning gas with the Insuflow device: a prospective randomized controlled multi-center study. JSLS. 1998;2(4):321–9.
70. Binnebosel M, et al. Influence of small intestinal serosal defect closure on leakage rate and adhesion formation: a pilot study using rabbit models. Langenbecks Arch Surg. 2011;396(1):133–7.
71. Wu MP, et al. Complications and recommended practices for electrosurgery in laparoscopy. Am J Surg. 2000;179(1):67–73.
72. Tucker RD. Laparoscopic electrosurgical injuries: survey results and their implications. Surg Laparosc Endosc. 1995;5(4):311–7.
73. Chino A, et al. A comparison of depth of tissue injury caused by different modes of electrosurgical current in a pig colon model. Gastrointest Endosc. 2004;59(3):374–9.
74. Joniau SG, et al. Complications and functional results of surgery for locally advanced prostate cancer. Adv Urol. 2012;2012:706309.
75. Yildirim M, et al. Rectal injury during radical prostatectomy. Ulus Travma Acil Cerrahi Derg. 2012;18(3):250–4.

Colon and Rectal Trauma

34

Matthew J. Martin and Carlos V.R. Brown

Key Points

- Colorectal injuries are commonly seen with penetrating abdominal trauma or high-velocity blunt mechanism trauma.
- Early diagnosis and intervention are critical, particularly if there is ongoing gastrointestinal spillage.
- Peritonitis or other hard signs of colon injury belong in the OR; otherwise, a CT scan is the evaluation study of choice.
- Injury management should be tailored to the patient and their injuries, and not by arbitrary categorization such as "right or left sided."
- Primary repair or anastomosis is the optimal strategy for most patients with colon injuries.
- Diverting or protective ostomy will always have a role in select high-risk injuries or patients.
- Damage control allows for control of bleeding and spillage and deferment of the decision for definitive management to a later time with a more stable patient.
- Diversion is appropriate for most major rectal injuries, but there is an increasing role for primary repair or anastomosis in select patients.
- Immediate evaluation is warranted for any suspicion of a post-colonoscopy perforation or bleeding.
- Most endoscopic injuries can be managed nonoperatively or with minimally invasive techniques if identified early.

M.J. Martin, MD, FACS (✉)
Department of Surgery, Legacy Emanuel Medical Center, Portland, OR, USA
Department of Surgery, Madigan Army Medical Center, 9040 Fitzsimmons Avenue, Tacoma, WA 98431, USA
e-mail: matthew.martin1@us.army.mil, docmartin2@yahoo.com

C.V.R. Brown, MD, FACS
Department of Surgery, University of Texas Southwestern – Austin, Austin, TX, USA
e-mail: cvrbrown@seton.org

Historical Aspects of Colon and Rectal Trauma

If you do a colostomy there will be someone to tell you why not primary anastomosis; if you do a primary anastomosis there will be someone to tell you why not colostomy.

– Moshe Schein, MD

Key Concept: Understanding the historical trends and key lessons in how colorectal injuries have been managed will help you make better decisions when faced with a challenging injury.

The entire field of abdominal surgery, and particularly surgery involving repair or reconstruction of the gastrointestinal tract, can trace its origins back to the basic principles and experiences gained from the management of traumatic injuries. Although once considered uniformly fatal, these injuries are now routinely managed with exceedingly low overall rates of surgical morbidity and mortality. This can be credited not only to advances in surgical capabilities and techniques but also to simultaneous advances in the development of safe anesthetic agents, effective antibiotics, and modern resuscitation principles.

There is a commonly used proverb that "the only winner in war is medicine," and arguably no field in medicine has benefited from the lessons learned during combat more than trauma and emergency surgery. In particular, the historical progression in the field of colon and rectal trauma represents a fascinating example of the exchange of ideas between military and civilian surgeons and the willingness to abandon widely held dogma based on accumulated evidence and

S.R. Steele et al. (eds.), *Complexities in Colorectal Surgery*,
DOI 10.1007/978-1-4614-9022-7_34, © Springer Science+Business Media New York 2014

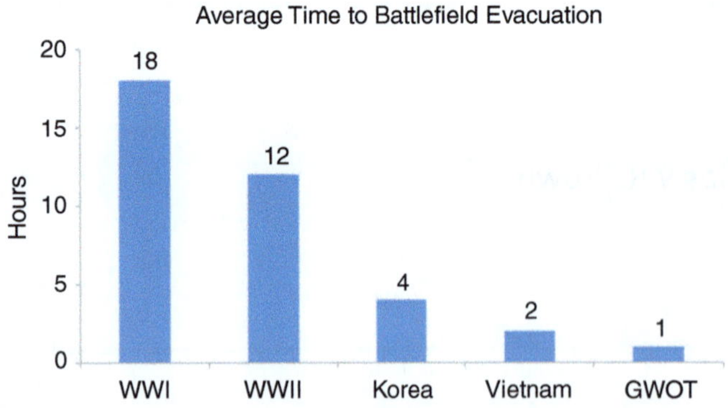

Fig. 34.1 Average time (in hours) from injury to arrival at a field hospital for major American conflicts (*GWOT* global war on terror) (Modified with permission from Perry et al. [4] © in 2004 Elsevier)

experience. While this has greatly benefitted the field of surgery, arguably the greatest beneficiary has been the injured or wounded patient. A recent large multicenter study of modern civilian colon trauma found a colon-related mortality rate of only 1.3 % [1], and several modern military series from combat operations in Iraq and Afghanistan have demonstrated similarly low morbidity and mortality rates [2, 3]. These stand in stark contrast to historical rates of morbidity and mortality with colorectal injuries well in excess of 50 % even with timely surgical intervention [4]. The overall declines in battlefield morbidity and mortality have mirrored the significant improvements in prehospital care and the time from injury to arrival at a field hospital with surgical capability (Fig. 34.1).

The historical trends and advancements in the management of colorectal trauma can largely be grouped around major conflicts and wars, when high volumes of penetrating abdominal wounds provided a large body of experiential data. As described in a historical analysis by V.J. Cirillo, the epidemiology of battlefield wounds and deaths can be roughly divided into two eras with World War I as the dividing line [5, 6]. Prior to and leading into World War I (Disease Era: 1775–1918), the most common causes of battlefield morbidity and mortality were not wounds or injuries, they were communicable disease, infection, and hypothermia. This epidemiology rapidly changed with World War II (Trauma Era: 1941–present), where improvements in medical care drastically reduced deaths due to disease and the development of modern weaponry heralded the rise of trauma as the primary cause of battlefield deaths.

Prior to World War I, the management of abdominal wounds was largely nonoperative, and the mortality approached 100 % if a bowel injury was present. Laparotomy was largely condemned as a treatment option, as summarized by MacCormac's experience from the Boer War (1899–1902) where he stated that "In this war a man wounded in the abdomen dies if he is operated upon and remains alive if he is left in peace" [7]. However, in the presence of evisceration with relatively easy access to the injured bowel, it was recognized that primary repair and return of the bowel to the abdominal cavity was advantageous [4]. With the understanding that repair of these injuries was clearly superior to observation alone, it was mainly a matter of waiting for the development of equipment and medications that would allow for safe anesthesia and postoperative recovery.

During World War I, the sheer volume of penetrating abdominal wounds coupled with advancements in casualty evacuation and prehospital trauma care led some surgeons to abandon nonoperative management in favor of laparotomy and primary repair of the injured colon [8, 9]. Although this approach was still associated with a considerable risk of repair failure, infection or sepsis, and death, there was a notable decrease in the overall battlefield mortality and particularly the mortality associated with abdominal wounds [10, 11]. During World War II, the next major paradigm shift in colorectal trauma management followed the publication of Ogilvie's classic analysis of the management of colon wounds from the North African campaign of 1942 [12]. He strongly advocated the use of fecal diversion for all colon injuries by either exteriorization of the wounded area of the colon or repair/resection with proximal diversion and credited this approach with the drastically reduced mortality rates compared to WWI [12, 13]. This approach became the formal doctrinal policy for surgeons of both the British and US medical forces, and proximal diversion was mandated for treatment of all colon wounds by the US Surgeon General in 1943 [13, 14]. For rectal injuries, the high risk of mortality from pelvic and retroperitoneal sepsis was significantly decreased during WWII by adopting the principles of wide local washout/debridement in addition to proximal diversion [4, 15]. This was most commonly accomplished by a posterior approach with excision of the coccyx to access the presacral space for washout and drain placement [15].

Further advances in the management of colorectal trauma over the next several decades arose from advances in surgical technique as well as improvements in prehospital care and evacuation during combat operations. Surgeons of the Korean and Vietnam War eras adopted a more anatomic-based approach to colon injuries, favoring resection and primary anastomosis for select right-sided injuries and exteriorization and/or colostomy for left-sided or rectal injuries [4]. One series from the Vietnam conflict reported excellent results with the use of a "closed colostomy" for isolated colon injuries, with primary repair of the injury followed by exteriorization of the repaired segment to observe for any postoperative suture line breakdown [16]. However, other series reported significantly worse outcomes with this approach, and exteriorization has been largely abandoned in favor of alternative techniques. For rectal trauma, the addition of distal washout of the rectum was reported to decrease infectious complications and completed the well-known “4 Ds” of rectal trauma: direct repair, divert, drain, and distal washout.

The prolonged peacetime experiences following the Vietnam War resulted in further refinements of management principles and operative techniques for colorectal trauma that are discussed in this chapter. This has also been the most productive time period in terms of generating controlled data on which to make evidence-based management decisions. In addition to retrospective case series, a number of higher-quality studies including prospective series, case–control studies, multicenter studies, and even randomized trials have been reported and have helped to drive further improvements in outcomes from colorectal injury. The overall trend of the past two decades can be summarized by these six principles:

1. Primary repair for most nondestructive, low-velocity type injuries.
2. Resection with anastomosis for most destructive and/or high-velocity injuries.
3. Elimination of routine proximal diversion for most colon injuries and select rectal injuries.
4. Decreased emphasis on anatomic location of injury as an important factor in management for colon injuries.
5. Adoption of damage control laparotomy principles allows for delay of decision making regarding diversion versus anastomosis in unstable or high-risk patients.
6. Tailored management of rectal injuries with individualized use of the “4 Ds,” with proximal diversion remaining the most common and important.

Most recently, there have been several excellent series detailing the experience with colorectal trauma in the conflicts in Iraq and Afghanistan over the past decade [2, 3, 17]. These series demonstrate that the trends observed in civilian practice of extending primary anastomosis without diversion to colon trauma have carried over to the military setting, with the majority of colon wounds being managed with primary repair or resection and anastomosis [2]. However, approximately one-third of patients were still managed with a diverting colostomy, demonstrating that proximal diversion remains an important and frequently used component in the arsenal of the combat surgeon. Analysis of these patients’ longer-term outcomes demonstrated the viability of primary repair or anastomosis, but also highlighted the higher risk of repair failure in the presence of associated abdominal injuries such as pancreas, stomach, spleen, diaphragm, and kidney [17]. With the realization that better data collection and analysis is critical to optimizing combat research, a dedicated Joint Surgical Transcolonic Injury or Ostomy Multi-Theater Assessment (J-STOMA) project and database has been established. The first published series of 977 patients from the J-STOMA database has provided valuable epidemiologic data and also identified a significant difference in mortality between patients with no fecal diversion (11 %) versus 4 % with fecal diversion [18].

A unique factor that also must be considered is that this is the first major combat experience where damage control principles have been widely adopted and utilized [19–21]. The adoption of damage control laparotomy techniques allows for a delay in the decision regarding anastomosis versus proximal diversion in the unstable or high-risk patient, which can then be performed at a later time in a more elective setting. Preliminary follow-up data from primary repair or anastomoses performed in the combat damage control setting have demonstrated acceptable morbidity rates and outcomes comparable to civilian patients undergoing damage control laparotomy [17, 19].

The radical overall change in the management of colorectal trauma is highlighted by the findings of a 1998 survey of US trauma surgeons regarding the management of these injuries [22]. The overwhelming majority (98 %) would use primary repair or resection with anastomosis for selected colon injuries, and almost one-third of respondents stated that they would “never” perform a colostomy for colon trauma. This stands in stark contrast to the World War II dictum of mandatory colostomy or exteriorization for all injuries. Although this is generally accepted to represent clear progress in the management of colorectal trauma, there is continued debate about whether the pendulum has swung too far in favor of primary anastomosis, particularly for war-related injuries [23]. Further controlled trials and reports of larger experiences with good long-term outcome data will undoubtedly help us to further clarify the optimal management techniques in both civilian and military settings.

Colon Trauma

Key Concept: Trauma surgery is all about rapid evaluation and prioritizing everything you do – starting from your physical exam and including resuscitation, imaging, and operative interventions.

Key Concept: Controlling life-threatening hemorrhage and stopping GI tract contamination are the top two priorities in abdominal trauma – and major bowel injuries often present with both. Failure to rapidly diagnose and intervene is lethal.

Many of the details of the surgical anatomy and techniques for various colorectal procedures are discussed in great detail by expert surgeons in other chapters of this text. Although there may certainly be many complicating factors such as anatomic distortion, poor visualization due to bleeding, and multiple simultaneous injuries in the trauma patient, the basic steps and technical considerations of the operation are no different than in most elective settings. The critical differences in successfully managing colorectal injuries are in the thought process and decision making – both preoperatively and in the

Table 34.1 Key elements of the initial trauma evaluation for colorectal trauma

History	Physical examination	Diagnostic and imaging studies
Abdominal pain or complaints	Overall impression ("sick" or "not sick")	Chest x-ray – free air, elevated or blurred diaphragm
Allergies and medications	Vital signs	FAST exam – free fluid in abdomen or pelvis
Prior abdominal surgery: particularly any prior bowel surgery, hernia repairs, mesh implantation, aortoiliac surgery	Focused abdominal exam: tenderness, distension, rebound, guarding, bruising, "seat-belt sign." Identify all prior incisions, any hernias	CT scan abdomen/pelvic: diagnostic study of choice in most patients. No oral contrast required for initial study. Consider follow-up CT with oral contrast or "triple contrast" for equivocal initial study or concerning clinical picture
Major comorbidities: vasculopathy, congestive heart failure, high-dose steroid use, immunosuppressants	Location of all open or penetrating wounds	"Triple-contrast" CT scan: may be useful for penetrating flank or back wounds with suspicion for retroperitoneal colon injury, but usually standard CT is adequate
Injury mechanism (from high to low risk) Penetrating, missile Penetrating, stab Blunt, high velocity Blunt, low velocity	Logroll and full back/flank exam	Abdominal x-rays: not useful as routine study in blunt trauma. Can be very useful in gunshot wounds for identifying location of fragments, estimating trajectories. Place radiolucent markers on all external wounds
	Pelvic and perineal exam	Diagnostic peritoneal lavage: mainly of historical interest, but can be used with equivocal CT findings (i.e., free fluid with no solid organ injury) in patients with unreliable exam
	Digital rectal exam (DRE)	Anoscopy, rigid proctoscopy: penetrating perineal trauma, open pelvic fracture, positive DRE, any other suspicion for rectal injury

operating room – that often need to be made rapidly with imperfect and incomplete information, in suboptimal and often chaotic settings, and under the pressure of time constraints (i.e., the "golden hour"). Therefore, this chapter will focus more on the key decision-making processes, common pitfalls, and optimal management strategies and less on the procedural details or surgical technique.

The fastest way to fail at managing the severely injured patient is to approach them with an elective surgical mindset. In the elective setting the priority is placed on being thorough and taking a "head to toe" systematic approach to evaluation in order to identify all pertinent medical and surgical issues. In the trauma setting, the exact opposite is true. A rapid, focused, and highly prioritized evaluation should be performed with the initial focus only on identifying potentially life- or limb-threatening injuries along with select and highly relevant aspects of the patient history. Attention can often be distracted by more dramatic but non-life-threatening injuries (i.e., open extremity fracture), and although it is difficult, these should be initially ignored (other than active hemorrhage) until completion of the primary survey and truncal exam. With respect to colorectal injury, the key aspects of the initial evaluation are shown in Table 34.1. This evaluation should focus on both identifying the presence of a colorectal injury as well as providing the key patient-related information that may alter your management decisions and risk: benefit analysis for primary repair versus diversion or another alternative.

Injury mechanism and location can be extremely helpful for gauging your level of suspicion of a bowel injury and for directing further workup. The highest level of suspicion should be for gunshot wounds to the trunk, particularly those that have clearly passed from anterior to posterior or crossed the midline from side to side. The default position for these wounds should be to assume that bowel injury is present and to perform a laparotomy. Perineal or trans-pelvic gunshot wounds and those with an associated pelvic fracture should be assumed to have a rectal injury until proven otherwise. Stab wounds to the abdomen, flank, back, or perineum carry a lower but still significant risk of colorectal injury and warrant a detailed exam, and often supplemental imaging, unless there are obvious signs of a bowel injury at presentation. The old approach of exploring the stab wound and performing a laparotomy if there is evidence of fascial penetration has largely been replaced with decision making based on the abdominal exam and use of imaging studies [24, 25]. For blunt trauma, the incidence of colorectal injury is significantly lower and much less common; therefore, it can be frequently misdiagnosed or overlooked completely. High-risk mechanisms are those that involve high velocity or forces of impact and include motorized vehicle crashes, falls from heights, or pedestrians struck by vehicles. Patients with lower mechanisms of blunt trauma such as falls from standing, low-speed motor vehicle collisions, or non-motorized vehicle crashes have exceedingly low risk of colon or rectal injuries and usually do not require additional studies if the history and exam is reassuring. A particular warning should be made for patients with a high-risk mechanism and an altered exam, typically from brain injury or due to alcohol or drug use. Supplemental imaging, usually with a CT scan, should be the standard, and a lower threshold for exploratory surgery should be maintained.

"Catatonia" and Early Decision Making

Key Concept: "I thought I would get a quick CT scan to rule out other injuries" is a commonly heard refrain at M&M conferences when explaining why a patient with operative abdominal injuries died in the CT scanner.

The sharp decline in civilian penetrating trauma volume and the increase in nonoperative management of most injuries have inadvertently created a widespread disease pathology among surgeons and surgical trainees that we have previously described as *catatonia* [26]. Defined as "the inability to make definitive management decisions without the use of detailed computed tomography imaging, coupled with a fear of the exploratory operation," this is a frequent cause of unnecessary delay to definitive operative intervention and a cause of preventable morbidity or mortality. An oft-heard excuse when explaining a major delay in operative intervention for a perforated colon is that the surgeon wanted "more information" about the injury or that the patient "needed resuscitation" before going to the operating room. In this chapter we emphasize the "golden rule" of the acute abdomen; any patient with an acute abdomen or peritonitis, or obvious signs of a bowel injury on initial exam or plain films, belongs in the operating room immediately. No prolonged imaging workup is required, and resuscitation can be done just as well in the operating room as it can anywhere else in the hospital. In the stable patient this approaches may save you time and resources; in the unstable or deteriorating patient with a colorectal injury, these approaches may save his or her life.

In the Operating Room

Once the decision has been made for operative intervention for a known or suspected colorectal injury, all of the basic principles of emergency surgery and ATLS apply. Although attention should be paid to hypothermia prevention and management with active warming devices (heated forced-air blanket), one exception to common practice that we believe should be omitted is the warming of the operating room to excessive ambient temperatures (>75 °F). This has been shown to be wholly ineffective at treating or preventing hypothermia and only results in discomfort of the operative team and likely additional contamination of the operative field due to sweat [27]. All patients should be expected to have a full stomach, so aspiration precautions during rapid sequence intubation are critical. Bleeding and ongoing blood loss should be anticipated, so emergency-release blood products (type O for packed cells and type AB for plasma) should be standing by and a type and cross should be performed as soon as possible. A Foley catheter should be placed barring any signs of urethral injury, although if there is a suspicion for bladder injury, then we recommend prepping in the genitals and placing a sterile catheter that can be accessed by the surgeon. This can be invaluable for manually distending the bladder with fluid and/or dye to identify injuries and to test for leaks after a repair.

It is important to optimize the operative exposure and visualization, and a few minutes to set up a self-retaining retractor (Bookwalter, Omni, etc.) will pay dividends in decreased overall operative times and frustration levels. This is particularly important for difficult exposure situations such as obesity or for pelvic dissections (sigmoid, rectum). This will also free the hands of the surgeon and assistant to perform more critical tasks. For the unstable or actively bleeding patient, a generous midline incision should be made at the start to allow rapid access to all quadrants of the abdominal cavity. For the stable patient, a smaller laparotomy incision may be made and then extended if necessary based on the injuries identified. Most right-sided colon injuries can be managed through a supra-umbilical midline incision, but left-sided or rectal injuries require inferior extension below the umbilicus toward the pubic symphysis. Descending or sigmoid colon injuries that require resection with anastomosis typically require the longest incisions to adequately mobilize the left colon (including the splenic flexure) and then perform an anastomosis in the lower abdomen or pelvis. If a large amount of hemoperitoneum is discovered on entering the abdominal cavity (even in a "stable" patient), then abandon any attempt at "minilaparotomy" and widely extend the incision from the xiphoid to several centimeters above the pubic symphysis.

Prepped Versus Unprepped Bowel

One of the most important factors that led to a revolution in the performance of colorectal surgery was the ability to decrease the risk of postoperative infectious complications. The high bacterial content of the colon has long been recognized as an area of concern with any intraoperative spillage, and the concept of increasing bacterial concentrations in the distal colon was a principal factor in promulgating the belief that left-sided injuries should be treated differently than right-sided injuries. For elective surgery, the standard of care has traditionally been to administer an oral mechanical bowel prep (with or without oral antibiotics) before surgery to both remove fecal material and to decrease the bacterial load in the event of intraoperative spillage [28]. In cases of emergent trauma with colorectal injury, the obvious lack of bowel prep before injury has been cited as one reason to treat these differently than elective operations and to forego primary repair or anastomosis in favor of diversion. Over the past decade, a large body of high-quality evidence has amassed that refutes the standard beliefs about the value of mechanical bowel preparation, with multiple randomized trials and several meta-analyses finding no benefit or even evidence of increased morbidity with bowel prep [29, 30].

The currently available data has led many surgeons to abandon or to more selectively utilize bowel prep for elective surgery, but it also provides reassurance for trauma surgeons that a preoperative bowel prep is not a requirement for a safe bowel repair or anastomosis. The two primary issues that a classic bowel prep was designed to address are (1) mechanical removal of fecal matter and (2) administration of antibiotic prophylaxis against infections due to fecal flora. For the vast majority of traumatic colorectal injuries, mechanical clearance of the colon is unnecessary and in fact would only serve to delay completion of the procedure. The second goal of infection prophylaxis is achieved with the administration of intravenous antibiotics that cover both aerobic and anaerobic organisms typical of fecal flora. Antibiotics should be administered as soon as there is evidence of the injury or a decision for laparotomy has been made. Although the optimal goal would be 30–60 min prior to the skin incision, this is often not realistic in trauma surgery. Re-dosing of antibiotics should be performed if the surgery is prolonged to near the normal dosing interval for the selected antibiotic or in cases where blood loss and transfusion are approaching one whole blood volume. Antibiotics should be continued for 24 h only, and there is no benefit (and potential harm) of continuing them longer even in the face of large volume contamination [31]. Appropriate single-agent therapy is as effective as multidrug regimens, and most centers use a B-lactam agent such as Unasyn or Zosyn. In class 4 cases with a delayed presentation and established infection, antibiotics should be continued as dictated by the location and nature of the infection.

Finally, an additional well-described option that can be utilized is the "on-table" bowel preparation or lavage [32]. This concept was initially espoused for all emergent colon surgery in order to achieve the same benefits as a standard preoperative bowel prep. However, it has fallen out of favor as the role of mechanical bowel preparation has been questioned and due to the difficulty of adequately lavaging the colon effectively and without spillage. The pros of an on-table lavage include the ability to debulk and clean the colon to facilitate easier repair or anastomosis, decompress a dilated colon, and remove a large stool burden that could cause future constipation or impaction. The cons include the lack of a proven benefit, the possibility of increased spillage and infections, and the need for making additional holes in the colon or small bowel to place the lavage catheter. We recommend consideration of on-table lavage only in situations of major colonic distension with a large amount of solid or liquid matter or significant solid fecal impaction that could impair recovery of motility or anastomotic healing. Some technical tips/tricks include as follows: (1) lavage the entire colon by opening the appendix and inserting a balloon-tipped catheter for instilling the fluid, then perform a standard appendectomy after catheter removal, and (2) insert a sterile ventilator tubing into the open proximal end of the colon to be lavaged and secure it with a large suture or umbilical tape (Fig. 34.2).

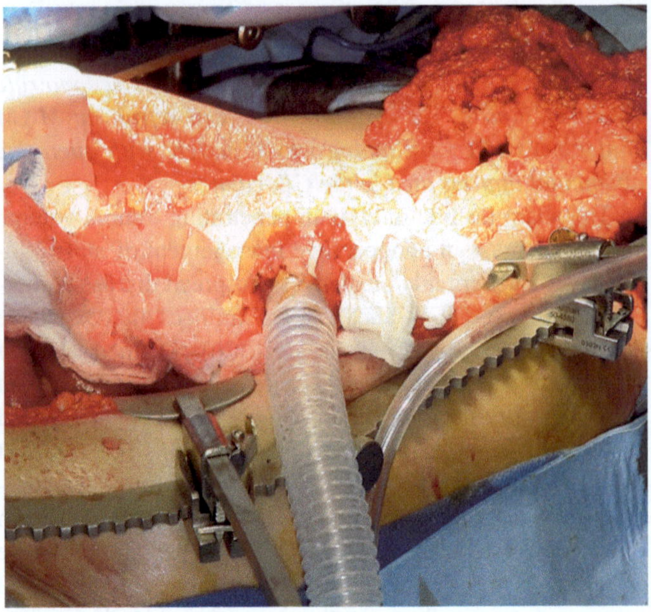

Fig. 34.2 On-table lavage of distal colon and rectum is performed using sterile ventilator tubing placed in the open end of the distal colon and secured with an umbilical tape

Also remember to use warmed fluids for the lavage in order to avoid causing or exacerbating systemic hypothermia.

Timing of Injury and Operative Decisions

Key Concept: Most traumatic colorectal injuries will present within the first few hours and a short delay should not impact management decisions. Longer delays with uncontrolled abdominal contamination should push you toward diversion and/or damage control techniques.

Key Concept: Delayed diagnosis of a contained injury with minimal associated symptoms should prompt consideration of nonoperative management – if the patient has already passed this "trial of life," then CLOSE *observation or percutaneous drainage may be all they need.*

One of the most important factors in determining the optimal approach to a colorectal injury is the duration of time that has elapsed between the initial injury, recognition of the injury, and intervention for the injury. Fortunately, for the vast majority of traumatic injuries to the colon or rectum, patients are immediately transported to a trauma hospital and the diagnosis is established on the initial evaluation and imaging. It also appears that minor delays in diagnosis or intervention (2–8 h) do not have much impact on postoperative patient outcomes, and this would typically not change any intraoperative decision making. This also applies to patients that present in a delayed fashion due to a partial-thickness injury that then progresses to full-thickness injury with perforation. As long as the change in status is quickly identified and intervention performed in a timely manner, there does not appear to be major added morbidity or mortality.

However, occasionally there may be a significant delay to either diagnose or intervene in a patient with a major colorectal injury, and this can result in severe morbidity or even mortality. Scenarios where this may occur include failure to recognize peritoneal signs or imaging findings at initial presentation, presence of factors that compromise the abdominal exam (such as severe head injury or intoxication), patient delay in seeking medical attention or in transfer to an appropriate facility, and masking of peritoneal signs by medications (i.e., steroids) or other patient factors. Delays of more than 8–12 h associated with fecal contamination will typically significantly alter both the local anatomy and the patient physiology, and as a result, the intraoperative decision making and choice of procedure will frequently have to be adapted based on the findings.

As a general principal, there should be a much more liberal use of proximal diversion rather than primary anastomosis or repair when there has been a long delay to operation in the setting of fecal contamination and peritonitis. Some of the key considerations and technical factors that may alter your approach in these cases include:

1. Prolonged fecal contamination can result in a SIRS response or even septic shock, and the patient may not tolerate prolonged surgery or reconstruction.
2. Pelvic sepsis after extraperitoneal rectal injuries can be rapidly fatal and may have little to no visible intra-abdominal pathology.
3. Bowel wall induration and edema may compromise staple or suture lines.
4. Massive small and/or large bowel distension may be present.
5. The mesentery is often thickened and shortened, limiting mobility and making even a simple colostomy difficult or impossible.

In select cases the patient may present with delayed recognition of a colorectal injury and minimal or localized associated signs or symptoms. In this case the patient has already demonstrated tolerance or control of the injury, and temporizing minimally invasive interventions may be all that are required. The classic *non-trauma* example of this would be perforated diverticulitis or appendicitis with a localized abscess that can be managed with antibiotics and a percutaneous drain. This is infrequently encountered in the trauma setting but may be seen more frequently with iatrogenic colorectal injury from endoscopy, biopsy, or other interventions. In these cases the optimal management strategy is usually to fully characterize the pathology with a high-quality CT scan, cover the patient with intravenous antibiotics, initiate bowel rest and NPO status, and ensure drainage of significant abscesses or fluid collections. This most often can be accomplished with image-guided percutaneous or transrectal drainage but may require laparoscopy or even laparotomy for difficult locations. Percutaneous drain placement may also be considered in the patient with a large amount of free air who is otherwise a good candidate for nonoperative management. Aspiration of the free air with or without placement of a drain can markedly improve the abdominal discomfort and provide an improved baseline for serial physical examinations.

Operative Management: Repair, Resect, or Divert?

Key Concept: Injury location used to drive management decisions for colon trauma, but this distinction has largely been abandoned and management should be based on the exact colon injury, associated injuries, and patient factors.

Key Concept: Remember to consider ALL *of the risks for repair versus diversion, including the morbidity associated with a second surgery for ostomy takedown. This risk analysis should most often favor primary repair or anastomosis, but a diverting or protective ostomy still has a clear role in high-risk injuries or patients.*

Once a full exploration has been completed and all bowel injuries identified, the first decision is whether the injury is amenable to primary repair or will require segmental or formal anatomic resection. The standard teaching is to categorize injuries as either destructive (>50 % of bowel circumference or devascularized) or nondestructive, with resection recommended for destructive and primary repair for nondestructive wounds. Although this is a good basic guideline, there are several other important factors to consider and these are outlined in Table 34.2. These include not only the size of the injury but the number and location of injuries as well as the adequacy of primary repair that may be achieved. An important technical point for missile wounds, particularly fragment or high-velocity gunshot wounds, is that the wound edges need to be debrided back to healthy

Table 34.2 Factors to guide primary repair versus resection for colon injury

Primary repair	Resection
Small size (nondestructive)	Destructive (>50 % circumference or devascularized)
Single injuries or multiple with adequate spacing	Multiple injuries with short spacing
Clean margins (after debridement of edges)	Inflamed or necrotic edges
Minimal or no mesenteric injury	Large mesenteric hematoma or laceration
Tension-free closure	Cannot be closed without tension
Healthy surrounding bowel	Major edema, inflammation, bowel wall hematoma
No major pathology present	Major pathology present (cancer, diverticulitis, etc.)
Closure leaves widely patent lumen	Closure would narrow lumen (>25 %)
Low velocity wound	High-velocity wound
At risk for short-gut syndrome with resection	Adequate bowel length after resection
No adjacent pancreatic injury or leak	Pancreatic injury/leak adjacent to injury

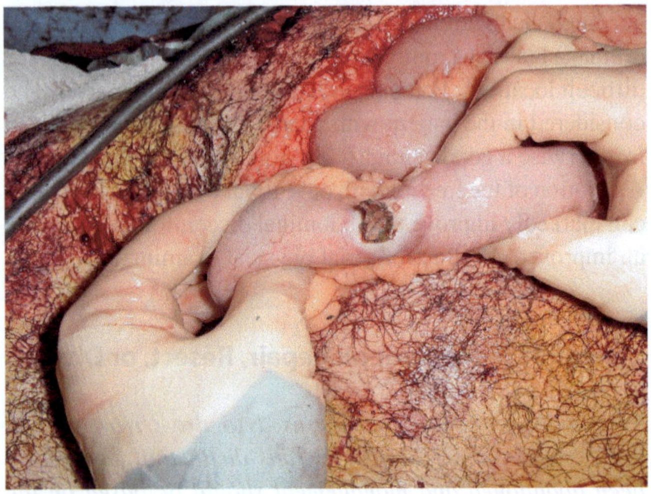

Fig. 34.3 Missile wound to bowel with small perforation but significant thermal injury to the surrounding bowel wall. This injury should be completely debrided and then repaired or resected

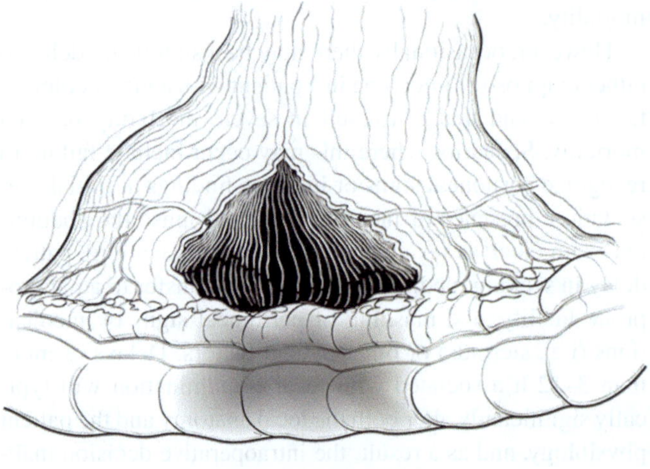

Fig. 34.4 Large tear of the mesenteric border of the bowel ("bucket-handle" deformity) from blunt deceleration forces. This usually requires resection of the now devascularized bowel segment to avoid subsequent ischemic complications (Reprinted with permission Martin and Beekley [26] © in 2011 Springer)

tissue before closure. These missiles will frequently cause extensive tissue damage or even direct thermal injury (Fig. 34.3) and will often break down within several days of closure if not adequately debrided. Thus, a small wound that initially appears appropriate for primary repair may actually require segmental resection once the full extent of tissue injury is identified and debrided. On the other hand, excessive debridement of surrounding tissue for high-velocity injuries has been advocated based on erroneous assumptions about the size and impact of the "temporary cavity" created by the missile. In addition to these overestimates of the size and force of cavitation, it is important to note that elastic tissues such as bowel tolerate stretch forces much better than inelastic tissue such as the liver [33]. Debridement of all clearly devitalized and any questionable tissue should be performed, but do not perform additional debridement of healthy tissues simply based on the injury mechanism or ballistics. The status of the mesentery is also an important factor as it relates to the adequacy of the blood supply to the injured area. A classically described injury seen in blunt trauma with rapid deceleration is a large tear of the mesentery without injury to the colon wall. This "bucket-handle" deformity can be misleading as the bowel will usually appear uninjured but should be resected due to the large area of devascularization (Fig. 34.4).

As discussed above in the historical overview of colorectal trauma, a dogma developed over time of categorizing the wounds into "right"- or "left"-sided injuries and basing the management off of this simple distinction. Right-sided injuries could undergo standard repair or resection with anastomosis, but left-sided injuries required exteriorization or proximal diversion. This was based on microbiological data showing increasing bacterial loads in the left colon and the observation of increased complications with left sided or more distal colon injuries. However, subsequent experience with both traumatic colon resections as well as emergent resection for diverticular disease demonstrated that left-sided repair or resection with primary anastomoses could be performed with an acceptably low risk of anastomotic leak or other major morbidity.

A major potential confounder of studies examining the question of right- versus left-sided colon injuries is the unequal distribution and severity of associated injuries. The right colon generally lies outside of the pelvis and is not intimately associated with any major vessels or organs except for the right kidney. Alternatively, the transverse colon lies over the body of the pancreas and the aorta/vena cava, while the sigmoid colon lies in the pelvis adjacent to the iliac vessels, bladder, ureter, sacral veins, and pelvic bones. Thus, left-sided colon injuries are much more likely to have associated vascular, pancreatic, and genitourinary injuries or a major pelvic fracture. The presence of these associated injuries will naturally increase the risk of blood loss, need for transfusion, duration of surgery, and systemic inflammatory response. As a result, morbidity and mortality is higher among this patient cohort, but most of this increase is likely independent of the colon injury. Some other key technical factors also play a likely role, including the difficulty of working in the narrower pelvis (left sided) versus the mid to upper abdomen (right sided) and the higher likelihood of anastomotic tension or ischemia with a colorectal anastomosis versus an ileocolic anastomosis.

Although still occasionally taught, the trauma community has largely abandoned the management of colon injuries according to the simplified right-left dichotomy. However, there is now a commonly held misunderstanding that the injury location is not important and that all colon injuries can be treated in a similar fashion regardless of location. Although the left-right distinction is no longer of primary importance, it is critical for the surgeon to appreciate the key issues and technical factors that will be encountered in different injury locations. Table 34.3 shows some of these

Table 34.3 Key considerations and patterns of associated injuries based on the location of the colon injury

Injury location	Key considerations and associated injuries
Cecum/ascending colon	Easiest area to mobilize and can be done rapidly with blunt hand dissection
	Assess for associated injury to right kidney and proximal ureter
	Large perinephric or retroperitoneal hematoma can displace ureter much more medially or anteriorly than normal
Hepatic flexure	Frequently associated injury to liver that is usually obvious
	Also carefully assess gallbladder and porta hepatis
	Diaphragm injuries frequently missed – remember to look and palpate over the dome
	Always inspect the duodenum and head of pancreas!
Transverse colon	If associated zone 1 retroperitoneal hematoma, worry about the aorta and vena cava first
	Always open the gastrocolic ligament widely as this aides mobilization but also exposes:
	(a) The posterior surface of the stomach – frequent site of missed gastric injuries
	(b) The body and tail of the pancreas – critical to drain or resect any injury, particularly if you are doing an adjacent colon anastomosis or primary repair
	(c) Posterior surface of the transverse colon mesentery
	Injuries at the root of the mesentery may involve the SMA/SMV, middle colics, or D4
Splenic flexure	May have a true lienocolic ligament or may be closely adherent to inferior pole of spleen
	Associated splenic injury common and usually obvious with hematoma or active bleeding
	If the hilar area of the spleen is involved, then carefully look for an injury to the pancreatic tail
	Diaphragm injuries frequently missed – look and palpate with spleen retracted inferomedially
Descending colon	Relatively easy to mobilize – sharply incise white line and the rest can be done bluntly
	Look for an associated zone 2 retroperitoneal hematoma = kidney or renovascular injury
	Assess for injury to proximal left ureter; hematomas can displace ureter as stated above
Sigmoid colon	Transition from abdominal cavity to the true pelvis – multiple critical structures in a small space
	Always identify ureter and assess for injury; drain all identified or suspected injuries
	Zone 3 hematoma = (1) pelvic fracture if blunt trauma or (2) iliac vessel injury if penetrating
	If you have any suspicion for pelvic vascular injury, get proximal control at distal aorta/cava first
Rectum	Can be injured by blunt shear forces or penetrating missiles, but also bone fragments from pelvic fractures – have a low threshold for proctoscopy with major pelvic fractures
	Intraperitoneal rectum should be treated like sigmoid colon injury
	Associated injuries to all pelvic structures should be considered, including distal ureters, iliac arteries and veins, bladder, uterus/vagina, prostate, spermatic cord
	Intravenous methylene blue can be helpful if injury to ureter is unclear
	Any gross hematuria is a bladder injury; placing a sterile Foley catheter can be helpful for inflating the bladder to identify an injury or after a bladder repair to test for leaks
	Of the "4 Ds" for rectal injuries, diversion is the most important in the majority of cases

SMA superior mesenteric artery, *SMV* superior mesenteric vein, *D4* fourth portion of duodenum important considerations according to the exact area of injury from the cecum to the rectum. Each of these individual colon and rectal injury types and locations has an associated "textbook" answer for what operation should be performed, but these do not take into account the wide variations in disease presentation, presence of multiple bowel injuries, presence of associated injuries, and the patient physiology at the time of operation. There are multiple standard and nonstandard surgical options that can be used alone or in combination, and it is critical to tailor your approach primarily to the patient and not only to the disease. We recommend a surgical approach based on the following general categorizations of the patient and the injuries present:

1. Low Risk: Surgical intervention on a stable patient, adequately resuscitated and physiology either normal or steadily improving, minimal to moderate contamination, no major associated injuries, and medically fit for surgery with no high-risk factors or major systemic disease
2. Moderate Risk: Immediate surgical intervention required due to patient instability, bleeding, or peritonitis. Moderate to large contamination, associated injuries but not immediately life threatening, hemorrhage controlled, non-coagulopathic, responding appropriately to resuscitation, and base deficit elevated (>5) but decreasing with resuscitation. Presence of comorbid disease, but medically controlled
3. High Risk: Emergent surgical intervention required and has >1 risk factor including ongoing large volume hemorrhage, receiving massive transfusion, coagulopathic (INR>1.5), metabolic acidosis (base deficit>5), large contamination, delayed diagnosis with fecal peritonitis, severe bowel edema, massive dilation, associated major vascular injury, or pancreatic injury. Presence of severe medical comorbid disease, high-dose steroid or other immunosuppressant therapy, elderly, active congestive heart failure, debilitated, malnutrition, and hostile abdomen

For low-risk patients, a standard primary repair or segmental resection should be performed, and continuity restored without the need for a colostomy or ileostomy. For moderate-risk patients, the majority can also safely undergo primary repair or resection with anastomosis and will not benefit from fecal diversion. In addition, placement of an ostomy will also subject them to the risks of a second surgery for ostomy takedown or the well-described possibility that they will never have their ostomy reversed [34]. A recent randomized trial in perforated diverticulitis demonstrated that only 58 % of end colostomies were eventually reversed [35]. For patients in the high-risk group, the decision for ostomy versus anastomosis can usually be deferred in favor of a damage control approach (see following section "Damage control laparotomy"). However, whether the decision is made initially or at a subsequent laparotomy, this is the patient population where a diverting ostomy should still be strongly considered. Although there is no level 1 evidence to support these decisions, a temporary diverting ostomy to allow both healing of the colon repair and recovery of the patient can be lifesaving. In addition, with more distal pelvic anastomoses (colorectal, ileorectal), the margin of error and tolerance to a leak is significantly decreased and could result in the need for a permanent ostomy. There are multiple intraoperative decisions and considerations that need to be made quickly and decisively, and that can have significant impact on both short- and long-term outcomes. Table 34.4 provides a partial list of these key decisions with associated factors and technical advice that should be considered.

If fecal diversion is felt to be indicated, then two additional (and in our opinion underutilized) options are available to the surgeon as a "compromise" solution between no diversion and standard ostomy placement. The first is to proceed with placement of a diverting ostomy with a plan for early reversal within 1–2 weeks of the initial surgery. This method allows for initial healing of the colon repair or anastomosis, and then a contrast study should be performed to demonstrate adequate healing without leak or stricture. This also allows time for the natural sorting-out process whereby patients will either progress appropriately following their trauma or develop additional complications or physiologic decline and thus eliminate them from consideration of an early ostomy reversal. A prospective randomized trial of this approach in patients with colon injuries demonstrated that early colostomy closure was safe and resulted in shorter operative times and less blood loss than delayed closure [36]. The second compromise option is to perform the definitive repair or anastomosis and then create a separate more proximal protective diverting colostomy or ileostomy. This concept has long been recognized in colorectal surgery for protection of low pelvic anastomoses or ileal pouch procedures and is also applicable to protecting the high-risk anastomosis in the trauma setting. The choice of the type and location of the ostomy should be mainly based on (1) completeness of fecal diversion, (2) ease of placement, and (3) ease of reversal. Other factors that should be considered include the body habitus and location of abdominal wall wounds and incisions that could alter the viable options available for siting the ostomy. Multiple studies have demonstrated that loop ostomies are clearly superior to end stomas in ease of placement and reversal and also provide adequate fecal diversion [36–38]. A recent prospective randomized trial in patients with feculent or purulent perforated diverticulitis demonstrated the superiority of this approach (primary colorectal anastomosis with protective loop ileostomy) versus a standard Hartmann's procedure [35]. The protective loop ileostomy approach was proven safe and was associated with significantly reduced major complications, hospital stay, and costs. In addition, the choice of ileostomy versus colostomy appears to be equivalent in

Table 34.4 Key intraoperative management issues and decisions in colorectal trauma

Key decision	Factors to consider	Technical issues/pearls
Primary repair or resection?	Size of injury Shape of injury (linear, round/stellate) Single or multiple Tissue quality Mesentery status (rents, hematomas, devascularized segment)	Debride injured or burned tissue Connect close injuries rather than leaving "bridges" Evacuate large mesenteric hematomas Close mesenteric tears Resect segment with "bucket-handle" mesenteric defect
Damage control?	Patient stability Transfusion requirement Acid/base getting better or worse? Multiple injuries? Another reason for a "second-look" (i.e., borderline bowel viability)	Make decision early in case Proceed if patient improving, terminate if getting worse Vacuum-assisted temporary closure works best Usually no need for other drains
Anastomosis or ostomy?	Patient baseline status (age, comorbidities, meds) Physiologic status Quality of the tissues Other injuries and proximity to anastomosis Body habitus, ability to properly site an ostomy	Consider difficulty and risk of ostomy takedown Be wary of anastomosis with an associated pancreatic injury! Obesity increases difficulty and complications with ostomy
Anastomosis: hand-sewn or stapled?	Operative time Other injuries to address Personal experience and comfort Tissue quality, edema Anatomic area and bowel alignment Available equipment	No difference in leak or complication rates in most series Hand-sewn potentially more secure with suboptimal tissue quality, bowel wall edema Laparoscopic staplers great for pelvis, hard-to-reach areas or sharp angles
Ostomy: loop, end, other?	High-risk anastomosis that needs protection? Need access to distal bowel segment? Body habitus Mesentery – shortened, edematous	Loop may reach skin easier with obesity or shortened mesentery May not get complete fecal diversion with a loop Remember the "end-loop" option (see text) Use an ostomy bar if any tension or obese patient Wrap ostomy in seprafilm for easier takedown
Leave a drain?	No indication for routine drainage of bowel anastomoses Widely drain any other adjacent injuries (pancreas, bladder, etc.) Other reasons: associated abscess cavity, control ascites in cirrhotic patient	Avoid direct contact of drain with anastomosis larger sump drains usually not beneficial Make exit site remote from incision and any ostomy
Place a feeding tube?	Degree of bowel injuries and surgery Estimated need for prolonged NPO status Estimated inability to take oral nutrition Need for feeding access as well as gastric decompression? Pancreatic or duodenal injury?	Generally avoid making additional holes in bowel in the trauma setting Stamm gastrostomy relatively safe and secure Higher complications with jejunostomy tubes with little benefit Consider intraoperative placement of nasojejunal tube

terms of the adequacy of diversion [38]. As the ileum is typically more mobile and of smaller caliber than the colon, a loop ileostomy is the technically easier option and provides more options for external siting. However, the surgeon must be cognizant that the risk of fluid and electrolyte problems due to high stoma output will be higher with ileostomy versus colostomy, and this can be particularly difficult to manage in elderly or debilitated patients. Our recommendation is that if a temporary protective ostomy is indicated, then a loop ileostomy (or end-loop ileostomy as shown in Fig. 34.5) is the best option and can easily be reversed without the need for laparotomy in most patients. An excellent alternative option, particularly in the patient who may need longer-term or even permanent diversion, is a loop transverse or sigmoid colostomy. Prior to ostomy reversal, all patients should undergo contrast imaging to document anastomotic healing and should have documentation of adequate anal sphincter function for fecal continence.

Level 1 and Prospective Evidence in Colorectal Trauma

There are few prospective randomized trials to guide any aspect of therapy in trauma, and this is particularly true in colorectal trauma. In addition, the level 1 studies that are available are severely limited by the variety of injuries included and the small sample sizes, making it difficult both to generalize these concepts and to apply them to any specific patient or injury. However, these classic studies have provided important evidence and driven widespread practice changes that once would have been considered heretical. Stone et al. [39] performed the first reported trial of 268 patients randomized to exteriorization or colostomy versus primary repair for small colon injuries. They demonstrated a tenfold reduced incidence of complications with primary repair and significantly increased hospital stay and costs associated with colostomy. In 1991 and 1995

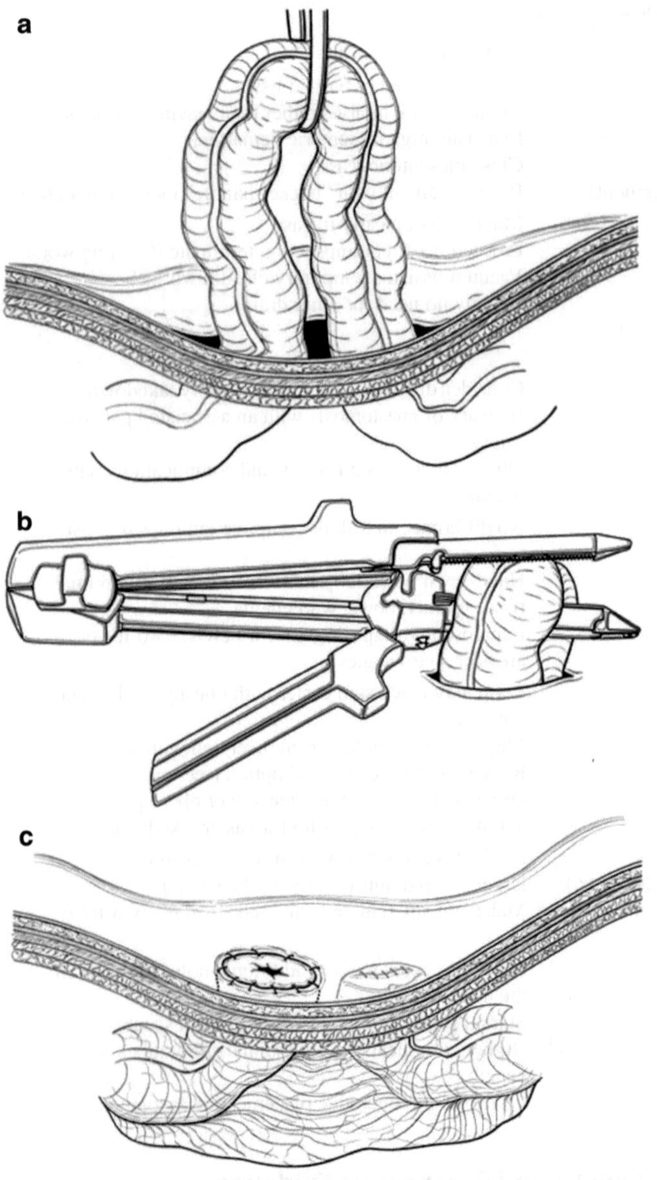

Fig. 34.5 Technique for end-loop ostomy (colon or ileum). (**a**) loop of bowel is delivered, (**b**) bowel is divided at the site of the planned ostomy, (**c**) proximal end is matured and the distal stapled end is secured in the subcutaneous position for easy future access and restoration of continuity (Reprinted with permission Martin and Beekley [26] © in 2011 Springer)

two randomized trials were reported that compared primary repair or anastomosis to proximal diversion (total 127 patients) [40, 41]. Both studies confirmed that primary repair or anastomosis was safe and effective and in fact was associated with lower complications than proximal diversion. In 2002 Kamwendo et al. [42] randomized patients to primary repair/anastomosis or colostomy and importantly included patients with delayed presentation, contamination, associated injuries, and shock. In addition to again confirming that primary repair was a safe option, they found that it remained superior to colostomy even among higher-risk patients with contamination.

No additional prospective randomized trials of the surgical management of colorectal injuries have been reported, but multiple prospective observational trials have provided valuable experiential evidence and recommendations [1, 43–48]. The majority of these have reported similar findings and conclusions that support the use of primary repair or anastomosis without diversion for all types of colonic injury. The largest and most widely cited of these is the multicenter observational study by the American Association for the Surgery of Trauma [1]. This trial reported on 297 patients that required colon resection for trauma, with 2/3 undergoing primary anastomosis and 1/3 managed with fecal diversion. Not surprisingly, this study found no difference between anastomosis and fecal diversion groups in morbidity or mortality. This study did examine many risk factors that are commonly proposed as indications for performing fecal diversion, such as hypotension, transfusion requirement, and severe contamination. Of note, although these were all associated with increased morbidity, this effect was independent of whether an ostomy or an anastomosis was performed, lending further support to performing primary repair or anastomosis in most scenarios. However, the low incidence of severe (destructive, high velocity, etc.) colon injuries in these trials limits any conclusions that can be drawn about this subgroup and the potential benefit of fecal diversion in select high-risk cases [44].

Rectal Trauma

Key Concept: Almost no patient actually requires all of the classic "4 Ds" of rectal injury (diversion, direct repair, drainage, distal washout). Diversion is often enough, with the other 3 Ds used selectively based on the rectal wound and associated injuries to soft tissue, bone, and pelvic structures.

Key Concept: Similar to the evolution of colon trauma, the utility of routine colostomy for rectal injuries is being challenged. This approach is safe for the right injury in the right patient, and with strict observation for complications or failure.

Rectal injury from trauma remains one of the most challenging entities that a surgeon will face, and proper management will dictate not only short-term morbidity and mortality but can affect longer-term issues such as fecal incontinence and pelvic floor dysfunction that can be severely disabling. Operating on the perineum or deep in the pelvis is uncommon for most general or trauma surgeons, and thus it is important to have a solid grasp of the fundamentals of management for rectal injuries. Arguably the best operative maneuver that you can do when faced with a challenging rectal injury is to call for help or advice from an experienced colleague or a colorectal specialist if available.

Anatomy Is Destiny

There is an oft-quoted aphorism that medical illustrators are eternal optimists, and this is particularly true for the rectum and other pelvic structures. Similar to the neck, the pelvis contains a large number of critical structures of the vascular, nervous, and aerodigestive tract in a relatively small and confined space. In addition, the pelvis contains important genitourinary system structures in close proximity to the rectum. Isolated injury of the rectum is relatively uncommon, and thus the surgeon is frequently faced with managing the rectal injury in the setting of concomitant vascular, genitourinary, or bony injuries. Operating in the deep pelvis is difficult in the average patient but can be extremely challenging in the setting of active bleeding or fecal spillage, large pelvic hematoma, obesity, and a narrow pelvic inlet (usually males). In addition to considerations of control and repair of the actual injuries, the anatomic relationships, perfusion, and innervation of the key pelvic structures are critical in determining such important outcomes as fecal continence, urinary continence, and sexual function. For these reasons and with the known natural history of rectal injuries, it is often best to minimize or entirely avoid violating anatomic planes and exploring the pelvis and instead ensure adequate control of spillage (proximal fecal diversion) and wide drainage (if needed).

Diagnosis

Most rectal injury is due to penetrating trauma, but approximately 10 % are due to blunt mechanism. In addition, there is a small, measurable injury rate due to transanal trauma (self-induced, sexual assault, or iatrogenic from medical devices such as enemas, rectal probes, or fecal drains) that will be discussed in a separate section of this chapter. Blunt mechanism injury to the liver bladder will almost always be seen in association with a major pelvic fracture or significant soft tissue damage to the perineum. Straddle and impalements-type injuries can also be seen. For penetrating trauma, any missile that crosses or enters the pelvis should be assumed to have hit the rectum until proved otherwise. This is one injury complex where a delay in diagnosis can be rapidly fatal due to pelvic sepsis and can result in permanent incontinence and need for a colostomy.

For the vast majority of blunt trauma patients with no obvious perineal or pelvic complaints and no other injuries in the pelvis, no additional workup beyond the physical exam is required. A digital rectal exam (DRE) looking for gross blood or a palpable injury should be performed. For patients with a known or suspected pelvic or perineal injury, a formal evaluation of the rectum and anus to rule out involvement should be performed. A patient that presents with a suspicious pattern of wounding (penetrating gluteal, trans-pelvic wound, multiple perineal fragments) or hematochezia should undergo rigid proctoscopy to identify an injury. A patient with blood in the rectum on proctoscopic exam without an identifiable proximal source has a rectal injury until proven otherwise and should be treated as such. In most of these instances with pelvic trauma, the patient will undergo a CT scan of the abdomen/pelvis, and this can provide additional valuable information about the presence and type of rectal injury. Particularly for penetrating trauma, a CT scan of the pelvis assists not only in looking for soft tissue injury or air around the rectum but also in trajectory of a penetrating wound. For those patients undergoing preoperative CT scans, look for perirectal edema or stranding, pelvic fragments, and air or fluid in the perirectal space, all of which may indicate rectal injury. Obtaining fine cuts between the entrance and exit wounds, or in the area of concern, can be very helpful for recreating the missile tract and deciding which structures are involved or nearby and could be injured. If the DRE is normal and the CT shows a trajectory away from the rectum, then no further evaluation is required. These initial CT scans are typically ordered with IV, but not oral or rectal contrast. If trajectory identified on the CT scan suggests possible injury, a more complete examination is warranted. Major blunt trauma patients will have at least an initial pelvic x-ray or more commonly (for major traumas) a CT scan performed. Any patient with a major pelvic fracture or an associated urological injury should also receive a more thorough exam to evaluate for a rectal injury.

For any of these patients at high risk (penetrating trauma with suspicious trajectory, major pelvic fractures, bladder injury, or history of transanal penetration), we typically perform a more thorough exam (digital rectal exam and rigid proctoscopy) in the operating room with proper sedation or general anesthesia to maximize patient comfort and adequacy of the exam. Of course, if intraperitoneal injury is suspected (peritoneal signs or indicated by CT scan) or diagnosed, then an exploratory laparoscopy or laparotomy is performed. The most critical distinction to make is whether the injury is in the intraperitoneal portion of the rectum or the extraperitoneal portion. This will alter the rest of your workup, management, surgical approach, and outcomes.

Management Options: Intraperitoneal Rectum

Once an intraperitoneal rectal injury has been identified by CT scan or abdominal exploration, the mainstay of therapy is primary repair or resection with anastomosis similar to colon injuries. Keeping in mind that most injuries are a result of penetrating trauma and in civilian practice will typically consist of stab wounds or low-velocity gunshot wounds, most intraperitoneal rectal injuries will be small and amenable to primary repair. Diverting loop colostomy is not required after primary repair of an intraperitoneal rectal injury in most cases. A larger, more destructive injury to the intraperitoneal rectum may require a segmental resection of the injured portion of rectum if it cannot be repaired primarily. Following segmental resection of the injured rectum a decision for anastomosis versus ostomy must be made. We recommend using the same risk scaling approach described above for colon injuries. Patients in the high-risk group and select patients with moderate risk should have an ostomy performed without anastomosis or an anastomosis with a protective proximal ostomy. Patients in the low-risk group and select moderate-risk patients can safely undergo anastomosis. An additional factor that should be considered is how low onto the rectum the resection had to be carried. If the injury required resection down to the mid or lower third of the rectum, then we would recommend an anastomosis with a protective loop ileostomy that can be reversed once the patient is fully recovered.

Management Options: Extraperitoneal Rectum

There has already been a "revolution" in the management of colon injuries marked by large-scale abandonment of routine fecal diversion for these injuries. However, for rectal injuries fecal diversion remains the mainstay of treatment, although there are small series now published that advocate for primary repair and eliminating the routine ostomy. The classic teaching for managing extraperitoneal rectal injuries involves the "4 Ds": diversion, direct repair, distal washout, and drain placement. These are aimed at treating the injury, the local contamination, and the anticipated development of perirectal abscess or repair leak. In our experience there are very few patients who require all 4 (or even 3) of these interventions, and the mainstay of care for most rectal injuries should be primary repair (if accessible) and proximal diversion.

Primary repair of an extraperitoneal rectal injury can be challenging due to the location and the presence of bleeding, hematoma, and other anatomic structures that may limit your ability to safely dissect down to the level of injury. It is also wise to avoid extensive mobilizations of the rectum unless absolutely necessary. A very distal injury that is inaccessible from the abdominal approach may be easily closed from inside the rectum with anoscopy or proctoscopy to assist with exposure. However, if the injury is not readily accessible from either end or if all you can visualize is a significant hematoma on proctoscopy, then do not aggressively attempt to violate those planes and dig out the site of injury. Simply pull up a diverting loop sigmoid colostomy or loop ileostomy for temporary fecal diversion and then observe the patient. The majority will heal spontaneously and can have bowel continuity restored within 1–3 months. If the patient does not have any other indication for a laparotomy, then the ileostomy or colostomy can easily be performed with laparoscopic techniques [49, 50]. There is no need to expose and resect ALL extraperitoneal injuries. They will typically heal after a period of diversion, and those that do not can be approached in the elective situation. Whatever you do, do not spend any amount of additional time trying to identify and repair an extraperitoneal rectal injury that will do just as well with diversion alone. This will only lead to prolonged operative times, increased blood loss, and onset of the lethal triad of acidosis, hypothermia, and coagulopathy, if it is not already present [26].

Another proposed option is to resect the damaged segment, perform a primary anastomosis, and then create a proximal diverting loop ileostomy [26]. This does leave an intervening column of stool in the segment distal to the ileostomy but usually this is of no consequence. If there is a concern or a very large stool burden, then an on-table lavage of the distal segment can be performed as described above. Although there is some debate about whether a loop ileostomy provides adequate diversion or protection of a distal anastomosis, we think that this is an excellent option for a patient with a medium risk for anastomotic complications. This concern can easily be addressed by modification of the standard loop ileostomy to create a stapled end-loop ileostomy (or colostomy) with the distal stapled end buried in the subcutaneous space for easy future identification and reversal [51, 52]. Subsequent reversal of the loop ileostomy can usually be done without the need for a laparotomy or even an additional incision [38, 50]. This is a significantly easier and lower-risk procedure (for both the patient and surgeon) compared with a repeat laparotomy with colostomy takedown and colorectal anastomosis [36].

The other 2 Ds – distal washout and drain placement – should be used infrequently. Distal washout can be performed if there is a large stool burden in the rectal canal or if there is a concern for fecal impaction that could affect bowel motility. A loop of sigmoid colon is chosen for colostomy formation and is delivered onto the anterior abdominal wall through a properly sited stoma aperture. Flow into the efferent limb of the stoma is prevented by stapling across the distal portion with a transverse firing of a TA-60 stapler. Prior to the firing of this stapler, a large-bore catheter is placed into the afferent limb of the stoma and saline is flushed through while an assistant keeps the anal sphincter open to prevent any resistance to flow (often with the use of a rigid proctoscope). This cleans out the distal rectum and makes presacral drainage unnecessary. Alternatively, ventilator tubing borrowed from anesthesia can be placed into the open bowel and secured with an umbilical tape to perform an on-table lavage (Fig. 34.2). The TA-60 stapler is then fired and the colostomy is matured.

Presacral drainage has been debated for years and its use has declined over the past decade. We feel that it is not necessary in the majority of cases and is commonly placed incorrectly when it is used. Perhaps the only case is for a large sacral injury with a lot of spillage, and then for only a short time initially to evacuate the fluid [26]. A prospective controlled trial in 1998 randomized patients with extraperitoneal rectal injury to presacral drain placement versus no drain, and they found no benefit of presacral drains in reducing any infectious complication [53]. The problem with presacral drainage is that you have to enter the presacral space from a perineal approach and you have to dissect into the area of injury. The drain must be placed in this area to be effective. Because of the difficulty with this approach, the drain is often malpositioned and ineffective.

Combined Anorectal Injuries

Most patients with major sphincter injuries or complex perineal wounds should be diverted, particularly if the wounds are associated with a pelvic fracture (open fracture). With anal sphincter injury, it may be tempting to delay their sphincter repair "for another time." However, early repair leads to the best chance for long-term outcome, and some reapproximation should be attempted as soon as the patient is stable (i.e., within several days of presentation). Life-threatening issues obviously take precedence, but do not forget about addressing the sphincter injury early as it could lead to major long-term morbidity and patient dissatisfaction if it is neglected or forgotten.

The Massive Perineal Wound

These will be some of the most difficult patients you will ever manage and can bleed to death from these wounds in a matter of minutes. We have seen these types of wounds not only in combat settings but also in industrial accidents and in motorcycle crashes with inadequate protective clothing. Although the soft tissue injury and destruction of the back and perineum is visually impressive (Fig. 34.6), it is important to remember that hemorrhage needs to be addressed first. These patients belong in the operating room as soon as possible and should almost never be delayed to obtain more imaging. The wound should be packed immediately on arrival and then wrapped with a binder or an elastic bandage to hold compression until you can get to the operating room. The abdominal exam, FAST exam, and pelvis x-ray should provide all the information you need to proceed to the OR for wound management with or without laparotomy. Most of these are going to require a laparotomy (or laparoscopy) for colonic diversion anyway, so the abdominal CT is redundant and unnecessary. If CT is absolutely necessary, you must be able to watch for hemorrhage from the perineum while the imaging is being done. The initial operation should focus on the damage control priorities of stopping hemorrhage and washing/debriding contamination and dead tissue. Identify key anorectal structures and tag them with visible sutures for future identification. A diverting colostomy should be performed with the expectation that it will likely be permanent if the anorectal complex has been destroyed. In select cases where it is clear that continuity and function will not be restored, a completion proctectomy may be indicated to remove this as a persistent source of wound infection and sepsis.

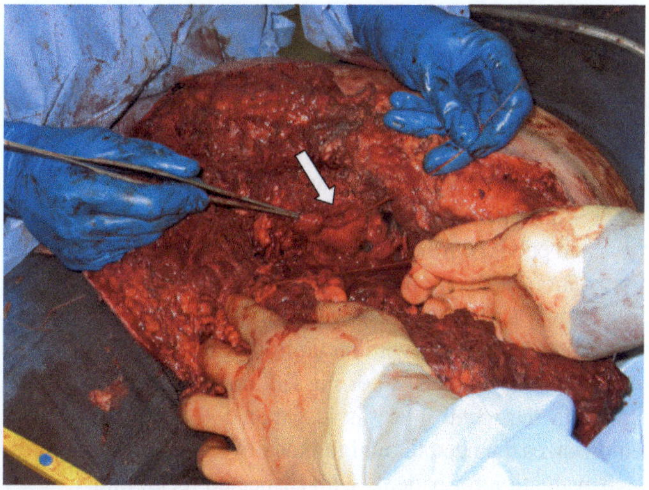

Fig. 34.6 Massive perineal blast wound with destruction of the sphincter complex and exposed distal rectum (*arrow*). These patients should be brought immediately to the operating room to prevent rapid exsanguination

Complications

The overall complication rate after rectal injury is 50 %. The most common complications directly attributable to a rectal injury are infectious – wound infection, abdominal or pelvic abscess, anastomotic leak, or even a devastating necrotizing infection. Unless the patient has a grossly contaminated pelvic fracture, prophylactic antibiotics are continued only for 24 h perioperatively. However, any signs of postoperative infection necessitate broad-spectrum antibiotics until the source can be localized and controlled. Assuming that there has been a repair/resection of the injury, many intraperitoneal or even extraperitoneal infections can be controlled with drainage (usually percutaneous using image guidance or even transrectal if low enough). However, early consideration of diversion must be given to failed primary repairs. As in any large intestinal operation, clinical signs and symptoms should guide early management. If there are ongoing signs of infection (fevers, increased white cell count, decreased urine output, etc.) not attributable to other injuries, then early reoperation is key. Diagnostic studies in the early preoperative period are often misleading or even falsely reassuring.

Outcomes

Overall mortality for all patients with rectal injuries can approach 25 %. Poor outcomes after rectal injury are usually related to associated injuries. As rectal injuries are most commonly a result of penetrating trauma, usually gunshot wounds, there is a high rate of associated vascular injuries of the abdomen and pelvis. Furthermore, after blunt trauma there is a high association of severe pelvic fracture. The presence of associated pelvic fracture or vascular injury will obviously worsen outcomes for patients with rectal injury. Unless the diagnosis of rectal injury is delayed or missed, mortality directly attributable to the rectal injury is less than 5 %. This once again emphasizes the need for a high index of suspicion and aggressive evaluation for patients with suspected rectal injury.

Damage Control Laparotomy

Key Concept: Damage control techniques are effective when applied EARLY and APPROPRIATELY – if you wait for severe acidosis, hypothermia, and coagulopathy, then you have missed your chance.

Key Concept: Damage control surgery does not mean sloppy or hurried surgery – frequently your best shot to do it right is at the first operation, and this will set the stage for a good or bad outcome.

A detailed description of the evolution, techniques, and details of damage control surgery is beyond the scope of this chapter. The key concept of DCL is to perform an abbreviated laparotomy that addresses only active bleeding and control of GI contamination and ruling out any other immediately life-threatening abdominal injuries. Detailed exploration, identification of all injuries, and reconstructions are deferred to a later time (usually 24–48 h later) in order to bring the patient to the ICU for resuscitation and optimization prior to a more prolonged surgery. Fortunately, DCL can be readily applied to any patient and does not require any complicated equipment, techniques, or supplies. The only thing that is required for success is good surgical judgment and understanding of when and how to initiate DCL. The classic indications described in the literature for DCL are altered patient physiology marked by acidosis, hypothermia, and coagulopathy. The key to successful DCL is to initiate it before these have developed or to immediately initiate DCL if these factors are already present at the initiation of surgery. This requires factoring in the patient's baseline condition, comorbidities, injury types and severity, and physiologic response to surgery and resuscitation. One of the most advantageous aspects of DCL is that it obviates the need for an immediate decision on primary anastomosis versus ostomy placement, and this decision can then be made at a later time with better information and a more stable patient.

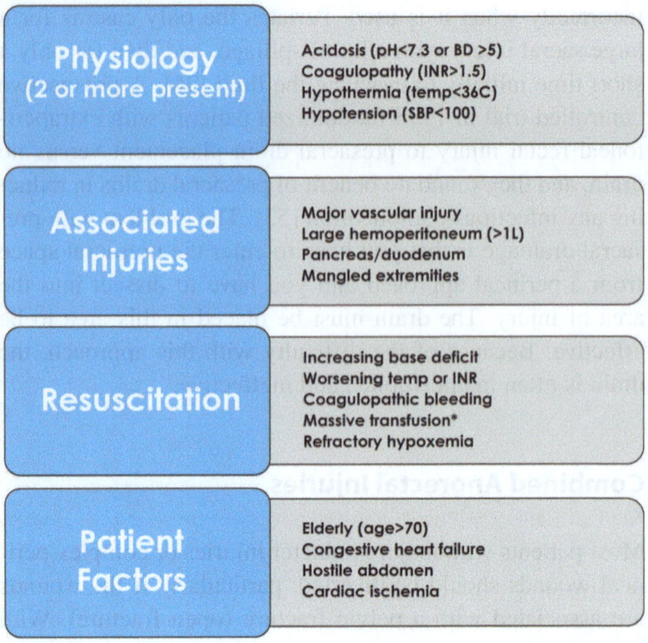

Fig. 34.7 Categorical listing of major factors to consider for damage control surgery

Figure 34.7 shows a list of the key factors that should be factored in to the decision to initiate (or terminate) damage control techniques. Arguably the most important of these is how the patient is responding to surgery and resuscitation. It is helpful to pause after 30–45 min and ask yourself "am I gaining or losing ground?" If the patient is unchanged or getting worse despite resuscitation, then DCL should be initiated. However, if the patient is clearly improving and you are satisfied that you have controlled all hemorrhage or other life-threatening issues, then continuing on and potentially completing the procedure as a single state laparotomy is warranted. This is best done by open and clear communication with the anesthesia provider, and we recommend making it a point to let them know when key points of the procedure are reached (i.e., bleeding is controlled, major injuries identified, starting the reconstruction or closure). Although many markers or "end points" of resuscitation have been proposed, we find that the most helpful and easily obtained global marker of the progress of the resuscitation is the arterial base deficit (BD). If an arterial line is not available, then a central venous base deficit is adequate. The absolute level will provide a measure of the severity of metabolic acidosis, but even more important will be to follow the trend of the BD with resuscitation.

The important technical aspects of the damage control procedure are stopping hemorrhage and controlling GI spillage. Although four-quadrant packing is commonly advocated, we find that haphazard throwing of sponges into the abdominal cavity is not effective and only delays identification and control of bleeding. If large volume hemoperitoneum is encountered on opening the abdomen, the first maneuver is to evacuate the blood and clot by scooping it out, suctioning, and placing sponges into and then immediately out of the abdomen to remove pools of blood. The general area of the ongoing bleeding is then usually obvious, and focused packing and assessment can then be performed of this quadrant. If it is not clear and/or the patient is in extremis, then pack all four quadrants and take a pause to allow for resuscitation before removing the packs.

The primary issue with colon injuries will obviously be GI contamination, but injuries to the mesentery can also result in significant bleeding. Active mesenteric bleeding can first be controlled with manual compression, and then 2-0 silk sutures or clamps can be applied. If the segment of bowel and mesentery is clearly going to require resection, then it may be faster to just control the bleeding by firing a stapler with a vascular load across it to both stop the hemorrhage and facilitate the segmental resection. Energy devices (such as harmonic scalpel or Enseal) are also very helpful to expedite division of longer areas of mesentery, particularly when working with a less experienced OR tech or resident. Control of GI contamination is the next priority, and we find that there is often time wasted in trying to control spillage from each injury as they are encountered by placing Babcock clamps or sutures for temporary closure. If there has already been gross spillage from the injuries, then there is little advantage to achieving temporary control unless there is active large volume spillage ongoing. We find that placing multiple clamps often gets in the way of full exploration and can result in further tearing of the bowel. Rapid temporary control (if needed) can be obtained by isolating the injured segment with occluding umbilical tapes or 0-silk ties (Fig. 34.8), and then more definitive repair or resection can

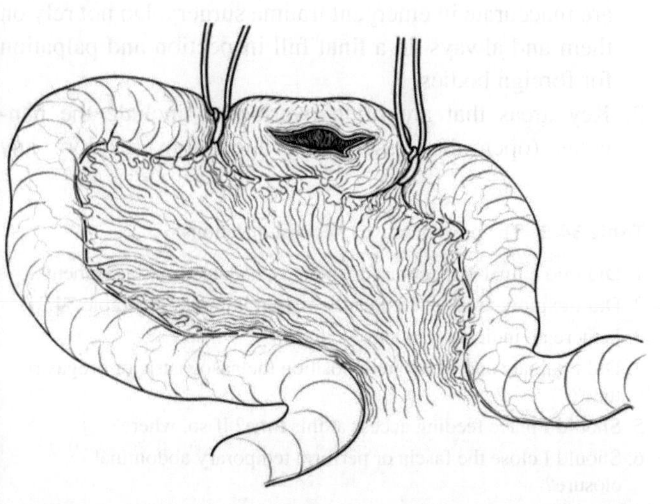

Fig. 34.8 Rapid control of bowel spillage during damage control surgery is obtained with umbilical tapes proximal and distal to injury (Reprinted with permission Martin and Beekley [26] © in 2011 Springer)

be performed immediately or at the second-look laparotomy. We favor a quick but thorough complete inspection of the small bowel and colon to identify and quantify all injuries present and then proceeding with either temporary or definitive closure and/or resection.

Some other key technical points or pearls that we recommend in the emergent or damage control setting for colon injuries:

1. Staplers can be used for primary repair of lacerations or perforations as well as segmental resections. Grasp the edges of the defect at the corners of the long axis of the wound with Allis clamps, lift and separate the clamps to elevate the injury and oppose the edges longitudinally, and fire a linear or TA stapler immediately under the clamps.
2. Laparoscopic linear staplers allow for greater reach and articulation than standard staplers, particularly for obese patients or working in the pelvis. Adding a buttressing material (i.e., Seamguard) is helpful for decreasing staple-line bleeding.
3. Energy devices are underused in the trauma setting and can provide more rapid and secure mesenteric and omental division. They are particularly useful for mesenteric division and mobilization along the distal sigmoid and proximal rectum.
4. Mesenteric pedicles should be clamped and ligated (or stapled) in large en-masse segments rather than the time-consuming elective approach of clamping each individual vessel.
5. Multiple injuries in relative proximity are often managed better by segmental resection than multiple primary repairs. Similarly, an anatomic colectomy (i.e., right hemicolectomy) with one anastomosis should be performed rather than multiple segmental resections and anastomoses.
6. Fascial closure should be performed at the earliest time possible in order to minimize the exposure of the patient to the risks associated with an open abdomen. All efforts should be focused on avoiding the highly morbid complication of an enteroatmospheric fistula (see Chap. 8).

Once your primary goals of the damage control laparotomy have been achieved, then a temporary abdominal closure (TAC) with vacuum assistance should be performed. The widespread availability of the Wound Vac System (Kinetic Concepts Inc., San Antonio, TX) has greatly facilitated and simplified TAC. The prepackaged TAC kit includes a thin plastic sheet with perforations that is placed over the exposed viscera followed by a sponge secured to the skin edges and then covered with an impermeable clear dressing, followed by application of suction. The same effect can be achieved with simple and commonly available supplies in the OR to create a "modified vac-pack": we use a sterile x-ray cassette cover with multiple perforations to cover the viscera, followed by Kerlix gauze or lap sponges to fill the wound and a chest tube or NG tube overlying the gauze. The dressing is covered with a sheet of Ioban and then suction is applied to the chest tube or NG tube. The advantages of TAC include speed and ease of application, protection of underlying viscera, control of wound fluid, avoidance of abdominal compartment syndrome, maintaining medial forces on the abdominal wall, and facilitation of repeat abdominal exploration(s). Although the terms DCL and TAC are frequently used interchangeably, it is important to note that TAC is a technique that facilitates damage control surgery but can also be applied outside of a damage control setting. TAC can also be useful in situations where a second-look laparotomy is desirable, such as borderline ischemic bowel and large contamination, or additional prolonged and complex reconstructions are required. TAC can also be used as a helpful temporizing measure in situations where the operating surgeon is faced with severe or complex injuries and lacks the expertise, equipment, or support to safely complete the definitive reconstructive. Leaving the abdomen open can provide the surgeon with time to consider all options, discuss with colleagues or seek out an expert opinion, or transfer the patient to a higher level of care.

The optimal timing for when to return the patient to the OR and perform subsequent explorations and definitive fascial closure remains an area of debate. Although the commonly voiced opinion is to let physiology dictate the timing of return, in practice most patients undergo scheduled return 24–48 h later unless they have not responded appropriately to resuscitation. Select patients may be returned earlier, and we have performed reexploration and definitive repairs + closure at 6–8 h later. At the second-look laparotomy, the decision for primary repair or anastomosis versus diverting ostomy is the same as previously described. A recent large, multicenter study from the Western Trauma Association demonstrated an overall leak rate of 7 % among patients with enteric injuries managed with an open abdomen [54]. Most of the patients underwent either immediate primary repair of small injuries or resection with delayed anastomosis for larger injuries. Although leak rates were significantly higher for left colon injuries, the authors recommend consideration of repair or anastomosis in all patients. This study also highlights the principle of aggressive attempts at fascial closure as early as possible, as the leak rate increased significantly (400 %) when the fascia was not closed by day 5. Similar findings have been reported from modern battlefield injuries and highlight that anastomoses can be selectively performed after DCL but that factors such as injury location and associated injuries must be factored in to the decision [17, 19].

Finally, although DCL and TAC are both useful techniques and likely save lives, there are associated risks and complications that must be considered in the risk-benefit analysis regarding their use. Leaving the abdomen open can increase fluid shifts and volume requirements, expose the bowel to injury and the risk of enteroatmospheric fistulae, require prolonging ventilator support, and necessitates multiple surgeries and general anesthetics. Leaving stapled-off ends of bowel for variable periods of time can result in further bowel distension and edema or necessitate resection of additional length to achieve the final anastomosis or ostomy. There is now some accumulating evidence that TAC is not a "free shot" and that this technique may result in increased morbidity when used too liberally or on lower-risk patients [55, 56].

The Postoperative Checklist

The preoperative "time-out" has become a widely utilized tool to improve operating room communication and optimize patient safety. Emergent surgery on a patient with major traumatic injuries is a perfect storm of factors that can lead to errors, oversights, and missed opportunities. We believe that an equally (or more) important concept for emergent abdominal surgery is the "postoperative time-out." At the conclusion of any major trauma laparotomy, particularly after repair or resection of injuries to the colon, we find it is helpful to run through a brief checklist of important but frequently overlooked items. This should be done before abdominal closure and transport out of the operating room and also gives the operating surgeon a chance to pause, take a deep breath, and survey the global situation after having been exclusively focused on individual abdominal injuries.

Table 34.5 lists the items that should at least be considered at this time. *Key points* for each of these items include:

1. Sponge and instrument counts are frequently not done or are inaccurate in emergent trauma surgery. Do not rely on them and always do a final full inspection and palpation for foreign bodies.
2. Key areas that are often overlooked include the pancreas (open the lesser sac), duodenum (explore any

Table 34.5 The postoperative checklist questions

1. Did I do a final inspection for sponges, needles, and instruments?
2. Did I explore areas of frequently missed injuries (see Table 34.3)?
3. Is there an indication to leave a drain?
4. Did I palpate and adequately position the nasogastric or orogastric tube?
5. Should I place feeding access at this time? If so, where?
6. Should I close the fascia or perform temporary abdominal closure?
7. Should I place retention sutures?
8. Should I close the skin or leave it open?
9. Does the patient have adequate intravenous access for resuscitation and monitoring?

para-duodenal hematoma), ureters, and diaphragm (look and palpate in both upper quadrants).

3. Drains are generally not indicated for bowel injury, but any associated injuries such as pancreas, duodenum, or genitourinary tract should be widely drained. We also find drain placement useful in patients with ascites (i.e., cirrhosis) to help control it during the early post-op period and wound healing phase.
4. Reach up and palpate for the NG/OG tube, and guide it into optimal position in the body of the stomach.
5. Most patients should not require feeding access, but if prolonged inability to take oral feeds is anticipated, then having enteral access can be critical. First choice should usually be to have anesthesia place a nasoduodenal or nasojejunal tube and guide it into position. A Stamm gastrostomy provides both feeding access and the ability to decompress the stomach and can obviate the need for prolonged NG tube placement. We avoid jejunostomy tubes unless there is some specific reason that the above options are not suitable.
6. See the discussion of damage control techniques.
7. Prophylactic external retention sutures are usually not indicated, but consider in patients with multiple risk factors for dehiscence: elderly, malnutrition, steroid use, smoker, large fecal soilage, ascites/cirrhosis, poor quality fascia, and closure under tension. Internal retention sutures (using #1 Vicryl or PDS suture) can provide reinforcement and avoid the skin breakdown problems seen with external sutures or plastic skin bridges.
8. We favor leaving the skin open and performing a delayed primary closure in cases with colorectal injuries and moderate to large fecal contamination, see trial by Velmahos et al. [57].
9. With emergent surgery the anesthesia provider may not have had time to obtain adequate venous access, place an arterial line, etc. This is usually easier to do (and more sterile) in the OR than later in the ICU or recovery room.

Colonoscopic Trauma

Key Concept: Bleeding and perforation are rare complications of colonoscopy that will be seen by most surgeons during their career. A high level of suspicion and use of diagnostic imaging is key to ensuring early diagnosis (<24 h).

Key Concept: Many of these injuries can be safely managed nonoperatively, and the remainder can usually be repaired or resected laparoscopically if recognized early. Damage control techniques may be required in cases with a delay to presentation or diagnosis (>48 h).

Colonoscopy has become a routine procedure for screening, surveillance, diagnosis, and intervention in a number of gastrointestinal diseases. It is most commonly performed to screen or survey for adenomatous polyps or adenocarcinoma and involves a thorough survey of the entire length of the colon and rectum. Although minor mucosal mechanical trauma from the scope is relatively common, more significant injuries including lacerations, full-thickness tears, or perforations are extremely uncommon. Although the overall incidence of significant colonoscopic injuries is low (less than 1 %), it is a high-volume procedure, and most surgeons will be faced with managing these injuries during their career. A reported series of over 230,000 colonoscopies demonstrated an overall incidence of 0.31 % for complications, with 0.03 % for perforations and 0.22 % for bleeding [58]. The incidence of bleeding and perforation are greatly increased (up to 3 %) when any type of endoscopic intervention is performed, typically polypectomy or biopsy [59]. In addition to direct colon trauma from the scope tip or instruments, other mechanisms of injury can include barotrauma from colon insufflation, thermal injury from cautery or coagulation devices, or stretch/tear injuries on the colon wall due to overaggressive advancing pressure or colonoscope looping. Retroflexion of the scope is an additional cause of injury and has been mainly reported in the perforations of the rectum [60]. In addition, significant injury to organs outside of the colon is possible, including major splenic lacerations and hemorrhage due to tension on the lienocolic attachments [61]. As the vast majority of bleeding complications can be managed either endoscopically or with angiography, the remainder of this section will focus on the management of perforation after colonoscopy.

Colonoscopic injury can occur anywhere along the length of the colon and can range from a partial-thickness injury with no symptoms to a large full-thickness laceration with peritonitis and hemodynamic instability. Particular areas of vulnerability include the cecum due to its relatively thin wall, the transverse and sigmoid colon due to their greater mobility and susceptibility to "looping" of the scope, and the sigmoid colon due to the higher incidence of pathology such as polyps or diverticula. The cecum and rectum are also susceptible to perforation from scope retroflexion [60]. The location of the perforation and the risk of peritonitis will also vary depending on whether the perforation is through a free intraperitoneal wall of the colon or into the mesentery or retroperitoneum of a fixed segment (ascending or descending colon, rectum). There is a well-defined entity of "post-polypectomy syndrome" that presents with abdominal pain, fever, and elevated white blood cell count and appears to be due to local peritoneal irritation from thermal burn during hot polypectomy. This typically resolves with observation only and the remainder of this section will focus on true full-thickness colonoscopic injuries and their management.

Reliable risk factors for identifying patients or procedures that present a higher risk of bleeding or perforation are difficult to identify due to the relative infrequency of these events. Several large, population-based analyses have identified older age, female gender, significant patient comorbidity, diverticulosis, presence of obstruction, performance of polypectomy or other interventions, and colonoscopy performed by a low-volume endoscopist as risk factors for bleeding or perforation [62, 63]. However, none of these variables have significant predictive value, and a high index of suspicion should be maintained for all colonoscopies, with immediate evaluation of patients presenting with significant pain or other abnormal complaints after the procedure. Although the overall risk of death within 30 days following colonoscopy is approximately 1 in 14,000, mortality rates as high as 15–20 % have been reported among patients with a perforation following colonoscopy [64–66]. One of the most important factors associated with morbidity and mortality after colonoscopic injury is the time to diagnosis. Immediate recognition and intervention for the perforation is optimal, but most perforations are not recognized during the procedure and rely on the later development of symptoms. Perforations that are diagnosed within 24 h of the procedure are associated with improved morbidity, decreased infectious complications, decreased need for emergent surgery and fecal diversion, and lower mortality [65, 67]. Early diagnosis (<24 h) has been found to be the strongest independent predictor of both morbidity and mortality on multivariate analysis [66].

A proposed algorithm for evaluation and management of these patients is presented in Fig. 34.9. In patients with clear peritonitis on exam or systemic manifestations of sepsis, the

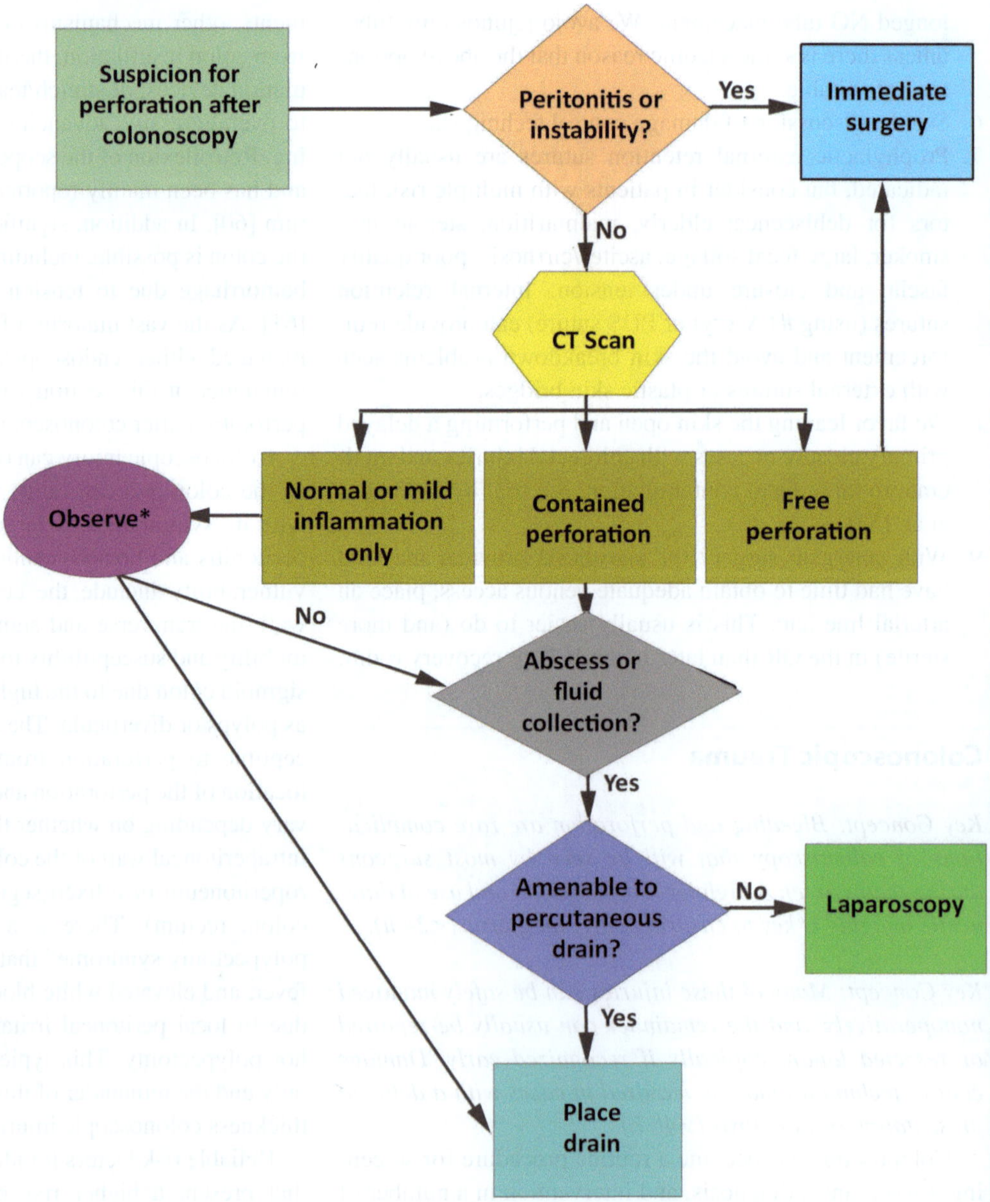

Fig. 34.9 Algorithm for evaluation and management of suspected post-colonoscopy perforation. *Observation should include hospital admission, bowel rest, serial examinations, and repeat imaging or surgery if condition worsens

safest option is to proceed immediately to the operating room for exploration and repair of the colon perforation. Other less common situations such as the presence of an obstructing mass or malignancy will usually be best handled by immediate operation. Resuscitation and broad-spectrum antibiotics should be started immediately and continued through the surgery. A frequent error that we have observed in the management of patients manifesting signs of sepsis from a colon perforation is to delay operation in favor of prolonged resuscitation in an attempt to restore normal physiology prior to operative intervention. This approach at best results in a delay to control of gastrointestinal spillage and at worst results in progression of sepsis to septic shock, multiorgan failure, and death. The first principle of abdominal sepsis is source control, and frequently patients will not begin responding to resuscitation until the colonic perforation is controlled and the fecal contamination is removed [68, 69].

Fortunately in most cases patients present with localized abdominal pain, distension, and general symptoms of fever or chills and malaise. Vital signs are often relatively normal or there may be a low-grade tachycardia. In this setting you have the luxury of time to proceed with an evaluation of the patient's physiologic and metabolic status, identification of the site and type of injury, and planning for either operative intervention or a nonoperative approach. Routine labs should be obtained including a white blood cell count, hematocrit, BUN/creatinine, and prothrombin time. It is also of vital importance to obtain a complete history regarding the colonoscopy procedure, and this is best obtained by a discussion with the responsible endoscopist in addition to review of the written report. There may have been particular areas of difficulty or concern during the procedure that are not revealed or emphasized on the final written report. If a polypectomy or biopsy was performed, then this would be the most likely area for a perforation, and important information would include the number and sites of polypectomy or biopsy, the method (snare, forceps, etc.), use of cautery or other energy devices, and the results of the pathology report if available. Another key piece of information is the presence of any underlying colon pathology such as malignancy, colitis, inflammatory bowel disease, or altered anatomy. This information could significantly alter the decision for operation versus observation, and the type and extent of surgery if operative intervention is required.

Abdominal x-rays are generally not helpful, but an upright chest x-ray can be useful to evaluate for the presence of free air and any intrathoracic reactive process such as pleural effusion or lobar consolidation/infiltrate. The gold standard study in these cases is a CT scan of the abdomen and pelvis with intravenous contrast. There is some debate about the need for enteral contrast, but we find that it can be very helpful in distinguishing a free intraperitoneal perforation from a contained or retroperitoneal process. As the primary site of interest is limited to the colon, rectal administration of water-soluble contrast at low pressures can be done in lieu of a more time-consuming (and often poorly tolerated) oral contrast prep. CT imaging of a colonic perforation will frequently not directly identify the injury, with diagnosis instead relying on understanding the local findings associated with bowel perforation. Free air and/or fluid is the most common finding and may be localized or diffuse. Contrast extravasation may be seen, but the absence of a leak at the time of the study does not rule out a perforation. Other signs include colonic wall thickening, mesenteric stranding and edema, complex mass or phlegmon, and an abscess [70]. Air or fluid in the extraperitoneal spaces can be seen with retroperitoneal colon or extraperitoneal rectal perforations and may even track superiorly around the kidneys.

After the initial patient evaluation and review of the imaging, it is important to classify the injury as a localized and contained process or a free perforation that is inadequately controlled in order to develop a plan of management (Fig. 34.9). If there is free contrast extravasation or other signs of an uncontrolled and active colon leak, then immediate operation is indicated. If there is a contained leak as evidenced by a localized abscess or fluid collection, then percutaneous drain placement and close observation can be initiated. Similarly, if the CT scan is normal or shows only mild inflammatory changes suggestive of a small or micro-perforation that has already sealed, then nonoperative management is also appropriate. It should be noted that nonoperative management or observation includes bowel rest, intravenous antibiotics, and serial patient assessments. If there is a decline in the examination or clinical status, then a reevaluation should be done with either repeat imaging or proceeding with operative exploration. Occasionally a patient may present with a large volume of free air and significant abdominal pain but no signs of an active leak or abscess on CT scan. We have found it helpful to percutaneously aspirate the free air (with or without drain placement) that can significantly improve the abdominal discomfort and allow more reliable serial examinations for nonoperative management. Although the duration from injury to presentation is an important factor in predicting outcomes, it should not be used as a primary factor when deciding on operative versus nonoperative management. If the patient presents in a delayed fashion and has minimal symptoms and reassuring imaging, then they can likely undergo nonoperative management as they have already passed a "trial of life." Similarly, those with obvious fecal contamination that has been ongoing for a prolonged period of time will require operative intervention. The main difference between the early and the late presenting patient is not in the indications for surgery, but in the type of surgery required and the available options.

Colonoscopic perforations that are recognized early have the benefit of little fecal contamination, minimal surrounding inflammation, and a prepped colon. These can usually be managed with a simple primary repair as described above for nondestructive colon injuries. This can be either sutured or stapled, with attention to not significantly narrowing the lumen. The repair should be covered with vascularized tissue whenever possible, such as omentum, peritoneum, or bowel serosa. Exceptions to this would be for larger injuries that are not amenable to primary repair, or if there is colonic pathology present (such as malignancy) that requires resection. In these cases, segmental or anatomic colectomy with a primary anastomosis should be performed. The abdominal cavity should be copiously irrigated and all contamination removed. Drain placement is not usually required, but if there is a defined cavity or abscess present, then it should be evacuated and a closed-suction drain placed. In cases of delayed presentation (>24–48 h) and significant fecal contamination and inflammation, even a small perforation can be incredibly difficult to manage definitively. The margins of the perforation and the surrounding colon will undoubtedly be thickened, inflamed, ischemic, or even necrotic. Often the bowel wall will not hold sutures or staples, resulting in tearing that enlarges the defect or creates additional defects. Do not count on a simple suture or staple line to hold up in this environment. The standard options for management include segmental resection and anastomosis, resection and diverting colostomy, or resection with anastomosis and a proximal protective ostomy. Sometimes you may need to use nonstandard or damage control options (see section "Damage control laparotomy") in the setting of a hostile abdomen, patient instability, or marked inflammation that precludes safe mobilization. One of the easiest options is to place a drainage tube (Foley or Mallenkot) into the perforation and bring it out through the nearest point of the abdominal wall. Tacking the involved area of the colon up to the abdominal wall may help to seal the area and create a controlled fistula. Another option if time is critical is to do a primary stapled or suture repair and then widely drain it, with the understanding that it will likely break down but the drains will convert it to a controlled colo-cutaneous fistula.

With the widespread acceptance of laparoscopic techniques for all areas of abdominal surgery, laparoscopy has a defined and increasing role in the management of colonoscopic injuries and perforations [71, 72]. First, laparoscopy provides a less invasive option than laparotomy for borderline cases where it is unclear if there is a free perforation or for placing drains in areas not amenable to percutaneous image-guided placement. For diagnosed perforations, laparoscopic repair is ideal if the diagnosis is made early (within 24 h), and there is no other contraindications to laparoscopy. For small perforations it may be more difficult to locate the site of injury laparoscopically; on-table colonoscopy with air insufflation can be helpful to identify the site of leak in these cases. Once identified, the area of perforation should be adequately mobilized and then repaired primarily. A hand-sewn repair is effective in the hands of a skilled advanced laparoscopist, but a repair using laparoscopic linear staplers can be significantly easier and faster. Even a standard segmental or full oncologic resection can be performed laparoscopically, but conversion to standard laparotomy should be done if there is any significant difficulty in locating or managing the injury. Finally, there also appears to be a role for laparoscopy in temporizing select patients that traditionally would have required emergent resection and colostomy. Large volume laparoscopic lavage and drain placement has been reported as a viable option for purulent and even feculent diverticulitis (Hinchey 3 and 4) and similarly could be used to temporize the patient with delayed presentation following a colonoscopic perforation [73–75]. We recommend that this option be only considered in hemodynamically stable patients without major cardiopulmonary dysfunction. The key technical points of this procedure are clearing all peritoneal contamination and widely lavaging the abdomen, but not disturbing adhesions or omentum around the area of perforation if it is sealed at the time of exploration. If the lavage is successful and the perforation appears controlled or sealed, then we recommend placement of two closed-suction drains, one adjacent to the area of injury and one in the pelvis to collect dependent fluid.

One of the less frequently discussed areas of endoscopy and surgery is how to deal with the patient and referring endoscopist when there has been a major complication. The first principle is to recognize that perforation is a risk of any endoscopic procedure whether it is performed by a novice or expert endoscopist and whether the colon is entirely normal or has major pathology. Adequate discussion of this risk during the consent process can go a long way toward preparing the patient in the event that this rare but potentially morbid complication does occur. The second principle is having a high index of suspicion and immediately evaluating any patient with abnormal pain or other symptoms after colonoscopy. Explaining your suspicions and this possibility during the workup may help gain the trust of the patient and family and prepare them for the ultimate diagnosis. If a perforation is diagnosed, then the two priorities should be having an open and honest discussion with the patient and family and obtaining a surgical consultation (for non-surgeons) or a second opinion if there are any doubts about the best management plan. Multiple studies have confirmed that a physician's demeanor and communication skills may have a much greater impact on the likelihood of patient dissatisfaction and malpractice claims than their medical skills or ability [76–78]. Malpractice risk has been related to patient dissatisfaction with the physicians' ability to establish rapport, provide access, meet patient expectations for care, and communicate effectively [78]. Empathy and active listening are critical, while denial or obfuscation can significantly harm or destroy a good patient-physician relationship. Clearly explaining the plan of management and the potential deviations from that plan will greatly help in managing expectations.

No matter how well the situation is handled, there is usually a significant component of guilt or regret on the part of the referring endoscopist and some element of blame from the patient and/or family. As a surgical consultant, you may come into this situation with the luxury of having no emotional investment or feelings of guilt related to the complication. In addition, the patient or family may view you as the savior or "hero" who is going to fix the problem created by the endoscopist. Although it is easy (and human nature) to enjoy this unwarranted adulation, it is important to not feed into this process at the further expense of the referring physician. Highlighting the epidemiology and risk factors for these complications as well as any positive aspects of the management to this point (rapid evaluation, early diagnosis) will benefit all involved. Alternatively, they may transfer some of their generalized anger or dissatisfaction with the referring physician or the complication to you. It is important to recognize that these are completely normal responses to a major adverse event and to allow them to express their feelings and try to constructively address their concerns. Allowing some time for processing and acceptance of the situation will usually calm down even the most inflamed and emotional situations. Finally, do not allow the extraneous situational or emotional factors to alter or compromise your treatments or recommendations.

Communication can also be difficult when there are multiple providers or care teams involved in managing the patient. A frequent source of patient dissatisfaction and suboptimal care is failure of the involved providers to present a clear and unified plan for managing the complication. Face-to-face discussion and agreement between the involved physicians is critical in order to provide clear and consistent guidance to the patient. Nothing is more frustrating to the patient, family, and nursing staff than to be given conflicting information or orders or to have frequent abrupt changes in the plan of care due to miscommunications. Any major disagreements or conflicts about the optimal plan of care should not be aired in front of the patient and family or in the medical record.

One of the best pieces of advice we have received for handling difficult situations such as these is: "Don't screw up a screw-up with a screw-up." In other words, there is a tendency to make poor or compromised decisions that are affected by guilt or emotions when handling patients who have had a major complication. Additionally, anger or mistrust from the patient or family members can impact decision making. This commonly manifests as a delay in proceeding with a needed intervention or in attempting a temporizing and often ineffectual treatment rather than the more definitive option. As a consultant, one of the most important contributions that you can bring to the case is a fresh and objective unbiased opinion. Although having to undergo emergency surgery after a supposedly "routine" colonoscopy may seem like the worst possible outcome, the results of inadequate treatment or further delay for a colon perforation can be much more morbid or even mortal. Highlight the positive aspects such as early diagnosis, control of the process, steps toward recovery of bowel function, and discharge plans. Keep the referring gastroenterologist (or other endoscopist) in the loop with the plan and copy them on operative reports and discharge summaries. Being supportive and nonjudgmental of the responsible endoscopist will go a long way toward maintaining a good working relationship and having an ally in the future if the roles are reversed.

Rectal Foreign Bodies

Key Concept: Rectal foreign bodies can be generally classified as voluntary or involuntary and sexual or nonsexual.

Key Concept: Prolonged attempts at bedside extraction should be avoided, and all difficult extractions should be performed in the operating room with a laparotomy set standing by if needed.

Key Concept: Counsel the patient and consent them for the possibility of laparotomy, bowel resection, and placement of an ostomy.

Overview

Rectal foreign bodies are not an uncommon problem encountered by the practicing general surgeon. A standard approach to clinical evaluation, diagnosis, and management will assist in successful foreign body removal with limited associated morbidity. Though patients of any age, ethnicity, and gender may present with a rectal foreign body, the majority are men in their 30s and 40s [79, 80]. The type of rectal foreign bodies varies considerably and may include blunt objects, sharp objects, or drug-containing packets. Rectal foreign bodies can be classified as voluntary or involuntary and placed for sexual or nonsexual purposes [79, 80]. Most often rectal foreign bodies are placed voluntarily during sexual activity but may be involuntary during rape or assault. Nonsexual placement of rectal foreign bodies includes voluntary placement during the practice of body-packing in order to hide or transport illegal drugs [81] or involuntary placement or ingestion by children or mentally ill adults. Regardless of the classification of rectal foreign body, the approach to diagnosis and management should be standardized and consistent.

Clinical Presentation and Diagnosis

The clinical presentation of rectal foreign bodies varies significantly and may be obscure due to patient embarrassment. Though some patients may report placement of the rectal foreign body, others will not be comfortable discussing the situation and may report only abdominal pain, rectal pain and/or bleeding, or obstipation [80, 82, 83]. Furthermore, presentation may be delayed (hours to days) after failed attempts to evacuate or remove the rectal foreign body prior to presenting to the emergency department. If possible, it is important to obtain an accurate history regarding type of foreign body, timing of placement, attempts at removal, and any symptoms concerning for rectal perforation (severe pain, fever, etc.).

Physical exam of a patient with a suspected or known rectal foreign body should focus on the abdominal and anorectal exams. The abdominal exam should be performed early in the evaluation, as the presence of diffuse peritonitis secondary to intraperitoneal rectal perforation requires prompt operative intervention. Even without peritonitis the abdominal exam may allow palpation of the rectal foreign body in the lower abdominal quadrants. After abdominal examination attention can be turned to the anorectal exam. External exam of the anus should be performed looking for bleeding or lacerations followed by a digital rectal exam. Though foreign objects lower in the rectal region may be palpable, those higher in the rectum will not. Digital rectal exam will also allow initial evaluation of the integrity of the external anal sphincter complex.

Laboratory tests are generally not helpful in the evaluation of a patient with a rectal foreign body. However, radiographic studies may add useful information while formulating a management plan. An acute abdominal series can reveal free intraperitoneal air on the upright chest x-ray and may add additional information as to the type of rectal foreign body. If a suspected foreign body cannot be palpated by digital rectal exam and cannot be seen of plain radiograph, a computed tomographic (CT) scan of the abdomen and pelvis should be performed. The CT scan will help evaluate for retained rectal foreign body and may provide clues for intraperitoneal or extraperitoneal rectal perforation. Findings suggestive of rectal perforation include bowel wall thickening, extraluminal air, mesenteric stranding, and fluid collections.

Treatment

Once a rectal foreign body has been diagnosed, the treatment plan is based on several factors including presence of diffuse peritonitis, type of rectal foreign body, and location of foreign object. In patients without diffuse peritonitis, the rectal foreign body can generally be removed using a transanal approach. This can most often be performed in the emergency department, in the high lithotomy position, with conscious sedation and a perianal nerve block using local anesthetic. If the foreign object cannot be removed with a local block and conscious sedation, the patient should be taken to the operating room for removal under general anesthetic [82]. Once adequate anesthetic and/or sedation have been achieved, both the patient and the anal sphincter should be relaxed. Following relaxation the anal canal should be gently dilated using two or three fingers; this will allow a thorough digital rectal examination, the essential first step in removing a retained rectal foreign body [80]. The digital rectal exam allows the surgeon to determine the precise location of the foreign object within the rectum and determine if it will be amenable to transanal removal.

If the foreign object is easily palpable on digital exam, it should be grasped by hand and removed. If it is more proximal within the rectum but still palpable, the foreign object can be grasped with a surgical instrument and brought distally toward the anal verge to grasp and remove. If the object cannot be brought distally within the rectum, gentle abdominal pressure can be applied in the left lower quadrant to aid in removal. Additionally, flexible endoscopy and a variety of snares may be used to extract foreign objects located more proximally in the rectum or sigmoid colon [83–85]. Foreign bodies that are difficult to grasp (round edges) or that have created a vacuum-type seal against the rectal mucosa may be challenging to remove with standard graspers. A Foley or other balloon-tipped catheter can be advanced alongside the object and then inflated to break the vacuum seal and aid in removal by gentle and gradual traction on the catheter. After removal of the foreign body, a rigid or flexible endoscopy should be performed to evaluate the integrity of the rectal mucosa. In addition, if there is any question of rectosigmoid perforation, a postoperative upright chest x-ray should be performed to evaluate for free intraperitoneal air.

If the rectal foreign body cannot be removed via the transanal route, a laparotomy is required. Upon exploration, if there is no evidence of rectal perforation, the foreign object can be milked distally from the sigmoid colon into the rectum to once again allow transanal removal. If the foreign body cannot be manipulated distally, a colotomy will be required to remove the object. The colotomy can be closed primarily and a diverting colostomy is not required. Laparotomy is also required for any patient with diffuse peritonitis or evidence of rectal perforation on plain radiography or CT scan. Managing a rectal perforation will depend on the severity and location (intraperitoneal versus extraperitoneal) of the perforation as described above for standard rectal trauma.

In the setting of intraperitoneal rectal perforation, the sigmoid colon and rectum are mobilized by taking down retroperitoneal attachments. Upon mobilization the rectum is inspected throughout its circumference to identify any and all injuries. Small perforations can be repaired primarily after debriding back to healthy tissue. The perforation should be closed transversely with a one- or two-layered closure based on surgeon preference. The peritoneal cavity is irrigated until free of gross spillage or contamination. Diverting colostomy, presacral drains, and rectal washout are not required. If an intraperitoneal injury is too severe or destructive to close, primarily the injured portion of rectum should be resected, the rectal stump stapled or oversewn, and a descending sigmoid colostomy matured through the left lower quadrant.

A proximal extraperitoneal rectal injury that is discovered or approached via the abdomen is repaired or resected in the same fashion as described above for intraperitoneal injuries. If an injury is not easily visualized during laparotomy, you should not perform extensive pelvic dissection or mobilization of the rectum just to fix an injury. Distal extraperitoneal injuries can be repaired via the transanal approach using 3-0 chromic suture. An attempt should be made to include all layers of the rectum in the closure, but if not possible, a water-tight closure of the rectal mucosa should be performed. An extraperitoneal injury that is not easily accessed via the transabdominal or transanal route can be managed by diverting colostomy alone.

Special Considerations

Sharp Versus Blunt Objects

Sharp objects (or blunt objects that have shattered) present a particular challenge as rectal foreign bodies. Not only do sharp foreign bodies pose a risk for additional damage to the rectal mucosa, but they also put the surgeon at risk for injury during removal. If there is a history or suspicion of a sharp object, the digital rectal exam should be deferred. Sharp objects should always be removed under direct visualization using a handheld anal retractor, rigid proctoscopy, or flexible endoscopy. Blunt rectal foreign bodies present a different sort of challenge. Though most can be removed as described previously, some blunt objects (particularly smooth objects) can be very difficult to grasp or to maneuver within the rectal canal. Use of a balloon catheter (as described above) or a suction device may assist in freeing the object and providing a point of fixation for removal [86].

Body Packing

Another type of rectal foreign body occurs during attempted internal concealment (body-packing) of illicit drugs (heroin, cocaine). The drugs are usually placed within condoms or other plastic materials and may be orally ingested or inserted transanally. Body-packing presents a unique challenge in the setting of rectal foreign body as rupture of the plastic material may lead to rapid mucosal absorption of the illicit drug and systemic toxicity. This possibility should be discussed with the anesthesia provider and preparations made to treat a systemic overdose. We also recommend that general anesthesia and muscle paralysis be utilized for these cases in order to minimize the difficulty of extraction and the potential for rupture of the container. This will also ensure that the airway is secured in the event of systemic absorption and overdose. Transanal extraction of drug-containing packets should be performed manually and surgical instruments should not be used as they may easily tear the plastic packets of drugs. If the packets of drugs cannot be removed or there are signs of obstruction, perforation, or systemic toxicity, laparotomy will be required for extraction of packets [80, 81].

Summary Pearls

Trauma to the colon and rectum may occur in isolation, as is most commonly the case in foreign body or colonoscopic injuries. On the other hand, it is often seen with associated injuries that may be more pressing. Regarding the bowel, you need to keep in mind the basic principles that govern the operative management for traumatic bowel injury – control hemorrhage and contamination, assess bowel viability, determine the need to resect versus repair, and decide on the method of reconstruction versus diversion. Rely on the condition of the patient, the environment you are in (i.e., combat versus civilian), and other cues to determine your course of action. While you should not be afraid to perform a primary anastomosis in properly selected patients, a stoma may also be the right decision. Use damage control principles, when appropriate, and more than anything else, recognize that sound surgical judgment is the key in the successful management of these patients.

References

1. Demetriades D, Murray JA, Chan L, Ordonez C, Bowley D, Nagy KK, et al. Penetrating colon injuries requiring resection: diversion or primary anastomosis? An AAST prospective multicenter study. J Trauma. 2001;50(5):765–75 [Multicenter Study].
2. Steele SR, Wolcott KE, Mullenix PS, Martin MJ, Sebesta JA, Azarow KS, et al. Colon and rectal injuries during Operation Iraqi Freedom: are there any changing trends in management or outcome? Dis Colon Rectum. 2007;50(6):870–7.
3. Cho SD, Kiraly LN, Flaherty SF, Herzig DO, Lu KC, Schreiber MA. Management of colonic injuries in the combat theater. Dis Colon Rectum. 2010;53(5):728–34.
4. Perry WB, Brooks JP, Muskat PC. The history of military colorectal trauma management. Semin Colon Rectal Surg. 2004;15(2):70–9.

5. Cirillo VJ. "More fatal than powder and shot": dysentery in the U.S. Army during the Mexican War, 1846–48. Perspect Biol Med. 2009;52(3):400–13.
6. Cirillo VJ. Two faces of death: fatalities from disease and combat in America's principal wars, 1775 to present. Perspect Biol Med. 2008;51(1):121–33.
7. MacCormac W. Some points of interest in connection with the surgery of war. Br Med J. 1895;ii:278–84.
8. Bennett JD. Abdominal surgery in war – the early story. J R Soc Med. 1991;84(9):554–7.
9. Derby AC. Wounds of the abdomen. Part 1: in war. Can J Surg. 1988;31(4):213–8.
10. Bowlby A, Wallace C. The development of British surgery at the front. Br Med J. 1917;1(2944):705–21.
11. Rignault DP. Abdominal trauma in war. World J Surg. 1992;16(5):940–6.
12. Ogilvie WH. Abdominal wounds in the Western Desert. Bull U S Army Med Dep. 1946;6(4):435–45.
13. Edwards DP. The history of colonic surgery in war. J R Army Med Corps. 1999;145(2):107–8.
14. Office of the Surgeon General: Circular Letter No. 178. 1943.
15. Welch CE. War wounds of the abdomen. N Engl J Med. 1947;237(6):187–94.
16. Middleton CJ, Wayne MA. Exteriorization of repaired missile wounds of the colon. J Trauma. 1973;13(5):460–2.
17. Vertrees A, Wakefield M, Pickett C, Greer L, Wilson A, Gillern S, et al. Outcomes of primary repair and primary anastomosis in war-related colon injuries. J Trauma. 2009;66(5):1286–91; discussion 91–3 [Comparative Study].
18. Glasgow SC, Steele SR, Duncan JE, Rasmussen TE. Epidemiology of modern battlefield colorectal trauma: a review of 977 coalition casualties. J Trauma. 2012;73:S503–8.
19. Sambasivan CN, Underwood SJ, Cho SD, Kiraly LN, Hamilton GJ, Kofoed JT, et al. Comparison of abdominal damage control surgery in combat versus civilian trauma. J Trauma. 2010;69 Suppl 1:S168–74.
20. Blackbourne LH. Combat damage control surgery. Crit Care Med. 2008;36(7 Suppl):S304–10.
21. Blackbourne LH. Defining combat damage control surgery. US Army Med Dep J. 2008:67–72.
22. Eshraghi N, Mullins RJ, Mayberry JC, Brand DM, Crass RA, Trunkey DD. Surveyed opinion of American trauma surgeons in management of colon injuries. J Trauma. 1998;44(1):93–7.
23. Welling DR, Hutton JE, Minken SL, Place RJ, Burris DG. Diversion defended – military colon trauma. J Trauma. 2008;64(4):1119–22.
24. Leppaniemi AK, Haapiainen RK. Selective nonoperative management of abdominal stab wounds: prospective, randomized study. World J Surg. 1996;20(8):1101–5; discussion 5–6.
25. Salim A, Sangthong B, Martin M, Brown C, Plurad D, Inaba K, et al. Use of computed tomography in anterior abdominal stab wounds: results of a prospective study. Arch Surg. 2006;141(8):745–50; discussion 50–2.
26. Martin MJ, Beekley A, editors. Front line surgery: a practical approach. 1st ed. New York: Springer; 2011.
27. Inaba K. Prospective evaluation of ambient operating room temperature on the core temperature of injured patients undergoing emergent surgery. J Trauma. 2012;73(6):1478–83.
28. Nichols RL, Broido P, Condon RE, Gorbach SL, Nyhus LM. Effect of preoperative neomycin-erythromycin intestinal preparation on the incidence of infectious complications following colon surgery. Ann Surg. 1973;178(4):453–62.
29. Slim K, Vicaut E, Launay-Savary MV, Contant C, Chipponi J. Updated systematic review and meta-analysis of randomized clinical trials on the role of mechanical bowel preparation before colorectal surgery. Ann Surg. 2009;249(2):203–9.
30. Fa-Si-Oen P, Roumen R, Buitenweg J, van de Velde C, van Geldere D, Putter H, et al. Mechanical bowel preparation or not? Outcome of a multicenter, randomized trial in elective open colon surgery. Dis Colon Rectum. 2005;48(8):1509–16.
31. Goldberg SR, Anand RJ, Como JJ, Dechert T, Dente C, Luchette FA, et al. Prophylactic antibiotic use in penetrating abdominal trauma: an Eastern Association for the Surgery of Trauma practice management guideline. J Trauma Acute Care Surg. 2012;73 (5 Suppl 4):S321–5.
32. Danne PD. Intra-operative colonic lavage: safe single-stage, left colorectal resections. Aust N Z J Surg. 1991;61(1):59–65.
33. Lindsey D. The idolatry of velocity, or lies, damn lies, and ballistics. J Trauma. 1980;20(12):1068–9.
34. Fallon Jr WF. The present role of colostomy in the management of trauma. Dis Colon Rectum. 1992;35(11):1094–102.
35. Oberkofler CE, Rickenbacher A, Raptis DA, Lehmann K, Villiger P, Buchli C, et al. A multicenter randomized clinical trial of primary anastomosis or Hartmann's procedure for perforated left colonic diverticulitis with purulent or fecal peritonitis. Ann Surg. 2012;256(5):819–26; discussion 26–7.
36. Velmahos GC, Degiannis E, Wells M, Souter I, Saadia R. Early closure of colostomies in trauma patients – a prospective randomized trial. Surgery. 1995;118(5):815–20.
37. Morris DM, Rayburn D. Loop colostomies are totally diverting in adults. Am J Surg. 1991;161(6):668–71.
38. Klink CD, Lioupis K, Binnebosel M, Kaemmer D, Kozubek I, Grommes J, et al. Diversion stoma after colorectal surgery: loop colostomy or ileostomy? Int J Colorectal Dis. 2011;26(4):431–6.
39. Stone HH, Fabian TC. Management of perforating colon trauma: randomization between primary closure and exteriorization. Ann Surg. 1979;190(4):430–6.
40. Chappuis CW, Frey DJ, Dietzen CD, Panetta TP, Buechter KJ, Cohn Jr I. Management of penetrating colon injuries. A prospective randomized trial. Ann Surg. 1991;213(5):492–7; discussion 7–8.
41. Sasaki LS, Allaben RD, Golwala R, Mittal VK. Primary repair of colon injuries: a prospective randomized study. J Trauma. 1995;39(5):895–901.
42. Kamwendo NY, Modiba MC, Matlala NS, Becker PJ. Randomized clinical trial to determine if delay from time of penetrating colonic injury precludes primary repair. Br J Surg. 2002;89(8):993–8.
43. Musa O, Ghildiyal JP, C Pandey M. 6 year prospective clinical trial of primary repair versus diversion colostomy in colonic injury cases. Indian J Surg. 2010;72(4):308–11.
44. Cornwell 3rd EE, Velmahos GC, Berne TV, Murray JA, Chahwan S, Asensio J, et al. The fate of colonic suture lines in high-risk trauma patients: a prospective analysis. J Am Coll Surg. 1998;187(1):58–63.
45. Edwards DP. Prospective audit of multiple penetrating injuries to the colon: further support for primary closure. J R Coll Surg Edinb. 1997;42(1):62.
46. Thomson SR, Baker A, Baker LW. Prospective audit of multiple penetrating injuries to the colon: further support for primary closure. J R Coll Surg Edinb. 1996;41(1):20–4.
47. Ivatury RR, Gaudino J, Nallathambi MN, Simon RJ, Kazigo ZJ, Stahl WM. Definitive treatment of colon injuries: a prospective study. Am Surg. 1993;59(1):43–9.
48. George Jr SM, Fabian TC, Voeller GR, Kudsk KA, Mangiante EC, Britt LG. Primary repair of colon wounds. A prospective trial in nonselected patients. Ann Surg. 1989;209(6):728–33; 733–4.
49. Almqvist PM, Bohe M, Montgomery A. Laparoscopic creation of loop ileostomy and sigmoid colostomy. Eur J Surg. 1995;161(12):907–9.
50. Lyerly HK, Mault JR. Laparoscopic ileostomy and colostomy. Ann Surg. 1994;219(3):317–22.
51. van der Sluis FF, Schouten N, de Graaf PW, Karsten TM, Stassen LP. Temporary end ileostomy with subcutaneously buried efferent

limb: results and potential advantages. Dig Surg. 2010;27(5): 403–8.
52. Prasad ML, Pearl RK, Orsay CP, Abcarian H. End-loop ileocolostomy for massive trauma to the right side of the colon. Arch Surg. 1984;119(8):975–6.
53. Gonzalez RP, Falimirski ME, Holevar MR. The role of presacral drainage in the management of penetrating rectal injuries. J Trauma. 1998;45(4):656–61.
54. Burlew CC, Moore EE, Cuschieri J, Jurkovich GJ, Codner P, Crowell K, et al. Sew it up! A Western Trauma Association multi-institutional study of enteric injury management in the postinjury open abdomen. J Trauma. 2011;70(2):273–7 [Multicenter Study].
55. Higa G, Friese R, O'Keeffe T, Wynne J, Bowlby P, Ziemba M, et al. Damage control laparotomy: a vital tool once overused. J Trauma. 2010;69(1):53–9.
56. Martin MJ, Hatch Q, Cotton B, Holcomb J. The use of temporary abdominal closure in low-risk trauma patients: helpful or harmful? J Trauma Acute Care Surg. 2012;72(3):601–6; discussion 6–8.
57. Velmahos GC, Vassiliu P, Demetriades D, Chan LS, Murray J, Salim A, et al. Wound management after colon injury: open or closed? A prospective randomized trial. Am Surg. 2002;68(9): 795–801.
58. Crispin A, Birkner B, Munte A, Nusko G, Mansmann U. Process quality and incidence of acute complications in a series of more than 230,000 outpatient colonoscopies. Endoscopy. 2009;41(12): 1018–25.
59. Damore 2nd LJ, Rantis PC, Vernava 3rd AM, Longo WE. Colonoscopic perforations. Etiology, diagnosis, and management. Dis Colon Rectum. 1996;39(11):1308–14.
60. Quallick MR, Brown WR. Rectal perforation during colonoscopic retroflexion: a large, prospective experience in an academic center. Gastrointest Endosc. 2009;69(4):960–3.
61. Gores PF, Simso LA. Splenic injury during colonoscopy. Arch Surg. 1989;124(11):1342.
62. Arora G, Mannalithara A, Singh G, Gerson LB, Triadafilopoulos G. Risk of perforation from a colonoscopy in adults: a large population-based study. Gastrointest Endosc. 2009;69(3 Pt 2):654–64.
63. Rabeneck L, Saskin R, Paszat LF. Onset and clinical course of bleeding and perforation after outpatient colonoscopy: a population-based study. Gastrointest Endosc. 2011;73(3):520–3.
64. Mai CM, Wen CC, Wen SH, Hsu KF, Wu CC, Jao SW, et al. Iatrogenic colonic perforation by colonoscopy: a fatal complication for patients with a high anesthetic risk. Int J Colorectal Dis. 2010;25(4):449–54.
65. Panteris V, Haringsma J, Kuipers EJ. Colonoscopy perforation rate, mechanisms and outcome: from diagnostic to therapeutic colonoscopy. Endoscopy. 2009;41(11):941–51.
66. La Torre M, Velluti F, Giuliani G, Di Giulio E, Ziparo V, La Torre F. Promptness of diagnosis is the main prognostic factor after colonoscopic perforation. Colorectal Dis. 2012;14(1):e23–6.
67. Rumstadt B, Schilling D. Optimizing time management after perforation by colonoscopy results in better outcome for the patients. Hepatogastroenterology. 2008;55(85):1308–10.
68. Pieracci FM, Barie PS. Management of severe sepsis of abdominal origin. Scand J Surg. 2007;96(3):184–96.
69. Berger D, Buttenschoen K. Management of abdominal sepsis. Langenbecks Arch Surg. 1998;383(1):35–43.
70. Singh JP, Steward MJ, Booth TC, Mukhtar H, Murray D. Evolution of imaging for abdominal perforation. Ann R Coll Surg Engl. 2010;92(3):182–8.
71. Thill V, Simoens C, Mendes da Costa P. Management of latrogenic perforation after gastrointestinal endoscopy. Hepatogastroenterology. 2010;57(104):1465–8.
72. Rumstadt B, Schilling D, Sturm J. The role of laparoscopy in the treatment of complications after colonoscopy. Surg Laparosc Endosc Percutan Tech. 2008;18(6):561–4.
73. Rogers AC, Collins D, O'Sullivan GC, Winter DC. Laparoscopic lavage for perforated diverticulitis: a population analysis. Dis Colon Rectum. 2012;55(9):932–8.
74. Liang S, Russek K, Franklin Jr ME. Damage control strategy for the management of perforated diverticulitis with generalized peritonitis: laparoscopic lavage and drainage vs. laparoscopic Hartmann's procedure. Surg Endosc. 2012;26(10):2835–42.
75. Toorenvliet BR, Swank H, Schoones JW, Hamming JF, Bemelman WA. Laparoscopic peritoneal lavage for perforated colonic diverticulitis: a systematic review. Colorectal Dis. 2010;12(9):862–7.
76. Mukherjee K, Pichert JW, Cornett MB, Yan G, Hickson GW, Diaz Jr JJ. All trauma surgeons are not created equal: asymmetric distribution of malpractice claims risk. J Trauma. 2010;69(3):549–54; discussion 54–6.
77. Hickson GB, Jenkins AD. Identifying and addressing communication failures as a means of reducing unnecessary malpractice claims. N C Med J. 2007;68(5):362–4.
78. Hickson GB, Federspiel CF, Pichert JW, Miller CS, Gauld-Jaeger J, Bost P. Patient complaints and malpractice risk. JAMA. 2002;287(22):2951–7.
79. Anderson KL, Dean AJ. Foreign bodies in the gastrointestinal tract and anorectal emergencies. Emerg Med Clin North Am. 2011;29(2):369–400, ix [Review].
80. Goldberg JE, Steele SR. Rectal foreign bodies. Surg Clin North Am. 2010;90(1):173–84, Table of Contents [Review].
81. Traub SJ, Hoffman RS, Nelson LS. Body packing – the internal concealment of illicit drugs. N Engl J Med. 2003;349(26): 2519–26.
82. Lake JP, Essani R, Petrone P, Kaiser AM, Asensio J, Beart Jr RW. Management of retained colorectal foreign bodies: predictors of operative intervention. Dis Colon Rectum. 2004;47(10):1694–8.
83. Ooi BS, Ho YH, Eu KW, Nyam D, Leong A, Seow-Choen F. Management of anorectal foreign bodies: a cause of obscure anal pain. Aust N Z J Surg. 1998;68(12):852–5.
84. Song D, Chen CS, Zeng XD, Dai XW. Nonoperative management for large rectal foreign body removal. Colorectal Dis. 2011;13(6):e163–4 [Case Reports].
85. van der Wouden EJ, Westerveld BD. Extraction of a rectal foreign body using a custom-made giant snare. Endoscopy. 2010;42 Suppl 2:E122 [Case Reports].
86. Billi P, Bassi M, Ferrara F, Biscardi A, Villani S, Baldoni F, et al. Endoscopic removal of a large rectal foreign body using a large balloon dilator: report of a case and description of the technique. Endoscopy. 2010;42 Suppl 2:E238 [Case Reports].

35 When Vascular Surgery Calls

Benjamin W. Starnes

Key Points

- Always seek out any information available on existing blood supply to the foregut, midgut, and hindgut.
- There are a myriad of minimally invasive procedures today that can be used to treat most vascular pathologies.
- For any thrombotic issues, pick an anticoagulation strategy and stick with it.
- Exposure and proximal/distal control remain integral first steps to approaching iliac vein injuries. If there are any problems, ligation of the vein is acceptable.

Background

The twenty-first century has seen dramatic changes in both the delivery of health care and the traditional training pathways for healthcare professionals. These changes have been evident in the field of vascular surgery perhaps more than any other surgical specialty. The endovascular revolution began in 1991 when Juan Carlos Parodi implanted the very first aortic stent graft in man for the repair of an abdominal aortic aneurysm [1]. Since that time, more and more patients who were previously deemed unfit for traditional open vascular surgery undergo minimally invasive approaches for correction of their underlying vascular pathology. This fact, coupled with an increase in the size of the population of people over age 80, has resulted in an explosion of vascular procedures in the United States and around the world.

Vascular surgeons traditionally completed a general surgery residency prior to specialty fellowship training. This gave vascular surgeons exposure to a wide variety of general surgery cases to include colon and rectal surgery. In the past 5 years, alternative training pathways or "Integrated" vascular 5-year residencies have diluted the experience of vascular trainees with a focus on only vascular surgery. Likewise, general surgery residencies have seen a decline in the *vascular* case volumes over the past decade. Thus, it has become increasingly important for the various surgical subspecialties to become codependent upon one another for the management of complex patients. The day will soon come when a vascular surgeon will no longer perform colectomy on a patient with ischemic colitis after elective aortic aneurysm repair. Similarly, surgeons routinely performing colon and rectal surgery may have little experience with vascular repairs or bypasses, such as dealing with profound ischemia or managing iliac vein injuries. The purpose of this chapter is to answer the question of what to do "When Vascular Surgery Calls." It is divided into several short sections covering unique topics common to the specialties of colorectal surgery and vascular surgery and will provide both general recommendations and useful tips and tricks for these not so uncommon scenarios.

The Physiology of Aortic Reconstruction

Increasingly, more and more aortic vascular procedures are performed using endovascular methods instead of traditional open surgical approaches. The physiologic changes that occur with each approach are starkly different. For example, managing a patient with ischemic colitis after open repair of a ruptured aortic aneurysm is much more challenging than the management of a patient with ischemic colitis after elective endovascular repair of an aortic aneurysm (EVAR).

Open Aortic Surgery

Key Concept: When consulted on a patient who recently underwent open aortic reconstruction, familiarize yourself

B.W. Starnes, MD
Division of Vascular Surgery, Department of Surgery, University of Washington, Seattle, WA, USA
e-mail: starnes@uw.edu

S.R. Steele et al. (eds.), *Complexities in Colorectal Surgery*,
DOI 10.1007/978-1-4614-9022-7_35, © Springer Science+Business Media New York 2014

with the blood flow to the superior mesenteric artery (SMA) and, more importantly, the internal iliac arteries both pre- and post-procedure.

Open aortic surgery typically involves either a transperitoneal or retroperitoneal approach. The retroperitoneum is routinely violated to expose the aorta and both common iliac arteries. The indication for the procedure will help guide subsequent management. For example, if the indication for the procedure was ischemia, such as aortoiliac occlusive disease or a completely thrombosed aorta, there has already been compromise to the inferior mesenteric artery (IMA) flow and pelvic circulation will become critical. The goal for the management of any patient with this type of presentation is for maintenance of circulation to the pelvis and, by default, the sigmoid colon via collaterals from the superior hemorrhoidal arteries. An aortobifemoral bypass should be carefully planned such that maximum perfusion to the pelvis is maintained.

The goals of therapy with open repair of an aortic aneurysm are different, to prevent death from subsequent rupture of the aneurysm. After clamping and opening of the aneurysm sac, several back-bleeding lumbar arteries are ligated from within the aneurysm sac, and, in most cases, the IMA is ligated from within. Bleeding from these vessels can be brisk and associated with a large amount of blood loss. Indications for reimplantation of an IMA are either sluggish back-bleeding noted at the time of surgery or the absence of back-bleeding from an obviously large and indispensible IMA (>3 mm in diameter). Brisk back-bleeding leads to simple suture ligation in a majority of cases. Colon ischemia is a feared complication of open aortic-based surgery and will be discussed later in a separate section within this chapter.

Endovascular Aortic Surgery

Key Concept: Just because a patient had a minimally invasive endovascular procedure to repair an aortic aneurysm, it doesn't mean they can't have ischemic colitis. Again, familiarize yourself with the blood flow to the superior mesenteric artery and the internal iliac arteries both pre-and post-procedure. The quality of blood flow to the inferior mesenteric artery pre-procedure becomes vitally important in decision-making.

Endovascular repair of either aortoiliac occlusive disease or an aortic aneurysm involves placement of sheaths and catheters through the common femoral arteries (Fig. 35.1). A variety of uncovered and covered stents can be used to either restore circulation or exclude pressurization of an aneurysm sac. Any type of catheter manipulation within an artery can cause distal embolization although fortunately, due to the robust collateral circulation of the bowel, this rarely leads to bowel infarction.

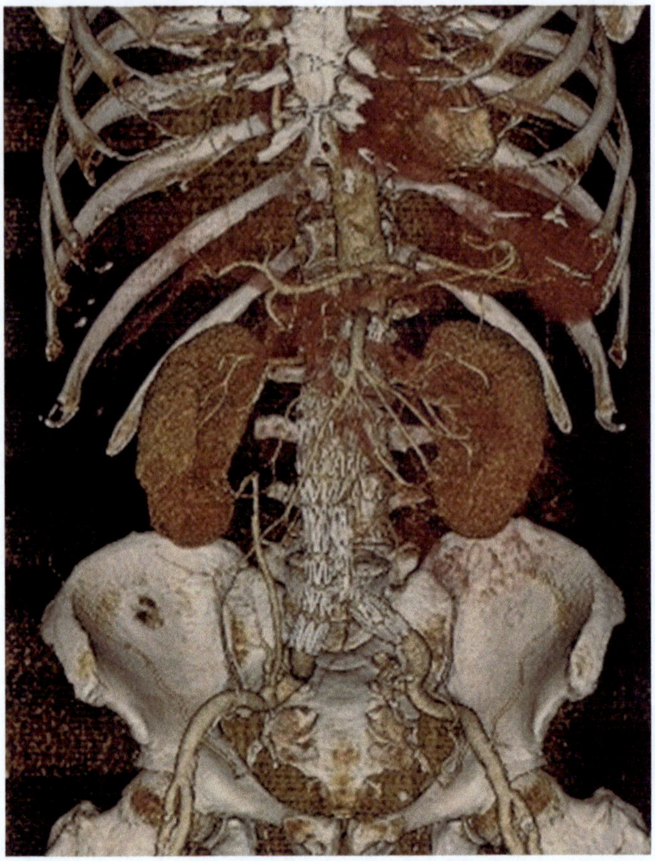

Fig. 35.1 Reconstructed CTA image showing successful implantation of an aortic stent graft to exclude an aortic aneurysm from the systemic circulation

Table 35.1 Suspected etiology for ischemic colitis after endovascular aneurysm repair (EVAR)

Suspected etiology for ischemic colitis after EVAR
1. An "indispensible" IMA (>3 mm on pre-op CTA) was covered
2. There is simultaneous SMA or celiac artery stenosis
3. A sheath injury to one or both internal iliac arteries has occurred
4. Embolization to the branches of the IMA occurred during manipulation within the sac

IMA inferior mesenteric artery, *SMA* superior mesenteric artery, *EVAR* endovascular aneurysm repair

For endovascular repair of an aortic aneurysm (EVAR), an upside-down Y-shaped prosthetic stent graft is placed within the aneurysm to exclude the aneurysm from circulation. The IMA will therefore be effectively "ligated," and this could lead to compromised blood flow to the sigmoid colon. Fortunately, ischemic colitis after EVAR is a rare event. In the rare situation that ischemic colitis is suspected after EVAR, attention should be focused on several potential vascular etiologies listed in Table 35.1.

If a vascular etiology is discovered during workup of ischemic colitis after EVAR, attempts should be made to correct that problem as quickly as possible. For example, in a

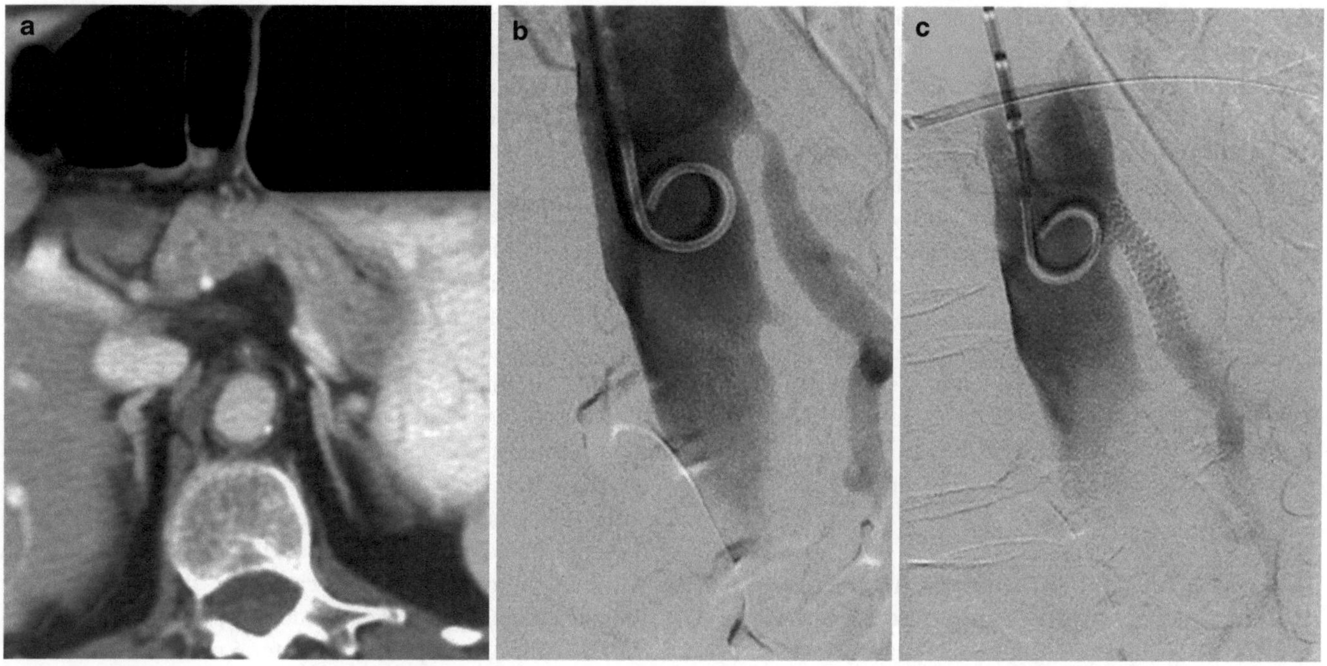

Fig. 35.2 A patient with left-sided colon cancer was noted to have critical SMA stenosis on preoperative CTA (Panel **a**). This lesion was preoperatively assessed with angiography (Panel **b**) and successfully stented (Panel **c**) prior to elective left hemicolectomy

patient with a known indispensible IMA (>3 mm in diameter and widely patent on preoperative CTA) who undergoes EVAR and develops ischemic colitis and a high-grade SMA stenosis is identified, the SMA should be stented using an endovascular approach (Fig. 35.2).

Colon Ischemia After Aortic-Based Surgery

Key Concept: Patients with ischemia limited to the mucosa can be safely monitored with serial endoscopic exams, whereas those with full-thickness necrosis should be treated urgently with colonic resection after confirmation of the findings on endoscopy. Remember, there is prosthetic material in the retroperitoneum!

Although uncommon after elective aortic-based surgery, the mortality associated with colon ischemia after open aortic aneurysm repair remains high (40–60 %) [2]. Early recognition of this situation is therefore essential. Colon ischemia is much more common after open repair of a ruptured aortic aneurysm (7–27 %) [3, 4] than either elective open (0.6–3 %) [5–9] or elective endovascular repair (1.3 %) [10].

Potential findings suggestive of ischemic colitis include shock and persistent acidosis, elevated lactate levels, fluid sequestration, or bloody diarrhea. Bloody bowel movements in the early postoperative period only occur in about 30 % of cases [7]. Early identification is crucial as progression to full-thickness necrosis can be associated with mortality rates as high as 80–100 % [11]. As stated previously, multiple robust collateral pathways exist for colonic perfusion, and the job of the vascular surgeon is to preserve as many of these collateral pathways as possible during the index operation.

Flexible sigmoidoscopy has been shown to be a reliable tool for diagnosing ischemic colitis after aortic-based surgery and is important for guiding subsequent therapy. Patients with ischemia limited to the mucosa can be safely monitored with serial endoscopic exams, bowel rest, avoidance of hypotension, and intravenous antibiotics. On the other hand, those with full-thickness necrosis should be treated urgently with colonic resection after confirmation of the findings on endoscopy. Fecal diversion and washout of the abdomen are required, ideally before soilage has occurred to prevent subsequent prosthetic graft infection.

Simultaneous Colon Mass and AAA

Key Concept: Multiple new options exist to treat patients presenting with this scenario. Don't ever feel obliged to perform two definitive operations simultaneously.

A classic board question in the 1990s revolved around what to do when a colon mass is found during elective AAA repair or, vice versa, what to do with a large aortic aneurysm during urgent colectomy for an obstructing colon cancer. The answers in the twenty-first century are a little bit easier, as minimally invasive techniques in vascular surgery have essentially eliminated the most feared risk of any combined strategy—graft infection. The first situation is now a rare event due to two facts: (1) the majority of patients being worked up for either situation have had an axial imaging study in the form of a CT scan, and with refinements in imaging techniques, either pathology can be easily diagnosed prior to any operation. (2) The majority of AAA repair are performed using endovascular techniques.

In the second scenario, a large aortic aneurysm found during urgent operation for obstructing colon cancer, the answer is even easier. Complete the colon operation and perform EVAR in the postoperative period in a staged fashion. This can often be performed during the same admission, as long as the patient is not bacteremic, even if there was intra-abdominal soilage during the first operation [12].

SMV or Portal Vein Thrombosis After Total Abdominal Colectomy (Laparoscopic or Open)

Key Concept: Patients with thrombosis of the superior mesenteric vein or portal vein following total abdominal colectomy have an underlying hypercoagulable condition until proven otherwise. The mainstay of therapy is anticoagulation.

The inferior mesenteric vein (IMV) is often routinely ligated during colonic resection, and subsequent thrombosis of this vein is associated with minimal morbidity. Portomesenteric venous thrombosis, however, is an uncommon but potentially lethal condition associated with either laparoscopic or open colon surgery. It is thought to occur more commonly in patients with specific thrombophilias or other predispositions to clotting. Portomesenteric venous thrombosis typically presents an average of 14 days after surgery, and the most common presenting symptom is abdominal pain [13]. Diagnosis can be made by either CT imaging (Fig. 35.3) with a classic "halo" sign in or around the portal

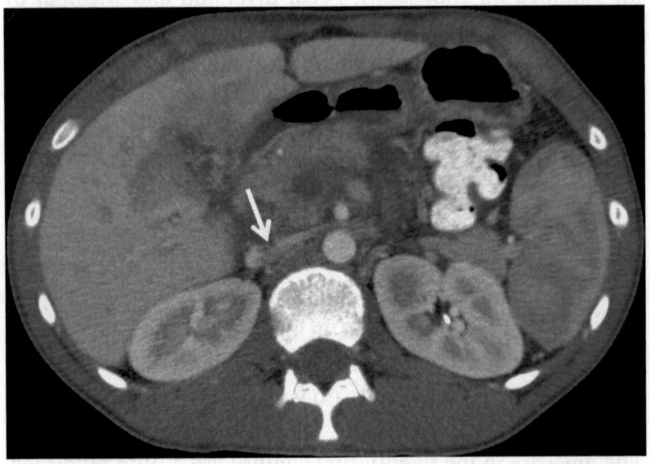

Fig. 35.3 SMV thrombosis (*arrow*) after elective laparoscopic colectomy

vein or by duplex examination. The latter exam can be confusing due to bowel wall edema or gas.

Treatment should be individualized based on extent of thrombosis and the presence of bowel ischemia. The mainstay of treatment for this disease process is systemic anticoagulation with heparin followed by warfarin therapy. Prior to anticoagulation, workup for a hypercoagulable condition should be done and include the following blood tests: prothrombin time (PT), partial thromboplastin time (PTT), international normalized ratio (INR), factor 5 Leiden, protein C, protein S, prothrombin G20210A mutation, antithrombin III, antiphospholipid antibodies, and homocysteine levels. Aggressive attempts at either open surgical thrombectomy or transhepatic thrombolysis should be approached with caution. The duration of warfarin therapy in these patients is controversial but in general, those patients who present with no provocation for the thrombotic episode and a documented hypercoagulable condition, therapy should be lifelong. If the thrombotic episode was provoked (i.e., surgical procedure), therapy should be for 6 months.

The Patient with Colorectal Cancer and Peripheral Vascular Disease

Key Concept: Follow the red blood cell from the aorta to the intestinal anastomosis. Successful bowel resections in patients with severe vascular disease require an understanding of macroperfusion.

Patients presenting with simultaneous colorectal malignancy and severe peripheral vascular disease are not uncommon. Unique combinations of disease should be sought out prior to any elective bowel resection in any patient with suspected vascular disease. Specifically, the status of the blood vessel feeding the anastomosis should be assessed. If a patient with vascular disease has a critical superior mesenteric artery stenosis or occlusion and the entire mesenteric circulation is dependent on the inferior mesenteric artery, an extended right hemicolectomy may lead to ischemic necrosis of the entire *small* bowel. A simple 15-min endovascular procedure to revascularize the superior mesenteric artery with angioplasty and stenting may be all that is needed to make the difference between an optimal and a poor outcome. Intraoperative retrograde SMA angioplasty and stenting has also been reported and may represent a salvage strategy for those patients with severe disease [14].

Prevention of Venous Thromboembolism

Key Concept: In any patient undergoing colectomy for cancer, strong consideration should be given for a full 30 days of postoperative VTE prophylaxis with low molecular weight heparins, in particular patients on chemotherapy, with obesity, or with residual cancer.

The overwhelming body of evidence from prospective, randomized clinical trials examining venous thromboembolism (VTE) prophylaxis has involved a treatment phase of between 5 and 7 days. Many of these studies were conducted when the hospital lengths of stay were much longer for any given surgical procedure. Current lengths of stay are much shorter, and this makes prophylaxis just as important and probably more difficult. Despite the current widespread use of laparoscopic surgical procedures, few data are available to provide specific recommendations for VTE prophylaxis in these patients. The more important indication for prophylaxis should depend on the underlying diagnosis. Approximately 20 % of first time VTE events are associated with malignancy [15]. Cancer patients have a fourfold increased risk for VTE compared to patients without this diagnosis, and the risk is even higher if the patient is currently receiving chemotherapy [16]. Furthermore, mortality secondary to VTE is more frequent in cancer patients. Considering all-cause in-hospital mortality for cancer patients, one in seven will die of VTE [17].

Regarding the duration of prophylaxis, a minimum of 7 days is recommended. Extended prophylaxis for 4–5 weeks with low molecular weight heparins (LMWHs) should be considered after abdominal or pelvic cancer surgery, particularly in patients with residual cancer, obesity, and a history of VTE [18, 19]. Two large randomized trials in patients undergoing abdominal operations for cancer demonstrated a significantly reduced incidence of deep vein thrombosis (DVT) with 30 days of LMWH prophylaxis versus 7 days of prophylaxis [20, 21]. In general surgery patients receiving low-dose prophylaxis, the risk of postoperative bleeding complications is around 6 %. The recommended doses of LMWHs for cancer patients are 40 mg of enoxaparin and 5,000 units of dalteparin. For other LMWHs, a general recommendation is to use doses higher than 3,400 units daily [18].

Intraoperative Iliac Vein Injuries

Key Concept: Don't panic! Grab a couple of sponge sticks and apply manual compression to the injury. Also remember the direction of blood flow. Apply pressure proximally first!

Intraoperative iliac vein injuries are fortunately infrequent but, when they occur to even the most seasoned of surgeons, can be an unforgettable event. Venous injuries frighten vascular surgeons more than arterial injuries. The reason for this is that the walls of veins are thin and can tear very easily, making them difficult to repair. The better course of valor in most circumstances is to ligate the injury, typically with 3-0 or 4-0 Prolene. Frequent mistakes I have seen involve clamping of the inferior vena cava prematurely because it is easy to dissect out, and the surgeons feel as if they are making progress in getting control. This should be the *last* maneuver. If you think there has been a lot of bleeding up until this point, just wait until you clamp the outflow. Your blood loss will double in 1 min. Remember in venous injuries that the direction of blood flow is *toward* the heart so that the term "proximal" is toward the feet in an iliac venous injury.

Common and internal iliac venous injuries can be difficult to expose. Sometimes, clamping and division of the common iliac artery, particularly on the right side, can be done to better expose a venous injury. This obviously requires arterial repair at the end of the case but can be lifesaving. Remember that this is a low-pressure system. Adequate exposure allows for proximal and distal control and attempt at repair for those facile and experienced with this procedure (Fig. 35.4). However, for those experienced, as long as the outflow is not compressed, simple packing and application of hemostatic agents is all that is needed until more experienced help arrives.

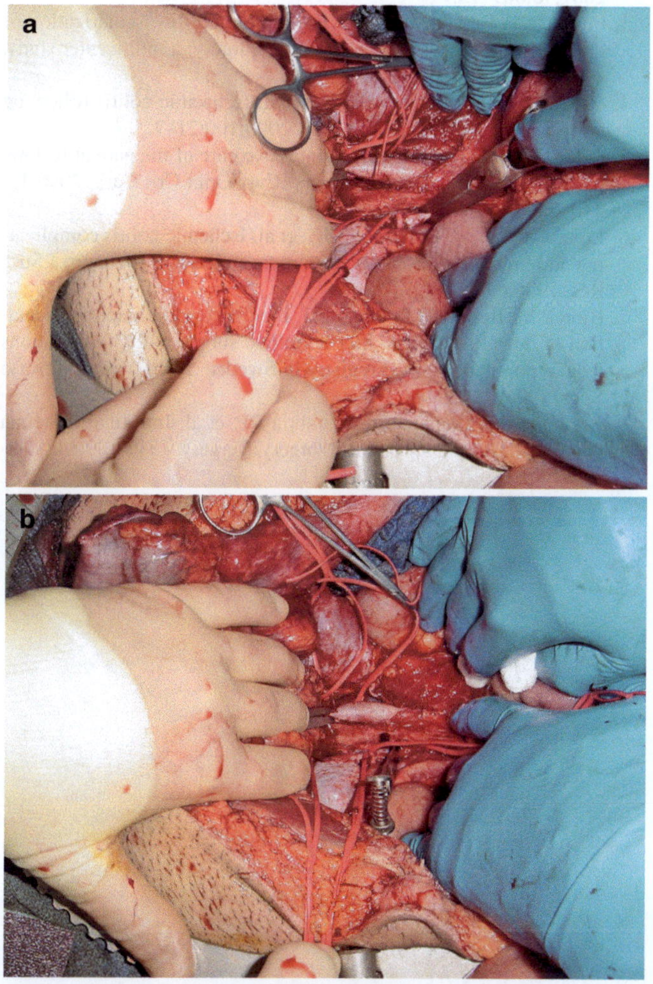

Fig. 35.4 (**a**, **b**) Two intraoperative images demonstrating proximal and distal control of an iliac vein injury. (Head is to right, feet to left, bulldog clamp on common iliac arteries, and veins and hypogastric with vessel loops. In (**b**), ischemic appearing rectosigmoid to the left of the white glove)

Summary Pearls

Vascular surgeons and colorectal surgeons mutually care for highly complex patients with a multitude of comorbidities. A general understanding of key concepts within each specialty may lead to better outcomes for patients either presenting with simultaneous colorectal pathology and vascular disease or colorectal or vascular complications resulting from respective surgical procedures. There are a myriad of minimally invasive procedures today that can be used to treat most vascular pathologies.

References

1. Parodi JC, Palmaz JC, Barone HD. Transfemoral intraluminal graft implantation for abdominal aortic aneurysms. Ann Vasc Surg. 1991;5:491–9.
2. Conrad MF, Crawford RS, Pedraza JD, et al. Long-term durability of open abdominal aortic aneurysm repair. J Vasc Surg. 2007;46:669–75.
3. Pittaluga P, Batt M, Hassen-Khodja R, et al. Revascularization of internal iliac arteries during aortoiliac surgery: a multicenter study. Ann Vasc Surg. 1998;12:537–43.
4. Van Damme H, Creemers E, Limet R. Ischaemic colitis following aortoiliac surgery. Acta Chir Belg. 2000;100:21–7.
5. Papia G, Klein D, Lindsay TF. Intensive care of the patient following open abdominal aortic surgery. Curr Opin Crit Care. 2006;12:340–5.
6. Longo WE, Lee TC, Barnett MG, et al. Ischemic colitis complicating abdominal aortic aneurysm surgery in the U.S. Veteran. J Surg Res. 1996;60:351–4.
7. Bjorck M, Bergqvist D, Troeng T. Incidence and clinical presentation of bowel ischaemia after aortoiliac surgery—2930 operations from a population-based registry in Sweden. Eur J Vasc Endovasc Surg. 1996;12:139–44.
8. Brewster DC, Franklin DP, Cambria RP, et al. Intestinal ischemia complicating abdominal aortic surgery. Surgery. 1991;109:447–54.
9. Levison JA, Halpern VJ, Kline RG, et al. Perioperative predictors of colonic ischemia after ruptured abdominal aortic aneurysm. J Vasc Surg. 1999;29:40–5.
10. Maldonado TS, Rockman CB, Riles E, et al. Ischemic complications after endovascular abdominal aortic aneurysm repair. J Vasc Surg. 2004;40(4):703–9.
11. Kehlet H, Moesgaard F. Prophylaxis against postoperative complications in gastroenterology. Scand J Gastroenterol Suppl. 1996;216:218–24.
12. Shalhoub J, Naughton P, Lau N, et al. Concurrent colorectal malignancy and abdominal aortic aneurysm: a multicentre experience and review of the literature. Eur J Vasc Endovasc Surg. 2009;37(5):544–56.
13. James AW, Rabl C, Westphalen AC, et al. Portomesenteric venous thrombosis after laparoscopic surgery: a systematic literature review. Arch Surg. 2009;144(6):520–6.
14. Pisimisis GT, Oderich GS. Technique of hybrid retrograde superior mesenteric artery stent placement for acute-on-chronic mesenteric ischemia. Ann Vasc Surg. 2011;25(1):132.E7–11.
15. Berquist D, Caprini JA, Dotsenko O, et al. Venous thromboembolism and cancer. Curr Probl Surg. 2007;44:157–216.
16. Heit JA, Mohr DN, Silverstein MD, et al. Predictors of recurrence after deep vein thrombosis and pulmonary embolism: a population-based cohort study. Arch Intern Med. 2000;160:761–8.
17. Shen VS, Pollak EW. Fatal Pe in cancer patients: is heparin prophylaxis justified? South Med J. 1980;73:841–3.
18. Geerts WH, Pineo GF, Heit JA, et al. Prevention of venous thromboembolism: the seventh accp conference on antithrombotic and thrombolytic therapy. Chest. 2004;126:338s–400.
19. Nicolaides AN, Breddin HK, Fareed J, et al. Prevention of venous thromboembolism. International consensus statement. Guidelines compiled in accordance with the scientific evidence. Int Angiol. 2001;20:1–37.
20. Bergqvist D, Agnelli G, Cohen AT, et al. Duration of prophylaxis against venous thromboembolism with enoxaparin after surgery for cancer. N Engl J Med. 2002;346:975–80.
21. Rasmussen MS, Jorgensen LN, Wille-Jorgensen P, et al. Prolonged prophylaxis with dalteparin to prevent late thromboembolic complications in patients undergoing major abdominal surgery: a multicenter randomized open-label study. J Thromb Haemost. 2006;4:2384–90.

Part VI

Beyond the Operating Room

Facing Our Failures

36

David A. Rothenberger and Howard M. Ross

Key Points

- Professionalism has evolved over the course of history, but only in the past century has the medical profession accepted the principles that a physician is accountable for patient outcomes, including failures, and that the public has the right to know those outcomes.
- More recently, it has been recognized that medical failures may also arise from system errors, inadequate communication, and poor organizational culture. Consequently, healthcare organizations are now also held accountable for their systems, processes, facilities, infrastructure, and teams of providers and staff who must be properly trained and deployed.
- More accurate methods to assess and track quality and safety are available, but honest self-reporting by providers and healthcare organizations is essential to assure all failures and vulnerabilities are evident. Only then can we optimally use lessons learned from our shortcomings to improve quality and safety outcomes.
- By following the principles of "Just Culture," healthcare organizations can effectively and equitably manage the many issues arising from medical failures, mitigate the emotional and physical toll on physicians and healthcare workers, and use their influence to modify the education and residency training programs to better prepare physicians to meet the public's demands for safety, transparency, and accountability.
- Specific immediate measures for physicians to take following a significant medical failure are outlined. Long-term recommendations to optimize full mental and physical recovery of physicians and other caregivers are detailed.

"Every surgeon carries about him a little cemetery, in which from time to time he goes to pray, a cemetery of bitterness and regret, of which he seeks the reason of his failures." [1]

Facing Our Failures

Key Concept: Many things you will encounter are not taught, but must be prepared for to help both you and your patient.

The unexpected ringing of the bedside phone jars you awake at 1:35 am. The tense voice of a nurse reports that your patient is not doing well and is being transferred to the intensive care unit. Never mind that when you last saw him 8 h ago, he had seemed to be making an uneventful recovery 4 days after a low anterior resection of a rectal cancer. Now, fully alert, you recognize this is a life-threatening complication. As you are driving the 15 min to the hospital, you speak to the ICU team and learn the patient's status is deteriorating rapidly. Options are weighed, orders are given, and you push the accelerator pedal harder as you mentally review the patient's other medical conditions, the operative details, the intraoperative decision-making, and the initial hospital

D.A. Rothenberger, MD, FACS, FASCRS (✉)
Department of Surgery,
University of Minnesota Medical School,
Minneapolis, MN, USA
e-mail: rothe002@umn.edu

H.M. Ross, MD, FACS, FASCRS
Division of Colon and Rectal Surgery,
Department of Clinical Surgery,
Temple University Health System,
Red Bank, NJ, USA
e-mail: howard.ross@tuhs.temple.edu

S.R. Steele et al. (eds.), *Complexities in Colorectal Surgery*,
DOI 10.1007/978-1-4614-9022-7_36, © Springer Science+Business Media New York 2014

course looking for a hint of what has happened…of what has gone wrong. At this point, fear and self-doubt creep into your consciousness….

Change the details and virtually all physicians can relate to such a scenario. We are, after all, human. Perfection is not possible and failures will occur. It goes without saying that the patient who is harmed by our shortcomings is the primary victim of medical failures, but that is not our focus here. Instead, our purpose is to help physicians and medical organizations understand how to mitigate the emotional turmoil associated with medical errors and how to learn from our failures and improve our outcomes. Regrettably, these subjects are lacking or minimized during medical school and residency training, and practicing physicians rarely discuss them in a supportive and useful way. Our intent is to at least partially fill this void. While this chapter applies to all care providers, it is written from the perspective of the physician and specifically for the surgeon.

Historical Context: Professionalism and Accountability

Key Concept: A historical review provides the context to understand how most physicians of today have come to accept the belief that professionalism and accountability are inextricably linked.

Until recently, medical practitioners were the antithesis of what we now call professionals, and accountability for outcomes was not a part of their ethos. More rigorous, scientific training and changing societal expectations compelled physicians to accept ever-increasing accountability for patient outcomes as part of their professional responsibility. As noted below, this fundamental change did not occur quickly or easily. In the early 1900s, a few visionary and tenacious physicians insisted that patient outcomes be reviewed openly and objectively so they could learn from each other's mistakes in a nonpunitive and educational forum. These principles were embodied in what became known as Morbidity and Mortality (M&M) conferences. At the time, this was a radical idea viewed by many physicians as a direct threat to their autonomy. Nonetheless, the idea was gradually embraced and in 1983, the Accreditation Council for Graduate Medical Education (ACGME) made M&M conferences a required component of all training programs.

Antiquity Through the Middle Ages

The notion that physicians are accountable for medical outcomes may have originated from the Hammurabi Law Code of the Babylonians, circa 1780 BC. The Code included 17 laws detailing a physician's responsibilities and establishing the concept of civil and criminal liability for improper and negligent medical care. It is the first known written attempt to regulate medical practice and to call for accountability: "…if a physician performed a major operation on a lord…and has caused the lord's death…they shall cut off his hand" [2].

The ancient Babylonians' effort to require accountability of medical practitioners was unique. Several millennia passed before subsequent societies and governments developed comparable codes. In medieval Europe, barber-surgeons, an illiterate group of men whose only training consisted of a short apprenticeship, provided bloodletting, crude wound care, teeth extraction, abscess drainage, and enema administration in addition to cutting hair and trimming beards. They had little or no formal surgical training and performed their very limited procedures without specialized knowledge or formal oversight.

Middle Nineteenth Century

As late as the mid-nineteenth century, elective surgery was extremely rare. The germ theory was still unknown, and anesthesia to control the associated pain was in its infancy and generally not available. Half the patients who underwent "serious procedures" such as an amputation died, usually from surgical infections. Most Civil War military surgeons learned the essentials of trauma surgery in battlefield locations working in isolation without help or supervision. Conducting a speedy operation was critical to survival of the operation, but there was little to be done to prevent a subsequent lethal infection. The dismal outcomes improved as the military developed more efficient evacuation and transportation of wounded soldiers to crude field hospitals where help was available and where ether and chloroform or a mixture of the two was used for a drip anesthetic. Military surgeons formed societies to track outcomes and share information that improved survival over the course of the prolonged and brutal Civil War [3]. Unfortunately, this concept of assessing outcomes to make changes to improve care of patients did not transfer to most civilian practices.

Late Nineteenth Century

The beginnings of what we might now call "modern surgery" date to the latter quarter of the nineteenth century when anesthesia and antisepsis were accepted in major medical centers in Europe. The most famous master surgeon of the time was Theodor Billroth, an Austrian, who had adopted Lister's antiseptic procedures and developed new operative techniques for major abdominal surgery that he performed safely and with excellent outcomes. His apprentices underwent several years of rigorous, scientific training. By contrast, formal medical training simply did not exist in America, and elective surgery was so rare that there were fewer than ten physicians in the entire country whose practice was restricted to surgery in 1889 ([4], p. 98). The future of surgery in America seemed bleak, and it is understandable that accountability for outcomes of elective surgery was a moot point in the chaotic, unregulated, low-volume surgical "system" of the late 1800s.

William Osler and William Stewart Halsted were charged to open the new Johns Hopkins Hospital in 1889 and its associated medical school in 1893 in Baltimore, Maryland. They insisted upon radical changes to bring "modern medical and surgical training" to the United States. Admission to medical school required that the student had first excelled while earning an undergraduate degree, and the medical school curriculum included laboratory experiments, anatomic dissections, reading original medical journal articles, and discussing the issues raised by the articles with the faculty. Osler and Halsted instituted the graduated responsibility residency system to train young physicians and surgeons at the newly opened hospital. The "pyramid system" used in surgery assured intense competition among trainees, as only a select few were allowed to complete the entire program ([4], p. 107). Their model was soon followed by a few other institutions, but most medical schools were still proprietary and of poor quality. Accountability for outcomes was not a concern for most.

Early Twentieth Century

Abraham Flexner, a research staff member of the Carnegie Foundation for the Advancement of Teaching, was directed to assess medical education in North America. To do so, he visited all 155 medical schools in the United States and Canada, most of which were proprietary, "for-profit" organizations. His comprehensive, scientific review, delivered in 1910, was highly critical of the nonscientific approach used in the American system of medical education. Flexner advocated formal analytic reasoning coupled with a strong clinical phase of training in academically oriented hospitals as the two essential elements needed to train physicians. He considered research an important but subsidiary element that could lead to improved patient outcomes. The changes he recommended to improve the standards, organization, and curriculum of North American medical schools had a profound impact causing many medical schools to close down and most of those remaining to enact fundamental reforms [5]. As a result, quality improved and medicine was, for the first time, growing into a respected profession in the United States. Accountability for outcomes was still a vague concept, but the future of surgery was no longer in doubt.

By the time of the Flexner Report, major hospitals were performing increasing numbers of complex operations. For example, at the Massachusetts General Hospital (MGH) in Boston, annual surgical volumes averaged 39 procedures between 1836 and 1846, but in 1914 more than 4,000 surgical procedures were done at MGH [3]. The strict requirements for a university undergraduate degree followed by rigorous medical school education and prolonged, focused residency training established surgeons as medical professionals who were dedicated to their patient's well-being and deserving of the patient's absolute trust. The public generally agreed that physician autonomy was an undisputed right and physicians defended such authority as essential to do their jobs including overseeing outcomes.

Accountability was generally left to autocratic chairs of departments and strong-willed hospital administrators who made unilateral decisions behind closed doors to both assign blame for events that went wrong and determine the consequences to the trainee or surgeon including dismissal. The patient, their family, or other representatives of the public rarely asked questions and were rarely, if ever, made aware of failures or allowed to be part of deliberations where poor results were discussed. This approach to accountability was not only arbitrary and inequitable but also convinced surgeons to remain silent and hide errors both from their superiors and from their patients rather than risk punishment or loss of authority.

In the early 1900s, Dr. Ernest Codman at Boston's MGH developed a case report system to track outcomes. He proposed a simple but profound idea, "The common sense notion that *every* hospital should follow *every* patient it treats, long enough to determine whether or not the treatment has been successful, and then to inquire, 'If not, why not?' with a view to preventing similar failures in the future" (italics from Codman) [6]. He was convinced that reviewing details of bad outcomes would improve patient care, prevent repetition of errors that lead to complications, and modify physician behavior and judgment. This approach required a fundamental shift in thinking about medical error and failures, a challenging adjustment for the autocratic medical establishment to accept. In fact, Codman resigned his position at MGH in 1914 because they refused to accept the "End Result" system or his suggestion that the system be used to evaluate surgeon competence and determine promotions. Nonetheless, Codman's ideas contributed to the increased standardization of hospital practices, and by 1917, at least some hospitals and physicians were willing to review autopsy findings together and to discuss their errors at so-called "morbidity and mortality" (M&M) conferences ([7], p. 269).

Middle Twentieth Century

The time from the 1920s to the 1980s is considered the golden age of surgery by some. There seemed to be no limit to what scientifically based and technically adept surgeons working with biomedical engineers could do to improve the lives of every person. No human condition seemed too daunting for innovative, surgical teams to tackle. Cancers could be cured, open-heart surgery evolved from rare and high risk to routine and relatively safe procedures, complex neurosurgery was done with low morbidity, joint replacements became commonplace, and organ transplantation was highly successful. Military surgeons and other investigators found ways to successfully manage major trauma, massive blood loss, shock, malnutrition, and infection.

As these new developments revolutionized patient care, they also increased the complexity and dangers of delivering that care. Physicians, prompted in part by their own recognition of the increased potential for error, by patient advocates, and by increasingly common and expensive malpractice lawsuits, slowly accepted more accountability for poor patient outcomes. M&M conferences, begun in 1917, evolved to become an accepted method for hospitals and training programs to meet their responsibility to be accountable for adverse outcomes. As a result, the ACGME made M&M conferences a required component of all training programs by 1983. The underlying objective was the same as that recommended by Codman, i.e., to enable confidential, peer review of adverse outcomes in an open, objective, non-punitive, and educational forum with the goal of improving patient outcomes [8, 9].

Assessing Safety and Quality: Highlights

Key Concept: In the past three decades, patient advocates increasingly raised concerns that our profession was failing to consistently provide high-quality, safe outcomes.

Critical analysis of national data confirmed their concerns and put pressure on physicians and researchers to find more reliable methods to meet the public's expectations of error-free care. Soon, new methods were developed to more accurately track outcomes in a risk-adjusted manner and compare one organization's results to others across the country. This effort led to countless new organizations devoted to improving safety and quality of medical care. Inevitably, new rules and regulations were written and new terminology emerged.

Public Perception and Influence

Until recently, Americans rarely questioned the authority, treatment decisions, or outcomes achieved by their physicians. They trusted their doctors and believed no other country could match the capabilities of the American healthcare system. While people generally understood that the practice of medicine is imperfect and that failures and complications are inevitable consequences of caring for sick patients, they also assumed that the medical world supervised a standardized, highly effective system to monitor results and prevent errors. The medical profession generally reinforced these societal assumptions, proudly pointing to M&M conferences, certifying examinations by various specialty boards, and numerous hospital rules and processes as examples of how the profession monitors its members to assure the public of safe, high-quality outcomes. Unfortunately, the safety net we had traditionally relied upon did not always keep pace with the evolution of modern medicine and its increased complexity and risk. Sporadic reports of tragic cases of errors resulting in major harm or death prompted some to question how this could occur in the American health system. For example, after the in-hospital death of an 18 year old in 1984, a lawsuit now referred to as the "Libby Zion case" was directed against a teaching hospital in New York. Contentious issues arising from the case included alleged lack of appropriate supervision of trainees and excessively long resident work hours resulting in poor decision-making because of fatigue [10]. Ultimately, a New York state regulation was passed to limit resident physicians' work to 80 h per week. In July 2003, the ACGME adopted similar regulations for all accredited medical training institutions in the United States [11].

VA-NSQIP

A major public challenge to the optimistic belief that American medicine was "best in the world" attracted the attention of Congress in the mid to late 1980s. There was a growing public perception that the surgical care provided in the 133 hospitals overseen by the Department of Veterans Affairs (VA) was characterized by excessive surgical mortality and morbidity. Public pressure forced Congress to review the matter. After confirming the safety concerns were legitimate, Congress passed Public Law 99–166 mandating the VA annually report its surgical outcomes on a risk-adjusted basis to account for patient comorbidities and compare them to national averages [12]. This was no small task since there was no risk adjustment model for surgical specialties nor were there national averages to use for comparison! To the great credit of the surgeons, statisticians, and other researchers at the VA, the National VA Surgical Risk Study (NVASRS) was launched in 44 VA medical centers to correct these two deficits and simultaneously improve surgical quality across their system. The success of their efforts led to establishment of an ongoing program, the National Surgical Quality Improvement Program (NSQIP) in 1994 [13]. The VA centers reported a 27 % decrease in operative mortality and a 45 % drop in morbidity rates from 1991 to 2000 as a result of their efforts, a resounding success by any standard [14].

Institute of Medicine Report

Somewhat surprisingly, the concerns about surgical quality in the VA had little impact on the private sector. Both the medical profession and the public apparently assumed the poor quality was confined to the VA system. Thus it is understandable that the 2000 Institute of Medicine (IOM) report, *To Err is Human* ([7], p. 31), shocked the lay public when it bluntly concluded that health care in the United States is not as safe as it should be – and can be. Using estimates from two major studies, they concluded that at least 44,000 people, and perhaps as many as 98,000 people, died in United States' hospitals each year as a result of medical errors that could have been prevented ([7], p. 31). Many failures were noted to be system errors and not the fault of a single healthcare worker or physician. Intensive care units, operating rooms, and emergency departments were the sites with the highest rates of preventable errors associated with major consequences. The 2000 IOM report drew attention not only to the loss of lives but also to the many other burdens incurred because of these preventable errors. This included tangible costs estimated at $17 billion to $37.6 billion per year and intangible items like the loss of trust and disability incurred by patients as well as the guilt, frustration, and loss of morale among well-intentioned physicians and other health professionals ([7], p. 41).

While many doctors and medical organizations initially responded to the 2000 IOM report with disbelief, our increasingly educated and technology-savvy citizenry trusted the IOM as a highly credible source. It is an independent, nonprofit, nongovernmental organization that uses unbiased, evidence-based, authoritative information to advise health and science professionals, policy-makers, leaders in society, and the public at large. Citizen and patient advocates endorsed the IOM report and demanded changes from the healthcare industry. Their advocacy coupled with additional studies confirming the conclusions of the 2000 IOM report forced our profession to acknowledge the fact that our healthcare system and our individual practices are not as error-free as we believed or as safe as our patients assumed. The safeguards, policies, and approaches we had relied on to provide our patients with optimal outcomes are insufficient. Simply put, we fail too often. It was clear that societal norms were changing and our profession and medical industry would be held fully accountable for our outcomes including failures. An increasingly skeptical public no longer trusted our profession to monitor itself in relative isolation behind closed doors. They expected individual physicians and healthcare organizations to find more reliable ways to achieve error-free care, to know their own outcomes, and to be transparent about their outcomes, both good and bad. This reality galvanized more researchers and clinicians to work together to achieve these goals.

ACS-NSQIP

Health services researchers recognized the need for hospitals and surgeons to have a reliable method to track surgical outcomes on a risk-adjusted basis to account for patient comorbidities and compare them to national averages. This information is essential if we are to assume responsibility to be accountable for both good and bad outcomes. Given the success of the VA-NSQIP experience, a pilot study was initiated at Emory University, the University of Michigan and the University of Kentucky [12]. It confirmed the methodology used by the VA for NSQIP was applicable to non-VA hospitals. As a result, the American College of Surgeons (ACS) with funding from the Agency for Healthcare Research and Quality began a pilot program in 2001 in 18 private and university hospitals to determine if morbidity and mortality would be decreased. The favorable outcomes led the ACS to enroll more academic medical centers and private hospitals into the program and to work with the Centers for Medicare and Medicaid Services (CMS) to improve surgical quality. Newer versions tailored to more surgical specialties are now available through ACS-NSQIP [15].

Role of M&M Conferences

Some hospital administrators and physicians suggest the costs of participating in NSQIP cannot be justified, especially since the time-honored, less expensive M&M conferences are already used to track outcomes. Orlander et al. [16] warned there is surprisingly little objective evidence that the M&M conferences are a reliable way to monitor outcomes and that too often, they evolve into a blame-seeking, punitive, and humiliating session. "Learning from one's errors is important, but confronting them is difficult and is particularly delicate when done in conference. If the effort is successful, it can serve as a model. If unsuccessful, it can instead convey the lesson that attempting to learn from error is at best unproductive and at worst unpleasant. Thus, the M&M conference is a double-edged sword, and particular attention should be given to the way that it is conducted."

Another potential problem with the M&M conference is underreporting of in-hospital and post-discharge complications and mortality. A retrospective comparison of these events as reported in M&M conferences for a general surgery division versus the rate determined by a Web-based reporting system used by a nurse reviewer based on the ACS-NSQIP platform showed that one of two deaths and three of four complications were not reported in the traditional surgical M&M. If accurate, this suggests other methods than M&M should be used to identify potential surgical morbidity and mortality [17].

Terminology

Key Concept: The increased focus on outcomes spawned the growth of innumerable organizations devoted to safety and quality.

Not surprisingly, the terminology related to safety, quality, and medical failures evolved and expanded as researchers and regulators from different organizations sought better ways to classify, analyze, report, and ultimately improve outcomes. Hospital administrators and clinical leaders now must deal with a plethora of quality organizations and regulatory agencies, each with their own processes and terminology, to maintain certification and meet various standards of safety and quality now open to public scrutiny. A comprehensive listing of such organizations and the terms and definitions each uses are beyond the scope of this chapter. The following are some of the more commonly used terms.

"Failure" is a general term defined as a lack of success or a falling short, while "complication" is more specific and refers to an undesired, unplanned secondary disease or condition that arises in the course of a primary disease or as a consequence of its treatment including a surgical operation. In 1993, Leape et al. [18] classified "medical errors" as being related to diagnostics, treatments, preventive services, or "other" issues. In 2000, the IOM defined "medical error" as the "failure of a planned action to be completed as intended (i.e., error of execution) or the use of a wrong plan to achieve an aim (i.e., error of planning)" ([7], p. 28). Today, the lexicon has expanded considerably to include "near misses," defined as an unplanned event that did not result in injury, illness, or damage – but had the potential to do so – and "events," some of which are labeled as "reportable," "serious reportable," "preventable," "never," and "sentinel." The Joint Commission in its Comprehensive Accreditation Manual for Hospitals (CAMH) [19], available for purchase online, defines a "sentinel event" as an "unexpected occurrence involving death or serious physical or psychological injury, or the risk thereof." Such an event requires immediate investigation and response including an action plan. Importantly, the CAMH makes it clear that the "terms 'sentinel event' and 'error' are not synonymous; not all sentinel events occur because of an error, and not all errors result in sentinel events." The CAMH outlines specific policies and standards related to sentinel events including the minimum scope of root cause analysis, and it defines which sentinel events are reviewable by the Joint Commission and which are not. None of these terms assigns accountability to a specific individual or a system failure. To do so requires an additional process such as a root cause analysis or peer review.

Understanding the Impact of Failure

Key Concept: None of the terms used to categorize failures captures the emotional or physical toll inflicted on the patient and their loved ones or the impact and remorse endured, usually silently, by the involved doctors, nurses, and other healthcare personnel.

The 2000 IOM report drew attention to such intangible costs often borne by all members of the healthcare team ([7], p. 41). Unfortunately, research to quantitate these costs and to learn how to mitigate the healthcare team's negative emotional response to error is limited.

Psychological Impact

Although it is difficult or impossible to quantitate the psychological toll of medical errors in dollars, no one doubts it is a very real burden that can be prolonged and overwhelming. There is nothing more psychologically painful, draining, and exasperating to the physician than a complication that has caused harm to a patient. When asked, senior surgeons often recall the hardest part and most painful memories of the first years in practice resulted from dealing with their personal reaction to a medical error. All surgeons know too well the dark thoughts and feelings of isolation and inadequacy that haunt the quiet of the wee hours after a serious complication. Recurring thoughts of what caused the problem and what could or should have been done differently are common. Often, there is no apparent cause for the event, but guilt and self-doubt may develop nonetheless. In cases where a preventable error occurred, shame, anger, and depression can result. Each of us faces these issues differently. The resilience needed for a physician to persevere and rebound after a medical failure that causes death or serious harm to a patient is poorly understood. Baseline mental and physical health and ability to access appropriate personal support are important predictors of full recovery.

Shanafelt et al. [20] queried members of the American College of Surgeons via an anonymous, cross-sectional survey in October, 2010. The survey included self-assessment of health habits, routine medical care practices, and personal wellness strategies as well as standardized assessments of burnout and quality of life. Their analysis of 7,197 respondents showed high overall and physical quality of life scores correlated with compliance to the Center for Disease Control aerobic exercise guidelines and with several personal wellness promotion strategies including talking with family, a significant other, or friends about feelings; protecting time away from work to spend with spouse, family, or friends; and participating in recreation/hobbies/exercise. Surgeons who had seen their primary care provider in the last 12 months (n=3,311, 46.2 %) were more likely to be up to date with all age-appropriate healthcare screening and had superior overall and physical quality of life scores. On multivariate analysis, surgeons placing greater emphasis on finding meaning in work, focusing on what is important in life, maintaining a positive outlook, and embracing a philosophy that emphasizes work/life balance were less likely to experience burnout.

Stress and Health

Physicians are often oblivious to the baseline stresses in our lives that make it difficult to maintain a healthy, balanced life. Driven and perfectionistic, we often act as though we are superhumans by taking on busier schedules than we can manage effectively while simultaneously expecting to achieve near perfection in everything we do – both professionally and personally. We ignore the literature documenting alcohol and substance abuse, depression, loss of job satisfaction, and suicide in our profession and assume these problems will not affect us.

Harms et al. [21] obtained useful baseline data from their analysis of nearly three decades of surgical residents from a single established general surgery training program to carefully define individual outcomes on personal and professional health and practice satisfaction. One hundred ten of 114 (97 %) former residents were contacted. Despite a high job satisfaction rate, surgeon health was compromised in up to 50 % by age 50, with a 20 % voluntary or involuntary retirement rate. Alcohol dependency occurred in 7.3 % of surgeons, which also contributed to the practice attrition rate. The success and length of a career in surgery were defined by postresidency factors rarely examined during training and included major and minor health issues, preventive health patterns/exercise, alcohol use dependency, and divorce. The authors did not specifically address the impact of surgical failures on these statistics, but Shanafelt et al. [22] found that for surgeons who reported an error during the preceding 3 months, there was a statistically significant adverse effect on mental quality of life, all three domains of burnout (emotional exhaustion, depersonalization, and personal accomplishment), and symptoms of depression.

Waterman et al. [23] reported a survey completed by 3,171 of 4,990 physicians in internal medicine, pediatrics, family medicine, and surgery and examined how errors affected five work and life domains. Physicians reported increased anxiety about future errors (61 %), loss of confidence (44 %), sleeping difficulties (42 %), reduced job satisfaction (42 %), and harm to their reputation (13 %) following errors. Physicians' job-related stress increased when they had been involved with a serious error. However, one-third of physicians involved only with near misses also reported increased stress. Physicians were more likely to be distressed after serious errors when they were dissatisfied with error disclosure to patients, perceived a greater risk of being sued, spent greater than 75 % time in clinical practice, or were female. Only 10 % agreed that healthcare organizations adequately supported them in coping with error-related stress. Despite such data, our profession and our healthcare organizations still do very little to accommodate schedules and encourage our trainees and colleagues to develop and maintain sound physical and mental health. Even more disturbing is that we do not have good mechanisms or training to identify when a colleague needs emotional support. Often there is little willingness to discuss one's feelings or to help develop coping strategies following a medical error. Those with responsibilities to trainees should be comfortable talking about the difficult aspects and stresses inherent in different medical specialties. For some trainees, high levels of life and death stress may not be tolerable even if given support and opportunity to develop coping skills. Such individuals may be best served if a faculty mentor advises them in a supportive way to choose less stressful ways to have a medical career or even to switch to a nonmedical field. This will help some make more appropriate career choices.

Fallibility, Vulnerability, and Transparency

We each know that today's medical world is complex, dangerous, and associated with risk. Notwithstanding our best intentions and the years of intensive training and expertise as well as the safeguards embedded in our systems, we or members of our team will make mistakes, some of which are preventable and some of which will harm or even kill the patient entrusted to our care. Although we can intellectually accept our fallibility, it does make us feel somewhat vulnerable, especially since we understand we will be held accountable for bad outcomes. The very words "failure," "complications," "errors," and "events" carry a highly negative connotation and elicit an emotional reaction in physicians that they are admitting error and negligence. These terms often evoke the specter that a regulatory body, the public, or even our own healthcare organization will use "accountability" as a pretext to find "someone to blame" when things "do not go perfectly." This makes it difficult both for an individual physician and for our profession collectively to objectively confront and process the issues associated with our failures. How can we realistically expect anyone in health care to be fully transparent in reporting mistakes and near misses to our patients and organizational representatives while understanding they both will hold us accountable and may discipline or prosecute us for a bad outcome? It is especially upsetting to physicians to be held accountable when systems issues and organizational culture not in our direct control are the root causes of a harm-producing error.

Failures, Organizational Culture, and Accountability

Key Concept: To prevent errors we must look beyond the individual provider to include the healthcare organization itself as the primary source of medical failures.

The organized study of medical failures in the past was typically confined to mortality and morbidity. Complications were usually attributed to an individual physician's error in judgment or technique. Our profession gradually accepted that we could learn from such mistakes by discussing them at a formal conference. As a result, the M&M conferences became a required component of all training programs by 1983. As outcomes researchers soon showed, medical failures were more common than previously acknowledged and most are preventable.

This harsh reality forced healthcare organizations to accept accountability for poor outcomes. They responded with a variety of technical solutions to "fix" the problems, but most learned it was necessary to make fundamental changes in their organizational culture to achieve their safety and quality goals.

Response to Systems Errors

The IOM report of 2000 [7] showed that poor outcomes are more often related to healthcare system and organizational shortcomings than to individual provider mistakes. These facts forced healthcare organizations to accept accountability for a majority of medical failures. In response to this new mandate, healthcare organizations began to emulate approaches that had worked in other high-risk, complex, high-performance industries. Technology had helped other industries achieve enviable reliability and safety records by minimizing human error. Hospitals and clinics invested heavily to deploy new technologies adapted to their environment. Examples include the electronic medical record, computerized order entry, smart infusion pumps, bar code and radiofrequency identification of instruments and sponges, verifying and reverifying patient identity, and innumerable checklists. They worked to correct or replace faulty systems, improve processes, and upgrade their facilities and equipment deficiencies. Additionally, hospitals and clinics invested major resources to develop and deploy robust informatics systems linked to their electronic medical records. Institutions employed a cadre of highly skilled data analysts and process improvement experts to assess their own outcomes.

Despite resource constraints, many healthcare organizations prioritized safety and quality as part of their responsibility to the public and the professionals who work in their environment. Simulation labs were built, but their use was more often limited to student and resident skill acquisition training than to training healthcare workers including physicians to function as a team. Teaching institutions recognized a special obligation to train the next generation of healthcare professionals to appropriately use data to drive quality. Many hired faculty with outcomes expertise and they joined ACS-NSQIP or other quality consortiums. To reap the full benefit of such programs, they invested in training and deploying nurse data abstractors as well as appropriate staff to help physicians interpret the data and intervene when deficiencies are identified.

While all these measures helped, they were not the panacea many had predicted. Failures continued to occur. The healthcare world had for the most part failed to take into account the impact of failure on physicians and others, and we failed to provide a safe environment in which to discuss and learn from our mistakes. It follows that when it is unacceptable or very difficult to honestly discuss errors amongst peers, physicians are likely to find it difficult or impossible to honestly discuss an error with a patient or their family. New approaches were needed to make real progress to assure the public we deserve their trust.

Medicine is not the first high-risk industry to face the paradox of balancing our human fallibility with the expectations of personal accountability and self-reporting, even though doing so makes us vulnerable to discipline. We know this is essential to improve outcomes by learning from our mistakes. Others including the airline industry and nuclear power industry have confronted the same issues. They found that shaming and punishing or even terminating people without changing the system does not solve the underlying problem. Instead, they learned to incorporate both system and human reliability into the design of their work knowing that neither can be perfect, but that together, the risk of error is decreased.

Just Culture

A consistent lesson learned from successful medical centers as well as other high-risk, high reliability industries is that developing the "right" organizational culture is essential to effect the changes needed to decrease the risk of failures. The "right" culture meets the expectation of full and transparent accountability for its outcomes and establishes norms of professional behavior, honest communication, and interdisciplinary teamwork. Doing this requires adopting principles and infrastructure to deal equitably and effectively with issues arising from both organizational and individual failure. Leaders must understand the potential devastating impact of medical failure on physicians and the entire provider team. Engagement of physicians, nurses, and staff is critical to drive these desired changes in culture, and it behooves the institution to identify, train, empower, and support physician champions. While external consultants may be helpful, they are unlikely to have the lasting impact that comes with using internal, trained and engaged physicians, nurses, and staff.

The needs of most healthcare organizations today can be met by adopting the framework of a "Just Culture" organization used by many other industries [24]. This term has evolved to mean a culture that holds the organization accountable for the systems and processes they design and/or use and for responding to inappropriate staff behaviors promptly and equitably. Human behaviors that can lead to poor outcomes are characterized in one of three categories: (1) human error, a mistake; (2) at-risk behavior, a choice where risk was not recognized or thought to be justified; and (3) reckless behavior, conscious disregard of unreasonable risk. Just Culture healthcare organizations hold their staff, including physicians, accountable for the quality of their behavior choices and for reporting both errors and system vulnerabilities. In the rare cases of possible reckless behavior, physicians may be subject to peer review or disciplinary procedures. Our profession's heritage of autonomy may partly explain why we too often continue to tolerate inappropriate, autocratic behavior that we know puts patients at risk. Abusive and domineering physicians undermine teamwork, inhibit a culture of safety, blame others for mistakes, and model behavior that trainees too often mimic since it falsely conveys power and confidence. A Just Culture organization puts an end to this tolerance [24].

Core Competencies

The ACGME recognized that training of young physicians had not kept pace with the complexity of modern medicine and surgery. As a result, in 1999, they approved six general competency domains, i.e., patient care, medical knowledge, practice-based learning and improvement, interpersonal and communication skills, professionalism, and systems-based practice. Each represents an area of skill and knowledge that must be mastered during training. Teamwork, quality, and accountability are integral features of these competencies, and each has the potential to improve patient outcomes and safety.

Kravet et al. [25] combined two ACGME mandates of the M&M conference and teaching the core competencies to address a major deficiency of the traditional M&M conference, i.e., its focus on identifying individual mistakes despite the recent clarity that most errors arise from system issues. They purposefully mixed traditional case-based M&M conferences with rounds focused on cases where root cause analysis identified specific system issues that caused a failure. They concluded, "The faculty members participating in our M&M grand rounds have truly been exemplary role models of humility, empathy, humanism, and professionalism. Their public sharing of medical errors, mishaps, and unexpected outcomes along with their commentaries of how the cases have affected them professionally and personally serve as wonderful opportunities for learning and reflection. Further, welcoming all clinicians and health team members has generated broad attendance and helped to foster a culture of teamwork, collaboration, and safety." They noted the need to have processes in place to follow up on issues and deficiencies identified during the conference. Without such follow-up, to correct deficiencies and improve patient outcomes, the organization risks losing credibility.

Safety and Teamwork

In health care, the "right" culture generally requires that the institution's top leaders devote time and resources to create a culture of safety and teamwork. Leape [26] identified six major changes needed in most hospitals to achieve that goal. These are the following: (1) move from looking at errors as individual failures to realizing they are caused by system failures; (2) move from a punitive environment to a Just Culture; (3) move from secrecy to transparency; (4) change from being doctor centered to being patient centered; (5) move our models of care from reliance on independent, individual performance excellence to interdependent, collaborative, interprofessional teamwork; and (6) make accountability universal and reciprocal, not top-down." Experts in human factors research, team building, and effective communication are in demand as consultants to help healthcare organizations develop both a culture of safety and systems of care delivery that support teamwork.

Cima and Deschamps [27] note that the majority of medical errors are the result of multiple linked but inadequate processes including "poorly designed systems of care delivery, poor information and knowledge transfer, ambiguous communication between providers and poor coordination of care." To overcome these deficiencies, they emphasize the need for surgeons to be specifically trained to be effective leaders in the operating room environment. They further advocate for surgical training to achieve competency in the four domains of behaviors found by Catchpole et al. [28] in order to contribute to high-performance operating teams and fewer surgical errors: leadership and management, teamwork and cooperation, problem solving and decision-making, and situational awareness.

Individual Accountability

All the emphasis on teamwork, communication, human factors, and system errors has led some to express concern that individual accountability is being lost. Whittemore [29], in his 2009 presidential address to the American Surgical Association, provided multiple examples of individual failure with catastrophic results both in medical and nonmedical industries. He then focused on the negative impact on safety and culture caused by our profession's failure to recognize and remediate nonprofessional, disruptive behaviors, and physical or psychiatric impairment in our colleagues.

The Joint Commission endorsed professionalism as one of the six ACGME core competencies and also introduced a new "Leadership Standard" effective January 1, 2009, that has two elements dealing with disruptive behavior [30]. One requires hospitals to have a code of conduct that defines acceptable and disruptive and inappropriate behaviors. The other requires leaders to create and implement a process for managing disruptive and inappropriate behaviors. Whittemore's lecture concluded by urging our profession to "go further by developing a more comprehensive process that should probably include some form of a 360° evaluation, both cognitive and functional performance testing and some form of real time observation, as is the case in virtually every other industry in which lives are potentially placed in harm's way" ([29], p. 361). Accepting this sort of oversight is our profession's next challenge, but the need to do so is inevitable given the increased complexity and risk inherent in delivery of modern medical care.

Recommendations When Failure Occurs

Key Concept: To successfully face your failures, look to actions in both the short term and long term.

As noted, medical failures vary widely and each is unique in terms of its root cause, its impact on the patient and family, and its effect on the physician(s), other healthcare team members and organizations involved. Preoperative informed consent including a discussion of what might go wrong and specific risks and complications has become more robust in recent years and can minimize surprise for the patient or family. Establishing a trusting relationship and open communication with the patient and family prior to surgery may limit involvement of the legal system if an event occurs. Today, it behooves any physician to confirm that the hospital(s) or medical center(s) in which they work has appropriate patient safety and quality mechanisms in place and a commitment to transparency and a Just Culture. Should an event occur, prepared organizations will have an organized team of clinical and administrative leaders, quality and risk management professionals, and other support personnel available to assist the physician better care for the involved patient, their family, and the team of caregivers. Parallel processes are implemented in a confidential manner that respects peer review protection. While clinical care is paramount, the emotional needs of all involved must be met as well. Physicians involved in training students, residents, and fellows have a special obligation and opportunity to demonstrate how to professionally manage the multiple issues arising from an unexpected, bad outcome. Trainees involved in such an event will observe your approach to the patient and family, the other healthcare team members, and your own personal response. If done correctly, you can provide an invaluable demonstration of the best our profession has to offer. Conversely, if a faculty member ducks the responsibility, cowers in self-pity and fear, or blames others, the trainee will be left with an indelible negative image of the profession he is hoping to join.

Immediate Steps

The following initial steps are suggested to guide the surgeon or other medical provider "facing a failure":

1. Optimize the medical and surgical care of the patient, and manage the event by ensuring the best resources and best know-how are made available to the patient. Though surgeons can manage most of their own complications, there are situations where you should seek consultations from local colleagues and/or transfer to a medical center of excellence and a physician whose unique expertise may mitigate the consequences of the event and improve the chance for full recovery for the patient. Three scenarios come to mind. One is an intraoperative complication outside your operative "comfort zone." For instance, repairing a bile duct injury, major vascular injury, ureteral transection, or distal rectal tear may not be part of your expertise. In such cases, the best response is to call for intraoperative emergency consultation from an experienced and skilled hepatobiliary surgeon, vascular surgeon, urologist, or colorectal surgeon, respectively. If no specialist is available in your community, it is usually better to stabilize and transfer the patient to a center where such expertise is available than to do a repair that is likely to fail and further complicate the situation. The second scenario is when the patient is not doing well postoperatively but you are uncertain what to do…order more tests, observe longer, or reoperate. Consultation with a colleague to review the course and examine the patient with "fresh eyes" can be life saving. A third scenario is when a postoperative complication occurs that requires nonoperative expertise or other surgical disciplines to manage the problem such as respiratory failure or acute myocardial infarction requiring surgery.
2. Communicate the event circumstances and disclose any injury honestly and clearly with the patient (if able to engage in communication) and with the patient's family and loved ones. If a reviewable event, let them know the

event will be evaluated. It is important to keep them fully informed on a regular basis as the consequences of the event unfold. The more serious the event and potential consequences, the more often one should personally talk to the patient and family.

3. Report the event internally to the appropriate representatives of the hospital/medical staff, your practice plan and to appropriate regulatory bodies, i.e., risk management, department head(s), or others who need to know.
4. Document in the patient's medical record (including the operative note if relevant) what occurred as objectively as possible; do not conjecture what might have happened. Never alter notes or obfuscate the truth.
5. Support and guide the team involved in the event by honestly discussing what happened, supporting their emotional needs and answering their questions. Explain your treatment and communication plans per items 1 and 2 above. Let them know if the event will be evaluated and what will be expected of them.
6. All involved in the event should be instructed to protect the patient's right to privacy and refrain from discussion outside of peer-review protected settings. This means they are not to discuss the event with noninvolved people or to discuss the event or speculate on its cause in "open" conversations where others may hear. Instruct all involved to report rumors if they hear of them to organizational support representative(s).
7. If you are concerned a member of the healthcare team is hiding details of an event or blaming you or someone else, speak to them professionally to encourage them to reveal the entire truth about the event. If the concern persists, speak to the appropriate physician or staff member(s) in charge of reviewing the event.
8. Work with the appropriate representatives of your organization to gather relevant data and a recollection of what happened in what sequence from all involved in the event as quickly and objectively as possible. Emphasize documenting "just the facts."
9. If appropriate, work with the representatives of your organization to hold a root cause analysis (RCA) as quickly as possible following the event before people's memory fades. Use the principles of Just Culture as the RCA is conducted and an action plan is developed.

Long-Term Recommendations

Following the immediate turmoil that accompanies a serious adverse event, the surgeon and other members of the team often continue to struggle with guilt, self-doubt, anger, and frustration. The physician may worry about their reputation and practice. Members of the team may not know the ultimate outcome or the findings of the root cause analysis, and they too may worry about their reputation and job security. The following steps taken over the long term will often mitigate the psychological burden that accompanies such an event:

1. Work to recognize and accept that complications may occur despite "complete" knowledge of the disease process, a sound treatment plan, and "perfect" technical execution. At the same time, it is important to be self-critical and, if mistakes were made, to acknowledge them and learn from them. Discussion with your trusted colleagues is often helpful to sort through the decision-making and technical aspects of a case where the outcome was not what you wanted. If needed, obtain additional skills training or scrub in with a colleague for complex cases until you regain the confidence needed to return to your surgical career.
2. Strive to maintain or develop personal coping strategies to deal with the residual stress and guilt following a surgical complication. Every day, physicians show courage as they make life and death decisions for their patients, but our willingness to admit we need emotional support is more daunting. If you recognize you are depressed or suicidal, seek professional help immediately.
3. Similarly, if you are concerned any member of your team is struggling emotionally, talk to them and encourage them to seek professional intervention.
4. Quality of life in a surgical career has been shown to be associated with health maintenance, so continue to exercise and eat well. If you need to "push the reset button," take some time away from the intensity of your work. Discuss your feelings with a spouse, significant other, or colleague while maintaining patient confidentiality.
5. It can be therapeutic to get involved to help your organization correct system errors that led to an event in your patient. At a minimum, it is important to advocate for appropriate changes to processes that put patients at risk and to be a physician champion for safety and for assuring your organization lives the principles embedded in the term Just Culture.
6. Encourage research to better identify stressors for the physician and other healthcare workers and better ways to manage them.
7. Encourage your organization and professional societies to develop better training so physicians can better recognize and fill unmet needs of our colleagues and coworkers to effectively deal with the emotional impact inflicted by medical errors.

Summary Pearls

Our understandings and methods of addressing the complex issues inherent in medical failures have changed radically in the past century in parallel with the evolution of the practice of medicine and surgery. The medical world now fully accepts accountability for outcomes as part of its professional responsibility, but we recognize the need to follow the principles of Just Culture to avoid the tendency to translate accountability as meaning identifying "someone to blame." No longer does the physician work in isolation and without oversight to provide the majority of care for a patient. Instead, we work to provide patient care within a highly regulated, complex, potentially dangerous system of interrelated and interdependent components where teamwork and communication are often as critical to successful outcomes as the surgeon's knowledge, judgment, and technical skill. Put another way, poor teamwork and miscommunication can sometimes negate the best the surgeon alone can offer the patient. It thus behooves each of us to do all we can to prevent failure. That said, we are fallible and must be prepared to manage failure when it occurs.

References

1. Leriche R. as quoted in: McDonald P. Colorectal quotations. J R Soc Med. 2005;98(2):77–8. PMCID: PMC1079390.
2. Hajar R. The air of history: early medicine to Galen (part I). Heart Views. 2012;13(3):120–8. http://dx.doi.org/10.4103/1995-705X.102164.
3. Bollet AJ. The truth about civil war surgery. Civil War Times. 2004 [cited 2012 Nov 1]; Published online at Historynet.com: 12 June 2006. Available from: http://www.historynet.com/the-truth-about-civil-war-surgery-2.htm.
4. Imber G. Genius on the edge: the bizarre double life of Dr. William Stewart Halsted. New York: Kaplan Publishing; 2011.
5. Cooke M, Irby DM, Sullivan W, Ludmerer KM. American medical education 100 years after the Flexner report. N Engl J Med. 2006;355(13):1339–44. http://dx.doi.org/10.1056/NEJMra055445. PMID: 17005951.
6. Brand RA. Ernest Amory Codman, MD, 1869–1940. Clin Orthop Relat Res. 2009;467(11):2763–5. Published online 2009 August 19. http://dx.doi.org/10.1007/s11999-009-1047-8. PMCID: PMC2758958
7. Kohn LT, Corrigan JM, Donaldson MS, editors. To err is human: building a safer health system. Committee on Quality of Health Care in America. Institute of Medicine. Washington: National Academy Press; 2000.
8. Campbell W. Surgical morbidity and mortality meetings. Ann R Coll Surg Engl. 1988;70(6):363–5. PMC: 2498614. PMID: 3207327.
9. Gawande A. Complications: a surgeon's notes on an imperfect science. New York: Metropolitan Books; 2002. p. 47–74. ISBN 0-8050-6319-6.
10. Spritz N. Oversight of physicians' conduct by state licensing agencies. Lessons from New York's Libby Zion case. Ann Intern Med. 1991;115(3):219–22. PMID 2058876.
11. Philibert I, Friedmann P, Williams WT, ACGME Work Group on Resident Duty Hours. New requirements for resident duty hours. JAMA. 2002;288(9):1112–4.
12. The American College of Surgeons National Surgical Quality Improvement Program (ACS NSQIP). [Internet]. 2012 [cited 2012 Dec 18]. Available from: http://site.acsnsqip.org/.
13. Khuri SF, Daley J, Henderson W, Hur K, Demakis J, Aust JB, et al. The Department of Veterans Affairs' NSQIP. The first national, validated, outcome-based, risk-adjusted, and peer-controlled program for the measurement and enhancement of the quality of surgical care. Ann Surg. 1998;228(4):491–507.
14. Khuri SF, Daley J, Henderson WG. The comparative assessment and improvement of quality of surgical care in the Department of Veterans Affairs. Arch Surg. 2002;137(1):20–7.
15. Birkmeyer JD, Shahian DM, Dimick JB, Finlayson SRG, Flum DR, Ko CY, et al. Blueprint for a new American College of Surgeons: National Surgical Quality Improvement Program. J Am Coll Surg. 2008;207(5):777–82.
16. Orlander JD, Barber TW, Fincke BG. Special theme articles: medical errors. The morbidity and mortality conference: the delicate nature of learning from error. Acad Med. 2003;77(10):1001–6. PMID: 12377674.
17. Hutter MM, Rowell KS, Devaney LA, Sokal SM, Warshaw AL, Abbott WM, et al. Identification of surgical complications and deaths: an assessment of the traditional surgical morbidity and mortality conference compared with the American College of Surgeons-National Surgical Quality Improvement Program. J Am Coll Surg. 2006;203(5):618–24. http://dx.doi.org/10.1016/j.jamcollsurg.2006.07.010. PMID: 17084322.
18. Leape LL, Lawthers AG, Brennan TA, Johnson WG. Preventing medical injury. QRB Qual Rev Bull. 1993;19(5):144–9. PMID: 8332330.
19. The Joint Commission. Comprehensive Accreditation Manual for Hospitals (CAMH): the official handbook. Oakbrook Terrace: The Joint Commission Resources; 2012. p. 2012.
20. Shanafelt TD, Oreskovich MR, Dyrbye LN, Satele DV, Hanks JB, Sloan JA, et al. The personal health habits and wellness practices of US surgeons. Ann Surg. 2012;255(4):625–33.
21. Harms BA, Heise CP, Gould JC, Starling JR. A 25-year single institution analysis of a health, practice, and fate of general surgeons. Ann Surg. 2005;242(4):520–6. PMID: 16192812.
22. Shanafelt TD, Balch CM, Bechamps G, Russell T, Dyrbye L, Satele D, et al. Burnout and medical errors among American surgeons. Ann Surg. 2010;251(6):995–1000. PMID: 19934755.
23. Waterman AD, Garbutt J, Hazel E, Dunagan WC, Levinson W, Fraser VJ, et al. The emotional impact of medical errors on practicing physicians in the United States and Canada. Jt Comm J Qual Patient Saf. 2007;33(8):467–76. PMID: 17724943.
24. Dekker S. Just culture: balancing safety and accountability. Burlington: Ashgate Publishing Company; 2007.
25. Kravet SJ, Howell E, Wright SM. Morbidity and mortality conference, grand rounds, and the ACGME's core competencies. J Gen Intern Med. 2006;21(11):1192–4. http://dx.doi.org/10.1111/j.1525-1497.2006.00523.x. PMCID: PMC1831665.
26. Leape LL. Errors in medicine. Clin Chim Acta. 2009;404(1):2–5.
27. Cima RR, Deschamps C. Role of the surgeon in quality and safety in the operating room environment. Gen Thorac Cardiovasc Surg. Published online: 19 July 2012. Available from: http://dx.doi.org/10.1007/s11748-012-0111-6.
28. Catchpole K, Mishra A, Handa A, McCulloch P. Teamwork and error in the operating room: analysis of skills and roles. Ann Surg. 2008;247(4):699–706. PMID: 18362635.
29. Whittemore AD. The competent surgeon: individual accountability in the era of "systems" failure. Ann Surg. 2009;250(3):357–62.
30. The Joint Commission: Behaviors that undermine a culture of safety. Sentinel Events Alert. 2008;40:1–4. Published online 9 July 2008. Available from: http://www.jointcommission.org/assets/1/18/SEA_40.PDF.

37 Teaching and Training for Laparoscopic Colorectal Resection

Bradley J. Champagne and Helen MacRae

Key Points

- Several barriers exist to improving the education and widespread adoption of laparoscopic colectomy.
- An honest assessment of an individual surgeon's extent of colorectal-based practice is likely required to ensure adequate training, and assessment of proficiency is achieved.
- More uniform completion of technical skills assessment along with appropriate and timely feedback during training is required to improve overall surgical education.

Introduction

Prospective randomized trials have demonstrated that laparoscopic colectomy (LC) for benign and malignant disease can be performed with acceptable morbidity and mortality, as well as reductions in the duration of hospital stay [1–5]. Furthermore, patients undergoing elective segmental colectomy by laparotomy have suffered significantly higher complication rates when compared to laparoscopy [6]. Outcomes and technical pearls for LC have been assessed in nearly 3,000 publications. However, an astonishing low percentage of articles in peer-reviewed journals address education for safe adoption of this technology. More specifically, studies evaluating training methods for LC consist of a mere 0.01 % (31/2998) of the current literature. There have been several hurdles to the progression of LC, but the lack of well-designed scientific evaluations of training and assessment with validated metrics has clearly contributed to problems with dissemination of this technology.

Industry has made substantial efforts to reduce the learning curve. One company has informally reported spending approximately ten million dollars over the last 9 years on education for LC. Despite this investment, and that of several surgical societies and training institutions, the majority (65 %) of elective colon resections in the United States are still performed by laparotomy [7]. In this chapter we will address the current barriers to more widespread adoption of laparoscopic colectomy and methods available for the training and assessment of both residents and attending surgeons in performance of these procedures.

Barriers

Key Concept: Different techniques, competing technology, changes in the surgical training environment, and a lack of consistent use of validated assessment tools all contribute to low rates of laparoscopic colectomy adoption.

One significant impediment to the widespread adoption of LC is a disagreement amongst opinion leaders teaching this technique as to the best method of performing LC. After three pivotal randomized trials showed equivalence for laparoscopic colectomy for colon cancer-related outcomes, there was an immediate international interest to establish this method as the standard of care for colon cancer resections. Over the ensuing years, experts espoused one of two fundamentally different techniques. Therefore, conventional laparoscopy (CL) and hand-assisted laparoscopic approaches (HAL) evolved separately, rather than together. This division was readily apparent at both national forums and traditionally

B.J. Champagne, MD (✉)
Division of Colon and Rectal Surgery, Department of Surgery, Case Western Reserve University School of Medicine, University Hospitals, 11100 Euclid Avenue/7 Lakeside 7th floor, Cleveland, OH 44106, USA
e-mail: brad.champagne@uhhospitals.org

H. MacRae, MD, FRCSC, FACS, FASCRS
Department of Surgery, Mount Sinai Hospital and University of Toronto, 451 Mount Sinai Hospital, Toronto, ON M5G 1X8, Canada

Colorectal Residency, Toronto, ON, Canada
e-mail: hmacrae@mtsinai.on.ca

S.R. Steele et al. (eds.), *Complexities in Colorectal Surgery*,
DOI 10.1007/978-1-4614-9022-7_37, © Springer Science+Business Media New York 2014

one-sided industry-sponsored mini-fellowships. This polarization amongst "experts" may have hindered training as surgeons and residents attempted to progress along the learning curve. As the HAL vs. CL debates waned, with advantages of each approach being accepted, surgeons performed and taught what they were comfortable with, and training the next generation became less ambiguous.

As surgeons continued to improve their ability at performing and teaching CL or HAL, robotics and single incision approaches for colorectal resection gained popularity. These technological "advancements" immediately became the new kids on the block, and we were immediately inundated with publications and presentations at regional and national meetings. Furthermore, some surgeons pushed their personal agendas forward, trying to claim their niche in the "latest and greatest" of laparoscopic colorectal resection. Industry has readily championed gaining any indication for these new devices, and as the debate amongst opinion leaders regarding the best approach forward takes precedence, education is again left on the sidelines. The theoretical and practical advantages of new technology in the appropriate spectrum should never be discouraged; however, constant re-evaluations of technique have impacted on training the next generation. National and institutional LC courses have become less focused on the most effective methods to learn and more concerned with satisfying industry's interest to gain exposure for their new equipment. This lack of consensus and commitment to an organized training strategy must be addressed. Diversity, in and of itself, is important to advance our surgical specialty; however, we must collaborate and make a conscious effort to ensure that advancements are not impediments to surgical education.

Another barrier in our efforts to offer elective laparoscopic colectomy to the majority of patients is our reluctance to categorize trainees. There are essentially four groups attempting to learn this technique: general surgery residents, colorectal residents, general surgeons, and colorectal surgeons, all of whom differ in their skill sets and long-term goals. The ever-changing landscape of general surgery residency, fluctuating requirements established by the American Boards of Surgery and Colorectal Surgery, and recent changes in health care uniquely impact each of these groups. Hospital administrators are now, more than ever, focused primarily on survival and reimbursement, impacting on teaching initiatives at most academic medical centers. Unfortunately, this new world of "do more with less" is unlikely to enhance minimally invasive colectomy training, unless specific initiatives are introduced to ensure training needs are appropriately addressed.

Lastly, and perhaps most importantly, methods for assessment of LC skills are practically nonexistent at most training programs. Numerous validated assessment tools have been evaluated and are available for LC, but are rarely implemented. Furthermore, the appropriate environment and subjects for their application remain unclear.

Who to Teach, and Why?

Key Concept: Surgeons and trainees must both be realistic about the volume of colorectal surgery that they are or will be performing in practice, and we need to maximize our efforts training these individuals appropriately.

Effective methods to teach laparoscopic colectomy (LC) are dependent on both the experience and expectations of the trainee. Two critical elements are required to be successful at mastering LC. These include a two-handed advanced laparoscopic skill set and being very familiar with colorectal anatomy through a high volume of cases. As we continue to teach residents at all levels and attending surgeons without discretion, it is essential to ask "Why?"

Colorectal Residents (Fellows)

An important group on whom to concentrate LC training are colorectal surgery trainees. Performing LC independently will be an essential component of their practice and an expectation required for fellowship certification. In 2008, the American Board of Colon and Rectal Surgery (ABCRS) introduced new minimum case requirements with a 3-year grace period. The 2012 graduating class was expected to complete their 1-year residency with at least 50 laparoscopic colon and rectal resections. This minimum requirement is an advancement and an acknowledgement of the importance of acquiring these skills. However, this falls somewhat short, as it currently does not distinguish between site and indication for resection. For open procedures, requirements are clearly defined for right, left, sigmoid, and rectal resection. Intuitively, this should hold true for a minimally invasive approach as well, but doesn't at the present time. The lack of specific parameters for laparoscopic cases may permit significant imbalance amongst finishing trainees.

Quantifying the number of LC cases needed in training to become proficient is challenging and likely is both resident and case dependent. Individual variation in skills exists across all professions and within colorectal surgery often fluctuates depending on the procedure (i.e., stoma vs. colon vs. pelvic operations). Several papers have reported a broad learning curve of 30–75 cases for experienced surgeons, yet the appropriate number and case mix for colorectal residents is essentially unstudied [8–10]. A recent survey of graduates of colon and rectal surgery residencies was performed to investigate this question. The survey sought to both quantify the number of cases performed during colorectal residency and qualify resident experience by evaluating comfort performing the procedure independently upon graduation. The authors found that 80 % of residents are very comfortable performing laparoscopic colectomies after performing 10 laparoscopic right and 30 laparoscopic left colectomies during their residency [11]. However a large proportion of residents in the survey did not perform enough cases to reach this benchmark. Fifty percent of residents performed less than ten cases during their year of colon and rectal surgery training, while only 1 in 6 residents perform greater than 30 of each type of surgery [11]. These trends demonstrate a wide discrepancy in laparoscopic experience of colon and rectal surgery residents and emphasize the need for more detailed operative standards. Furthermore, there is some debate on the importance of having a minimum number at all. Although some surgeons may demonstrate "mastery" of a particular operation after five procedures while others demonstrate mastery at 50, it is most important that the appropriate level of skill is eventually achieved. Conversely, another trainee who has performed 100 operations, but continues to lack the ability to successfully and safely perform the procedure, likely should not be accredited either. This highlights the need for a more detailed and validated operative assessment and demonstration of proficiency.

The variation amongst colorectal residencies in exposure to LC will likely decrease as more attending colorectal surgeons at training programs attempt to develop minimally invasive skills. Therefore, the primary objective going forward should be geared towards improving objective assessment. Validated assessment tools will be discussed in detail below. Program directors should strive to improve collaboration and develop consensus on a structured, mandatory assessment tool for the performance of LC. The recent introduction of a technical skills assessment (COSATS) that may 1 day become part of the ABCRS certifying exam will likely introduce an element of accountability in all areas of technical competence. Laparoscopic colectomy will almost assuredly be an integral part of this examination; yet ultimately, individual programs have the primary responsibility to ensure their trainees have adequate technical skill by incorporating a validated objective tool within their program.

General Surgery Residents

Structured curricula have been introduced during general surgery residency for learning basic laparoscopic procedures (i.e., FLS), yet there are few reports on dedicated programs for advanced techniques. Laparoscopic colorectal resection is an index case for advanced skills training; however, recent data from the ACGME resident case log system has demonstrated that graduates lack the appropriate volume to reach proficiency [12, 13]. More specifically, surgical chief residents averaged less than 9 LC cases during their final training year and 13 during their entire residency. The ongoing impact of this limitation is somewhat concerning when considering the recent data that 98 % of the colectomies for diverticulitis in the United States are performed by general surgeons who complete less than ten colectomies per year [14].

This environment has created concern regarding the likelihood of successful development of competence in essential colorectal surgery cases by trainees during their residency [15–17]. General surgery program directors are attempting to adjust to a new climate of education and an expanding curriculum, but reduced resources and economic pressures have made the transition challenging. Some now view fellowships as the time where graduates have their opportunity to "learn" specialized skill sets. Furthermore, we are starting to witness the introduction of "fellowships" in general surgery (i.e., "super-chief" years) in attempt to ease this transition.

Academic surgeons must also ask "Why" should we teach general surgery residents advanced laparoscopic colorectal procedures? It is very unlikely that these trainees will be proficient at a laparoscopic sigmoid colectomy or low anterior resection at the completion of training. Furthermore, the majority of residents are pursuing additional fellowship training. Should we only teach those residents that plan on performing advanced laparoscopy as part of their practice? The answer to this question is probably "yes," but significant changes in residency curriculum would have to change on a widespread scale before this philosophy is embraced. Most notably, residency programs should consider both introducing elective rotations for senior level trainees in their area of interest and/or offering mini-mentorships with specific faculty. Or perhaps offer a structured curriculum with different areas of expertise being built into the program's core curriculum based on an individual trainee's interests? This system seems more appropriate in our current era of duty hour restrictions, but would require endorsement from the American Board of Surgery and the ACGME. Until then, all academic surgeons, as surgical educators by definition, should strive to maximize specific goals with each resident.

Attending Surgeons

Teaching LC to existing faculty members and community surgeons encompasses a different set of challenges. Senior colorectal surgeons may have excessive knowledge of the appropriate anatomy and steps of the operation, but may often lack in the two-handed laparoscopic skill set required to successfully perform the procedure. On the other hand, practicing general surgeons typically have two-handed laparoscopic experience, but typically are less familiar with the details of colorectal disease and tissue planes. Most practicing surgeons have considerable existing time constraints, necessitating prioritizing learning needs and willingness to invest time in meeting them. Therefore, prior to tackling the massive hurdle of learning LC, a surgeon must be honest with himself or herself. It is critical for general surgeons to have a reasonable volume of open colorectal procedures before attempting to develop LC skills. If other members or partners in their group are performing the majority of colorectal procedures, it may be more efficient to promote the advancement of that individual's practice, rather than multiple surgeons having insufficient volumes. Without the opportunity for repetition and deliberate practice, LC cannot be learned appropriately. This situation must also be recognized and not exploited by our partners in industry by enrolling all willing surgeons in "hands-on" courses.

Colorectal attending surgeons that trained prior to the era of minimally invasive techniques must also be realistic. They likely have the volume of colorectal cases but must commit the time to developing two-handed laparoscopic skills and proficiency in LC techniques. They must also recognize whether the laparoscopic or open technique is most suitable for their practice and minimize the impact of their attempt to learn new skills on the operative experience of their trainees.

Effective Training Methods

Key Concept: Effective surgical training requires time spent prior to the operation learning the skills and discussing the case, in the operation with real-time feedback and open discussion and nonthreatening and honest feedback postoperatively.

Introduction

The three essential elements to achieve successful outcomes in surgery are preoperative, operative, and postoperative detailed patient care. If one of these steps is neglected, patients are at increased risk for complications. This model should be embraced and applied to surgical education. The technical demands and protracted learning curve specifically for LC can be reduced when this three-phase approach is considered. Preoperative preparation, improved intraoperative communication, and immediate objective postoperative assessment with a validated tool will enhance training. Gary Dunnington and his colleagues at SIU (Southern Illinois University) describe this approach as "capturing the teachable moment" and outline their system as B.I.D. ("briefing, intraoperative teaching, and debriefing") [18]. The immediate discussion below will pertain to residents and fellows, as attending surgeons are trained separately through advanced laparoscopic courses. That will be addressed at the end of the chapter.

Preoperative Preparation

Successful preparation for LC requires the trainee to embrace both traditional and nonclinical methods. The necessary approach to reduce the aforementioned barriers and to increase the volume of quality cases performed by residents is often debated. However, surgical educators uniformly agree that nonclinical technical skills exercises, designed to optimize a resident's experience with each operation, will play a critical role. The American College of Surgeons Review Committee for Surgical Education has made it mandatory that all surgical training programs have a means of training outside the operating room [19]. Therefore, simulation and surgical skills laboratories will continue to play a role in training for general and procedure-specific laparoscopic cases (Fig. 37.1). In its broadest terms, simulation is defined as the act of imitating the behavior of some situation or some process by means of something suitably analogous. Therefore, the majority of nonclinical technical skill exercises, regardless of the model, qualify as "simulation." Current platforms vary considerably in level of fidelity, from box trainers to technologically advanced virtual reality (VR) programs.

Simple box trainers for laparoscopic skills such as the validated MISTELS (McGill Inanimate System for Training and Evaluation of Laparoscopic Skills) are effective at the junior trainee level and should be readily incorporated into any laboratory curricula. VR platforms have also been shown to improve performance in the operating room. More specifically, dedicated practice with VR simulators has correlated with improved operative times and efficiency of movement for clinical laparoscopic cholecystectomy [20]. Seymour et al. evaluated 16 residents of varying levels and compared clinical laparoscopic cholecystectomy outcomes between residents who received training on a VR system and those who did not. They found no difference in baseline assessments between the two groups, but found that residents who trained on the simulator were faster, made fewer errors, and were less likely to injure the gallbladder in the operating room [20]. Grantcharov et al. also evaluated 16 residents and compared training on a VR simulator to a control group. They found improved economy of movements and fewer errors in residents who were trained on a VR simulator [21]. Beyer and colleagues evaluated transfer of skills from simulators to the operating room using the Global Operative Assessment of Laparoscopic Skills (GOALS), a validated laparoscopic skills assessment model [22]. Their prospective trial involving 19 residents found improved GOAL scores in residents who were trained on a simulator when compared to those who were not.

Simbionix (Cleveland, OH) offers a VR (LAP Mentor) model for laparoscopic sigmoid colectomy that more accurately portrays resection in the operating room than previous hybrid systems [23]. Of the five types of validity, face, content, and construct have been established for general procedures with the LAP Mentor VRS [24, 25]. More recently, construct validity, i.e., the ability of the simulator to distinguish between different levels of skills, was established for

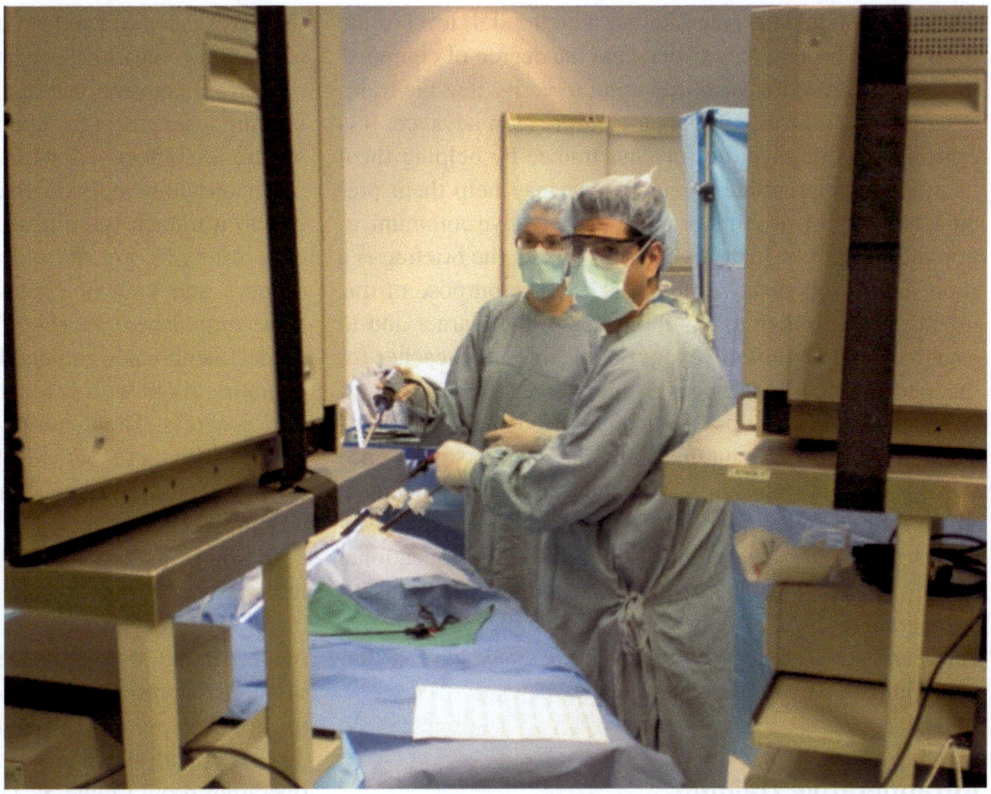

Fig. 37.1 Laparoscopic colectomy in a porcine model

certain metrics specifically with the laparoscopic sigmoid model [26]. In this study, the metrics assessing the instrument path length, the accuracy of the medial peritoneal mobilization, and the quality of the IMA dissection demonstrated the strongest ability to differentiate between general surgeons and laparoscopic colorectal surgeons. However, construct validity was not established for technical errors, as the model could not distinguish between experts and novice surgeons.

The successful application for procedure-specific training with VR systems has recently been demonstrated in two randomized trials. Grantcharov et al. developed a comprehensive ex vivo preoperative training curriculum that improved performance for LC [27]. Calatayud et al. tested "warm-up" with a VR system prior to laparoscopic cholecystectomy and found that OSATS global rating scales were better after practice [28]. The colectomy study involved preparation with simulation, cognitive training, and participation in a cadaver lab. In this study, residents were PGY-2 through 4, having previously completed FLS and possessing some advanced laparoscopic experience. Using an entire curriculum that addressed multiple aspects of performance, which included procedure-specific simulation, overall LC skills were enhanced. This impressive approach was successful; however, having all trainees perform this labor intense program prior to the procedure may not be practical. The cost and time requirements of the model are likely not likely sustainable in most training programs outside of a trial. However, this well-designed trial most importantly demonstrates that preparation can improve performance for LC. Each academic institution may choose to incorporate one of these preparation models or a variation on this theme. The VR studies for basic laparoscopic skills training have routinely incorporated a proficiency-based model, whereby trainees have proficiency targets to meet, rather than time on task as a training goal [20, 27]. For the cognitive component of procedures, different modalities have been used. For example, in an effort to simplify this "rehearsal" and hasten the learning curve for laparoscopic right colectomy, we designed an ongoing multicenter trial with an edited 15-min "voice-over" instructional video for residents to review before performing laparoscopic right colectomy. The results are unknown, but the early feedback has been encouraging.

In addition to simulation and nontraditional preparation, several very basic but underutilized modalities should be considered to improve the educational quality of each LC case for the trainee. Residents must fulfill their responsibility by coming to the operating room with a detailed knowledge of the relevant anatomy, the indications for surgery, steps of the procedure, and the potential complications. Additionally, they should possess, to a certain degree, the skills required to do a portion of the case. As faculty, we often know how to access the best video or atlas that most accurately depicts the appropriate steps of the procedure. Ideally, a curriculum-based approach will include resources for residents to access to enable them to efficiently acquire this knowledge [27].

The trainer should become familiar with the skill level of the resident and be sure they understand the degree of complexity for each case. It is also important to verify that the trainees are being informed about case coverage in advance. It is critical to be an advocate for your trainee by helping them identify the appropriate resources that may help them prepare. Lastly, and most importantly, preoperative communication must improve. In the SIU B.I.D. model, the briefing is a short interaction at the scrub sink [19]. The purpose of this interaction is to both assess the needs of the learner and to establish learning objectives for both learner and teacher for that particular case. This conversation forces a review of past experiences and helps formulate needs and deficits. Furthermore, learners automatically integrate the experience making it more retrievable at a later date. Unfortunately it seems that this interaction seldom occurs. In a recent survey of nearly 5,000 residents, only 18 % felt that the educational goals of the case or details of the procedure are discussed preoperatively [29]. Adoption of this simple yet effective communication strategy, outlined above, may have a dramatic impact on your current trainees.

Intraoperative Training

Preoperative preparation and postoperative assessment for laparoscopic colectomy may be underutilized, but they are both definable and have been evaluated. General intraoperative teaching methods and procedure specific approaches are nebulous. More specifically, each LC entails numerous variables that can hinder consistent and effective training. Three of these variables routinely inhibit a trainee's ability to master laparoscopic colorectal resection, and two are specific to laparoscopy. First, several attending surgeons are not comfortable with their own ability to perform LC. Second, the window between the correct and inaccurate dissection plane is similar to open surgery, but the trainer's ability to control precision and prevent potential problems is slightly compromised with laparoscopy. These two variables are prevalent in academic surgery, but will likely wane in time as the generation of minimally invasive surgeons continues to progress. Lastly, several faculty surgeons frankly have no interest in teaching residents the basics or details of laparoscopic colorectal resection. Unfortunately, the reasons or excuses for this are plentiful and were outlined above (individual, systemic, time constraints, error avoidance, report cards, etc.).

Several conventional and previously studied methods of training residents in the operating room have been described but are less effective for LC. *Scaffolding* involves conscious or unconscious individualized support during surgery relative to a trainee's abilities [30–32]. This style was historically effective, yet the reduction of case volume amongst trainees and lack of consistent faculty-trainee interaction have diminished its role. The Halstedian apprenticeship model also relies significantly on experience acquired in the operating room with graduated responsibility for trainees as they progress. The majority of trainers accomplished in LC learned with these methods, but have failed to recognize that the new landscape of residency likely requires more focused educational opportunities to achieve the same result.

A significant amount of the communication during LC is ineffective. As first assistants, trainers have lost the ability to direct with an instrument or their finger and therefore depend on verbal and nonverbal cues. Roberts et al. provided in an in-depth theoretical analysis of communication in the operating room in an effort to highlight teachable moments [33]. They thoughtfully categorize four types of interaction in the operating room (Table 37.1) [33]. *Instrumental* interactions are the most common form of interaction in the operating room. The goal of the faculty surgeon with these interactions is simply to perform the case as efficiently and safely as possible, with little attention to teaching. All surgeons desire safe and efficient outcomes for their patients; however, to also incorporate teaching surgeons must replace *instrumental only* interactions with *instrumental/teaching* communication, when appropriate. This goal is achievable when an appropriate understanding of mutual expectations and familiarity is established before the procedure. This discussion should also include an explanation by the attending regarding their method of instruction on the two-dimensional monitor that both are viewing. This will decrease *banter* and noneffective interactions.

In addition to improving communication both preoperatively and during the case, surgical educators agree that deliberate practice is critical to master a technical skill. Ericcson explains deliberate practice as identifying an area of performance that is to be improved and then providing immediate detailed feedback during performance [34]. This

Table 37.1 Concepts of intraoperative surgeon-resident interaction outlined by Roberts and colleagues

Intraoperative communication category	Description
Instrumental	Goal of interaction is to move the case forward Termed instrumental because the surgeon often uses the learner like an instrument, as a means to an end
Pure teaching	Intended primarily to benefit the learner through providing educational value
Instrumental and teaching	Intended to achieve the pragmatic goal of moving the case forward while also conferring teaching
Banter	Conversation unrelated to the procedure

From Roberts and Williams [18]

approach is most useful for LC cases when the procedure is deconstructed into steps. Having the trainee master the dissection of the inferior mesenteric artery prior to attempting the pelvic dissection is an example of this. However, the operating room with the inherent variability in disease and patient anatomy, as well as other constraints, may diminish the ability of residents to engage in deliberate practice. Thus, mastery of skills that have ex vivo models available for practice should be transferred to a skills laboratory, reserving operating room learning for fine-tuning of performance.

Guidance and/or supervision in the operating room is critical to learning LC skills; however, it may be suboptimal. A national survey of 125 surgical residency programs addressed resident satisfaction with teaching and showed that 40 % of residents *sometimes* felt "over-supervised" in the operating room and 21 % *always* felt "over-supervised," both contributing to decreased satisfaction [35]. Optimally, the supervising faculty reduces the amount of guidance as trainees ascend along the learning curve and demonstrate improved skills, safety, and confidence. The amount of supervision in the operating room is largely influenced by the complexity of the case, resident experience, attending skill, and desire to teach. This variability will always exist, but the group at Southern Illinois University (SIU) attempted to analyze and investigate operative supervision [36]. To accomplish their goal they used an operative performance rating system and blinded external experts to rate the amount of guidance for videotaped procedures [36]. As expected, the researchers found variability amongst the supervising surgeons and witnessed a reduction in guidance with upper level residents. Furthermore, they discovered that the faculty surgeon typically underestimates the amount of supervision that they provide [36]. This finding requires further exploration and dramatically influences to the ability of faculty to objectively assess a resident's operative performance and ability to ultimately perform the operation independently. This problem is likely enhanced during performance of LC. An experienced faculty member can practically operate with a trainee's hands and tactfully expose the correct plane of dissection. These nonverbal clues are further assisted when the trainer holds the camera and subconsciously orients the line of dissection in the center of the monitor. Ideally, as the trainee becomes more accomplished, a second learning curve develops. This second tier of difficulty is readily exposed when the trainer is replaced with a junior resident. The junior resident is capable of holding the camera and another instrument, but all of the nonverbal guidance and direction are absent. Therefore, as we prepare our trainees to operate independently, we must find a balance between maintaining patient safety and fostering independence. This in essence is the art of surgical education.

Assessment

The structured stepwise approach to LC and ability to video record cases make this an ideal procedure for objective assessment. Prior to the development of validated scoring tools, studies evaluating the performance of trainees in the operating room for LC lacked detail about the complexity of the case, the role of the trainee, and appropriate end points. Conversion rates and operative times were used to assess performance, yet they are likely more reflective of the attending surgeon, not the resident.

After the OSATS (objective structured assessment of technical skill) was developed and validated [37], numerous applications and variations of this tool were introduced for almost every subspecialty (Fig. 37.2). We have now been inundated with validated scoring systems containing both generic and procedure specific metrics, with several measures developed specifically for LC. Unfortunately, it has been demonstrated that substantial time often elapses between performance in the operating room and the completion of an evaluation tool [38]. Ideally, the faculty should complete a technical evaluation at the end of every case, or at least within 24 h. As faculty, we must become familiar with the validated specialty-specific tools for LC that are available for the assessment of trainees. Utilization of a validated assessment tool not only stimulates a post-procedure conversation but also ultimately involves procedure-specific feedback as well areas for improvement and practice.

The GAS (general assessment scale) developed specifically for LC is a great example of this concept (Fig. 37.3) [39]. This validated tool creatively incorporates the amount of verbal/nonverbal support needed for the trainee to complete the steps of the procedure [39]. GAS is ideal for the

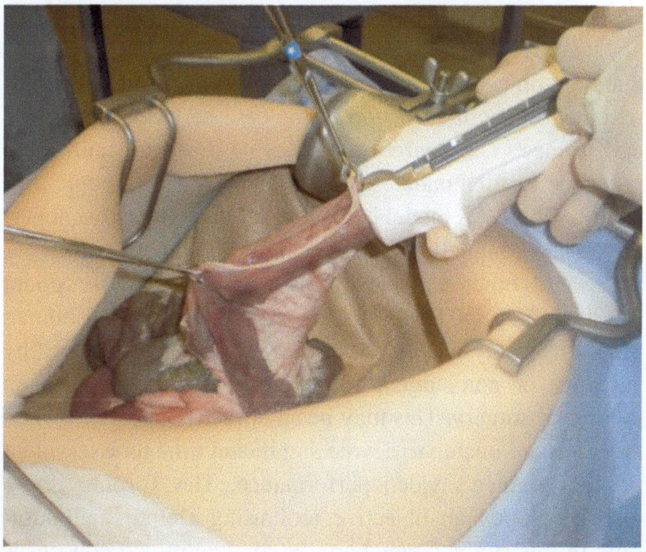

Fig. 37.2 Simulation model for bowel anastomosis

National Training Programme
in Laparoscopic Colorectal Surgery

FORM A

GLOBAL ASSESSMENT BY TRAINER (GAS)

A. PRECEPTOR

A1 Name of Preceptor ☐☐☐☐☐☐☐☐☐☐☐☐☐☐☐☐☐☐☐☐☐☐☐☐☐

A2 Name of Trainee ☐☐☐☐☐☐☐☐☐☐☐☐☐☐☐☐☐☐☐☐☐☐☐☐☐

A3 Patient ID ☐☐☐☐☐☐☐☐☐☐☐☐☐☐☐☐☐☐☐☐☐☐☐☐☐

B4 Operating date ☐☐/☐☐/☐☐☐☐

B. ASSESSMENT

1 Not performed, step had to be done by trainer
2 Partly performed, step had to be partly done by trainer
3 Performed, with substantial verbal support
4 Performed with minor verbal support
5 Competent performance, safe (without guidance)
6 Proficient performance, couldn't be better

EXPOSURE						
B1 Correct theater setup	1☐	2☐	3☐	4☐	5☐	6☐
B2 Appropriate patient positioning	1☐	2☐	3☐	4☐	5☐	6☐
B1 Safe access technique	1☐	2☐	3☐	4☐	5☐	6☐
B4 Exposure of operating field	1☐	2☐	3☐	4☐	5☐	6☐
VASCULAR						
B5 Safe dissection of vascular pedicle	1☐	2☐	3☐	4☐	5☐	6☐
B6 Dissection of mesentry (retrocolic)	1☐	2☐	3☐	4☐	5☐	6☐
B7 Safe identification of ureter or duodenum	1☐	2☐	3☐	4☐	5☐	6☐
MOBILISATION						
B8 Dissection of hepatic or splenic flexure	1☐	2☐	3☐	4☐	5☐	6☐
B9 Mesorectal dissection (where applicable)	1☐	2☐	3☐	4☐	5☐	6☐
B10 Safe dissection of bowel	1☐	2☐	3☐	4☐	5☐	6☐
ANASTOMOSIS						
B11 Safe evacuation of specimen	1☐	2☐	3☐	4☐	5☐	6☐
B12 Anastomosis	1☐	2☐	3☐	4☐	5☐	6☐
OVERALL PERFORMANCE						
B13 Overall Performance	1☐	2☐	3☐	4☐	5☐	6☐

C. ASSESSING THE ASSESSMENT

C1 How dificult was this operation (1=very easy, 6=very difficult)	1☐	2☐	3☐	4☐	5☐	6☐

C1 How useful was this form for the assessment of this particular case?

Not useful ☐ Mainly not useful☐ Partly not useful☐ Partly useful☐ Mainly useful☐ Very useful☐

C2 How long did it take you to fill in this form? ☐☐ minutes

Version 1/ 16.09.2008 REC Ref number 04/Q040354

Fig. 37.3 National Training Programme in Laparoscopic Colorectal Surgery (Modified from Miskovic et al. [39])

assessment of trainees and can be effectively modified for any laparoscopic colorectal resection or resident level. It produces an objective score but also can be used to foster communication about each step of the case between the faculty and trainee. The degree of nonverbal communication and guidance is often underestimated during a laparoscopic procedure. The GAS model helps remind the trainee that supervision and completing the case can be all perception!

Several other validated tools exist for the assessment LC, including OCHRA [40] (Observational clinical human reliability analysis). This software program can be used by surgeons or non-surgeons to evaluate operative videos in colorectal surgery. This may be an attractive approach when surgeons are unable to devote significant time to assessment of their trainee's video performance. The Toronto group also developed an objective tool using Delphi methodology. In this study, Grantcharov et al. determined consensus for the essential steps to be included on a tool designed to measure technical competence for LC [41]. The reliability and validity of this model will require further validation, but it has potential for the evaluation of training and practicing surgeons.

To effectively incorporate meaningful assessment tools into residency, department chairs, general surgery program directors, and colorectal program directors must mandate their usage and study their effectiveness. The lack of consensus on a national scale and even within colorectal surgery is a major impediment. Agreement on a validated comprehensive assessment tool for LC will require considerable investment. However, without formative assessment, technical deficiencies will persist, and both general and colorectal residents will continue to struggle with LC. Procedure-based assessments are mandated in training programs in the United Kingdom. These operation-specific tools cover all components of a procedure from the preoperative assessment and consent to the operative steps. This strategy is excellent for formative feedback, yet multiple evaluations of the resident on each procedure are required for reliable assessment (Fig. 37.4).

Laparoscopic Courses, Training Attending Surgeons

Key Concept: Unique barriers exist when expanding training to attending surgeons, especially with regard to determining competence with short "hands-on" courses.

Over the last decade innumerable laparoscopic colectomy "hands-on" courses have been offered at academic institutions and society meetings. The average annual budget for the two largest companies sponsoring these programs has been reported at approximately $500,000/year. Early success was measured by determining if the attendees returned to their home institution and attempted LC [42]. However, data tracking either long-term adoption of LC into practice or patient outcomes for these cases has never been reported. Over the years, SAGES and ASCRS provided "guidelines" for these postgraduate courses, but the enforcement or adherence to these recommendations has not been evaluated. The guidelines highlight the importance of performing greater than 25 resections per year and the need for follow-up mentorship. Ho et al. recently reported that approximately 46 % of surgeons attending courses at their institution over the years have no access to mentors [43]. The authors recommended tele-mentoring as a potential avenue to improve training for those attending LC courses; however, currently the medicolegal implications and reimbursement for this type of approach have not been addressed.

Optimizing the training experience for an attending surgeon attempting to learn LC at a 2-day course also requires significant preparation. Surgeons with a variety of

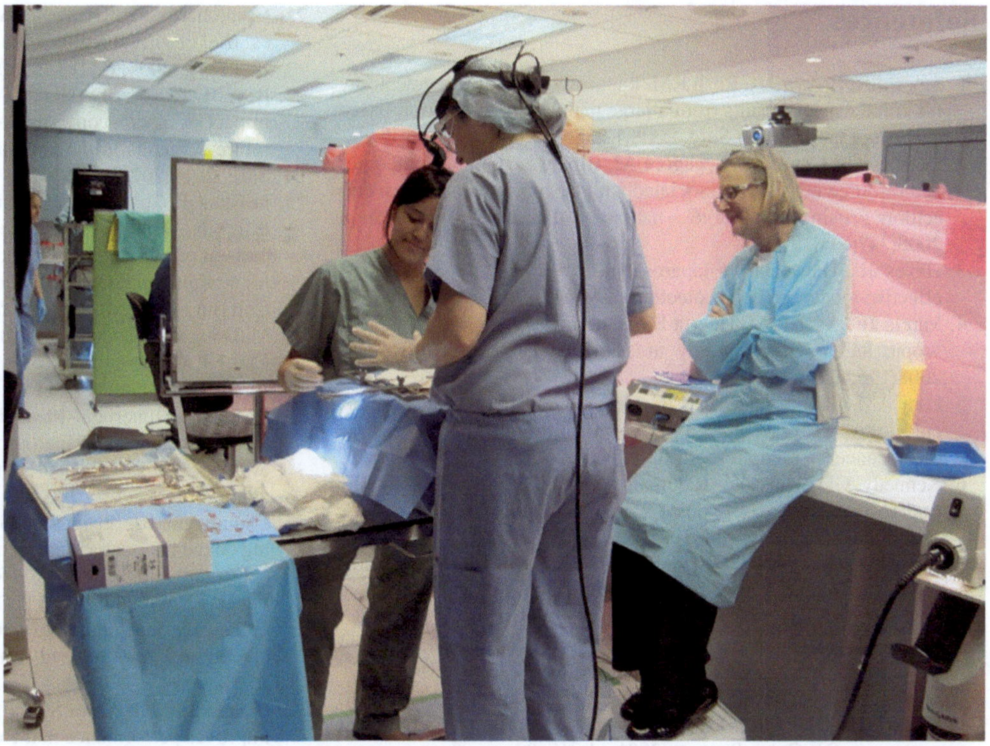

Fig. 37.4 Attending surgeon evaluation and constructive feedback at a skill station

backgrounds and skill often participate in the same sessions. Course directors and their industry partners rarely scrutinize the participants prior to the day of the course, and the needs of each attending surgeon vary tremendously. It is not uncommon, within the same course, to have one surgeon learning how to use both hands with another inquiring about low rectal transection and single incision techniques. This can be improved by performing a more careful survey of potential attendees and categorizing applicants based on experience and goals.

Both cadaveric and porcine models have been used successfully during these workshops. Cadaver labs offer a more realistic anatomical approach, but they are expensive and at times inconsistent. The porcine model is excellent for laparoscopic sigmoid colectomy, but they lack a right colon, limiting the overall experience. Participants continue to rate the "live OR" experience as the most meaningful section of the course. Furthermore, attendees frequently request the actual videos and power point lectures that are given during their visit. If the course director's goal is to optimize uptake of LC, these resources should be made readily available for participants.

In addition to pre-course surveys, participants should agree to send their follow-up operative videos for blinded assessment. Previous studies have shown that surgeons consistently overestimate their own performance during or after their participation in a course [44]. Industry should budget longitudinal mentoring with both video assessment and potentially a second visit from either the trainee or trainer. The validated CAT (Competency Assessment Tool) and OCHRA, both described by Miskovic et al., could be used for the objective assessment of videos with this method [45].

Summary Pearls

Maintaining a standard of excellence for LC requires a comprehensive and consistent approach to surgical education. Faculty in academic institutions must continue to fight for the appropriate resources and incentives needed to train the next generation of surgeons. The impact of health care on education with the inevitable push to provide less expensive but equivalent and more efficient care must be carefully considered.

Recent studies with simulation have shown promise for training as a pre-procedure "warm-up" and also for potential assessment. However, we must continue to ask, "At what cost?" If less expensive, but as effective methods exist, they should be utilized. Faculty surgeons must also strive to vastly improve day-to-day communication with trainees before the procedure, intraoperatively, and with assessment postoperatively. Several validated metrics and tools of assessment exist for LC, but as a surgical specialty we must collaborate and reach consensus to improve their widespread utilization. Lastly, the technological advancements particular to minimally invasive surgery must also be scrutinized more effectively. As leaders in the world of surgical education, we must ensure that our trainees are not overlooked in place of personal or professional gains.

References

1. Steele SR, Brown TA, Rush RM. Laparoscopic vs. open colectomy for colon cancer: results from a large nationwide population-based analysis. J Gastrointest Surg. 2008;12:583–91.
2. Delaney CP, Change E, Senagore AJ, Broder M. Clinical outcomes and resource utilization associated with laparoscopic and open colectomy using a large national database. Ann Surg. 2008;247(5):819–24.
3. Hayes JL, Hansen P. Is laparoscopic colectomy for cancer cost effective relative to open colectomy? ANZ J Surg. 2007;77:782–6.
4. Varela JE, Asolati M, Huerta S, Anthony T. Outcomes of laparoscopic and open colectomy at academic centers. Am J Surg. 2008;196:403–6.
5. Lacy AM, Garcia-Valdecasas JC, Delgado S. Laparoscopic-assisted colectomy vs. open colectomy for treatment of non-metastatic colon cancer: a randomized trial. Lancet. 2002;359:2224–9.
6. Kennedy GD, Heise C, Rajamanickam V, Harms B, Foley EF. Laparoscopy decreases postoperative complication rates after abdominal colectomy. Ann Surg. 2009;249:596–601.
7. Kang CY, Chaudhry OO, Halabi WJ, et al. Outcomes of laparoscopic colorectal surgery: data from the Nationwide Inpatient Sample 2009. Am J Surg. 2012;204(6):952–7.
8. Senagore AJ, Luchtefeld MA, Mackeigan JM. What is the learning curve for laparoscopic colectomy? Am Surg. 1995;61:681–5.
9. Schlata CM, Mamazza J, Seshadri PA, Cadeddu M, Gregoire R, Poulin EC. Defining a learning curve for laparoscopic colorectal resections. Dis Colon Rectum. 2001;44:217–22.
10. Dincler S, Koller MT, Steurer J, Bachmann LM, Christen D, Buchmann P. Multidimensional analysis of learning curves in laparoscopic sigmoid resection: eight year results. Dis Colon Rectum. 2003;46:1371–3.
11. Stein SL, Sulberg J, Champagne BJ. Learning laparoscopic colectomy during colorectal residency: what does it take and how are we doing? Surg Endosc. 2012;26:488–92.
12. Charron P, Campbell R, DeJesus S, Gallagher J, Williamson P, Ferrara A. The gap in laparoscopic colorectal experience between colon and rectal and general surgery residency training programs. Dis Colon Rectum. 2007;50:2023–31.
13. Alkhoury F, Martin JT, Contessa J, et al. The impact of laparoscopy on the volume of open cases in general surgery training. J Surg Educ. 2010;67(5):316–9.
14. Weber WP, Guller U, Jain NB, et al. Impact of surgeon and hospital caseload on the likelihood of performing laparoscopic vs open sigmoid resection for diverticular disease: a study based on 55,949 patients. Arch Surg. 2007;142:253–9.
15. Pugh CM, Darosa DA, Santacaterina S, Clark RE. Faculty evaluation of simulation-based modules for assessment of intraoperative decision making. Surgery. 2011;149(4):534–42.
16. Stain SC, Biester TW, Hanks JB, et al. Early tracking would improve the operative experience of general surgery residents. Ann Surg. 2010;252(3):445–9; discussion 449–51.
17. Drolet BC, Sangisetty S, Tracy TF, et al. Surgical residents' perceptions of 2011 accreditation council for graduate medical education duty hour regulations. JAMA Surg. 2013;148(5):427–33.
18. Roberts NK, Williams RG. The briefing, intraoperative teaching, debriefing model for teaching in the operating room. J Am Coll Surg. 2008;10:299–303.
19. Roberts KE, Bell RL, et al. Evolution of surgical skills training. World J Gastroenterol. 2006;12(20):3219–24.
20. Crochet P, Aggarwal R, Dubb SS, et al. Deliberate practice on a virtual reality laparoscopic simulator enhances the quality of surgical technical. Ann Surg. 2011;253(6):1216–22.
21. Grantcharov TP, Kristiansen VB, Bendix J, et al. Randomized clinical trial of virtual reality simulation for laparoscopic skills training. Br J Surg. 2004;91(2):146–50.
22. Beyer L, Troyer JD, Mancini J, Bladou F, Berdah SV, Karsenty G. Impact of laparoscopy simulator training on the technical skills of future surgeons in the operating room: a prospective study. Am J Surg. 2011;202(3):265–72.
23. LeBlanc F, Champagne BJ, Augestad KM, Neary PC, Senagore AJ, Ellis CN, Delaney CP, Colorectal Surgery Training Group. A comparison of human cadaver and augmented reality simulator models for straight laparoscopic colorectal skills acquisition training. J Am Coll Surg. 2012;211(2):250–5.
24. McDougall EM, Corica FA, Boker JR, Sala LG, Stoliar G, Borin JF, Chu FT, Clayman RV. Construct validity testing of a laparoscopic surgical simulator. J Am Coll Surg. 2006;202:779–87.
25. Zhang A, Hünerbein M, Dai Y, Schlag PM, Beller S. Construct validity testing of a laparoscopic surgery simulator (Lap Mentor): evaluation of surgical skill with a virtual laparoscopic training simulator. Surg Endosc. 2008;22:1440–4.
26. Champagne BJ, Shanmugan S, Leblanc F, et al. Virtual reality training on the GI mentor laparoscopic sigmoid model: what metrics have construct validity. Dis Colon Rectum. 2013 (in press).
27. Palter VN, Grantcharov TP. Development and validation of a comprehensive curriculum to teach an advanced minimally invasive procedure: a randomized controlled trial. Ann Surg. 2012;256(1):25–32.
28. Calatayud MD, Arora S. Warm-up in a virtual reality environment improves performance in the operating room. Ann Surg. 2010;251:1181–5.
29. Snyder RA, Tarpley MJ, Tarpley JL, Davidson M, Brophy C, Dattilo JB. Teaching in the operating room: results of a national survey. J Surg Educ. 2012;69(5):643.
30. DeGrave WS, Dolmans DH, Van Der Vleuten CP. Profiles of effective tutors in problem-based learning: scaffolding student learning. Med Educ. 1999;33(12):901–6.
31. Carter BN. The fruition of Halsted's concept of surgical training. Surgery. 1952;32:518–27.
32. Whitson BA, Hoang CD, Jie T, Maddaus MA. Technology-enhanced interactive surgical education. J Surg Res. 2006;136(1):13–8.
33. Roberts NK, Brenner MJ, et al. Capturing the teachable moment: a grounded theory study of verbal teaching interactions in the operating room. Surgery. 2012;151:643–50.
34. Kim MJ, Boehler ML. Skills coaches as part of the educational team: a randomized controlled trial of teaching of a basic surgical skill in the laboratory setting. Am J Surg. 2010;199:94–8.
35. Chen X, Williams R, et al. How do supervising surgeons evaluate guidance provided in the operating room? Am J Surg. 2012;203:44–8.
36. Sanfey HA, Dunnington GL. Basic surgical skills testing for junior residents: current views of general surgery program directors. J Am Coll Surg. 2011;212:406–12.
37. Martin JA, Regehr G, et al. Objective structured assessment of technical skill (OSATS) for surgical residents. Br J Surg. 1997;84(2):273–8.
38. Kim MJ, Williams RG, Boehler ML, et al. Refining the evaluation of operating room performance. J Surg Educ. 2009;66(6):352–6.
39. Miskovic D, Wyles S, et al. Development, validation and implementation of a monitoring tool for training in laparoscopic colorectal surgery in the English National Training Program. Surg Endosc. 2011;25:1136–42.
40. Miskovic D, Ni M, et al. Observational clinical human reliability analysis for competency assessment in laparoscopic colorectal surgery at the specialist level. Surg Endosc. 2012;26:796–803.
41. Palter VN, Graafland M, Schijven MP, Grantcharov TP. Designing a proficiency-based, content validated virtual reality curriculum for

laparoscopic colorectal surgery: a Delphi approach. Surgery. 2012; 151(3):391–7.
42. Ross HM, Simmang CL, Fleshman JW, Marcello PW. Adoption of laparoscopic colectomy: results and implications of ASCRS hands-on course participation. Surg Innov. 2008;15(3):179–83.
43. Ho VP, Trencheva K, Stein SL, Milsom JW. Mentorship for participants in a laparoscopic colectomy course. Surg Endosc. 2012;26(3): 722–6.
44. Sarker SJ, Telfah MM, Onuba L, et al. Objective assessment of skills acquisition during laparoscopic surgery courses. Surg Innov. 2013;20(5):530–8
45. Miskovic D, Ni M, Wyles SM, Kennedy RH, et al. Is competency assessment at the specialist level achievable? A study for the national training programme in laparoscopic colorectal surgery in England. National Training Programme in Laparoscopic Colorectal Surgery in England. Ann Surg. 2013;257(3):476–82.

The Surgeon Investigator: Balancing Research and Clinical Practice

38

Nancy N. Baxter

Key Points

- Set the stage for success: negotiate for what you need and set expectations realistically based on resources available.
- Actively seek out mentorship and manage the mentoring relationship.
- Set priorities and block off time for research—avoid letting clinical time creep into research time.
- Understand the metrics of success at your institution.

Introduction

Surgeons bring a unique perspective to research; clinical input can be particularly relevant in framing appropriate questions with the potential for impact. Involvement of clinicians in the research process increases the potential that research findings are translated into practice. Research is for many a particularly rewarding part of a career; however, attempting to balance a career as a surgeon and an investigator is challenging. Although research is often considered a requirement of academic appointments, many surgeon investigators are not well supported. There are of course many paths to success; however, many of the barriers to success are common and if not always avoidable can at least be anticipated.

Getting Started

Key Concept: *You need to set yourself up for success from the very beginning. In light of this, research is similar to many other endeavors—you need to have proper training, adequate time allocation, and support and have clear (and documented) communication with your supervisors regarding what is expected of both your clinical and research production.*

As with most operations, advanced planning increases the likelihood of a good outcome. Prior to starting your academic position, three key elements will strongly affect your likelihood of success.

Training

In today's very competitive grant environment, research training is a virtual requirement for success as a surgeon investigator. Although highly motivated surgeons without research training become productive researchers, becoming a principal investigator with peer-reviewed funding without research training is difficult. Some surgeons have obtained advanced degrees while in surgical residency or fellowship and while this is clearly advantageous; for those who have not, obtaining adequate research training is a necessary first step and may need to be completed during the first years of an academic appointment. This can be an advantage. If you are at a new institution, enrolling in an advanced degree will help integrate you in the research community, enabling a new researcher to make important connections outside their direct specialty. Additionally, thesis work can be designed to develop seamlessly into a program of research. However, requirements for an advanced degree will add yet more demands on time, and maintaining a balance in an early career will be even more challenging.

Negotiation

Although your success is important to those who have hired you, heads of departments and divisions have many competing objectives—you are only one small piece in a very large puzzle. It is therefore essential to optimally use opportunities

N.N. Baxter, MD, PhD, FRCSC, FACS
Division of General Surgery,
University of Toronto, St Michael's Hospital,
30 Bond St., 16CC-040, Toronto, ON MSB 2H9, Canada
e-mail: baxtern@smh.ca; baxtern@smh.toronto.on.ca

S.R. Steele et al. (eds.), *Complexities in Colorectal Surgery*,
DOI 10.1007/978-1-4614-9022-7_38, © Springer Science+Business Media New York 2014

to negotiate for resources. Protected time and research support are key components of success and should be part of job negotiations for surgeon investigators at any level. This may be a challenge for new surgeons searching for their first job; however, mistakes made at the negotiating table can haunt for years. Junior level faculty are often overwhelmed by clinical volume, and unless there is a meaningful and supported plan to put time aside for research, managing a successful balance between clinical duties and research is unlikely. Although surgeon investigators can expect to work on research at night and on weekends, having night and weekends as one's only "protected" research time is not tenable. Equally, being given protected time for research without salary support for these nonclinical duties results in an unfunded mandate that often becomes a low priority in a busy practice. Ideally, the proportion of time set aside for research should be specified and a realistic mechanism to achieve this protected time should be made explicit. It is key that this plan is supported not only by your division head but also by clinical colleagues and is reflected in work schedules and duty hours. Expectations with respect to clinical revenues should be commensurate with the portion of time given to clinical work. Although there is an expectation that most investigators will eventually obtain support for their research time through external funding, salary support for research time must be part of any recruitment package. Given the current funding environment, the standard 3 years of salary support is no longer appropriate; 5 years of support is more realistic.

In general, surgical researchers at the beginning of their careers do not come to a first job with an established funding source for research projects (if you do, negotiate for more as you should be highly attractive to many academic institutions!). Your initial research must therefore be supported until independent funding can be obtained. Although, in general, such support is given in the form of "start-up money" for an investigator to use based on their own best judgement, support may also be given in kind, particularly from senior researchers. Ask for what you need; some research is inherently more expensive than others particularly if purchasing equipment is required. If your researcher has such needs, go into negotiations prepared to argue your case with a clear outline of the costs of your research. Otherwise, if possible, find some information about typical start-up packages at your institution and other institutions. This will give you a benchmark of what is considered acceptable and certainly don't ask for less. Some administrators may consider clinical research less costly; however, this has not been my experience. Clinical research often requires involvement of research assistants, analysts, clinical trials nurses, etc., and hiring personnel for research can be quite expensive.

Protected time, salary support, and research funding (amount and duration) should be specified in your contract. Although having a lawyer review your contract may cause some discomfort, in many circumstances, it is advisable.

Managing Expectations

Universities differ greatly in how success is defined—have a clear understanding from the outset how your productivity will be assessed by the chief of your department and university. For example, some institutions may consider obtaining early investigator funding at the national level (i.e., a K award) as the main marker of success for the early career researcher, while others may accept a certain number of research publications per year. Be absolutely sure that the level of research productivity expected is consistent with the amount of protected time and research support that you have been given. If you are offered 20 % protected time, expectations should be *considerably* lower than if you have 50 % or 70 % of your time supported. With anything less than 40 % protected research time, expectations of K awards and/or peer-reviewed grant funding are completely unrealistic.

Universities have appointment reviews and tenure timelines; it is essential to understand the process and begin planning early. At a minimum, have a crystal clear understanding of the expectations for your first review, when this will be conducted, who will attend, and what the ramifications of the review might be. If you need to pursue additional training, ensure that your tenure timeline will be extended, as you are unlikely to be extremely productive when taking courses or obtaining an advanced degree.

Ongoing communication is also critical. In particular if university or departmental commitments for protected time and/or start-up monies are not met, this must be communicated and rectified early. If issues develop that affect your ability to achieve the amount of protected time promised, for example, the departure of a clinical partner, it is important that this is noted and documented and expectations of research productivity changed.

How to Establish a Research Career While Starting Your Practice

Key Concept: You will spend more time, and ultimately be much more successful, doing what you really feel passionate about. Understanding not only your goals but also the resources of your institution will help maximize your efficiency, while developing a clinical practice and research agenda.

Starting your research career is daunting. Most of us have a very clear vision of the clinical aspects of our career, what operations we will be doing, what types of patients we will be seeing, etc. The plans for our research careers, however, are often considerably less concrete and may need to change markedly depending on the resources and opportunities available. While this is an exciting time, when researchers are full of energy, enthusiasm, and willingness to try new things, an inability to find focus may result in a failure to launch.

Transitioning to Independence

Surgical training is long and arduous; the structure is highly hierarchical and creative thinking is not generally encouraged. In contrast, research success often depends on developing novel and creative ideas in collegial groups with a considerably less vertical power structure. It can be very challenging to transition from training to independence in both the clinical and research world. Developing a research agenda can be difficult and the source of much angst. Starting in a new environment can be particularly hard as research partnerships and collaborations need to be started from scratch. In contrast, staying at the institution where you trained, while comfortable, may pose problems in establishing independence from previous supervisors. This can be a very challenging period—in the best of circumstances, when many doors are open, at least some must be closed. In less fortunate circumstances, all doors may seem closed and an individual may need to do a lot of knocking to get anywhere.

It is critical to begin to develop a research agenda; however, this can only be achieved by taking time for self-reflection: honestly ask yourself what your research goals and passions are. Some researchers see a career with a specific disease focus, for example, evaluating a molecular pathway for a specific malignancy; some researchers are issue-focused, for example, evaluating quality of surgical care in populations; while finally, others may be focused on specific methodology, for example, evaluating the conduct of systematic reviews. There are a number of key factors to developing a successful program of research. First, it is essential to take advantage of the opportunities and resources at your academic institution. Be flexible—can your research interests match those of established well-respected researchers in your institution, even if this means some changes in your research focus? Working closely with established researchers will increase your chance of success. Be open to new ideas and be opportunistic. Continue to follow paths that result in success and consider not persevering on those that seem to result in failure. It is however important to maintain passion for the research you are doing—you must be confident in the potential for your work or you will soon find more rewarding things to do.

For surgeons, it is important to remember that some research may resonate with the scientific community but not the clinical community. Advancing in your surgical societies is important for career satisfaction and academic promotion; therefore, consider planning your research strategically; if your main body of research is likely to be of most interest to the basic science community, consider developing some discrete research projects of interest to clinicians in your field. Actively think about maintaining a balanced research portfolio.

Mentorship

Key Concept: Few scientists are successful without good mentorship; for those that do succeed without a mentor, the path is difficult. Yet, choosing the right *mentor for you versus* any *mentor is likely more important.*

Effective mentoring has been demonstrated to influence research productivity [1] and most academic institutions try, with variable success, to foster the development of mentorships for junior faculty. Although it is important to establish good mentoring relationships early in an academic career, there is little advice about how to accomplish this.

An effective mentor can be thought of as a coach, with the ability to listen actively and insightfully as key attributes. In general, effective mentors have power—they are senior and successful in their fields with the ability to provide opportunities to their mentees [2]. Importantly, a mentor should generally not have a direct supervisory role over the mentee; supervisors have inherent conflict between the needs of the individual and the needs of the division or department, whereas an ideal mentor remains objective and honest and has only the best interest of the mentee at heart. Of course, mentor-mentee relationships as in all relationships have chemistry; when choosing a mentor, it is important to consider not just the status of an individual but also your compatibility with that person in terms of common interests and personality. Once a relationship is established, being a good mentee is essential to maintaining your mentor's investment. Demonstrate that you actively listen and take advice even when this may be difficult. Just as selecting a mentor with adequate time to invest in the relationship is important, demonstrating respect for your mentor's time is critical; be reliable and prepared. To get the most out of a mentoring relationship, plan regular meetings no less than quarterly, and particularly at the beginning of your career, monthly meetings are better. Set goals, objectives, and timelines with your mentor and work towards your objectives at each meeting.

Because most institutions do not recognize the contributions of mentors in any significant way, in general mentors are motived by less concrete factors. Recognizing the contribution of your mentor and understanding what motivates him/her are keys to enhancing the relationship. The best mentors are altruistic and recognize the need to contribute to the next generation of leaders. For many, enthusiasm is infectious and the dynamism and energy of early researchers can be inspiring to those who have been doing research for some time. Manage up—if you have developed an effective mentor-mentee relationship, maintain it by ensuring your mentor is satisfied with your progress and participation. However, it is important to ensure that the main goal of the relationship is to be of assistance to you, the mentee; sharing ideas does not mean sharing intellectual property; you own your ideas—not your mentor. Additionally, providing guidance should not be interpreted being in control; the goal is not for you to do your mentor's work. Managing boundaries is important, and while most mentors understand their role, be aware that not every mentoring relationship ends positively.

Finding an effective mentor can be a real challenge, particularly for academic surgeons. Expecting a single individual to be capable of mentoring a surgeon at the beginning of their career, often in a subspecialized area of surgery with specific research interests, is frankly unrealistic. Start with self-assessment; determine the key aspects of your career that would be enhanced by effective mentoring. If there is a surgeon at your institution capable of mentoring you in all the areas of need, consider yourself lucky. Otherwise, consider a number of mentors with the appropriate skills and expertise in each of these key areas. For example, having a clinical mentor who is a skilled surgeon in your specialty, a research mentor who is a well-regarded academic expert in your field of research, and an academic mentor who can give you feedback and guidance about departmental and university politics and policy would potentially be an effective mentoring team. Formal mentorship programs, where a new recruit is assigned a mentor, may not work as well as relationships that develop through the initiative of the mentee [2]. If there is a formal mentorship program at your institution, take advantage of it. However, ask for a number of mentor options and speak with suitable potential mentors to determine if there is a good fit. This approach has a greater likelihood for success. Be active in your pursuit of mentorship; evaluate who in your academic community would have the skills and ability to be a mentor to you. Ask others who they would recommend as mentors in your research area at your institution. Consider approaching potential mentors with a direct request or consider a courtship—perhaps engage a potential mentor in short-term collaboration to see if the appropriate chemistry develops.

In the current era of connectivity, distance mentoring may meet specific mentoring needs. While an "e-mentor" should not replace a mentor at your institution, developing a supportive and advisory relationship outside your institution may be essential, particularly if you have a novel program of research for your institution or are relatively isolated in your surgical field. "e-mentorship" can also be an effective way to maintain existing mentoring relationships when you transition to a staff position, or change academic positions. Many societies offer the mentoring programs, matching mentors and mentees at different institutions. These can be very useful, particularly for high-level career advice and networking.

Remember there are other forms of mentorship that can be highly effective and have a lasting career impact. Peer mentoring, where a relationship develops between individuals at a similar career stage, is often highly effective. The peer mentoring relationship is bidirectional, i.e., at times, an individual is the mentor in the relationship, while at other times, the same individual is the mentee. Peers are able to share learning, coach each other through specific tasks, and provide support. Peer-peer relationships may be characterized by a less constrained interchange of ideas and concerns, as they are less hierarchical than traditional mentoring relationships. However, peers often compete for resources, opportunities, and success, and therefore, the peer mentoring relationship needs to be managed carefully.

With continuous progress in surgical technique and technology, reverse mentoring is real and an important way for a new academic surgeon to establish their expertise, demonstrate value to their department, and develop good will among surgical colleagues. If you have been brought to your department with the goal of bring a new technique (surgical or research), consider sharing your expertise with other departmental members. In many cases, it will be important to be sensitive and wait for the right moment to express a willingness to help a more senior colleague learn something new. If you will be playing the role of a reverse mentor, be explicit about this—develop a plan and set goals, objectives, and limitations. In this way, you can avoid potential abuse of your time and talents while ensuring you are given adequate credit for your efforts. Before undertaking this, develop support at the departmental or divisional level and be acknowledged appropriately. Most importantly, be generous and kind; remember that 1 day you may be in need of reverse mentoring yourself. Finally, if the mentor-mentee relationship is not working for either of you, it is best to simply part ways early rather than struggle through in a nonproductive and often discordant relationship.

Setting Priorities and Managing Your Time

Key Concept: You cannot accomplish everything all at once. Instead of spinning your wheels, develop a wish/task list, prioritize it, and be flexible to adjust along the way or say "no."

David Sackett wrote that setting priorities is a critical element to a research career that determines success as a clinician scientist [3]. He suggests conducting a priority setting exercise that consists of generating and documenting four lists:

- *List 1*: *Things I'm doing that I want to quit.*
- *List 2*: *Things I'm not doing that I want to start.*
- *List 3*: *Things I want to keep doing.*
- *List 4*: *How I plan to shorten List 1 and lengthen List 2 over the next 6 months.*

These lists should be revisited at least once every 6 months with the expectation that list 1 is SHORTER and list 2 is LONGER. From experience, this can be extraordinarily difficult to do in practice, but is important to achieve long-term goals. When starting a career, there may be many demands made on your time outside of your clinical work: committee work, teaching, etc. This is not to even mention your personal and family responsibilities. Acceptance of some divisional, departmental, or university duties is almost certainly expected as part of good citizenship. Be strategic; try to align committee participation with your research or clinical goals, for example, participation on the endoscopy committee may allow you to lead a quality improvement initiative. Ask mentors about what opportunities to seek and what time sinks to avoid. Importantly, enthusiastic and competent clinicians are always in demand and thus learning to say no is important, or you will find yourself overextended and failing to live up to commitments. Making commitments when distracted or rushed is almost always regretted—give yourself time for decisions and only accept when you will be able to meet the obligations; establish a reputation for follow-through. Once your schedule is full, when asked to take on a new commitment, there are several things you should consider. First, is this an absolute "must do"? There are many different reasons why something is a "must do"—this may be a once in a lifetime opportunity, a role with highly strategic potential, or something required by your department head. If the activity is not a "must do" but is something you would like to do, do not commit until you understand the time commitment, evaluated your schedule, and determined what activity you will stop doing to make the time. Importantly, the activities you plan to stop should not be spending time with your family, taking vacation, or exercising!

Managing your time is very challenging as there will be many competing demands; busy clinician scientists often fall into the trap of using designated research time as "flexible" time (i.e., time that can be used for clinical activities if necessary). This can become a slippery slope that results in clinical duties routinely being scheduled into research time. Block out research time in your schedule. A half day should be the minimum time blocked; it is almost impossible to think or write in a creative and meaningful way in an hour set aside here or there. Within your research time, designate time for specific activities—this helps to move projects forward and enables advanced planning. If you plan to apply for a grant, you should be scheduling time to work on the grant MANY months in advance. When possible, plan your clinical schedule around important research activities; for example, try to avoid having your OR day on the day of the week important research rounds are given at your institution. There may be days that have you scheduled for research time, but lack the focus to make progress, for example, on a day you are particularly worried about a sick patient or you were on call the night before. I like to have "busy work" ready for times like these—tasks that need to be done, but do not require a great deal of focus or mental energy, for example, updating your CV and completing administrative tasks for grants.

Publishing

Key Concept: *Publishing is expected of a surgical investigator. Remember to have projects at various stages along the pipeline, and choose your journals wisely when submitting manuscripts for publication.*

One of the main benchmarks to academic success is of course publishing in peer-reviewed journals. Because publications are so important, it is essential to plan your program of research to ensure that you publish early in your research career. Because major projects started at the beginning of an academic appointment may take years to come to fruition, developing smaller projects that would lead to a research product sooner is strategically very important. The creation of a well-balanced research portfolio will help with appointment reviews and with grant applications. A good policy is to at all times have at least one manuscript submitted to a journal or in press, one manuscript in preparation for submission, one "short" research project in progress, and one multiyear research project ongoing.

Academic progress is measured by both the quantity and quality of research product. It is easy to count the number of articles published, as this is definitely considered a metric of success anywhere. However, universities and programs are aware that not all peer-reviewed publications are equal; the journal of publication is therefore considered a prime indicator of the quality of the academic product. Although the highest profile publications in your area of research or clinical activity are likely well known to you, they may not be well known to university promotion committees. Many universities now require that the Impact Factor of each journal be indicated in the publication record of your CV. It is therefore critical for early investigators to understand what the Impact Factor is and how potential target journals for your research product may differ substantially based on this metric.

The Impact Factor is published annually by Thomson Reuters as part of the Science Citation Index [4] and is available through library services at most academic institutions.

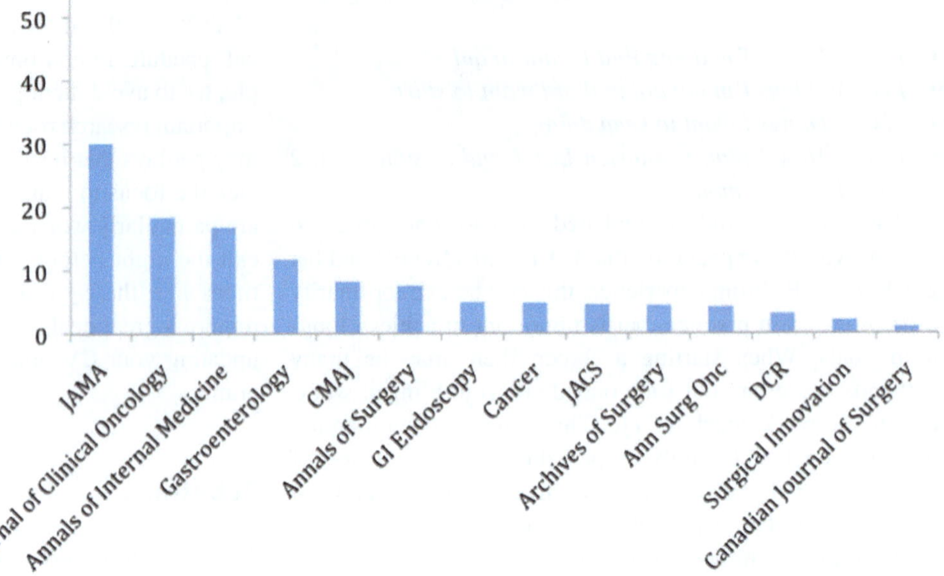

Fig. 38.1 2011 Impact Factor for select journals publishing my work within the past 5 years

Although not the sole method of determining the relative rank of journals, it is the overwhelmingly dominant metric. The Impact Factor is a measure of the average number of citations for articles in a given journal; the Impact Factor for journals in the year 2013 will be calculated in the following manner:

A. Total number of articles published in journal in 2011
B. Total number of articles published in the journal in 2012
C. Total number of citations in the medical literature in 2013 to articles published in the journal in 2011 or 2012

$$2013 \text{ ImpactFactor} = C/(A+B)$$

Figure 38.1 presents the Impact Factor for some of the journals I have published in over the past 5 years. Several things are notable; first, the highest ranked surgical journal, *Annals of Surgery* (Impact Factor 7.492), does not have a particularly high Impact Factor when compared to other journals. The journals with the highest Impact Factor tend to be general medical journals such as the *New England Journal of Medicine* (53.298) and *JAMA* (30.026). These are journals with a wide readership and are highly influential. However, even among medical specialties, the Impact Factor for *Annals of Surgery* is not particularly high. For example, if I have surgical research of broad interest to the surgical and oncology community, I would at least consider sending my manuscript for consideration to the *Journal of Clinical Oncology* (Impact Factor 18.372) before sending it to *Annals of Surgery*.

When selecting a journal, I have three considerations:

1. Who will want to publish my work? Is the work novel or likely to have general interest and impact? If the answer to these questions is yes, then I will submit my work to a journal with a broad readership and a high Impact Factor. If my research is of importance to a narrow group of readers or is more confirmatory or exploratory in nature, I will select a journal accordingly. I generally decide where my work will be a long shot, where my work will have a reasonable chance of being accepted, and where my work will be likely to be accepted. If there is no urgency to publish, in particular there is no chance another research will publish something very similar, I will begin by submitting to the highest impact journal that might possibly be interested. In general, the editors of high impact journals reject a large number of publications without sending for review—often, a rejection comes within a week or two and does not delay time to publication substantively. Once rejected, I will send my manuscript to the journal that where I think the work has a reasonable chance of being accepted, and so on. If my manuscript is accepted with minor or no revisions, I consider this a signal that perhaps I underestimated the potential impact and importance of my work.
2. Who needs to read and be aware of my work? If it is particularly important that surgeons in my subspecialty are aware of my findings, I may consider publishing in a lower impact journal to reach a specific audience. Subspecialty journals may have a tremendous impact within the scope of practice of readers of the journal. For example, important research on the surgical management of complex perianal fistula due to Crohn's disease is likely to have more impact on practice if published in a subspecialty journal that is highly read by the target audience (such as *Diseases of the Colon and Rectum*, Impact Factor 3.132) than in a higher impact journal such as *Gastroenterology* (Impact Factor 11.675), which is not routinely read by the target audience.

3. Have I been happy with service at the journal in the past? The important factors I consider include the ease of the submission process and the timeliness of rejection notices, reviews, and notification of acceptance. Also, it is very important that accepted manuscripts do not wait for many months prior to publication. There are thousands of indexed journals to choose from and I will think twice about sending to a journal that has provided poor service in the past.

There are of course other measures of research significance, and I do not propose to value the Impact Factor of a journal as the only or best metric. While the Impact Factor is an important measure, it is flawed. Journals with a large number of review articles tend to have a comparatively high Impact Factor as this type of article is frequently cited. For example, the journal *CA: A Cancer Journal for Clinicians*, a publication of the American Cancer Society, publishes annual cancer statistics for the United States and solicited review articles. Because these annual cancer statistics are frequently cited, the Impact Factor of this journal is 101.78, nearly twice that of *New England Journal of Medicine*. Clearly, the impact of publication articles published in this journal is not twice that of articles published in the *New England Journal of Medicine*. Additionally, subspecialty journals will never achieve the Impact Factor of journals of broad interest to the medical community despite the fact that articles published in subspecialty journals may change the care of a large number of patients.

Finally, it is much more common to publish in a journal with a high Impact Factor than to publish an article that has high impact. The Impact Factor for a given journal is often driven by a relatively small number of articles published in that year; many articles will have a low number of citations, while a few articles will have a very high number. Because institutions are aware of the limitations of the Impact Factor, academic promotion committees may ask for other measures of research success. Currently, one of the more common measures is the h-index [5]. The h-measure is an evaluation of research impact and productivity for an individual researcher as a measure of research impact. To calculate the h-index, all articles written by an individual author are ordered according to the number of citations to that article. The h-index is based on the distribution of these ordered articles. A scientist with an h-index of x has x articles published that have been cited at least x times. For example, according to Google Scholar, my h-index is 33, meaning that I am an author on 33 articles that have been cited at least 33 times. Note that this measure attempts to balance both quantity and quality. While Hirsh suggested some h-index benchmarks for promotion, for promotion to associate professor, it is likely more important to have a good understanding of the benchmarks at your institution. Calculate the h-factor for faculty that have recently been promoted—this will give some indication of where you stand in comparison to your peers.

Of note, there are limitations to the h-index. The measure does not consider the number of authors on a paper or the order of authorship. Additionally, as it takes time for citations to occur, the h-index will naturally increase as the time actively publishing increases. Finally, some noble laureates actually have a relatively poor h-index as they have produced a small number of publications, although they were of seminal importance. Despite the limitations, it is important to be aware of your h-factor particularly when you are considering promotion as many schools at least consider this metric with the goal of applying more objective criteria to decision-making. While it is quite possible that the specific metric of academic success will change over time, it is almost certain that academic institutions will continue to use measures that enable benchmarking; being aware of what metrics are in use at your institutions is key.

Obtaining Funding

Key Concept: Funding not only is a metric of success, it allows you to continue your role long term as a surgical investigator. Plan ahead, as obtaining funding is often a long process, and set realistic and achievable goals.

Obtaining peer-reviewed funding is essential to maintain your research team and to continue your salary support for research once your 3–5 years of institutional salary support is over. Additionally, obtaining funding for your research is an important measure of academic success, and at many institutions, it is the most important measure. Obtaining funding has always been highly competitive; however, in the current era of fiscal restraint, there are even more challenges.

The first step to success in obtaining funding for your research is to develop your strategic plan for funding. As part of your plan, consider the two major types of funding: salary support awards and research funding awards. Set feasible goals; if you have been given 20 % protected time, it is not possible for you to obtain a major mentored career award and unlikely that you will be successful as a principal investigator on an R01. Obtaining institutional funds or specialty society grants for projects and becoming active in cooperative groups conducting research in your area would be very feasible. In contrast, if you have been given 50 % or more protected time for research, you will be expected to obtain funding for salary and research support, and obtaining NIH support may be an important benchmark for consideration of promotion at your institution—expect to spend considerable time applying for funding!

When you start applying for funds, start small; institutions and societies often have money for small grants for new investigators. In fact, some societies even have grants to support researchers transitioning from training to their first appointment—these may need to be applied for while still in

Table 38.1 National Institutes of Health submission and funding information for R01 equivalent grants and K awards over time [6]

Year	Type of application	Number submitted	Number awarded	% successful
2003	R01 new	13,539	2,303	17.0 %
	R01 1st resubmission	4,128	1,630	39.5 %
	K awards	2,147	938	43.7 %
2012	R01 new	19,259	1,662	8.6 %
	R01 1st resubmission	5,373	2,001	37.2 %
	K awards	2,940	930	31.6 %

training, so these opportunities are easy to miss without advance planning. Speak to the grant and award officers at your institution to determine what funds are available for new faculty. Scan the websites of societies relevant to your specialty and research interests—think broadly as societies such as the American Society of Clinical Oncology will provide career development support to surgeons. Determine the application dates and requirements for each funding opportunity and understand the grant application process at your institution—some require submission days to weeks before the deadline. Create a calendar with this information and for awards you want to apply for in the next 12 months, and block time specifically for grant development in your schedule. Remember that the number of years of eligibility for early career awards varies greatly between granting agencies; the expectations for awards with a longer period of eligibility will of course be much greater, so it may be useful to have a stepwise approach. For example, start with an application to a specialty society for a career development award instead of applying for a mentored career award (K awards) from the NIH in your first year in practice. While mentored career development award applications to the NIH have a higher funding rate than grant application for research (Table 38.1) [6], still less than one-third of grants are funded. It is better to wait until you have a successful track record of obtaining smaller grants and career awards, have a number of publications, and have pilot data to support an application for the larger grants. Determine if your school has a grant for institutional K awards—these are mentored career development awards supported by the NIH but administered through individual institutions. If your institution has such an award and your research fits the goals of the program, then speak with those administering the program. If you are eligible to apply, then apply, even if no surgeons have been funded through the program before. For these awards, you are competing with an internal pool of candidates and the likelihood of success is higher than for a K08 or K23.

You should be applying for grants for research funding in concert with applications for career development awards. Although mentored career development awards are valuable, a K award is not an absolute criterion for research success; salary support is critical and you can obtain this through peer-reviewed funding for research. Of course, an R01 should not be your first grant application—start with institutional and specialty societies to build credibility and generate pilot data.

Because it is so important to receive research funding, it is worth developing grant writing skills. Many great ideas have not been funded because applications were poorly written. Ask mentors for successful grant applications and read them carefully. Take a course in grant writing—even if you have written successful applications in the past, you can always learn more from the experts. Additionally, use the resources at your institution—many have editing services that are highly useful and will make an application look extremely professional. Additionally, many institutions have an internal review system; researchers in your institution review your grant and provide feedback prior to submission of your application. Of course, both editing and internal reviews require time and advance planning is key to having materials available for review prior to the day before the submission deadline. Here are some general tips for grant writing that I have learned in both writing and reviewing a large number of grants:

1. **Talk to the program officers**. These individuals are often researchers and are interested in fostering new investigators. Call them, particularly if you are not sure if your grant idea would be a good fit for their institute or program.
2. **Understand the grant requirements precisely**. If your grant goes over the page limit, it may not be reviewed at all or the extra pages not distributed to reviewers. If you do not use an approved font, your grant may be rejected altogether. Pay attention to detail—a reviewer will not have confidence that you can complete a research project if you cannot write a grant properly. Get help—your grant administration office or department should be able to help with budgets, formatting advice, etc.
3. **Understand the review criteria**. The criteria the reviewers are to use to rate grants are in general specified in the application details. If one of the review criteria is innovation, be sure to include a statement or section describing why your grant is innovative. Specifically use the words described in the review criteria. Don't make the reviewer guess why your grant might be innovative (or novel, or have impact, etc.); tell them why in an explicit fashion.

4. **When writing a grant do not start by writing the introduction**. Start by writing the specific aims for the grant and have these reviewed by the entire study team. This may actually require a number of drafts. Once the specific aims are decided upon, draft the methods section. Only when this is complete, then write the introduction. This way you can ensure that the introduction addresses all relevant information specific to your aims and methods.
5. **Don't *overestimate* your reviewer**. You will likely be reviewed by a nonexpert in your specific area of research. Do not assume extreme familiarity with your material. Bring a reviewer through your grant in a stepwise fashion and avoid jargon. Send your grant to an experienced researcher outside of your field who is not on your study team to review and give feedback.
6. **Don't *underestimate* your reviewer**. It is also possible your reviewer may be an expert in your field, or you may have a motivated reviewer with expert "Google" capability. Do not overstate findings, and do not omit major controversies. If you do and are discovered, you will lose all credibility.
7. **Build an appropriate team with all skills necessary**. For a junior investigator, it is reasonable and preferable to have a more senior investigator as a coinvestigator (or even as a coprincipal investigator); describe how you will receive mentorship from the senior investigator through regular study meetings, etc. Determine all the skills that will be necessary to complete the project and be sure there is a team member with established skills in that area. Don't include unnecessary coinvestigators—each coinvestigator should have a specific and critical role in the conduct of the researcher.
8. **Don't bite off more than you can chew**. New investigators often submit research proposals with excellent ideas that are just too ambitious to achieve. When considering funding for an investigator with a limited track record, research panels will strongly consider the likelihood of successful completion. As such, a focused, specific research question is more likely to receive funding than a grand plan. Build credibility over time.

Unfortunately, most grants do not receive funding. Importantly, most successful grants are resubmissions (Table 38.1), so do not give up on an application simply because you did not obtain funding the first time around. When considering resubmission, pay very close attention to the reviewers' comments. A review that includes terms like innovative, important, and novel indicates that there is real potential for success on resubmission. Are the problems the reviewers identified fixable? Do they ask for more pilot data, an expansion of the research team, and do they think the grant is overly ambitious? These are issues that can be addressed. On the other hand, if they indicate the methodology is fatally flawed or the work is not feasible, unless there has been a fundamental misunderstanding on the part of the reviewers, it is time to go back to the drawing board. When rewriting your grant, be responsive to the reviewers whenever possible and be polite when drafting the response to reviewers' section—you may have the same reviewer assigned to you and it is best to avoid making your reviewer angry. Ultimately, you hopefully will be able to receive support. It may come all at once or take more time, but have several different avenues available for funding, especially as options become increasingly scarce (Table 38.2).

Key Concept: Similar to other aspects in life, maintaining balance in your surgical career for both clinical practice and research, as well as personal life, is a difficult but necessary endeavor to ultimately achieve success and happiness.

Financial issues continue to plague the surgeon investigator. In this era of diminishing resources and reimbursement for both university and community medical centers, oftentimes the funding originally dedicated to research is the first to be cut. Additionally, not only are there shortfalls with research budgets, but there are also diminishing funds available for researchers' salaries as well. More and more, you as the surgeon investigator will be faced with a decision to pursue your research with no consideration, plan, or even opportunity for financial reimbursement for your efforts. Your hospital administration may have primary metrics in place based on your projected numbers of cases or RVUs they want you to meet. There will be constant competition with volume-based incentives that will make up the bulk of your salary. Even your allocated research time will seem to diminish as administrative and adjunct (i.e., hospital committees, educational) requirements mount. On the other

Table 38.2 My research award timeline

	2002	2003	2004	2005	2006
Salary support				CIHR New Investigator (K-equivalent)	
Research support			ASCO CDA	R01 R21 equivalent	Ministry of Health Early Researcher Award

Legend: *ASCO* American Society of Clinical Oncology, *CDA* Career Development Award, *CIHR* Canadian Institutes of Health Research hand, you may not want to dedicate so much time to your research that your surgical skills diminish and you are unable to stay sharp clinically. While you must navigate these waters carefully, it is important to keep in mind what truly brings you professional and personal happiness and do your best to prioritize your time and efforts accordingly.

Summary Pearls

For many of us, there is nothing more rewarding than having the opportunity to pursue a lifetime surgical career both clinically and in research. While balancing your research and clinical demands is becoming increasingly more difficult, it is possible to achieve success and happiness in both arenas. Keys to doing this, however, are proper planning well in advance, as well as managing your expectations and those of your partners and institution. Having the knowledge and understanding of how you can best obtain funding, how your efforts will be measured, and, most importantly, what fulfills you personally will go a long way towards a successful career as a surgical investigator.

References

1. Sambunjak D, Straus S, Marušić A. Mentoring in academic medicine: a systematic review. JAMA. 2006;296:1103–15.
2. Sambunjak D, Straus SE, Marusic A. A systematic review of qualitative research on the meaning and characteristics of mentoring in academic medicine. J Gen Intern Med. 2010;25: 72–8.
3. Sackett D. On the determinants of academic success as a clinician-scientist. Clin Invest Med. 2001;24(2):94–100.
4. The Thomson Reuters impact factor. Available at: http://thomsonreuters.com/products_services/science/free/essays/impact_factor/. Accessed 29 Mar 2013.
5. Hirsch JE. An index to quantify an individual's scientific research output. Proc Natl Acad Sci U S A. 2005;102(46):16569–72.
6. NIH research portfolio online reporting tools. Available at: http://report.nih.gov/success_rates/. Accessed 31 Mar 2013.

Medicolegal and Ethical Dilemmas

39

Jason D. Keune and Ira J. Kodner

Key Points

- While medicolegal reform is likely necessary, the way forward is still unknown.
- Basic patterns of malpractice claims exist and you should practice ways to minimize them.
- Informed consent goes beyond just telling your patient the procedures and risks.
- Ensure your patients have some form of advanced directives—they are good for everyone.
- Ethical principles in surgery are complex and unique to our specialty.
- Understand the potential role that conflict of interests may have in you and your fellow medical professionals.

Introduction

The issue of medical professional liability is perhaps the most prominent medicolegal problems facing today's colorectal surgeon. The matter tends to wax and wane as an issue of importance, often rising to prominence in political debate at times when healthcare reform is debated. The predominant reasons why colorectal surgeons are interested in the medicolegal realm are that malpractice insurance premiums often form a substantial portion of a practice's budget and knowing what to do when a malpractice lawsuit arises. Other medicolegal problems facing colorectal surgeons include the matter of expert witness testimony. There is currently no standard on who can become an expert witness, but some are calling for the implementation of such standards. Finally, the issue of informed consent straddles the medicolegal and ethical worlds. While obtaining informed consent is firmly ensconced in what is considered to be an ethical practice of surgery, the way that informed consent plays out in the courts is ever changing.

Malpractice

Key Concept: *Malpractice issues translate tremendous costs. While potential reforms are possible, several issues still loom large, namely, regulating expert witness guidelines and providing alternatives to the present system, while still protecting the patient.*

The American Medical Association has long advocated for reforms that protect physicians from malpractice lawsuits. The Congressional Budget Office has estimated that the poorly functioning medical professional liability system (MPL) is costing the US taxpayer $62.4 billion and several groups within Congress have called for its reform [1]. This amount represents only the cost to federal programs, and the cost to the private healthcare industry, which is not known, is likely just as great. As with any divisive political issue, there are two sides to the debate, with the AMA and the typically Republican members of Congress arguing that the cost is too great for the federal budget to bear and that lawsuits are overly burdensome on physicians, who should spend their time caring for patients and not constantly defending themselves in court. The argument from those that oppose reform of the MPL is that such federal limitations on the court system would be unconstitutional. Of note, the Supreme Court ruling on the Affordable Care Act of 2011 (ACA) upheld all the portions having to do with malpractice reform.

J.D. Keune, MD, MBA
Department of Surgery, Washington University School of Medicine, Barnes-Jewish Hospital, 660 S. Euclid Ave, Campus Box 8109, St. Louis, MO 63110, USA
e-mail: keunej@wudosis.wustl.edu

I.J. Kodner, MD, FACS (✉)
Department of Surgery, Washington University School of Medicine, Barnes-Jewish Hospital, 660 S. Euclid Ave, St. Louis, MO 63110, USA
e-mail: ijkodner@aol.com; kodner@wudosis.wustl.edu

S.R. Steele et al. (eds.), *Complexities in Colorectal Surgery*,
DOI 10.1007/978-1-4614-9022-7_39, © Springer Science+Business Media New York 2014

Table 39.1 Recommended qualifications for the physician who acts as an expert witness

The physician expert witness must have had a current, valid, and unrestricted state license to practice medicine at the time of the alleged occurrence
The physician expert witness should have been a diplomate of a specialty board recognized by the American Board of Medical Specialties at the time of the alleged occurrence and should be qualified by experience or demonstrated competence in the subject of the case
The specialty of the physician expert witness should be appropriate to the subject matter in the case
The physician expert witness who provides testimony for a plaintiff or a defendant in a case involving a specific surgical procedure (or procedures) should have held, at the time of the alleged occurrence, privileges to perform those same or similar procedures in a hospital accredited by the Joint Commission or the American Osteopathic Association
The physician expert witness should be familiar with the standard of care provided at the time of the alleged occurrence and should have been actively involved in the clinical practice of the specialty or the subject matter of the case at the time of the alleged occurrence
The physician expert witness should be able to demonstrate evidence of continuing medical education relevant to the specialty or the subject matter of the case
The physician expert witness should be prepared to document the percentage of time that is involved in serving as an expert witness. In addition, the physician expert witness should be willing to disclose the amount of fees or compensation obtained for such activities and the total number of times he or she has testified for the plaintiff or defendant

From Ref. [5]

Alternatives to the court system have been proposed. The ACA included a provision that reserves $50 million of grant funding for development, implementation, and evaluation of such alternatives. A certificate of merit program would require a pre-court hearing to determine whether a case has merit before proceeding to trial. Another alternative is a health court that would have a panel of health experts decide cases rather than the lay juries that currently do [2]. Under the ACA, states will make proposals to the Department of Health and Human Services with demonstration projects that will be required to resolve disputes and promote efforts to improve patient safety. For the colorectal surgeon, one concern regarding the MPL is the medical malpractice insurance premium. Recent data indicate that insurance premiums for malpractice insurance have stayed even for the past several years, even improving in some circumstances [3].

Very closely associated with the MPL system is the need for expert witness testimony within the field of colorectal surgery. The surgeon who acts as expert witness is one of the most important figures in a medical malpractice trial. Indeed, justice depends highly on the quality of the expert opinion given. A recent study looking at the expenses incurred for processing and resolving medical malpractice claims identified fees to expert witnesses as the greatest expense second only to payment of trial lawyers. The study also showed that payments to expert witnesses had grown since 2005, as a percentage of total claim resolution cost. Though the study did not distinguish colorectal surgeons as a subgroup, it did show that expert witnesses in general surgery were involved in 25,012 claims closed from 1985 to 2008, representing 32 % on average of the total costs incurred in these closed claims [3].

The American College of Surgeons regularly renews its statement regarding surgeons acting as expert witnesses. The most recent statement, updated in April 2011, is given in Tables 39.1 and 39.2 [4]. Yet, these are only recommendations, left to the discretion of the individual to act accordingly. How and if this is carried out in reality may be a completely different story.

Common Malpractice Claims

Key Concept: You should be aware of the more common malpractice claims as well as how (potentially) best to avoid them.

In 1993, Kenneth Kern reviewed the most common claims filed in the field of colorectal surgery over the prior two decades. He found that the majority of claims were filed within the categories of failure to timely diagnose disease (43 %), iatrogenic colon injury (24 %), iatrogenic medical complications during diagnosis or treatment (15 %), sphincter injury with fecal incontinence resulting from anorectal surgery or midline episiotomy (10 %), and lack of informed consent (8 %) [5]. Since this study, there has been no update of this data, though the distribution of colorectal disease as well as the types of complications that are at risk of litigation are similar.

Other studies have looked at the risk of lawsuit after colon cancer is discovered 1–4 years after colonoscopies that ostensibly cleared the colon of cancer risk [6] and the risk of missing cancers on barium or Hypaque colon examinations [7]. In 1993, Gerstenberger and Plumeri examined 610 endoscopy-associated and 486 gastroenterology-associated malpractice claim files of the Physicians Insurers Association of America data-sharing project. "Improper performance" was alleged in 54 % of claims and "diagnosis error" in 24 % of claims. Of the claims focusing on diagnostic error, 61 % pertained to missed malignancies, of which 69 % were colorectal. In contrast, 95 % of the claims focusing on improper performance claimed perforation or direct injury to the gastrointestinal tract [8].

Several authors have put forth recommendations on avoiding lawsuits. Amongst the most common recommendations are represented by David Beck [9]: (1) good communication and interpersonal skills, (2) proper documentation,

Table 39.2 Recommended guidelines for behavior of the physician acting as an expert witness

Physicians have an obligation to testify in court as expert witnesses when appropriate. Physician expert witnesses are expected to be impartial and should not adopt a position as an advocate or partisan in the legal proceedings
The physician expert witness should review all the relevant medical information in the case and testify to its content fairly, honestly, and in a balanced manner. In addition, the physician expert witness may be called upon to draw an inference or an opinion based on the facts of the case. In doing so, the physician expert witness should apply the same standards of fairness and honesty
The physician expert witness should be prepared to distinguish between actual negligence (substandard medical care that results in harm) and an unfortunate medical outcome (recognized complications occurring as a result of medical uncertainty)
The physician expert witness should review the standards of practice prevailing at the time and under the circumstances of the alleged occurrence
The physician expert witness should be prepared to state the basis of his or her testimony or opinion and whether it is based on personal experience, specific clinical references, evidence-based guidelines, or a generally accepted opinion in the specialty. The physician expert witness should be prepared to discuss important alternate methods and views
Compensation of the physician expert witness should be reasonable and commensurate with the time and effort given to preparing for deposition and court appearance. It is unethical for a physician expert witness to link compensation to the outcome of a case
The physician expert witness is ethically and legally obligated to tell the truth. Transcripts of depositions and courtroom testimony are public records and subject to independent peer reviews. Moreover, the physician expert witness should willingly provide transcripts and other documents pertaining to the expert testimony to independent peer review if requested by his or her professional organization. The physician expert witness should be aware that failure to provide truthful testimony exposes the physician expert witness to criminal prosecution for perjury, civil suits for negligence, and revocation or suspension of his or her professional license

From Ref. [5]

and (3) ensuring accurate informed consent. Good communication with patients has become more difficult in the present era, with time pressures to see more patients over a set period of time, with many procedures being performed in the outpatient setting, and with inpatient stays becoming shorter. Beck emphasizes the need for physicians to listen to patients, to remember and use the patient's name, to use lay terminology, to take the time to answer all of the patient's questions, and to make sure that his contact information is available.

Complete and accurate documentation is crucial in defending claims and may even serve as a deterrent to a potential claim, when a plaintiff's attorney reviews a potential case and finds that the documentation is so complete that it would be difficult to convince a jury that what happened is anything other than what is documented. Charles F. Gay, Jr., JD has published a list of suggestions that can be helpful with regard to documentation—the list is shown in Table 39.3 [10].

Table 39.3 Helpful hints at documenting properly and accurately

1. If you are the treating or primary physician, make a daily entry on the chart
2. Always sign, date, and time each entry
3. Chart at the earliest time
4. If a situation prevents you from charting until later, state why and that the record times are best estimates
5. Chart all consultations
6. Write legibly and spell correctly. Use accepted medical abbreviations
7. Never alter the medical records
8. Never black out or white out any entry on a chart. Should you make a mistake in charting, place a single line through the erroneous entry and label the entry "error in charting." Follow the hospital policy on charting. An addendum is acceptable if placed in sequence with the date and time made
9. Chart professionally. Do not impugn or insult the patient. Do not impugn, insult, or criticize colleagues, co-workers, or support staff
10. Always designate the dose, site, route, and time of medication administration
11. Do not chart incident reports in your notes
12. Chart objectively rather than subjectively and avoid ambiguous terms
13. Document use of all restraints, safeguards, and patient positioning
14. Document all patient noncompliance
15. Document all patient education, discharge instructions, and patient responses
16. Document the patient's status on transfer or discharge
17. Ensure the patient's name is on each page of the medical chart
18. Do not chart in advance

With permission from Terry Hicks

Informed Consent

Key Concept: Informed consent is a process that allows respect for a patient's autonomy to be preserved and can be broken down into seven elements. Except in certain emergency settings, informed consent should be obtained from a patient every time a procedure is performed.

Most of you recognized that informed consent should be comprised of a detailed description of the procedure and accompanied by the procedure's inherent risks, benefits, and alternatives. Yet, it should really go beyond that. Beauchamps and Childress have broken informed consent down into seven elements as shown in Table 39.4 [11].

The threshold elements describe the preconditions necessary for appropriate informed consent. The notion of competence, at its core, means the "ability to perform a task [12]." In one sense, in order to exercise autonomy at all, a person must be competent. The determination of whether a

Table 39.4 Seven elements of informed consent

I. Threshold elements (preconditions)
1. Competence (to understand and decide)
2. Voluntariness (in deciding)
II. Transformation elements
3. Disclosure (of material information)
4. Recommendation (of a plan)
5. Understanding (of 3 and 4)
III. Consent elements
6. Decision (in favor of a plan)
7. Authorization (of the chosen plan)

From Beauchamp and Childress [13]. With permission of Oxford University Press, USA

patient is competent rests on his cognitive abilities both to comprehend information and to consider the consequences of actions. The judging of competence in marginal cases is a complex task that is beyond the scope of this chapter. The other threshold element is voluntariness, that is, the condition in which decision-making can be considered free from outside coercive influence.

The transformation elements are a second preliminary requirement for informed consent. Disclosure of material information is a central component of the informed consent process and is often thought of as the major condition on which a good informed consent is based. Beauchamps and Childress have outlined the core information that should be disclosed in an informed consent, including the fifth element, recommendation [13]:

- Those facts or descriptions that patients or subjects usually consider material in deciding whether to refute or consent to the proposed intervention or research
- Information the professional believes to be material
- The professional's recommendation
- The purpose of seeking consent
- The nature and limits of consent as act of authorization

The last transformation element is a demonstrated understanding of the disclosure and the recommendation.

Next, the consent elements comprise the action portion of the informed consent process. A decision must be made by the patient, with a caveat that the decision is voluntary, as specified in the preconditions. Finally, for the informed consent process to be complete, the patient must signify, usually in the form of a document, his or her authorization that the procedure may be carried out.

Ethics

Key Concept: The practice of surgery involves unique ethical challenges. In part, this is secondary to the fact that surgeons take on a different level of responsibility than most physicians when they encounter patients.

The field of ethics in surgery encompasses a wide range of topics and ideals—too large to concisely state in this chapter. Yet, it is important to recognize not only the role that ethics play daily in surgery but how surgery can be particularly challenging. Often, the surgeon may meet the patient only once prior to heading off to the operating room for a large and very invasive procedure. The doctor-patient relationship has to be established in this short first meeting, as it often is the start to a longer-term relationship. After the operative procedure, the surgeon and team take full responsibility for the procedure itself, the postoperative care, and, most often, the long-term follow-up of the patient—including management of any complications that might arise. The established relationship that results from this interaction is intense since it comes about very quickly and often under adverse circumstances.

Another challenge is the fact that surgeons cannot easily "redo" their work, as many in other professions can. This luxury of time is afforded to attorneys who can appeal their cases, movie directors who can reshoot a scene, and accountants who can amend a return that has already been filed. Indeed, most non-surgeon physicians function on a different timescale than surgeons and can more easily change a course of action if the treatment selected is not working. For surgeons who work under the pressure of time, it is imperative that you do what you think is best, using your judgment, medical knowledge and expertise, and previous experience. You ought to be as scrupulous as possible in assuring that bioethical and legal guidelines are followed since this is what good patient care consists in.

Treating Yourself, a Family Member, or Friend

Key Concept: Understand the complex factors at play when embarking on this situation and ask yourself honestly, "Am I the right person for the job?" (more than just technically or knowledgeably).

We have previously considered the ethical problems that arise when a surgical problem arises in a surgeon's beloved friend or family member [14]. The problem with such situations is knowing whether or not it is possible to assume the same level of objectivity as when you operate on a stranger. The postoperative management of such a patient may become difficult to pull off if tough choices must be made. The first consideration that can be made is one of *beneficence*. It is possible that the surgeon in question is the best possible person to perform the operation—such a situation may arise for a trauma surgeon who sees his brother in the trauma bay after a stabbing to the chest. Since all of the other trauma surgeons are at home, beneficence dictates that the surgeon should operate, given that he is the only one who can perform a lifesaving operation. A second consideration is one of *nonmaleficence*. The conflict of interest that arises in situations such as this may cause one interest (such as the prolongation of a life) to outweigh another more clinically important interest (such as the best course of action for the patient). Furthermore, respect for *autonomy* may come into play as patients may be hesitant to question their physician-relative that may lead them to consent to more risky procedures than they would otherwise undertake. It is difficult to guarantee autonomous consent, free from coercion in such an instance.

LaPuma and Priest have addressed this topic in the literature with seven questions a physician who is considering treating a relative ought to consider prior to making a decision [15]. First, the physician should consider whether he is trained to meet his relative's needs. Second, he should wonder whether his closeness to the relative would prevent him from probing his relative's intimate history and coping with bad news, if need be. Third, the physician should wonder whether he is objective enough to prevent his giving, "too much, too little, or inappropriate care." Fourth, he should consider whether his involvement might exacerbate intrafamilial conflicts. Fifth, the physician ought to wonder whether his relative might better comply with treatment prescribed by an unrelated physician. Sixth, he should examine whether he would allow a physician to whom he may refer his relative to actually care for him or her. Finally, the physician should be readily accountable to both his peers and the public for the care he gives his relative.

The treating of family members is a problem that was known historically. In 1794, Thomas Percival wrote, in reference to the topic, "The natural anxiety and solicitude which he experiences at the sickness of a wife, child, or anyone who by the ties of consanguinity is rendered particularly dear to him, tend to obscure his judgment and produce timidity and irresolution in his practice [16]." Little has changed with reference to this view, with the current American Medical Association position being, "physicians generally should not treat themselves or members of their immediate families … [except] in emergency settings or isolated settings where there is no qualified physician available [17]."

Refusing Treatment

Key Concept: Refusal of care is a patient's right (with sound mind and proper understanding). With any confusion, you should likely opt in favor of lifesaving treatment.

Another ethical dilemma commonly besetting the colorectal surgeon arises when a patient or a patient's family refuses a treatment that has been recommended. This situation becomes particular when the patient has sound decision-making capacity and refuses potentially life-sustaining treatment. In the Nancy Cruzan case, the US Supreme Court upheld the right of person of sound mind to refuse lifesaving medical treatment including resuscitation, blood transfusion, ventilators, and artificial hydration and nutrition. The court defended its decision with the statement, "the right of every individual to the possession and control of his own person, free from all restraint or interference of others, unless by clear and unquestionable authority of law under the liberty interest, protected by the Due Process clause of the Fourteenth Amendment of the Constitution." Every refusal of lifesaving treatment by a patient should be accompanied by an evaluation of decision-making capacity and a consequent assurance that the patient fully understands the consequences should he refuse treatment. If uncertainty exists, physicians are right to opt in favor of the lifesaving treatment.

A more common and familiar scenario in which a patient might refuse life-sustaining treatment is when the patient is acting from religious belief. Jehovah's Witnesses, for example, will often refuse to accept blood transfusions. In the setting of major surgery, this refusal is often associated with a major risk of death, making the decision to operate on such patients a difficult one. In all cases, though, the patient's autonomy must prevail over almost every other consideration when the patient is competent and is not a minor. In cases where the physician considers the patient to not be competent to make such a major decision, she may seek a court order permitting the blood transfusion. If a reasonable argument that the negative effects, whatever aspect that might be, of transfusion are outweighed by the positive, courts may permit the transfusion of blood. In the setting of minors, parents may attempt to block the transfusion of blood products. This is probably the most common situation in which a court order is sought, and the one that court orders to transfuse is most commonly granted.

The matter of decisional capacity deserves further examination. Impaired decisional capacity may be found in minors, mentally handicapped persons, those with organic brain disease or in toxic states, and those with psychiatric conditions. The treatment of minors with respect to decisional capacity varies from state to state. Several different situations can arise in which minors can be declared to have sufficient decisional capacity to provide informed consent, notably, when they are emancipated, when they present with conditions that are previously categorized as minor treatment statutes, and when they are designated as "mature" minors [18]. Another complexity in decisional capacity arises when a patient has a progressively deteriorating mental condition such as Alzheimer's disease. A simple diagnosis of mild Alzheimer's does not mean that a patient has lost decisional capacity. In fact, such patients have capacity to make most of their medical decisions. The problem exists when the patient deteriorates to the point at which the decisional capacity comes into question. The status of disease, paired with the complexity of the decision at hand, can make the matter of adequate decisional capacity difficult to discern in such patients.

Advanced Directives

Key Concept: Having knowledge of a patient's advanced directives will not only help you out with difficult decisions but most often will also help family members understand what your patient wants for themselves and allow the desired treatment.

When a patient does not have decisional capacity, a problem arises about who should make decisions for the patient regarding care. Advanced directives are instructions that are provided by patients that provide direction to caretakers about how decisions should be made should they become impaired [19]. Surgeons quite frequently find themselves at the bedside of a dying patient who has lost such decisional capacity, so facility with such issues is paramount. For surgeons, several other factors also make knowledge about advanced directives and decisional capacity important. First, we respect the notion that medical decisions should be rooted in autonomy; patients should be able to decide what medical therapies they undergo. If incapacitated, then surgeons can continue to respect patient autonomy through the use of advanced directives. Surgeons do not often have the type of established physician-patient relationship that a primary care doctor might have. Finally, surgeons often provide invasive therapy and treat morbid problem with a high risk of mortality. These features all promote the idea that surgeons should be familiar with advanced directives.

There are several standard ways that patients can express their preferences through an advanced directive. The first is through a living will. A living will is a document created by a patient that details what the patient's preferences are at if death should become imminent and the patient should become incapacitated. For some, a living will is simply a statement that the patient would like to die a natural death and indicate unwillingness to be kept alive by heroic measures or, by contrast, that the patient would like to be kept alive as long as possible, despite whatever may happen. Others, however, give specific directions as to which medical therapies should and should not be used, from pain medication to enteral feeding to hydration. In many states, the activation of a living will requires the patient to be in imminent danger of death before the terms are activated.

A second method by which a patient's preferences can be expressed is by appointment of a durable power of attorney for health care. A durable power of attorney is a surrogate decision-maker who steps in when a patient no longer has decisional capacity. The "durable" aspect refers to the fact that the power of attorney will be able to continue to make decisions for the patient, should they become incapacitated.

If there is not a designated power of attorney and no document exists detailing what should be done should a patient become incapacitated, the problem then exists of finding a surrogate decision-maker. States differ as to just how a surrogate decision-maker should be identified, but a defined hierarchy usually is specified, e.g., spouse, adult children, and siblings. Such a surrogate decision-maker, once identified, should be interested in acting in the best interest of and according to the wishes and values of the patient (see below). It is generally thought that a durable power of attorney, or a family member who knows the patient well, is superior to a living will in that a person who is familiar with the patient's preferences can respond to the nuances in treatment and often tortuous twists and turns that can be faced when morbidly ill.

Designation of a durable power of attorney or a family member with familiarity about the patient's preferences as a surrogate decision-maker is often not enough. The spectrum of options available to a patient can be quite vast, and often, the decision-maker will not know what the patient would want. What should be done then? Two standards apply in this situation. First, the *substituted judgment* standard may be applied. In applying substituted judgment, the decision-maker bases the decision on his knowledge of the patient, and of other, perhaps similar decisions that the patient has made in the past. The decision-maker then decides what to do based on what he thinks the patient would want if he were competent. Often though, decision-makers do not feel comfortable making such an estimation, possibly because their knowledge about the patient is not that intimate. In this setting, decision-makers can use the other standard, that of the "best interest." In the best interest standard, decision-makers decide based on what, in the decision-makers opinion, would be best for the patient, without trying to determine what the patient would want.

Several other problems arise in surrogate decision-making. The matter of when the advance directive should be activated is an important one. Take, for example, an elderly woman who has undergone a colectomy for cancer and on postoperative day three develops a severe pneumonia, which requires intubation. The patient, now incapacitated, cannot make decisions regarding her care, but, unless the patient becomes moribund, this is not the right time to resort to a living will. Instead, standard, aggressive care should be provided. In general, it is wise to err on the side of life and on the side of standards of care. In such situations, consultation from the hospital's ethics committee can be valuable.

In 1991, the Physician Order for Life-Sustaining Treatment (POLST) Paradigm Initiative was brought into existence as an alternative to the advanced directive [20]. It was recognized that the diversity and lack of uniformity amongst advanced directives lead to uneven realization of patients' end-of-life preferences [21]. The POLST Paradigm Initiative was a task force centered at Oregon Health & Science University comprised of stakeholders from across the spectrum of health care. The result was the development of a standardized form, released in 1995, known as "the POLST form" which could serve as an actual set of portable physician orders and would be placed in the front of a patient's chart. A sample POLST form is shown in Fig. 39.1 [22].

HIPAA PERMITS DISCLOSURE TO HEALTH CARE PROFESSIONALS & ELECTRONIC REGISTRY AS NECESSARY FOR TREATMENT

Physician Orders for Life-Sustaining Treatment (POLST)

Follow these orders until orders change. These medical orders are based on the patient's **current** medical condition and preferences. Any section not completed does not invalidate the form and implies full treatment for that section. With significant change of condition new orders may need to be written.
Guidance for Health Care Professionals. http://www.ohsu.edu/polst/programs/documents/Guidebook.pdf.

Patient Last Name:	Patient First Name	Middle Int.
Date of Birth: (mm/dd/yyyy) ______ ______ ______	Gender: ☐ M ☐ F	Last 4 SSN: ☐☐☐☐
Address: (street / city / state / zip)		

A *Check One*

CARDIOPULMONARY RESUSCITATION (CPR): ***Patient has no pulse and is not breathing.***

☐ **Attempt Resuscitation/CPR**
☐ **Do Not Attempt Resuscitation/DNR**

When not in cardiopulmonary arrest, follow orders in **B** and **C**.

B *Check One*

MEDICAL INTERVENTIONS: ***If patient has pulse and/or is breathing.***

☐ **Comfort Measures Only** (Allow Natural Death). Relieve pain and suffering through the use of any medication by any route, positioning, wound care and other measures. Use oxygen, suction and manual treatment of airway obstruction as needed for comfort. ***Patient prefers no transfer to hospital*** *for life-sustaining treatments.* ***Transfer*** *if comfort needs cannot be met in current location.*
Treatment Plan: Maximize comfort through symptom management.

☐ **Limited Additional Interventions** In addition to care described in Comfort Measures Only, use medical treatment, antibiotics, IV fluids and cardiac monitor as indicated. No intubation, advanced airway interventions, or mechanical ventilation. May consider less invasive airway support (e.g. CPAP, BiPAP). ***Transfer*** *to hospital if indicated. Generally avoid the intensive care unit.*
Treatment Plan: Provide basic medical treatments.

☐ **Full Treatment** In addition to care described in Comfort Measures Only and Limited Additional Interventions, use intubation, advanced airway interventions, and mechanical ventilation as indicated. ***Transfer to hospital*** *and/or intensive care unit if indicated.*
Treatment Plan: Full treatment including life support measures in the intensive care unit.

Additional Orders: ______________________________

C *Check One*

ARTIFICIALLY ADMINISTERED NUTRITION: ***Offer food by mouth if feasible.***

☐ No artificial nutrition by tube.
☐ Defined trial period of artificial nutrition by tube.
☐ Long-term artificial nutrition by tube.

Additional Orders: ______________________________

D

DOCUMENTATION OF DISCUSSION:

☐ Patient (Patient has capacity)
☐ Parent of minor
☐ Court-Appointed Guardian
☐ Health Care Representative or legally recognized surrogate
☐ Surrogate for patient with developmental disabilities or significant mental health condition (Note: Special requirements for completion. See reverse side.)
☐ Other______________________________

Signature of Patient or Surrogate

Signature: ***recommended***	Name (print):	Relationship (write "self" if patient):

This form will be sent to the POLST Registry unless the patient wishes to opt out, if so check opt out box ☐

E

SIGNATURE OF PHYSICIAN / NP/ PA

My signature below indicates to the best of my knowledge that these orders are consistent with the patient's **current** medical condition and preferences.

Print Signing Physician / NP / PA Name: ***required***	Signer Phone Number:	Signer License Number: *(optional)*
Physician / NP / PA Signature: ***required***	Date: ***required***	Office Use Only

SEND FORM WITH PATIENT WHENEVER TRANSFERRED OR DISCHARGED, SUBMIT COPY TO REGISTRY

Fig. 39.1 A sample POLST form (From: POLST Paradigm Forms[23])

HIPAA PERMITS DISCLOSURE TO HEALTH CARE PROFESSIONALS & ELECTRONIC REGISTRY AS NECESSARY FOR TREATMENT

Information for patient named on this form PATIENT'S NAME: ________________________

The POLST form is **always voluntary** and is usually for persons with advanced illness or frailty. POLST records your wishes for medical treatment in your current state of health. Once initial medical treatment is begun and the risks and benefits of further therapy are clear, your treatment wishes may change. Your medical care and this form can be changed to reflect your new wishes at any time. However, no form can address all the medical treatment decisions that may need to be made. The Oregon Advance Directive is recommended for all capable adults, regardless of their health status. An Advance Directive allows you to document in detail your future health care instructions and/or name a Health Care Representative to speak for you if you are unable to speak for yourself.

Contact Information

Surrogate (optional):	Relationship:	Phone Number:	Address:

Health Care Professional Information

Preparer Name:	Preparer Title:	Phone Number:	Date Prepared:
PA's Supervising Physician:		Phone Number:	
Primary Care Professional:			

Directions for Health Care Professionals

Completing POLST

- Completing a POLST is always voluntary and cannot be mandated for a patient.
- Should reflect current preferences of persons with advanced illness or frailty. Also, encourage completion of an Advance Directive.
- Verbal / phone orders are acceptable with follow-up signature by physician/NP/PA in accordance with facility/community policy.
- Use of original form is encouraged. Photocopies, faxes, and electronic registry forms are also legal and valid.
- A person with developmental disabilities or significant mental health condition requires additional consideration before completing the POLST form; refer to *Guidance for Health Care Professionals* at http://www.ohsu.edu/polst/programs/documents/Guidebook.pdf.

Sending to Oregon POLST Registry (Required unless "Opt Out" box is checked)

For the Oregon POLST Registry the following must be completed:

- Patient's full name
- Date of birth
- Section A
- MD / DO / NP / PA signature
- Date signed

Send a copy of both sides of this POLST form to the Oregon POLST Registry.

FAX or eFAX:
503- 418-2161
or
Mail:
Oregon POLST Registry
CDW-EM
3181 SW Sam Jackson Park Rd.
Portland, OR 97239

Date Submitted _______ /_______ /_______

MAY PUT REGISTRY ID STICKER HERE:

Registry Phone: 503-418-4083
*Please allow up to 10 days from receipt for processing into the Registry. Mailed confirmation packets may take four weeks for delivery.

Reviewing POLST

This POLST should be reviewed periodically and if:

- The patient is transferred from one care setting or care level to another, or
- There is a substantial change in the patient's health status, or
- The patient's treatment preferences change, or
- The patient's primary care professional changes.

Voiding POLST

- A person with capacity, or the valid surrogate of a person without capacity, can void the form and request alternative treatment.
- Draw line through sections A through E and write "VOID" in large letters if POLST is replaced or becomes invalid.
- Send a copy of the voided form to the POLST Registry as above (required).
- If included in an electronic medical record, follow voiding procedures of facility/community.

For permission to use the copyrighted form contact the OHSU Center for Ethics in Health Care. Information on the POLST program is available online at **www.polst.org** or at **polst@ohsu.edu**.

SEND FORM WITH PATIENT WHENEVER TRANSFERRED OR DISCHARGED, SUBMIT COPY TO REGISTRY

Fig 39.1 (continued)

In contrast to a patient's advance directive, which is ideally formulated well in advance of any illness, and addresses potential illness, the POLST form serves as an actual physician order and is formulated in the context of an advanced chronic illness. POLST is most appropriately used when life expectancy is less than 1 or 2 years and the need for advanced life support is highly likely and predictable. POLST programs are currently in use or development in well more than half of US states [23]. In one study of a stratified, random sample of 90 Medicaid-eligible nursing facilities in Oregon, Wisconsin, and West Virginia [24], it was found that residents with POLST forms were more likely to have orders about life-sustaining treatment preferences beyond cardiopulmonary resuscitation than residents without (98.0 % vs. 16.1 %, $P<0.001$). Furthermore, there were no differences in symptom assessment or management between residents with and without POLST forms. Residents with POLST forms indicating orders for comfort measures only were less likely to receive medical interventions (e.g., hospitalization) than residents with POLST full treatment orders ($P=0.004$), residents with traditional do-not-resuscitate orders ($P<0.001$), or residents with traditional full code orders ($P<0.001$). These findings are consistent with the goals of POLST and suggest a successful implementation of this paradigm.

Conflicts of Interest (COI)

Key Concept: A conflict of interest is a state in which there exists a dynamic interaction between two differing interests of the same person, such that his interest in one impacts his ability to realize, and possibly execute, a pure motive in the other. Be aware of your surroundings and fully disclose all potential conflicts.

Another common ethical problem faced by colorectal surgeons is the problem of financial conflicts of interest. As federal research funding available to surgeons diminishes, the idea of obtaining extramural support from the biomedical and pharmaceutical industry becomes attractive. In addition, colorectal surgeons in practice, especially those in academic practice, are common targets of marketing efforts by such companies. Many institutions in the field of medicine and biomedical research, such as the American Medical Association [25], PhRMA [26], and the National Institutes of Health [27], as well as most universities have also published guidelines that serve to give their members guidance with regard to financial COI and relationships with industry. Guidelines for the management of conflicts of interest have also been put forth by the Institute of Medicine [28] and the Association of American Medical Colleges [29].

One of us (JDK) has recently published a summary and categorization of 4 years of disclosures (2006–2009) given by presenters at the annual Clinical Congress of the American College of Surgeons. We found that in the 3,122 disclosures made by 490 individuals, "colorectal surgeon" was the most common profession and the most common type of disclosure was "consulting." This may be that they are actually the highest or, perhaps, the group most likely to disclose relationships. Regardless, the company with the highest number of disclosures was Covidien. Disclosers used 195 different terms to describe their relationships, making the need for a standardized nomenclature necessary [30]. In another recent study, only 71 % of disclosers at a national meeting of orthopedic surgeons believed that their relationships involved any "conflict" [31].

The conflict of interest problem is a specific case within a broader category of ethical problems that has grown in importance over the last several decades: institutional bioethics. In 1995, Ezekiel Emanuel wrote that the focus of bioethics could be shifted from "articulating principles and rules that apply to individual cases to devising institutional structures that can ensure ethical behavior [32]." The response to Emanuel's call in the intervening time has been scarce. Institutions are difficult to classify morally—do they represent collections of individuals, or are they entities that deserve the rights of individuals? Also, the number and variety of institutions that physicians interact with is large. What happens to a physician's individual moral responsibility if an institution requires an individual physician to do something that it has deemed "ethical"? Who would take on responsibility if an unforeseen harm is done to a patient as a result of guidelines being properly followed, if simple rule following is to be encouraged—the physician or the institution? Aside from ethical guidelines, all institutions have guidelines of many other types that can restrict certain behaviors in individuals and empower others.

The real problem with physician conflicts of interest comes about when one of the two interests is financial and the other is the well-being of the patient. There is an overarching view in society that physicians should have no interests interfering with their relationship with the patient. Financial conflicts are viewed as particularly deplorable. The American "healthcare system" would not be recognizable, however, without the massive private industry component that produces drugs and devices and manages health systems. At times, it seems that there is no interface between this private industry component and patients, other than physicians. At present, the role of institutions in medicine to mediate this relationship is still being worked out.

The other concern in financial conflicts of interest is that physicians that receive payments from industry cannot manage this interest weighed against the well-being of the patient. The question that needs to be answered is: "is it possible to have a conflict of interest and yet be free from the type of bias that would negatively impact patient care?" Also, the fact that financial conflicts of interest are focused on as compared to other interests such as academic promotion, advancement of original ideas in diagnosis or therapy, and balance between family and work life should be addressed. One reason for the focus on financial conflicts of interest is that money is fungible and quantifiable. Is there something more about financial conflicts of interest to warrant a nearly exclusive focus on this conflict of interest? There is no term to describe conflicts of interest, properly managed, but the proper management of all conflicts of interest seems to be common to the successful practice of surgery.

In surveys, most physicians report some financial relationship with industry [33, 34]. Such relationships were historically accepted as a necessary part of the progression of biomedical science, though serious accusations of imprudent management on the parts of both physicians and industry started arising in over the last decade [35–38]. Yet, what about now? Is disclosure what is needed to provide appropriate accountability for this problem? As Justice Louis Brandies famously put it, and Senator Charles Grassley echoed it, "Sunlight is said to be the best of disinfectants [39, 40]," For several years prior to the passage of the Patient Protection and Affordable Care Act (PPACA), attempts at legislation of the physician financial conflicts of interest problem were attempted by members of the US Congress, led by Charles Grassley, who has made openness and disclosure across industries a focus of his legislative effort. On March 23, 2010, the PPACA became law and includes a section known as the "Physician Payment Sunshine Provision [41]." The provision requires drug, biologic, and medical device companies to report all payments and other transfers of value to physicians and teaching hospitals. The minimum value required for reporting is $10 per instance or $100 per year. The first reports will be due on March 31, 2013. Table 39.5 is extracted from the PPACA and shows what financial relationships will be counted. It will be intriguing to see what effect this large-scale disclosure has on this relationship between institutions and individuals in surgery.

Financial conflicts of interest amongst surgeons represent a special case. A continuous and long-lasting relationship between physicians and industry is needed for the innovation and production of safe surgical devices that has marked the progress of surgery of the last several decades. Given that the means of production in the United States is in the private sector, there is therefore, by necessity, a relationship between device manufacturers and actively operating surgeons. Innovation and device development is difficult to conceive of without such a relationship.

Summary Pearls

This chapter represents simply a few of the highlights regarding medicolegal and ethical situations you will face. Not everything needs to be a dilemma. Foremost, do the right thing for your patient with a clean conscious and no ulterior motives. By simply adhering to that principle, you will likely be able to avoid major problems. When you do have an issue,

Table 39.5 Financial relationships that will require disclosure under the Patient Protection and Affordable Care Act (PPACA)

SEC. 1128G o42 U.S.C. 1320a–7 h. TRANSPARENCY REPORTS AND REPORTING OF PHYSICIAN OWNERSHIP OR INVESTMENT INTERESTS.
(a) TRANSPARENCY REPORTS.—
(1) PAYMENTS OR OTHER TRANSFERS OF VALUE.—
(A) IN GENERAL.—On March 31, 2013, and on the 90th day of each calendar year beginning thereafter, any applicable manufacturer that provides a payment or other transfer of value to a covered recipient (or to an entity or individual at the request of or designated on behalf of a covered recipient), shall submit to the Secretary, in such electronic form as the Secretary shall require, the following information with respect to the preceding calendar year:
(i) The name of the covered recipient.
(ii) The business address of the covered recipient and, in the case of a covered recipient who is a physician, the specialty and National Provider Identifier of the covered recipient.
(iii) The amount of the payment or other transfer of value.
(iv) The dates on which the payment or other transfer of value was provided to the covered recipient.
(v) A description of the form of the payment or other transfer of value, indicated (as appropriate for all that apply) as— (I) cash or a cash equivalent; (II) in-kind items or services; (III) stock, a stock option, or any other ownership interest, dividend, profit, or other return on investment; or (IV) any other form of payment or other transfer of value (as defined by the Secretary).
(vi) A description of the nature of the payment or other transfer of value, indicated (as appropriate for all that apply) as— (I) consulting fees; (II) compensation for services other than consulting; (III) honoraria; (IV) gift; (V) entertainment; (VI) food; (VII) travel (including the specified destinations); (VIII) education; (IX) research; (X) charitable contribution; (XI) royalty or license; (XII) current or prospective ownership or investment interest; (XIII) direct compensation for serving as faculty or as a speaker for a medical education program; (XIV) grant; or (XV) any other nature of the payment or other transfer of value (as defined by the Secretary).
(vii) If the payment or other transfer of value is related to marketing, education, or research specific to a covered drug, device, biological, or medical supply, the name of that covered drug, device, biological, or medical supply.
(viii) Any other categories of information regarding the payment or other transfer of value the Secretary determines appropriate."

From: Patient Protection and Affordable Care Act/Title VI. H.R. 3590 the United States Senate. Title VI. http://en.wikisource.org/wiki/Patient_Protection_and_Affordable_Care_Act/Title_VI
From The Patient Protection and Affordable Care Act (PPACA) [41]

talk to your peers, support group, or the ethics board of your hospital to get other opinions. Through it all, you are not alone. What you will likely find out is that you face similar issues that many of your fellow surgeons face on a daily basis as well.

References

1. Wah RM. Letter. "From the AMA: medical malpractice reform." The New York Times. 15 Oct 2011.
2. Medical liability reform – demonstration grants. American College of Physicians. 2011. Accessed online on 16 Aug 2012 at: http://www.acponline.org/advocacy/where_we_stand/access/internists_guide/iii12-medical-liability-reform-demo.pdf.
3. Carroll AE, Parikh PD, Buddenbaum JL. The impact of defense expenses in medical malpractice claims. J Law Med Ethics. 2012;40(1):135–42.
4. The American College of Surgeons. Statement on the physician acting as an expert witness. Bulletin of the American College of Surgeons, 4th edn, Vol. 96, 2011.
5. Kern KA. Medical malpractice involving colon and rectal disease: a 20-year review of United States civil court litigation. Dis Colon Rectum. 1993;36(6):531–9.
6. Rex DK, Bond JH, Feld AD. Medical-legal risks of incident cancers after clearing colonoscopy. Am J Gastroenterol. 2001;96(4):952–7.
7. Barloon TJ, Shumway J. Medical malpractice involving radiologic colon examinations: a review of 38 recent cases. AJR Am J Roentgenol. 1995;165(2):343–6.
8. Gerstenberger PD, Plumeri PA. Malpractice claims in gastrointestinal endoscopy: analysis of an insurance industry data base. Gastrointest Endosc. 1993;39(2):132–8.
9. Beck DE. Chapter 14. Medicolegal aspects of coloprotologic practice. In: Wexner SD, Zbar AP, Pescatori M, editors. Complex anorectal disorders. London: Springer; 2005.
10. Gay Jr CF. Medicolegal issues. In: Hicks TC, Beck DE, Opelka FG, Timmcke AE, editors. Complications of colorectal surgery. Baltimore: Williams & Wilkins; 1996. p. 468–77.
11. Beauchamp TL, Childress JF. Principles of biomedical ethics. 6th ed. New York: Oxford University Press; 2008. p. 120–1.
12. Culver CM, Gert B. Philosophy in medicine. New York: Oxford University Press; 1982. p. 123–6.
13. Beauchamp TL, Childress JF. Principles of biomedical ethics. 6th ed. New York: Oxford University Press; 2009. p. 121.
14. Kerrigan J, Rovelstad S, Kodner IJ, La Puma J, Keune JD. All in the family: how close is too close? The ethics of treating loved ones. Surgery. 2011;149(3):433–7.
15. La Puma J, Priest ER. Is there a doctor in the house? An analysis of the practice of physicians' treating their own families. JAMA. 1992;267(13):1810–2.
16. American Medical Association. Of the duties of physicians to each other, and to the profession at large: of the duties of physicians in reward to professional services to each other. In: Code of medical ethics. Chicago: American Medical Association; 1847, chap 2, article II.
17. AMA Code of Ethics. Opinion 8.19-Self-treatment or treatment of immediate family members. Accessed online on 2 Sept 2012 at: http://www.ama-assn.org/ama/pub/physician-resources/medical-ethics/code-medical-ethics/opinion819.page?.
18. Baren JM. Ethical dilemmas in the care of minors in the emergency department. Emerg Med Clin North Am. 2006;24(3):619–31.
19. Jaworska A. Advance directives and substitute decision-making. In: Zalta EN, editor. The Stanford encyclopedia of philosophy (Summer 2009 ed.). http://plato.stanford.edu/archives/sum2009/entries/advance-directives/.
20. History of the POLST paradigm initiative. Center for Ethics in Health Care. Oregon Health and Science University. 2008. Accessed online on 13 Sept 2012 at: http://www.ohsu.edu/polst/developing/history.htm.
21. Perkins HS. Controlling death: the false promise of advance directives. Ann Intern Med. 2007;147:51–7.
22. POLST Paradigm Forms. Physician orders for life sustaining treatment website. Accessed online at: http://www.ohsu.edu/polst/programs/sample-forms.htm. on 19 Sept 2012.
23. State Contact List. Physician orders for life sustaining treatment website. Accessed online at: http://www.ohsu.edu/polst/programs/state+programs.htm. on 19 Sept 2012.
24. Hickman SE, Nelson CA, Perrin NA, Moss AH, Hammes BJ, Tolle SW. A comparison of methods to communicate treatment preferences in nursing facilities: traditional practices versus the physician orders for life-sustaining treatment program. J Am Geriatr Soc. 2010;58(7):1241–8.
25. American Medical Association. Conflict of interest policy and statement on disclosure of affiliations. 1999. Accessed online on 21 Dec 2009 at: www.ama-assn.org/ama1/pub/upload/mm/37/coi-policy.doc.
26. The Pharmaceutical Research and Manufacturers of America (PhRMA). Code on interactions with healthcare professionals. 2009. Accessed online on 21 Dec 2009 at: http://www.phrma.org/files/attachments/PhRMA%20Marketing%20Code%202008.pdf.
27. The National Institutes of Health Ethics Program. Conflict of interest. 2008. Accessed online on 21 Dec 2009 at: http://ethics.od.nih.gov/topics/coi.htm.
28. Institute of Medicine. Conflict of interest in medical research, education, and practice. Washington: National Academies Press; 2009. Accessed online on 30 Oct 2009 at: http://www.iom.edu/en/Reports/2009/Conflict-of-Interest-in-Medical-Research-Education-and-Practice.aspx.
29. The AAMC Task Force on Industry Funding of Medical Education. Industry funding of medical education report of an AAMC task force. Accessed online on 30 Oct 2009 at: http://services.aamc.org/publications/showfile.cfm?file=version114.pdf&prd_id=232.
30. Keune JD, Vig S, Hall BL, Matthews BD, Klingensmith ME. Taking disclosure seriously: disclosing financial conflicts of interest at the American College of Surgeons. J Am Coll Surg. 2011; 212(2):215–24.
31. Okike K, Kocher MS, Wei EX, Mehlman CT, Bhandari M. Accuracy of conflict-of-interest disclosures reported by physicians. N Engl J Med. 2009;361(15):1466–74.
32. Emanuel EJ. Medical ethics in the era of managed care: the need for institutional structures instead of principles for individual cases. J Clin Ethics. 1995;6(4):335–8.
33. Campbell EG, Gruen RL, Mountford J, Miller LG, Cleary PD, Blumenthal D. A national survey of physician-industry relationships. N Engl J Med. 2007;356(17):1742–50.
34. Campbell EG, Weissman JS, Ehringhaus S, Rao SR, Moy B, Feibelmann S, Goold SD. Institutional academic industry relationships. JAMA. 2007;298(15):1779–86.
35. Harris G. Top psychiatrist didn't report drug maker's pay, files show. The New York Times. 4 Oct 2008.
36. Meier B, Duff W. Medical school says former army surgeon hid ties to Medtronic. The New York Times. 14 July 2009.
37. Giles J. Exposing the links between doctors and Big Pharma. New Scientist. Feb 2009.
38. Martinez B. Spitzer charges Glaxo concealed Paxil data. The Wall Street Journal. 3 June 2004.
39. Brandeis L. What publicity can do. Harper's Weekly. 20 Dec 1913.
40. Woodward C. New US law applies 'sunshine' to physician payments and gifts from drug, device industries. CMAJ. 2010;182(10): E467–8.
41. The Patient Protection and Affordable Care Act (PPACA). Public Law 111–148. 23 Mar 2010.

Economic Issues Impacting Surgical Care Delivery

40

Anthony J. Senagore

Key Points

- Changes in healthcare require the surgeon to have a much broader knowledge of the financial impact of their individual clinical care in order to maintain fiscal responsibility.
- Clinical decision-making directly impacts contribution margin and cash flow at several levels within the healthcare system.
- Resource utilization and implementation of new technology must be considered in light of the clinical benefit to the patient and balanced against overall costs to the system.
- The surgeon should begin to understand the concept of warranty of care, which assesses the frequency of complications based upon clinical presentation and balances the cost of mitigation and treatment.

Introduction

This chapter will attempt to provide an overview of the topic of cost structure related to surgical practice and variations across practice patterns, especially given the impending significant transformation of the US healthcare system. The following discussion is meant to be a very utilitarian approach to the issue rather than the more traditional concept of cost-effectiveness that is aimed at population-level discussions. The hope would be that you will gain some introspection related to the role of the provider in the cost structure of care delivery rather than a keener understanding of a population-centric analysis of the value of a service. The terms we will focus on are aimed at an understanding of the impact of clinical decision-making on contribution margin and cash flow to support the business intelligence at the provider, division, department, and hospital levels. It is no longer possible for clinical leaders to be lacking in a comprehensive understanding of the incremental impact of resource utilization, as well as the implementation of new technologies. These decisions will strongly influence institutional profitability and, therefore, ultimate viability in the more competitive world of the Accountable Care Organization.

While surgeons will continue to assess care plans and innovation within the constructs of procedural indications, risk factors, and short- and long-term outcomes, it is the additional impact on contribution margin that is rarely assessed. It is only the excess revenue above cost of care delivery that will provide financing for new technology and recruitment of talent at an institutional level. This discussion will focus on a description of how hospitals and physicians are reimbursed for their activities, a process for assessing the typical costs of care, and finally a construct for assessing the potential financial risks/benefits for assessing and either adopting or forgoing new technologies and procedures.

Diagnosis-Related Groups (DRGs)

Key Concept: While the current tiered DRG system is designed to include similar patients, differences in resource utilization within like groupings may not be accurately reflected and reimbursed.

The Health Care Financing Administration (Medicare) implemented the prospective payment system in 1983 in the United States [1]. The purpose of the system was to ensure access to care for beneficiaries, while simultaneously providing a mechanism to control increases in healthcare costs for the program. The system is based on a system that incorporates one or more operative procedures on an organ

A.J. Senagore, MD, MS, MBA
Division of Colorectal Surgery, Department of Surgery, Central Michigan College of Medicine, Saginaw, MI 48601, USA
e-mail: anthony.senagore@cmich.edu

S.R. Steele et al. (eds.), *Complexities in Colorectal Surgery*,
DOI 10.1007/978-1-4614-9022-7_40, © Springer Science+Business Media New York 2014

system into a single grouping for payment. The four goals of the DRG system were the following: (1) inclusion of patient characteristics should be limited to data routinely collected on the hospital billing form, (2) a manageable number of DRGs should encompass the patients managed in inpatient care, (3) each DRG should contain patients with a similar pattern of resource intensity, and (4) each DRG should contain patients who are clinically similar [1]. Currently, the majority of these groupings exist in a 3-tier format under the MS-DRG system to contrast those patients designated with or without major comorbidities/complications (CC versus non-CC) versus those with more severe major complications/comorbidities (MCC) within a given organ system. As an example under the current CMS hospital fee schedule, DRG 331 (colectomy; non-CC) is reimbursed at approximately a base rate of $8,310 compared to DRG 330 (colectomy with CC) that is reimbursed $15,400. Alternatively, DRG 329 (colectomy with MCC) that would include cases like perforated diverticulitis is reimbursed approximately $22,000. The final payment is a bit more complex because a case weight multiplier is used, as well as adjustments for a variety of issues such as outlier status or post-acute care transfer. This level of calculation is beyond the scope of this article. It is interesting to note, however, that a re-operative colectomy could fall into either 331 or 330 depending on comorbidities and postoperative complications yet are equally complex for the surgeon. Therefore, a healthy patient with a locally recurrent colon cancer with abdominal wall involvement might be reimbursed as a DRG 331 (and hopefully discharged without serious mishap). It is likely that the patient would require an extensive resection; however, in the absence of blood transfusions, a prolonged ileus, a significant surgical site infection, or some other postoperative misadventure, it might not rise to the level of DRG 330. This would be in spite of the fact that a prolonged operative time will be required and considerably more operative resources (possibly even expensive biologic mesh for abdominal wall reconstruction) will be consumed compared to a routine first time colectomy. Another example is the report of Pessaux et al. [2], regarding re-operative hepatic resection. They reviewed 42 patients submitted to 55 repeat hepatectomies (42 s, 11 third, and 2 fourth hepatectomies). There was no intraoperative or postoperative mortality; however, the morbidity rates doubled from first to third hepatectomy (9.5–18.2 %). Operative duration was considerably longer after a second or third hepatectomy compared to the first. Therefore, the implication is that resource consumption would be higher; however, reimbursement might not reflect this fact. As a result, the common mantra of "we seek to deliver tertiary and quaternary care" should be assessed carefully because without the "easier" cases, an institution could find itself in an unsustainable business model. Remember the MS-DRG system is designed to provide the entire spectrum of care based upon the typical mix of patients within a family, not for complete reimbursement for each tier.

A more parochial debate is occurring now with respect to robotic-assisted laparoscopic resections (RALR). Despite a paucity of debated defining advantages of RALR over more standard laparoscopic approaches, there is consistent evidence that RALR adds significantly to healthcare expenditures. These costs are related not only to device acquisition but also to increased operative time and consumables costs [3–10]. Interestingly, a recent analysis of robotic-assisted prostatectomy could only identify a financial benefit related to incremental admission volume due to reduced LOS for other surgical procedures, but only when compared to open not laparoscopic prostatectomy [11]. This issue is made even more compelling by the general lack of supporting data in favor of RALR in colorectal surgery, including recent meta-analyses which assessed a variety of outcomes including return of bowel function, hospital stay, oncological outcomes, anastomotic leakage, or postoperative morbidity and mortality—none of which were improved with the aid of the robot [4, 12–14]. We will return to a further assessment of the impact of resource utilization on DRG performance later when we reflect on the concept of warranty.

Impact of Bundled Care and Episode of Care Methodologies

Key Concept: The current strategy for reimbursement based on expected outcomes for a given procedure, which includes penalties for the development of complications, is (in part) a flawed concept, rooted in poor methodology, and is in many cases inconsistent with the available data.

The implementation of a "bundled care" payment structure for colon resection is based upon the concept that the performance of the procedure has a longer duration of impact than simply the index hospital stay. The corollary implication is that someone is capable of fully and accurately assigning components of the care process to the colectomy and determining what time frame is appropriate. The process would preferably begin with the definition of the optimal cost structure of the "perfect outcome" for the "ideal patient" (i.e., healthy patient, short length of stay, appropriate resource consumption, and no complications or readmission). From this base case cost structure, one would then have to adjust the cost structure to account for risk adjustment, true costs of complications, impact of post-discharge resources (i.e., home care, subacute nursing facility), and readmission. One of the major failings of the current process of defining all complications as either "potentially avoidable" or "never events" detracts from the opportunity for a fair assessment of payment. The missing component of this discussion is the failure to acknowledge either of the two facts: (1) across a population of colectomy patients, there remains a predictable complication rate with variation around a mean, and (2) cost structure and effectiveness of mitigation strategies must be included in the total reimbursement to allow the provider to meet this cost.

An elegant attempt at creating a clinically relevant structure around the cost implications of complications was developed by Clavien et al., and subsequently modified in which a proposed classification of negative outcomes of surgery and a severity grading system for complications based upon the cost of managing the complications, sequelae, and failures to cure [16]. This system graded severity on the magnitude of re-intervention and whether there was permanent disability or death [16]. Dindo et al. modified this system by expanding the previous 5 grades to 7 levels of severity [16]. Precision was added by defining whether the complication required general anesthetic, ICU admission was needed, and/or the extent of organ failure was present [2]. These and other modifications have been subsequently reviewed and redefined as the "Accordion Classification" for the purpose of expanding or contracting definitions across studies of different size and complexity [17]. Although an elegant and clinically relevant tool for clinicians to compare outcomes across various study groups, the system does not provide an economic framework for evaluating cost related to specific outcomes or focused prevention strategies. A refined approach would also require a methodology to capture post-discharge diagnoses and costs of treatment for utility in a bundled care format. Aside from the lack of a clinically relevant economic definition of complications, the current methods of reimbursement create diametrically opposed incentives for either under- or overreporting certain events. As mentioned earlier, the Centers for Medicare & Medicaid Services diagnosis-related group (MS-DRG) method of payment attempts to both risk adjust clinically and define broad groups of resource consumption [1]. The current system for colectomy consists of MS-DRG 331, MS-DRG 330, and MS-DRG 329 [1]. This system, however, potentially rewards certain hospital-acquired complications of surgical care, while simultaneously punishing certain costs associated with processes of care that actually reduce complications [18]. Conversely, a per diem payment strategy previously embraced by many commercial payers impedes innovation in care plans by forcing providers to calculate a length of stay that supports their cost structure while simultaneously maintaining more bed capacity than might be required with enhanced recovery. A final pitfall of the current system is a lack of a specific and consistent methodology for intra-institutional and cross institution cost and quality comparisons, including comparisons of the ACS NSQIP system to either the University Health Consortium or the Solucient® risk adjustment methodologies within the same institution [19, 20]. Further complicating the issue is the recent initiatives by the Centers for Medicare & Medicaid Services to deny supplemental payments for the so-called "never" events [21]. While rudimentary in implementation, the risk exists that complications that may not actually be predicted nor mitigated will not be compensated and adversely impact reimbursement in patient care. This will only exacerbate the current cost shifting in medical care delivery. Examples of this issue are the multiple publications which were unable to find a benefit related to implementation of the SCIP measures in reducing surgical site infections [22–25]. While no one can argue against the goal, clearly the data would suggest that the cost of reporting outcomes, devising the implementation process, and the resources of the care plan may well have outstripped any benefit to the patient or the healthcare system while negatively impacting cost at the institutional level. In fact, a recent publication demonstrated that despite real reductions in reimbursement, there has been no reduction in the reported incidence of these so-called preventable infectious complications [26]. These data raise the specter that reductions in reimbursement without clear assignment of risk adjustment risk equally punishing both poor performers and providers assuming care of patients at greatest risk.

A Concept of Warranty Cost

Key Concept: Utilizing the risk-adjusted evidence-informed case rate (ECR) type of analysis, an institution could more accurately define contracting needs, resource acquisition/allocation, and provider compensation for their organization.

If the primary goal of healthcare reform is to control cost increases, while simultaneously providing information for the consumer to accurately compare healthcare value, then a transparent, transferrable, and accurate measurement tool is required. As previously defined by Fry et al., this system should allow for the easy, reliable, and consistent reporting of information from the medical record that has been accurately monetized to the cost of a deliverable episode of care [27]. This group further demonstrated that an administrative dataset can be relatively easily modified by the addition of present on admission diagnosis codes (i.e., congestive heart failure, insulin-dependent diabetes mellitus) and readily available laboratory data to support accurate risk-stratified measurements of clinical outcomes in colectomy patients [28]. The benefit of this system would be to identify patient-centric diagnoses that drive both cost and clinical outcome more precisely. The same benefit could be achieved by refinement of postoperative diagnoses associated with complications. They identified, for a required hospital care cost of $4,723, appropriate risk adjustment increased cost by an average of $1,219 per case. Furthermore, addressing adverse outcomes (AO, defined as an inpatient death or a risk-adjusted postoperative length of stay outlier) required an additional $2,339 for death and an additional $282 per case allocated to the stop-loss pool to cover extraordinary costs of catastrophic AOs. As this type of analysis is refined, institutions and consumers could better assess true quality tempered by the impact of the type of patients managed. An urban institution managing patients with a greater burden of poorly controlled medical conditions would deserve a greater margin of warranty payment compared to an institution caring for a population with minimal comorbid disease burden. Similarly, the warranty cost of true "tertiary/quaternary" care would be appropriately higher. This concept is often defined as evidence-informed case rate (ECR), which has been defined by previous work in cancer care, chronic care, interventional cardiology, and orthopedic care [29, 30]. The work of de Brandt et al. suggested that we define the cost of care for a colectomy by focusing on resection type rather than the specific pathology, while analyzing the quantity and types of typical services and the types of available services caused by undesired complications [30].

This exercise could easily be adopted by any institution/department as the data regarding the major drivers of cost differential for the population managed by the institution and the variability across providers should be available in the billing system. Using colectomy as an example, the institution would begin with the "best case" patient (as discussed earlier) focusing on the group with the lowest cost structure at their institution. From this base case, one could easily assess the incremental cost of additional resources related to mitigation of complications, the cost of specific complications and the frequency of those events, and finally provider-specific variations for similar service. This process can easily be performed using the internal administrative data collected from the information system used to populate the UB 2004 form for bill submission, which provides a readily available low-cost model to guide cost analysis and outcomes that drive margin and quality. As an example, one could assess the institutional benefit for adopting Entereg for the prevention of postoperative ileus by assessing their base rate of postoperative ileus within the colectomy population, their success in reducing postoperative ileus with the drug, and the cost of the drug. Barletta performed this exercise and determined that the business case for adoption of Entereg was best aimed at the open colectomy population [31]. On the contrary, it would not be useful in the minimally invasive setting, especially following an enhanced recovery protocol. This type of introspection simultaneously allows the institution to focus quality improvement, reduce unnecessary cost, and provide a reduction in warranty cost all based on its internal performance. The rigor of this exercise allows the providers to understand the local "best case" and the population they treat without resorting to misinformed value judgments about which alterations in care plans would most fit the specific needs of the organization. For example, a smaller community hospital primarily managing an elective colon cancer population would clearly be exposed to a different base cost structure than a tertiary care facility tasked with managing a greater population of patients requiring multivisceral resection for advanced disease.

A theoretical fully loaded cost model based upon the ECR process discussed above is shown in Table 40.1. The model does not directly include risk adjustment because the best case was defined economically, assuming that whatever clinical decisions were made resulted from the combination of both patient-centric and surgeon-centric characteristics. The PROMETHEUS group found only a weak correlation between the severity index of provider's patients (a measure of how costly and prone to complications that provider's population is) and that provider's profit margins [15, 29]. This conclusion is a further support of the analysis provided by Fry and the hypothetical analysis in this chapter, which all demonstrated that only certain diagnoses truly influence cost of care. Utilizing the ECR type of analysis, an institution could more accurately define contracting needs, resource acquisition/allocation, and provider compensation for their organization. In addition, the organization would be able to articulate their value proposition to payers and consumers or alternatively understand opportunities for improvement to enhance competitiveness. The data in Table 40.1 demonstrate a base cost of $7,621 for laparoscopic colectomy and $8,721 for open. The data offer some interesting insights at an institutional level, beginning with the fact that for whatever reason the team chose a laparoscopic approach, the result was still a lower cost.

Expanding the discussion further, one can assess the "ultimate" warranty cost for their own institution (or the amount of money ideally collected on each patient that would allow the institution to cover expenses of the few who develop a complication). In this case (Table 40.2), the total warranty cost ranges from $111 to $2,172 for the elective and open procedures based upon technique. This cost is determined by applying the cost impact of managing the various complications across the entire population managed. Therefore, if a team could further reduce the frequency or cost of managing an issue, the warranty cost could be further reduced. This might include a broader use of laparoscopic procedures with appropriate training or alternatively defining cases better managed in an open fashion to avoid long case time or cost of conversion. This hypothetical analysis demonstrates that for this institution's colectomy population, elderly patients and urgent or emergent colectomy were all associated with significant increases in warranty cost primarily due to the increased number of

Table 40.1 The table demonstrates the cost associated with elective laparoscopic and open segmental colectomy and the mean episode costs associated with urgent/emergent procedures and the various complication patterns

Elective admit/no complications	$7,621(*N*=99)	$8,719(*N*=92)
Urgent admit/no complications	$7,708(*N*=7)	$9,343(*N*=29)
Elective admit/≥3 complications	$26,490(*N*=2)	$19,416(*N*=5)
Urgent admit/≥3 complications	$20,654 (*N*=3)	$49,251(*N*=12)
Elective admit/UROR	$42,946 (*N*=1)	$14,316(*N*=2)
Urgent admit/UROR	$(*N*=0)	$49,241(*N*=4)
Elective admit/POI	$9,638(*N*=5)	$14,065(*N*=13)
Urgent admit/POI	$(*N*=0)	$12,193(*N*=4)
Elective admit/POI/POA	$12,072(*N*=1)	$12,037(*N*=5)
Urgent admit/POI/POA	$0(*N*=0)	$19,856(*N*=3)

≥3 complications, unplanned return to operating room (*UROR*), postoperative ileus (*POI*), and postoperative anemia (*POA*)

Table 40.2 The table demonstrates the base case cost (elective laparoscopic segmental colectomy) and the incremental cost increases associated with open colectomy and the effect of frequency and episode mean cost of complications

Elective admit/no complications	$7,621	$1,098/$285
Urgent admit/no complications	$87/$2	$1,722/$141
Elective admit/≥3 complications	$18,869/$106	$11,795/$166
Urgent admit/≥3 complications	$12,946/$109	$41,630/$1,407
Elective admit/UROR	$35,325//$100	$6,695/$38
Urgent admit/UROR	$(*N*=0)	$41,620/$469
Elective admit/POI	$2,017/$28	$6,444/$236
Urgent admit/POI	$(*N*=0)	$4,572/$52
Elective admit/POI/POA	$4,365/$12	$4,416/$62
Urgent admit/POI/POA	$(*N*=0)	$12,235/$103
Total warranty elective	$246	$787
Total warranty urgent	$111	$2,172

≥3 complications, unplanned return to operating room (*UROR*), postoperative ileus (*POI*), and postoperative anemia (*POA*)
The warranty cost is defined by the episode cost × the number of episodes divided by the total patient population of 355

complications occurring per patient. Elderly patients typically have a greater preponderance of present on admission conditions that adversely impact the physiologic response to acute illness and surgical intervention and may be only minimally modifiable prior to surgery. The incidence of colonic pathology requiring urgent or emergent surgical intervention is also higher in this population, further augmenting the risk exposure to the provider. Interestingly, the analysis also confirmed that the most costly outcomes are usually multifactorial and unlikely to be mitigated by a globally implemented set of process measures. Instead, it would be more profitable to assess specific components of resource consumption by treatments implemented on a case-by-case basis. Although none of these factors can be directly mitigated, it would be relatively easy to model these risk factors for any potential payer-based population. Recognition of the impact of unavoidable patient characteristics (i.e., severe aortic stenosis in a patient with an obstructing rectal cancer) within a surgical procedure population could avoid forcing providers to accept significant risk without fair compensation or alternatively to "cherry-pick" the population to treat. It is unreasonable to expect the provider to accept the entire risk of managing complicated patients with acute surgical pathology, or worse yet, be the recipient of only the highest risk patients from a given payer without expecting a premium in return. Alternatively, if the payer/provider relationship allowed for nonselective referral, the ECR payment rate could be negotiated based upon the specific demographics and history of the beneficiary pool. Clearly, this would result in an advantageous position versus the current, and often adversarial, fee negotiations that are focused only on lower price—or worse yet, the assumption of poor care. One final concept was that both postoperative ileus and perioperative anemia were important cost drivers, while surgical site infection had no impact on cost structure. This is similar to the work from Wick et al., who demonstrated that consistent improvement in process measure implementation and reporting did not alter the infection rate [22]. Deep organ space infection did complicate the cost of care model; however, the true impact was always related to urgent operations, indicating that acute physiology played a greater role than any current process measure. Importantly, anastomotic leak and the associated downstream complications were considered separately from isolated SSI in this model. This is an important distinction, because any alleged measures for reducing SSI will not likely decrease the anastomotic leak rate. Yet, SSI routinely follows leak development. In addition, attributing outrageously high costs to SSI rather than the complex septic physiology related to anastomotic leaks blurs any rational discussion of cost-effective implementation of SSI reduction strategies [24–26]. The analysis further supports the ECR premise that the average cost per complication had an even stronger negative correlation on cost and margin—the greater the "defect," the greater the cost of that defect and the providers' financial risk [29]. Implementation of specific understanding of outcome and cost metrics may be the optimal way to truly "bend the cost curve" for surgical care in the United States. This approach is more precise compared to a concept that all complications can be avoided, or the imprecise application of strategies either unproven or unhelpful in reducing these complications. Providers who can demonstrate superior care and lower cost, documented by a more balanced scorecard approach, would arm consumers with a better framework for decision-making regarding their surgical care.

Summary Pearls

The colorectal surgeon will have to develop a solid understanding of the components of care, the variations of process implementation, and the population they care for in their practice to create a successful economic model for value-based purchasing. The market pressures created by the Accountable Care Organization can have a positive influence on the continued innovation of care directed by the surgeon. Success in the future will require an attention to detail in the care of their patients and a wise use of technology.

References

1. "Medicare program; changes to the hospital inpatient prospective payment systems for acute care hospitals and fiscal year 2010 rates; and changes to the long term care hospital prospective payment system and rate years 2010 and 2009 rates; final rule." Federal Register 74. 2009;(165):43754–4236. Available online at: www.cms.gov/AcuteInpatientPPS. Accessed Feb 2013.
2. Pessaux P, Lermite E, Brehant O, Tuech JJ, Lorimier G, Arnaud JP. Repeat hepatectomy for recurrent colorectal liver metastases. J Surg Oncol. 2006;93(1):1–7.
3. Abbou CC, Hoznek A, Salomon L, et al. Laparoscopic radical prostatectomy with a remote controlled robot. J Urol. 2001;165(6 Pt 1): 1964–6.
4. Lin S, Jiang HG, Chen ZH, Zhou SY, Liu XS, Yu JR. Meta-analysis of robotic and laparoscopic surgery for treatment of rectal cancer. World J Gastroenterol. 2011;17(47):5214–20.
5. Park JS, Choi GS, Park SY, Kim HJ, Ryuk JP. Randomized clinical trial of robot-assisted versus standard laparoscopic right colectomy. Br J Surg. 2012;99(9):1219–26.
6. Link RE, Bhayani SB, Kavoussi LR. A prospective comparison of robotic and laparoscopic pyeloplasty. Ann Surg. 2006;243(4):486–91.
7. Baik SH, Kwon HY, Kim JS, et al. Robotic versus laparoscopic low anterior resection of rectal cancer: short-term outcome of a prospective comparative study. Ann Surg Oncol. 2009;16(6):1480–7.
8. Delaney CP, Lynch AC, Senagore AJ, Fazio VW. Comparison of robotically performed and traditional laparoscopic colorectal surgery. Dis Colon Rectum. 2003;46(12):1633–9.
9. Barbash GI, Glied SA. New technology and health care costs – the case of robot-assisted surgery. N Engl J Med. 2010;363(8):701–4.
10. D'Annibale A, Morpurgo E, Fiscon V, Trevisan P, Sovernigo G, Orsini C, Guidolin D. Robotic and laparoscopic surgery for treatment of colorectal diseases. Dis Colon Rectum. 2004;47(12): 2162–8.
11. Leddy LS, Lendvay TS, Satava RM. Robotic surgery: applications and cost effectiveness. Open Access Sur. 2010;3:99–107.
12. Memon S, Heriot AG, Murphy DG, Bressel M, Lynch AC. Robotic versus laparoscopic proctectomy for rectal cancer: a meta-analysis. Ann Surg Oncol. 2012;19(7):2095–101.
13. Ortiz-Oshiro E, Sanchez-Egido I, Moreno-Sierra J, Perez CF, Diaz JS, Fernandez-Represa JA. Robotic assistance may reduce conversion to open in rectal carcinoma laparoscopic surgery: systematic review and meta-analysis. Int J Med Robot. 2012;8(3):360–70.
14. Trastulli S, Farinella E, Cirocchi R, et al. Robotic resection compared with laparoscopic rectal resection for cancer: systematic review and meta-analysis of short-term outcome. Colorectal Dis. 2012;14(4):e134–56.
15. PROMETHEUS Payment Inc [Internet]. Philadelphia: PROMETHEUS Payment Inc.; 2008. [cited 20 May 2009]. Available from: http://www.PROMETHEUSpayment.org. Accessed Feb 2013.
16. Dindo D, Demartines N, Clavien PA. Classification of surgical complications-a new proposal with evaluation in a cohort of 6336 patients and results of a survey. Ann Surg. 2004;240:205–13.
17. Strassberg SD, Linehan DC, Hawkins WG. The accordion severity grading system of surgical complications. Ann Surg. 2009;250: 177–86.
18. Senagore AJ, Brannigan A, Kiran RP, Brady K, Delaney CP. Diagnosis-related group assignment in laparoscopic and open colectomy: financial implications for payer and provider. Dis Colon Rectum. 2005;48(5):1016–20.
19. Steinberg SM, Popa MR, Bethel MJ, Michalek JA, Ellison EC. Comparison of risk adjustment methodologies in surgical quality improvement. Surgery. 2008;144(4):662–7; discussion 662–7.
20. Hall BL, Hirbe M, Waterman B, Boslaugh S, Dunagan WC. Comparison of mortality risk adjustment using a clinical data algorithm (American College of Surgeons National Surgical Quality Improvement Program) and an administrative data algorithm (Solucient) at the case level within a single institution. J Am Coll Surg. 2007;205(6):767–77.
21. Berenguer CM, Ochsner Jr MG, Lord SA, Senkowski CK. Analysis of centers for Medicaid and Medicare services 'never events' in elderly patients undergoing bowel operations. Am Surg. 2010; 76(8):841–5.
22. Wick EC, Gibbs L, Indorf LA, Varma MG, Garcia-Aguilar J. Implementation of quality measures to reduce surgical site infection in colorectal patients. Dis Colon Rectum. 2008;51:1004–9.
23. Englesbe MJ, Brooks L, Kubus J, Luchtefeld M, Lynch J, Senagore A, Eggenberger JC, Velanovich V, Campbell Jr DA. A statewide assessment of surgical site infection following colectomy: the role of oral antibiotics. Ann Surg. 2010;252(3):514–9; discussion 519–20.
24. Morse BC, Boland BN, Blackhurst DW, Roettger RH. Improving surgical site infections: using national surgical quality improvement program data to institute surgical care improvement project protocols in improving surgical outcomes. J Am Coll Surg. 2010;210(5):737–41.
25. Stulberg JJ, Delaney CP, Neuhauser DV, Aron DC, Fu P, Koroukian SM. Adherence to surgical care improvement project measures and the association with postoperative infections. JAMA. 2010;303(24): 2479–85.
26. Lee GM, Kleinman K, Soumerai SB, Tse A, Cole D, Fridkin SK, Horan T, Platt R, Gay C, Kassler W, Goldmann DA, Jernigan J, Jha AK. Effect of nonpayment for preventable infections in U.S. hospitals. N Engl J Med. 2012;367(15):1428–37.
27. Fry DE, Pine M, Jones BL, Meimban RJ. Surgical warranties to improve quality and efficiency in elective colon surgery. Arch Surg. 2010;145(7):647–52.
28. Fry DE, Pine M, Jordan HS, Elixhauser A, Hoaglin DC, Jones B, Warner D, Meimban R. Combining administrative and clinical data to stratify surgical risk. Ann Surg. 2007;246:875–85.
29. de Brantes F, Camillus J. Evidence-informed case rates: a new health care payment model [Internet]. New York: Commonwealth Fund; 2007 [cited 20 May 2007]. Available from: de Brantes F, D'Andrea G, Rosenthal MB. Should health care come with a warranty? Many goods and services come with warranties; should health care? Analysis of one payment model shows promise and challenges. Health Affairs. 2009;28(4): w678–87 (published online 16 June 2009; 10.1377/hlthaff.28.4.w678). Accessed Feb 2013.
30. de Brantes F, Camillus J. Evidence-informed case rates: a new health care payment model [Internet]. New York: Commonwealth Fund; 2007 [cited 20 May 2007]. Available from: http://www.commonwealthfund.org/publications/publications_show.htm?doc_id=478278. Accessed Feb 2013.
31. Barletta JF, Asgeirsson T, El-Badawi KI, Senagore AJJ. Introduction of alvimopan into an enhanced recovery protocol for colectomy offers benefit in open but not laparoscopic colectomy. J Laparoendosc Adv Surg Tech A. 2011;21(10):887–91.

Defining Competence and the Role of the Board

41

David J. Schoetz Jr.

Key Points

- Educational techniques must evolve to reflect changes in the learners while preserving basic principles.
- Maintenance of certification is indeed a lifelong process, reflecting the need for continued application to one's profession in order to improve the overall care of patients.
- The American Board of Colon and Rectal Surgery is the central organization in defining and implementing evolving educational opportunities.

Competence is "the quality of being competent or capable of performing an allotted function" [1]. Training of physicians has always had as its primary goal, the formulation of an end product that is capable of providing safe and effective care, while recognizing that continued acquisition of knowledge and skills following the completion of the initial training period is an essential part of professionalism. It has long been accepted that the lifelong application of knowledge and practice of both the art and science of one's chosen specialty will continually enhance and improve individual performance to the benefit of each patient.

Key Concept: Defining competence for surgical trainees is a process in evolution and extends beyond the traditional metric of case numbers and subjective assessment.

It is fair to say that the definition of competence has been elusive enough that residency training programs have been willing to declare competence of each trainee on the day that they complete their residency but no longer. Achievement of board certification has not equated to competence to practice (by the Boards' own admission). While in some part motivated by medicolegal concerns for potential shared complicity in tort litigation on the part of training programs and program directors, the much more significant concern has been the inability to accurately and reproducibly define the parameters of competence within each medical specialty.

For colon and rectal surgery, and other technically focused specialties (be they surgical or medical), this has evolved into the application of cumulative case numbers as a presumed surrogate for technical competence. There is no question that there is an empirical value to performance of procedures, but the number alone does not adequately describe individual resident performance, with all of the subtle nuances of each individual situation for each resident. Consequently, there is a movement to define the minimal technical requirements for each individual procedure within the domain of each specialty. The ACGME has initiated the Milestone Project, which is an attempt to define specific outcomes for each specialty as defined by expert educators in the field. These data will be evaluated on an ongoing basis and will be incorporated into the new annual program reporting for each program [2]. While creative and encouraging, it should be pointed out that these outcomes are in the early stages of being defined and have not yet been demonstrated to be associated with competence. Furthermore, they are subjective evaluations of technical performance and may not be as robust as other more easily quantifiable measures such as communication, system-based performance, and practice-based learning.

Key Concept: Changes ranging from how we manage certain disease processes to the level of responsibility given to trainees has impacted general surgery training and increased the need for additional training beyond residency.

D.J. Schoetz Jr., MD
Division of Surgery, Department of Colon and Rectal Surgery, Lahey Clinic, Tufts University School of Medicine, 41 Mall Road, Burlington, MA 01805, USA
e-mail: david.j.schoetz@lahey.org

The opinions expressed in this manuscript represent the opinions of the author and are in no way a reflection of the official policies or opinions of the American Board of Colon and Rectal Surgery.

S.R. Steele et al. (eds.), *Complexities in Colorectal Surgery*,
DOI 10.1007/978-1-4614-9022-7_41, © Springer Science+Business Media New York 2014

At present, all colon and rectal surgeons must be fully trained general surgeons. It is this fact that has, until recently, allowed for achievement of sufficient specialty training in one additional year of colorectal residency. General surgery has been under enormous stress to provide satisfactory training in 5 years, and this has resulted in a concerted effort to redefine the training of general surgeons. Lewis and Klingensmith have neatly and comprehensively reviewed these stresses in a recent forum at the American Surgical Association [3]. The authors outline the changes in the practice of general surgery that have occurred over the past 20 years, the net effect of which is to reduce the volume of some operations that were previously the staples of general surgical training. Of particular importance for the specialty of colon and rectal surgery is the increasing percentage of abdominal operations performed laparoscopically; this, combined with the vanishing numbers of surgical procedures for peptic ulcer disease and complex biliary tract disease, percutaneous vascular procedures, and the increasingly non-operative management of abdominal trauma, has focused attention on complex minimally invasive colorectal procedures as necessary for training general surgeons. This, combined with the non-ACGME industry-funded postresidency fellowships in bariatrics and other advanced minimally invasive procedures (and some non-ACGME-sponsored colorectal fellowships as well), has spawned a desire on the part of the American Board of Surgery to consider a subspecialty of advanced gastrointestinal tract surgery as a way to compete with existing training paradigms.

Other issues of concern to general surgery include the fact that about 80 % of graduating general surgery residents pursue additional training beyond the basic 5-year training period, predominantly because they do not feel confident to practice independently [3] and because they believe that additional training provides a competitive advantage in the workplace [4]. Consequently, the real total duration of general surgery training is currently 6–7 years for the majority of general surgery graduates.

Finally, many factors have conspired to eliminate traditional residency concepts of graduated responsibility, both in decision making and operating. Today's chief resident has often not been solely responsible for a decision to operate or for an unsupervised operative intervention. Some of these factors will never return to Halsteadian ideals. Perhaps there was not sufficient supervision in the past, to the patients' detriment in some cases. However, the end result of this evolution is often a new graduate who is ill-prepared for independent function as a practicing surgeon.

Key Concept: *Paradigm shifts for attending surgeons, residents, and curricula that mirror the evolving modern training environment are required to maximize educational opportunities and minimize inefficiency.*

Approaches to altering the educational directions of residency training are severalfold [3]. Curriculum redesign must be undertaken to reflect changes in practice and then be treated as a dynamic and fluid situation, changing with the evolution of practice. Abandoning outdated portions of the curriculum will free up time for the resident to learn what is essential. Furthermore, there must be an acknowledgement that service demands on the part of the residents creates inefficiencies of learning that must be challenged and streamlined wherever possible. Physician extenders and other nonresident resources must be used more liberally to cover the service needs traditionally provided by residents; current and anticipated economic constraints will challenge the ability to do so, since traditionally service and education have been inexorably intertwined.

Individual self-directed learning rather than group lectures will become the norm, particularly with more stresses (and presumably further reductions) on maximum allowable work hours. Adult learning theory suggests that today's residents are least inspired by traditional lectures and most by interactive self-directed tools. Consequently, sophisticated learning resources such as the Surgical Council on Resident Education (SCORE®) portal should be made available to all residents, as should other validated teaching vehicles. Self-assessment is essential to monitor individual resident performance, and comparisons among residents and programs will improve the value of these exercises.

There needs to be a greater focus on improving the teaching skills of surgical attendings. The old concept of "stealing the case" while not providing constructive feedback to the operating resident cannot continue. Residents need to be directed toward those procedures that will enhance their education; only devoted attendings can provide this constructive instruction. Those attending who cannot provide appropriate direction will be deleted from teaching services. Each technical interaction should be followed by a debriefing exercise, even if to say "well done in all aspects." Regular formative evaluations must be a required part of each resident interaction.

Key Concept: *Despite present-day technical limitations, simulation will likely have a large role in training future generations of surgeons.*

Simulation is currently a very popular strategy to assist in and accelerate training of students and residents (and surgeons at all levels). Probably the most compelling reason for the use of simulation is to provide a certain level of technical proficiency without actual patient risk exposure [5]. Many technical skills can be perfected on low-fidelity bench top training devices. Fundamentals of Laparoscopic Surgery (FLS) was developed by the Society of Gastrointestinal and Endoscopic Surgery (SAGES), endorsed by the American College of Surgeons and the Association of Program Directors in Surgery, and is now required for each surgical trainee prior to certification by the American Board of Surgery (and thus all colon and rectal residents). Fundamentals of Endoscopic Surgery (FES) is currently being validated and presumably will follow the same path, being ultimately required for certification. Most recently there has been exploration of a program of Fundamentals of Robotic Surgery.

Repetitive practice in the simulation environment results in skills acquisition that expedites technical performance in both the operating room and the endoscopy suite. In other areas, such as central line and peripheral intravenous line insertion, urinary catheter placement, tube thoracostomies, lumbar puncture, airway management, and other mechanical procedures that can be taught and practiced, there have been developed curricula and training exercises as well as mannequins for those in need of developing and honing individual skills.

Limitations of computer power presently limit high-fidelity simulators for teaching all but the most focused technical procedures. At present, there is virtually no haptic feedback; consequently these simulators provide primarily visual feedback for technical maneuvers and are more applicable to endoscopy and laparoscopy with its many permutations (robotics, NOTES). Certainly the enthusiasm for high-fidelity simulation will result in much more sophisticated devices in the future. One needs to be circumspect in considering resource allocation, since these new devices tend to be expensive and often are purchased before validation. It would not be difficult to accumulate attractive but relatively unhelpful simulators.

Key Concept: A collaborative effort across several surgical organizations has and will play a role in determining the ideal evolution in training. Similar to other surgical subspecialties, residents desiring colon and rectal surgery residencies may one day embark on pre-specialty-focused training during their general surgery residency.

With these demands as a developing background, colon and rectal surgery has for some time examined the need to change its training paradigm to assure that residents receive sufficient training in the specialty. Changes in general surgery training continue to challenge the colon and rectal surgeons to define their own curriculum. Several years ago a group was convened comprised of representatives from the American Board of Colon and Rectal Surgery (ABCRS), the American Society of Colon and Rectal Surgeons (ASCRS), the Residency Review Committee (RRC), and the Association of Program Directors for Colon and Rectal Surgery (PDA) to examine training. As a result, the curriculum of colon and rectal surgery was defined. The ASCRS in conjunction with the PDA then utilized the curriculum to create the *ASCRS Textbook of Colon and Rectal Surgery*, now in its second edition [6]. The ABCRS developed a set of minimum numbers of cases required for each applicant for board certification; these were implemented over a relatively brief period of time.

As a result of the deliberations of the Blue Ribbon Committee, the ABCRS in 2008 brought a request to the American Board of Surgery (ABS) asking that those residents pursuing a career in colon and rectal surgery be trained in 2 rather than 1 year; it was the feeling of the Blue Ribbon Committee for colon and rectal surgery that a 2-year residency period would improve the overall training experience of colon and rectal surgeons. This could also be in the form of a "hybrid" chief year, with at least 6 months of colon and rectal surgery and 6 months of traditional general surgery chief residency. The trainees from the 4+2 of 4+1+1 training programs would be able to achieve certification by ABS. A sizable percentage of practicing colon and rectal surgeons, for various reasons, perform a considerable amount of traditional general surgery [7], and thus it was the feeling of the leadership of the specialty that preservation of double board certification was important to colon and rectal surgeons. This request was denied at the time by the ABS, presumably because they were in the process of defining their own curriculum.

Subsequently, data were generated from the American Board of Surgery and used to generate a hypothetical training model in which 6 months of early specialty-directed tracking were allowed; the residents self-selected cases in their chosen subspecialty field. The individual overall resident case experience did not suffer while the subspecialty experience was enriched [8]. These data were subsequently confirmed by actual case log numbers from applicants for the ABS qualifying examination, in which coexisting fellowships did not adversely affect resident case numbers and, in some instances, actually increased them. Furthermore, the data demonstrated that self-directed specialty pre-fellowship operative training was already a reality [9].

In fact, relatively recently the ABS has recognized a "flexibility option" that would allow a resident to focus on a single-specialty area for 12 months of the last 3 years of general surgery residency [3]. To date, few have availed themselves of this option. General surgery program directors feel that there would be a logistical impediment to providing a satisfactory operative breadth for all of the residents in a given program, and since incoming residents are not often chosen for their ultimate career goals, the organizational aspects of this are indeed potentially daunting.

From a colon and rectal surgery training point of view, residents would be forced to make earlier career decisions for pursuing a career in colorectal surgery. Since general surgery residents currently decide on pursuing a colorectal residency in their PGY-3 or PGY-4 year [10], in order to allow residents to make earlier decisions and track into the specialty, substantive exposure to colorectal surgery would have to be accomplished earlier in the general surgery residency. Currently the matching process occurs during the PGY-5 general surgery year; early tracking would probably require another matching process that would allow interested general surgery residents to match in a general surgery program with a desired colorectal training program at the same institution. This would be a potential manpower and Medicare residency funding nightmare for general surgery program directors. For the foreseeable future, it is likely that a small number of pilot programs will be piloted in institutions with both general surgery and colorectal residencies in order to compare outcomes to those of traditional training schemes.

Key Concept: The ABCRS remains a central figure in helping guide the future training and accreditation of colon and rectal surgeons.

Throughout all of these discussions on the proposed evolution of the specialty, the American Board of Colon and Rectal Surgery has been integrally involved. The American Board of Medical Specialties (ABMS) was established to share examination techniques among various specialties in order to standardize the curriculum within each specialty and to improve the overall quality of patient care by better and more standardized education. Independence of each individual board was assured [11]. The American Board of Proctology (now ABCRS) won a hard-fought and often bitter battle for independence from the American Board of Surgery and became the 18th (of 24) member of the ABMS. It is the tenacity of our forbearers that has placed colon and rectal surgery in control of its own destiny; this is something that should never be relinquished nor compromised.

Primary board certification was considered the ultimate successful achievement after completion of the residency training period. Certainly, most residents are repeatedly counseled regarding the need to achieve board certification. More recently, many specialties use board passage rates as a measure of the quality of a particular training program. Minimum pass rates will be used in the New Accreditation System of the ACGME and the individual Residency Review Committees.

Each board has its own examination procedure. For colon and rectal surgery, as for general surgery, there is a qualifying examination (written). Passage of the written allows one to take the certifying examination (oral). All colon and rectal residents must pass the ABS examination in order to take the test for colon and rectal surgery. Many wonder whether this format should change; it is the belief of ABCRS, and other boards with a similar format, that the two parts of the examination test different aspects of each candidate. The written examination, subject to strict psychometric scrutiny, tests factual knowledge felt to be a prerequisite for satisfactory practice. The oral examination, on the other hand, reflects the ability of the candidate to apply this knowledge in patient management situations under some stress. These two parts of the examination, combined with case logs and performance assessments by the program director, are certainly not a perfect system but have evolved over time to be a basic reflection of the skills felt to be necessary to be a safe practitioner of the specialty.

Key Concept: Recertification and maintenance of certification are methods to help ensure the credibility and competency of all colon and rectal surgeons.

For a long time the completion of the examination and achievement of certification resulted in a lifelong certificate, never having to repeat the process throughout one's subsequent professional life. Since the aim of board certification is to continue to provide quality care for the public, the responsibility for continuous professional development was (and continues to be) the responsibility of each diplomate. Provision of a "lifetime" certificate was felt for some time to be disingenuous by the public, and well-publicized continuing medical education "junkets" were rather patently less rigorous educational activities than vacations. It is fair to say that some acted in a less than professional manner in not truly keeping abreast of developments in their fields. In an attempt to maintain some control over the board process, the concept of intermittent "recertification" was introduced by each of the boards. Colon and rectal surgery had its first recertification examination in 1991 with an initial required frequency of every 10 years [11]. The American Board of Surgery had initiated time-limited certificates in 1976, with a similar 10-year interval.

Those with time-unlimited certificates are commonly referred to as "grandfathered," without an absolute requirement to recertify. The ABCRS strongly urges these individuals to voluntarily enter the process. As of May 2011, there were 454 people with time-unlimited certificates (28 % of all diplomates); 41 % of these are under age 62 years [11]. While there is not a legal requirement to do so, voluntarily entering the process would demonstrate a commitment to the public trust afforded to those who actively practice colon and rectal surgery.

Recertification has substantially evolved with the development of maintenance of certification (MOC). The ABMS adopted the six competencies of the ACGME Outcome project and incorporated them as the cornerstone of the MOC process, which is characterized by four essential components [12]:

1. *Professional standing* every 5 years – full licensure in the state in which one practices, documentation of privileges in colon and rectal surgery, and a letter of recommendation by the chief of surgery at one's hospital
2. *Lifelong learning and self-assessment*
3. *Cognitive expertise* every 10 years
4. *Evaluation of performance in practice* – ongoing participation in outcomes databases or quality assessment programs (e.g., SCIP, NSQIP, UHC)

Work continues on defining the parameters of MOC. Because of the continued need for double board certification and the excellent relationship between ABCRS and ABS, a reciprocity arrangement has been reached to allow sharing of MOC parts one, two, and four between the two boards. The examination will need to be taken separately for each specialty.

Part four, practice-based improvement, has been the most difficult to describe, characterize, and implement. In the ideal world, each individual surgeon's outcomes should be incorporated into the process. Comparative effectiveness research could then shape not only individual improvements but also population-based evolutions of best practices. This effort will require a number of resource reallocations and a reasonably uniform acceptance by all members of the specialty and others caring for similar conditions; nevertheless, this will accomplish what MOC part 4 was ultimately designed to do.

Key Concept: The manner in which we initially examine candidates upon completion of a colon and rectal surgery residency, as well as board-certified surgeon in the MOC process, will also evolve in an attempt to more accurately define competency.

Notably absent from the initial certification process and the MOC evaluation is an assessment of technical proficiency. While the Fundamentals of Laparoscopic Surgery are indeed a minimum technical performance standard, they are certainly not sufficient to evaluate a practicing colon and rectal surgeon. Furthermore, during one's professional career, it would be advised to reassess skills on a periodic basis. Finally, some individuals take a period of time away from clinical practice and wish to reenter after a period of inactivity. For all of these reasons, the ASCRS, in conjunction with the ABCRS and the PDA, have initiated a project to create the Colorectal Objective Structured Assessment of Technical Skills (COSATS). These are a group of eight skills that should be able to be accomplished by a practicing colorectal surgeon. The first testing demonstrated validity comparing a small group of general surgery chief residents to matched colorectal residents. The second effort, completed recently, tested nearly 40 colon and rectal residents. It is the belief of the ABCRS that the COSATS will become part of the requirements for initial certification and, by periodic testing, the MOC process as well. Certainly the Fundamentals of Endoscopic Surgery will also be a requirement. As other validated tools of technical performance become available, they will each be evaluated for their value in the ongoing assessment of performance.

Communication skills may best be evaluated by utilization of standardized patients in a simulation environment. Construction of both exercises for training and high-stakes assessment will evolve and will need to be considered for inclusion in the ongoing evaluation of colorectal surgeons.

Summary Pearls

It is abundantly clear that board certification has changed forever and that the logical place to focus the ongoing efforts of continuous quality assessment should reside with the board. No longer will it be acceptable to complete a residency, take a test or two and never again be accountable to those whom we serve. While the process is lengthy and potentially difficult, the ultimate reward reflects the original motivations for the establishment and success of the board movement.

References

1. Competence (n.d.). The American Heritage® Stedman's Medical Dictionary. Retrieved 23 Oct 2012, from Dictionary.com website: http://dictionary.reference.com/browse/competence.
2. Available at: http://www.acgme.org/acgmeweb/Portals/0/PFAssets/PublicationsNewsletters/CRS_Newsletter_Apr12.pdf. Accessed 28 Dec 2012.
3. Lewis FR, Klingensmith ME. Issues in general surgery residency training – 2012. Ann Surg. 2012;256:553–9.
4. Yeo H, Viola K, Berg D, et al. Attitudes, training experiences, and professional expectations of US general surgery residents. JAMA. 2009;302:1301–8.
5. deMontbrun SL, MacRae H. Simulation in surgical education. Clin Colon Rectal Surg. 2012;25:156–65.
6. Beck D, Roberts PL, Saclarides TJ, Senagore AJ, Stamos MJ, Wexner S, editors. The ASCRS textbook of colon and rectal surgery. 2nd ed. New York: Springer Publ; 2011.
7. Chu KM, Schoetz DJ. What impact might general surgery practice patterns of colon and rectal surgeons have on future training? Dis Colon Rectum. 2007;50:1250–4.
8. Stain S, Biester TW, Hanks JB, Ashley SW, Valentine RJ, Bass BL, Buyske J. Early tracking would improve the operative experience of general surgery residents. Ann Surg. 2010;252:445–51.
9. Hanks JB, Ashley SW, Mahvi DM, Meredith WJ, Stan SC, Biester TW, Borman KR. Feast of famine? The variable impact of coexisting fellowships on general surgery resident operative volumes. Ann Surg. 2011;254:476–85.
10. Schmitz CC, Rothenberger DA, Trudel JL, Wolff BG. Career decisions and the structure of training. An American Board of Colon and Rectal Surgery survey of colorectal residents. Ann Surg. 2009;250:62–7.
11. Schoetz DJ. The American Board of Colon and Rectal Surgery: past, present and future. Clin Colon Rectal Surg. 2012;25:166–70.
12. Available at : http://www.abcrs.org/recertification/. Accessed 13 Jan 2013.

Knowing When to Say "When" 42

Alan G. Thorson

Key Points

- The best and least traumatic retirements result from key planning long before retirement is expected, including financial planning for postretirement income and developing a diversity of interests that will hold your attention when the practice of medicine is no longer feasible.
- Surgeons need to be the primary assessors of their competency, and any decline thereof, as they progress through their active practice years and be the ones to recognize the need to begin the transition process.
- There is life after medicine.

When one door closes, another one opens, but we often look so long and regretfully at the closed door that we fail to see the one that has opened for us.

–Alexander Graham Bell (Scientist)

Introduction

Walking away gracefully. The perfect end to a storied career at the right time. No matter the stage of your career, it is something that you've likely thought about, or for some, hopefully experienced. We all want to exit on top, go out in style. The clichés are bountiful because it is a crucial aspect to our professional lives. Sports are littered with examples. Would you rather be John Elway "riding off in the sunset" following two consecutive NFL championships or Michael Jordan—arguably the greatest NBA player in history—who may be more known mockingly for his three retirements and inability to give it up than his multiple on and off-the-court accomplishments? And what about all the "end of the bench" players who simply fade away? Does it make their accomplishments or careers any less significant? These questions probably have different answers for each of you, as well as varying degrees of relevance. We would all likely agree that caring for patients and the opportunity to practice surgery are what brought us and kept us in our chosen paths. Yet, how do we measure success and how do we know when to call it quits? For some, a career is left unfulfilled without having "X" number of publications, becoming chief/chair of surgery or president of a society. For others, it is simply doing your best, enjoying life and family, or serving in any capacity to make your hospital a better place. Regardless of ambitions, each of us eventually will end our surgical practice. The question is will we know when to say "when?"

The decision to retire from a practice of colon and rectal surgery merits discussion as a complexity in surgery due to the inherent controversies and inconsistencies that exist within that decision. Many issues arise that may impact the timing of retirement. Although the following discussion is not meant to be comprehensive, an evaluation of these issues will go a long way in determining when retirement might be desirable or even necessary. Such issues are represented by both internal and external forces. Those internal forces include the paradox of a patient's reliance on their physician coexisting with a physician's reliance on their patients. These might also be termed soft factors, emotional in nature or products of passion. External forces include all of the physical and mental changes that occur naturally with aging as well as economic and workforce implications for the individual's practice and profession. These represent hard factors.

For any profession, the decision to retire can be, but isn't always, difficult. Some individuals have predetermined dates for retirement and have well-planned goals and objectives to allow them to meet their desired ends. They may actually be anxious to retire to move on to other interests and personal

A.G. Thorson, MD, FACS
Division of Colon and Rectal Surgery, Department of Surgery, Creighton University School of Medicine, The University of Nebraska College of Medicine, 9850 Nicholas Street, Ste 100, Omaha, NE 68114, USA
e-mail: agthorson@msn.com

S.R. Steele et al. (eds.), *Complexities in Colorectal Surgery*,
DOI 10.1007/978-1-4614-9022-7_42, © Springer Science+Business Media New York 2014

goals. Soft factors have the least impact on these individuals. The hard factors have been recognized and dealt with long ago. Others have laid the foundations necessary for a comfortable retirement and are simply awaiting the appropriate confluence of events to make the final decision. They are prepared for retirement but still derive a great deal of satisfaction with their current practice. The hard factors have been dealt with in this group as well, and the soft factors are manageable. Yet for others, the decision is much harder. They may or may not have dealt with the hard factors affecting their decision, and the soft factors may lead to irrational choices and decisions when it comes to self-evaluation and suitability for continued practice.

Soft Factors

Professionals are used to serving. As physicians, our lives have been devoted to serving our patients and communities, and retirement may have implications for life and death issues—literally and figuratively. Concerns for our patients are real. Patients who have lost their primary care physician through illness, retirement, career change, or systems change express feelings of loss, abandonment, frustration, and anger directly related to losing their physicians. They describe concerns about the difficulty of getting prescription medications, lack of continuity of care related to medical records, and loss of continuity with preventive care [1]. At least some of these feelings undoubtedly transfer to colon and rectal surgeons and loss also, particularly for issues relating to preventive colonoscopy and cancer follow-up. I can only imagine the strength of some of these feelings in hereditary colorectal cancer families where in many cases long-term transgenerational relationships are established. For some physicians, the recognition of such patient perceptions and reliance may delay a decision to retire, as they do not want to "hurt" their patients.

Then there is the physician's reliance upon their patients and colleagues. Many physicians need the daily feedback from their patients; for without it, they feel a sense of emptiness or they may feel unfulfilled. Their commitment to their patients over the years has left them with little time to develop other interests and hobbies. When they look at retirement, they see only a life without purpose and subsequently fear entering that stage of their life.

Hard Factors

Age as a Factor

In addition to this internal turmoil, there are a host of external forces that contribute to retirement decisions. For individuals practicing within health systems, retirement may be forced upon them through indirect actions or incentive changes. Age may be a factor in a system's decision to terminate a surgeon for a number of reasons including the desire of a health system to hire someone younger with the capacity for higher production and the prospects for longer employment. As a French proverb states, "A surgeon should be young, a physician old." There may be a perception that newly trained surgeons will be more likely to adopt the newest treatments that a system may desire for a number of reasons including marketing and patient recruitment.

Presently in the United States, for employed surgeons, the use of the surgeon's chronologic age as a determinant of when he or she must retire is clearly in violation of the Age Discrimination in Employment Act (ADEA). Nevertheless, it is still possible to establish economic incentives or other environmental constructs that "encourage" retirement in the absence of documented age-related competency issues. Such competency issues are difficult to prove given the fact that there is no agreement on what skills we should test or how to test them. Although it is safe to say that age does ultimately affect competency, various studies have given mixed results depending on the population being tested and a host of variables within those populations that can impact outcome. Age alone is a poor test, no doubt, but the issue of competency deserves closer scrutiny.

A study of senior and younger surgeons attending annual meetings of the American College of Surgeons compared computerized cognitive tasks measuring visual sustained attention, reaction time, visual learning, and memory administered to both practicing and retired surgeons. The majority of practicing senior surgeons performed at or near the level of younger surgeons on all cognitive tasks, as did almost half of the retired surgeons. The authors concluded that older age does not inevitably preclude cognitive proficiency. Furthermore, the variability in performance across age groups suggests the need for formal measures of objective cognitive functioning to detect changes in performance to aid in retirement decisions [2], measures that have not yet been developed.

The story behind cognitive decline with age involves complex interactions between different types of intelligence [3] leading to variations in practice that, up to a point, may actually have beneficial effects [4]. Adults as old as in their 70s may have an advantage in cumulative information acquired through a lifetime of clinical practice (known as professional expertise and wisdom) but may take twice as long to process the same tasks as adults in their 20s [5]. In this situation, an older physician may have an advantage in efficient diagnostic skills through pattern recognition, while experiencing a decline in analytical skills, with subsequent overreliance on clinical first impressions [6]. Studies supportive of this have demonstrated that senior physicians experiencing competency issues have shown errors related to premature diagnostic conclusions following incomplete history and data gathering, coupled with limited differential considerations [7].

Despite the ultimate conclusion of the natural aging process, the timing of that process is highly variable. As mentioned, other studies show that many older physicians can compete effectively with at least a significant cohort of their younger colleagues [2, 8]. Many factors may modify the impact of age on competency including innate intelligence, continuous self-improvement and education [9], self-directed learning and practice at technical skills [4], as well as maintenance of healthy lifestyles through proper diet and nutrition, participation in health screenings, avoidance of tobacco products, and by staying physically active [10].

Other External Forces

Other external forces that can impact a decision to retire include the status of financial planning for retirement. Although hard data are difficult to obtain, some surgeons will find themselves poorly prepared for retirement from a financial standpoint as a result of poor spending habits with expenditures outstripping their income, due to bad financial advice or bad investment decisions, multiple marriages, or by simply going through their savings. Some simply never initiate a savings program. Some place themselves in a situation where they feel they never have enough.

For those in solo practices, there are the costs of closing a business to consider. These include the impact on personnel and the need to give proper notice, the maintenance or storage (if not electronic) of records which may be necessary for up to 20 years and the provision for continued care of patients—making sure notice is given to provide sufficient time to select another surgeon. There may be equipment and facilities to sell or leases to adjust to match planned retirement. Such issues and the time needed to resolve them may delay retirement for some individuals.

For those in small group practices, consideration must be given to the impact that retirement might have on overhead and production in the practice of the partners or associates that remain behind. Malpractice and the cost of tail coverage may also alter retirement plans if consideration has not been given to these issues before retirement is contemplated.

Unfortunately, for others a life event that was entirely unexpected (i.e., accident, health issue) has completely changed the landscape. Finally, though not often discussed, a small number of surgeons have had the ill-fated "luck" to experience one or several bouts of untoward patient outcomes for which credentialing problems have arisen, resulting in a mandated curtailment of privileges. All of these factors weigh not only into the process but also the options that are available as well.

Competency

Never retire. Michelangelo was carving the Rondanini just before he died at eighty-nine. Verdi finished his opera Falstaff at eighty.

–W. Gifford-Jones (British Physician)

Many surgeons will retire well within the confines of a safe practice environment, long before significant declines of cognitive or technical skills occur. Some will push retirement back as far as they can for one or more of the considerations mentioned previously and maintain competency well into a more advanced age. Although Dr. Gifford-Jones would like to believe that all physicians should practice "til the end, reality suggests a different path." Once past age 65, the percentage of still practicing physicians who will push the competency envelope, both physically and mentally, begins a steep rise and necessitates careful monitoring [11–13]. From that point on, competency may be the most critical element to consider in the overall assessment of the need to retire. But who will do that assessment?

As previously discussed, we do not presently have formal measures of objective cognitive functioning to detect changes in performance that could aid in retirement decisions. Blasier, writing on the aging surgeon, proposed a two-pronged approach to this dilemma: (1) mandatory measures that compel a surgeon to stop operating and (2) education to increase surgeon and societal awareness of this potential problem and to encourage surgeons to use heightened insight into their own limitations [14]. Regarding the first, as pointed out, mandatory measures involving age as a primary end point are severely restricted by the ADEA. Furthermore, without the ability to test effectively, that leaves only the education of surgeons, other health-care providers, and society about the potential problem as a proposed solution.

Unfortunately, the solutions for education also have issues. Leaving recognition to self-reporting is not taking an unbiased approach to the situation. Similarly, establishing a system of proctoring is cumbersome and subject to additional bias in that colleagues that could serve as proctors might be too lenient while competitors too harsh. Also, relying on surgeons to evaluate their colleague in the operating room outside of a very formal process probably will not capture subtle changes of early decline and small lapses in judgment, which will likely occur long before there are gross deviations visible to other health-care personnel. Such minor initial alterations are also not likely to be picked up by standard hospital quality assurance programs. Furthermore, it can be extremely difficult for the evaluator. Providing an honest assessment and feedback is hard enough at times. In this situation, being the "bearer of bad news," especially when previous relationships exist, may mean substantial alterations in a mentor's practice or the end of another surgeon's career. If self-reporting is what is left, then the surgeon will need to recognize that his skills will fade, that appropriate planning can make retirement very satisfying and that retirement is not the end of life [14].

To be able to self-report, surgeons will have to be taught to recognize the signs of early decline. These include, but are not limited to, loss of manual dexterity, increasing operating times for uncomplicated operations, inability to complete complex operations without assistance, lack of attention to detail in the taking of histories and interpretation of laboratory data, jumping to conclusions too quickly in differential diagnosis and prior to consideration of broader differentials, and increasing needs for brighter illumination and magnification.

In the absence of self-recognition and subsequent reporting, the responsibility for reporting falls back onto colleagues who become aware of such problems either through personal direct observation or by communications with nurses and technicians who share their direct observations with concern. If possible, open discussion with the offending surgeon should be the first approach. If this is not possible or such interaction fails in the face of obvious decline, then reporting to the appropriate review or licensing body is required.

Technical Skills

It is time I stepped aside for a less experienced and less able man.

–Scott Elledge (Author)

Determining which is the ideal ending for you will depend, in part, on how you found yourself at this point in your career and the circumstances surrounding this critical decision. As stated, for some this is simply the culmination of a long and successful practice. "The time is right." You have given your life to surgery and your patients, and there is no more fitting time to retire from your established practice. Yet, something else may have brought you more emergently to this junction in your career than you would have liked or planned for—difficulties in the operating room. A decline in technical skills from the standpoint of patient safety is definitely a part of competency. What you used to be able to do now takes longer or requires help; worse, your technical performance directly results increasingly in poor patient outcomes. As even the best technical surgeon or the "perfect" operation can still result in untoward outcomes, this may not be readily recognized initially. Yet, each individual surgeon must perform an honest self-assessment of his/her own ability to complete a case properly and safely—our profession depends on it.

Beyond this, there are other issues that might surface in the face of health-care reform and the desire of health systems to offer the latest glitzy product to their patients. If safety or improved outcome is not a factor, but a more senior surgeon simply does not want spend the necessary time and effort learning a new complex technology with limited applicability to his remaining planned practice time, then there is not a medical role for termination or retirement. However, a surgeon taking this road must recognize and accept that if the new technology is desirable, their patient referral pattern may shift based on market economics, which may reach beyond either real or only perceived health-care benefits. For colorectal surgeons, this may hit especially close to home, as the transition from open colectomy to laparoscopic approaches, and future platforms such as robotics, may have already influenced practice patterns and personal considerations regarding the need to acquire additional skills.

Transition

Don't simply retire from something; have something to retire to.

–Harry Emerson Fosdic (American Pastor)

One option for a retiring colon and rectal surgeon is to slow down or modify your practice. Modification might take the form of eliminating inpatient or abdominal surgery in favor of outpatient anorectal surgery, endoscopy, or any combination thereof. Such a course would require the surgeon to have backup care available through remaining partners or other arrangements for those situations where an unexpected outcome of an outpatient procedure resulted in the need for inpatient care. The patients should be informed of such arrangements prior to any outpatient procedure in case such an incident should occur. One advantage of such an approach is that an outpatient practice as described could very well generate adequate revenue to minimize any change in practice dynamics for partners or colleagues in a multi-physician practice. There would be potential issues with regard to on-call status that would need to be discussed with those who would be picking up that coverage, though often this is less of an issue when planned well ahead of time.

Another option that some surgeons find preferable is just to slow down without any change in overall patient mix. This is usually a more complex process. Such an approach has many additional connotations, as it would assume a percentage drop in revenue correlating with the anticipated or desired drop in volume. Additional issues to consider in this circumstance include changes to on-call schedules that could shift such responsibilities on to other physicians and may require changes in hospital staff privileges. The involved medical liability carrier may not recognize part-time as a lower tier premium. If so, the liability premium may become a much larger percentage of overall overhead.

The same issue could occur with a group practice where lost productivity may not be accompanied by a reduction in expenses, thus increasing overhead percentage or shifting it to remaining practice members. Such potential impacts on others must be recognized and dealt with in a mutually agreeable way, early on, to avoid unnecessary conflicts. In a solo practice, setting such changes would still occur but would have to be dealt with on an individual basis. In some cases, these resulting changes in overhead may preclude the ability to slow down in this way.

For some surgeons, teaching serves as an excellent transition from active practice to retirement. The advantages include continuing to participate in the profession of medicine while keeping in contact with colleagues and lifetime interests in medicine. This may involve anything from seeing an outpatient clinic with residents, taking on medical students, or simply providing lectures to the community hospital. This can be an important step especially for those surgeons who have not developed meaningful outside interests or hobbies that can hold their interest once they leave medical practice.

Some surgeons will find it in their interests to make themselves available for quality reviews as a way to satisfy their desire to stay in tune with their lifelong profession. Usually these arrangements last for only a relatively short period of time as it is frequently preferable to have reviewers actively engaged in practice, or recently so engaged, to ensure that they are up-to-date with current standards. However, the process can serve as a good transition. Other reviewer positions are sometimes available for various accrediting organizations, providing an added benefit through the opportunity for some travel.

Finally, volunteering can assist in making such a transition easier to accept. This might or might not be in the medical field. In your personal situation, if you are retiring at the peak of your game, you may be interested volunteering your surgical services at a clinic for underserved patients either at home or overseas. If you have made a decision to retire only because you are concerned about your technical skills, you might consider volunteering in nonsurgical roles in such areas. If you are leaving medicine due to questions of competency, then consider other volunteer opportunities that are replete in almost any community across America and internationally. You may have other skills, nonmedical skills, which can be utilized to keep you feeling good about the work you do while helping others in need.

In the words of Ralph Waldo Emerson, "It is one of the most beautiful compensations of life that no man can sincerely try to help another without helping himself." You can't volunteer without receiving some of the benefit personally. There is no sweeter compensation than that. Volunteering is a way to grow yourself, to improve yourself and your community and your nation for you and for your children and your children's children. How beautiful is that? How critically important is that?

Preparation

Half our life is spent trying to find something to do with the time we have rushed through life trying to save.
–Will Rogers (Actor and Social Commentator)

Preparation for retirement should begin the first day on the job following completion of residency. Financial planning is critical. If you do not have expertise in managing financial matters, you need to get an advisor to help in this area. If educational debt is involved you need to assess the best timeline for paying it off, while simultaneously beginning a savings program for retirement income. An entire financial plan is important to include the actual timing to pay off debts, the starting of savings, the advantages and disadvantages of buying or renting a home, and how such choices will affect your overall financial stability over the years. If you have not budgeted in the past, you need to learn how. A little sacrifice up front can make a world of difference when retirement hits. And for most surgeons, the amount of time in active practice before retirement is roughly only equal to the time you have spent in education and training so far. It goes fast. There is no time for planning delay.

If you have special outside interests or hobbies, don't lose them during your practice years, as you will need them at the other end of the road. If medicine is your only hobby, then prepare yourself for medical hobbies when you retire. Position yourself so you can teach, do quality reviews, make accreditation visits, mentor students, or even serve as a docent for available museums with medical exhibits or involving opportunities for education about period medical care in Civil War or Frontier reenactments. Use your imagination. Medicine is more than just hospital wards and medical clinics.

The End Game

I promise to keep on living as though I expected to live forever. Nobody grows old by merely living a number of years. People grow old only by deserting their ideals. Years may wrinkle the skin, but to give up interest wrinkles the soul.
–Douglas MacArthur (American General)

Be prepared to be family again. Whether it is you alone or with your partner or a family too, it is time to finally give them the attention they deserve and thus the attention you deserve. Enjoy the ability to plan without fear of interruption. And make plans while you have time. The wisest physicians retire at the top of their game. They leave practice while people are asking them to stay, not when they are being asked to leave. They retire into an environment that provides ample opportunity for any number of choices with regard to the transition. Those that wait until they are being asked to leave risk not only being unable to practice medicine any longer, they risk not being able to do anything else either.

If you have always felt you needed to practice until you dropped dead because you felt you owed it back for all of the education and training you received, admit you were wrong. The best thing you can do for your patients is to retire before you risk missing an important diagnosis because you were not quite all there or before that operation is no longer the elegant procedure you once did. Putting a patient through that is no benefit to your patients. And it is of no benefit to you either.

Since the time you decided to go into medicine, you have been about trying to be the best. You pledged to be perfect, to do what is right and best for your patients. To finish that pledge, you need to retire before you stop doing that "best," being the "best." When you finally do retire, you need to be able to be proud that you did your best in that choice also.

References

1. Freeman T, Brown JB, Reid G, Stewart M, Thind A, Vingilis E. Patients' perceptions on losing access to FPs: qualitative study. Can Fam Physician. 2013;59(4):e195–201.
2. Drag LL, Bieliauskas LA, Langenecker SA, Greenfield LJ. Cognitive functioning, retirement status, and age: results from the Cognitive Changes and Retirement among Senior Surgeons study. J Am Coll Surg. 2010;211(3):303–7.
3. Adler RG, Constantinou C. Knowing—or not knowing—when to stop: cognitive decline in ageing doctors. Med J Aust. 2008; 189(11–12):622–4.
4. Lee L, Weston W. The aging physician. Can Fam Physician. 2012;58(1):17–8.
5. Durning SJ, Artino AR, Holmboe E, Beckman TJ, van der Vleuten C, Schuwirth L. Aging and cognitive performance: challenges and implications for physicians practicing in the 21st century. J Contin Educ Health Prof. 2010 Summer;30(3):153–60.
6. Eva KW, Cunnington JP. The difficulty with experience: does practice increase susceptibility to premature closure? J Contin Educ Health Prof. 2006 Summer;26 (3): 192–8.
7. Caulford PG, Lamb SB, Kaigas TB, Hanna E, Norman GR, Davis DA. Physician incompetence: specific problems and predictors. Acad Med. 1994;69(10 Suppl):S16–8.
8. Eva KW. The aging physician: changes in cognitive processing and their impact on medical practice. Acad Med. 2002;77(10 Suppl): S1–6.
9. Johnson FE, Novell LA, Coplin MA, Longo WE, Vernava AM, Wade TP, Virgo KS. How practice patterns in colon cancer patient follow-up are affected by surgeon age. Surg Oncol. 1996;5(3): 127–31.
10. Hamer M, Chida Y. Physical activity and risk of neurodegenerative disease: a systematic review of prospective evidence. Psychol Med. 2009;39(1):3–11. Review.
11. Greenfield LJ, Proctor MC. When should a surgeon retire? Adv Surg. 1999;32:385–93.
12. Rovit RL. To everything there is a season and a time to every purpose: retirement and the neurosurgeon. J Neurosurg. 2004;100(6): 1123–9.
13. Trunkey DD, Botney R. Assessing competency: a tale of two professions. J Am Coll Surg. 2001;192(3):385–95.
14. Blasier RB. The problem of the aging surgeon: when surgeon age becomes a surgical risk factor. Clin Orthop Relat Res. 2009;467(2): 402–11.

Index

S.R. Steele et al. (eds.), *Complexities in Colorectal Surgery*,
DOI 10.1007/978-1-4614-9022-7, © Springer Science+Business Media New York 2014

N

O

P

T

U

V

W

X

Y

Z

FSC
www.fsc.org
MIX
Papier aus verantwortungsvollen Quellen
Paper from responsible sources
FSC® C105338

If you have any concerns about our products, you can contact us on
ProductSafety@springernature.com

In case Publisher is established outside the EU, the EU authorized representative is:
Springer Nature Customer Service Center GmbH
Europaplatz 3, 69115 Heidelberg, Germany

Printed by Libri Plureos GmbH
in Hamburg, Germany